W9-DIG-819

http://connection.LWW.com

Get Connected!

Connect to a one-of-a-kind resource for students!

connection

Access everything you need at connection

- **E-mail updates** notify you of recent changes on the site and of content updates to the texts.

- **Chat rooms** enable on-line discussions for you to efficiently discuss specific topics with your peers and professor.

- **Message boards** make communication a snap.

- **Create-your-own-website**, using **connection's** easy-to-use format, stores the syllabus, notes, and schedule.

And just for the student...

- **Calendar of events** to keep up with the latest in the field of nursing pharmacology.

- **Internet links** direct you to online resources for additional information on nursing fundamentals.

Register in 3 easy steps...

1. Simply log on to the **connection** website and access the Resource Center for Karch: **Focus on Nursing Pharmacology, 2nd Edition**.

2. Enter your name and e-mail address, and set-up a user name and password.

3. Now you have immediate access to all the benefits of **connection**.

Connect today.
http://connection.LWW.com/go/karch

Lippincott
LIPPINCOTT WILLIAMS & WILKINS

G452-01-P   N1NXG452

Focus on
NURSING
PHARMACOLOGY

Focus on
NURSING
PHARMACOLOGY

SECOND EDITION

Amy M. Karch, RN, MS
Assistant Professor of Clinical Nursing
University of Rochester School of Nursing
Rochester, New York

LIPPINCOTT WILLIAMS & WILKINS
A **Wolters Kluwer** Company
Philadelphia · Baltimore · New York · London
Buenos Aires · Hong Kong · Sydney · Tokyo

Acquisitions Editor: Margaret Zuccarini
Managing Editor: Barclay Cunningham
Editorial Assistant: Helen Kogut
Production Editor: Nicole Walz
Senior Production Manager: Helen Ewan
Managing Editor / Production: Erika Kors
Art Director: Carolyn O'Brien
Design Coordinator: Brett MacNaughton
Design: BJ Crimm
Senior Manufacturing Manager: William Alberti
Indexer: Ann Cassar
Compositor: Peirce Graphic Services
Printer: Quebecor—Versailles

2nd Edition

Copyright © 2003 by Lippincott Williams & Wilkins.
Copyright © 2000 by Lippincott Williams & Wilkins. All rights reserved. This book is protected by copyright. No part of it may be reproduced, stored in a retrieval system, or transmitted, in any form or by any means—electronic, mechanical, photocopy, recording, or otherwise—without prior written permission of the publisher, except for brief quotations embodied in critical articles and reviews and testing and evaluation materials provided by publisher to instructors whose schools have adopted its accompanying textbook. Printed in the United States of America. For information write Lippincott Williams & Wilkins, 530 Walnut Street, Philadelphia PA 19106.

Materials appearing in this book prepared by individuals as part of their official duties as U.S. Government employees are not covered by the above-mentioned copyright.

9 8 7 6 5 4 3 2 1

Library of Congress Cataloging-in-Publication Data
Karch, Amy Morrison, 1949-
    Focus on nursing pharmacology / Amy M. Karch.—2nd ed.
      p. ; cm.
    Includes bibliographical references and index.
    ISBN 0-7817-3538-6 (alk. paper)
     1. Pharmacology. 2. Nursing. I. Title: Nursing pharmacology. II. Title.
    [DNLM: 1. Pharmaceutical Preparations—Nurses' Instruction. 2. Drug Therapy—
Nurses' Instruction. 3. Pharmacology—Nurses' Instruction. QV 4 K183f2003]
    RM300 .K37 2003
    615'.1—dc21

                       2002073151

Care has been taken to confirm the accuracy of the information presented and to describe generally accepted practices. However, the authors, editors, and publisher are not responsible for errors or omissions or for any consequences from application of the information in this book and make no warranty, express or implied, with respect to the content of the publication.

The authors, editors, and publisher have exerted every effort to ensure that drug selection and dosage set forth in this text are in accordance with the current recommendations and practice at the time of publication. However, in view of ongoing research, changes in government regulations, and the constant flow of information relating to drug therapy and drug reactions, the reader is urged to check the package insert for each drug for any change in indications and dosage and for added warnings and precautions This is particularly important when the recommended agent is a new or infrequently employed drug.

Some drugs and medical devices presented in this publication have Food and Drug Administration (FDA) clearance for limited use in restricted research settings. It is the responsibility of the health care provider to ascertain the FDA status of each drug or device planned for use in his or her clinical practice.

LWW.com

DEDICATION

Dedicated to my many students, past and present, who have taught me how to teach and kept me inspired and enthusiastic about the wonders of learning . . . and to my family, who have offered support, tolerance, and love when it was needed the most.

Reviewers

Joy E. Ache-Reed, RN, MSN
Assistant Professor of Nursing
Indiana Wesleyan University
Marion, Indiana

Eileen Augento, MA, ANP, CDE
Assistant Professor
Long Island University
Brooklyn, New York

N. June Baker, RN, BSN, MSN, APN
Instructor
GBC
Elko, Nevada

Diane Brown, MSN, RN, CCRN
Full time Faculty
University of Akron
Akron, Ohio

Bonita E. Broyles, RN, BSN, MA, EdD
Faculty, Second Level Coordinator
Piedmont Community College
Roxboro, North Carolina

Diane Cline, RN, MSN
Nursing Professor
Victor Valley College
Victorville, California

Cynthia L. Dakin, RN, MSN, PhD (c)
Clinical Specialist
Northeastern University
School of Nursing
Boston, Massachusetts

Karen Freas Gapper, MSN, RN
Associate Professor
Queensborough Community College
Bayside, New York

Joan Parker Frizzell, PhD, RN
Assistant Professor
La Salle University
School of Nursing
Philadelphia, Pennsylvania

Steve Gelone, PharmD
Associate Professor of Pharmacy
Temple University School of Pharmacy
Philadelphia, Pennsylvania

Joanne D. Gilroy, MS, FNP-C, CNM
Syracuse University
College of Nursing
Syracuse, New York

Frances S. Izzo, RN, CS, CCRN
Associate Professor of Nursing
Nassau Community College
Garden City, New York

Peggy Jenkins, MS, BS, CCRN
Associate Professor of Nursing
Hartwick College
Oneonta, New York

Rene Johnson, MSN, BSN
Instructor of Nursing, Bachelor of Science in
Nursing Program
Oklahoma Panhandle State University
Goodwell, Oklahoma

Judith Ann Kilpatrick, MSN, RNC
Lecturer
Widener University
Chester, Pennsylvania

Barbara Lange, RN, BSN
Assistant Professor
Elizabethtown Community College
Elizabethtown, Kentucky

Karen Lavallee, RN, C, CS, ARNP, MS
Professor
New Hampshire Technical Institute
Concord, New Hampshire

Linda McIntosh, RN, LPC, MSN, MS
Clinical Instructor
School of Nursing
North Carolina A & T State University
Greensboro, North Carolina

x REVIEWERS

Carolyn McKenzie, RN, MSN
Nursing Faculty
Randolph Community College
Asheboro, North Carolina

Samuel Joyce Mejia, BSN, MS,
Faculty
San Jacinto College
Pasadena, Texas

Patricia J. Neafsey, BS, MS, PhD, RD
Associate Professor
University of Connecticut
School of Nursing
Storrs, Connecticut

Staci Pacetti, PharmD
Fellow in Infectious Diseases
Temple University School of Pharmacy
Philadelphia, Pennsylvania

Phyllis M. Parks-Veal, BS, PharmD
Assistant Professor
Georgia College and State University
Milledgeville, Georgia

Andrew M. Peterson, PharmD, BCPS
Assistant Professor of Clinical Pharmacy
Philadelphia College of Pharmacy
University of the Sciences in Philadelphia
Philadelphia, Pennsylvania

Mary Catherine Rawls, RN, BSN, MSN
Professor of Nursing
Castleton State College
Castleton, Vermont

Tina Rotzler
Technology Coordinator
Hartwick College
Oneonta, New York

Sandy Schnicker
LPN Instructor
Cape Girardeau Career and Technology Center
Cape Girardeau, Missouri

Marsha K. Sharp, RN, MSN
Assistant Professor of Nursing
Elizabethtown Community College
Elizabethtown, Kentucky

Judy S. Siefert, RN, MSN
Chairperson
Alvin Community College
Alvin, Texas

Geralyn Valleroy- Frandsen, MSN, RN
Assistant Professor of Nursing
Maryville University
Saint Louis, Missouri

Donna B. Vaughn, RN, MS
Professor
Department of Vocational Nursing Education
Del Mar College
Corpus Christi, Texas

Cheryl A. Williams, MS, RN, ANP
Assistant Professor, Nursing Faculty
University of Massachusetts
Boston, Massachusetts

Preface

Pharmacology is a difficult course to teach in a standard nursing curriculum, whether it is a diploma, associate, baccalaureate, or graduate program. Teachers are difficult to find, and time and money often dictate that the invaluable content of such a course is incorporated into other courses. As a result, the content is often lost. At the same time, changes in medical care delivery—more outpatient and home care, shorter hospital stays, and more self-care—have resulted in additional legal and professional responsibilities for nurses, making them more responsible for the safe and effective delivery of drug therapy. Pharmacology should not be such a formidable obstacle in nursing curriculum. The study of drug therapy incorporates physiology, pathophysiology, chemistry, and nursing fundamentals—subjects that are already taught in most schools. A textbook that approaches pharmacology as an understandable, teachable, and learnable subject would greatly facilitate the incorporation of this subject into nursing curricula. Yet many nursing pharmacology texts are large and burdensome, mainly because they have needed to cover not only the basic pharmacology but also the particulars included in each area considered.

The concept for this text is based on the availability of many annually published nursing drug guides, which cover all the information that a nursing student or nurse should need to know about each individual drug and which then can serve as the ideal companion to a basic nursing pharmacology text. The changes in the area of drug therapy are occurring so rapidly, it is essential to have an annual update on all the new standards and options for therapy. By removing much of the laborious and constantly changing information on each drug and referring students to a nursing drug guide (which could then be used directly in patient care and care planning), the nursing pharmacology text becomes a succinct, practical book that allows students to learn the concepts involved in the study of pharmacology without overwhelming them with thousands of specific drug details.

With this goal in mind, *Focus on Nursing Pharmacology* provides a concise, user-friendly, and uncluttered text for the modern student. This difficult subject is presented in a streamlined, understandable, teachable, and learnable manner. Because this book is designed to be used in conjunction with a handbook of current drug information, it avoids clutter by focusing on "need-to-understand" content and concepts and by directing the student to refer to a nursing drug guide for more specific, current, and up-to-the minute drug details.

The text reviews and integrates previously learned knowledge of physiology, chemistry, and nursing fundamentals into chapters focused on helping students conceptualize what is important to know about each group of drugs.

Line art and tabular information summarize pertinent concepts, thereby facilitating student learning. Special features further focus student learning on clinical application, critical thinking, patient teaching and review questions for each chapter. In addition, a CD-ROM containing more than 700 drug monographs is included with the text, providing a "comfortable" source of specific drug detail when the student is ready to assimilate that detail.

ORGANIZATION

The organization of *Focus on Nursing Pharmacology* is based on the "simple to complex" approach, much like the syllabus for a basic nursing pharmacology course. Because students learn best "from the bottom up," Part 1 begins with an overview of basic nursing pharmacology. Building upon this foundation, Part 2 introduces the teaching of drug classes, starting with the chemotherapeutic agents—both antimicrobial and antineoplastic drugs. Because the effectiveness of these drugs depends on their interference with the most basic element of body physiology—the cell—students can easily understand the pharmacology of this class. Mastering the pharmacotherapeutic effects of this drug class helps establish a firm grasp of the basic principles taught in Part 1. Once the easiest pharmacological concepts are understood, the student is prepared to move on to the more challenging physiologic and pharmacologic concepts.

In Part 3, the immune system drugs are taught because recent knowledge about the immune system has made it the cornerstone of modern therapy. All of the immune system drugs act in ways that the immune system would itself if it were able. Recent immunological research has contributed to much greater understanding of this system, making it important to position information about drugs affecting this system close to the beginning of the text, instead of at the end as has been customary.

Parts 4 and 5 of the text address drugs that affect the nervous system, the basic functioning system of the body. Following the nervous system, and closely related to it, is the endocrine system and associated drug classes in Part 6. The sequence of these parts introduces students to the concept of control, teaches them about the interrelatedness of these two systems, and prepares them for understanding many aspects of shared physiological function and the inevitable linking of the two systems into one: the neuroendocrine system.

Parts 7, 8, and 9 discuss drugs affecting the reproductive, cardiovascular, and renal systems, respectively. The sequencing of cardiovascular and renal drugs is logical because most of the augmenting cardiovascular drugs (such as diuretics) affect the renal system. Part 10 covers respiratory system drugs, which provide the link between the left and right ventricles of the heart. Part 11 addresses drugs acting on the gastrointestinal system. The GI system stands on its own; it does not share many actions or interactions with any other system.

TEXT FEATURES

The features in *Focus on Nursing Pharmacology* are designed to skillfully support the text discussion, encouraging the student to look at the whole patient and to focus on the essence of information that is important to learn about each drug class, thereby enhancing the student's learning potential.

TERMS

- **Chapter pedagogy** includes a drug list, key term list, chapter introduction, bulleted chapter summary, bibliography and review questions to guide student learning, focusing on the seminal information presented in each chapter. In the Nursing Considerations section, italics highlight the rationale for each nursing intervention. In the chapter drug list, a ℗ appears next to each drug that is considered to be the prototype for its specific class. A glossary at the end of the text defines all key terms.
- **Drugs in Focus in-text drug summary tables** clearly identify the drugs within a class, highlighting them by generic and brand names, usual dosage and usual indications. A ℗ appears next to each drug that is considered to be the prototype for its specific class in these tables.
- **Web link icons** alert the student to electronic sources of drug information and drug therapy for specific diseases.
- **Nursing Challenges** teach the student the salient and sometimes life-preserving nursing interventions for a specific drug or drug therapy.
- **Cultural/Gender Considerations** encourage the student to consider the patient as a unique individual with a special set of characteristics that not only can influence variations in drug effectiveness, but also can impact the patient's perspective on drug therapy.
- **Lifespan Considerations** present a concise summary of points to consider when using the drugs of each class with children, adults, and older patients.
- **Nursing Care Guides** present general guidelines related to the nursing management of drug therapy for a particular class of drugs.
- **Patient Teaching Checklists** provide a basic framework for creating a customized patient education plan.
- **Case Studies** illustrate clinical application of drugs, drug effects, and patient variations for a specific drug.

A Patient Teaching CD-ROM presents drug-specific teaching points for more than 700 drugs for easy reference. It allows the student to formulate a customized patient teach-

ing plan for any of the 700 drugs. In addition, it contains information on Canadian drug names and laws and appendix-like information on vitamins, parenterals, and other drugs.

A Dosage Calculations CD-ROM provides practice questions in an interactive electronic format. It offers feedback in ratio proportion and formula methods.

ANCILLARY PACKAGE

For Students

- Student Study Guide—is organized chapter by chapter to match the text and provides creative interactive learning experiences to enhance the 'real' learning your students will enjoy when using this text and study guide package. Many activities involve learning to use drug information resources available on the Web and so work to expand the power of your students to access and critique the availability and quality of drug information on the Web.
- Patient Teaching CD-ROM—provides drug-specific teaching points for more than 700 drugs. Students can simply click the mouse to instantly create a customized client teaching printout for any drug monograph. This exciting electronic feature is an invaluable aid that will provide customized teaching materials and support the teaching experiences for your students.
- Dosage Calculations CD-ROM—offers NCLEX-style practice questions, with explanations of the correct answers in ratio proportion and formula methods. An electronic dosage calculator is included for use with selected questions.

For Faculty

- Instructor's Manual—provides tips and guidance helpful in preparing for class and implementing the contents of this creative new text package. Gleaned from many years of teaching nursing pharmacology, these tips will prove helpful in spicing up your class presentation, help to stimulate interactive learning experiences for your students, and work together with the text, study guide, and CD-ROM to fully enhance the learning potential of your students. Power Point presentations for each chapter provide a great audio-visual link for lectures.
- Testbank—available on disk, this testbank of more than 750 completely new NCLEX-style test items is available in ASCII format and capable of full manipulation in your own word-processing software. This feature provides the opportunity for adding, changing, and rearranging test items to meet your specific teaching and testing needs.

TO THE STUDENT USING THIS TEXT

As you begin your study of pharmacology, don't be overwhelmed or confused by all of the details. The study of drugs fits perfectly into your study of the human body—anatomy, physiology, chemistry, nutrition, psychology, and sociology. Approach the study of pharmacology from the perspective of putting all of the pieces together; this can be not only fun but challenging! Work to understand the concepts and all of the details will fall into place, be easy to remember, and apply to the clinical situation. This understanding will help you in creating the picture of the whole patient as you are learning to provide comprehensive nursing care. This text is designed to help you accomplish all of this in a simple and concise manner. Good luck!

Amy M. Karch, RN, MS

Acknowledgments

I would like to thank the many people who have worked so hard to make this book a reality: the many students and colleagues who have, for so long, pushed for a pharmacology book that was straight-forward and user friendly; my editor at Lippincott Williams & Wilkins, Margaret Zuccarini, who had the vision and the drive to see this project through and who has become a mentor and a friend; Helen Kogut, our editorial assistant, who somehow manages to keep everything in order and flowing smoothly and who is my anchor at LWW; editors Leslie Mosby and Barclay Cunningham, who worked hard to insert new ideas and comprehension; Nicole Walz, project editor, who smoothed the book's way through the production process; Doris Wray, who works her technical magic and who is the sane voice of reason; my wonderful husband, Fred Karch, who not only tolerates moods, deadlines, lack of sleep and endless questions, but who manages to bring the sunshine when things seem to be impossible; to Tim, Jyoti, Mark, Cortney, and Kathryn who continue to thrive and grow and have become the wonderful, supportive people in my life; and to Duncan, who has no idea what joy and peace his friendly, wagging tail brings.

Contents

1

Introduction to Nursing Pharmacology

CHAPTER

1

Introduction to Drugs

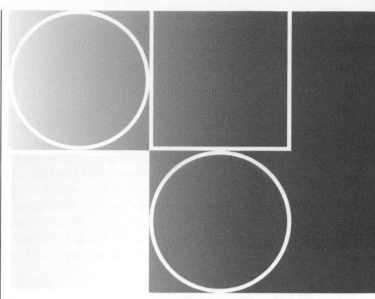

Key Terms
adverse effects
brand name
chemical name
drugs
Food and Drug Administration (FDA)
generic drugs
generic name
genetic engineering
orphan drugs
over-the-counter (OTC) drugs
pharmacology
pharmacotherapeutics
phase I study
phase II study
phase III study
phase IV study
preclinical trials
teratogenic

3

The human body works through a complicated series of chemical reactions and processes. **Drugs** are chemicals that are introduced into the body to cause some sort of change. When drugs are administered, the body begins a sequence of processes designed to handle the new chemicals. These processes, which involve breaking down and eliminating the drugs, in turn affect the body's complex series of chemical reactions.

For many reasons, understanding how drugs act on the body to cause changes and applying that knowledge in the clinical setting are important aspects of nursing practice. For instance, patients today often follow complicated drug regimens and receive potentially toxic drugs. Many also manage their own care at home. The nurse is in a unique position regarding drug therapy, because nursing responsibilities include the following:

- Administering drugs
- Assessing drug effects
- Intervening to make the drug regimen more tolerable
- Providing patient teaching about drugs and the drug regimen

Knowing how drugs work makes these tasks easier to handle, thus enhancing drug therapy.

This text is designed to provide the pharmacological basis for understanding drug therapy. The physiology of a body system and the related actions of many drugs on that system are presented in a way that allows clear understanding of how drugs work and what to anticipate when giving a particular type of drug. Thousands of drugs are available for use, and it is impossible to memorize all of the individual differences among drugs in a class.

This text addresses general drug information. The nurse can refer to *Lippincott's Nursing Drug Guide* (*LNDG*), or to another drug guide, to obtain the specific details required for safe and effective drug administration. Drug details change constantly, and the practicing nurse should rely on an up-to-date and comprehensive drug guide in the clinical setting.

A nursing care guide in each text chapter serves as a model for developing nursing care guides for any drugs being administered (Table 1–1). The various sections of each drug monograph in *LNDG* also can be used to develop other care guides or teaching plans. See Figure 1–1 for an example of a drug monograph. The CD-ROM found at the back of this book contains patient teaching guides for all of the drugs found in *LNDG*. The nurse can use this text as a resource for basic concepts of pharmacology and a nursing drug guide as an easy-to-use reference in the clinical setting.

Understanding how to read a drug label is essential. Drug labels have specific features that identify the drug, and it is important to become familiar with each aspect of a drug label (Figure 1–2).

PHARMACOLOGY

Pharmacology is the study of the biological effects of chemicals. In clinical practice, health care providers focus on how chemicals act on living organisms. Nurses deal with **pharmacotherapeutics,** or clinical pharmacology, the branch of pharmacology that uses drugs to treat, prevent, and diagnose disease. Clinical pharmacology addresses two key concerns: the drug's effects on the body, and the body's response to the drug.

Because a drug can have many effects, the nurse must know which ones may occur when a particular drug is administered. Some drug effects are therapeutic, or helpful. But others are undesirable or potentially dangerous. These negative effects are called **adverse effects.** (See Chapter 3 for a detailed discussion of adverse effects.)

SOURCES AND EVALUATION OF DRUGS

Drugs are available from varied sources, both natural and synthetic. The drugs listed in this book have been through rigorous testing and are approved for sale to the public, either with or without a prescription from a health care provider.

Sources of Drugs

Chemicals that might prove useful as drugs can come from many natural sources, such as plants, animals, or inorganic compounds, or they may be developed synthetically. To become a drug, a chemical must have a demonstrated therapeutic value or efficacy without severe toxicity or damaging properties.

Plants

Plants and plant parts have been used as medicines since prehistoric times. Even today, plants are an important source of chemicals that are developed into drugs. For example, digitalis products used to treat cardiac disorders and various opiates used for sedation are still derived from plants. Table 1–2 provides examples of drugs derived from plant sources.

Drugs also may be processed using a synthetic version of the active chemical found in a plant. An example of this type of drug is dronabinol (*Marinol*), which contains the active ingredient delta-9-tetrahydrocannabinol found in marijuana. It helps prevent nausea and vomiting in cancer patients but does not have all of the adverse effects that occur when the marijuana leaf is smoked. Marijuana leaf is a controlled substance with high abuse potential and has no legal or accepted medical use. The synthetic version of the active ingredient allows for an accepted form to achieve the desired therapeutic effect in cancer patients.

Sometimes a drug effect occurs from ingestion of plant-derived food. For instance, the body converts natural licorice to a false aldosterone, resulting in fluid retention and hy-

TABLE 1-1 Sample Nursing Care Plan from *Lippincott's Nursing Drug Guide* for a Patient Receiving Oral Linezolid

Assessment	Nursing Diagnoses	Implementation	Evaluation
HISTORY (contraindications/cautions) Hypertension Hyperthyroidism Blood dyscrasias Hepatic dysfunction Pheochromocytoma Phenylketonuria Carcinoid syndrome Pregnancy Lactation Known allergy to: linezolid **MEDICATION HISTORY** (possible drug–drug interactions) Pseudoephedrine SSRIs MAOIs Antiplatelet drugs **DIET HISTORY** (possible drug–food interactions) Foods high in tyramine **PHYSICAL ASSESSMENT** (screen for contraindications and to establish a baseline for evaluating effects and adverse effects) Local: Culture site of infection CNS: Affect, reflexes, orientation CV: P, BP, peripheral perfusion GI: Bowel sounds, liver evaluation Skin: Color, lesions Hematologic: CBC with differential, liver function tests	Potential alteration in nutrition, less than body requirements, related to GI effects Potential alteration in comfort related to GI effects, headache Risk for altered tissue perfusion related to bone marrow effects Knowledge deficit related to drug therapy	Safe and appropriate administration of drug: Culture infection site to ensure appropriate use of drug Provision of safety and comfort measures: • Monitor BP periodically • Monitor platelet counts before and periodically during therapy • Alleviation of GI upset • Ready access to bathroom facilities • Nutritional consult • Safety provisions if dizziness and CNS effects occur • Avoidance of tyramine-rich foods Patient teaching regarding: Drug Side effects to anticipate Warnings Reactions to report Support and encouragement to cope with disease, high cost of therapy, and side effects Provision of emergency and life-support measures in cases of acute hypersensitivity	Monitor for therapeutic effects of drug: resolution of infection. If resolution does not occur, reculture site. Monitor for adverse effects of drug: • GI upset—nausea, vomiting, diarrhea • Liver function changes • Pseudomembranous colitis • Blood dyscrasias—changes in platelet counts • Fever • Rash • Sweating • Photosensitivity • Acute hypersensitivity reactions Evaluate effectiveness of patient teaching program: patient can name drug, dose of drug, use of drug, adverse effects to expect, reactions to report Evaluate effectiveness of comfort and safety measures Monitor for drug–drug, drug–food interactions as appropriate Evaluate effectiveness of life-support measures if needed

From Karch, A. M. (2002). *2002 Lippincott's nursing drug guide.* Philadelphia: Lippincott Williams & Wilkins.

Generic name

Pronunciation guide

Brand name

FDA pregnancy category

Therapeutic drug classes

Action of drug on the body

Uses for the drug
Evaluation points–
resolution or stabilization
of those conditions

Conditions limiting use of drug
Assessment points–
history of these conditions,
physical assessment
indicating these conditions

Forms and dosages available
for use

Recommended dose of drug
for adults, pediatrics, etc.

linezolid

(lah nez' oh lid)

Zyvox, Zyvox for Oral Suspension,
Zyvox IV Injection

Pregnancy Category C

Drug classes
Antibiotic
Oxazolidinones

Therapeutic actions
Bacteriostatic and bacteriocidal; interferes
with protein synthesis on the bacterial
ribosome: effective in vancomycin-
resistant *Enterococcus* (VRE),
Staphyloccus, and methicillin-resistant *S.
aureus* (MRSA and penicillin-resistant
pneumococci and *S. aureus*; is a reversible,
nonselective MAO inhibitor.

Indications
• Treatment of infections due to
vancomycin-resistant *Enterococcus
faecnom*
• Treatment of nosocomial and community-
acquired pneumonia due to *S. aureus* and
penicillin-susceptible *Streptococcus
pneumoniae*
• Treatment of skin and skin structure
infections including those caused by
methicilin-resistant *S. aureus*

Contraindications/cautions
• Contraindicated in presence of allergy to
linezolid; pregnancy, lactation;
phenylketonuria (oral form).
• Use caution in the presence of bone
marrow suppression, hepatic dysfunction,
hypertension, hyperthyroidism,
pheochromocytoma, carinoid syndrome.

Dosage
Note: No dosage adjustment is needed if
switching between oral and IV forms.
Available Forms: Tablets—400, 600 mg;
oral suspension—100 mg/5 mL; IV
solution—2 mg/mL
ADULT
• *VRE, MRSA, pneumonia, complicated
skin and skin structure infections*: 600
mg IV or PO q12h for 10–14d.

• *Uncomplicated skin and skin structure
infections*: 400 mg PO q12h for 10–14d.

PEDIATRIC: Safety and efficacy not
established.

Pharmacokinetics

Route	Onset	Peak
Oral	Rapid	1–2h

Metabolism: Hepatic, $T_{1/2}$:5 h
Distribution: Crosses placenta; passes into
breast milk
Excretion: Urine

IV facts
Preparation: Use premixed solution—
available in 100, 200 and 300 mL forms;
store at room temperature, protect from
light, leave overwrap in place until ready to
use.
Infusion: Infuse over 30–130 min, switch
to oral form as soon as appropriate. May be
infused into line using 5% Dextrose
Injection, 0.9% Sodium Chloride, or
Lactated Ringer's.
Incompatibilites: Do not introduce
additives into this solution; do not mix in
solution or at Y-connection with any other
drugs. If other drugs are being given
through the same line, the line should be
flushed before and after linezolid
administration.

Adverse effects
• GI: *Nausea*, vomiting, dry mouth,
diarrhea, anorexia, gastritis, stomatitis,
pseudomembranous colitis
• CNS: *Headache*, dizziness, *insomnia*,
fatigue, somnolence, depression,
nervousness
• Hematologic: Altered prothrombin time,
thrombocytopenia
• Other: Fever, rash, sweating,
photosensitivity, tendinitis

Clinically important interactions
✳ **Drug-drug** • Risk of hypertension
and related adverse effects if combined
with drugs containing pseudoephedrine,
SSRIs, MAOIs; use caution and monitor
patient carefully if any of these
combinations are used

Action of body on the drug—
points for assessment
(hepatic and renal function),
cautions, and contraindications

Nursing actions for safe and
appropriate administration of
the drug in IV form
Implementation—nursing
actions

Effects of drug on the body—
therapeutic but can be
expected
Assessment point—
baselines for these systems
Nursing Diagnoses—
potential alterations resulting
from these effects
Evaluation—
presence/absence of these
effects

Anticipated interactions
Assessment points—history
of use of these agents,
physical response
Evaluation—changes from
anticipated therapeutic
response related to drug
interactions

FIGURE 1-1. Example of a drug monograph from *Lippincott's Nursing Drug Guide.*

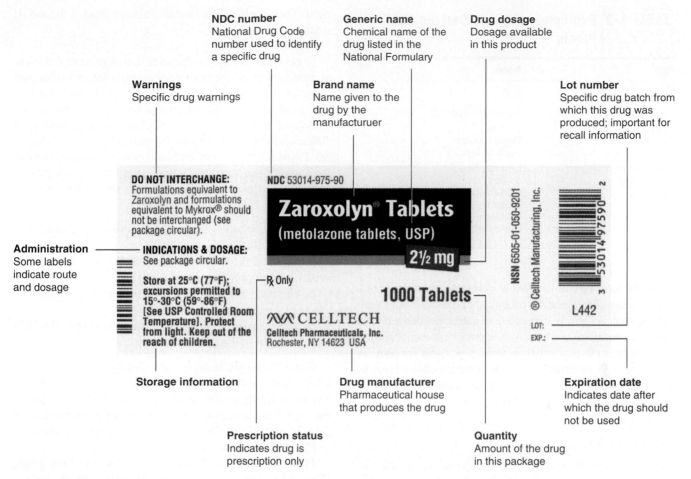

NDC number
National Drug Code
number used to identify
a specific drug

Generic name
Chemical name of the
drug listed in the
National Formulary

Drug dosage
Dosage available
in this product

Warnings
Specific drug warnings

Brand name
Name given to the
drug by the
manufacturuer

Lot number
Specific drug batch from
which this drug was
produced; important for
recall information

Administration
Some labels
indicate route
and dosage

DO NOT INTERCHANGE:
Formulations equivalent to
Zaroxolyn and formulations
equivalent to Mykrox® should
not be interchanged (see
package circular).

NDC 53014-975-90

Zaroxolyn® Tablets
(metolazone tablets, USP)

2½ mg

INDICATIONS & DOSAGE:
See package circular.

Rx Only

Store at 25°C (77°F);
excursions permitted to
15°-30°C (59°-86°F)
[See USP Controlled Room
Temperature]. Protect
from light. Keep out of the
reach of children.

1000 Tablets

CELLTECH
Celltech Pharmaceuticals, Inc.
Rochester, NY 14623 USA

NSN 6505-01-050-9201
® Celltech Manufacturing, Inc.

L442

LOT:
EXP.:

Storage information

Drug manufacturer
Pharmaceutical house
that produces the drug

Expiration date
Indicates date after
which the drug should
not be used

Prescription status
Indicates drug is
prescription only

Quantity
Amount of the drug
in this package

(Courtesy of CellTech Pharmaceuticals)

FIGURE 1–2. Reading a drug label (sample drug label courtesy of Celltech Pharmaceuticals, Rochester, NY).

pokalemia or low serum potassium levels if large amounts of licorice are eaten. However, people seldom think of licorice as a drug.

Finally, plants have become the main component of the growing alternative therapy movement. Chapter 6 discusses the alternative therapy movement and its impact on today's drug regimens.

Animal Products

Animal products are used to replace human chemicals that are not produced because of disease or genetic problems. Until recently, insulin for treating diabetes was obtained exclusively from cow and pig pancreas tissue. Now **genetic engineering**—the process of altering DNA—permits scientists to produce human insulin by altering *Escherichia coli* bacteria, making insulin a better product without some of the impurities that come with animal products.

Thyroid drugs and growth hormone preparations also may be obtained from animal thyroid and hypothalamus tissues. But many of these preparations are now created synthetically, and the synthetic preparations are considered to be purer and safer than preparations derived from animals.

Inorganic Compounds

Salts of various elements can have therapeutic effects in the human body. Aluminum, fluoride, iron, and even gold are used to treat various conditions. The effects of these elements usually were discovered accidentally when a cause–effect relationship was observed. Table 1–3 shows examples of some elements used for their therapeutic benefit.

Synthetic Sources

Today, many drugs are developed synthetically after chemicals in plants, animals, or the environment have been screened for signs of therapeutic activity. Scientists use genetic engineering to alter bacteria to produce chemicals that are therapeutic and effective. Other technical advances allow scientists to alter a chemical with proven therapeutic effectiveness to make it better. Sometimes, a small change in a chemical's structure can make that chemical more useful as a drug—more potent, more stable, less toxic. These technological advances have led to the development of groups of similar drugs, all of which are derived from an original prototype, but each of which has slightly different properties, making a particular drug more desirable in a specific situation. Throughout this

TABLE 1-2 | Examples of Drugs Derived from Plants

Plant	Product
Riccinus communis	Seed Oil Castor oil (*Neolid*)
Digitalis purpurea (foxglove plant)	Leaves Dried leaves Digitalis leaf
Papaver somniferum (poppy plant)	Unripe capsule Juice Opium (paregoric) Morphine (*Roxanol*) Codeine Papaverine (*Pavabid*)

book, the icon ⓟ will be used to designate those drugs of a class that are considered the prototype of the class. For example, the cephalosporins are a group of antibiotics derived from the same chemical structure. Alterations in the chemical rings or attachments to that structure make it possible for some of these drugs to be absorbed orally, whereas others must be given parenterally. Some of these drugs cause severe toxic effects (eg, renal toxicity), but others do not.

Drug Evaluation

After a chemical that might have therapeutic value is identified, it must undergo a series of scientific tests to evaluate its actual therapeutic and toxic effects. This process is tightly controlled by the **Food and Drug Administration (FDA),** an agency of the U. S. Department of Health and Human Services that regulates the development and sale of drugs. FDA-regulated tests are designed to ensure the safety and reliability of any drug approved in this country. For every 100,000 chemicals that are identified as being potential drugs, only about 5 end up being marketed.

Phases of Drug Development

Before receiving final FDA approval to be marketed to the public, drugs must pass through several stages of develop-

TABLE 1-3 | Examples of Elements Used for their Therapeutic Effects

Element	Therapeutic Use
Aluminum	Antacid to decrease gastric acidity Management of hyperphosphatemia Prevention of the formation of phosphate urinary stones
Fluoride	Prevention of dental cavities Prevention of osteoporosis
Gold	Treatment of rheumatoid arthritis
Iron	Treatment of iron deficiency anemia

ment. These include preclinical trials and phase I, II, and III studies.

Preclinical Trials

In **preclinical trials,** chemicals that may have therapeutic value are tested on laboratory animals for two main purposes: (1) to determine whether they have the presumed effects in living tissue, and (2) to evaluate any adverse effects.

Animal testing is important because unique biological differences can cause very different reactions to the chemical. These differences can be found only in living organisms, so computer-generated models alone are often inadequate.

At the end of the preclinical trials, some chemicals are discarded for the following reasons:

• The chemical lacks therapeutic activity when used with living animals.
• The chemical is too toxic to living animals to be worth the risk of developing into drugs.
• The chemical is highly **teratogenic** (causing adverse effects to the fetus).
• The safety margins are so small that the chemical would not be useful in the clinical setting.

Some chemicals, however, are found to have therapeutic effects and reasonable safety margins. This means that the chemicals are therapeutic at doses that are reasonably different from doses that cause toxic effects. Such chemicals will pass the preclinical trials and advance to phase I studies.

Phase I Studies

Phase I studies use human volunteers to test the drugs. These studies are more tightly controlled than preclinical trials and are performed by specially trained clinical investigators. The volunteers are fully informed of possible risks and may be paid for their participation.

Usually, the volunteers are healthy, young men. Women are not good candidates for phase I studies because the chemicals may exert unknown effects on a woman's ova. Since women are born with all of the ova they are ever going to have, there is too much risk involved in taking a drug that might destroy or alter the ova. Men produce sperm daily, so there is less potential for complete destruction or alteration of the sperm.

Some chemicals are therapeutic in other animals but have no effects in humans. Investigators in phase I studies scrutinize the drugs being tested for effects in humans. They also look for adverse effects and toxicity. At the end of phase I studies, many chemicals are dropped from the process for the following reasons:

• They lack therapeutic effect in humans.
• They cause unacceptable adverse effects.
• They are highly teratogenic.
• They are too toxic.

Some chemicals move to the next stage of testing despite undesirable effects. For example, the antihypertensive drug minoxidil (*Loniten*) was found to effectively treat malignant hypertension, but it caused unusual hair growth on the palms and other body areas. However, because it was so much more effective at the time of its development than any other antihypertensive drug, it proceeded to phase II studies. (Now, its hair-growing effect has been channeled for therapeutic use into various hair-growth preparations such as *Rogaine*.)

Phase II Studies

Phase II studies allow clinical investigators to try the drug in patients who have the disease that the drug is meant to treat. Patients are told about the possible benefits of the drug and are invited to participate in the study. Those who consent to participate are fully informed about possible risks and are monitored very closely, often at no charge to them, to evaluate the drug's effects. Usually, phase II studies are performed at various sites across the country—in hospitals, clinics, and doctors' offices—and are monitored by representatives of the pharmaceutical company studying the drug.

At the end of phase II studies, a drug may be removed from further investigation for the following reasons:

- It is less effective than anticipated.
- It is too toxic when used with patients.
- It produces unacceptable adverse effects.
- It has a low benefit-to-risk ratio, meaning that the therapeutic benefit it provides does not outweigh the risk of potential adverse effects that it causes.
- It is no more effective than other drugs already on the market, making the cost of continued research and production less attractive to the drug company.

A drug that continues to show promise as a therapeutic agent receives additional scrutiny in phase III studies.

Phase III Studies

Phase III studies involve use of the drug in a vast clinical market. Prescribers are informed of all the known reactions to the drug and precautions required for its safe use. Prescribers observe patients very closely, monitoring them for any adverse effects. Sometimes, prescribers ask patients to keep journals and record any symptoms they experience. Prescribers then evaluate the reported effects to determine whether they are caused by the disease or by the drug. This information is collected by the drug company that is developing the drug and is shared with the FDA. When a drug is used widely, totally unexpected responses may occur. A drug that produces unacceptable adverse effects or unforeseen reactions is usually removed from further study by the drug company. In some cases, the FDA may have to request that a drug be removed from the market.

Food and Drug Administration Approval

Drugs that finish phase III studies are evaluated by the FDA, which relies on committees of experts familiar with the specialty area in which the drugs will be used. Only those drugs that receive FDA committee approval may be marketed. Figure 1–3 recaps the various phases of drug development discussed.

It is estimated that the entire drug development and approval process can take 5 to 6 years, resulting in a so-called drug lag in the United States. In some instances, a drug that

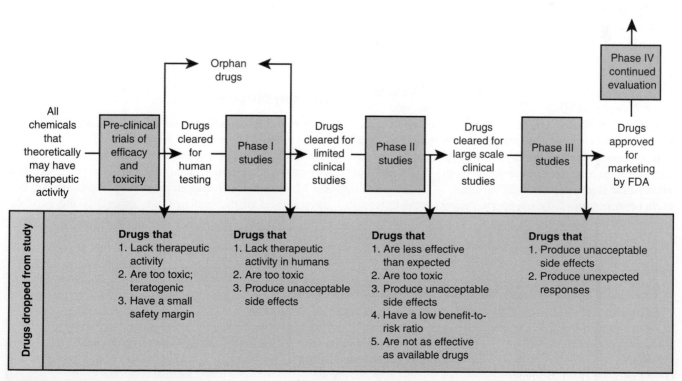

FIGURE 1–3. Phases of drug development.

is available in another country may not become available here for years. The FDA regards public safety as primary in drug approval, so the process remains strict. However, it can be accelerated in certain instances involving the treatment of deadly diseases. For example, some drugs (including delavirdine [*Rescriptor*] and efavirenz [*Sustiva*]) that were thought to offer a benefit to patients with acquired immune deficiency syndrome (AIDS), a potentially fatal immune disorder, were pushed through because of the progressive nature of AIDS and the lack of a cure. All literature associated with these drugs indicates that long-term effects and other information about the drug may not yet be known.

In addition to the drug lag issue, there also are concerns about the high cost of drug approval. In 1998, the estimated cost of taking a chemical from discovery to marketing as a drug was about $50 to $60 million. Because of this kind of financial investment, pharmaceutical companies are unwilling to risk approval of a drug that might cause serious problems and prompt lawsuits.

Continual Evaluation

An approved drug is given a **brand name** (trade name) by the pharmaceutical company that developed it. The **generic name** of a drug is the original designation that the drug was given when the drug company applied for the approval process. **Chemical names** are names that reflect the chemical structure of a drug. Some drugs are known by all three names. It can be confusing to study drugs when so many different names are used for the same compound. In this text, the generic and chemical names always appear in straight print, and the brand name is italicized (eg, minoxidil [*Rogaine*]). See Box 1–1 for examples of drug names.

After a drug is approved for marketing, it enters a phase of continual evaluation or **phase IV study.** Prescribers are obligated to report to the FDA any untoward or unexpected adverse effects associated with drugs they are using, and the FDA continually evaluates this information. Some drugs cause unexpected effects that are not seen until wide distribution occurs. Sometimes, those effects are therapeutic. For example, patients taking the antiparkinsonism drug amantadine (*Symmetrel*) were found to have fewer cases of influenza than other patients, leading to the discovery that amantadine is an effective antiviral agent.

In other instances, the unexpected effects are dangerous. In 1998, the antihypertensive drug mibefradil (*Posicor*) was pulled from the market not long after its release because patients taking it were found to have more cardiac morbidity. In 1997, the diet drug dexfenfluramine (*Redux*) was removed from the market only months after its release because patients developed serious heart problems. These problems were not seen in any of the premarket studies.

LEGAL REGULATION OF DRUGS

The FDA regulates the development and sale of drugs. Local laws further regulate the distribution and administration of drugs. In most cases, the strictest law is the one that prevails. Nurses should become familiar with the rules and regulations in the area in which they practice. These regulations can vary from state to state, and even within a state.

Over the years, the FDA has become more powerful, usually in response to a drug disaster affecting many people. In the 1930s, the drug Elixir of Sulfanilamide was distributed in a vehicle of ethylene glycol that had never been tested in humans. It turned out that ethylene glycol is toxic to humans, and hundreds of people died while many others became very ill. This led to the Federal Food, Drug and Cosmetic Act of 1938, which gave the FDA power to enforce standards for testing drug toxicity and monitoring labeling.

In the 1960s, the drug thalidomide (*Thalidomid*) was used as a sleeping aid by pregnant women, resulting in the birth of many babies with limb deformities. The public outcry resulted in the Kefauver–Harris Act of 1962, which gave the FDA regulatory control over the testing and evaluating of drugs and set standards for efficacy and safety.

Other laws have given the FDA control over monitoring of potentially addictive drugs and responsibility for monitoring, to some extent, the sale of drugs that are available without prescription.

Table 1–4 provides a summary of these laws.

Pregnancy Categories

As part of the standards for testing and safety, the FDA requires that each new drug be assigned to a pregnancy category (Box 1–2). The categories indicate a drug's potential or actual teratogenic effects, thus offering guidelines for use of that particular drug in pregnancy. Research into the development of the human fetus, especially the nervous system, has led many health care providers to recommend

---

BOX 1-1

Examples of Generic, Chemical, and Brand Names of Drugs

levothyroxine sodium	←	**generic name**	→	colfosceril palmitate
L-thyroxine, T₄	←	**chemical name**	→	dipalmitoylphosphatidylcholine
Eltroxin, Levothroid, Synthroid	←	**brand names**	→	*Exosurf Neonatal*

TABLE 1-4	Federal Legislation Affecting the Clinical Use of Drugs	

Year Enacted	Law	Impact
1906	Pure Food and Drug Act	Prevented the marketing of adulterated drugs; required labeling to eliminate false or misleading claims
1938	Federal Food, Drug and Cosmetic Act of 1938	Mandated tests for drug toxicity and provided means for recall of drugs; established procedures for introducing new drugs; gave FDA the power of enforcement
1951	Durham–Humphrey Amendment	Tightened control of certain drugs; specified drugs to be labeled "may not be distributed without a prescription"
1962	Kefauver–Harris Act	Tightened control over the quality of drugs; gave FDA regulatory power over the procedure of drug investigations; stated that efficacy as well as safety of drugs had to be established
1970	Controlled Substances Act	Defined drug abuse and classified drugs as to their potential for abuse; provided strict controls over the distribution, storage, and use of these drugs
1983	Orphan Drug Act	Provided incentives for the development of orphan drugs for treatment of rare diseases

BOX 1-2
FDA Pregnancy Categories

The Food and Drug Administration (FDA) has established five categories to indicate the potential for a systemically absorbed drug to cause birth defects. The key differentiation among the categories rests on the degree (reliability) of documentation and the risk–benefit ratio.

Category A: Adequate studies in pregnant women have not demonstrated a risk to the fetus in the first trimester of pregnancy, and there is no evidence of risk in later trimesters.

Category B: Animal studies have not demonstrated a risk to the fetus but there are no adequate studies in pregnant women, *or* animal studies have shown an adverse effect, but adequate studies in pregnant women have not demonstrated a risk to the fetus during the first trimester of pregnancy, and there is no evidence of risk in later trimesters.

Category C: Animal studies have shown an adverse effect on the fetus but there are no adequate studies in humans; the benefits from the use of the drug in pregnant women may be acceptable despite its potential risks, *or* there are no animal reproduction studies and no adequate studies in humans.

Category D: There is evidence of human fetal risk, but the potential benefits from the use of the drug in pregnant women may be acceptable despite its potential risks.

Category X: Studies in animals or humans demonstrate fetal abnormalities or adverse reaction; reports indicate evidence of fetal risk. The risk of use in a pregnant woman clearly outweighs any possible benefit.

Regardless of the designated Pregnancy Category or presumed safety, *no* drug should be administered during pregnancy unless it is clearly needed.

that no drug should be used during pregnancy because of potential effects on the developing fetus. In cases in which a drug is needed, it is recommended that the drug of choice be one for which the benefit outweighs the potential risk.

Controlled Substances

The Controlled Substances Act of 1970 established categories for ranking of the abuse potential of various drugs. This same act gave control over the coding of drugs and the enforcement of these codes to the FDA and the Drug Enforcement Agency (DEA), a part of the U. S. Department of Justice. The FDA studies the drugs and determines their abuse potential; the DEA enforces their control. Drugs with abuse potential are called *controlled substances*. Box 1–3 contains descriptions of each category, or schedule.

The prescription, distribution, storage, and use of these drugs is closely monitored by the DEA in an attempt to decrease substance abuse of prescribed medications. Each prescriber has a DEA number, which allows the DEA to monitor prescription patterns and possible abuse. A nurse should be familiar with not only the DEA guidelines for controlled substances but also the local policies and procedures, which might be even more rigorous.

GENERIC DRUGS

When a drug receives approval for marketing from the FDA, the drug formula is given a time-limited patent, in much the same way as an invention is patented. The length of time for which the patent is good depends on the type of chemical involved. When the patent runs out on a brand-name drug, the drug can be produced by other manufacturers. **Generic drugs** are chemicals that are produced by companies that just manufacture drugs. Because they do not have the research, the advertising, or, sometimes, the quality control departments that pharmaceutical companies have, they can produce the generic drugs more cheaply.

In the past, some quality-control problems were found with generic products. For example, the binders used in a generic drug might not be the same as those used in the brand-name product; as a result, the way the body breaks down and uses the drug may differ. In that case, the bioavailability of the drug is different from that of the brand-name product.

Many states require that a drug be dispensed in the generic

BOX 1-3
DEA Schedules of Controlled Substances

The Controlled Substances Act of 1970 regulates the manufacturing, distribution, and dispensing of drugs that are known to have abuse potential. The Drug Enforcement Agency (DEA) is responsible for the enforcement of these regulations. The controlled drugs are divided into five DEA schedules based on their potential for abuse and physical and psychological dependence.

Schedule I (*C-I*): High abuse potential and no accepted medical use (heroin, marijuana, LSD)

Schedule II (*C-II*): High abuse potential with severe dependence liability (narcotics, amphetamines, and barbiturates)

Schedule III (*C-III*): Less abuse potential than schedule II drugs and moderate dependence liability (nonbarbiturate sedatives, nonamphetamine stimulants, limited amounts of certain narcotics)

Schedule IV (*C-IV*): Less abuse potential than schedule III and limited dependence liability (some sedatives, antianxiety agents, and non-narcotic analgesics)

Schedule V (*C-V*): Limited abuse potential. Primarily small amounts of narcotics (codeine) used as antitussives or antidiarrheals. Under federal law, limited quantities of certain schedule V drugs may be purchased without a prescription directly from a pharmacist. The purchaser must be at least 18 years of age and must furnish suitable identification. All such transactions must be recorded by the dispensing pharmacist.

Prescribing physicians and dispensing pharmacists must be registered with the DEA, which also provides forms for the transfer of schedule I and II substances and establishes criteria for the inventory and prescribing of controlled substances. State and local laws are often more stringent than federal law. In any given situation, the more stringent law applies.

form if one is available. This requirement helps keep down the cost of drugs and health care. Some prescribers, however, specify that a drug prescription be "dispensed as written" (DAW)—that is, that the brand-name product be used. By doing so, the prescriber ensures the quality control and bioavailability expected with that drug. These elements may be most important in drugs that have narrow safety margins, such as digoxin (*Lanoxin*), a heart drug, and warfarin (*Coumadin*), an anticoagulant. The initial cost may be higher, but some prescribers believe that, in the long run, the cost to the patient will be less.

ORPHAN DRUGS

Orphan drugs are drugs that have been discovered but are not financially viable and therefore have not been "adopted" by any drug company. Orphan drugs may be useful in treating a rare disease, or they may have potentially dangerous adverse effects. Orphan drugs are often abandoned after preclinical trials or phase I studies. The Orphan Drug Act of 1983 provided

tremendous financial incentives to drug companies to adopt these drugs and develop them. These incentives help the drug company put the drug through the rest of the testing process, even though the market for the drug in the long run may be very small (as in the case of a drug to treat a rare neurological disease that affects only a small number of people). Some drugs in this book have orphan drug uses listed.

OVER-THE-COUNTER DRUGS

Over-the-counter (OTC) drugs are products that are available without prescription for self-treatment of a variety of complaints. Some of these agents were approved as prescription drugs but later were found to be very safe and useful for patients without the need of a prescription. Some were not rigorously screened and tested by the current drug evaluation protocols because they were developed and marketed before the current laws were put into effect. Many of these drugs were "grandfathered" into use because they had been used for so long. The FDA is currently testing the effectiveness of many of these products and, in time, will evaluate all of them.

Though OTC drugs have been found to be safe when "taken as directed," there are several problems related to OTC drug use that nurses should consider:

- Taking these drugs could mask the signs and symptoms of underlying disease, making diagnosis difficult.
- Taking these drugs with prescription medications could result in drug interactions and interfere with drug therapy.
- Not taking these drugs as directed could result in serious overdoses.

Many patients do not consider OTC drugs to be medications and therefore do not report their use. Nurses should always include specific questions about OTC drug use when taking a drug history and should provide information in all drug-teaching protocols about avoiding OTC use while taking prescription drugs.

SOURCES OF DRUG INFORMATION

The fields of pharmacology and drug therapy change so quickly that it is important to have access to sources of information about drug doses, therapeutic and adverse effects, and nursing-related implications. Textbooks provide valuable background and basic information to help in the understanding of pharmacology, but in clinical practice it is important to have access to up-to-the-minute information. Several sources of drug information are readily available.

Package Inserts

All drugs come with a package insert prepared by the manufacturer according to strict FDA regulations. The package insert contains all of the chemical and study information that led to the drug's approval. Package inserts sometimes are difficult to understand.

Reference Books

The *Physician's Drug Reference (PDR)* is a compilation of the package insert information from drugs used in this country, along with some drug advertising. This information is cross-referenced. The book may be difficult to use.

Drug Facts and Comparisons provides a wide range of drug information, including comparisons of drug costs, patient information sections, and preparation and administration guidelines. This book is organized by drug class and can be more user-friendly than the *PDR*.

AMA Drug Evaluations contains detailed monographs in an unbiased format including many new drugs and drugs still in the research stage.

Lippincott's Nursing Drug Guide (LNDG) has drug monographs organized alphabetically and includes nursing implications and patient teaching points.

Journals

Medical Letter is a monthly review of new drugs, drug classes, and specific treatment protocols. *American Journal of Nursing* offers information on new drugs, drug errors, and nursing implications.

Internet Information

Box 1–4 lists some informative Internet sites for obtaining drug information, patient information, or therapeutic information related to specific disease states.

BOX 1-4
Internet Information

Ways to get started and to evaluate sites with drug information on the Internet

GOOD PLACES TO BEGIN (SEARCH TOOLS AND PLACES TO BROWSE)
Alta Vista:
  http://www.altavista.com
Cliniweb:
  http://www.ohsu.edu/cliniweb
Hardin Meta Directory of Internet Health Sources:
  http://www.lib.uiowa.edu/hardin/md/index.html
MetaCrawler:
  http://www.metacrawler.com
Yahoo Search:
  http://www.yahoo.com

LEARNING MORE ABOUT THE INTERNET
Learn the Net:
  http://learnthenet.com
To find an Internet service provider (ISP):
  http://www.thelist.com
Evaluating websites:
  http://hitiweb.mitretek.org/docs/policy.html

GOVERNMENT SITES
Agency for Health Care Research and Quality (AHRQ):
  http://www.ahcpr.gov
CancerNet (National Cancer Institute):
  http://www.cancer.gov
Centers for Disease Control:
  http://www.cdc.gov
Drug Formulary:
  http://www.intmed.mcw.edu/drug.html
Food and Drug Administration:
  http://www.fda.gov
Healthfinder:
  http://www.healthfinder.gov
National Institutes of Health:
  http://www.nih.gov

National Institute for Occupational Safety and Health:
  http://www.cdc.gov/niosh
National Library of Medicine:
  http://www.nlm.nih.gov
Office of Disease Prevention and Health Promotion:
  http://www.odphp.osophs.dhhs.gov

NURSING AND HEALTH CARE SITES
American Diabetes Association:
  http://www.diabetes.org
American Nurses Association:
  http://www.ana.org
Cumulative Index to Nursing and Allied Health Literature:
  http://www.cinahl.com
International Council of Nurses:
  http://www.icn.ch
Joint Commission on Accreditation of Healthcare Organizations:
  http://www.jcaho.org
Journal of American Medical Association:
  http://www.jama.ama-assn.org
Lippincott's Nursing Center:
  http://www.nursingcenter.com
Mayo Health Oasis:
  http://www.mayohealth.org
Medscape:
  http://www.medscape.com
Merck & Co. (search the *Merck Manual*):
  http://www.merck.com
New England Journal of Medicine:
  http://www.nejm.org
Nurse Practitioner resources:
  http://nurseweb.ucsf.edu/www/arwwebpg.htm
RxList:
  http://www.rxlist.com

CHAPTER SUMMARY

- Drugs are chemicals that are introduced into the body to bring about some sort of change.
- Drugs can come from many sources: plants, animals, inorganic elements, and synthetic preparations.
- The FDA regulates the development and marketing of drugs to ensure safety and efficacy.
- Preclinical trials involve testing of potential drugs on laboratory animals to determine their therapeutic and adverse effects.
- Phase I studies test potential drugs on healthy, human subjects.
- Phase II studies test potential drugs on patients who have the disease the drugs are designed to treat.
- Phase III studies test drugs in the clinical setting to determine any unanticipated effects or lack of effectiveness.
- FDA pregnancy categories indicate the potential or actual teratogenic effects of a drug.
- DEA controlled substance categories indicate the abuse potential and associated regulation of a drug.
- Generic drugs are sold under their chemical names, not brand names; they may be cheaper but are not necessarily as safe as brand-name drugs.
- Orphan drugs are chemicals that have been discovered to have some therapeutic effect but that are not financially advantageous to develop into drugs.
- OTC drugs are available without prescription for the self-treatment of various complaints.

Review Questions

1. Clinical pharmacology studies
   a. the biological effects of chemicals.
   b. drugs used to treat, prevent, or diagnose disease.
   c. plant components that can be used as medicines.
   d. binders and other vehicles for delivering medication.
2. Phase I drug studies involve
   a. the use of laboratory animals to test chemicals.
   b. patients with the disease the drug is designed to treat.
   c. mass marketing surveys of drug effects in large numbers of people.
   d. healthy, human volunteers who are often paid for their participation.
3. The generic name of a drug is
   a. the name assigned to the drug by the pharmaceutical company developing it.
   b. the chemical name of the drug based on its chemical structure.
   c. the original name assigned to the drug at the beginning of the evaluation process.
   d. often used in advertising campaigns.

4. An orphan drug is a drug that
   a. has failed to go through the approval process.
   b. is available in a foreign country but not in this country.
   c. has been discovered but is not financially viable and therefore has not been "adopted" by any drug company.
   d. is available without a prescription.
5. OTC (over-the-counter) drugs
   a. are nontoxic and can be used freely without problems.
   b. are not really medications and should not be included in a patient drug history.
   c. were all once prescription drugs that are now safe for unsupervised use.
   d. are drugs that are available without prescription for the self-treatment of many different ailments.
6. The FDA pregnancy categories
   a. indicate a drug's potential or actual teratogenic effects, offering guidelines for use of a particular drug in pregnancy.
   b. are used for research purposes only.
   c. list drugs that are more likely to have addicting properties.
   d. are tightly regulated by the DEA.
7. The storing, prescribing, and distributing of controlled substances—drugs that are more apt to be addictive—are monitored by
   a. the FDA.
   b. the Department of Commerce.
   c. the FBI.
   d. the DEA.
8. Generic drugs are
   a. drugs sold by generic name, not a brand name.
   b. always as safe and effective as the brand-name product.
   c. always cheaper than the brand-name product.
   d. available without a prescription.

BIBLIOGRAPHY

Anderson, P. O. (2000). *Handbook of critical drug data* (9th ed.). Hamilton, IL: Drug Intelligence.
Cardinale, V. (1998). Consumers looking for more answers, clearer directions. *Drug Topics Supplement, 142*(11), 23a.
McEvoy, B. R. (2002). *Drug facts and comparisons*. St. Louis: Facts and Comparisons.
Fitzgerald, M. (1994). Pharmacological highlights: Principles of pharmacokinetics. *Journal of the American Academy of Nursing Practice, 6*(12), 581.
Food and Drug Administration. (1994). FDA Launches MEDWATCH program: Monitoring adverse drug reactions. *NP News, 2*, 1, 4.
Gilman, A., Hardman, J. G., & Limbird, L. E. (Eds.) (2002). *Goodman and Gilman's the pharmacological basis of therapeutics* (10th ed.). New York: McGraw-Hill.
The medical letter on drugs and therapeutics. (2002). New Rochelle, NY: Medical Letter.

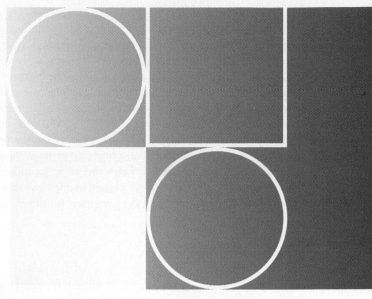

Drugs and the Body

Key Terms

absorption

biotransformation

chemotherapeutic agents

critical concentration

distribution

excretion

first-pass effect

half-life

pharmacodynamics

pharmacokinetics

placebo effect

receptor sites

selective toxicity

To understand what happens when a drug is administered, the nurse must understand **pharmacodynamics,** or how the drug affects the body, and **pharmacokinetics,** or how the body acts on the drug. These processes form the basis for the guidelines that have been established regarding drug administration—for example, why certain agents are given intramuscularly (IM) and not intravenously (IV), why some drugs are taken with food and others are not, and the usual dose to use. Knowing the basic principles of pharmacodynamics and pharmacokinetics helps the nurse to anticipate therapeutic and adverse drug effects and to intervene in ways that ensure the most effective drug regimen for the patient.

PHARMACODYNAMICS

Pharmacodynamics is the science dealing with interactions between the chemical components of living systems and the foreign chemicals, including drugs, that enter those systems. All living organisms function by a series of complicated, continual chemical reactions. When a new chemical enters the system, multiple changes in and interferences with cell functioning may occur. To avoid such problems, drug development works to provide the most effective and least toxic chemicals for therapeutic use.

DRUG ACTIONS

Drugs usually work in one of four ways:

1. To replace or act as substitutes for missing chemicals.
2. To increase or stimulate certain cellular activities.
3. To depress or slow cellular activities.
4. To interfere with the functioning of foreign cells, such as invading microorganisms or neoplasms. (Drugs that act in this way are called **chemotherapeutic agents.**)

There are several possible ways that drugs can achieve these results, which are described in this chapter.

Receptor Sites

Many drugs are thought to act at specific areas on cell membranes called **receptor sites.** The receptor sites react with certain chemicals to cause an effect within the cell. In many situations, nearby enzymes break down the reacting chemicals and open up the receptor site for further stimulation.

To better understand this process, think of how a key works in a lock. The specific chemical (the key) approaches a cell membrane and finds a perfect fit (the lock) at a receptor site (Figure 2–1). The interaction between the chemical and the receptor site affects enzyme systems within the cell. The activated enzyme systems then produce certain effects, such as increased or decreased cellular activity, changes in cell membrane permeability, or alterations in cellular metabolism.

Some drugs interact directly with receptor sites to cause the same activity that natural chemicals would cause at that site. These drugs are called *agonists* (see Figure 2–1). For example, insulin reacts with specific insulin receptor sites to change cell membrane permeability, thus promoting the movement of glucose into the cell.

Other drugs act to prevent the breakdown of natural chemicals that are stimulating the receptor site. For example, monoamine oxidase (MAO) inhibitors block the breakdown of norepinephrine by the enzyme MAO. (Normally, MAO breaks down norepinephrine, removes it from the receptor site, and recycles the components to form new norepinephrine.) The blocking action of MAO inhibitors allows norepinephrine to stay on the receptor site, stimulating the cell longer and leading to prolonged norepinephrine effects. Those effects can be therapeutic (eg, relieving depression) or adverse (eg, increasing heart rate and blood pressure).

Selective serotonin reuptake inhibitors (SSRIs) work similarly to MAO inhibitors in that they also exert a blocking action. Specifically, they block removal of serotonin from receptor sites. This action leads to prolonged stimulation of brain cells, which is thought to provide relief from depression.

Some drugs react with receptor sites to block normal stimulation, producing no effect. For example, curare (a drug used on the tips of spears in the Amazon to paralyze prey and cause death) occupies receptor sites for acetylcholine, which is necessary for muscle contraction and movement. Curare prevents muscle stimulation, causing paralysis. Curare is said to be a *competitive antagonist* of acetylcholine (see Figure 2–1).

Still other drugs react with specific receptor sites on a cell and, by reacting there, prevent the reaction of another chemical with a different receptor site on that cell. Such drugs are called *noncompetitive antagonists* (see Figure 2–1).

For some drugs, the actual mechanisms of action are unknown. But speculation exists that many drugs use receptor site mechanisms to bring about their effects.

Drug–Enzyme Interactions

Drugs also can cause their effects by interfering with the enzyme systems that act as catalysts for various chemical reactions. Enzyme systems work in a cascade effect, with one enzyme activating another and eventually causing a cellular reaction. If a single step in one of the many enzyme systems is blocked, normal cell function is disrupted. Acetazolamide (*Diamox*) is a diuretic that blocks the enzyme carbonic anhydrase, which subsequently causes alterations in the hydrogen ion and water exchange system in the kidney as well as the eye.

Selective Toxicity

Ideally, all chemotherapeutic agents would act only on enzyme systems that are essential for the life of a pathogen or

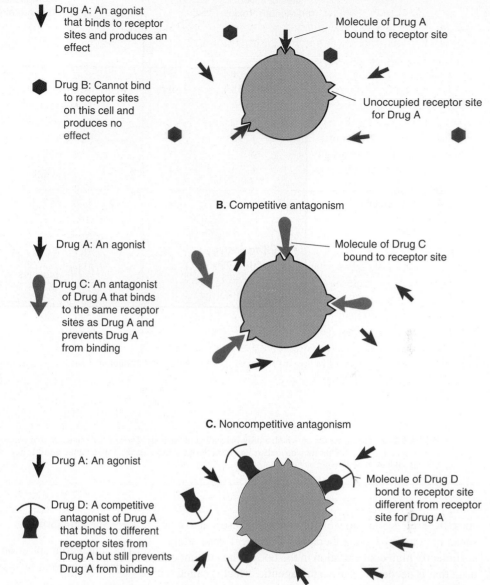

A. Agonist interaction with receptor site on cell

Drug A: An agonist that binds to receptor sites and produces an effect

Drug B: Cannot bind to receptor sites on this cell and produces no effect

Molecule of Drug A bound to receptor site

Unoccupied receptor site for Drug A

B. Competitive antagonism

Drug A: An agonist

Drug C: An antagonist of Drug A that binds to the same receptor sites as Drug A and prevents Drug A from binding

Molecule of Drug C bound to receptor site

C. Noncompetitive antagonism

Drug A: An agonist

Drug D: A competitive antagonist of Drug A that binds to different receptor sites from Drug A but still prevents Drug A from binding

Molecule of Drug D bond to receptor site different from receptor site for Drug A

FIGURE 2-1. Receptor theory of drug action. (**A**) Agonist interaction with receptor site on cell: molecules of drug A react with specific receptor sites on cells of effector organs and change the cells' activity. (**B**) Competitive antagonism: drug A and drug C have an affinity for the same receptor sites and compete for these sites; drug C has a greater affinity, occupies more of the sites, and antagonizes drug A. (**C**) Noncompetitive antagonism: drug D reacts with a receptor site that is different from the receptor site for drug A but still somehow prevents drug A from binding with its receptor sites. Drugs that act by inhibiting enzymes can be pictured as acting similarly to the receptor site antagonists illustrated in **B** and **C**. Enzyme inhibitors block the binding of molecules of normal substrate to active sites on the enzyme.

neoplastic cell and would not affect healthy cells. The ability of a drug to attack only those systems found in foreign cells is known as **selective toxicity.** Penicillin, an antibiotic used to treat bacterial infections, has selective toxicity. It affects an enzyme system unique to bacteria, causing bacterial cell death without disrupting normal human cell functioning.

Unfortunately, most other chemotherapeutic agents also destroy normal human cells, causing many of the adverse effects associated with antipathogen and antineoplastic chemotherapy. Cells that reproduce or are replaced rapidly (eg, bone marrow cells, gastrointestinal [GI] cells, hair follicles) are more easily affected by these agents. Consequently, the goal of many chemotherapeutic drug regimens is to deliver a dose that will be toxic to the invading cells yet cause the least amount of toxicity to the host.

PHARMACOKINETICS

Pharmacokinetics involves the study of absorption, distribution, metabolism (biotransformation), and excretion of drugs. In clinical practice, pharmacokinetic considerations include the onset of drug action, drug half-life, timing of the peak effect, duration of drug effects, metabolism or biotransformation of the drug, and the site of excretion. Figure 2–2 outlines these processes, which are described in the following sections.

Critical Concentration

After a drug is administered, its molecules first must be absorbed into the body, then make their way to the reactive tis-

FIGURE 2–2. The processes by which a drug is handled in the body. *Dashed lines* indicate that some portion of a drug and its metabolites may be reabsorbed from the excretory organs. The dynamic equilibrium of drug pharmacokinetics is shown.

sues. If a drug is going to work properly on these reactive tissues, and thereby have a therapeutic effect, it must attain a sufficiently high concentration in the body. The amount of a drug that is needed to cause a therapeutic effect is called the **critical concentration.**

Drug evaluation studies determine the critical concentration required to cause a desired therapeutic effect. The recommended dosage of a drug is based on the amount that must be given to eventually reach the critical concentration. Too much of a drug will produce toxic effects, and too little will not produce the desired therapeutic effects.

Loading Dose

For some drugs that take a prolonged period to reach a critical concentration, if their effects are needed quickly, a loading dose is recommended. Digoxin (*Lanoxin*), a drug used to increase the strength of heart contractions, and many of the xanthine bronchodilators (eg, aminophylline, theophylline) used to treat asthma attacks are often started with a loading dose (a higher dose than that usually used for treatment) to reach the critical concentration. The critical concentration then is maintained at the recommended dosing schedule.

Dynamic Equilibrium

The actual concentration that a drug reaches in the body results from a dynamic equilibrium involving several factors:

• Absorption from the site of entry
• Distribution to the active site
• Biotransformation (metabolism) in the liver
• Excretion from the body

These factors are key elements in determining the amount of drug needed (dose) and the frequency of dose repetition (scheduling) required to achieve the critical concentration for the desired length of time. When administering a drug, the nurse needs to consider the phases of pharmacokinetics so that the drug regimen can be made as effective as possible.

Absorption

In order to reach reactive tissues, a drug must first make its way into the circulating fluids of the body. **Absorption** refers to what happens to a drug from the time it is introduced to the body until it reaches the circulating fluids and tissues. Drugs can be absorbed from many different areas in the body: through the GI tract either orally or rectally, through mucous membranes, through the skin, through the lung, or through muscle or subcutaneous tissues (see Figure 2–2).

Drugs can be absorbed into cells through various processes, which include passive diffusion, active transport, and filtration. Passive diffusion is the major process through which drugs are absorbed into the body. Passive diffusion occurs across a concentration gradient. When there is a greater concentration of drug on one side of a cell membrane, the drug will move through the membrane to the area of lower concentration. This process does not require any cellular energy. It occurs more quickly if the drug molecule is small, is soluble in water and in lipids (cell membranes are made of lipids and proteins—see Chapter 7), and has no electrical charge that could repel it from the cell membrane.

Unlike passive diffusion, active transport is a process that uses energy to actively move a molecule across a cell membrane. The molecule may be large, or it may be moving against a concentration gradient. This process is not very important in the absorption of drugs, but it is often involved in drug excretion in the kidney.

Filtration is another process the body commonly uses in drug excretion. Filtration involves movement through pores in the cell membrane, either down a concentration gradient or as a result of the pull of plasma proteins (when pushed by hydrostatic, blood, or osmotic pressure).

Administration

The oral route is the most frequently used administration route in clinical practice. Oral administration is not invasive, is cheaper, and is the safest way to deliver drugs. Patients can easily continue their drug regimen at home when they are taking oral medications.

Oral administration subjects the drug to a number of barriers aimed at destroying ingested foreign chemicals. The acidic environment of the stomach is one of the first barriers to foreign chemicals. The acid breaks down many compounds and inactivates others. This fact is taken into account by pharmaceutical companies when preparing capsules or tablets of drugs. The binders that are used often are designed to break down in a certain acidity and release the active drug to be absorbed.

When food is present, stomach acidity is higher and the stomach empties more slowly, thus exposing the drug to the acidic environment for a longer period. Certain foods that increase stomach acidity, such as milk products, alcohol, and protein, also speed the breakdown of many drugs. Other foods may chemically bind drugs or block their absorption. To decrease the effects of this acid barrier and the direct effects of certain foods, oral drugs ideally should be given 1 hour before or 2 hours after a meal.

Some drugs that cannot survive in sufficient quantity when given orally need to be injected directly into the body. Drugs that are injected IV reach their full strength at the time of injection, avoiding initial breakdown. These drugs are more apt to cause toxic effects, because the margin for error in dosage is much smaller. Drugs that are injected IM are absorbed directly into the capillaries in the muscle and sent into circulation. This takes time, because the drug must be picked up by the capillary and taken into the veins. Because men have more vascular muscles than women do, IM drugs in men reach a peak level faster than in women. Subcutaneous (SC) injections deposit the drug just under the skin, where it is slowly absorbed into circulation. Timing of absorption varies with SC injection, depending on the fat content of the injection site and the state of local circulation.

Table 2–1 outlines the various factors that affect drug absorption.

First-Pass Effect

Drugs that are taken orally are usually absorbed from the small intestine directly into the portal venous system (the blood vessels that flow through the liver on their way back to the heart). Aspirin and alcohol are two drugs that are known to be absorbed from the lower end of the stomach. The portal veins deliver these absorbed molecules into the liver, which immediately transforms most of the chemicals delivered to it by a series of liver enzymes. These enzymes break the drug into metabolites, some of which are active

TABLE 2-1 | Factors That Affect Absorption of Drugs

Route	Factors Affecting Absorption
IV (intravenous)	None: direct entry into the venous system
IM (intramuscular)	Perfusion or blood flow to the muscle Fat content of the muscle Temperature of the muscle: cold causes vasoconstriction and decreases absorption; heat causes vasodilation and increases absorption
SC (subcutaneous)	Perfusion or blood flow to the tissue Fat content of the tissue Temperature of the tissue: cold causes vasoconstriction and decreases absorption; heat causes vasodilation and increases absorption
PO (oral)	Acidity of stomach Length of time in stomach Blood flow to gastrointestinal tract Presence of interacting foods or drugs
PR (rectal)	Perfusion or blood flow to the rectum Lesions in the rectum Length of time retained for absorption
Mucous membranes (sublingual, buccal)	Perfusion or blood flow to the area Integrity of the mucous membranes Presence of food or smoking Length of time retained in area
Topical (skin)	Perfusion or blood flow to the area Integrity of skin
Inhalation	Perfusion or blood flow to the area Integrity of lung lining Ability to administer drug properly

and cause effects in the body and some of which are deactivated and can be readily excreted from the body. As a result, a large percentage of the oral dose is destroyed at this point and never reaches the tissues. This phenomenon is known as the **first-pass effect.** The recommended dose for oral drugs can be considerably higher than the recommended dose for parenteral drugs, taking the first-pass effect into account.

Injected drugs and drugs absorbed from sites other than the GI tract undergo a similar biotransformation when they pass through the liver. Because some of the active drug already has had a chance to reach the reactive tissues before reaching the liver, the injected drug is more effective at a lower dose than the oral equivalent.

Distribution

The portion of the drug that gets through the first-pass effect is delivered to the circulation for transport throughout the body. **Distribution** involves the movement of a drug to the body's tissues (see Figure 2–2). As with absorption, factors that can affect distribution include the drug's lipid solubility and ionization and the perfusion of the reactive tissue.

For example, tissue perfusion is a factor in treating a diabetic patient who has a lower leg infection and needs antibiotics to destroy the bacteria in the area. In this case, systemic drugs may not be effective because part of the disease process involves changes in the vasculature and decreased blood flow to some areas, particularly the lower limbs. If there is not adequate blood flow to the area, little antibiotic can be delivered to the tissues and little antibiotic effect will be seen.

In the same way, patients who are in a cold environment may experience vasoconstriction in the extremities, preventing blood flow to those areas. The circulation would be unable to deliver drugs to those areas, and the patient would receive little therapeutic effect from drugs intended to react with those tissues.

Many drugs are bound to proteins and are not lipid soluble. These drugs cannot be distributed to the central nervous system (CNS) because of the effective blood–brain barrier (see later discussion), which is highly selective in allowing lipid-soluble substances to pass into the CNS.

Protein Binding

Most drugs are bound to some extent to proteins in the blood to be carried in circulation. The protein–drug complex is relatively large and cannot enter into capillaries and then into tissues to react. The drug must be freed from the protein's binding site at the tissues.

Some drugs are tightly bound and are released very slowly. These drugs have a very long duration of action, because they are not freed to be broken down or excreted and therefore are very slowly released into the reactive tissue. Some drugs are loosely bound; they tend to act quickly and to be excreted quickly. Some drugs compete with each other for protein binding sites, altering effectiveness or toxicity when the two drugs are given together.

Blood–Brain Barrier

The blood–brain barrier is a protective system of cellular activity that keeps many things (eg, foreign invaders, poisons) away from the CNS. Drugs that are highly lipid soluble are more likely to pass through the blood–brain barrier and reach the CNS. Drugs that are not lipid soluble are not able to pass the blood–brain barrier. This fact can be of clinical significance in the treatment of a brain infection with antibiotics. Almost all antibiotics are not lipid soluble and cannot cross the blood–brain barrier. Effective antibiotic treatment can occur only when the infection is bad enough to alter the blood–brain barrier and allow antibiotics to cross.

Although many drugs can cause adverse CNS effects, these are often the result of indirect drug effects and not the actual reaction of the drug with CNS tissue. For example, alterations in glucose levels and electrolyte changes can interfere with nerve functioning and produce CNS effects.

Placenta and Breast Milk

Many drugs readily pass through the placenta and affect the developing fetus in pregnant women. As stated earlier, it is best not to administer any drugs to pregnant women because of the possible risk to the fetus. Drugs should be given only when the benefit clearly outweighs any risk.

Many other drugs are secreted into breast milk and therefore have the potential to affect the neonate. Because of this possibility, the nurse must always check the ability of a drug to pass into breast milk when giving a drug to a nursing mother.

Biotransformation (Metabolism)

The body is well prepared to deal with a myriad of foreign chemicals. Enzymes in the liver, in many cells, in the lining of the GI tract, and even circulating in the body detoxify foreign chemicals to protect the fragile homeostasis that keeps the body functioning (see Figure 2–2). Almost all of the chemical reactions that the body uses to convert drugs and other chemicals into nontoxic substances are based on a few processes that work to make the chemical less active and more easily excreted from the body.

Liver Enzyme Systems

The liver is the single most important site of drug metabolism or **biotransformation,** the process by which drugs are changed into new, less active chemicals. Think of the liver as a sewage treatment plant. Everything that is absorbed from the GI tract first enters the liver to be "treated." The liver detoxifies many chemicals and uses others to produce needed enzymes and structures.

The hepatic cells' intracellular structures are lined with enzymes, which are packed together in what is called the *hepatic microsomal system.* Because orally administered drugs enter the liver first, the enzyme systems immediately work on the absorbed drug to biotransform it. As explained earlier, this first-pass effect is responsible for neutralizing most of the drugs that are taken. Phase I biotransformation involves oxidation, reduction, or hydrolysis of the drug via the cytochrome P450 system of enzymes. These enzymes are found in most cells but are especially abundant in the liver. Phase II biotransformation usually involves a conjugation reaction that makes the drug less polar and more readily excreted by the kidney.

The presence of a chemical that is metabolized by a particular enzyme system often increases the activity of that enzyme system. This process is referred to as *enzyme induction*. Only a few basic enzyme systems are responsible for metabolizing most of the chemicals that pass through the liver. Increased activity in an enzyme system speeds the metabolism of the drug that caused the enzyme induction as well as any other drug that is metabolized via that same enzyme system. This explains why some drugs cannot be taken together effectively: the presence of one drug speeds the metabolism of others, preventing them from reaching their therapeutic levels. Some drugs inhibit an enzyme system, making it less effective. As a consequence, any drug that is metabolized by that system will not be broken down for excretion, and the blood levels of that drug will increase, often to toxic levels. These actions also explain why liver disease is often a contraindication or a reason to use caution when administering certain drugs. If the liver is not functioning effectively, the drug will not be metabolized as it should be, and toxic levels could develop rather quickly. Table 2–2 gives some examples of drugs that induce or inhibit the cytochrome P450 system.

Excretion

Excretion is the removal of a drug from the body. The skin, saliva, lungs, bile, and feces are some of the routes used to excrete drugs. The kidneys, however, play the most important role in drug excretion (see Figure 2–2). Drugs that have been made water soluble in the liver are often readily excreted from the kidney by *glomerular filtration*—the passage of water and water-soluble components from the plasma into the renal tubule.

Other drugs are secreted or reabsorbed through the renal tubule by active transport systems. The acidity of the urine can play an important part in the excretions. The active transport systems that move the drug into the tubule often do so by exchanging it for acid or bicarbonate molecules. This is an important concept to remember when trying to clear a drug rapidly from the system or trying to understand why a drug is being given at the usual dose but is reaching toxic levels in the system. The patient's kidney functioning and urine acidity are important things to consider before administering a drug. Kidney dysfunction can lead to toxic levels of a drug in the body because the drug cannot be excreted.

Figure 2–3 outlines the pharmacokinetic processes that are undergone by a drug administered orally.

Half-Life

The **half-life** of a drug is the time it takes for the amount of drug in the body to decrease to one-half of the peak level it previously achieved. For instance, if a patient takes 20 mg of a drug with a half-life of 2 hours, 10 mg of the drug will remain 2 hours after administration. Two hours later, 5 mg will be left (one-half of the previous level); in 2 more hours, only 2.5 mg will remain. This information is important in determining the appropriate timing for a drug dose or determining the duration of a drug's effect on the body.

The half-life is determined by a balance of all of the factors working on that drug: absorption, distribution, biotrans-

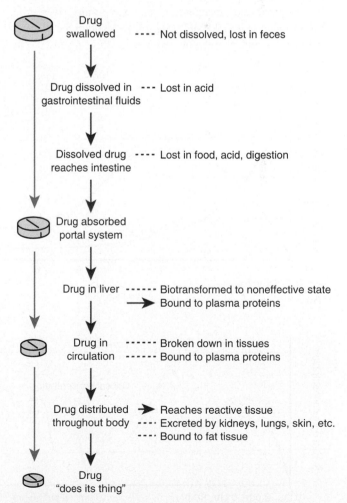

FIGURE 2–3. Pharmacokinetics affect the amount of a drug that reaches reactive tissues. Very little of an oral dose of a drug actually reaches reactive sites.

TABLE 2-2	Examples of Drugs that Alter the Effects of the Cytochrome P450 Enzyme System in the Liver

Drugs that Induce or Increase Activity	Drugs that Inhibit or Decrease Activity
Nicotine (cigarette smoking)	Ketoconazole (*Nizoral*)
Alcohol (drinking)	Mexiletine (*Mexitil*)
Glucocorticoids (*Cortone,* others)	Quinidine (*Quinaglute*)

formation, and excretion. The absorption rate, the distribution to the tissues, the speed of biotransformation, and how fast a drug is excreted are all taken into consideration when determining the half-life of the drug. The half-life that is indicated in any drug monograph is the half-life for a healthy person. Using this information, the half-life of a drug for a patient with kidney or liver dysfunction (which could prolong the biotransformation and the time required for excretion of a drug) can be estimated and changes made in the dosage schedule by the prescriber.

The timing of drug administration is important to achieve the most effective drug therapy. Nurses can use their knowledge of drug half-life to explain the importance of following a schedule of drug administration in the hospital or at home. Figure 2–4 shows the effects of drug administration on the critical concentration of a drug.

FACTORS INFLUENCING DRUG EFFECTS

When administering a drug to a patient, the nurse must be aware that the human factor has a tremendous influence on what actually happens to a drug when it enters the body. No two people react in exactly the same way to any given drug. Even though textbooks and drug guides explain the pharmacodynamics and pharmacokinetics of a drug, it must be re-

membered that such information usually is based on studies of healthy, adult males. Things may be very different in the clinical setting. Consequently, before administering any drug, the nurse must consider a number of factors. These are discussed in detail in the following sections and summarized in Box 2–1.

Weight

The recommended dosage of a drug is based on drug evaluation studies and is targeted at a 150-pound person. People who are much heavier than that may require larger doses to get a therapeutic effect from a drug because they have increased tissues to perfuse and increased receptor sites in some reactive tissue. People who are much lighter than the norm may require smaller doses of a drug. Toxic effects may occur at the recommended dosage if the person is very small.

Age

Age is a factor primarily in children and older adults. Children metabolize many drugs differently than adults do, and they have immature systems for handling drugs. Many drugs come with recommended pediatric dosages, and others can be converted to pediatric dosages using one of several conversion formulas (Box 2–2).

Older adults undergo many physical changes that are a part

FIGURE 2-4. Influence of biologic half-life, route of administration, and dosage regimen on serum drug levels. **(A)** Influence of route of administration on time course of drug levels after administration of a single dose of a drug. The *dashed lines* indicate how the biologic half-life of the drug may be determined from the curve of drug concentration after an intravenous dose. At time 0, immediately after the injection, there were 4 units of drug in each milliliter of serum. The drug concentration fell to half this amount, 2 units/mL, after 1 hour, the drug's biologic half-life. **(B)** Influence of dosage regimen on serum drug levels (drug given four times daily, at 10 AM and at 2, 6, and 10 PM). The drug accumulates as successive doses are given throughout each day; the drug is being given at a rate greater than the patient's body can eliminate it. This dosage regimen has been chosen so that the patient will have a therapeutic level of the drug for a significant portion of the day, yet never have a toxic level of the drug.

BOX 2-1

Factors Affecting the Body's Response to a Drug

Weight
Age
Gender
Physiological factors—diurnal rhythm, electrolyte balance, acid–base balance, hydration
Pathological factors—disease, hepatic dysfunction, renal dysfunction, gastrointestinal dysfunction, vascular disorders, low blood pressure
Genetic factors
Immunological factors—allergy
Psychological factors—placebo effect, health beliefs, compliance
Environmental factors—temperature, light, noise
Drug tolerance
Cumulative effects

of the aging process. Their bodies may respond very differently in all aspects of pharmacokinetics—less effective absorption, less efficient distribution because of fewer plasma proteins and less efficient perfusion, altered biotransformation or metabolism of drugs because of liver changes with age, and less effective excretion owing to less efficient kidneys. Many drugs now come with recommended geriatric dosages. Other drugs may also need decreased dosages in the elderly.

When administering drugs to a patient at either end of the age spectrum, the nurse should monitor closely for desired effects. If the effects are not what would normally be expected, a dosage adjustment should be considered.

Gender

Physiological differences between men and women can influence a drug's effect. When giving IM injections, for example, it is important to remember that men have more vascular muscles, so the effects of the drug will be seen sooner in men than in women.

Women have more fat cells than men do, so drugs that deposit in fat may be slowly released and cause effects for a prolonged period. For example, gas anesthetics have an affinity for depositing in fat and can cause drowsiness and sedation sometimes weeks after surgery.

Women who are given any drug should always be questioned about the possibility of pregnancy, because, as stated previously, the use of drugs in pregnant women is not recommended unless the benefit clearly outweighs the potential risk to the fetus.

Physiological Factors

Physiological differences such as diurnal rhythm of the nervous and endocrine systems, acid–base balance, hydration,

and electrolyte balance can affect the way that a drug works on the body and the way that the body handles the drug. If a drug does not produce the desired effect, review the patient's acid–base and electrolyte profile and the timing of the drug.

Pathological Factors

Drugs are usually used to treat disease or pathology. However, the disease that the drug is intended to treat can change the functioning of the chemical reactions within the body and thus change the response to the drug.

Other pathological conditions can change the basic pharmacokinetics of a drug. For example, GI disorders can affect the absorption of many oral drugs. Vascular diseases and low blood pressure alter the distribution of a drug, preventing it from being delivered to the reactive tissue and rendering it nontherapeutic. Liver or kidney diseases affect the way that a drug is biotransformed and excreted and can lead to toxic reactions when the usual dose is given.

Genetic Factors

Genetic differences can sometimes explain patients' varied responses to a given drug. Some people lack certain enzyme systems necessary for metabolizing a drug, whereas others have overactive enzyme systems and break down drugs very quickly. Still others have differing metabolisms or slightly different enzymatic makeups that alter their chemical reactions and the effects of a given drug. Predictable differences in the pharmacokinetics and pharmacodynamic effects of drugs can be anticipated with people of particular cultural backgrounds because of their genetic makeup. Such differences are highlighted throughout this book.

Immunological Factors

People can develop an allergy to a drug. After exposure to its proteins, a person can develop antibodies to a drug; with future exposure to the same drug, that person may experience a full-blown allergic reaction. Sensitivity to a drug can range from dermatological effects to anaphylaxis, shock, and death. (Drug allergies are discussed in detail in Chapter 3.)

Psychological Factors

The patient's attitude about a drug has been shown to have a real effect on how that drug works. A drug is more likely to be effective if the patient thinks it will work than if the patient believes it will not work. This is called the **placebo effect.**

The patient's personality also influences compliance with the drug regimen. Some people who believe that they can influence their health actively seek health care and willingly follow a prescribed regimen. These people usually trust the medical system and believe that their efforts will be positive. Other people do not trust the medical system; they may be-

BOX 2-2
Formulas for Calculating Dosages

PEDIATRIC DOSAGES

Children often require different doses of drugs than adults because children's bodies often handle drugs very differently from adults' bodies. The "standard" drug dosages listed in package inserts and references such as the PDR refer to the adult dosage. In some cases, a pediatric dosage is suggested, but in many cases it will need to be calculated based on the child's age, weight, or body surface. The following are some standard formulae for calculating the pediatric dose.

Fried's Rule

$$\text{infant's dose } (< 1 \text{ y}) = \frac{\text{infant's age (in mo)}}{150 \text{ mo}}$$
$$\times \text{ average adult dose}$$

Young's Rule

$$\text{child's dose } (1\text{–}12 \text{ y}) = \frac{\text{child's age (in yrs)}}{\text{child's age (in yrs)} + 12}$$
$$\times \text{ average adult dose}$$

The surface area of a child is determined using a nomogram which determines surface area based on height and weight measurements.

Pediatric dosage calculations should be checked by two persons. Many institutions have procedures for double checking the dosage calculation of those drugs (eg, digoxin) used most frequently in the pediatric area.

Clark's Rule

$$\text{child's dose} = \frac{\text{weight of child (lb)}}{150 \text{ lb}}$$
$$\times \text{ average adult dose}$$

Surface Area Rule

$$\text{child's dose} = \frac{\text{surface area of child (in square meters)}}{1.73}$$
$$\times \text{ average adult dose}$$

Height		Surface Area	Weight	
feet	centimeters	in square meters	pounds	kilograms

Nomogram for estimating surface area of infants and young children. To determine the surface area of the patient, draw a straight line between the point representing the height on the left vertical scale and the point representing the weight on the right vertical scale. The point at which this line intersects the middle vertical scale represents the patient's surface area in square meters.

lieve that they have no control over their own health and may be unwilling to comply with any prescribed therapy. Knowing a patient's health-seeking history and feelings about health care is important in planning an educational program that will work for that particular patient. It is also important to know this information when arranging for necessary follow-up procedures and evaluations.

As the caregiver most often involved in drug administration, the nurse is in a position to influence the patient's attitude about drug effectiveness. Frequently, the nurse's positive attitude, combined with additional comfort measures, can improve the patient's response to a medication.

Environmental Factors

The environment can affect the success of drug therapy. Some drug effects are helped by a quiet, cool, nonstimulating environment. For example, sedating drugs are given to help a patient relax or to decrease tension. Cutting down on external stimuli to decrease tension and stimulation will help the drug be more effective. Other drug effects may be influenced by temperature. For example, antihypertensives that are working well during cold, winter months may become too effective in warmer environments, when natural vasodilation to release heat tends to lower the blood pressure. If a patient's response to a medication is not as expected, the nurse might look for changes in environmental conditions.

Tolerance

Some drugs become tolerated by the body over time. Tolerance may come about because of increased biotransformation of the drug, increased resistance to its effects, or other pharmacokinetic factors. Drugs that are tolerated no longer cause the same reaction, and they need to be taken in increasingly larger doses to achieve a therapeutic effect. An example of this type of drug is morphine, an opiate used for pain relief. The longer morphine is taken, the more tolerant the body becomes to the drug, so that larger and larger doses are needed to relieve pain. Clinically, this situation can be avoided by giving the drug in smaller doses or in combination with other drugs that may also relieve pain. *Cross-tolerance,* or resistance to drugs within the same class, may also occur in some situations.

Cumulation

If a drug is taken in successive doses at intervals that are shorter than recommended, or if the body is not able to eliminate a drug properly, the drug can accumulate in the body, leading to toxic levels and adverse effects. This can be avoided by following the drug regimen precisely. In reality, with many people managing their own therapy at home, strict compliance with a drug regimen seldom occurs. Some people take all of their medications first thing in the morn-

ing, so that they won't forget to take the pills later in the day. Others realize that they forgot a dose and then take two to make up for it. Many interruptions of everyday life can interfere with strict adherence to a drug regimen. If a drug is causing serious adverse effects, review the drug regimen with the patient to find out how the drug is being taken, and then educate the patient appropriately.

Drug–Drug Interactions

When two or more drugs are taken together, there is a possibility that the drugs will interact with each other to cause unanticipated effects in the body. Usually this is an increase or decrease in the desired therapeutic effect of one or all of the drugs or an increase in adverse effects.

Clinically significant drug–drug interactions occur with drugs that have small margins of safety. If there is very little difference between a therapeutic dose and a toxic dose of the drug, interference with the drug's pharmacokinetics or pharmacodynamics can produce serious problems. For example, drug–drug interactions can occur in the following situations:

- *At the site of absorption:* One drug prevents or accelerates absorption of the other drug. For example, the antibiotic tetracycline is not absorbed from the GI tract if calcium or calcium products are present in the stomach.
- *During distribution:* One drug competes for the protein binding site of another drug, so the second drug cannot be transported to the reactive tissue. For example, aspirin competes with the drug methotrexate (*Rheumatrex*) for protein binding sites. Because aspirin is more competitive for the sites, the methotrexate is bumped off, resulting in increased release of methotrexate and increased toxicity to the tissues.
- *During biotransformation:* One drug stimulates or blocks the metabolism of the other drug. For example, warfarin (*Coumadin*), an oral anticoagulant, is biotransformed more quickly if it is taken at the same time as barbiturates, rifampin, or many other drugs. Because the warfarin is biotransformed to an inactive state more quickly, higher doses will be needed to achieve the desired effect.
- *During excretion:* One drug competes for excretion with the other drug, leading to accumulation and toxic effects of one of the drugs. For example, digoxin (*Lanoxin*) and quinidine (*Quinaglute*) are both excreted from the same sites in the kidney. If they are given together, the quinidine is more competitive for these sites and is excreted, resulting in increased serum levels of digoxin, which cannot be excreted.
- *At the site of action:* One drug may be an antagonist of the other drug, or may cause effects opposite those of the other drug, leading to no therapeutic effect. This is seen, for example, when an antihypertensive drug is taken with an allergy drug that also increases blood pressure. The effects on blood pressure are negated, and there is a loss of the antihypertensive effectiveness of the drug.

Whenever two or more drugs are being given together, the nurse should first consult a drug guide for a listing of clinically significant drug–drug interactions. Sometimes problems can be avoided by spacing the drugs apart or adjusting their dosages. Check the monograph of any drug that is being given to monitor for clinically important drug–drug interactions.

Drug–Food Interactions

Certain foods can interact with drugs in much the same way that drugs can interact with each other. For the most part, this interaction occurs when the drug and the food are in direct contact in the stomach. Some foods increase acid production, speeding the breakdown of the drug molecule and preventing absorption and distribution of the drug. Some foods chemically react with certain drugs and prevent their absorption into the body. The antibiotic tetracycline cannot be taken with iron products for this reason. Tetracycline also binds with calcium to some extent and should not be taken with foods or other drugs containing calcium.

As stated earlier, oral drugs are best taken on an empty stomach. If the patient cannot tolerate the drug on an empty stomach, the food selected to be taken with the drug should be something that is known not to interact with it. Drug monographs usually list important drug–food interactions and give guidelines to avoid problems and optimize the drug's therapeutic effects.

Drug–Laboratory Test Interactions

As explained previously, the body works through a series of chemical reactions. Because of this, administration of a particular drug may alter tests that are done on various chemical levels or reactions as part of a diagnostic study. This drug–laboratory test interaction is caused by the drug being given and not necessarily by a change in the body's responses or actions. It is important to keep these interactions in mind when evaluating a patient's diagnostic tests. If one test result is off and does not fit in with the clinical picture or other test results, consider the possibility of a drug–laboratory test interference. For example, dalteparin (*Fragmin*), a low-molecular-weight heparin used to prevent deep vein thrombosis after abdominal surgery, may cause increased levels of the liver enzymes aspartate aminotransferase (AST) and alanine aminotransferase (ALT) with no injury to liver cells or hepatitis.

ACHIEVING THE OPTIMAL THERAPEUTIC EFFECT

As overwhelming as all of this information may seem, most patients can follow a drug regimen to achieve optimal therapeutic effects without serious adverse effects. Avoiding problems is the best way to treat adverse or ineffective drug effects. The nurse should incorporate basic history and phys-

ical assessment factors into any care plan, so that obvious problems can be spotted and handled promptly. If a drug just does not do what it is expected to do, the nurse should further examine the factors that are known to influence drug effects (see Box 1–1). Frequently, the drug regimen can be modified to deal with that influence. Rarely is it necessary to completely stop a needed drug regimen because of adverse or intolerable effects. The nurse is the caregiver in the best position to assess problems early, intervene appropriately, and prevent the occurrence of serious problems.

CHAPTER SUMMARY

- Pharmacodynamics is the study of the way that drugs affect the body.
- Most drugs work by replacing natural chemicals, by stimulating normal cell activity, or by depressing normal cell activity.
- Chemotherapeutic agents work to interfere with normal cell functioning, causing cell death. The most desirable chemotherapeutic agents are those with selective toxicity to foreign cells and foreign cell activities.
- Drugs frequently act at specific receptor sites on cell membranes to stimulate enzyme systems within the cell and to alter the cell's activities.
- Pharmacokinetics, the study of the way the body deals with drugs, includes absorption, distribution, biotransformation, and excretion of drugs.
- The goal of established dosing schedules is to achieve a critical concentration of the drug in the body. This critical concentration is the amount of the drug necessary to achieve the drug's therapeutic effects.
- Arriving at a critical concentration involves a dynamic equilibrium among the processes of drug absorption, distribution, metabolism or biotransformation, and excretion.
- Absorption involves moving a drug into the body for circulation. Oral drugs are absorbed from the small intestine, undergo many changes, and are affected by many things in the process. IV drugs are injected directly into the circulation and do not need additional absorption.
- Drugs are distributed to various tissues throughout the body depending on their solubility and ionization. Most drugs are bound to plasma proteins for transport to reactive tissues.
- Drugs are metabolized or biotransformed into less toxic chemicals by various enzyme systems in the body. The liver is the primary site of drug metabolism or biotransformation. The liver uses the cytochrome P450 enzyme system to alter the drug and start its biotransformation.
- The first-pass effect is the breakdown of oral drugs in the liver immediately after absorption. Drugs given by other routes often reach reactive tissues before passing through the liver for biotransformation.
- Drug excretion is removal of the drug from the body. This occurs mainly through the kidneys.

- The half-life of a drug is the period of time it takes for an amount of drug in the body to decrease to one-half of the peak level it previously achieved. The half-life is affected by all aspects of pharmacokinetics. Knowing the half-life of a drug helps in predicting dosing schedules and duration of effects.
- The actual effects of a drug are determined by the pharmacokinetics, the pharmacodynamics, and many human factors that can change the drug's effectiveness.
- To provide the safest and most effective drug therapy, the nurse must consider all of the interacting aspects that influence drug concentration and effectiveness.

Review Questions

1. Chemotherapeutic agents are drugs that
   a. are used only to treat cancers.
   b. replace normal body chemicals that are missing due to disease.
   c. interfere with the functioning of foreign cells, such as invading microorganisms or neoplasms.
   d. stimulate a cell's normal functioning.
2. Receptor sites
   a. are a normal part of enzyme substrates.
   b. are protein areas on cell membranes that react with specific chemicals to cause an effect within the cell.
   c. can usually be stimulated by many different chemicals.
   d. are responsible for all drug effects in the body.
3. Selective toxicity is
   a. the ability of a drug to seek out a specific bacterial species or microorganism.
   b. the ability of a drug to cause only specific adverse effects.
   c. the ability of a drug to cause fetal damage.
   d. the ability of a drug to attack only those systems found in foreign or abnormal cells.
4. Pharmacokinetics involves the study of
   a. absorption, distribution, biotransformation, and elimination of drugs.
   b. the way that drugs affect the body.
   c. receptor site activation and suppression.
   d. drug–drug interactions.
5. The absorption of a drug taken orally can be affected by
   a. the blood flow to muscle beds.
   b. the acidity of the gastric juices, often influenced by the presence of food.
   c. the weight and age of the patient.
   d. the temperature of the peripheral environment.
6. Much of the biotransformation that occurs when a drug is taken occurs as part of
   a. the protein binding effect of the drug.
   b. the functioning of the renal system.
   c. the first-pass effect through the liver.
   d. the distribution of the drug to the reactive tissues.
7. The half-life of a drug
   a. is determined by a balance of all of the factors working on that drug—absorption, distribution, biotransformation, and excretion.
   b. is a constant factor for all drugs taken by a patient.
   c. is influenced by the fat distribution of the patient.
   d. can be calculated with the use of a body surface nomogram.
8. Drug–drug interactions are important considerations in clinical practice that could result in
   a. bizarre drug effects on the body.
   b. the need to adjust drug dosage or timing of administration to ensure effective drug therapy.
   c. a need for more drugs in the drug regimen.
   d. a new therapeutic effect not encountered with either drug alone.

BIBLIOGRAPHY

Batt, A. M., et al. (1994). Drug metabolizing enzymes related to laboratory medicine: Cytochrome P-450 and UDP glucuronosyltransferases. *Clinica Chimica Acta, 226,* 171–190.
DeMaagd, G. (1995). High-risk drugs in the elderly population. *Geriatric Nursing, 16*(5), 198–207.
Edwards, J. (1997). Guarding against adverse drug events. *American Journal of Nursing, 97*(5), 26–31.
Gilman, A., Hardman, J. G., & Limbird, L. E. (Eds.) (2002). *Goodman and Gilman's the pharmacological basis of therapeutics* (10th ed.). New York: McGraw-Hill.
Kelly, J. (1995). Pharmacodynamics and drug therapy. *Professional Nursing, 10*(12), 792–796.
O'Mahoney, M. S. & Woodhouse, K. W. (1994). Age, environmental factors and drug metabolism. *Pharmacology and Therapeutics, 61,* 279–287.
Pirmohamed, M., et al. (1996). The role of active metabolites in drug toxicity. *Drug Safety, 11,* 114–144.
The medical letter on drugs and therapeutics. (2002). New Rochelle, NY: Medical Letter.
Wetterberg, L. (1994). Light and biological rhythms. *Journal of Internal Medicine, 235,* 5–19.
Wissmann, J. (1996). Strategies for teaching critical thinking in pharmacology. *Nurse Educator, 21,* 42–46.

C H A P T E R

3

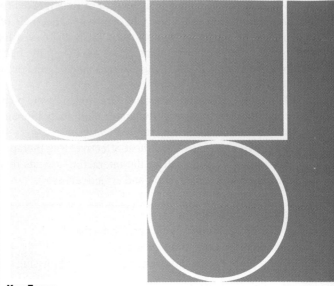

Key Terms
blood dyscrasia
dermatological reactions
drug allergy
hypersensitivity
poisoning
stomatitis
superinfections

Toxic Effects
of Drugs

A̲ll drugs are potentially dangerous. Even though chemicals are carefully screened and tested in animals and in people before they are released as drugs, drug products often cause unexpected or unacceptable reactions when they are given. Drugs are chemicals, and the human body operates by a vast series of chemical reactions. Consequently, many effects can be seen when just one chemical factor is altered. Today's potent and amazing drugs can cause a great variety of reactions, many of which are more severe than ever seen before.

ADVERSE EFFECTS

Adverse effects are undesired effects that may be unpleasant or even dangerous. They can occur for many reasons, including the following:

- The drug may have other effects on the body besides the therapeutic effect.
- The patient is sensitive to the drug being given.
- The drug's action on the body causes other responses that are undesirable or unpleasant.
- The patient is taking too much or too little of the drug, leading to adverse effects.

The nurse, as the caregiver who most frequently administers medications, must be constantly alert for signs of drug reactions of various types. Patients and their families need to be taught what to look for when patients are taking drugs at home. Some adverse effects can be countered with specific comfort measures or precautions. Knowing that these effects may occur and what actions can be taken to prevent or cope with them may be the most critical factor in helping the patient to comply with drug therapy.

Adverse drug effects can be of several types: primary actions, secondary actions, and hypersensitivity.

Primary Actions

One of the most common occurrences in drug therapy is the development of adverse effects from simple overdosage. In such cases, the patient suffers from effects that are merely an extension of the desired effect. For example, an anticoagulant may act so effectively that the patient experiences excessive and spontaneous bleeding. This type of adverse effect can be avoided by monitoring the patient carefully and adjusting the prescribed dose to fit that particular patient's needs.

In the same way, a patient taking an antihypertensive drug may become dizzy, weak, or faint when taking the "recommended dose" but be able to adjust to the drug therapy with a reduced dose. These effects can be caused by individual response to the drug, high or low body weight, age, or underlying pathology that alters the effects of the drug.

Secondary Actions

Drugs can produce a wide variety of effects in addition to the desired pharmacological effect. Sometimes the drug dose can be adjusted so that the desired effect is achieved without producing undesired secondary reactions. But sometimes this is not possible, and the adverse effects are almost inevitable. In such cases, the patient needs to be informed that these effects may occur and counseled about ways to cope with the undesired effects. For example, many antihistamines are very effective in drying up secretions and helping breathing, but they also cause drowsiness. The patient who is taking antihistamines needs to know that driving a car or operating dangerous machinery could pose a serious problem because of the drowsiness and therefore should be avoided.

Hypersensitivity

Some patients are excessively responsive to either the primary or the secondary effects of a drug. This is known as **hypersensitivity,** and it may result from a pathological or underlying condition. For example, many drugs are excreted through the kidneys; a patient who has kidney problems may not be able to excrete the drug and may accumulate the drug in the body, causing toxic effects.

Hypersensitivity also can occur if a patient has an underlying condition that makes the drug's effects especially unpleasant or dangerous. For example, a patient with an enlarged prostate who takes an anticholinergic drug may develop urinary retention or even bladder paralysis when the drug's effects block the urinary sphincters. This patient needs to be taught to empty the bladder before taking the drug. A reduced dosage also may be required to avoid potentially serious effects on the urinary system.

DRUG ALLERGY

A **drug allergy** occurs when the body forms antibodies to a particular drug, causing an immune response when the person is re-exposed to the drug. A patient cannot be allergic to a drug that has never been taken, although patients can have cross-allergies to drugs within the same drug class as one formerly taken. Many people state that they have a drug allergy because of the effects of a drug. For example, one patient stated that she was allergic to the diuretic furosemide (*Lasix*). On further questioning, the nurse discovered that the patient was "allergic" to the drug because it made her urinate frequently—the desired drug effect, but one that the patient thought was a reaction to the drug. Patients who state that they have a drug "allergy" should be further questioned as to the nature of the allergy. Many patients do not receive needed treatment because the response to the drug is not understood.

Drug allergies fall into four main classifications: anaphylactic reactions, cytotoxic reactions, serum sickness, and delayed reactions (Table 3–1). The nurse, as the primary caregiver involved in administering drugs, must constantly assess for potential drug allergies and must be prepared to intervene appropriately.

DRUG-INDUCED TISSUE AND ORGAN DAMAGE

Drugs can act directly or indirectly to cause many types of adverse effects in various tissues, structures, and organs (Figure 3–1). These drug effects account for many of the cautions that are noted before drug administration begins. The possible occurrence of these effects also accounts for the fact that the use of some drugs is contraindicated in patients with a particular history or underlying pathology. The specific contraindications and cautions for the administration of a given drug are noted with each drug type discussed in this book and in the individual monographs of various drug guides. These effects occur frequently enough that the nurse should be knowledgeable about the presentation of the drug-induced damage and about appropriate interventions that should be used if they occur.

Dermatological Reactions

Dermatological reactions are adverse reactions involving the skin. These can range from a simple rash to potentially fatal exfoliative dermatitis. Many adverse reactions involve the skin because many drugs can deposit there or cause direct irritation to the tissue. Procainamide (*Pronestyl*), a drug used to treat cardiac arrhythmias, causes a characteristic skin rash in many patients.

Assessment. Hives, rashes, and other dermatological lesions may be seen. Severe reactions may include exfoliative dermatitis, which is characterized by rash and scaling, fever, enlarged lymph nodes, enlarged liver, and the potentially fatal erythema multiforme exudativum (Stevens–Johnson syndrome), which is characterized by dark red papules appearing on the extremities with no pain or itching, often in rings or disk-shaped patches.

Interventions. In mild cases, or when the benefit of the drug outweighs the discomfort of the skin lesion, provide frequent skin care; instruct the patient to avoid rubbing, tight

TABLE 3-1 | Types of Drug Allergies

Allergy Type	Assessment	Interventions
ANAPHYLACTIC REACTION This allergy involves an antibody that reacts with specific sites in the body to cause the release of chemicals, including histamine, that produce immediate reactions (mucous membrane swelling and constricting bronchi) that can lead to respiratory distress and even respiratory arrest.	Hives, rash, difficulty breathing, increased BP, dilated pupils, diaphoresis, "panic" feeling, increased heart rate, respiratory arrest	Administer epinephrine, 0.3 mL of a 1:1000 solution SC for adults or 0.01 mg/kg of 1:1000 SC for pediatric patients. Massage the site to speed absorption rate. Repeat the dose every 15–20 min, as appropriate. Notify the prescriber and/or primary caregiver and discontinue the drug. Be aware that prevention is the best treatment. Counsel patients with known allergies to wear Medic-Alert identification and, if appropriate, to carry an emergency epinephrine kit.
CYTOTOXIC REACTION This allergy involves antibodies that circulate in the blood and attack antigens (the drug) on cell sites, causing death of that cell. This reaction is not immediate but may be seen over a few days.	Complete blood count showing damage to blood-forming cells (decreased hematocrit, decreased white blood cell count, decreased platelets); liver function tests showing elevated liver enzymes; renal function test showing decreased renal function	Notify the prescriber and/or primary caregiver and discontinue the drug. Support the patient to prevent infection and conserve energy until the allergic response is over.
SERUM-SICKNESS REACTION This allergy involves antibodies that circulate in the blood and cause damage to various tissues by depositing in blood vessels. This reaction may occur up to a week or more after exposure to the drug.	Itchy rash, high fever, swollen lymph nodes, swollen and painful joints, edema of the face and limbs	Notify the prescriber and/or primary caregiver and discontinue the drug. Provide comfort measures to help the patient cope with the signs and symptoms (cool environment, skin care, positioning, ice to joints, administer antipyretics or anti-inflammatory agents, as appropriate).
DELAYED ALLERGIC REACTION This reaction occurs several hours after exposure and involves antibodies that are bound to specific white blood cells.	Rash, hives, swollen joints (similar to the reaction to poison ivy)	Notify the prescriber and/or primary caregiver and discontinue drug. Provide skin care and comfort measures that may include antihistamines or topical corticosteroids.

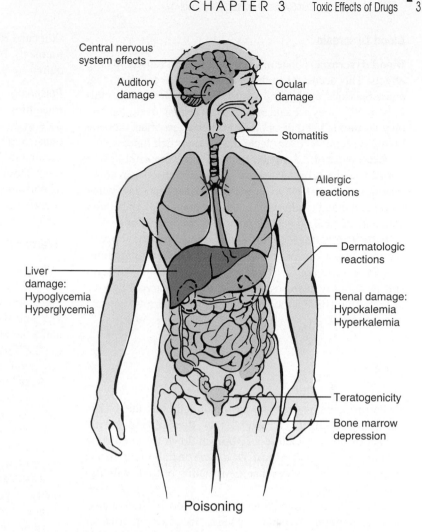

Central nervous system effects

Auditory damage

Ocular damage

Stomatitis

Allergic reactions

Dermatologic reactions

Liver damage:
Hypoglycemia
Hyperglycemia

Renal damage:
Hypokalemia
Hyperkalemia

Teratogenicity

Bone marrow depression

Poisoning

FIGURE 3-1. Variety of adverse effects associated with drug use.

or rough clothing, and harsh soaps or perfumed lotions; and administer antihistamines, as appropriate. In severe cases, discontinue the drug and notify the prescriber and/or primary caregiver. Be aware that, in addition to these interventions, topical corticosteroids, antihistamines, and emollients are frequently used.

Stomatitis

Stomatitis, or inflammation of the mucous membranes, can occur because of a direct toxic reaction to the drug or because the drug deposits in the end capillaries in the mucous membranes, leading to inflammation. Fluorouracil (*Adrucil*), an antineoplastic agent, causes mouth sores or stomatitis in most of the patients who take it.

Assessment. Symptoms can include swollen gums, inflamed gums (gingivitis), swollen and red tongue (glossitis), difficulty swallowing, bad breath, and pain in the mouth and throat.

Interventions. Provide frequent mouth care with a nonirritating solution. Offer nutrition evaluation and development of a tolerated diet, which usually involves frequent, small

meals. If necessary, arrange for a dental consultation. Note that antifungal agents and/or local anesthetics are sometimes used.

Superinfections

One of the body's protective mechanisms is the wide variety of bacteria that live within or on the surface of the body. This bacterial growth is called the *normal flora*. The normal flora protect the body from invasion by other bacteria, viruses, fungi, and so on. Several kinds of drugs (especially antibiotics) destroy the normal flora, leading to the development of **superinfections** or infections caused by the usually controlled organisms.

Assessment. Symptoms can include fever, diarrhea, black or hairy tongue, inflamed and swollen tongue (glossitis), mucous membrane lesions, and vaginal discharge with or without itching.

Interventions. Provide supportive measures (frequent mouth care, skin care, access to bathroom facilities, small and frequent meals). Administer antifungal therapy as appropriate. In severe cases, discontinue the drug responsible for the superinfection.

Blood Dyscrasia

Blood dyscrasia is bone marrow suppression caused by drug effects. This occurs when drugs that can cause cell death (eg, antineoplastics, antibiotics) are used. Bone marrow cells multiply rapidly; they are said to be rapidly turning over. Because they go through cell division and multiply so often, they are highly susceptible to any agent that disrupts cell function.

Assessment. Symptoms include fever, chills, sore throat, weakness, back pain, dark urine, decreased hematocrit (anemia), low platelet count (thrombocytopenia), low white blood cell count (leukopenia), and a reduction of all cellular elements of the complete blood count (pancytopenia).

Interventions. Monitor blood counts. Provide supportive measures (rest, protection from exposure to infections, protection from injury, avoidance of activities that might result in injury or bleeding). In severe cases, discontinue the drug or stop administration until the bone marrow recovers to a safe level.

Toxicity

Liver Injury

Oral drugs are absorbed and passed directly into the liver in the first-pass effect. This exposes the liver cells to the full impact of the drug before it is broken down for circulation throughout the body. Most drugs are metabolized in the liver, so any metabolites that are irritating or toxic will also affect liver integrity.

Assessment. Symptoms may include fever, malaise, nausea, vomiting, jaundice, change in color of urine or stools, abdominal pain or colic, elevated liver enzymes (eg, aspartate aminotransferase [AST], alanine aminotransferase [ALT]), alterations in bilirubin levels, and changes in clotting factors (eg, partial thromboplastin time).

Interventions. Discontinue the drug and notify the prescriber and/or primary caregiver. Offer supportive measures (small, frequent meals; skin care; cool environment; rest periods).

Renal Injury

The glomerulus in the kidney has a very small capillary network that filters the blood into the renal tubule. Some drug molecules are just the right size to get plugged into the capillary network, causing acute inflammation and severe renal problems. Some drugs are excreted from the kidney unchanged; they have the potential to directly irritate the renal tubule and alter normal absorption and secretion processes. Gentamicin (*Garamycin*), a potent antibiotic, is frequently associated with renal toxicity.

Assessment. Elevated blood urea nitrogen (BUN), elevated creatinine concentration, decreased hematocrit, electrolyte imbalances, fatigue, malaise, edema, irritability, and skin rash may be seen.

Interventions. Notify the prescriber and/or primary caregiver and discontinue the drug as needed. Offer supportive measures (eg, positioning, diet and fluid restrictions, skin care, electrolyte therapy, rest periods, controlled environment). In severe cases, be aware that dialysis may be required for survival.

Poisoning

Poisoning occurs when an overdose of a drug damages multiple body systems, leading to the potential for fatal reactions. Assessment parameters vary with the particular drug. Treatment of drug poisoning also varies, depending on the drug. Throughout this book, specific antidotes or treatments to poisoning are identified, if known. Emergency and life support measures often are needed in severe cases.

Alterations in Glucose Metabolism

Hypoglycemia

Some drugs affect metabolism and the use of glucose, causing a low serum blood glucose concentration, or hypoglycemia. Glipizide (*Glucotrol*) and glyburide (*DiaBeta*) are antidiabetic agents which have the desired action of lowering the blood glucose level, but which can lower blood glucose too far, causing hypoglycemia.

Assessment. Symptoms may include fatigue; drowsiness; hunger; anxiety; headache; cold, clammy skin; shaking and lack of coordination (tremulousness); increased heart rate; increased blood pressure; numbness and tingling of the mouth, tongue, and/or lips; confusion; and rapid and shallow respirations. In severe cases, seizures and/or coma may occur.

Interventions. Restore glucose, intravenously (IV) or orally if possible. Provide supportive measures (eg, skin care, environmental control of light and temperature, rest). Institute safety measures to prevent injury or falls. Offer reassurance to help the patient cope with the experience.

Hyperglycemia

Some drugs stimulate the breakdown of glycogen or alter metabolism in such a way as to cause high serum glucose levels, or hyperglycemia. Ephedrine (generic), a drug used as a bronchodilator and antiasthma drug and to relieve nasal congestion, can break down stored glycogen and cause an elevation of blood glucose by its effects on the sympathetic nervous system.

Assessment. Fatigue, increased urination (polyuria), increased thirst (polydipsia), deep respirations (Kussmaul's respirations), restlessness, increased hunger (polyphagia), nausea, hot or flushed skin, and fruity odor to breath may be observed.

Interventions. Administer insulin therapy to decrease blood glucose as appropriate. Provide support to help the patient deal with signs and symptoms (eg, access to bathroom facilities, controlled environment, reassurance, mouth care).

Electrolyte Imbalances

Hypokalemia

Some drugs affecting the kidney can cause low serum potassium levels (hypokalemia) by altering the renal exchange system. For example, loop diuretics function by causing the loss of potassium as well as sodium and water. Potassium is essential for the normal functioning of nerves and muscles.

Assessment. Symptoms include a serum potassium concentration ($[K^+]$) lower than 3.5 mEq/L, weakness, numbness and tingling in the extremities, muscle cramps, nausea, vomiting, diarrhea, decreased bowel sounds, irregular pulse, weak pulse, orthostatic hypotension, and disorientation. In severe cases, paralytic ileus (absent bowel sounds, abdominal distention, and acute abdomen) may occur.

Interventions. Replace serum potassium and carefully monitor serum levels and patient response. Provide supportive therapy (eg, safety precautions to prevent injury or falls, orientation of the patient, comfort measures for pain and discomfort).

Hyperkalemia

Some drugs that affect the kidney, such as the potassium-sparing diuretics, can lead to potassium retention and a resultant increase in serum potassium levels (hyperkalemia). Other drugs that cause cell death or injury, such as many antineoplastic agents, also can cause the cells to release potassium, leading to hyperkalemia.

Assessment. Symptoms include a serum potassium level higher than 5.0 mEq/L, weakness, muscle cramps, diarrhea, numbness and tingling, slow heart rate, low blood pressure, decreased urine output, and difficulty breathing.

Interventions. Institute measures to decrease the serum potassium concentration, including use of sodium polystyrene sulfonate. Offer supportive measures to cope with discomfort. Institute safety measures to prevent injury or falls. Monitor cardiac effects and be prepared for cardiac emergency. In severe cases, be aware that dialysis may be needed.

Sensory Effects

Ocular Toxicity

The blood vessels in the retina are very tiny and called "end arteries." That is, they stop and do not interconnect with other arteries feeding the same cells. Some drugs are deposited into these tiny arteries, causing inflammation and tissue damage. Chloroquine (*Aralen*), a drug used to treat some rheumatoid diseases, can cause retinal damage and even blindness.

Assessment. Blurring of vision, color vision changes, corneal damage, and blindness may be observed.

Interventions. Monitor the patient's vision carefully when the patient is receiving known oculotoxic drugs. Consult with the prescriber and/or primary caregiver and discontinue the drug as appropriate. Provide supportive measures, especially if vision loss is not reversible. Monitor lighting and exposure to sunlight.

Auditory Damage

Tiny vessels and nerves in the eighth cranial nerve are easily irritated and damaged by certain drugs. The macrolide antibiotics can cause severe auditory nerve damage. Aspirin, one of the most commonly used drugs, is often linked to auditory ringing and eighth cranial nerve effects.

Assessment. Dizziness, ringing in the ears (tinnitus), loss of balance, and loss of hearing may be observed.

Interventions. Monitor the patient's perceptual losses or changes. Provide protective measures to prevent falling or injury. Consult with the prescriber to decrease dose or discontinue the drug. Provide supportive measures to cope with drug effects.

Neurological Effects

General Central Nervous System Effects

Although the brain is fairly well protected from many drug effects by the blood–brain barrier, some drugs do affect neurological functioning, either directly or by altering electrolyte or glucose levels. β-Blockers, used to treat hypertension, angina, and many other conditions, can cause feelings of anxiety, insomnia, and nightmares.

Assessment. Symptoms may include confusion, delirium, insomnia, drowsiness, hyperreflexia or hyporeflexia, bizarre dreams, and hallucinations.

Interventions. Provide safety measures to prevent injury. Caution the patient to avoid dangerous situations such as driving a car or operating dangerous machinery. Orient the patient and provide support. Consult with the prescriber to decrease drug dose or discontinue the drug.

Atropine-like (Cholinergic) Effects

Some drugs mimic the effects of the parasympathetic nervous system by directly or indirectly stimulating cholinergic receptors. Donepezil (*Aricept*), a drug used to treat Alzheimer's disease, causes many cholinergic effects. Many cold remedies and antihistamines also cause cholinergic effects.

Assessment. Dry mouth, altered taste perception, dysphagia, heartburn, constipation, bloating, paralytic ileus, urinary hesitancy and retention, impotence, blurred vision, cycloplegia, photophobia, headache, mental confusion, nasal congestion, palpitations, decreased sweating, and dry skin may be seen.

Interventions. Provide sugarless lozenges and mouth care to help mouth dryness. Arrange for bowel program as appropriate. Have the patient void before taking the drug, to aid voiding. Provide safety measures if vision changes occur. Arrange for medication for headache and nasal congestion as appropriate. Advise the patient to avoid hot environments and to take protective measures to prevent falling and to prevent dehydration, which may be caused by exposure to heat owing to decreased sweating.

Parkinson-like Syndrome

Drugs that directly or indirectly affect dopamine levels in the brain can cause a syndrome that resembles Parkinson's disease. Many of the antipsychotic and neuroleptic drugs can cause this effect. In most cases, the effects go away when the drug is withdrawn.

Assessment. Lack of activity, akinesia, muscular tremors, drooling, changes in gait, rigidity, extreme restlessness or "jitters" (akathisia), or spasms (dyskinesia) may be observed.

Interventions. Discontinue the drug, if necessary. Know that treatment with anticholinergics or antiparkinson drugs may be recommended if the benefit of the drug outweighs the discomfort of its adverse effects. Provide small, frequent meals if swallowing becomes difficult. Provide safety measures if ambulation becomes a problem.

Neuroleptic Malignant Syndrome

General anesthetics and other drugs that have direct central nervous system effects can cause neuroleptic malignant syndrome, a generalized syndrome that includes high fever.

Assessment. Extrapyramidal symptoms, hyperthermia, autonomic disturbances, and fever may be observed.

Interventions. Discontinue the drug, if necessary. Know that treatment with anticholinergics or antiparkinson drugs may be required. Provide supportive care to lower the body temperature. Institute safety precautions as needed.

Teratogenicity

Many drugs that reach the developing fetus or embryo can cause death or congenital defects, which can include skeletal and limb abnormalities, CNS alterations, heart defects, etc. The exact effects of a drug on the fetus may not be known. In some cases, a predictable syndrome occurs when a drug is given to a pregnant woman. In any situation, a pregnant woman who is given a drug should be advised of the possible effects on the baby. Before a drug is administered to a pregnant patient, the actual benefits should be weighed against the potential risks. All pregnant women should be advised not to self-medicate during the pregnancy.

Interventions. Provide emotional and physical support for dealing with fetal death or birth defects.

Box 3–1 summarizes all of the adverse effects that have been described throughout this chapter.

CHAPTER SUMMARY

- No drug does only what is desired of it. All drugs have adverse effects associated with them.
- Adverse drug effects can range from allergic reactions to tissue and cellular damage. The nurse, as the health care provider most associated with drug administration, needs to assess each situation for potential adverse effects and intervene appropriately to minimize those effects.
- Adverse effects can be extensions of the primary action of a drug or secondary effects that are not necessarily desirable but are unavoidable.
- Allergic reactions can occur when a person makes antibodies to a drug or drug protein. If the person is exposed to

---

BOX 3-1
Summary of Adverse Drug Effects

Extension of primary action
Occurrence of secondary action
Allergic reactions
    Anaphylactic reactions
    Cytotoxic reactions
    Serum-sickness reactions
    Delayed allergic reactions
Tissue and organ damage
    Dermatologic reactions
    Stomatitis
    Superinfections
    Blood dyscrasia
    Toxicity
        Liver injury
        Renal injury
        Poisoning
    Alterations in glucose metabolism
        Hypoglycemia
        Hyperglycemia
    Electrolyte imbalances
        Hypokalemia
        Hyperkalemia
    Sensory effects
        Ocular toxicity
        Auditory damage
    Neurological effects
        General CNS effects
        Atropine-like (cholinergic) effects
        Parkinson-like syndrome
        Neuroleptic malignant syndrome (NMS)
    Teratogenicity

---

that drug another time, an immune response may occur. Allergic reactions can be of various types. The exact response should be noted to avoid future confusion in patient care.

- Tissue damage can include skin problems, mucous membrane inflammation, blood dyscrasia, superinfections, liver toxicity, hypoglycemia or hyperglycemia, renal toxicity, electrolyte disturbances, various central nervous system problems (ocular toxicity, auditory damage, atropine-like effects, Parkinson-like syndrome, neuroleptic malignant syndrome), teratogenicity, and overdose poisoning.

Review Questions

1. An example of a drug allergy is
   a. dry mouth occurring with an antihistamine.
   b. increased urination occurring with a thiazide diuretic.
   c. hives and difficulty breathing after an injection of penicillin.
   d. skin rash associated with procainamide use.
2. A patient taking glyburide (an antidiabetic drug) has his morning dose and then does not have a chance to eat for several hours. An adverse effect that might be expected from this would be
   a. teratogenic effects.

b. a skin rash.

c. anticholinergic effects.

d. hypoglycemia.

3. A patient with a severe infection is given gentamicin, the only antibiotic shown to be effective in culture and sensitivity tests. A few hours after the drug is started IV, the patient becomes very restless and develops edema. Blood tests reveal abnormal electrolytes and elevated BUN. This reaction was most likely caused by

a. an anaphylactic reaction.

b. renal toxicity associated with gentamicin.

c. superinfection related to the antibiotic.

d. hypoglycemia.

4. A patient is taking a drug that is known to be toxic to the liver. The patient is being discharged to home. Points related to liver toxicity of the drug that the patient should be advised to report immediately include

a. fever, changes in the color of urine or stool, and malaise.

b. rapid, deep respirations and increased sweating.

c. dizziness, drowsiness, and dry mouth.

d. rash, black or hairy tongue, and white spots in the mouth or throat.

5. Patients receiving antineoplastic drugs that disrupt cell function often have adverse effects involving cells that turn over rapidly in the body. These cells include

a. ovarian cells.

b. liver cells.

c. cardiac cells.

d. bone marrow cells.

6. Pregnant women should be advised of the potential risk to the fetus any time they take a drug during pregnancy. Fetal problems related to drug therapy can include

a. fetal death.

b. nervous system disruption.

c. skeletal and limb abnormalities.

d. all of the above.

BIBLIOGRAPHY

Barditch-Crovo, P. (1995). Adverse reactions to therapy for HIV infections. *Emergency Medical Clinics of North America, 13,* 133–146.

Brody, T. M., et al. (1994). *Human pharmacology: Molecular to clinical* (2nd ed.). St. Louis: C.V. Mosby.

Drug facts and comparisons. (2002). St. Louis: Facts and Comparisons.

Food and Drug Administration. (1994). FDA Launches MEDWATCH program: Monitoring adverse drug reactions. *NP News, 2,* 1, 4.

Gilman, A., Hardman, J. G., & Limbird, L. E. (Eds.) (2002). *Goodman and Gilman's the pharmacological basis of therapeutics* (10th ed.). New York: McGraw-Hill.

The medical letter on drugs and therapeutics. (2002). New Rochelle, NY: Medical Letter.

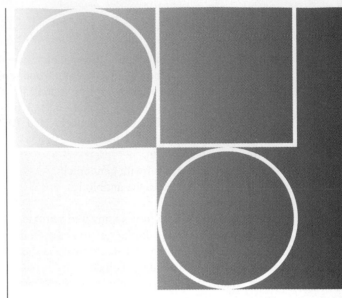

CHAPTER 4

Nursing Management

Key Terms
assessment
nursing
nursing diagnosis
nursing process

The delivery of medical care today is in a constant state of change, and sometimes crisis. The population is aging, resulting in more chronic disease and more complex care issues. The population also is transient, resulting in unstable support systems and fewer at-home care providers and helpers. At the same time, medicine is undergoing a technological boom, including greater use of computed tomography (CT) scans, nuclear magnetic resonance imaging (MRI) scans, experimental drugs, and so on. Patients are being discharged earlier from acute care facilities, or they are not being admitted at all for procedures that used to be treated in-hospital with follow-up support and monitoring provided. Patients also are becoming more responsible for their own care and for adhering to complicated medical regimens at home.

NURSING: ART AND SCIENCE

Nursing is a unique and complex science as well as a nurturing and caring art. In the traditional sense, nursing has been viewed as ministering to and soothing the sick. In the current state of medical changes, nursing also has become increasingly technical and scientific. Nurses have had to assume increasing responsibilities that involve not only nurturing and caring but also assessing, diagnosing, and intervening with patients to treat, to prevent, and to educate in order to help patients cope with various health states.

The nurse deals with the whole person, including physical, emotional, intellectual, social, and spiritual aspects. The nurse needs to consider how a person responds to treatment, disease, and the changes in lifestyle that may be required. The nurse is the key health care provider who is in a position to assess the whole patient, to administer therapy as well as medications, to teach the patient how best to cope with the therapy so as to ensure the most favorable outcome, and to evaluate the effectiveness of the therapy. Being able to do this requires broad knowledge in the basic sciences (anatomy, physiology, nutrition, chemistry, pharmacology), the social sciences (sociology, psychology), education, and many other disciplines.

THE NURSING PROCESS

Although not all nursing theorists completely agree on the process that defines the practice of nursing, most do include certain key elements in the **nursing process.** These elements are the basic components of the decision-making or problem-solving process:

- **Assessment** (gathering information)
- **Nursing diagnosis** (analyzing the information gathered to arrive at some conclusions)
- Interventions (actions undertaken to meet the patient's needs, such as administration of drugs, education, and comfort measures)

- Evaluation (determining the effects of the interventions that were performed)

In general, the nursing process provides an effective method for handling all of the scientific and technical information as well as the unique emotional, social, and physical factors that each patient brings to a given situation. With respect to drug therapy, use of the nursing process ensures that the patient receives the best, most efficient, scientifically based, holistic care. Box 4–1 outlines the steps of the nursing process, which are discussed in detail in the following paragraphs.

Assessment

The first step of the nursing process is the systematic, organized collection of data about the patient. Because the

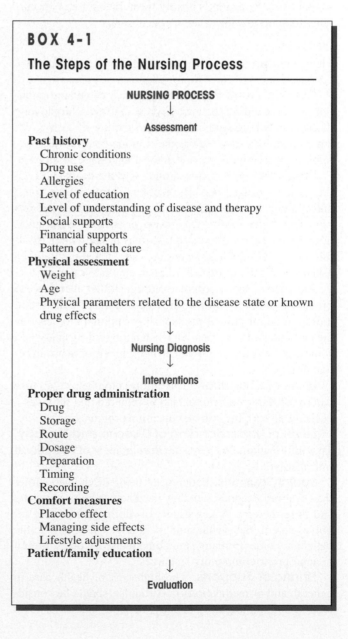

BOX 4-1

The Steps of the Nursing Process

NURSING PROCESS
↓
Assessment

Past history
   Chronic conditions
   Drug use
   Allergies
   Level of education
   Level of understanding of disease and therapy
   Social supports
   Financial supports
   Pattern of health care
Physical assessment
   Weight
   Age
   Physical parameters related to the disease state or known drug effects
↓
Nursing Diagnosis
↓
Interventions

Proper drug administration
   Drug
   Storage
   Route
   Dosage
   Preparation
   Timing
   Recording
Comfort measures
   Placebo effect
   Managing side effects
   Lifestyle adjustments
Patient/family education
↓
Evaluation

nurse is responsible for holistic care, these data must include information about physical, intellectual, emotional, social, and environmental factors. These data provide the nurse with the facts needed to plan educational and discharge programs, arrange for appropriate consultations, and monitor the physical response to treatment or to disease.

In clinical practice, the process of assessment never ends. The patient is not in a steady state, but rather a dynamic state, adjusting to physical, emotional, and environmental influences. Each nurse develops a unique approach to the organization of the assessment, an approach that is functional and useful in the clinical setting and that makes sense to that nurse and in the particular clinical situation.

Drug therapy is a complex and important part of health care, and the principles of drug therapy should be incorporated into every patient assessment plan. The particular information that is needed varies with each drug, but the concepts involved are similar. Two key areas that need to be assessed are the patient's history (past illnesses and the current problem) and his or her physical status.

Past History

The patient's past experiences and illnesses can influence a drug's effect.

Chronic Conditions. The presence of certain conditions (eg, renal disease, heart disease, diabetes, chronic lung disease) may be contraindications to the use of a drug. Or, these conditions may require that caution be used when administering a certain drug or that the drug dosage be adjusted.

Drug Use. Prescription drugs, over-the-counter (OTC) drugs, street drugs, alcohol, nicotine, alternative therapies, and caffeine may have an impact on a drug's effect. Patients often neglect to mention OTC drugs or alternative therapies, not considering them to be actual drugs or not willing to admit their use to the health care provider. Patients should be asked specifically about OTC drug or alternative therapy use.

Allergies. Past exposure to a drug or other allergens can provoke a future reaction or provide a caution for the use of a drug, food, or animal product. It is important to describe the particular allergic reaction when noting a drug allergy. In some cases, the reaction is not an allergic response but an actual drug effect.

Level of Education. This information helps the nurse determine the level of explanation required and provides a basis for developing patient education programs.

Level of Understanding of Disease and Therapy. This information also helps the development of educational information.

Social Supports. Patients are being discharged earlier than ever before, and often they need help at home with care and drug therapy. A key aspect of discharge planning involves determining what support, if any, is available to the patient at home. In many situations, it also involves referral to appropriate community resources.

Financial Supports. The high cost of health care in general, and of medications in particular, should be considered when initiating drug therapy. In some situations, a less expensive drug might be considered in place of a very expensive drug. Because of financial constraints, a patient may not follow through with a prescribed drug regimen. In such cases, the nurse may refer the patient to appropriate resources that might offer financial assistance.

Pattern of Health Care. Knowing how a patient seeks health care gives the nurse valuable information to include in the educational plan. Does this patient routinely seek follow-up care, or does he or she wait for emergency situations? Does the patient tend to self-treat many complaints, or is every problem brought to a health care provider?

Physical Assessment

Weight. A patient's weight helps determine whether the recommended drug dosage is appropriate. Because the recommended dosage typically is based on a 150-pound adult male, patients who are much lighter or much heavier need a dosage adjustment.

Age. Patients at the extremes of the age spectrum—children and older adults—often require dosage adjustments based on the functional level of the liver and kidneys and the responsiveness of other organs.

Physical Parameters Related to the Disease State or Known Drug Effects. Assessing these factors before drug therapy begins provides a baseline level to which future assessments can be compared to determine the effects of drug therapy. The specific parameters that need to be assessed depend on the disease process being treated and on the expected therapeutic and adverse effects of the drug therapy. For example, if a patient is being treated for chronic pulmonary disease, the respiratory status and reserve need to be assessed, especially if a drug is being given that has known effects on the respiratory tract. In contrast, a thorough respiratory evaluation would not be warranted in a patient with no known pulmonary disease who is taking a drug with no known effects on the respiratory system. Because the nurse has the greatest direct and continual contact with the patient, the nurse has the best opportunity to detect minute changes that ultimately determine the course of drug therapy—therapeutic success or discontinuation because of adverse or unacceptable responses.

NOTE: Review the monographs in the drug guide being used for the specific parameters that need to be assessed in relation to the particular drug being discussed. This assessment provides not only the baseline information needed before giving that drug but also the data required to evaluate the effects of that drug on the patient. This information should supplement the overall nursing assessment of the patient, which includes social, intellectual, financial, environmental, and other physical data.

Nursing Diagnosis

Once data have been collected, the nurse must organize and analyze that information to arrive at a nursing diagnosis. A nursing diagnosis is simply a statement of the patient's status from a nursing perspective. This statement directs appropriate nursing interventions. A nursing diagnosis shows actual or potential alterations in patient function based on the assessment of the clinical situation. Because drug therapy is only a small part of the overall patient situation, nursing diagnoses that are related to drug therapy must be incorporated into a total picture of the patient.

In the nursing considerations sections of this book, the nursing diagnoses listed are those that reflect potential alteration of function based only on the particular drug's actions (ie, therapeutic and adverse effects). No consideration is given to environmental or disease-related problems. These diagnoses, culled from the North American Nursing Diagnosis Association (NANDA) list of accepted nursing diagnoses, are only a part of the overall nursing diagnoses related to the patient's situation. See Box 4–2 for a list of the accepted NANDA nursing diagnoses.

Interventions

The assessment and diagnosis of the patient situation direct specific nursing interventions. Three types of interventions are frequently involved in drug therapy: drug administration, provision of comfort measures, and patient/family education.

Proper Drug Administration

There are seven points to consider in the safe and effective administration of a drug:

1. *Drug:* Know that it is standard nursing practice to ensure that the drug being administered is the correct dose and the correct drug, and that it is being given at the correct time and to the correct patient.
2. *Storage:* Be aware that some drugs require specific storage environments (eg, refrigeration, protection from light).
3. *Route:* Determine the best route of administration; this is frequently established by the formulation of the drug. Nurses can often have an impact in modifying the route to arrive at the most efficient, comfortable method for the patient based on the patient's specific situation. When establishing the prescribed route, check the proper method of administering a drug by that route.
4. *Dosage:* Calculate the drug dosage appropriately, based on either the available drug form, the patient's body weight or surface area, or the patient's kidney function.
5. *Preparation:* Know the specific preparation required before administering any drug. For example, oral drugs may need to be shaken or crushed. Parenteral drugs may need to be reconstituted or diluted with specific solutions. Topical drugs may require specific handling, such as the use of gloves during administration or shaving of a body area before application.
6. *Timing:* Recognize that the administration of one drug may require coordination with the administration of other drugs, foods, or physical parameters. As the caregiver most frequently involved in administering drugs, the nurse must be aware of and juggle all of these factors, as well as educate the patient to do this on his or her own.
7. *Recording:* After assessing the patient, making the appropriate nursing diagnoses, and delivering the correct drug, by the correct route, in the correct dose, and at the correct time, document that information in accordance with the local requirements for recording medication administration.

Box 4–3 summarizes points to consider for proper drug administration.

Comfort Measures

Nurses are in a unique position to help the patient cope with the effects of drug therapy.

Placebo Effect

The anticipation that a drug will be helpful (placebo effect) has been proven to have tremendous impact on the actual success of drug therapy. Therefore, the nurse's attitude and support can be a critical part of drug therapy; a back rub, a kind word, and a positive approach may be as beneficial as the drug itself.

Managing Adverse Effects

Interventions can be directed at decreasing the impact of the anticipated adverse effects of a drug and promoting patient safety. Such interventions include environmental control (eg, temperature, light), safety measures (eg, avoiding driving, avoiding the sun, using side rails), and physical comfort (eg, skin care, laxatives, frequent meals).

Lifestyle Adjustment

Some drug effects require that a patient change his or her lifestyle to cope effectively. For example, patients taking diuretics may have to rearrange their day so as to be near toilet facilities when the drug works. Patients taking monoamine oxidase inhibitors (MAOIs) must adjust their diet to prevent serious adverse effects from interaction of the drug with certain foods. In some cases the change in lifestyle that is needed can have a tremendous impact on the patient and can affect coping and compliance with any medical regimen.

NOTE: Special points regarding drug administration and related comfort measures are noted with each drug class discussed in this book. Refer to the individual drug monographs in the drug guide being used for more detailed interventions regarding a specific drug.

Patient and Family Education

With patients becoming increasingly responsible for their own care, it is essential that they have all of the information necessary to ensure safe and effective drug therapy at home. In fact, many states now require that patients be given written information. Key elements that should be included in any drug education program are the following:

1. *Name, dose, and action of drug:* Many patients see more than one health care provider; knowing this information is crucial to ensuring safe and effective drug therapy and avoiding drug–drug interactions.
2. *Timing of administration:* Teach patients when to take the drug with respect to frequency, other drugs, and meals.

BOX 4-2
NANDA-Approved Nursing Diagnoses

This list contains the nursing diagnoses approved by the North American Nursing Diagnoses Association (NANDA) for use and testing (2001–2002)

Exchanging
Imbalanced Nutrition: More Than Body Requirements
Imbalanced Nutrition: Less Than Body Requirements
Risk for Imbalanced Nutrition: More Than Body
  Requirements
Risk for Infection
Risk for Altered Body Temperature
Hypothermia
Hyperthermia
Ineffective Thermoregulation
Autonomic Dysreflexia
Risk for Autonomic Dysreflexia
Constipation
Perceived Constipation
Diarrhea
Bowel Incontinence
Risk for Constipation
Impaired Urinary Elimination
Stress Urinary Incontinence
Reflex Urinary Incontinence
Urge Urinary Incontinence
Functional Urinary Incontinence
Total Urinary Incontinence
Risk for Urge Urinary Incontinence
Urinary Retention
Ineffective Tissue Perfusion (Specify type: Renal, Cerebral,
  Cardiopulmonary, Gastrointestinal, Peripheral)
Risk for Fluid Volume Imbalance
Excess Fluid Volume
Deficient Fluid Volume
Risk for Deficient Fluid Volume
Decreased Cardiac Output
Impaired Gas Exchange
Ineffective Airway Clearance
Ineffective Breathing Pattern
Impaired Spontaneous Ventilation
Dysfunctional Ventilatory Weaning Response (DVWR)
Risk for Injury
Risk for Suffocation
Risk for Poisoning
Risk for Trauma
Risk for Aspiration
Risk for Disuse Syndrome
Latex Allergy Response
Risk for Latex Allergy Response
Ineffective Protection
Impaired Tissue Integrity
Altered Oral Mucous Membrane
Impaired Skin Integrity
Risk for Impaired Skin Integrity
Impaired Dentition
Decreased Intracranial Adaptive Capacity
Disturbed Energy Field

Communicating
Impaired Verbal Communication

Relating
Impaired Social Interaction
Social Isolation
Risk for Loneliness
Ineffective Role Performance
Deficient Parenting
Risk for Deficient Parenting
Risk for Impaired Parent/Infant/Child Attachment
Sexual Dysfunction
Interrupted Family Processes
Caregiver Role Strain
Risk for Caregiver Role Strain
Dysfunctional Family Processes: Alcoholism
Parental Role Conflict
Ineffective Sexuality Patterns

Valuing
Spiritual Distress
Risk of Spiritual Distress
Readiness for Enhanced Spiritual Well-Being

Choosing
Ineffective Coping
Impaired Adjustment
Defensive Coping
Ineffective Denial
Disabled Family Coping
Compromised Family Coping
Readiness for Enhanced Family Coping
Readiness for Enhanced Community Coping
Ineffective Community Coping
Ineffective Therapeutic Regimen Management
Noncompliance (Specify)
Ineffective Family Therapeutic Regimen Management
Ineffective Community Therapeutic Regimen Management
Effective Therapeutic Regimen Management
Decisional Conflict (Specify)
Health-Seeking Behaviors (Specify)

Moving
Impaired Physical Mobility
Risk for Peripheral Neurovascular Dysfunction
Risk for Perioperative-Positioning Injury
Impaired Walking
Impaired Wheelchair Mobility
Impaired Transfer Ability
Impaired Bed Mobility
Activity Intolerance
Fatigue
Risk for Activity Intolerance
Disturbed Sleep Pattern
Sleep Deprivation
Deficient Diversional Activity
Impaired Home Maintenance
Ineffective Health Maintenance
Delayed Surgical Recovery
Adult Failure to Thrive
Feeding Self-Care Deficit
Impaired Swallowing
Ineffective Breastfeeding
Interrupted Breastfeeding
Effective Breastfeeding
Ineffective Infant Feeding Pattern

BOX 4-2 (CONTINUED)

NANDA-Approved Nursing Diagnoses

Bathing/Hygiene Self-Care Deficit
Dressing/Grooming Self-Care Deficit
Toileting Self-Care Deficit
Delayed Growth and Development
Risk for Delayed Development
Risk for Disproportionate Growth
Relocation Stress Syndrome
Risk for Disorganized Infant Behavior
Disorganized Infant Behavior
Readiness for Enhanced Organized Infant Behavior

Perceiving
Disturbed Body Image
Disturbed Self-Esteem
Chronic Low Self-Esteem
Situational Low Self-Esteem
Disturbed Personal Identity
Disturbed Sensory Perception (Specify: Visual, Auditory, Kinesthetic, Gustatory, Tactile, Olfactory)
Unilateral Neglect
Hopelessness
Powerlessness

Knowing
Deficient Knowledge (Specify)
Impaired Environmental Interpretation Syndrome
Acute Confusion
Chronic Confusion
Disturbed Thought Processes
Impaired Memory

Feeling
Acute Pain
Chronic Pain
Nausea
Dysfunctional Grieving
Anticipatory Grieving
Chronic Sorrow
Risk for Other-Directed Violence
Risk for Self-Mutilation
Risk for Self-Directed Violence
Post-Trauma Syndrome
Rape-Trauma Syndrome
Rape-Trauma Syndrome: Compound Reaction
Rape-Trauma Syndrome: Silent Reaction
Risk for Post-Trauma Syndrome
Anxiety
Death Anxiety
Fear

New Nursing Diagnoses
Risk for Relocation Stress Syndrome
Risk for Suicide
Self-Mutilation
Risk for Powerlessness
Risk for Situational Low Self-Esteem
Wandering
Risk for Falls

Nursing Diagnoses revised and approved at the 2000 Biennial Conference on the Classification of Nursing Diagnoses.

---

3. *Special storage and preparation instructions:* Some drugs require particular handling procedures; inform patients how to carry out these requirements.
4. *Specific OTC drugs or alternative therapies to avoid:* Many patients do not consider OTC drugs or herbal or alternative therapies to be actual drugs and may inadvertently take them along with their prescribed medications, causing unwanted or even dangerous drug–drug interactions. Prevent these situations by explaining which drugs or therapies should be avoided.

BOX 4-3

Points to Consider for Proper Drug Administration

Correct drug and patient
Correct storage of drug
Correct and most effective route
Correct dosage
Correct preparation
Correct timing
Correct recording of administration

5. *Special comfort or safety measures:* Teach patients how to cope with anticipated adverse effects to ease anxiety and avoid noncompliance with drug therapy. Also educate patients about the importance of follow-up tests or evaluation.
6. *Safety measures:* Instruct all patients to keep drugs out of the reach of children. Remind all patients to inform any health care provider they see about the drugs they are taking; this can prevent drug–drug interactions and misdiagnoses based on drug effects.
7. *Specific points about drug toxicity:* Give patients a list of warning signs of drug toxicity. Advise patients to notify their health care provider if any of these effects occur.
8. *Specific warnings about drug discontinuation:* Some drugs with a small margin of safety and drugs with particular systemic effects cannot be stopped abruptly without dangerous effects. Alert patients who are taking these drugs to this problem and encourage them to call their health care provider immediately if they cannot take their medication for any reason (eg, illness, financial constraints).

Box 4–4 summarizes points to consider in patient/ family education.

BOX 4-4

Points to Consider in Patient/Family Education

Name, dose and action of drug
Timing of administration
Special storage and preparation information
Specific over-the-counter drugs and herbal or alternative therapies to avoid
Special comfort measures
Safety measures that need to be observed
Specific points about drug toxicity
Specific warnings to report to health care provider

NOTE: Refer to the CD-ROM at the back of this book for teaching guides that can be used for patients in the actual clinical setting.

Evaluation

Evaluation is part of the continual process of patient care that leads to changes in assessment, diagnosis, and intervention. The patient is continually evaluated for therapeutic response, the occurrence of adverse drug effects, and the occurrence of drug–drug, drug–food, drug–alternative therapy, or drug–laboratory test interactions. The efficacy of the nursing interventions and the education program must be evaluated. In some situations, the nurse evaluates the patient simply by reapplying the beginning steps of the nursing process and analyzing for change (Figure 4–1). In some cases of drug therapy, specific therapeutic drug levels also need to be evaluated.

CHAPTER SUMMARY

- Nursing is a complex art and science that provides for nurturing and care of the sick as well as prevention and education services.

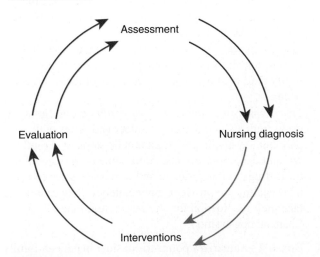

FIGURE 4-1. The continual, dynamic nature of the nursing process.

- The nursing process is a problem-solving process involving assessment, nursing diagnosis, interventions, and evaluation. It is an ongoing, dynamic process that provides safe and efficient care.
- Nursing assessment must include information on the history of past illnesses and the current complaint, as well as a physical examination; this provides a database of baseline information to ensure safe administration of a drug and to evaluate the drug's effectiveness and adverse effects.
- Nursing diagnoses use the data gathered during the assessment to determine actual or potential problems that require specific nursing interventions.
- Nursing interventions should include proper administration of a drug; comfort measures to help the patient cope with the drug effects; and patient and family education regarding the drug effects, ways to avoid adverse effects, warning signs to report, and any other specific information about the drug that will facilitate patient compliance.
- Evaluation is a continual process that assesses the situation and leads to new diagnoses or interventions as the patient reacts to the drug therapy.
- A nursing care guide and patient education materials can be prepared for each drug being given, using information about a drug's therapeutic effects, adverse effects, and special considerations.

Review Questions

1. A patient reports to you that she has a drug allergy. In exploring the allergic reaction with the patient, the following might indicate an allergic response:
   a. increased urination.
   b. dry mouth.
   c. rash.
   d. drowsiness.
2. It is important to obtain a medical history from a patient before beginning drug therapy because
   a. many medical conditions alter the pharmacokinetics and pharmacodynamics of a drug.
   b. it is part of the nursing protocol.
   c. a baseline is needed for evaluating drug effects.
   d. it is the first step in the nursing process.
3. Physical assessment of a patient being started on a laxative might include all of the following except
   a. liver function tests.
   b. abdominal examination.
   c. skin color and lesion.
   d. lung auscultation.
4. A nursing diagnosis
   a. directs medical care.
   b. helps the patient become more compliant.
   c. shows actual or potential alteration in patient function.
   d. determines insurance reimbursement in most cases.
5. A patient receiving an antihistamine complains of dry mouth and nose. An appropriate comfort measure for this patient would be
   a. use of a humidifier and an increase in fluid consumption.

b. voiding before taking the drug.

c. avoiding exposure to the sun.

d. a back rub.

6. When establishing the nursing interventions appropriate for a given patient

  a. the patient should not be actively involved.

  b. the family or other support systems should not be consulted.

  c. teaching is important only if the patient seems compliant.

  d. an evaluation of all of the data accumulated should be incorporated to achieve an effective care plan.

7. The evaluation step of the nursing process

  a. is often not necessary.

  b. is important only in the acute setting.

  c. is a continual process that redirects nursing interventions as needed.

  d. includes making nursing diagnoses.

8. A patient has been through a teaching format for digoxin (generic), a drug used to increase the effectiveness of the heart's contractions. Which of the following statements would indicate that the teaching was effective?

  a. "I need to take my pulse every morning before I take my pill."

  b. "Sometimes I forget my pills, but I usually make up the missed ones once I remember."

  c. "This pill might help my hay fever."

  d. "I don't remember the name of it, but it is the white one."

BIBLIOGRAPHY

Bickley, L. (1998). *Bates' guide to physical examination and history taking* (8th ed.). Philadelphia: Lippincott Williams & Wilkins.

Buchanan, L. M. (1994). Therapeutic nursing intervention knowledge development and outcome measures for advanced practice. *Nursing and Health Care, 15*(4), 190–195.

Carpenito, L. J. (1999). *Handbook of nursing diagnoses* (8th ed.). Philadelphia: Lippincott Williams & Wilkins.

Carpenito, L. J. (1999). *Nursing care plans and documentation* (3rd ed.). Philadelphia: Lippincott Williams & Wilkins.

Carpenito, L. J. (1999). *Nursing diagnosis: Application in clinical practice* (8th ed.). Philadelphia: Lippincott Williams & Wilkins.

Cohen, M. (1994). Medication errors . . . misprinted doses: FDA Precautions. *Nursing, 94*(3), 14.

McCloskey, J., & Bulechek, G. (Eds.). (1996). *Nursing interventions classification* (2nd ed.). St. Louis: C. V. Mosby.

Redman, B. (1997). *The practice of patient education* (8th ed.). St. Louis: Mosby–Year Book.

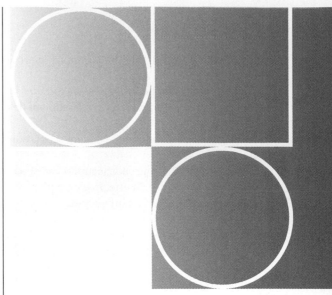

Key Terms
apothecary system
Clark's Rule
conversion
Fried's Rule
metric system
ratio and proportion
Young's Rule

Dosage Calculations

To determine the correct dose of a particular drug for a patient, one should take into consideration the patient's sex, weight, age, and physical condition, as well as the other drugs that the patient is taking. Frequently, the dose that is needed for a patient is not the dose that is available, and it is necessary to convert the dosage form available into the prescribed dosage. Doing the necessary mathematical calculations to determine what should be given is the responsibility of the prescriber who orders the drug, the pharmacist who dispenses the drug, and the nurse who administers the drug. This provides for a good set of checks on the dosage being given before the patient actually receives the drug. In many institutions, drugs arrive at the patient care area in unit-dose form, prepackaged for each individual patient. The nurse who will administer the drug may come to rely on the prepackaged unit-dose that is sent from the pharmacy and may not even recalculate or recheck the dose to match the order that was written. But mistakes still happen, and the nurse, as the person who is administering the drug, is legally and professionally responsible for any error that might occur. It is necessary for practicing nurses to know how to convert drug orders into available forms of a drug to ensure that the right patient is getting the right dose of a drug.

MEASURING SYSTEMS

At least four different systems are currently used in drug preparation and delivery: the **metric system,** the **apothecary system,** the household system, and the avoirdupois system. With the growing number of drugs available and increasing awareness of medication errors that occur in daily practice, efforts have been made to decrease the dependence on so many different systems. In 1995, the United States Pharmacopeia Convention established standards requiring that all prescriptions, regardless of the system that was used in the drug dosage, include the metric measure for quantity and strength of drug. It was also established that drugs may be dispensed only in the metric form. Prescribers are not totally converted to this new standard, and the nurse must be able to covert what is ordered into the available form to ensure patient safety. It is important to be able to perform **conversions** within each system of measure and between systems of measure.

Metric System

The metric system is the most widely used system of measure. It is based on the decimal system, so all units are determined as multiples of 10. This system is used worldwide and makes the sharing of knowledge and research information possible. The metric system uses the gram as the basic unit of solid measure and the liter as the basic unit of liquid measure. Table 5–1 lists the standard units of the metric system.

Apothecary System

The apothecary system is a very old system of measure that was specifically developed for use by apothecaries or pharmacists. The apothecary system uses the minim as the basic unit of liquid measure and the grain as the basic unit of solid measure. This system is much harder to use than the metric system and is rarely seen in most clinical settings. Occasionally a prescriber will write an order in this system and the dosage will have to be converted to an available form. An interesting feature of this system is that it uses Roman numerals placed after the unit of measure to denote amount. For example, 15 grains would be written "gr xv." Table 5–1 lists the standard units of the apothecary system.

Household System

The household system is the measuring system that is found in recipe books. Many people are familiar with the teaspoon

TABLE 5-1 Basic Units of Measure of the Metric, Apothecary, and Household Measuring Systems

System	Solid Measure	Liquid Measure
Metric	gram (g) 1 milligram (mg) = 0.001 g 1 microgram (μg) = 0.000001 g 1 kilogram (kg) = 1000 g	liter (L) 1 milliliter (mL) = 0.001 L 1 mL = 1 cubic centimeter = 1 cc
Apothecary	grain (gr) 60 gr = 1 dram (dr) 8 dr = 1 ounce (oz)	minim (min) 60 min = 1 fluidram (f dr) 8 f dr = 1 fluidounce (f oz)
Household	pound (lb) 1 lb = 16 ounces (oz)	pint (pt) 2 pt = 1 quart (qt) 4 qt = 1 gallon (gal) 16 oz = 1 pt = 2 cups (c) 32 tablespoons (tbsp) = 1 pt 3 teaspoons (tsp) = 1 tbsp 60 drops (gtt) = 1 tsp

and the cup as units of measure. This system uses the teaspoon as the basic unit of fluid measure and the pound as the basic unit of solid measure. Although efforts have been made in recent years to standardize these measuring devices, wide variations have been noted in the capacity of some of these units. Patients need to be advised that flatware teaspoons and drinking cups vary tremendously in the volume that they contain. A flatware teaspoon could hold up to two measuring teaspoons of quantity. When a patient is using a liquid medication at home, it is important to clarify that the measures indicated in the instructions refer to a standardized measuring device. Table 5–1 lists the standard units of the household system.

Avoirdupois System

The avoirdupois system is another older system that was very popular when pharmacists routinely had to compound medications on their own. This system uses ounces and grains, but they measure differently than those of the apothecary and household systems. The avoirdupois system is seldom used by prescibers but may be used for bulk medications that come directly from the manufacturer.

Other Systems

Some drugs are measured in units other than those already discussed. These measures may reflect chemical activity or biological equivalence. One of these measures is the unit (U). A unit usually reflects the biological activity of the drug in 1 mL of solution. The unit is unique for the drug it measures; a unit of heparin would not be comparable to a unit of insulin. Milliequivalents (mEq) are used to measure electrolytes (eg, potassium, sodium, calcium, fluoride). The milliequivalent refers to the ionic activity of the drug in question; the order is usually written for a number of milliequivalents instead of a volume of drug. International units (IU) are sometimes used to measure certain vitamins or enzymes. These are also unique to each drug and cannot be converted to another measuring form.

CONVERTING BETWEEN SYSTEMS

The simplest way to convert measurements from one system to another is to set up a **ratio and proportion** equation. The ratio containing two known equivalent amounts is placed on one side of an equation, and the ratio containing the amount you wish to convert and its unknown equivalent is placed on the other side. To do this, it is necessary to first check a table of conversions to determine the equivalent measure in the two systems you are using. Table 5–2 presents some accepted conversions between systems of measurement. It is a good idea to post a conversion guide in the medication room or on the medication cart for easy access. When conversions are used frequently, it is easy to remember them. When conversions are not used frequently, it is best to look them up.

Try the following conversion using Table 5–2. Convert 6 f oz (apothecary system) to the metric system of measure. According to Table 5–2, 1 f oz is equivalent to 30 mL. Use this information to set up a ratio:

$$\frac{1 \, f \, oz}{30 \, mL} = \frac{6 \, f \, oz}{X}$$

The known ratio, 1 f oz (apothecary system) is equivalent to 30 mL (metric system), is on one side of the equation. The other side of the equation contains 6 f oz, the amount (apothecary system) that you want to convert, and its unknown (metric system) equivalent, X. Because the fluid-ounce measurement is in the numerator (top number) on the left side of the equation, it must also be in the numerator on the right side of the equation. This equation would read as follows: One fluidounce is to thirty milliliters as six fluid-ounces is to how many milliliters?

The first step in the conversion is to cross multiply (multiply the numerator from one side of the equation times the denominator from the other side, and vice-versa):

$$\frac{1 \, f \, oz}{30 \, mL} = \frac{6 \, f \, oz}{X}$$

$$1 \, f \, oz \times X = 6 \, f \, oz \times 30 \, mL$$

This could also be written

$$(1 \, f \, oz)(X) = (6 \, f \, oz)(30 \, mL)$$

After multiplying the numbers, you have

$$1 \, (f \, oz) \, X = 180 \, (f \, oz)(mL)$$

Next, rearrange the terms to let the unknown quantity stand alone on one side of the equation:

TABLE 5-2	Some Commonly Accepted Conversions Between Systems of Measurement

Metric System	Apothecary System	Household System
SOLID MEASURE		
1 kg		2.2 lb
454 g		1.0 lb
1 g = 1000 mg	15 gr (gr xv)	
60 mg	1 gr (gr i)	
30 mg	1/2 gr (gr ss)	
LIQUID MEASURE		
1 L = 1000 mL		about 1 qt
240 mL	8 f oz (f oz viii)	1 c
30 mL	1 f oz (f oz i)	2 tbsp
15–16 mL	4 f dr (f dr iv)	1 tbsp = 3 tsp
8 mL	2 f dr (f dr ii)	2 tsp
4–5 mL	1 f dr (f dr i)	1 tsp = 60 gtt
1 mL	15–16 min (min xv or min xvi)	
0.06 mL	1 min (min i)	

$$X = \frac{180 \ (mL)(f \ oz)}{1 \ f \ oz}$$

Whenever possible, cancel out numbers as well as units of measure. In this example, canceling out leaves

$$X = 180 \ mL$$

By canceling out, you are left with the appropriate amount and unit of measure. The answer to the problem is that 6 f oz is equivalent to 180 mL.

Try another conversion. Convert 32 gr (apothecary system) to its equivalent in the metric system, expressing the answer in milligrams. First, find the conversion on Table 5–2: 1 gr is equal to 60 mg. Set up the ratio:

$$\frac{1 \ gr}{60 \ mg} = \frac{32 \ gr}{X}$$

Cross multiply:

$$(1 \ gr)(X) = (32 \ gr)(60 \ mg)$$

$$1 \ (gr) \ X = 1920 \ (gr)(mg)$$

Rearrange:

$$X = \frac{1920 \ (gr)(mg)}{1 \ gr}$$

Finally, cancel out units and numbers:

$$X = 1920 \ mg$$

Therefore, 32 gr is equivalent to 1920 mg.

CALCULATING DOSAGE

As mentioned earlier, because there are several systems of measurement available that might be used when ordering a drug and because drugs are made available only in certain forms or dosages, it may be necessary to calculate what the patient should be receiving when interpreting a drug order.

Oral Drugs

Frequently, tablets or capsules for oral administration are not available in the exact dose that has been ordered. In these situations, the nurse who is administering the drug must calculate the number of tablets or capsules that should be given to make up the ordered dose. The easiest way to determine this is once again to set up a ratio and proportion equation. The ratio containing the two known equivalent amounts is put on one side of the equation, and the ratio containing the unknown value is put on the other side. The known equivalent is the amount of drug available in one tablet or capsule; the unknown is the number of tablets or capsules that are needed for the prescribed dose:

$$\frac{\text{amount of drug available}}{\text{one tablet or capsule}} = \frac{\text{amount of drug prescribed}}{\text{number of tablets or capsules to give}}$$

The phrase "amount of drug" serves as the unit, so this information must be in the numerator of each ratio.

Try this example: An order is written for 10 grains of aspirin (gr x, aspirin). The tablets that are available each contain 5 grains. How many tablets should be given? First, set up the equation:

$$\frac{5 \ gr}{1 \ tablet} = \frac{10 \ gr}{X}$$

Cross multiply the ratio:

$$5 \ (gr) \ X = 10 \ (gr)(tablet)$$

Rearrange and cancel units and numbers:

$$X = \frac{10 \ (gr)(tablet)}{5 \ (gr)}$$

$$X = 2 \ tablets$$

Try another example: An order is written for 0.05 g *Aldactone* to be given orally (PO). The *Aldactone* is available in 25-mg tablets. How many tablets would you have to give? First, you will need to convert the grams to milligrams.

$$\frac{1 \ g}{1000 \ mg} = \frac{0.05 \ g}{X}$$

Cross multiply:

$$1 \ (g) \ X = (0.05 \times 1000) \ (g)(mg)$$

Simplify:

$$X = \frac{50 \ (g)(mg)}{1 \ (g)}$$

$$X = 50 \ mg$$

The order has been converted to the same measurement as the available tablets. Now solve for the number of tablets that you will need, letting X be the desired dose.

$$\frac{25 \ mg}{1 \ tablet} = \frac{50 \ mg}{X}$$

$$25 \ (mg) \ X = (50 \times 1) \ (mg)(tablet)$$

$$X = \frac{50 \ (mg)(tablet)}{25 \ (mg)}$$

$$X = 2 \ tablets$$

Sometimes the desired dose will be a fraction of a tablet or capsule, $\frac{1}{2}$ or $\frac{1}{4}$. Some tablets come with score markings that allow them to be cut. Pill cutters are readily available in most pharmacies to help patients cut tablets appropriately. One must use caution when advising a patient to cut a tablet. Many tablets today come in a matrix system that allows for slow and steady release of the active drug. These drugs cannot be cut, crushed, or chewed. A drug reference should always be consulted before cutting a tablet. However, as a quick reference, any tablet that is designated as having delayed or sustained release may very well be one that cannot be cut. Capsules can be very difficult to divide precisely, and some of them also come with warnings that they cannot be cut, crushed, or chewed. If the only way to deliver the correct dose to a patient is by cutting one of these preparations, a different drug or a different approach to treating the patient should be tried.

Other oral drugs come in liquid preparations. Many of the drugs used in pediatrics and for adults who might have difficulty swallowing a pill or tablet are prepared in a liquid form. Some drugs that do not come in a standard liquid form can be prepared as a liquid by the pharmacist. If the patient is not able to swallow a tablet or capsule, check for other available forms and consult with the pharmacist about the possibility of preparing the drug in a liquid as a suspension or a solution. The same principle used to determine the number of tablets needed to arrive at a prescribed dose can be used to determine the volume of liquid that will be required to administer the prescribed dose. The ratio on the left of the equation shows the known equivalents, and the ratio on the right side contains the unknown. The phrase "amount of drug" must appear in the numerator of both ratios, and the volume to administer is the unknown (X).

$$\frac{\text{amount of drug available}}{\text{volume available}} = \frac{\text{amount of drug prescribed}}{\text{volume of administer}}$$

Try this example: An order has been written for 250 mg sulfisoxazole. The bottle states that the solution contains 125 mg/5 mL. How much of the liquid should you give?

$$\frac{125 \text{ mg}}{5 \text{ mL}} = \frac{250 \text{ mg}}{X}$$

Cross multiply:

$$125 \text{ (mg) X} = (250 \times 5) \text{ (mg)(mL)}$$

Simplify:

$$X = \frac{1250 \text{ (mg)(mL)}}{125 \text{ mg}}$$

So the desired dose is

$$X = 10 \text{ mL}$$

Even if you are working in an institution that provides unit-dose medications, practice your calculation skills occasionally to make sure that you can figure out the dose of a drug to give. Power can be lost, computers can go down, and the ability to determine conversions is a skill that anyone who administers drugs should have in reserve.

Parenteral Drugs

All drugs administered parenterally must be administered in liquid form. The person administering the drug needs to calculate the volume of the liquid that must be given to administer the prescribed dose. The same formula can be used for this determination that was used for determining the dose of an oral liquid drug:

$$\frac{\text{amount of drug available}}{\text{volume available}} = \frac{\text{amount of drug prescribed}}{\text{volume to administer}}$$

Try this example: An order has been written for 75 mg meperidine to be given intramuscularly (IM). The vial states that it contains meperidine, 1.0 mL = 50.0 mg. Set up the equation just as before:

$$\frac{50 \text{ mg}}{1 \text{ mL}} = \frac{75 \text{ mg}}{X}$$

$$50 \text{ (mg) X} = (75 \times 1) \text{ (mg)(mL)}$$

$$X = \frac{75 \text{ (mg)(mL)}}{50 \text{ (mg)}}$$

$$X = 1.5 \text{ mL}$$

Intravenous Solutions

Intravenous (IV) solutions are used to deliver a prescribed amount of fluid, electrolytes, vitamins, nutrients, or drugs directly into the bloodstream. Although most institutions now use electronically monitored delivery systems, it is still important to be able to determine the amount of an IV solution that should be given using standard calculations. Most IV delivery systems come with a standard control called a microdrip, by which each milliliter delivered contains 60 drops. Macrodrip systems, which deliver 15 drops/mL, are also available; they are usually used when a large volume must be delivered quickly. In giving IV drugs, the microdrip system is most commonly encountered. Check the packaging of the IV tubing if you have any doubts or are unfamiliar with the packaging. The ratio that is used to determine how many drops of fluid to administer per minute is the following:

$$\text{drops/minute} = \frac{\text{mL of solution prescribed per hour}}{60 \text{ minutes/1 hour}} \times \text{drops delivered per mL}$$

That is, the number of drops per minute, or the rate that you will set by adjusting the valve on the IV tubing, is equal to the amount of solution that has been prescribed per hour times the number of drops delivered per mL divided by 60 minutes in an hour.

Try this example: An order has been written for a patient to receive 400 mL of 5% dextrose in water (D5W) over a period of 4 hours in a standard microdrip system (ie, 60 drops/mL). Calculate the correct setting (drops per minute).

$$X = \frac{400 \text{ mL/4 h} \times 60 \text{ drops/mL}}{60 \text{ min/h}}$$

Simplify:

$$X = \frac{100 \text{ mL/h} \times 60 \text{ drops/mL}}{60 \text{ min/h}}$$

$$X = \frac{6000 \text{ drops/h}}{60 \text{ min/h}}$$

Therefore,

$$X = 100 \text{ drops/min}$$

Now calculate the same order for an IV set that delivers 15 drops/mL:

$$X = \frac{400 \text{ mL/4 h} \times 15 \text{ drops/mL}}{60 \text{ min/h}}$$

$$X = \frac{100 \text{ mL/h} \times 15 \text{ drops/mL}}{60 \text{ min/h}}$$

$$X = \frac{1500 \text{ drops/h}}{60 \text{ min/h}}$$

$$X = 25 \text{ drops/min}$$

If a patient has an order to be given an IV drug, the same principle can be used to calculate the speed of the delivery.

For example, an order is written for a patient to receive 50 mL of an antibiotic over 30 minutes. The IV set used dispenses 60 drops/mL, which allows greater control. Calculate how fast the delivery should be.

$$X = \frac{50 \text{ mL/0.5 h} \times 60 \text{ drops/mL}}{60 \text{ min/h}}$$

$$X = \frac{100 \text{ mL/h} \times 60 \text{ drops/mL}}{60 \text{ min/h}}$$

$$X = \frac{6000 \text{ drops/h}}{60 \text{ min/h}}$$

$$X = 100 \text{ drops/min}$$

Pediatric Considerations

Children require different dosages of most drugs than adults do. The "standard" drug dosage that is listed on package inserts and in many references refers to the dose that has been found to be most effective in the adult male. An adult's body handles drugs differently and may respond to drugs differently than a child's. A child's body may handle a drug differently in all areas of pharmacokinetics—absorption, distribution, metabolism, and excretion. The responses of the child's organs to the effects of the drug also may vary because of the immaturity of the organs. Most of the time a child requires a smaller dose of a drug to achieve the comparable critical concentration. On rare occasions, a child may require a higher dose of a drug. For ethical reasons, drug research per se is not done on children. Over time, however, enough information can be accumulated from experience with the drug to have a recommended pediatric dosage. The drug guide that you have selected to use in the clinical setting will have the pediatric dose listed if this information is available. Sometimes there is no recommended dosage but a particular drug is needed for a child. In these situations, there are established formulas that can be used to estimate the appropriate dosage. These methods of determining a pediatric dose take into consideration the child's age, weight, or body surface.

Fried's Rule applies to a child younger than 1 year of age. The rule assumes that an adult dose would be appropriate for a child who is 12.5 years (150 months) old. Fried's Rule states

$$\text{child's dose (age} <1 \text{ year)} = \frac{\text{infant's age (in months)}}{150 \text{ months}}$$
$$\times \text{ average adult dose}$$

Young's Rule, which applies to children age 1 to 12 years of age, states

$$\text{child's dose (age 1–12 years)} = \frac{\text{child's age (in years)}}{\text{child's age (in years)} + 12}$$
$$\times \text{ average adult dose}$$

Clark's Rule uses the child's weight to calculate the appropriate dose and assumes that the adult dose is based on a 150-lb person. It states

$$\text{child's dose} = \frac{\text{weight of child (in pounds)}}{150 \text{ pounds}}$$
$$\times \text{ average adult dose}$$

The child's surface area may also be used to determine the approximate dosage that should be used. To do this, the child's surface area is determined with the use of a nomogram (Figure 5–1). The height and weight of the child are taken into consideration in this chart. The following formula is then used:

FIGURE 5–1. The West nomogram for calculating body surface area (BSA). Draw a straight line connecting the child's height (left scale) to the child's weight (right scale). The BSA value, which is calculated in square meters, is found at the point where the line intersects the SA column. The formula for estimating a child's dose is: Child's BSA (in m²) × adult dose ÷ 1.73. Normal values are shown in the box.

$$\text{child's dose} = \frac{\text{surface area in square meters}}{1.73}$$

$$\times \text{average adult dose}$$

For example, a 3-year-old child weighing 30 lb is to receive a therapeutic dose of aspirin. The average adult dose is 5 gr, and the dose to be given is the unknown (X). The calculation may be made from the child's age, by Young's Rule:

$$X = \frac{3\ y}{3 + 12\ y} \times 5\ gr$$

$$X \times \frac{15\ (y)(gr)}{15\ y}$$

$$X = 1\ gr$$

Alternatively, the calculation may be based on the child's weight, using Clark's Rule:

$$X = \frac{30\ lb}{150\ lb} \times 5\ gr$$

$$X = \frac{150\ (gr)(lb)}{150\ lb}$$

$$X = 1\ gr$$

With small children, even a tiny dosage error can be critical. When working in pediatrics, it is important to become familiar with at least one of these methods of determining the drug dose to use. Many institutions require that two nurses check critical pediatric dosages. This is a good practice when working with small children. Box 5–1 summarizes the pediatric conversion formulas.

BOX 5-1

Formulas Used for Calculating Pediatric Dosages

FRIED'S RULE

$$\text{child's dose (age} < 1 \text{ year)} = \frac{\text{infant's age (in months)}}{150 \text{ months}}$$

$$\times \text{average adult dose}$$

YOUNG'S RULE

$$\text{child's dose (age 1–12 years)} = \frac{\text{child's age (in years)}}{\text{childs age (in years)} + 12}$$

$$\times \text{average adult dose}$$

CLARK'S RULE

$$\text{child's dose} = \frac{\text{weight of child (in pounds)}}{150 \text{ pounds}} \times \text{average adult dose}$$

SURFACE AREA CALCULATION

$$\text{child's dose} = \frac{\text{surface area in square meters}}{1.73} \times \text{average adult dose}$$

CHAPTER SUMMARY

- At least four different systems are currently used in drug preparation and delivery. These include the metric system, the apothecary system, the household system, and the avoirdupois system.
- The metric system is the most widely used system of measure. The United States Pharmacopeia Convention established standards requiring that all prescriptions, regardless of the system that was used in the drug dosage, include the metric measure for quantity and strength of drug. All drugs are dispensed in the metric system.
- It is important to know how to convert dosages from one system to another. The method of ratio and proportion, which uses basic principles of algebra to find an unknown, is the easiest method of converting doses within and between systems.
- Children require different dosages of most drugs than adults do because of the way that their bodies handle drugs and the way that drugs affect their tissues and organs.
- Standard formulas can be used to determine the approximate dose that should be given to a child when the average adult dose is known. These include Fried's Rule (which considers age less than 1 year), Clark's Rule (which considers the child's weight), Young's Rule (which considers weight and age greater than 1 year), and the surface area rule, which requires the use of a nomogram to determine body surface area.

Review Questions

1. Digoxin 0.125 mg is ordered for a patient who is having trouble swallowing. The bottle of digoxin elixir reads 0.5 mg/2 mL. How much would you give?
   a. 5 mL
   b. 0.5 mL
   c. 1.5 mL
   d. 1 mL
2. The usual adult dose of *Benadryl* is 50 mg. What would be the safe dose for a child weighing 27 lb?
   a. 0.9 mg
   b. 1.8 mg
   c. 9.0 mg
   d. 18 mg
3. An order is written for 700 mg ampicillin PO. The drug is supplied in liquid form as 1 g/3.5 mL. How much of the liquid should be given?
   a. 5 mL
   b. 2.5 mL
   c. 6.2 mL
   d. 2.45 mL
4. An order is written for 1000 mL of normal saline to be administered over 10 hr. The drop factor on the IV tubing states 15 drops/mL. What is the IV flow rate?
   a. 50 mL/hr at 50 drops/min
   b. 100 mL/hr at 25 drops/min
   c. 100 mL/hr at 100 drops/min
   d. 100 mL/hr at 15 drops/min

5. The average adult dose of meperidine is 75 mg. What dose would be appropriate for a 10-month-old infant?
   a. 50 mg
   b. 5 mg
   c. 25 mg
   d. 0.5 mg
6. A patient needs to take 0.75 g tetracycline PO. The drug comes in 250-mg tablets. How many tablets should the patient take?
   a. 2 tablets
   b. 3 tablets
   c. 4 tablets
   d. 30 tablets
7. Aminophylline is supplied in a 500 mg/2.5 mL solution. How much would be given if an order were written for 100 mg aminophylline IV?
   a. 5 mL
   b. 1.5 mL
   c. 2.5 mL
   d. 0.5 mL

8. Heparin 800 U is ordered for a patient. The heparin is supplied in a multidose vial that is labeled 10,000 U/mL. How many cubic centimeters of heparin would be needed to treat this patient?
   a. 0.8 cc
   b. 0.08 cc
   c. 8.0 cc
   d. 0.4 cc

BIBLIOGRAPHY

Broussard, M. C., & Pire, S. (1996). Medication problems in the elderly: A home healthcare nurse's perspective. *Home Healthcare Nurse, 14,* 441–443.

Gilman, A. G., Hardman, J. G., & Limbird, L. E., (Eds.). (2002). *Goodman and Gilman's the pharmacological basis of therapeutics* (10th ed.). New York: McGraw-Hill.

Lee, M. (1996). Drugs and the elderly: Do you know the risks? *American Journal of Nursing, 96* (7), 25–32.

Morrison, G. (1996). Drug dosing in the intensive care unit: The patient with renal failure. In J. M. Rippe, R. S. Irwin, & M. P. Fink, *Intensive care medicine* (3rd ed.). Boston: Little, Brown.

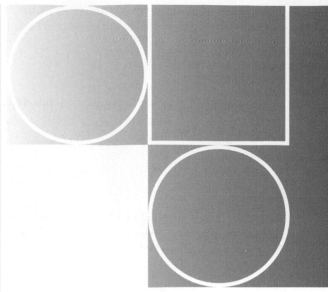

Key Terms
alternative therapies
cost comparisons
Internet
off-label uses
self-care

Drug Therapy in the 21st Century

The dawning of the 21st century has come with myriad new considerations and pressures in the health care industry. For the first time, consumers have access to medical and pharmacological information from many sources. Consumers are taking steps to demand specific treatments and considerations. Alternative therapies are being offered and advertised at record pace, and this is causing people to rethink their approach to medical care and the medical system. At the same time, financial pressures have led to early discharge of patients from health care facilities and to provision of outpatient care for patients who, in the past, would have been hospitalized and monitored closely. Health care providers are being pushed to make decisions about patient care and prescriptions based on finances in addition to medical judgment. The nurse is caught in the middle of all of this change. Patients are demanding information and may not understand it when they get it. Patient teaching and home care provisions are vital to the success of any health regimen. The nurse is frequently in the best position to listen, teach, and explain some of this confusing information to the patient and to facilitate the care of the patient in the health system.

CONSUMER AWARENESS

Access to information has become so broad in the past decade that consumers are often overwhelmed with details, facts, and choices that affect their health care. Gone is the era when the health care provider was seen as omniscient and always right. The patient now comes into the health care system burdened with the influence of advertising, the Internet, and a growing alternative therapy industry. Many patients no longer calmly accept whatever medication is selected for them. They often come with requests and demands, and they partake of a complex system of over-the-counter (OTC) and alternative medicines that further complicate the safety and efficacy of standard drug therapy.

Media Influence

In the past 10 years there has been an explosion of drug advertising in the mass media. It became legal to advertise prescription drugs directly to the public in the 1990s, and it is now impossible to watch television, listen to the radio, or flip through a magazine without confronting numerous drug advertisements.

Federal guidelines determine what can be said in an advertisement, but in some cases this further confuses the issue for many consumers. If a drug advertisement states what the drug is used for, it must also state contraindications, adverse effects, and precautions. Because, in many cases, listing the possible adverse effects is not a good selling point, many advertisements are pure business ploys to get consumers to be interested in the drug and to request it from their health care providers (even if they don't know what the drug is used for). It is not unusual to see a smiling, healthy-looking person romping through a field of beautiful flowers on a sunny day with a cute baby or puppy in tow. The ad might simply state how wonderful it is to be outside on a day like today—contact your health care provider if you, too, would like to take drug X. Numerous calls to caregivers each day are requests for this drug that makes you feel young, happy, and energetic. Although most people now know what the erectile dysfunction drug *Viagra* is used for, some of the ads for this drug simply show a happy, older couple smiling and dancing the night away and encourage viewers to ask their health care providers about *Viagra*. What older person wouldn't want a drug that makes you feel so happy and energetic?

Parenting magazines, which are often found in pediatricians' offices, are full of advertisements for antibiotics and asthma medications. These ads picture smiling, cute children and encourage readers to check with their pediatricians about the use of these drugs. If the drug's indication is mentioned, the second page of the ad may well have the U.S. Food and Drug Administration (FDA)–approved drug insert printed out, in extremely tiny print and in full medical lingo. Most readers have trouble reading the words on these required pages. Even if the words are legible, they frequently don't have any meaning for the reader. The pediatrician or nurse may spend a great deal of time explaining why a particular drug is not indicated for a particular child and may actually experience resistance on the part of the parent who wants the drug for his or her child.

As the marketing power for prescription drugs continues to grow, the health care provider must be constantly aware of what patients are seeing, what the ads are promising, and the real data behind the indications and contraindications for these "hot" drugs. It is a continuing challenge to stay up to date and knowledgeable about drug therapy.

The media also look for headlines in current medical research or reports. It is not unusual for the media to take a headline or research title and make news. Sometimes the interpretation of the medical report is not accurate, and this can influence a patient's response to suggested therapy or provide a whole new set of demands or requests for the health care provider. Many of the standard talk shows include a medical segment that presents just a tiny bit of information, frequently out of context, which opens a whole new area of interest for the viewer. Some health care providers have learned to deal with the "disease of the week" as seen on these shows; others can be unprepared to deal with what was presented and may lose credibility with the patient.

The Internet

The **Internet** and World Wide Web are now readily accessible to most consumers. People who do not have Internet access at home will find it readily available at the local library or at work or even in computer centers that allow community access. The information available over the Internet is completely overwhelming to most people. A person can spend hours looking up information on a drug—including pharmaceutical company information sites, chat rooms with other people who are taking the drug, on-line pharmacies, lists of government regulations, and research reports about the drug and its effectiveness. Many people do not know how to evaluate the information that they can access. Is it accurate or anecdotal? Patients often come into the health care system with pages of information downloaded from the Internet that they think pertains to their particular situation. The nurse or physician can spend a tremendous amount of time deciphering and interpreting the information and explaining it to the patient. Some tips that might be helpful in determining the usefulness or accuracy of information being accessed are found in Box 6–1.

OVER-THE-COUNTER DRUGS

OTC medications have allowed people to take care of simple medical problems without seeking advice from their health care providers. OTC drugs are drugs that have been deemed to be safe when used as directed. Many of them were "grandfathered in" as drugs when stringent testing and evaluation systems became law and have not been tested or evaluated to the extent that new drugs are today. Aspirin, one of the nonprescription standbys for many years, falls into this category. Slowly, the FDA is looking at all of these drugs to determine effectiveness and safety. Other OTC drugs are former prescription drugs that have been tested and found to be safe for use by the general public. Each year several prescription drugs are reviewed for possible OTC status. In 2000, lovastatin, an antihyperlipidemic drug, was considered for OTC

status. It eventually was decided that the public would have a hard time self-prescribing this drug, because high lipid levels can be determined only with a blood test and present no signs and symptoms, so its OTC status was not approved. Some recently approved OTC drugs are cimetidine, to decrease gastric upset and heartburn, and various vaginal antifungal medications for treating yeast infections.

The availability of OTC drugs gives patients freedom for **self-care,** but there are some drawbacks to the use of OTC drugs that should be considered. The use of OTC drugs can mask the signs and symptoms of an underlying problem, making it difficult to arrive at an accurate diagnosis if the condition persists. These drugs are safe when used as directed, but many times the directions are not followed or even read. The idea that "If one makes me feel better, two will make me feel really good" is not always safe in the use of these drugs. Many people are not aware of which drugs are in these preparations and can inadvertently overdose when taking one preparation for each symptom they have. Table 6–1 gives an example of the ingredients that are found in some common cold/allergy preparations. Patients who take doses of different preparations to cover their various symptoms could easily wind up with an unintended overdose or toxic reaction.

Many OTC drugs interact with prescription drugs, with possibly serious effects for the patient. Many patients do not consider OTC drugs to be "real" drugs and do not mention their use when reporting a drug history to the health care provider. Every patient drug teaching session should include information on which particular OTC drugs must be avoided or advice to check with the health care provider before taking any other medications. When taking a drug history, it is important to specifically ask whether the patient is taking any OTC drugs or any other medications. Serious adverse or toxic effects can be avoided if this information is known.

Alternative Therapies and Herbal Medicine

Another aspect of the increasing self-care movement is the rapidly growing alternative or herbal therapies market. Herbal or **alternative therapies** are found in ancient records and have often been the basis for discovery of an active ingredient that is later developed into a regulated medication. Today, alternative therapies can also include nondrug measures such as imaging and relaxation.

Currently, these products are not controlled or tested by the FDA, and therefore the advertising surrounding these products is not as restricted or as accurate as it would be with classic drugs. Consumers are urged to use the "natural" approach to medical care and to self-treat with a wide variety of products. Numerous Internet sites point out all of the natural treatments that can be used to cure various disorders. Television ads and magazine spreads push the use of these products in place of prescribed medications. Many people who want to gain control of their medical care or who do not want to take "drugs" for their diabetes or depression or fatigue are drawn to these products. The Dietary Supplement Health and Education Act of 1994, updated in 2000, states that herbal products, vitamins and minerals, and amino acids

---

BOX 6-1

Some Guidelines for Evaluating Internet Sites

Address identification
  .com—commercial, advertising, selling, business site
  .edu—education site: school system, university, college
  .gov—government site
  .net—part of a linked network system, may include any of the above
  .org—sponsored by an organization, including professional, charitable, and educational groups

Site evaluation
  Navigation—Is the site easy to access and navigate or confusing?
  Contributors—Who prepared the site? Is it reviewed? Is it purely commercial? What are the qualifications of the person(s) maintaining the site?
  Dates—Is the site updated frequently? When was the site last updated?
  Accuracy/reliability—Is the information supported by other sites? Is the information accurate and in agreement with other sources you have reviewed? Does the site list other links that are reasonable and reliable?

TABLE 6-1	Ingredients Found in Some Common Cold and Flu OTC preparations[a]	
Drug	**Ingredients**	**Advertised use**
Vicks Formula 44 Cough & Decongestant	Pseudoephedrine, dextromethorphan	Cough, stuffy nose
Vicks 44D Cough & Head Congestion	Pseudoephedrine, dextromethorphan	Cough, sinus pressure
Vicks 44M Cold, Flu & Cough	Pseudoephedrine, chorpheniramine, dextromethorphan	Cough, aches, stuffy head, flu
Vicks Nyquil Liquicaps	Pseudoephedrine, doxylamine, dextro-methorphan	Cough, aches, need to sleep, stuffy head
Thera-Flu Nondrowsy Formula	Pseudoephedrine, dextromethorphan	Stuffy head, need to stay awake, cough, aches

[a]A patient could take one preparation for cough, a second to cover sinus pressure, a third to cover the aches and pains, and a fourth to stay awake or fall asleep—when the total amounts the patient is taking are considered, a serious overdose of pseudoephedrine or dextromethorphan could easily occur.

are classified as dietary supplements and are not required to go through premarketing testing. The advertising that is permitted for these products does not allow direct claims to cure, treat, diagnose, or prevent a specific disease but does allow for nondisease claims such as "for muscle enhancement," "for hot flashes," or "for memory loss." Table 6–2 lists common alternative therapies and their suggested uses.

Several issues need to concern the health care provider when a patient elects to self-treat with alternative therapies. The active ingredients in these products have not been tested by the FDA and often, when test results are available, have been tested on only a very small number of people with no reproducible results. When a patient decides to take bilberry to control diabetes, for example, the reaction that will occur is not really known. In some patients the blood glucose level might decrease; in others, it might increase. The incidental ingredients in many of these products are unknown. Because many of these products are produced directly from plants or from a natural state, the fertilizer used for the plant, the time of year when the plant was harvested, and the other ingredients that are compounded with the product have a direct effect on its efficacy. Saw palmetto, an herb that has been used successfully to alleviate the symptoms of benign prostatic hypertrophy, is available in a wide variety of preparations from different manufacturers. A random sampling of these products performed in 2000 revealed that the content of the identified active ingredient varied from 20% to 400% of the recommended dose (*Medical Letter*, February 2001 [1097]). It is difficult to guide patients to the correct product with such a wide range of variability.

Patients often do not mention the use of alternative therapies to the health care provider. Some patients believe that the health care provider would disapprove of the use of these products and do not want to discuss it; others believe that these are just natural products and do not need to be mentioned. With the increasing use of these products, however, several drug interactions have been reported to the FDA that can cause serious complications for patients who are taking prescription medications. Diabetic patients who decide to use juniper berries, ginseng, garlic, fenugreek, coriander, dandelion root, or celery to "help maintain their blood glucose level" may run into serious problems with hypoglycemia when they also use their prescription antidiabetic drugs. If the patient does not report use of these alternative therapies to the health care provider, extensive medical tests and dosage adjustments might be done to no avail. St. John's wort, a highly advertised and popular alternative therapy, has been found to interact with oral contraceptives, digoxin (a heart medication), the selective serotonin reuptake inhibitors (used for depression), and the antivirals used to treat acquired immunodeficiency syndrome (AIDS). Patients using St. John's wort for the symptoms of depression who are also taking Prozac for depression may experience serious adverse effects and toxic reactions. If the health care provider is not told about the use of St. John's wort, treatment of the toxicity can become very complicated.

Asking patients specifically about the use of any herbal or alternative therapies should become a routine part of any health history. If a patient presents with an unexpected reaction to a medication, ask the patient about any herbal or natural remedies he or she may be using. If a patient reports the use of an unusual or difficult to find remedy, try looking it up on the Internet at *http://nccam.nih.gov*, a site with generalized information about complementary and alternative medicines.

OFF-LABEL USES

When a drug is approved by the FDA, the therapeutic indications for which the drug is approved are stated. Once a drug becomes available, it is sometimes used for indications that are not part of the approved indications. This is called **off-label** use of the drug. It is commonly done for those groups of patients for which there is little premarketing testing, pediatric and geriatric groups especially. With the ethical issues involved in testing drugs on children, the use of particular drugs in children often occurs by trial and error when the drug is released with adult indications. Dosing calculations and nomograms become very important in determining the approximate dose that should be used for a child.

Drugs used to treat various psychiatric problems are often not approved for that use. The fact that little is really known about the way the brain works and what happens when the

TABLE 6-2 Alternative and Complementary Therapies

Many natural substances are used by the public for self-treatment of many complaints. These substances, derived from folklore of various cultures, often have ingredients that have been identified and have known therapeutic activities. Some of these substances have unknown mechanisms of action, but over the years have been reliably used to relieve specific symptoms. There is an element of the placebo effect in using some of these substances. The power of believing that something will work and that there is some control over the problem is often very beneficial in achieving relief from pain or suffering. Some of these substances contain yet unidentified ingredients, which, when discovered, may prove very useful in the modern field of pharmacology. Because these products are not regulated or monitored, there is always a possibility of toxic effects. Some of these products may contain ingredients that interact with prescription drugs. A history of use of these alternative therapies may explain unexpected reactions to some drugs.

Substance	Reported Use
alfalfa	Topical: healing ointment, relief of arthritis pain Oral: arthritis treatment, strength giving
aloe leaves	Topical: treatment of burns, healing of wounds Oral: treatment of chronic constipation
anise	Oral: relief of dry cough, treatment of flatulence
apple	Oral: control of blood glucose, constipation
arnica gel	Topical: relief of pain from muscle or soft tissue injury
ashwagandha	Oral: enhancement of mental and physical functioning; general tonic; used to protect cells during cancer chemotherapy and radiation therapy Avoid use during pregnancy and lactation.
astragalus	Oral: increases stamina and energy; improves immune function and resistance to disease Do not use with fever or acute infection.
bilberry	Oral: treatment of diabetes; cardiovascular problems; lowers cholesterol and triglycerides; treatment of diabetic retinopathy; treatment of cataracts, night blindness
birch bark	Topical: treatment of infected wounds, cuts Oral: as tea for relief of stomach ache
blackberry	Oral: as tea for generalized healing; treatment of diabetes
black cohosh root	Oral: treatment of premenstrual syndrome (PMS), menopausal disorders, rheumatoid arthritis Contains estrogen-like components. Do not use with hormone replacement therapy or oral contraceptives; avoid use in pregnancy and lactation.
bromelain	Oral: treatment of inflammation, sports injuries, upper respiratory tract infection, PMS, and adjunctive therapy in cancer treatments Associated with nausea, vomiting, diarrhea, menstrual disorders.
burdock	Oral: treatment of diabetes; atropine-like side effects; uterine stimulant
camomile	Topical: treatment of wounds, ulcer, conjunctivitis Oral: treatment of migraines, gastric cramps, relief of anxiety Contains coumarin—monitor patients taking anticoagulants very closely. May cause depression; monitor patients on antidepressants. Cross reaction with ragweed allergies may occur.
catnip leaves	Oral: treatment of bronchitis, diarrhea
cat's claw	Oral: treatment of allergies, arthritis; adjunct in the treatment of cancers and AIDS Do not use with pregnancy or lactation, in transplant recipients; increased risk of bleeding episodes if taken with oral anticoagulants.
cayenne pepper	Topical: treatment of burns, wounds, relief of toothache pain.
celery	Oral: lowers blood glucose, acts as a diuretic; may cause potassium depletion
chaste-tree berry	Oral: progesterone-like effects; used to treat PMS and menopausal problems, to stimulate lactation Use caution with hormone replacement therapy and oral contraceptives.
chicken soup	Oral: breaks up respiratory secretions, bronchodilator, relieves anxiety
chicory	Oral: treatment of digestive tract problems, gout; stimulates bile secretions
Chinese angelica (dong quai)	Oral: general tonic; treatment of anemias, PMS, menopause, antihypertensive, laxative Use caution with flu, hemorrhagic diseases. Monitor patients taking antihypertensives or vasodilators for toxic effects. Use caution with hormone replacement therapy.
chong cao fungi	Oral: antioxidant, promotes stamina, sexual function Avoid use in children.
coleus forskohlii	Oral: treatment of asthma, hypertension, eczema Use caution with antihypertensives or antihistamines, severe additive effects can occur. Avoid use with hypotension or in people with peptic ulcers.
comfrey	Topical: treatment of wounds, cuts, ulcers Oral: gargle for tonsillitis
coriander	Oral: weight loss, lowers blood glucose

TABLE 6-2 | Alternative and Complementary Therapies (continued)

Substance	Reported Use
dandelion root	Oral: treatment of liver and kidney problems; decreases lactation (after delivery or with weaning); lowers blood glucose
dehydroepiandrosterone (DHEA)	Oral: slows aging, improves vigor—"Fountain of Youth"; androgenic side effects
Di huang	Oral: treatment of diabetes mellitus
dried root bark of lycium Chinese mill	Oral: lowers cholesterol, lowers blood glucose
echinacea (cone flower)	Oral: treatment of colds, flu; stimulates the immune system, attacks viruses; causes immunosuppression May be liver toxic. Do not use longer than 8 wk. Do not give with liver toxic drugs or immunosuppressants. Avoid use with antifungals; serious liver injury could occur. Avoid use in patients with systemic lupus erythematosus, tuberculosis, AIDS.
elder bark and/or flowers	Topical: gargle for tonsillitis, pharyngitis Oral: treatment of fever, chills
ephedra	Oral: increases energy, relieves fatigue. *Warning:* associated with serious complications, withdrawn in some states
ergot	Oral: treatment of migraine headaches, treatment of menstrual problems, hemorrhage
eucalyptus	Topical: treatment of wounds Oral: decreases respiratory secretions, suppresses cough
evening primrose	Oral: treatment of PMS, menopause, rheumatoid arthritis, diabetic neuropathy Do not use with phenothiazines, antidepressants; increases risk of seizures; avoid use in patients with epilepsy, schizophrenia
fennel	Oral: treatment of colic, gout, flatulence; enhances lactation
fenugreek	Oral: lowers cholesterol levels; reduces blood glucose; aids in healing
feverfew	Oral: treatment of arthritis, fever, migraine Use caution with anticoagulants; may increase bleeding. Avoid use before or immediately after surgery because of bleeding risk.
fish oil	Oral: treatment of coronary diseases, arthritis, colitis, depression, aggression, attention deficit disorder
gamboge	Oral: appetite suppressant, lowers cholesterol, promotes weight loss
garlic	Oral: treatment of colds, diuretic; prevention of coronary artery disease, intestinal antiseptic; lowers blood glucose, anticoagulant Use caution with diabetic patients, oral anticoagulants Known to affect blood clotting. Do not use with warfarin.
ginger	Oral: treatment of nausea, motion sickness, postoperative nausea (may increase risk of miscarriage) Affects blood clotting. Do not give with anticoagulants.
ginkgo	Oral: vascular dilation; increases blood flow to the brain, improving cognitive function; used in treating Alzheimer's disease; antioxidant Can inhibit blood clotting. Do not give with aspirin or NSAIDs. Can interact with phenytoin, carbemazepine, phenobarbital. Tricyclic antidepressants, monoamine oxidase inhibitors (MAOIs) use caution.
ginkobe	Oral: increases cerebral blood flow, improves concentration and memory
ginseng	Oral: aphrodisiac, mood elevator, tonic, antihypertensive; decreases cholesterol levels; lowers blood glucose; do not use for >3 mo; adjunct in cancer chemotherapy and radiation therapy May cause irritability if combined with caffeine. Inhibits clotting. Do not use with anticoagulants, aspirin, NSAIDs. May cause headaches, manic episodes if used with phenelzine, MAOIs. Additive effects of estrogens and corticosteroids. May also interfere with digoxin's cardiac effects. Monitor patients closely.
goldenrod leaves	Oral: treatment of renal disease, rheumatism, sore throat, eczema
goldenseal	Oral: lowers blood glucose, aids healing; treatment of bronchitis, colds, flu-like symptoms, cystitis. High doses may cause paralysis. Affects blood clotting; do not give with anticoagulants.
gotu kola	Topical: treatment of cellulitis, scleroderma, open wounds, pressure sores
grape seed extract	Oral: treatment of allergies, asthma; improves circulation, decreases platelet aggregation Use caution with oral anticoagulants, may increase bleeding.
green tea leaf	Oral: antioxidant, used as a preventative for cancer and cardiovascular disease Use caution with oral anticoagulants; may increase bleeding.
guayusa	Oral: lowers blood glucose; weight loss

(table continues on page 58)

TABLE 6-2 Alternative and Complementary Therapies (continued)

Substance	Reported Use
hawthorn	Oral: treatment of angina, arrhythmias, blood pressure problems; decreases cholesterol Use with caution with digoxin, angiotensin-converting enzyme inhibitors; may potentiate effects.
hop	Oral: sedative; aids healing; alters blood glucose
horehound	Oral: expectorant; treatment of respiratory problems, GI disorders
horse chestnut seed	Oral: treatment of varicose veins, hemorrhoids Use caution with oral anticoagulants; may increase bleeding.
Java plum	Oral: treatment of diabetes mellitus
juniper berries	Oral: increases appetite, aids digestion, diuretic, urinary tract disinfectant; lowers blood glucose
kava	Oral: treatment of nervous anxiety, stress, restlessness; tranquilizer Do not use with alprazolam—may cause coma. Do not use with Parkinson's disease or history of stroke. Do not combine with St. John's wort, antianxiety drugs, or alcohol.
kudzu	Oral: reduces cravings for alcohol; being researched for use with alcoholics
ledum tincture	Topical: treatment of insect bites, puncture wounds; dissolves some blood clots and bruises
licorice	Oral: prevents thirst, soothes coughs; treats "incurable" chronic fatigue syndrome; treatment of duodenal ulcer. Acts like aldosterone. Blocks spironolactone effects. Can lead to digoxin toxicity because of effects of lowering aldosterone. Use extreme caution. Contraindicated with renal or liver disease, hypertension, coronary artery disease, pregnancy, lactation. Do not combine with thyroid drugs, antihypertensives, oral contraceptives.
ma huang	Oral: treatment of colds, nasal congestion, asthma. Contains ephedrine. Do not use with antihypertensives, diabetes, MAOIs, or digoxin. Serious side effects could occur.
mandrake root	Oral: treatment of fertility problems
marigold leaves/flowers	Oral: relief of muscle tension, increases wound healing
melatonin	Oral: relief of jet lag, treatment of insomnia
milk thistle	Oral: treatment of hepatitis, cirrhosis, fatty liver due to alcohol or drugs
milk vetch	Oral: improves resistance to disease; adjunct therapy in cancer chemotherapy and radiation therapy
mistletoe leaves	Oral: weight loss; relief of signs and symptoms of diabetes
momordica charantia (Karela)	Oral: blocks intestinal absorption of glucose; lowers blood glucose; weight loss
nightshade leaves/roots	Oral: stimulates circulatory system; treatment of eye disorders
parsley seeds/leaves	Oral: treatment of jaundice, asthma, menstrual difficulties, conjunctivitis
passionflower vine	Oral: sedative/hypnotic May increase sedation with other CNS depressants, MAOIs. Avoid alcohol while using this drug.
peppermint leaves	Oral: treatment of nervousness, insomnia, dizziness, cramps, coughs Topical: rubbed on forehead to relieve tension headaches
psyllium	Oral: treatment of constipation; lowers cholesterol Can cause severe gas and stomach pain; may interfere with nutrient absorption. Avoid use with warfarin, digoxin, lithium—absorption of drug may be blocked. Do not combine with laxatives.
raspberry	Oral: healing of minor wounds; control and treatment of diabetes
rosemary	Topical: relief of rheumatism, sprains, wounds, bruises, eczema Oral: gastric stimulation, relief of flatulence, stimulation of bile release, relief of colic
Rue extract	Topical: relief of pain associated with sprains, groin pulls, whiplash
saffron	Oral: treatment of menstrual problems, abortifacient
sage	Oral: lowers blood pressure; lowers blood glucose
SAMe (adomet)	Oral: promotion of general well being and health Associated with frequent GI complaints and headache.
sarsaparilla	Oral: treatment of skin disorders, rheumatism
saw palmetto	Oral: treatment of benign prostatic hyperplasia Do not use with estrogen replacement or birth control pills—may greatly increase side effects. May decrease iron absorption. Do not combine with finasteride; toxicity could occur.
schisandra	Oral: health tonic, liver protectant; adjunct in cancer chemotherapy and radiation therapy Do not use in pregnancy, causes uterine stimulation.

TABLE 6-2 Alternative and Complementary Therapies (continued)

Substance	Reported Use
St. John's wort	Oral: treatment of depression, PMS symptoms; antiviral Topical: treatment of puncture wounds, insect bites, crushed fingers or toes Avoid tyramine-containing foods; hypertensive crisis is possible. Can increase sensitivity to light; do not combine with drugs that cause photosensitivity. Severe photosensitivity can occur in light-skinned people. Serious drug interactions have been reported with selective serotonin reuptake inhibitors (SSRIs), MAOIs, kava, digoxin, theophylline, AIDS antiviral agents, oral contraceptives. Avoid these combinations.
sweet violet flowers	Oral: treatment of respiratory disorders, emetic
tarragon	Oral: weight loss; prevents cancer; lowers blood glucose
tea tree oil	Topical: antifungal, antibacterial; used in the treatment of burns and insect bites, as a mouth wash
thyme	Topical: liniment, treatment of wounds, gargle Oral: antidiarrhetic, relief of bronchitis and laryngitis Can increase sensitivity to light; do not combine with drugs that cause photosensitivity. Do not use MAOIs or with SSRIs—can cause serious side effects.
tumeric	Oral: antioxidant, anti-inflammatory; used to treat arthritis May cause GI distress. Do not use with known biliary obstruction. May cause increased bleeding with oral anticoagulants.
valerian	Oral: sedative/hypnotic; reduces anxiety, relaxes muscles Can cause severe liver damage. Do not use with barbiturates, alcohol, CNS depressants, or antihistamines; can cause serious sedation.
went rice	Oral: cholesterol and triglyceride lowering effects Do not use in pregnancy, liver disease, alcoholism, or acute infections.
white willow bark	Oral: treatment of fevers
xuan seng	Oral: lowers blood glucose; slows heart rate; treatment of congestive heart failure
yohimbe	Oral: treatment of erectile dysfunction Can affect blood pressure, CNS stimulant; has cardiac effects.

Reprinted with permission from Karch, A. (2001). *2002 Lippincott's nursing drug guide*. Philadelphia: Lippincott Williams & Wilkins.

chemicals in the brain are altered has led to a polypharmacy approach in psychiatry—mixing and juggling drugs until the effect that is wanted is achieved. That same combination might not work in another patient with the same diagnosis because of brain and chemical differences in that patient. The nurse needs to be cognizant of off-label uses of drugs. The liability issues surrounding many of these uses are very fuzzy, and the nurse should be clear about the intended use, why the drug is being tried, and its potential for problems. The off-label use of drugs is widespread and often leads to discovery of a new use for a drug. If the use makes no sense to you, however, question it before you administer the drug.

HEALTH CARE CRISIS

The cost of medical care and drugs has skyrocketed in the past few years. This is partly from the demand to have the best possible, most up-to-date, and safest care and drug therapies. The research and equipment requirements to meet these demands are huge. At the same time, the rising cost of health insurance to pay for all of this is a major complaint for employers and consumers. As a result, health maintenance organizations (HMOs) have surged in popularity. These groups run the medical care system like a business, with the financial aspects of business becoming the overriding concern; decisions are often made by nonmedical personnel with a keen eye on the bottom line. Patients are being discharged from hospitals far earlier than ever before, as a cost-saving move, and many are not even admitted to hospitals for surgical or invasive procedures that used to require several days of hospitalization and monitoring. As a result, there is less monitoring of the patient, and more responsibility for care falls on the patient or the patient's significant others. Teaching the patient about self-care, drug therapies, and what to expect is even more crucial now. The nurse is the one who most often is responsible for this teaching.

Health Maintenance Organizations and Regulations

HMOs provide a centralized control system to provide patients with their medical care within a budget. In many communities, the HMO provides a centralized building with participating physicians and services housed in one area. Consumers are often provided with all of their health care at this facility and find the HMO insurance cost less expensive than traditional medical insurance. The tradeoff is often a loss of choice. The health care providers in the organization are the only ones who can be consulted. The HMO may regulate access to emergency facilities, types and timing of tests allowed, and procedures covered. Accessibility to prescription drugs is also controlled. The formulary for each HMO differs. Sometimes only generic products are covered and newer drugs must be paid for by the patient; in other instances, a tier system exists and the patient may urge the provider to choose a drug from a lower tier, at a lower cost. Many health care providers believe that their ability to make decisions is limited by such regulations and that decisions are often made by nonmedical personnel at the other end of a telephone, who have no contact with the patient. The regulatory power of HMOs is being challenged in various court cases and through legislation and may change dramatically in the coming years.

Cost Considerations

Despite the insurance coverage a patient may have for prescription medications, it is often necessary for the health care provider to choose a drug therapy based on the costs of the drugs available. With more and more of the population reaching retirement age and depending on a fixed income, costs are a real issue. Sometimes this may mean not selecting a first-choice drug but settling for a drug that should be effective. Patients who take antibiotics must be reminded to take the full course and not to stop the drug when they feel better, saving the remaining pills for the next time they feel sick, hoping to avoid the costs of another health care visit and a new prescription. This practice has contributed to the problem of resistant bacteria, which is becoming more dangerous all the time.

Patients also need to be advised not to split tablets in half unless specifically advised to do so. Some drugs can be split, and it is cheaper to order the larger size and have the patient cut the tablet. Some patients think that by cutting the drug in half they will have coverage for twice the time allowed by the prescription and will not be as dependent on the drug. With the new matrix delivery systems used for many medications, however, splitting the drug can cause it to become toxic or ineffective. Patients should be specifically alerted to avoid cutting drugs when it could be dangerous, especially if they are being advised to cut other tablets to be economical. The cost of treating the toxic reactions may far exceed the cost of the original drug.

Generic drug availability in many cases reduces the cost of a drug. Generic drugs are preparations that are off patent and therefore can be sold by their generic name, without the cost associated with brand name products. Generic drugs are tested for bioequivalence with the brand name product, and resulting information is available to prescribers. When a drug has a small margin of safety (a small difference between the therapeutic and the toxic dose), a prescriber may feel more comfortable ordering the drug by brand name, to ensure that the dosage and binders are what the prescriber expects. When "DAW" (dispense as written) is on a prescription, the prescription is filled with the brand-name drug—such as Lanoxin instead of digoxin, or Coumadin instead of warfarin. In some situations, the generic drug is not less expensive than the brand-name drug, so using only generic drugs does not guarantee that the patient is getting the least expensive preparation. Many pharmacies post the costs of commonly used drugs, and patients may do **cost comparisons** and request that a different

drug be prescribed. The nurse is often the person who is in the middle of this issue and must be able to explain the reason for the drug choice or request that the prescriber consider an alternative treatment.

Table 6–3 presents an example of a cost comparison of some β-blockers commonly used to treat hypertension. When deciding which drug to use, the patient or nurse may need to consider the range of costs. **Facts and Comparisons** provides a cost comparison of drugs in each class, and **The Medical Letter** provides cost comparisons of drugs that are reviewed in each issue.

Home Care

The home care industry is one of the most rapidly growing offshoots of the changes in costs and medical care delivery. Patients go home directly from surgery with the responsibility for changing dressings, assessing wounds, and monitoring their own recovery. Patients are being discharged from hospitals because the hospital days allowed for a particular diagnosis have run out. These patients may be responsible for their own monitoring, rehabilitation, and drug regimens. At the same time, the population is aging and may be less accepting of all of this responsibility. Home health aides, visiting nurses, and home care programs are taking over some of the responsibilities that used to be handled in the hospital.

TABLE 6-3 | Cost Comparison of β-blockers Used for the Treatment of Hypertension

	Dosage (mg)	Average cost for a 30-day supply
Acebutolol	200–1200	
Generic		$21.30
Sectral		$37.50
Atenolol	25–100	
Generic		$ 8.70
Tenormin		$32.40
Betaxolol	5–40	
Generic		$24.60
Kerlone		$28.80
Bisoprolol	5–20	
Generic		$36.30
Zebeta		$37.80
Carvedilol	12.5–50	$92.40
Metoprolol	50–200	
Generic		$ 7.80
Lopressor		$21.90
Nadolol	20–240	
Generic		$18.30
Corgard		$41.40
Propranolol	40–240	
Generic		$ 8.40
Inderal		$21.60
Timolol	10–40	
Generic		$16.20
Blocadren		$31.80

Adapted from (2001). Choosing a beta blocker, *Medical Letter, 43,* 9.

The responsibility of meeting the tremendous increase in teaching needs of patients frequently resides with the nurse. Patients need to know exactly what medications they are taking (generic and brand names), the dose of each medication, and what each is supposed to do. They also need to know what they can do to alleviate some of the adverse effects that are expected with each drug (eg, small meals if gastrointestinal upset is common, use of a humidifier if secretions will be dried and make breathing difficult); which OTC drugs or alternative therapies they need to avoid while taking their prescribed drugs; and what to watch for that would indicate a need to call the health care provider. With patients who are taking many drugs at the same time, this information should be provided in writing, in language that is clear and understandable. Many pharmacies provide written information with each drug that is dispensed, but trying to organize these sheets of information into a useable and understandable form is difficult for many patients. The nurse is often the one who needs to sort this out and organize, simplify, and make sense of the provided information. The cost of dealing with toxic or adverse effects is often much higher, in the long run, than the cost of the time spent teaching and explaining things to the patient.

The projections for trends in health care indicate even greater expansion of the home health care system, with hospitals being used for only the most critically ill patients. The role of the nurse in this home health system is crucial—as teacher, assessor, diagnostician, and patient advocate.

CHAPTER SUMMARY

- The 21st century poses new challenges for patients and health care providers, including information overload, demands for specific treatments, increased access to self-care systems, and financial pressures to provide cost-effective care.
- The mass media bombard consumers with medical reviews, research updates, and advertising for prescription drugs. If the use of a drug is stated, the adverse effects and cautions also must be stated. If the use is not stated, the drug advertisement is free to use any images and suggestions to sell the drug.
- Increasing access to the Internet and World Wide Web has increased consumer access to drug information, advertising, and even purchasing without a mediator of this information. Determining the reliability of an Internet site is a challenge for the consumer and the health care provider.
- OTC drugs and herbal and alternative therapies allow patients to make medical decisions and self-treat many common signs and symptoms. Problems arise when they are used inappropriately, when they interact with prescription drugs, or when they mask signs and symptoms, making diagnosis difficult.
- The health care crisis in this country has led to the emergence of HMOs and tight regulations on medical therapy and drug therapy alternatives. The choice of a drug to be used may be determined by the HMO formulary or by cost comparison

with other drugs in the same or a similar class. Cost comparison is a major consideration in the use of many drugs.
- Off-label uses of drugs occur when a drug has been released and is available for use. The use of a drug for an indication that is not approved by the FDA occurs commonly in pediatric and in psychiatric medicine, where testing is limited or made ineffective by individual differences.
- Home care is one of the most rapidly growing areas of medical care. Patients are increasingly more responsible for managing their own medical regimens from home with dependence on home health providers and teaching and support from knowledgeable nurses.

Review Questions

1. Drugs can be advertised in the mass media only if
   a. the FDA indication is clearly stated.
   b. the actual use is never stated.
   c. adverse effects and precautions are stated if the use is stated.
   d. all adverse effects are clearly stated.
2. Herbal treatments and alternative therapies
   a. are considered drugs and regulated by the FDA.
   b. are considered dietary supplements and not regulated by the FDA.
   c. have no restrictions on claims and advertising.
   d. contain no drugs, only natural substances.
3. The Internet provides useful information to patients and is
   a. tightly regulated as to content by the FDA.
   b. difficult to evaluate as to reliability of information.
   c. reliable and factual in any printed claim.
   d. a good place to get drugs without a prescription.
4. OTC drugs are drugs that are
   a. deemed to be safe when used as directed.
   b. harmless to the public.
   c. too old to be tested.
   d. cheaper to use than prescription drugs.
5. Health histories should include specific questions about the use of OTC drugs and alternative therapies because
   a. many insurance policies cover these drugs.
   b. patients should be reprimanded about the use of these products.
   c. patients often do not consider them to be drugs and do not report their use.
   d. patients should never use these products when taking prescription drugs.
6. The home health care industry is booming because
   a. there is a shortage of hospital beds.
   b. patients feel safer at home and prefer to be cared for at home.
   c. patients are going home sooner and becoming responsible for their own care sooner than in the past.
   d. the nursing shortage makes it difficult to care for patients in hospitals.
7. The cost of drug therapy is a major consideration in most areas because
   a. generic drugs are always cheaper.

b. the high cost of drugs combined with more fixed-income consumers puts constraints on drug use.

c. pharmacies usually carry only one drug from each class.

d. patients like to shop around and get the best drug for their money.

BIBLIOGRAPHY

Anderson, P. O. (2000). *Handbook of critical drug data* (9th ed.). Hamilton, IL: Drug Intelligence.

Cardinale, V. (1998). Consumers looking for more answers, clearer directions. *Drug Topics Supplement, 142* (11), 23a.

DerMarderosina, A. (Ed.). (2000). *The review of natural products.* St. Louis: Facts and Comparisons.

Drug facts and comparisons. (2002). St. Louis: Facts and Comparisons.

Gilman, A. G., Hardman, J. G., & Limbird, L. E., (Eds.). (2002). *Goodman and Gilman's the pharmacological basis of therapeutics* (10th ed.). New York: McGraw-Hill.

Karch, A. (2002). *2003 Lippincott's nursing drug guide.* Philadelphia. Lippincott Williams & Wilkins.

The medical letter on drugs and therapeutics. (2001). New Rochelle, NY: Medical Letter.

Chemotherapeutic Agents

Introduction to Cell Physiology

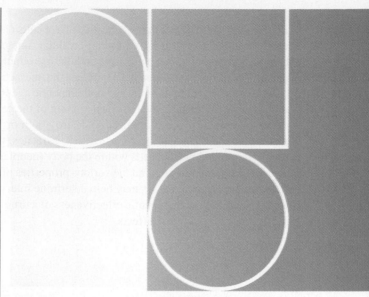

Key Terms

cell cycle

cell membrane

cytoplasm

diffusion

endocytosis

exocytosis

histocompatibility antigens

lipoprotein

lysosomes

mitochondria

nucleus

organelles

osmosis

ribosomes

Chemotherapeutic drugs are agents that affect cells (1) by altering cellular function or disrupting cellular integrity, causing cell death, or (2) by preventing cellular reproduction, eventually leading to cell death. To understand the actions and the adverse effects caused by chemotherapeutic agents, it is important to understand the basic functioning of the cell.

Chemotherapeutic drugs are used to destroy both organisms that invade the body (bacteria, viruses, parasites, protozoa, fungi) and abnormal cells within the body (neoplasms or cancers). By keeping in mind the various properties of the cell and cell processes, nurses may help determine interventions that increase the therapeutic effectiveness of a drug and limit the undesired adverse effects.

THE CELL

The cell is the basic structural unit of the body. The cells that make up living organisms, which are arranged into tissues and organs, all have the same basic structure. Each cell has a nucleus, a cell membrane, and cytoplasm, which contains a variety of organelles (Figure 7–1).

Cell Nucleus

The **nucleus** of a cell contains all of the genetic material that is necessary for cell reproduction and for regulation of cellular production of proteins. Each cell is "programmed" by the genes for the production of specific proteins that allow

the cell to carry out its function, maintain cell homeostasis or stability, and promote cell division. The nucleus is encapsulated in its own membrane and remains distinct from the rest of the cytoplasm. A small spherical mass, called the nucleolus, is located within the nucleus. Within this mass are dense fibers and proteins that will eventually become **ribosomes,** the sites of protein synthesis within the cell.

The nucleus also contains genes, or sequences of DNA, that control basic cell functions and allow for cell division. Genes are responsible for the formation of messenger RNA and transcription RNA, which are involved in production of the proteins unique to the cell. The DNA necessary for cell division is found on long strains called chromatin. These structures line up and enlarge during the process of cell division.

Cell Membrane

The cell is surrounded by a thin barrier called the **cell membrane,** which separates the intracellular fluid from the extracellular fluid. The membrane is essential for cellular integrity and is equipped with many mechanisms for maintaining cell homeostasis.

Lipoproteins
The cell membrane, which consists of lipids and proteins, is a **lipoprotein** structure. The two components are arranged in a freely moving double layer. The membrane is largely composed of lipids—phospholipids, glycolipids, and cholesterol. The phospholipids, which are bipolar in nature, line up with their polar regions pointing toward the interior or ex-

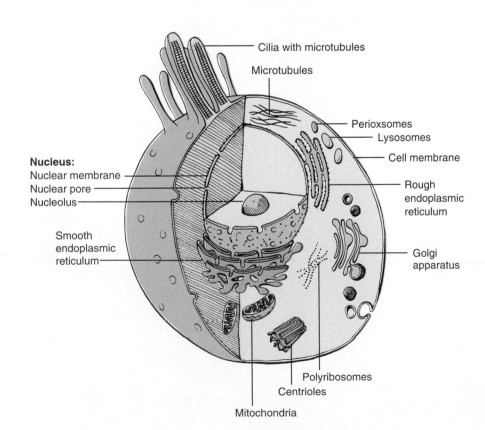

Cilia with microtubules

Microtubules

Perioxsomes

Lysosomes

Cell membrane

Rough endoplasmic reticulum

Golgi apparatus

Nucleus:
Nuclear membrane
Nuclear pore
Nucleolus

Smooth endoplasmic reticulum

Polyribosomes

Centrioles

Mitochondria

FIGURE 7–1. General structure of a cell and the location of its organelles.

terior of the cell and their nonpolar region lying within the cell membrane. The polar regions mix well with water, and the nonpolar region repels water. These properties allow the membrane to act as a barrier, keeping the cytoplasm within the cell and regulating what can enter the cell (Figure 7–2). The freely moving nature of the membrane allows it to adjust to the changing shape of the cell.

Receptor Sites

Embedded in the lipoprotein membrane are a series of peripheral proteins with several functions. As discussed in Chapter 2, one type of protein located on the cell membrane is known as a receptor site. This protein reacts with specific chemicals outside the cell to stimulate a reaction within a cell. For example, the receptor site for insulin reacts with the hormone insulin to cause activation of adenosine triphosphate (ATP) within the cell. This reaction alters the cell's permeability to glucose. Receptor sites are very important in the functioning of neurons, muscle cells, endocrine glands, and other cell types, and they play a very important role in clinical pharmacology.

Identifying Markers

Other surface proteins are surface antigens, or genetically determined identifying markers. These proteins provide the **histocompatibility antigens** or human leukocyte antigens (HLAs) that the body uses to identify a cell as a self-cell (ie, a cell belonging to that individual). The body's immune system recognizes these proteins and acts to protect self-cells and to destroy non–self-cells. When an organ is transplanted from one person to another, a great effort is made to match as many histocompatibility antigens as possible to reduce the chance that the "new" body will reject the transplanted organ.

Histocompatibility antigens can be changed in several ways: by cell injury, with viral invasion of a cell, with age, and so on. If the markers are altered, the body's immune system reacts to the change and can ignore it, allowing neoplasms to grow and develop. The immune system may also attack the cell, leading to many of the problems associated with autoimmune disorders and chronic inflammatory conditions.

Channels

Channels or pores within the cell membrane are made by proteins in the cell wall that allow the passage of small substances in or out of the cell. Specific channels have been identified for sodium, potassium, calcium, chloride, bicarbonate, and water, and other channels may also exist. Some drugs are designed to affect certain channels specifically. For example, calcium channel blockers prevent the movement of calcium into a cell through calcium channels.

Cytoplasm

The cell **cytoplasm** lies within the cell membrane. This complex area, which contains many **organelles** (structures with specific functions), is the site of activities of cellular metabolism and special cellular functions. The organelles within the cytoplasm include the mitochondria, the endoplasmic reticulum, free ribosomes, the Golgi apparatus, and the lysosomes.

Mitochondria

The **mitochondria** are rod-shaped power plants within each cell that produce energy in the form of ATP, which allows the cell to function. Mitochondria are plentiful in very active cells such as muscle cells and are relatively scarce in inactive cells such as bone cells. Mitochondria, which can reproduce when a cell is very active, are always very abundant in cells that consume energy. For example, cardiac muscle cells, which must work continually to keep the heart contracting, contain a great number of mitochondria. Milk-producing cells in breast tissue, which are normally quite dormant, contain very few mitochondria. If a woman is lactating, however, the mitochondria become more abundant to meet the demands of the milk-producing cells. The mitochondria can take carbohydrates, fats, and proteins from the cytoplasm and make ATP via the Krebs cycle, which depends on oxygen. Cells use the ATP to maintain homeostasis, produce proteins, and carry out specific functions. If oxygen is not available, lactic acid builds up as a byproduct of cellular respiration. Lactic acid leaves the cell and is transported to the liver for conversion to glycogen and carbon dioxide.

Endoplasmic Reticulum

Much of the cytoplasm of a cell is made up of a fine network of channels known as cisternae, which are interconnected channels that form the endoplasmic reticulum. The undulating surface of the endoplasmic reticulum provides a large surface for chemical reactions within the cell. Many granules that contain enzymes and ribosomes, which produce protein, are scattered over the surface of the endoplasmic reticulum. Production of proteins, nonproteins, hormones, and other substances takes place there. The breakdown of many toxic substances may also occur in these channels.

Free Ribosomes

Other ribosomes that are not bound to the surface of the endoplasmic reticulum exist throughout the cytoplasm. These

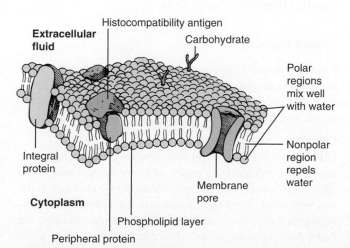

FIGURE 7–2. Structure of the lipid bilayer of the cell membrane. (Adapted from Bullock, B. L. [2000]. *Focus on pathophysiology.* Philadelphia: Lippincott Williams & Wilkins.)

free-floating ribosomes produce proteins that are important to the structure of the cell and some of the enzymes that are necessary for cellular activity.

Golgi Apparatus

The Golgi apparatus is a series of flattened sacs that may be part of the endoplasmic reticulum. These structures prepare hormones or other substances for secretion by processing them and packaging them in vesicles to be moved to the cell membrane for excretion from the cell. In addition, the Golgi apparatus may produce lysosomes and store other synthesized proteins and enzymes until they are needed.

Lysosomes

Lysosomes are membrane-covered organelles that contain specific digestive enzymes that can break down proteins, nucleic acids, carbohydrates, and lipids. These organelles form a membrane around any substance that needs to be digested and secrete the digestive enzymes directly into the isolated area, protecting the rest of the cytoplasm from injury. The lysosomes are responsible for digesting worn or damaged sections of a cell, which they accomplish by encapsulating the area and self-digesting it. If a cell dies and the membrane ruptures, the release of lysosomes causes the cell to self-destruct.

This phenomenon can be seen with old lettuce in the refrigerator. The side of the lettuce head that has been "lying down" for a prolonged period becomes brown and wet as the lettuce cells die and self-digest when their lysosomes are released. If the lettuce is not used, the released lysosomes begin to digest any healthy lettuce that remains, with eventual destruction of the entire head. Lysosomes are important in ecology. Dead trees, animals, and other organisms self-digest and disappear.

CELL PROPERTIES

Cells have certain properties that allow them to survive. **Endocytosis** involves incorporation of material into the cell. Pinocytosis, a form of endocytosis, refers to the engulfing of specific substances that have reacted with a receptor site on the cell membrane. This process allows cells to absorb nutrients, enzymes, and other materials. Phagocytosis is a similar process; it allows the cell, usually a neutrophil or macrophage, to engulf a bacterium or a foreign protein and destroy it within the cell by secreting digestive enzymes into the area. **Exocytosis** is the opposite of endocytosis. This property allows a cell to move a substance to the cell membrane and then secrete the substance outside the cell. Hormones, neurotransmitters, enzymes, and other substances that are produced within a cell are excreted into the body by this process (Figure 7–3).

Homeostasis

The main goal of a cell is to maintain homeostasis, which means keeping the cytoplasm stable within the cell membrane. Each cell uses a series of active and passive transport systems to achieve homeostasis, and the exact system used

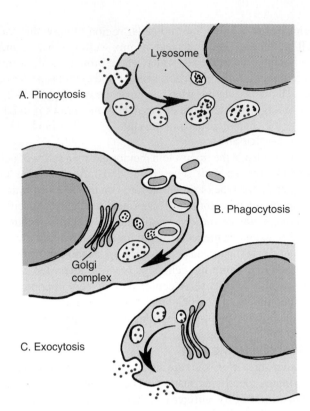

FIGURE 7–3. Schematic representation of endocytosis and exocytosis. Pinocytosis (**A**) is the movement of nutrients and needed substances into the cell through specific receptors on the cell surface. Phagocytosis (**B**) involves the destruction of engulfed proteins or bacteria. Exocytosis (**C**) is the movement of substances (waste products, hormones, neurotransmitters) out of the cell.

depends on the type of cell and its reactions with the immediate environment. For a cell to produce the energy needed to carry out cellular metabolism and other processes, the cell must have a means to obtain necessary elements from the outside environment. In addition, it must have a way to dispose of waste products that could be toxic to its cytoplasm. To accomplish this, the cell moves substances across the cell membrane, either by passive transport or by active (energy-requiring) transport (Figure 7–4).

Passive Transport

Passive transport happens without the expenditure of energy and can occur across any semipermeable membrane. There are essentially three types of passive transport: diffusion, osmosis, and facilitated diffusion.

Diffusion

Diffusion is the movement of a substance from a region of higher concentration to a region of lower concentration. The difference between the concentrations of the substance in the two regions is called the *concentration gradient* of the substance; usually, the greater the concentration gradient, the faster the substance moves. Movement into and out of a cell is regulated by the cell membrane. Some substances move through channels or pores in the cell membrane. Small substances and materials with no ionic charge move most freely

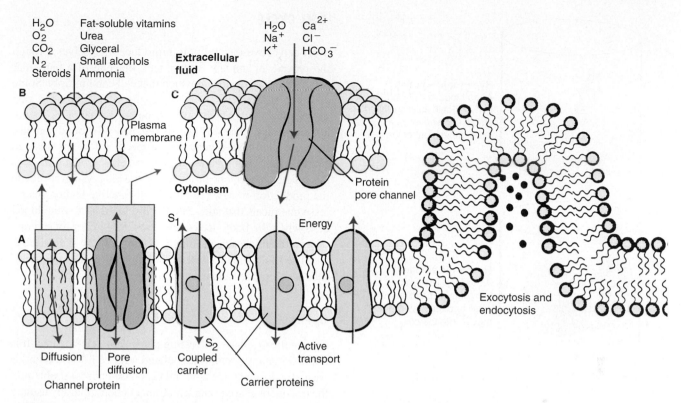

H₂O   Fat-soluble vitamins
O₂   Urea
CO₂   Glyceral
N₂   Small alcohols
Steroids Ammonia

FIGURE 7-4. Schematic representation of transport across a cell membrane **(A)**, which includes *diffusion* through the cell membrane **(B)** and *pore diffusion* through a protein channel **(C)**.

through the channels. Substances with a negative charge move more freely than substances with a positive charge. Substances that move into and out of a cell by diffusion include sodium, potassium, calcium, carbonate, oxygen, bicarbonate, and water.

When a cell is very active and is using energy and oxygen, the concentration of oxygen within the cell decreases. The concentration of oxygen outside the cell remains relatively high, so oxygen moves across the cell membrane (down the concentration gradient) to supply needed oxygen to the inside of the cell. Cells use this process to maintain homeostasis during many activities that occur in the life of a cell.

Osmosis

Osmosis, a special form of diffusion, is the movement of water across a semipermeable membrane from an area that is low in dissolved solutes to one that is high in dissolved solutes. The water is attempting to equalize the dilution of the solutes. This diffusion of water across a cell membrane from an area of high concentration (of water) to an area of low concentration creates pressure on the cell membrane, called *osmotic pressure.* The greater the concentration of solutes in the solution to which the water is flowing, the higher the osmotic pressure.

A fluid that contains the same concentration of solutes as human plasma is called an *isotonic* solution. A fluid that contains a higher concentration of solutes than human plasma is a *hypertonic* solution, and it draws water from cells. A fluid that contains a lower concentration of solutes than human plasma does is *hypotonic;* it loses water to cells. If a human red blood

cell, which has a cytoplasm that is isotonic with human plasma, is placed into a hypertonic solution, it shrinks and shrivels because the water inside the cell diffuses out of the cell into the solution. If the same cell is placed into a hypotonic solution, the cell swells and bursts because water moves from the solution into the cell (Figure 7–5).

Facilitated Diffusion

Sometimes a substance cannot move freely on its own in or out of a cell. Such a substance may attach to another molecule, called a carrier, to be diffused. This form of diffusion, known as *facilitated diffusion,* does not require energy, just the presence of the carrier. Carriers may be hormones, enzymes, or proteins. Because the carrier required for facilitated diffusion is usually present in a finite amount, this type of diffusion is limited.

Active Transport

Sometimes a cell requires a substance in greater concentration than found in the environment around it or needs to maintain its own cytoplasm in a situation that would normally allow chemicals to leave the cell. When this happens, the cell must move substances against the concentration gradient using active transport, which requires energy. When a cell is deprived of oxygen because of a blood supply problem or insufficient oxygenation of the blood, systems of active transport begin to malfunction, placing the cell's integrity in jeopardy.

One of the best known systems of active transport is the

Hypertonic solution
A red blood cell placed in hypertonic solution will shrink and shrivel up as water moves out of the cell.

Hypotonic solution
A red blood cell placed in hypotonic solution will swell and burst as water moves into the cell.

FIGURE 7–5. Red blood cell response to hypertonic and hypotonic solutions.

sodium–potassium pump. Cells use active transport to maintain a cytoplasm with a higher level of potassium and a lower level of sodium than the extracellular fluid contains. This allows the cell to maintain an electrical charge on the cell membrane, which gives many cells the electrical properties of excitation (the ability to generate a movement of electrons) and conduction (the ability to send this stimulus to other areas of the membrane). Some drugs use energy to move into cells by active transport. Drugs are frequently bonded with a carrier when they are moved into the cell. Cells in the kidney use active transport to excrete drugs from the body as well as to maintain electrolyte and acid–base balances.

CELL CYCLE

Most cells have the ability to reproduce themselves through the process of mitosis. The genetic makeup of a particular cell determines the rate at which that cell can multiply. Some cells reproduce very quickly (eg, the cells lining the gastrointestinal tract, which have a generation time of 72 hours), and some reproduce very slowly (eg, the cells found in breast tissue, which have a generation time of a few months). In some cases, certain factors influence cell reproduction. Erythropoietin, a hormone produced by the kidney, can stimulate the production of new red blood cells. Active leukocytes release chemicals that stimulate the production of white blood cells when the body needs new ones. Regardless of the rate of reproduction, each cell has approximately the same life cycle. The life cycle of a cell, called the **cell cycle,** consists of four active phases and a resting phase (Figure 7–6).

G_0 Phase

During the G_0 phase, or resting phase, the cell is stable. It is not making any proteins associated with cell division and is basically dormant. Cells in the G_0 phase cause a problem in the treatment of some cancers. Cancer chemotherapy usually works on active, dividing cells, leaving resting cells fairly untouched. When the resting cells are stimulated to become active and regenerate, the cancer can return, which is why cancer chemotherapeutic regimens are complicated and extended over time and why a 5-year cancer-free period is usually the basic guide for considering a cancer to be cured.

G_1 Phase

When a cell is stimulated to emerge from its resting phase, it enters what is called the G_1 phase, which lasts from the time of stimulation from the resting phase until the formation of DNA. During this period, the cell synthesizes the substances

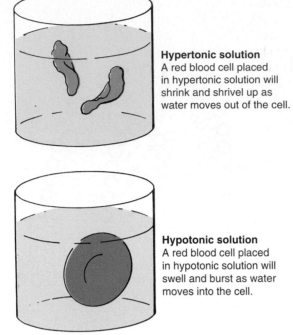

FIGURE 7–6. Diagram of the cell cycle, showing G_0, G_1, S, G_2, and M phases. (Adapted from Bullock, B. L. [2000]. *Focus on pathophysiology.* Philadelphia: Lippincott Williams & Wilkins.

that are needed for DNA formation. The cell is actively collecting materials to make these substances and producing the building blocks for DNA.

S Phase

The next phase, called the S phase, involves the actual synthesis of DNA, which is an energy-consuming activity. The cell remains in this phase until the amount of cellular DNA has doubled.

G₂ Phase

After the cellular DNA has doubled in preparation for replication, the G_2 phase begins. During this phase, the cell produces all the substances that are required for the manufacture of the mitotic spindles.

M Phase

After the cell has produced all the substances necessary for the formation of a new cell, or daughter cell, it undergoes cell division. This occurs during the M phase of the cell cycle. During this phase, the cell splits to form two identical daughter cells, a process called *mitosis*.

▢▮◖▮ WEB LINKS

Students may want to consult the following Internet sources:

Information on cell physiology, theories of cell formation, ongoing cellular research:
http://www.historyoftheuniverse.com/cell.html
Information on cell structure, properties, division:
http://www.life.uiuc.edu/plantbio/cell

CLINICAL SIGNIFICANCE OF CELL PHYSIOLOGY

Knowledge of the basic structure and function of the cell may help in understanding the therapeutic and toxic effects of the various classes of chemotherapeutic agents. Drugs may alter the cell membrane, causing the cell to rupture and die. Or they may deprive the cell of certain nutrients, altering the proteins that the cell produces and interfering with normal cell functioning and cell division. Because most chemotherapeutic agents do not possess complete selective toxicity, they also affect the normal cells of patients to some extent.

CHAPTER SUMMARY

- The cell is the basic structural unit of all living organisms.
- The cell is composed of a nucleus, which contains genetic material and controls the production of proteins by the cell; a cytoplasm, which contains various organelles important to cell function; and a cell membrane, which separates the inside of the cell from the outside environment.
- The cell membrane functions as a fluid barrier made of lipids and proteins. The arrangement of the lipoprotein membrane controls what enters and leaves the cell.
- Proteins on the cell membrane surface can act either as receptor sites for specific substances or as histocompatibility markers that identify the cell as a self-cell.
- Channels or pores in the cell membrane allow for easier movement of specific substances needed by the cell for normal functioning.
- Mitochondria are rod-shaped organelles that produce energy in the form of ATP for use by cells.
- Ribosomes are sites of protein production within the cell cytoplasm. The specific proteins produced by a cell are determined by the genetic material within the cell nucleus.
- The Golgi apparatus packages particular substances for removal from the cell (eg, neurotransmitters, hormones).
- Lysosomes are packets of digestive enzymes located in the cell cytoplasm. These enzymes are responsible for destroying injured or nonfunctioning parts of the cell and for cellular disintegration when the cell dies.
- Endocytosis is the process of moving substances into a cell by extending the cell membrane around the substance and engulfing it. Pinocytosis refers to the engulfing of necessary materials, and phagocytosis refers to the engulfing and destroying of bacteria or other proteins by white blood cells.
- Exocytosis is the process of removing substances from a cell by moving them toward the cell membrane and then changing the cell membrane to allow passage of the substance out of the cell.
- Cells maintain homeostasis by regulating the movement of solutes and water into and out of the cell.
- Diffusion, which does not require energy, is the movement of solutes from a region of high concentration to a region of lower concentration across a concentration gradient.
- Osmosis, which, like diffusion, does not require energy, is the movement of water from an area low in solutes to an area high in solutes. Osmosis exerts a pressure against the cell membrane that is called osmotic pressure.
- Active transport, an energy-requiring process, is the movement of particular substances against a concentration gradient. Active transport is important in maintaining cell homeostasis.
- Cells replicate at differing rates depending on the genetic programming of the cell. All cells go through a life cycle consisting of the following phases: G_0, the resting phase; G_1, which involves the production of proteins for DNA synthesis; S, which involves the synthesis of DNA; G_2, which involves manufacture of the materials needed for mitotic spindle production; and M, the mitotic phase, in which the cell splits to form two identical daughter cells.
- Chemotherapeutic drugs act on cells to cause cell death or alteration. All properties of the drug that affect cells should be considered when administering a chemotherapeutic agent.

Review Questions

1. The basic unit of human structure is
   a. the mitochondria.
   b. the nucleus.
   c. the nucleolus.
   d. the cell.
2. The cell membrane is composed of
   a. a phospholipid structure.
   b. channels of protein.
   c. a cholesterol-based membrane.
   d. Golgi apparati.
3. The saying, "One rotten apple can spoil the whole barrel," refers to the cell-degrading properties of
   a. calcium channels.
   b. lysosomes.
   c. histocompatibility receptors.
   d. nuclear spindles.
4. The ribosomes are important sites for
   a. digestion of nutrients.
   b. excretion of waste products.
   c. production of proteins.
   d. hormone receptors.
5. A human cell placed in salty sea water will
   a. burst from water entering the cell.
   b. shrivel and die from water leaving the cell.
   c. not be affected in any way.
   d. break apart from the salt effect.
6. The sodium–potassium pump maintains a negative charge on the cell membrane by
   a. osmosis.
   b. diffusion.
   c. active transport.
   d. facilitated diffusion.
7. All cells progress through basically the same cell cycle, including
   a. two phases.
   b. four active phases and a rest phase.
   c. three periods of rest and a splitting phase.
   d. four active phases.
8. The amount of time that a cell takes to progress through the cell cycle is determined by
   a. the acidity of the environment.
   b. the genetic makeup of the cell.
   c. the location of the cell in the body.
   d. the number of ribosomes in the cell.

BIBLIOGRAPHY

Bullock, B. S. (2000). *Focus on pathophysiology.* Philadelphia: Lippincott Williams & Wilkins.

Fox, S. (1991). *Perspectives on human biology.* Dubuque, IA: Wm. C. Brown Publishers.

Ganong, W. (1999). *Review of medical physiology* (19th ed.). Norwalk, CT: Appleton & Lange.

Guyton, A., & Hall, J. (1999). *Textbook of medical physiology.* Philadelphia: W. B. Saunders.

Gilman, A., Hardman, J. G., & Limbird, L. E. (Eds.) (2002). *Goodman and Gilman's the pharmacological basis of therapeutics* (10th ed.). New York: McGraw-Hill.

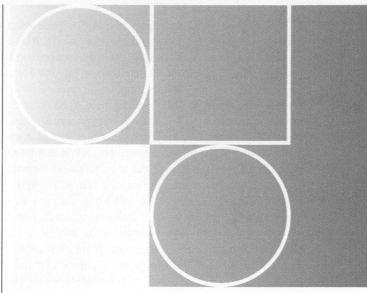

CHAPTER **8**

Anti-infective Agents

73

Key Terms

culture
prophylaxis
resistance
sensitivity testing
spectrum

bacitracin
chloramphenicol
meropenem

polymyxin B
spectinomycin
vancomycin

Anti-infective agents are drugs that are designed to act selectively on foreign organisms that have invaded and infected the body of a human host. Ideally, these drugs would be toxic to the infecting organisms only, and would have no effect on the host cells. In other words, they would possess *selective toxicity*—the ability to affect certain proteins or enzyme systems that are used by bacteria but not by human cells. Although human cells are different from the cells of invading organisms, they are somewhat similar, and no anti-infective drug has yet been developed that does not affect the host.

This chapter focuses on the principles involved in the use of anti-infective therapy. The following chapters discuss specific agents that are used to treat particular infections: antibiotics, which are used to treat bacterial infections; antivirals; antifungals; antiprotozoals, which are used to treat infections caused by specific protozoa, including malaria; anthelmintics, which are used to treat infections caused by worms; and antineoplastics, which are used to treat cancers, diseases caused by abnormal cells.

ANTI-INFECTIVE THERAPY

For centuries, people used various naturally occurring chemicals in an effort to treat disease. Often this was a random act that proved useful. For instance, the ancient Chinese found that applying moldy soybean curds to boils and infected wounds helped prevent infection or hastened cure. Their finding was, perhaps, a precursor to the penicillins used today.

The use of drugs to treat systemic infections is a relatively new concept. The first drugs used to treat systemic infections were developed in the 1920s. Paul Ehrlich was the first scientist to work on developing a synthetic chemical that would be effective only against infection-causing cells, not human cells. His research led the way for scientific investigation into anti-infective agents. In the late 1920s, scientists discovered penicillin in a mold sample; in 1935, the sulfonamides were introduced. Since then, the number of anti-infectives available for use has grown tremendously. However, many of the organisms that these drugs were designed to treat are rapidly learning to repel the effects of anti-infectives, so much work remains to deal with these emergent strains.

Mechanisms of Action

Anti-infective agents may act on the cells of the invading organisms in several different ways. The goal is interference with the normal function of the invading organism to prevent it from reproducing and to cause cell death without affecting host cells. Various mechanisms of action are briefly described here. The specific mechanism of action for each drug class is discussed in the chapters that follow.

• Some anti-infectives interfere with biosynthesis of the bacterial cell wall. Because bacterial cells have a slightly different composition than human cells, this is an effective way to destroy the bacteria without interfering with the host (Box 8–1). The penicillins work in this way.
• Some anti-infectives prevent the cells of the invading organism from using substances essential to their growth and development, leading to an inability to divide and eventually to cell death. The sulfonamides, the antimycobacterial drugs, and trimethoprim work in this way.
• Many anti-infectives interfere with the steps involved in protein synthesis, a necessary function to maintain the cell and allow for cell division. The aminoglycosides, the macrolides, and chloramphenicol work in this way.
• Some anti-infectives interfere with DNA synthesis in the cell, leading to inability to divide and cell death. The fluoroquinolones work this way.
• Other anti-infectives alter the permeability of the cell membrane to allow essential cellular components to leak out, causing cell death. Some antibiotics, antifungals, and antiprotozoal drugs work in this manner (Figure 8–1).

Anti-infective Activity

The anti-infectives that are used today vary in their effectiveness against invading organisms; that is, the **spectrum** of activity varies. Some are so selective in their action that they are effective against only a few microorganisms with a very specific metabolic pathway or enzyme. These drugs are said to have a narrow spectrum of activity (Box 8–2). Other drugs interfere with biochemical reactions in many different kinds of microorganisms, making them useful in the treatment of a wide variety of infections. Such drugs are said to have a broad spectrum of activity.

BOX 8-1
Anti-infective Mechanism: Interference With Cell Wall Synthesis

Bacitracin (*Baci-IM, AK-Tracin, Baciguent*) is an antibiotic that interferes with the cell wall synthesis of susceptible staphylococcal bacteria. Adverse effects include nephrotoxicity and superinfection. Because of the development of resistant strains and more potent antibiotics, bacitracin is now indicated only for the treatment of respiratory infections in infants caused by susceptible staphylococci, treatment of eye infections, prevention of infections in minor skin wounds, and treatment of minor skin infections caused by susceptible strains of staphylococci. Bacitracin is available in intramuscular, ophthalmic, and topical preparations.
    Usual dosage

Infants <2.5 kg: 900 U/kg per day IM in three divided doses
Infants >2.5 kg: 1,000 U/kg per day IM in two to three divided doses
Ophthalmic use: ½-inch ribbon to affected eye, b.i.d. to q3–4h
Topical use: apply to affected area one to five times per day

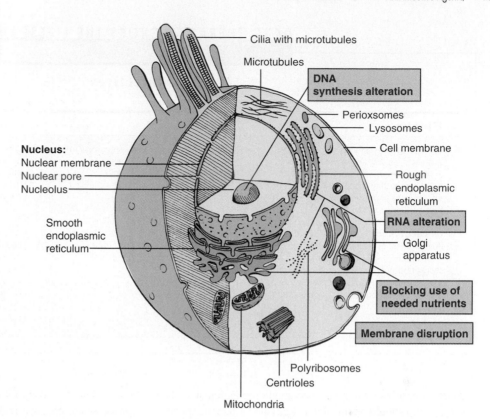

Cilia with microtubules
Microtubules
DNA synthesis alteration
Perioxsomes
Lysosomes
Cell membrane
Rough endoplasmic reticulum
RNA alteration
Golgi apparatus
Blocking use of needed nutrients
Membrane disruption
Nucleus:
Nuclear membrane
Nuclear pore
Nucleolus
Smooth endoplasmic reticulum
Polyribosomes
Centrioles
Mitochondria

FIGURE 8-1. Anti-infectives can affect cells by disrupting the cell membrane, interfering with DNA synthesis, altering RNA, or blocking the use of essential nutrients.

Some anti-infectives are so active against the infective microorganisms that they actually cause the death of the cells they affect. These drugs are said to be bactericidal. Some anti-infectives are not as aggressive against invading organisms; they interfere with the ability of the cells to reproduce or divide. These drugs are said to be bacteriostatic. Several drugs are both bactericidal and bacteriostatic, often depending on the concentration of the drug that is present. Many of the adverse effects noted with the use of anti-infectives are associated with the aggressive properties of the drugs and their effect on the cells of the host as well as those of the pathogen.

Human Immune Response

The goal of anti-infective therapy is reduction of the population of the invading organism to a point at which the human immune response can take care of the infection. If a drug were aggressive enough to eliminate all traces of any invading pathogen, it might be toxic to the host as well. The immune response (see Chapter 15) involves a complex interaction among chemical mediators, leukocytes, lymphocytes, antibodies, and locally released enzymes and chemicals. When this response is completely functional and all of the necessary proteins, cells, and chemicals are being produced by the body, it can isolate and eliminate foreign proteins, including bacteria, fungi, and viruses. However, if a person is immunocompromised for any reason (eg, malnutrition, age, acquired immune deficiency syndrome [AIDS], use of immunosuppressant drugs), the immune system may be incapable of dealing effectively with the invading organisms. It is difficult to treat any infections in such patients for two reasons: (1) anti-infective drugs cannot totally eliminate the pathogen without causing severe toxicity in the host, and (2) these patients do not have the immune response in place to deal with even a few invading organisms. Immunocompromised patients present a real challenge to health care providers. In helping these people cope with infections, prevention of infection and proper nutrition are often as important as drug therapy.

BOX 8-2
Narrow-Spectrum Antibiotic

Spectinomycin (*Trobicin*) is an example of an antibiotic with very specific effects. This drug interferes with protein synthesis, leading to cell death, only in susceptible strains of *Neisseria gonorrhoeae*. Spectinomycin is not known to be effective against any other bacterial species, and its use is limited to the treatment of specific gonococcal infections. The drug is given as one 2-g IM injection, which may be increased to a 4-g IM injection in areas where bacterial resistance is prevalent.

Resistance

Because anti-infectives act on specific enzyme systems or biological processes, many microorganisms that do not use that system or process are not affected by a particular anti-infective drug. These organisms are said to have a natural or intrinsic **resistance** to that drug. When prescribing a drug for treatment of

DRUG THERAPY ACROSS THE LIFESPAN

Anti-infectives

Children	Adults	Older Adults
Use anti-infectives with caution; early exposure can lead to early sensitivity. Controversy is widespread regarding the use of antibiotics to treat ear infections, a common pediatric problem. Some believe that the habitual use of antibiotics for what might well be a viral infection has contributed greatly to the development of resistant strains. Children can have increased susceptibility to the gastrointestinal and nervous system effects of anti-infectives; monitor hydration and nutritional status carefully.	Adults often demand anti-infectives for a "quick cure" of various signs and symptoms. Drug allergies and the emergence of resistant strains can be a big problem with this group. Pregnant and nursing women must use extreme caution in the use of anti-infectives. Many of them can affect the unborn baby and also cross into breast milk, leading to toxic effects in the neonate.	Older patients often do not present with the same signs and symptoms of infection that are seen in younger people. Culture and sensitivity tests are important to determine the type and extent of many infections. The older patient is susceptible to severe adverse gastrointestinal, renal, and neurological effects and must be monitored for nutritional status and hydration during drug therapy. Anti-infectives that adversely affect the liver and kidneys must be used with caution in older patients, who may have decreased organ function.

an infection, this innate resistance should be anticipated. The selected drug should be one that is known to affect the specific microorganism that is causing the infection.

Since the advent of anti-infective drugs, microorganisms that were once very sensitive to the effects of particular drugs have begun to develop acquired resistance to the agents (Box 8–3). This can result in a serious clinical problem. The emergence of resistant strains of bacteria and other organisms poses a threat: anti-infective drugs may no longer control potentially life-threatening diseases, and uncontrollable epidemics may occur.

Acquiring Resistance

Microorganisms develop resistance in a number of ways, including the following:

- Producing an enzyme that deactivates the antimicrobial drug. For example, some strains of bacteria that were once controlled by penicillin now produce an enzyme called penicillinase, which inactivates penicillin before it can affect the bacteria. This occurrence led to the development of new drugs that are resistant to penicillinase.
- Changing cellular permeability to prevent the drug from entering the cell, or altering transport systems to exclude the drug from active transport into the cell.
- Altering binding sites on the membranes or ribosomes, which then no longer accept the drug.
- Producing a chemical that acts as an antagonist to the drug.

Most commonly, the development of resistance depends on the degree to which the drug acts to eliminate the invading microorganisms that are most sensitive to its effects. The cells that remain may be somewhat resistant to the effects of the drug, and, over time, these cells form the majority in the population. These cells differ from the general population of

the species because of slight variations in their biochemical processes or biochemicals. The drug does not cause a mutation of these cells; it simply allows the somewhat different

---

BOX 8-3

Bacterial Resistance to an Anti-infective Drug

Vancomycin (*Vancocin, Vancoled*) is an antibiotic that interferes with cell wall synthesis in susceptible bacteria. It was developed in response to the need for a drug that could be used both for patients who are intolerant to or allergic to penicillin and/or cephalosporins and for patients with staphylococcal infections that no longer respond to penicillin or cephalosporins.

This anti-infective drug can be used orally or intravenously to treat life-threatening infections when less toxic drugs cannot be used. It is used orally as prophylaxis against bacterial endocarditis in patients who cannot take penicillins or cephalosporins and to treat staphylococcal infections in people who do not respond to either of these groups of drugs.

Because vancomycin can be highly toxic, its use is reserved for very special situations. It can cause renal failure, ototoxicity, superinfections, and a condition known as "red man syndrome," which is characterized by sudden and severe hypotension, fever, chills, paresthesias, and erythema or redness of the neck and back. When it is the only antibiotic that is effective against a specific bacteria, however, the benefits outweigh the risks.

Usual dosage:

Adult: 500 mg to 1 g PO or IV q6h for 7–10 d
Pediatric: 40 mg/kg per day PO or IV in four divided doses; do not exceed 2 g/d

cells to become the majority or dominant group after elimination of the sensitive cells. Other microbes may develop resistance through actual genetic mutation. A mutant cell survives the effects of an antibiotic and divides, forming a new colony of resistant microbes with a genetic composition that provides resistance to the anti-infective agent.

Preventing Resistance

Because the emergence of resistant strains of microbes is a serious public health problem that continues to grow, health care providers must work together to prevent the emergence of resistant pathogens. Exposure to an antimicrobial agent leads to the development of resistance, so it is important to limit the use of antimicrobial agents to the treatment of specific pathogens known to be sensitive to the drug being used.

Drug dosage is important in preventing the development of resistance. Doses should be high enough, and the duration of drug therapy should be long enough, to eradicate even slightly resistant microorganisms. The recommended dosage for a specific anti-infective agent takes this issue into account. Around-the-clock dosing eliminates the peaks and valleys in drug concentration and helps maintain a constant therapeutic level to prevent the emergence of resistant microbes during times of low concentration. The duration of drug use is critical to ensure that the microbes are completely, not partially, eliminated and are not given the chance to grow and develop resistant strains.

It has proved to be difficult to convince people who are taking anti-infective drugs that the timing of doses and the length of time they continue to take the drug are important. Many people stop taking a drug once they start to feel better and then keep the remaining pills to treat themselves at some time in the future when they do not feel well. This practice favors the emergence of resistant strains.

Health care providers should also be cautious about the indiscriminate use of anti-infectives. Antibiotics are not effective in the treatment of viral infections or illnesses such as the common cold. However, many patients demand prescriptions for these drugs when they visit practitioners because they are convinced that they need to take something to feel better. Health care providers who prescribe anti-infectives without knowing the causative organism and which drugs might be appropriate are promoting the emergence of resistant strains of microbes. With many serious illnesses, including pneumonias, for which the causative organism is suspected, antibiotic therapy may be started as soon as a culture is taken and before the results are known. Health care providers also tend to try newly introduced, more powerful drugs when a more established drug may be just as effective. Use of a powerful drug in this way leads to the rapid emergence of resistant strains to that drug, perhaps limiting its potential usefulness when it might be truly necessary.

TREATMENT OF SYSTEMIC INFECTIONS

Many infections that once led to lengthy, organ-damaging, or even fatal illnesses are now managed quickly and effi-ciently with the use of systemic anti-infective agents. Before the introduction of penicillin to treat streptococcal infections, many people developed rheumatic fever with serious cardiac complications. Today, rheumatic fever and the resultant cardiac valve defects are seldom seen. Several factors should be considered before beginning one of these chemotherapeutic regimens to ensure that the patient obtains the greatest benefit possible with the fewest adverse effects. These factors include identification of the correct pathogen and selection of a drug that is most likely to (1) cause the least complications for that particular patient and (2) be most effective against the pathogen involved.

Identification of the Pathogen

Identification of the infecting pathogen is done by **culture** of a tissue sample from the infected area. Bacterial cultures are performed in a laboratory, where a swab of infected tissue is allowed to grow on an agar plate. Staining techniques and microscopic examination are used to identify the offending bacterium. When investigators search for parasitic sources of infection, stool can be examined for ova and parasites. Microscopic examination of other samples is also used to detect fungal and protozoal infections. The correct identification of the organism causing the infection is an important first step in determining which anti-infective drug should be used.

Sensitivity of the Pathogen

In many situations, health care providers use a broad-spectrum anti-infective agent that has been shown likely to be most effective in treating an infection with certain presenting signs and symptoms. In other cases of severe infection, a broad-spectrum antibiotic is started after a culture is taken but before the exact causative organism has been identified. Again, experience influences selection of the drug, based on the presenting signs and symptoms. In many cases, it is necessary to perform **sensitivity testing** on the cultured microbes. Sensitivity testing shows which drugs are capable of controlling the particular microorganism. This testing is especially important with microorganisms that have known resistant strains. In these cases, culture and sensitivity testing identify the causal pathogen and the most appropriate drug for treating the infection.

Combination Therapy

In some situations, a combination of two or more types of drugs effectively treats the infection. When the offending pathogen is known, combination drugs may be effective in interfering with its cellular structure in different areas or developmental phases. Combination therapy may be used for several reasons:

- Combination therapy may allow the health care provider to use a smaller dosage of each drug, leading to fewer adverse effects but still having a therapeutic impact on the pathogen.

- Some drugs are synergistic, which means that they are more powerful when given in combination.
- Many microbial infections are caused by more than one organism, and each pathogen may react to a different anti-infective agent.
- Sometimes, the combined effects of the different drugs delay the emergence of resistant strains. This is important in the treatment of tuberculosis (a mycobacterial infection), malaria (a protozoal infection), and some bacterial infections. However, resistant strains seem more likely to emerge when fixed combinations are used over time, at least in some cases. Individualizing the combination seems to be more effective in destroying the pathogen without allowing time for the emergence of strains that are resistant to the drugs.

ADVERSE REACTIONS TO ANTI-INFECTIVE THERAPY

Because anti-infective agents affect cells, it is always possible that the host cells will also be damaged (Box 8–4). No anti-infective agent has been developed that is completely free of adverse effects. The most commonly encountered adverse effects associated with the use of anti-infective agents are direct toxic effects on the kidney, gastrointestinal (GI) tract, and nervous system. Hypersensitivity reactions and superinfections also can occur.

Kidney Damage

Kidney damage occurs most frequently with drugs that are metabolized by the kidney and then eliminated in the urine.

Such drugs, which have a direct toxic effect on the fragile cells in the kidney, can cause conditions ranging from renal dysfunction to full-blown renal failure. When patients are taking these drugs (eg, aminoglycosides), they should be monitored closely for any sign of renal dysfunction. To prevent any accumulation of the drug in the kidney, patients should also be well hydrated throughout the course of the drug therapy.

Gastrointestinal Toxicity

GI toxicity is very common with many of the anti-infectives. Many of these agents have direct toxic effects on the cells lining the GI tract, causing nausea, vomiting, stomach upset, or diarrhea, and such effects are sometimes severe (Box 8–5). There is also some evidence that the death of the microorganisms releases chemicals and toxins into the body, which can stimulate the chemoreceptor trigger zone (CTZ) in the medulla and induce nausea and vomiting.

In addition, some anti-infectives are toxic to the liver. These drugs can cause hepatitis and even liver failure. When patients are taking drugs known to be toxic to the liver (eg, many of the cephalosporins), they should be monitored closely and the drug should be stopped at any sign of liver dysfunction.

Neurotoxicity

Some anti-infectives can damage or interfere with the function of nerve tissue, usually in areas where drugs tend to accumulate in high concentrations (Box 8–6). For example, the aminoglycoside antibiotics collect in the eighth cranial nerve and can cause dizziness, vertigo, and loss of hearing. Chloro-

---

BOX 8-4
Serious Adverse Effects of Antibiotic Treatment

Chloramphenicol (*Chloromycetin*), an older antibiotic, prevents bacterial cell division in susceptible bacteria. Because of the potential toxic effects of this drug, its use is limited to serious infections for which no other antibiotic is effective. Chloramphenicol produces a "gray syndrome" in neonates and premature babies, which is characterized by abdominal distention, pallid cyanosis, vasomotor collapse, irregular respirations, and even death. In addition, the drug can cause bone marrow depression, including aplastic anemia, which may result in death. These effects are seen even with the use of the ophthalmic and otic forms of the drug. Although the use of chloramphenicol is severely limited, it has stayed on the market because it is needed to treat serious infections caused by bacteria that are not sensitive to any other antibiotic. It is available in oral, intravenous, ophthalmic, and otic forms.
    Usual dosage

Adult or pediatric: 50 mg/kg per day PO or IV in divided doses
Ophthalmic: instill ointment or solution as prescribed
Otic: 2–3 gtt into affected ear t.i.d.

BOX 8-5
Severe Gastrointestinal Toxicity Resulting From Anti-infective Treatment

Meropenem (*Merrem IV*), an intravenous antibiotic, inhibits the synthesis of bacterial cell walls in susceptible bacteria. It is used to treat intra-abdominal infections and some cases of meningitis caused by susceptible bacteria. Meropenem almost always causes very uncomfortable gastrointestinal effects; in fact, use of this drug has been associated with potentially fatal pseudomembranous colitis. It also results in headache, dizziness, rash, and superinfections. Because of its toxic effects on gastrointestinal cells, it is used only to treat those infections with proven sensitivity to meropenem and reduced sensitivity to less toxic antibiotics.
    Usual dosage

Adult: 1 g IV q8h
Pediatric < 3 mo: not recommended
Pediatric >3 mo: 20–40 mg/kg IV q8h (if >50 kg, 1–2 g IV q8h)
Geriatric: lower dose in accordance with creatinine clearance level

<table>
</table>

BOX 8-6

Nerve Damage Caused by an Anti-infective Agent

Polymyxin B (generic), an older antibiotic, uses a surfactant-like reaction to enter the bacterial cell membrane and disrupt it, leading to cell death in susceptible gram-negative bacteria. This drug is available for intramuscular, intravenous, or intrathecal use and an ophthalmic agent for the treatment of infections caused by susceptible bacteria. Because of the actions of polymyxin B on cell membranes, it can be toxic to the human host, leading to nephrotoxicity, neurotoxicity (facial flushing, dizziness, ataxia, paresthesias, and drowsiness), and drug fever and rashes. Therefore, it is reserved for use in acute situations in which the invading bacteria have been proven to be sensitive to polymixin B and less sensitive to other, less toxic antibiotics.

Usual dosage

Adult and pediatric: 15,0000–25,000 U/kg per day IV (may be divided into two doses) *or*
25,000–30,000 U/kg per day IM divided into four to six doses *or*
50,000 U intrathecal q.d. for 3–4 d, then every other day for at least 2 wk

quine, which is used to treat malaria and some other rheumatoid disorders, can accumulate in the retina and optic nerve and cause blindness. Other anti-infectives can cause dizziness, drowsiness, lethargy, changes in reflexes, and even hallucinations when they irritate specific nerve tissues.

Hypersensitivity Reactions

Allergic or hypersensitivity reactions reportedly occur with many antimicrobial agents. Most of these agents, which are protein bound for transfer through the cardiovascular system, are able to induce antibody formation in susceptible people. With the next exposure to the drug, immediate or delayed allergic responses may occur. Some of these drugs have demonstrated cross-sensitivity (eg, penicillins, cephalosporins), and care must be taken to obtain a complete patient history before administering one of these drugs. It is important to determine what the allergic reaction was and when the patient experienced it (eg, after first use of drug, after years of use). Some patients report having a drug allergy, but closer investigation indicates that their reaction actually constituted an anticipated effect or a known adverse effect to the drug. Proper interpretation of this information is important to allow treatment of a patient with a drug to which the patient reported a supposed allergic reaction but which would be very effective against a known pathogen.

Superinfections

One offshoot of the use of anti-infectives, especially broad-spectrum anti-infectives, is destruction of the normal flora.

When the normal flora is destroyed, opportunistic pathogens that were kept in check by the "normal" bacteria have the opportunity to invade tissues and cause infections. These opportunistic infections are called *superinfections*. Common superinfections include vaginal or GI yeast infections, which are associated with antibiotic therapy, and infections caused by *Proteus* and *Pseudomonas* throughout the body, which are a result of broad-spectrum antibiotic use. If patients receive drugs that are known to induce superinfections, they should be monitored closely and the appropriate treatment for any superinfection should be started as soon as possible.

PROPHYLAXIS

Sometimes it is clinically useful to use anti-infectives as a means of **prophylaxis,** to prevent infections before they occur. For example, when patients anticipate traveling to an area where malaria is endemic, they may begin taking antimalarial drugs before the journey and periodically during the trip. Patients who are undergoing GI or genitourinary surgery, which might introduce bacteria from those areas into the system, often have antibiotics ordered immediately after the surgery and periodically thereafter, as appropriate, to prevent infection. Patients with known cardiac valve disease, valve replacements, and other conditions are especially prone to the development of subacute bacterial endocarditis because of the vulnerability of their heart valves. These patients use prophylactic antibiotic therapy as a precaution when undergoing invasive procedures, including dental work. Refer to the American Heart Association's recommended schedule for this prophylaxis.

CHAPTER SUMMARY

- Anti-infectives are drugs designed to act on foreign organisms that have invaded and infected the human host with selective toxicity, which means that they affect biological systems or structures that are found in the invading organisms but not in the host.
- The goal of anti-infective therapy is interference with the normal function of invading organisms to prevent them from reproducing and promotion of cell death without negative affects on the host cells. The infection should be eradicated with the least toxicity to the host and the least likelihood for development of resistance.
- Anti-infectives can work by altering the cell membrane of the pathogen, by interfering with protein synthesis, or by interfering with the ability of the pathogen to obtain needed nutrients.
- Anti-infectives also work to kill invading organisms or to prevent them from reproducing, thus depleting the size of the invasion to one that can be dealt with by the human immune system.
- Pathogens can develop resistance to the effects of anti-infectives over time when (1) mutant organisms that do not respond to the anti-infective become the majority of the

pathogen population or (2) the pathogen develops enzymes to block the anti-infectives or alternative routes to obtain nutrients or maintain the cell membrane.

- An important aspect of clinical care involving anti-infective agents is preventing or delaying the development of resistance. This can be done by ensuring that the particular anti-infective agent is the drug of choice for the specific pathogen involved and that it is given in high enough doses for sufficiently long periods to rid the body of the pathogen.

- Culture and sensitivity testing of a suspected infection ensures that the correct drug is being used to treat the infection effectively. Culture and sensitivity testing should be performed before an anti-infective agent is prescribed.

- Anti-infectives can have several adverse effects on the human host, including renal toxicity, multiple GI effects, neurotoxicity, hypersensitivity reactions, and superinfections.

- Some anti-infectives are used as a means of prophylaxis when patients expect to be in situations that will expose them to a known pathogen, such as travel to an area where malaria is endemic, or oral or invasive GI surgery in a person who is susceptible to subacute bacterial endocarditis.

Review Questions

1. Spectrum of activity of an anti-infective indicates
   a. the acidity of the environment in which they are most effective.
   b. the cell membrane type that the anti-infective affects.
   c. the anti-infective's effectiveness against different invading organisms.
   d. the resistance factor that bacteria have developed to this anti-infective.

2. Bacterial resistance to an anti-infective is not the result of
   a. natural or intrinsic properties of the bacteria.
   b. changes in cellular permeability or cellular transport systems.
   c. the production of chemicals that antagonize the drug.
   d. initial exposure to the anti-infective.

3. The emergence of resistant strains of microbes is a serious public health problem. Health care providers can work to prevent the emergence of resistant strains by
   a. encouraging the patient to stop the antibiotic as soon as the symptoms are resolved, to prevent overexposure to the drug.
   b. encouraging the use of antibiotics when patients feel they will help.
   c. limiting the use of antimicrobial agents to the treatment of specific pathogens known to be sensitive to the drug being used.
   d. using the most powerful drug available to treat an infection, to ensure eradication of the microbe.

4. Sensitivity testing of a culture shows
   a. the drugs that are capable of controlling that particular microorganism.
   b. the patient's potential for allergic reactions to a drug.
   c. the offending microorganism.
   d. an immune reaction to the infecting organism.

5. GI toxicity is a very common adverse effect seen with anti-infective therapy. A patient experiencing GI toxicity might complain of
   a. elevated blood urea nitrogen (BUN).
   b. difficulty breathing.
   c. nausea, vomiting, or diarrhea.
   d. yellowish skin or sclera.

6. Superinfections can occur when anti-infective agents destroy the normal flora of the body. *Candida* infections are commonly associated with antibiotic use. A patient with this type of superinfection would exhibit
   a. difficulty breathing.
   b. vaginal discharge or white patches in the mouth.
   c. elevated BUN.
   d. dark lesions on the skin.

7. An example of an anti-infective used as a means of prophylaxis would be
   a. amoxicillin used to treat tonsillitis.
   b. penicillin used to treat an abscess.
   c. an antibiotic used before dental surgery.
   d. norfloxacin used to treat a bladder infection.

8. An important characteristic of any anti-infective drug is
   a. a broad spectrum of activity.
   b. a narrow spectrum of activity.
   c. resistance.
   d. selective toxicity.

BIBLIOGRAPHY

Cohen, F. L., & Tartasky, D. (1997). Microbial resistance to drug therapy: a review. *American Journal of Infection Control, 25*(1), 51–64.

Degnan, R. (1997). Pharmacology in practice: Antibiotics. *RN, 60*(10), 49–55.

Drug facts and comparisons. (2002). St. Louis: Facts and Comparisons.

Gilman, A., Hardman, J. G., & Limbird, L. E. (Eds.) (2002). *Goodman and Gilman's the pharmacological basis of therapeutics* (10th ed.). New York: McGraw-Hill.

Karch, A. M. (2002). *2003 Lippincott's nursing drug guide.* Philadelphia: Lippincott Williams & Wilkins.

Porth, C. M. (2001). *Pathophysiology: Concepts of altered health states* (5th ed.). Philadelphia: Lippincott Williams & Wilkins.

The medical letter on drugs and therapeutics. (2002). New Rochelle, NY: Medical Letter.

CHAPTER **9**

Antibiotics

Key Terms
aerobic
anaerobic
antibiotic
bactericidal
bacteriostatic
gram negative
gram positive
synergy

81

Aminoglycosides
amikacin
Ⓟ gentamicin
kanamycin
neomycin
netilmicin
streptomycin
tobramycin

Cephalosporins
Ⓟ cefaclor
cefadroxil
cefazolin
cefdinir

cefepime
cefixime
cefmetazole
cefonicid
cefoperazone
cefotaxime
cefotetan
cefoxitin
cefpodoxime
cefprozil
ceftazidime
ceftibuten
ceftizoxime

ceftriaxone
cefuroxime
cephalexin
cephapirin
cephradine
loracarbef

Fluoroquinolones
Ⓟ ciprofloxacin
gatifloxacin
levofloxacin
lomefloxacin
moxifloxacin
norfloxacin

ofloxacin
sparfloxacin
trovafloxacin
Macrolides
azithromycin
clarithromycin
dirithromycin
(P) erythromycin
Lincosamides
(P) clindamycin
lincomycin
Monobactam Antibiotics
aztreonam
Penicillins
(P) amoxicillin
ampicillin

carbenicillin
mezlocillin
penicillin G benzathine
penicillin G potassium
penicillin G procaine
penicillin V
piperacillin
ticarcillin
Penicillinase-resistant Antibiotics
(P) cloxacillin
dicloxacillin
nafcillin
oxacillin
Sulfonamides
sulfadiazine
sulfisoxazole
(P) sulfasalazine

Tetracyclines
demeclocycline
doxycycline
minocycline
oxytetracycline
(P) tetracycline
Antimycobacterial Antibiotics
Antituberculosis Drugs
capreomycin
cycloserine
ethambutol
ethionamide
(P) isoniazid
pyrazinamide
rifabutin
rifampin
rifapentine
Leprostatic Drugs
clofazimine
(P) dapsone

Antibiotics are chemicals that inhibit specific bacteria. Those substances that prevent the growth of bacteria are said to be **bacteriostatic,** and those that kill bacteria directly are said to be **bactericidal.** Several antibiotics are both bactericidal and bacteriostatic, depending on the concentration of the particular drug. Antibiotics are used to treat a wide variety of systemic and topical infections. Many new infections appear each year, and researchers are challenged to develop new antibiotics to deal with each new threat. Antibiotics are made in three ways: by living microorganisms, by synthetic manufacture, and in some cases, through genetic engineering. Discussed in this chapter are the major classes of antibiotics: aminoglycosides, cephalosporins, fluoroquinolones, lincosamides, macrolides, monobactams, penicillins and penicillinase-resistant drugs, sulfonamides, tetracyclines, and the disease-specific antimycobacterials, including the antituberculosis and leprostatic drugs.

BACTERIA AND ANTIBIOTICS

Bacteria can invade the human body through many routes: respiratory, gastrointestinal (GI), skin, and so on. Once bacteria invade the body, the body becomes the host for the bacteria, supplying nutrients and enzymes that the bacteria need for reproduction. Unchallenged, the invading bacteria can multiply and send out other bacteria to further invade tissue.

The human immune response is activated when bacteria invade. Many of the signs and symptoms of an infection are related to the immune response to the invader as the body tries to rid itself of the foreign cells. Fever, lethargy, slow-wave sleep induction, and the classic signs of inflammation (ie, redness, swelling, heat, and pain) all indicate that the body is responding to an invader.

The goal of antibiotic therapy is to decrease the population of the invading bacteria to a point at which the human immune system can effectively deal with the invader. To determine which antibiotic will effectively treat a specific infection, the causative organism must be identified. Culture and sensitivity testing is performed to identify the invading bacterial species by growing it in the laboratory and then determining the antibiotic to which that particular organism is most sensitive (ie, which antibiotic best kills or controls the bacteria). Antibiotics have been developed to interfere with specific proteins or enzyme systems, so they are effective only against bacteria that use those proteins or enzymes.

Gram-positive bacteria are those whose cell wall retains a stain, known as Gram's stain, or resists decolorization with alcohol during culture and sensitivity testing. Gram-positive bacteria are commonly associated with infections of the respiratory tract and soft tissues. An example of a gram-positive bacterium is *Streptococcus pneumoniae,* a common cause of pneumonia. In contrast, **gram-negative** bacteria are those whose cell walls lose a stain or are decolorized by alcohol. These bacteria are frequently associated with infections of the genitourinary (GU) or GI tract. An example of a gram-negative bacterium is *Escherichia coli,* a common cause of cystitis. **Aerobic** bacteria depend on oxygen for survival, whereas **anaerobic** bacteria (eg, those bacteria associated with gangrene) do not use oxygen.

If culture and sensitivity testing is not possible, either because the source of the infection is not identifiable or because the patient is too sick to wait for treatment, clinicians attempt to administer a drug with a broad spectrum of activity against gram-positive or gram-negative bacteria or against anaerobic bacteria. Antibiotics that interfere with a biochemical reaction common to many organisms are known as broad-spectrum antibiotics. These drugs are often given at the beginning of treatment until the exact organism and sensitivity can be established. Because these antibiotics have such a wide range of effects, they are frequently associated with adverse effects. Human cells have many of the same properties as bacterial cells and can be affected in much the same way, so damage may occur to the human cells as well as the bacterial cells.

In choosing an antibiotic, clinicians also look for a drug with selective toxicity, or the ability to strike foreign cells with little or no effect on human cells. There is no perfect antibiotic that is without effect on the human host, and this factor should be considered in antibiotic selection. Because various antibiotics have anticipated adverse effects, they may be contraindicated in some patients, such as those who are immunocompromised, have severe GI disease, or are debilitated. The antibiotic of choice is one that affects the causative organism and leads to the fewest adverse effects for the patient involved.

DRUG THERAPY ACROSS THE LIFESPAN

Antibiotics

Children

Children are very sensitive to the gastrointestinal and central nervous system (CNS) effects of most antibiotics, and more severe reactions can be expected when these drugs are used in children. It is important to monitor the hydration and nutritional status of children who are adversely affected by drug-induced diarrhea, anorexia, nausea, and vomiting. Superinfections can be a problem for small children as well. For example, thrush (oral candidiasis) is a common superinfection that makes eating and drinking difficult.

Many antibiotics do not have proven safety and efficacy in pediatric use, and extreme caution should be used when giving them to children. The fluoroquinolones, for instance, are associated with damage to developing cartilage and are not recommended for growing children.

Pediatric dosages of antibiotics should be double-checked to make sure that the child is receiving the correct dose, thereby improving the chance of eradicating the infection and decreasing the risk of adverse effects.

Antibiotic treatment of ear infections, a common pediatric problem, is controversial. Ongoing research suggests that judicious use of decongestants and anti-inflammatories may be just as successful as the use of antibiotics without the risk of development of resistant bacterial strains.

Parents, not wanting to see their child sick, may demand antibiotics as a cure-all whenever their child is fussy or feverish. Parent education is very important in helping to cut down the unnecessary use of antibiotics in children.

Adults

Adults are of a generation that believes that antibiotics are a cure-all for any discomfort and fever. It is very important to educate adults that antibiotics are useful only against specific bacteria and can actually cause problems when used unnecessarily for viral infections, such as the common cold.

Adults need to be cautioned to take the entire course of the medication; not to store up unused pills for future infections; and not to share antibiotics with symptomatic friends.

Pregnant and nursing women should not take antibiotics unless the benefit clearly outweighs the potential risk to the fetus or neonate. Tetracyclines, for example, are associated with pitting of enamel in developing teeth and of calcium deposits in growing bones. These drugs can cause serious problems for neonates. Women of child-bearing age should be advised to use barrier contraceptives if any of these drugs are used.

Many antibiotics interfere with the effectiveness of oral contraceptives, and unplanned pregnancies can occur.

Older Adults

In many instances, older adults do not present with the same signs and symptoms of infections as other patients. Therefore, assessing the problem and obtaining appropriate specimens for culture is especially important with this population.

Older patients may be more susceptible to the adverse effects associated with antibiotic therapy. Their hydration and nutritional status should be monitored closely, as should the need for safety precautions if CNS effects occur. If hepatic or renal dysfunction is expected (particularly in very old patients, those who may depend on alcohol, and those who are taking other hepatotoxic or nephrotoxic drugs), the dosage may need to be lowered and the patient should be monitored more frequently.

Elderly patients also need to be cautioned to complete the full course of drug therapy, even when they feel better, and not to save pills for self-medication at a future time.

In some cases, antibiotics are given in combination to promote **synergy,** so that their combined effect is greater than their effect if they are given individually. Use of synergistic antibiotics allows the patient to take a lower dose of each antibiotic to achieve the desired effect. Another possible benefit of combined therapy is that a lower dose of one of the antibiotics can be used, which helps reduce the adverse effects of that particular drug and makes it more useful in certain clinical situations. Or, one drug may "help" another become more effective (Box 9–1).

In some situations, antibiotics are used as a means of *prophylaxis,* or prevention of potential infection. Patients who will soon be in a situation that commonly results in a specific infection (eg, patients undergoing GI surgical procedures, which may introduce GI bacteria into the bloodstream or peritoneum) may be given antibiotics before they are exposed to the bacteria. Usually a large, one-time dose of an antibiotic is given to destroy any bacteria that enter the host immediately and thereby prevent a serious infection.

BACTERIA AND RESISTANCE TO ANTIBIOTICS

Bacteria have survived for hundreds of years because they can adapt to their environment. They do this by altering their cell wall or enzyme systems to become resistant to (ie, protect themselves from) unfavorable conditions or situations. Many species of bacteria have developed resistance to certain antibiotics. For example, bacteria that were once very sensitive to penicillin have developed an enzyme called penicillinase, which effectively inactivates many of the penicillin-type drugs. New drugs had to be developed to treat infections involving these once-controlled bacteria effectively. Because these newer drugs are resistant to penicillinase, they can no longer be inactivated by the bacteria. Other drugs have been developed specifically to treat resistant infections. It is very important to use these drugs only when the identity and sensitivity of the offending bacterium have been established. Indiscriminate use of these new drugs can lead to the development of more resistant strains for which there is no effective antibiotic (Box 9–2).

The longer an antibiotic has been in use, the greater the chance of development of a resistant strain. Efforts to control the emergence of resistant strains involve intensive education programs that advocate the use of antibiotics only when necessary and effective, and not for treatment of viral infections such as the common cold.

In addition, the use of antibiotics may result in the development of superinfections or overgrowth of resistant pathogens such as bacteria, fungi, or yeasts, because antibiotics (particularly broad-spectrum agents) destroy bacteria in the flora that normally work to keep these opportunistic invaders in check. When "normal" bacteria are destroyed or greatly reduced in number, there is nothing to prevent the invaders from occupying the host. In most cases the superinfection is an irritating adverse effect (eg, vaginal yeast infection, candidiasis, diarrhea), but in some cases, the superinfection can be more severe than the infection originally being treated. Treatment of the su-

---

BOX 9-1

Using Combination Drugs to Fight Resistant Bacteria

Clavulanic acid protects certain β-lactam antibiotics from breakdown in the presence of penicillinase enzymes.

A combination of amoxicillin and clavulanic acid (*Augmentin*) is commonly used to allow the amoxicillin to remain effective against certain strains of resistant bacteria (usual dosage, 250–500 mg PO q8h for adults or 20–40 mg/kg per day PO in divided doses for children). The theory behind the combination of ticarcillin and clavulanic acid (*Timentin*) is similar.

Sulbactam is another drug that increases the effectiveness of antibiotics against certain resistant bacteria (usual dosage, 3.1 g IM q4–6h for adults; safety not established for children). When combined with ampicillin in the drug *Unasyn,* sulbactam inhibits many bacterial penicillinase enzymes, broadening the spectrum of the ampicillin. In this combination, sulbactam is also slightly antibacterial (usual adult dosage, 0.5–1 g sulbactam with 1–2 g ampicillin IM or IV q6–8h).

BOX 9-2

Antibiotics Developed Specifically for Treating Resistant Strains

A new class of antibiotics, called streptogramins, became available in 1999. Two drugs in this new class, quinupristin and dalfoprostin, are available only in a combination form called *Synercid*. Together, they work synergistically and have been effective in treating vancomycin-resistant enterococci (VRE), resistant *Staphylococcus aureus,* and resistant *Staphylococcus epidermidis*. The drug is approved for VRE and methicillin-sensitive *S. aureus* (MSSA) infections.

The drug also seems to be active against penicillin-resistant pneumococcus. The usual dosage of this drug, for patients 16 years of age and older, is 7.5 mg/kg IV q12h for 7 days. The drug should not be used unless the bacterium is clearly identified as being resistant to other antibiotics and sensitive to this one. Indiscriminant use of this new drug can lead to the development of even more invasive and resistant bacteria.

Linezolid (*Zyvox*) was introduced in 2000. This drug is indicated specifically for treatment of infections caused by vancomycin-resistant and methicillin-resistant strains of bacteria. It is available in intravenous and oral forms. The usual adult dosage is 600 mg PO, or it may be administered IV q12h for 10 to 14 d. This drug must also be used cautiously and only when a sensitive bacterial species has been clearly identified. These drugs are part of a wide variety of compounds that are being investigated to deal with the increasing problem of resistant bacteria.

perinfection leads to new adverse effects and the potential for different superinfections. A vicious cycle of treatment and resistance is the result.

AMINOGLYCOSIDES

The aminoglycosides are a group of powerful antibiotics used to treat serious infections caused by gram-negative aerobic bacilli. Because most of these drugs have potentially serious adverse effects, newer, less toxic drugs have replaced aminoglycosides in the treatment of less serious infections.

Amikacin (*Amikin*) is available for short-term intramuscular (IM) or intravenous (IV) use for serious gram-negative infections. The potential for nephrotoxicity and ototoxicity with amikacin is very high, so the drug is used only as long as absolutely necessary.

Gentamicin (*Garamycin*) is available in many forms: ophthalmic, topical, IV, intrathecal, impregnated beads on surgical wire, and liposomal injection. It covers a wide variety of infections, including pseudomonal diseases and once-rare infections seen in patients with acquired immunodeficiency syndrome (AIDS).

Kanamycin (*Kantrex*), which is available in parenteral and oral forms, is used to treat hepatic coma when ammonia-producing bacteria in the GI tract cause serious illness. It is also used as an adjunctive therapy to decrease GI bacterial flora. Kanamycin should not be used for longer than 7 to 10 days because of its potential toxic effects, which include renal damage, bone marrow depression, and GI complications.

Neomycin (*Mycifradin*) is a slightly milder aminoglycoside that is used to suppress GI bacteria preoperatively and to treat hepatic coma. In topical form, neomycin is used to treat skin wounds and infections.

Netilmicin (*Netromycin*) is reserved for short-term IV or IM treatment of very serious infections.

Streptomycin (generic), once a popular drug, is very toxic to the eighth cranial nerve and kidney. Today it is used as the fourth drug in combination therapy for tuberculosis. It can be used in severe infections if the organism has been shown to be sensitive to streptomycin and no less toxic drugs can be used.

Tobramycin (*Nebcin, Tobrex*) is used for short-term IM or IV treatment of very serious infections. This drug is also available in an ophthalmic form for the treatment of ocular infections caused by susceptible bacteria.

Therapeutic Actions and Indications

The aminoglycosides are bactericidal. They inhibit protein synthesis in susceptible strains of gram-negative bacteria, which in turn leads to loss of functional integrity of the bacterial cell membrane, causing cell death (Figure 9–1). These drugs are used to treat serious infections caused by susceptible strains of gram-negative bacteria, including *Pseudomonas aeruginosa, E. coli, Proteus* species, the *Klebsiella–Enterobacter–Serratia* group, *Citrobacter* species, and *Staphylococcus* species such as *S. aureus*. Aminoglycosides are indicated for the treatment of serious infections that are susceptible to penicillin when penicillin is contraindicated, and they can be used in severe infections before culture and sensitivity tests have been completed.

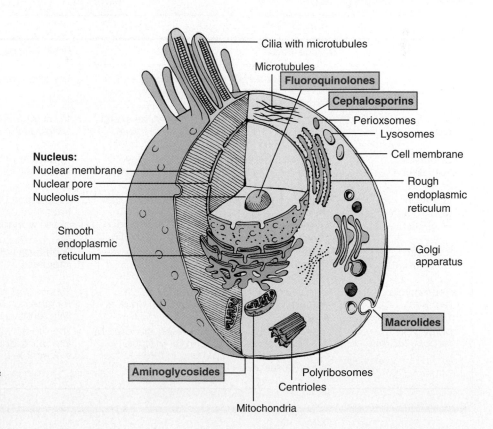

FIGURE 9-1. Sites of cellular action of aminoglycosides, cephalosporins, fluoroquinolones, and macrolides. Aminoglycosides disrupt the cell membrane. Cephalosporins cause bacteria to build weak cell walls when dividing. Fluoroquinolones interfere with DNA enzymes necessary for growth and reproduction. Macrolides change protein function by binding to the cell membrane to cause cell death or prevent cell division.

Pharmacokinetics

The aminoglycosides are poorly absorbed from the GI tract but rapidly absorbed after IM injection, reaching peak levels within 1 hour. They are widely distributed throughout the body, crossing the placenta and entering breast milk. They should be used with great caution during pregnancy and lactation because of potential toxic effects on the neonate.

Aminoglycosides are excreted unchanged in the urine and have an average half-life of 2 to 3 hours. Urine function should be tested daily when these drugs are used, because they depend on the kidney for excretion and are toxic to the kidney; renal function can change daily while a patient is receiving the drug.

Contraindications and Cautions

Aminoglycosides are contraindicated in the following conditions:

- Known allergy to any of the aminoglycosides
- Renal or hepatic disease that could be exacerbated by toxic aminoglycoside effects and that could interfere with drug metabolism and excretion, leading to higher toxicity
- Pre-existing hearing loss, which could be intensified by toxic drug effects on the auditory nerve
- Active infection with herpes or mycobacterial infections that could be worsened by the effects of an aminoglycoside on normal defense mechanisms

- Myasthenia gravis or parkinsonism, which often are exacerbated by the effects of a particular aminoglycoside on the nervous system
- Lactation, because aminoglycosides are excreted in breast milk and potentially could cause serious effects in the baby. Caution should be used during pregnancy, because aminoglycosides are used only to treat severe infections, and the benefits of the drug should be carefully weighed against potential adverse effects on the fetus.

Adverse Effects

The many serious adverse effects associated with aminoglycosides limit their usefulness. Central nervous system (CNS) effects include ototoxicity possibly leading to irreversible deafness; vestibular paralysis resulting from drug effects on the auditory nerve; confusion; depression; disorientation; and numbness, tingling, and weakness related to drug effects on other nerves.

Renal toxicity, which may progress to renal failure, is caused by direct drug toxicity in the glomerulus, meaning that the drug molecules cause damage (eg, obstruction) directly to the kidney. Bone marrow depression may result from direct drug effects on the rapidly dividing cells in the bone marrow, leading to immune suppression and resultant superinfections, fever, and so on.

DRUGS IN FOCUS
Aminoglycosides

Drug Name	Dosage/Route	Usual Indication
amikacin (*Amikin*)	15 mg/kg per day IM or IV divided into two or three equal doses; reduce dosage in renal failure	Treatment of serious gram-negative infections
Ⓟ gentamicin (*Garamycin*)	Adult: 3 mg/kg per day IM or IV in three equal doses q8h; reduce dosage in renal failure Pediatric: 2–2.5 mg/kg per day q8h IV or IM	Treatment of *Pseudomonas* infections and a wide variety of gram-negative infections
kanamycin (*Kantrex*)	7.5 mg/kg q12h IM or 15 mg/kg per day IV divided into two to three equal doses given slowly	Treatment of hepatic coma and to decrease GI normal flora
neomycin (*Mycifradin*)	Adult: 15 mg/kg per day in divided doses q6h IM Pediatric: 50–100 mg/kg per day in divided doses PO for hepatic coma; do not use IM	Suppression of GI normal flora preoperatively; treatment of hepatic coma; topical treatment of skin wounds
netilmicin (*Netromycin*)	Adult: 1.5–3.25 mg/kg IM or IV q12h; reduce dosage in renal failure Pediatric: 2.7–4 mg/kg IM or IV q12h	Short-term IV treatment of very serious infections
streptomycin (generic)	Adult: 1–2 g/d IM in divided doses q6–12h Pediatric: 20–40 mg/kg per day IM in divided doses q6–12h	Fourth drug in combination therapy regimen for tuberculosis; treatment of severe infections with sensitive organisms
tobramycin (*Nebcin, Tobrex*)	Adult: 3 mg/kg per day in three equal doses IM or IV q8h; reduce dosage in renal failure Pediatric: 6–7.5 mg/kg per day in three to four equal doses q6–8h IV or IM	Short-term IV or IM treatment of serious infections; ocular infections caused by susceptible bacteria

GI effects include nausea, vomiting, diarrhea, weight loss, stomatitis, and hepatic toxicity. These effects are a result of direct GI irritation, loss of bacteria of the normal flora with resultant superinfections, and toxic effects in the mucous membranes and liver as the drug is metabolized.

Cardiac effects can include palpitations, hypotension, and hypertension. Hypersensitivity reactions include purpura, rash, urticaria, and exfoliative dermatitis.

Clinically Important Drug–Drug Interactions

If aminoglycosides are taken in combination or with potent diuretics, the incidence of ototoxicity, nephrotoxicity, and neurotoxicity increases. This combination should be avoided if at all possible.

If these antibiotics are given with anesthetics, nondepolarizing neuromuscular blockers, succinylcholine, or citrate anticoagulated blood, increased neuromuscular blockade with paralysis is possible. If a patient who has been receiving an aminoglycoside requires surgery, the fact that the aminoglycoside has been given should be indicated prominently on the chart. After surgery, the patient will require extended monitoring and support.

In addition, most aminoglycosides have a synergistic bactericidal effect when given with penicillins, cephalosporins, carbenicillin, or ticarcillin. In certain conditions, this synergism is used therapeutically to increase the effectiveness of treatment.

Nursing Considerations for Patients Receiving Aminoglycosides

Assessment: History and Examination

Screen for the following possible contraindications or cautions for use of the drug: known allergy to any aminoglycoside (obtain specific information about the nature and occurrence of allergic reactions); history of renal or hepatic disease; pre-existing hearing loss; active infection with herpes, vaccinia, varicella, or fungal or mycobacterial organisms; myasthenia gravis; parkinsonism; infant botulism; and current pregnancy or lactation status.

Physical assessment should be performed to establish baseline data for assessing the effectiveness of the drug and the occurrence of any adverse effects associated with drug therapy. Perform culture and sensitivity tests at the site of infection. Conduct orientation and reflex assessment as well as auditory testing to evaluate any CNS effects of the drug. Also assess vital signs: respiratory rate and adventitious sounds to monitor for signs of infection or hypersensitivity reactions; temperature to assess for signs and symptoms of infection; blood pressure to monitor for cardiovascular effects of the drug. Renal and hepatic function tests should be done to determine baseline function of these organs and, possibly, the need to adjust dosage.

Nursing Diagnoses

Patients who receive aminoglycosides may have the following nursing diagnoses related to drug therapy:

- Acute Pain related to GI, CNS effects of drug
- Disturbed Sensory Perception (Auditory) related to CNS effects of drug
- Risk for Infection related to bone marrow suppression
- Excess Fluid Volume related to nephrotoxicity
- Deficient Knowledge regarding drug therapy

Implementation

The accompanying Nursing Challenge describes information about antibiotic use that should be provided as part of patient education.

- Check culture and sensitivity reports *to ensure that this is the drug of choice for this patient.*
- Ensure that the patient receives the full course of the aminoglycoside as prescribed, divided around the clock, *to increase effectiveness and decrease the risk for development of resistant strains of bacteria.*

NURSING CHALLENGE
Using Antibiotics Properly

As part of the patient education plan, nurses should include information about the risks and dangers of antibiotic abuse by incorporating some of the following points:

- Explain clearly that a particular antibiotic is effective against only certain bacteria and that a culture needs to be taken to identify the bacteria.
- Explain that bacteria can develop resistant strains that will not be affected by antibiotics in the future, so use of antibiotics now may make them less effective in situations in which they are really necessary.
- Ensure that patients understand the importance of taking the full course of medication as prescribed, even if they feel better. Stopping an antibiotic midway through a regimen often leads to the development of resistant bacteria. Using all of the medication will also prevent patients' saving unused medication to self-treat future infections or to share with other family members.
- Tell patients that allergies may develop with repeated exposures to certain antibiotics. In addition, explain to patients that saving antibiotics to take later, when they think they need them again, may lead to earlier development of an allergy, which will negate important tests that could identify the bacteria making them sick.
- Offer other medications, such as antihistamines, decongestants, or even chicken soup, to patients who request antibiotics; this may satisfy their need for something to take. Explaining that viral infections do not respond to antibiotics usually offers little consolation to patients who are suffering from a cold or the flu.

The publicity that many emergent, resistant strains of bacteria have received in recent years may help to get the message across to patients about the need to take the full course of an antibiotic and to use antibiotics only when they are the appropriate drug of choice.

- Monitor the site of infection and presenting signs and symptoms (eg, fever, lethargy) throughout the course of drug therapy. *Failure of these signs and symptoms to resolve may indicate the need to reculture the site. Arrange to continue drug therapy for at least 2 days after all signs and symptoms resolve.*
- Monitor the patient regularly for signs of nephrotoxicity, neurotoxicity, and bone marrow suppression *to effectively arrange for discontinuation of drug or decreased dosage, as appropriate, if any of these toxicities occurs.*
- Provide safety measures *to protect the patient if CNS effects, such as confusion, disorientation, or numbness and tingling, occur.*
- Provide small, frequent meals as tolerated to maintain nutrition, offer frequent mouth care, and offer ice chips or sugarless candy to suck *to provide relief and if stomatitis and sore mouth are problems, and to provide adequate fluids to replace fluid lost with diarrhea.*
- Ensure that the patient is hydrated at all times during drug therapy *to minimize renal toxicity from drug exposure.*
- Ensure that the patient is instructed about the appropriate dosage regimen and possible adverse effects *to enhance patient knowledge about drug therapy and to promote compliance.*

The patient should

Take safety precautions, such as changing position slowly and avoiding driving and hazardous tasks, if CNS effects occur.

Try to drink a lot of fluids and to maintain nutrition (very important) even though nausea, vomiting, and diarrhea may occur.

Avoid exposure to other infections (eg, crowded areas, people with known infectious diseases).

Report difficulty breathing, severe headache, loss of hearing or ringing in the ears, or changes in urine output to the health care provider.

Evaluation

- Monitor patient response to the drug (resolution of bacterial infection).
- Monitor for adverse effects (orientation and affect, hearing changes, bone marrow suppression, renal toxicity, hepatic dysfunction, GI effects).
- Evaluate the effectiveness of the teaching plan (patient can name drug, dosage, possible adverse effects to watch for, and specific measures to help avoid adverse effects).
- Monitor the effectiveness of comfort and safety measures and compliance with the therapeutic regimen.

CEPHALOSPORINS

The cephalosporins were first introduced in the 1960s. These drugs are similar to the penicillins in structure and in activity.

Over time, four generations of cephalosporins have been introduced, each group with its own spectrum of activity, described as follows.

First-generation cephalosporins are largely effective against the same gram-positive bacteria that are affected by penicillin G as well as the gram-negative bacteria *Proteus mirabilis, E. coli,* and *Klebsiella pneumoniae.* (*PEcK* is an easy way to remember which bacteria are susceptible to the first-generation cephalosporins.)

Second-generation cephalosporins are effective against those strains as well as *Haemophilus influenzae, Enterobacter aerogenes,* and *Neisseria* species. (Remember *HENPeCK.*) The second-generation drugs are less effective against gram-positive bacteria.

Third-generation cephalosporins are relatively weak against gram-positive bacteria but are more potent against the gram-negative bacilli as well as *Serratia marcescens.* (Remember *HENPeCKS.*)

Fourth-generation cephalosporins are just now being developed. The first drug of this group, cefepime (*Maxipime*), is active against gram-negative and gram-positive organisms, including cephalosporin-resistant staphylococci and *P. aeruginosa.*

Therapeutic Actions and Indications

The cephalosporins are both bactericidal and bacteriostatic, depending on the dose used and the specific drug involved. In susceptible species, these agents basically interfere with the cell wall–building ability of bacteria when they divide. That is, they prevent the bacteria from biosynthesizing the framework of their cell walls. The bacteria with weakened cell walls swell and burst as a result of the osmotic pressure within the cell (see Figure 9–1).

Cephalosporins are indicated for the treatment of infections caused by susceptible bacteria. Selection of an antibiotic from this class depends on the sensitivity of the involved organism, the route of choice, and sometimes the cost involved. It is important to reserve cephalosporins for appropriate situations, because cephalosporin-resistant bacteria are appearing in increasing numbers. Before therapy begins, a culture and sensitivity test should always be performed to evaluate the causative organism and appropriate sensitivity to the antibiotic being used.

Pharmacokinetics

Some of the cephalosporins are well absorbed from the GI tract: cephalexin, cephradine, cefaclor, cefditoren, cefixime, cefprozil, cefadroxil, ceftibuten, cefuroxime, cefpodoxime, cefdinir, and loracarbef. The others are absorbed well after IM injection or IV administration.

The cephalosporins are primarily metabolized in the liver and excreted in the urine. Caution must be used in patients with hepatic or renal impairment, because either condition could alter drug metabolism and excretion. These drugs cross the placenta and enter breast milk. They should be used during pregnancy and lactation only if the benefits clearly outweigh the potential risk of toxicity to the fetus or neonate.

DRUGS IN FOCUS
Cephalosporins

Drug Name	Dosage/Route	Usual Indications
First-generation Cephalosporins		
cefadroxil (*Duricef*)	Adult: 1–2 g PO in a single or two divided doses; reduce dosage in renal impairment Pediatric: 30 mg/kg per day PO in divided doses q12h	Indicated for urinary tract infections (UTIs) pharyngitis, and tonsillitis caused by group A β-hemolytic streptococci as well as skin infections
cefazolin (*Kefzol, Zolicef*)	Adult: 250–500 mg IM or IV q4–8h; reduce dosage in renal impairment Pediatric: 25–50 mg/kg per day IM or IV in three or four divided doses	Respiratory tract, skin, GU, biliary tract, bone, joint, and myocardial infections as well as sepsis
cephalexin (*Keflex, Bioflex*)	Adult: 250 mg PO q.i.d. Pediatric: 25–50 mg/kg per day PO in divided doses	Respiratory, skin, bone, and GU infections; used for otitis media in children
cephapirin (*Cefadyl*)	Adult: 500 mg to 1 g IM or IV q4–6h; reduce dosage in renal impairment Pediatric: 40–80 mg/kg per day IM or IV in four divided doses	Respiratory tract, skin, GU, biliary tract, bone, joint, and myocardial infections as well as sepsis and osteomyelitis
cephradine (*Velosef*)	Adult: 250–500 mg PO q6–12h; reduce dosage in renal impairment Pediatric: 25–100 mg/kg per day PO in divided doses q4–6h	Respiratory tract, skin, GU, biliary tract, bone, joint, and myocardial infections as well as sepsis and osteomyelitis; useful in situations in which a switch from parenteral to oral route is expected (eg, preoperative prophylaxis followed by oral postoperative prophylaxis)
Second-generation Cephalosporins		
Ⓟ cefaclor (*Ceclor*)	Adult: 250 mg PO q8h—do not exceed 4 g/d; must be taken every 8–12 h around the clock Pediatric: 20 mg/kg per day PO in divided doses q8h; do not exceed 1 g/d	Respiratory tract infections, skin infections, UTIs, otitis media, typhoid fever, anthrax exposure
cefmetazole (*Zefazone*)	Adult: 2 g IV q6h for 5–14 d; reduce dosage in renal impairment Pediatric: safety not established	Used for severe infections; preoperative prophylaxis for cesarean section and abdominal, vaginal, biliary, or colorectal surgery
cefonicid (*Monocid*)	Adult: 1 g/d IM or IV; reduce dosage in renal impairment Pediatric: safety not established	Used for severe infections; preoperative prophylaxis for cesarean section and abdominal, vaginal, biliary, or colorectal surgery
cefotetan (*Cefotan*)	Adult: 1–2 g/d IM or IV in divided doses q12h for 5–10 d; reduce dosage in renal impairment Pediatric: safety not established	Used for severe infections; preoperative prophylaxis for cesarean section and abdominal, vaginal, biliary, or colorectal surgery
cefoxitin (*Mefoxin*)	Adult: 1–2 g IM or IV q6–8h; reduce dosage with renal impairment Pediatric: 80–160 mg/kg per day IM or IV in divided doses q4–6h	Used for severe infections; preoperative prophylaxis for cesarean section and abdominal, vaginal, biliary or colorectal surgery; more effective in gynecological and intra-abdominal infections than some other agents
cefprozil (*Cefzil*)	Adult: 250–500 mg PO q12h for 10 d—reduce dosage with renal impairment; should be taken every 12 h for 10 d Pediatric: 7.5–20 mg/kg PO q12h for 10 d; for child 6 mo to 2 years of age, 15 mg/kg PO q12h for 10 d	Pharyngitis, tonsillitis, otitis media, sinusitis, secondary bronchial infections, and skin infections
cefuroxime (*Ceftin, Zinacef*)	Adult: 250 mg PO b.i.d.; 750 mg to 1.5 g IM q8h; reduce dosage with renal impairment Pediatric: 125 mg PO b.i.d.; 50–100 mg/kg per day IM or IV in divided doses q6–8h	Wide range of infections, as listed for other second-generation drugs; also used to treat Lyme disease and preferred in situations involving an anticipated switch from parenteral to oral drug use

Drugs in Focus continues on page 90

DRUGS IN FOCUS (CONTINUED)
Cephalosporins

Drug Name	Dosage/Route	Usual Indications
loracarbef (*Lorabid*)	Adult: 200–400 mg PO q12h; reduce dosage with renal impairment Pediatric: 15–30 mg/kg per day in divided doses q12h PO; should be taken every 12 hours for 7–14 d	Pharyngitis, tonsillitis, otitis media, sinusitis, UTIs, secondary bronchial infections, and skin infections

Third-generation Cephalosporins

Drug Name	Dosage/Route	Usual Indications
cefdinir (*Omnicef*—a suspension form is available for children)	Adult: 300 mg PO q12h for 10 d; reduce dosage with renal impairment Pediatric: 7 mg/kg PO q12h	Respiratory infections, otitis media, sinusitis, laryngitis, bronchitis, skin infections
cefixime (*Suprax*)	Adult: 400 mg/d PO; reduce dosage with renal impairment Pediatric: 8 mg/kg per day PO; may be given as a single daily dose, making compliance easier	Uncomplicated UTIs, respiratory infections, otitis media, uncomplicated gonorrhea
cefoperazone (*Cefobid*)	Adult: 2–4 g/d IM or IV in divided doses q12h; reduce dosage with hepatic impairment Pediatric: safety not established	Moderate to severe skin, urinary tract, and respiratory tract infections; pelvic inflammatory disease; intra-abdominal infections; peritonitis; septicemia
cefotaxime (*Claforan*)	Adult: 2–8 g/d IM or IV in divided doses q6–8h; reduce dosage with renal impairment Pediatric: 50–180 mg/kg per day IM or IV in divided doses q4–6h	Moderate to severe skin, urinary tract, and respiratory tract infections; pelvic inflammatory disease; intra-abdominal infections; peritonitis; septicemia; bone infections; CNS infections; preoperative prophylaxis
cefpodoxime (*Vantin*)	Adult: 100–400 mg PO q12h; reduce dosage with renal impairment Pediatric: 5 mg/kg per dose PO q12h—given every 12h for 7–14 d	Respiratory infections, UTI's, gonorrhea, skin infections, and otitis media
ceftazidime (*Ceptaz, Tazicef*)	Adult: 1 g q8–12h IM or IV; reduce dosage with renal impairment Pediatric: 30–50 mg/kg q8–12h IM or IV	Moderate to severe skin, urinary tract, and respiratory tract infections; intra-abdominal infections; septicemia; bone infections; CNS infections
ceftibuten (*Cedax*—available in a suspension form for children)	Adult: 400 mg PO q.d. for 10 d; reduce dosage with renal impairment Pediatric: 9 mg/kg per day PO for 10 d *Note:* once-a-day dosing increases compliance	Pharyngitis, tonsillitis, exacerbations of bronchitis, otitis media
ceftizoxime (*Cefizox*)	Adult: 1–2 g IM or IV q8–12h; reduce dosage with renal impairment Pediatric: 50 mg/kg IM or IV q6–8h	Respiratory, gynecological, pelvic inflammatory, intra-abdominal, skin, and bone and joint infections; also used for sepsis and meningitis
ceftriaxone (*Rocephin*)	Adult: 1–2 g/d IM or IV in divided doses b.i.d.—q.i.d. Pediatric: 50–75 mg/kg per day IV or IM in divided doses q12h	Moderate to severe skin, urinary tract, and respiratory tract infections; pelvic inflammatory disease; intra-abdominal infections; peritonitis; septicemia; bone infections; CNS infections; preoperative prophylaxis; unlabeled use for treatment of Lyme disease

Fourth-generation Cephalosporin

Drug Name	Dosage/Route	Usual Indications
cefditoren (*Spectracef*)	Adult and Children >12 yr: 200–400 mg PO b.i.d.; reduce dosage with renal impairment	Acute exacerbations of chronic bronchitis; pharangitis and tonsillitis; skin and skin structure infections
cefepime (*Maxipime*)	Adult: 0.5–2 g IM or IV q12h; must be injected for greatest effectiveness q12h for 7–10 d; reduce dosage with renal impairment Pediatric: 50 mg/kg per dose q12h IV or IM for 7–10 d	Moderate to severe skin, urinary tract, and respiratory tract infections

Contraindications and Cautions

These drugs should not be used in patients with known allergies to cephalosporins or penicillins, because cross-sensitivity is common. In addition, caution must be used in patients with renal failure.

Adverse Effects

The most common adverse effects of the cephalosporins involve the GI tract and include nausea, vomiting, diarrhea, anorexia, abdominal pain, and flatulence (common). Pseudomembranous colitis, a potentially dangerous disorder, has also been reported with some cephalosporins. A particular drug should be discontinued immediately at any sign of violent, bloody diarrhea or abdominal pain.

CNS symptoms include headache, dizziness, lethargy, and paresthesias. Nephrotoxicity is also associated with the use of cephalosporins, most particularly in patients who have a predisposing renal insufficiency. Other adverse effects include superinfections, which occur frequently because of the death of protective bacteria of the normal flora. Patients receiving parenteral cephalosporins should also be monitored for the possibility of phlebitis with IV administration or local abscess at the site of an IM injection.

Clinically Important Drug–Drug Interactions

The concurrent administration of cephalosporins with aminoglycosides increases the risk of nephrotoxicity. Patients who receive this combination should be monitored frequently, including evaluation of serum blood urea nitrogen (BUN) and creatinine levels.

Patients who receive oral anticoagulants in addition to cephalosporins may experience increased bleeding. They should be taught how to monitor for blood loss (eg, bleeding gums, easy bruising) and should be aware that the dose of the oral anticoagulant may need to be reduced.

When a patient consumes alcohol while receiving cephalosporins or up to 72 hours after discontinuation of the drug, in many cases a disulfiram-like reaction occurs. A disulfiram-like reaction causes unpleasant symptoms such as flushing, throbbing headache, nausea and vomiting, chest pain, palpitations, dyspnea, syncope, vertigo, blurred vision, and, in extreme reactions, cardiovascular collapse, convulsions, or even death. Patients should be warned about this possible reaction and urged to refrain from drinking beverages or medications containing alcohol for 72 hours after the drug is stopped.

Nursing Considerations for Patients Receiving Cephalosporins
Assessment: History and Examination

Screen for the following possible contraindications or cautions for use of the drug: known allergy to any cephalosporin, penicillin, or any other allergens, because cross-sensitivity often occurs (obtain specific information about the nature and occurrence of the allergic reactions); history of renal disease, which could exacerbate nephrotoxicity related to the cephalosporin; and current pregnancy or lactation status.

Physical assessment should be performed to establish baseline data for assessing the effectiveness of the drug and the occurrence of any adverse effects associated with drug therapy. Perform culture and sensitivity tests at the site of infection. Examine skin for any rash or lesions to provide a baseline for possible adverse effects. Note respiratory status—including rate, depth, and adventitious sounds—to provide a baseline. Check renal function test results, including BUN and creatinine clearance, to assess the status of renal functioning and to detect the possible need to alter dosage. Monitor hepatic function to assess the body's ability to metabolize the drug. Examine injection sites to provide a baseline for determining adverse reactions or abscess formation.

Nursing Diagnoses

Patients receiving a cephalosporin may have the following nursing diagnoses related to drug therapy:

- Acute Pain related to GI, CNS effects of drug
- Risk for Infection related to repeated injections
- Deficient Fluid Volume and Imbalanced Nutrition: Less than Body Requirements, related to diarrhea
- Deficient Knowledge regarding drug therapy

Implementation

- Check culture and sensitivity reports *to ensure that this is the drug of choice for this patient.*
- Monitor renal function test values before and periodically during therapy *to arrange for appropriate dosage reduction as needed.*
- Ensure that the patient receives the full course of the cephalosporin as prescribed, divided around the clock *to increase effectiveness and to decrease the risk of development of resistant strains.*
- Monitor the site of infection and presenting signs and symptoms (eg, fever, lethargy) throughout the course of drug therapy. *Failure of these signs and symptoms to resolve may indicate the need to reculture the site. Arrange to continue drug therapy for at least 2 days after the resolution of all signs and symptoms.*
- Provide small, frequent meals as tolerated, frequent mouth care, and ice chips or sugarless candy to suck if stomatitis and sore mouth are problems, *to relieve discomfort and provide nutrition,* and adequate fluids *to replace fluid lost with diarrhea.*
- Monitor patient for any signs of superinfection *to arrange for treatment if superinfection occurs.*
- Monitor injection sites regularly and *provide warm compresses and gentle massage to injection sites if painful or swollen. If signs of phlebitis occur, remove IV line and reinsert in a different vein.*
- Initiate safety measures, including adequate lighting, siderails on the bed, and assistance with ambulation *to protect the patient from injury if CNS effects occur.*
- Be sure to instruct the patient about the appropriate dosage schedule and about possible side effects *to enhance patient knowledge about drug therapy and to promote compliance.*

The patient should

Take safety precautions, including changing position slowly and avoiding driving and hazardous tasks, if CNS effects occur.

Try to drink a lot of fluids and to maintain nutrition (very important) even though nausea, vomiting, and diarrhea may occur.

Report difficulty breathing, severe headache, severe diarrhea, dizziness, or weakness to the health care provider.

Avoid consuming alcoholic beverages while receiving cephalosporins and for at least 72 hours after completing the drug course, because serious side effects could occur.

Evaluation

- Monitor patient response to the drug (resolution of bacterial infection).
- Monitor for adverse effects (orientation and affect; renal toxicity; hepatic dysfunction; GI effects; and local irritation, including phlebitis at injection and IV sites).
- Evaluate the effectiveness of the teaching plan (patient can name drug, dosage, possible adverse effects to expect, and specific measures to help avoid adverse effects).
- Monitor the effectiveness of comfort and safety measures and the patient's compliance with the regimen.

FLUOROQUINOLONES

The fluoroquinolones are a relatively new class of antibiotics with a broad spectrum of activity. These drugs, which are all made synthetically, are associated with relatively mild adverse reactions. The most widely used fluoroquinolone is ciprofloxacin (*Cipro*), which is effective against a wide spectrum of gram-negative bacteria. It is available in injectable, oral, and topical forms. In 2001 it was approved for prevention of anthrax infection in areas that might be exposed to germ warfare. It is also effective against typhoid fever. Other fluoroquinolones include the following agents.

Gatifloxacin (*Tequin*) is an agent that is available in oral and IV forms for treatment of a variety of sensitive urinary and respiratory tract infections in adults.

Levofloxacin (*Levaquin*), which is available in oral and IV forms, may be used to treat respiratory, urinary tract, skin, and sinus infections caused by susceptible gram-negative bacteria. Because of its parenteral availability, it may be preferred for severe infections or for use when the patient cannot take oral drugs.

Lomefloxacin (*Maxaquin*) is an oral drug that can be used to treat lower respiratory tract infections as well as many urinary tract infections. It is the drug of choice for preoperative and postoperative prophylaxis to prevent urinary tract infections after transurethral procedures or transrectal prostate biopsies.

Moxifloxacin (*Avelox*), an oral agent, is used to treat sinusitis, bronchitis, and pneumonia in adults.

Norfloxacin (*Noroxin*) is recommended only for treatment of various urinary tract infections caused by susceptible gram-negative bacteria.

Ofloxacin (*Floxin, Ocuflox*) can be given IV or orally to treat respiratory, skin, and urinary tract infections as well as pelvic inflammatory disease. In addition, this drug is available as an ophthalmic agent for the treatment of ocular infections caused by susceptible bacteria.

Sparfloxacin (*Zagam*) is an oral agent used to treat community-acquired pneumonia and acute bronchitis caused by susceptible bacteria.

Trovafloxacin (*Trovan*) and alatrofloxacin (*Trovan IV*), which are available in IV and oral forms, may be used to treat a wide spectrum of infections caused by susceptible gram-negative respiratory, intra-abdominal, urinary tract, gynecological, and skin bacteria. Strains that have become resistant to the very frequently used ciprofloxacin may still be sensitive to these fluoroquinolones.

Therapeutic Actions and Indications

The fluoroquinolones enter the bacterial cell by passive diffusion through channels in the cell membrane. Once inside, they interfere with the action of DNA enzymes necessary for the growth and reproduction of the bacteria (see Figure 9–1). This leads to cell death because the bacterial DNA is damaged and the cell cannot be maintained. At the moment, the fluoroquinolones have the advantage of a unique way of disrupting bacterial activity. There is little cross-resistance with other forms of antibiotics. However, misuse of these drugs in the short time the class has been available has led to the existence of resistant strains of bacteria. Because so many resistant strains are emerging, infected tissue should always be cultured to determine the exact bacterial cause and sensitivity. These drugs have been associated with lesions in developing cartilage and therefore are not recommended for use in children younger than 18 years of age.

The fluoroquinolones are indicated for treating infections caused by susceptible strains of gram-negative bacteria including *E. coli, P. mirabilis, K. pneumoniae, Enterobacter cloacae, Proteus vulgaris, Proteus rettgeri, Morganella morgani, Moraxella catarrhalis, H. influenzae, P. aeruginosa, Citrobacter freundii, S. aureus, Staphylococcus epidermidis,* some *Neisseria gonorrhoeae,* and group D streptococci. These infections frequently include urinary tract, respiratory tract, and skin infections.

Pharmacokinetics

The fluoroquinolones are absorbed from the GI tract, metabolized in the liver, and excreted in the urine and feces. Caution must be used in patients with renal or hepatic impairment, which could interfere with the metabolism and excretion of the drugs. They are widely distributed in the body. The fluoroquinolones cross the placenta and enter breast milk; they should be used during pregnancy and lactation only if the benefit outweighs the potential risk to the neonate.

Contraindications and Cautions

Fluoroquinolones are contraindicated in patients with known allergy to any fluoroquinolone and in pregnant or lactating women, because the drugs have unknown effects on fetuses and infants. Caution should be used in the presence of renal dysfunction, which could interfere with drug excretion, and seizures, which could be exacerbated by the drugs' effects on cell membrane channels.

Adverse Effects

Several adverse effects are associated with fluoroquinolones. The most common are headache, dizziness, insomnia, and depression, related to possible effects on the CNS membranes. GI effects include nausea, vomiting, diarrhea, and dry mouth, related to direct drug effect on the GI tract and possibly to stimulation of the chemoreceptor trigger zone (CTZ) in the CNS.

Immunological effects include bone marrow depression, which may be related to drug effects on the cells of the bone marrow that rapidly turn over. Other adverse effects include fever, rash, and photosensitivity, a potentially serious adverse effect that can cause severe skin reactions. Patients should be advised to avoid sun and ultraviolet light exposure and to use protective clothing and sunscreens.

Clinically Important Drug–Drug Interactions

When fluoroquinolones are taken concurrently with iron salts, sucralfate, mineral supplements, or antacids, the therapeutic effect of the fluoroquinolone is decreased. If this drug combination is necessary, administration of the two agents should be separated by at least 4 hours.

If fluoroquinolones are taken with drugs that increase the QTc interval or cause torsades de pointes (quinidine, procainamide, amiodarone, sotalol, bepridil, erythromycin, terfenadine, astemizole, cisapride, pentamidine, tricyclics, phenothiazines), severe to fatal cardiac reactions are possible. These combinations should be avoided, but if they must be used, patients should be hospitalized with continual cardiac monitoring.

Combining fluoroquinolones with theophylline leads to increased theophylline levels because the two drugs use similar metabolic pathways. The theophylline dose should be decreased by one half, and serum theophylline levels should be monitored carefully.

DRUGS IN FOCUS
Fluoroquinolones

Drug Name	Dosage/Route	Usual Indications
(P) ciprofloxacin (*Cipro*)	Adult: 100–500 mg b.i.d. PO for up to 6 wk; reduce dosage in renal failure Pediatric: not recommended because of potential effects on developing cartilage	Treatment of infections caused by a wide spectrum of gram-negative bacteria
gatifloxacin (*Tequin*)	Adult: 200–400 mg q.d. PO of IV for up to 14 d; reduce dosage with renal impairment	Treatment of adults with sensitive respiratory and urinary tract infections
levofloxacin (*Levaquin*)	Adult: 250–500 mg PO or IV q.d.; reduce dosage in renal impairment	Treatment of respiratory, urinary tract, skin, and sinus infections caused by susceptible gram-negative bacteria in adults
lomefloxacin (*Maxaquin*)	Adult: 400 mg PO q.d. for 10–14 d; reduce dosage with renal impairment	Treatment of lower respiratory tract and urinary tract infections in adults; preoperative and postoperative prophylaxis for transurethral prostate biopsies
moxifloxacin (*Avelox*)	Adult: 400 mg PO q.d. for 5–10 d; reduce dosage in renal impairment	Treatment of adults with sinusitis, bronchitis, or community-acquired pneumonia
norfloxacin (*Noroxin*)	Adult: 400 mg PO q12h for up to 28 d; reduce dosage in renal impairment	Treatment of urinary tract infections
ofloxacin (*Floxin, Ocuflox*)	Adult: 200–400 mg q12h PO or IV for up to 10 d; reduce dosage in renal impairment	Treatment of respiratory, skin, and urinary tract infections; pelvic inflammatory disease; ocular infections
sparfloxacin (*Zagam*)	Adult: 400 mg PO on day 1, then 200 mg PO q.d.; reduce dosage in renal impairment	Treatment of community-acquired pneumonia and chronic bronchitis
trovafloxacin (*Trevan*) alatrofloxacin (*Trovan IV*)	Adult: 200–300 mg q.d. PO or IV; switch to oral form as soon as possible	Treatment of a wide spectrum of gram-negative infections, including strains that may be resistant to ciprofloxacin

In addition, when fluoroquinolones are combined with nonsteroidal anti-inflammatory drugs (NSAIDs), an increased risk of CNS stimulation is possible. If this combination is used, patients should be monitored closely, especially those who have a history of seizures or CNS problems.

Nursing Considerations for Patients Receiving Fluoroquinolones

Assessment: History and Examination

Screen for the following possible contraindications or cautions for use of the drug: known allergy to any fluoroquinolone (obtain specific information about the nature and occurrence of allergic reactions); history of renal disease that could interfere with excretion of the drug; and current pregnancy or lactation status, because of potential adverse effects on the fetus or infant.

Physical assessment should be performed to establish baseline data for assessing the effectiveness of the drug and the occurrence of any adverse effects associated with drug therapy. Perform culture and sensitivity tests at the site of infection. Examine the skin for any rash or lesions to provide a baseline for possible adverse effects. Conduct assessment of orientation, affect, and reflexes to establish a baseline for any CNS effects of the drug. Perform renal function tests, including BUN and creatinine clearance, to evaluate the status of renal functioning and to assess necessary changes in dosage.

Nursing Diagnoses

The patient receiving a fluoroquinolone may have the following nursing diagnoses related to drug therapy:

- Acute Pain related to GI, CNS, skin effects of drug
- Deficient Fluid Volume and Imbalanced Nutrition: Less than Body Requirements, related to GI effects of drug
- Deficient Knowledge regarding drug therapy

Implementation

- Check culture and sensitivity reports *to ensure that this is the drug of choice for this patient.*
- Monitor renal function tests before initiating therapy *to appropriately arrange for dosage reduction if necessary.*
- Ensure that the patient receives the full course of the fluoroquinolone as prescribed *to eradicate the infection and to help prevent the emergence of resistant strains.*
- Monitor the site of infection and presenting signs and symptoms (eg, fever, lethargy, urinary tract signs and symptoms) throughout the course of drug therapy. *Failure of these signs and symptoms to resolve may indicate the need to reculture the site. Arrange to continue drug therapy for at least 2 days after resolution of all signs and symptoms.*
- Provide small, frequent meals as tolerated, frequent mouth care, and ice chips or sugarless candy to suck if dry mouth is a problem *to relieve discomfort and provide nutrition, and adequate fluids to replace those lost with diarrhea.*
- Implement safety measures, including adequate lighting, use of siderails, and assistance with ambulation *to protect patient from injury if CNS effects occur.*
- Ensure that the patient receives instructions about the appropriate dosage schedule and possible adverse effects *to enhance patient knowledge about drug therapy and to promote compliance.*

The patient should

Take safety precautions, including changing position slowly and avoiding driving and hazardous tasks, if CNS effects occur.

Try to drink a lot of fluids and to maintain nutrition (very important), although nausea, vomiting, and diarrhea may occur.

Avoid ultraviolet light and sun exposure, using protective clothing and sunscreens.

Report difficulty breathing, severe headache, severe diarrhea, severe skin rash, fainting spells, and heart palpitations to the health care provider.

Evaluation

- Monitor patient response to the drug (resolution of bacterial infection).
- Monitor for adverse effects (orientation and affect, GI effects, photosensitivity).
- Evaluate the effectiveness of the teaching plan (patient can name drug, dosage, possible adverse effects to expect, and specific measures to help avoid adverse effects).
- Monitor the effectiveness of comfort and safety measures and compliance with the therapeutic regimen.

MACROLIDES

The macrolides are antibiotics that interfere with protein synthesis in susceptible bacteria. The macrolides include the following drugs.

Erythromycin (*E-Mycin, ERYC,* and others), the first macrolide to be developed, proved to be a good alternative for patients who were allergic to penicillins. It is the drug of choice for the treatment of Legionnaire's disease, infections caused by *Corynebacterium diphtheriae,* ureaplasma, syphilis, mycoplasmal pneumonias, and chlamydial infections. It is readily absorbed from the GI tract and is metabolized in the liver with excretion mainly in the bile to feces. The half-life of erythromycin is 1.6 hours. It crosses the placenta and enters breast milk; it therefore should be used during pregnancy and lactation only if the benefit clearly outweighs the risk to the fetus or the neonate.

Azithromycin (*Zithromax*) is used for treating mild to moderate respiratory infections and urethritis in adults and is effective in treating otitis media, pharyngitis, and tonsillitis in children. It is absorbed from the GI tract and mainly excreted unchanged in the urine, making it necessary to monitor renal function when a patient is taking this drug. The half-life of azithromycin is 68 hours. It crosses the placenta and enters breast milk and therefore should be used during pregnancy and lactation only if the benefit clearly outweighs the risk to the neonate.

Clarithromycin (*Biaxin*) is an expensive oral agent that is effective in treating several respiratory, skin, sinus, and maxillary infections. In addition, it is effective against mycobacteria. It is readily absorbed from the GI tract and is metabolized in the liver for excretion in the urine. It is necessary to monitor renal function when a patient is taking this drug, because it is excreted by the renal system. The half-life of clarithromycin is 3 to 7 hours. It crosses the placenta and enters breast milk and therefore should be used during pregnancy and lactation only if the benefit clearly outweighs the risk to the neonate.

Dirithromycin (*Dynabac*) is effective in treating susceptible upper and lower respiratory tract infections, skin infections, and pharyngitis/tonsillitis. It is absorbed from the GI tract, being converted from the prodrug dirithromycin to erythromycylamine in the intestinal wall. Most of the drug is excreted through the feces. It has a half-life of 2 to 36 hours. It also has the advantage of once-a-day dosing, which increases compliance in many cases. Dirithromycin crosses the placenta and enters breast milk; it should be used during pregnancy and lactation only if the benefit clearly outweighs the risk to the fetus or neonate.

Therapeutic Actions and Indications

The macrolides, which may be bactericidal or bacteriostatic, exert their effect by binding to the bacterial cell membrane and changing protein function (see Figure 9–1). This action can prevent the cell from dividing or cause cell death, depending on the sensitivity of the bacteria and the concentration of the drug.

Macrolides are indicated for treatment of the following conditions: acute infections caused by susceptible strains of *S. pneumoniae, Mycoplasma pneumoniae, Listeria monocytogenes,* and *Legionella pneumophila;* infections caused by group A β-hemolytic streptococci; pelvic inflammatory disease caused by *N. gonorrhoeae;* upper respiratory tract infections caused by *H. influenzae* (with sulfonamides); infections caused by *C. diphtheriae* and *Corynebacterium minutissimum* (with antitoxin); intestinal amebiasis; and infections caused by *Chlamydia trachomatis.*

In addition, macrolides may be used as prophylaxis for endocarditis before dental procedures in patients with valvular heart disease who are allergic to penicillin. Topical macrolides are indicated for the treatment of ocular infections caused by susceptible organisms and for acne vulgaris, and they may also be used prophylactically against infection in minor skin abrasions and for the treatment of skin infections caused by sensitive organisms.

Contraindications and Cautions

Macrolides are contraindicated in patients with a known allergy to any macrolide, because cross-sensitivity occurs. Ocular preparations are contraindicated for viral, fungal, or mycobacterial infections of the eye, which could be exacerbated by loss of bacteria of the normal flora.

Caution should be used in patients with hepatic dysfunction that could alter the metabolism of the drug; in those with renal disease that could interfere with the excretion of some of the drugs; in lactating women, because macrolides secreted in breast milk can cause diarrhea and superinfections in the infant; and in pregnant women, because of potential adverse effects on the developing fetus.

DRUGS IN FOCUS
Macrolides

Drug Name	Dosage/Route	Usual Indications
azithromycin (*Zithromax*)	Adult: 500 mg PO as a single dose on day 1, then 250 mg PO q.d. to a total dose of 1.5 g Pediatric: 10 mg/kg PO as a single dose on day 1, then 5 mg/kg PO on days 1–5	Treatment of mild to moderate respiratory infections and urethritis in adults and otitis media and pharyngitis/tonsillitis in children
clarithromycin (*Biaxin*)	Adult: 250–500 mg q12h PO for 7–14 d; reduce dosage with renal impairment Pediatric: 15 mg/kg per day PO given q12h for 10 d	Treatment of various respiratory, skin, sinus, and maxillary infections; effective against mycobacteria
dirithromycin (*Dynabac*)	Adult: 500 mg PO q.d. Pediatric: safety for use in children <12 years of age not established	Treatment of respiratory tract and skin infections
Ⓟ erythromycin (*E-Mycin, Eryc*)	Adult: 15–20 mg/kg per day IV or PO Pediatric: 30–50 mg/kg per day PO in divided doses	Treatment of infections in people allergic to penicillin, Legionnaires' disease, infections caused by *Corynebacterium diphtheriae, Ureaplasma* species, syphilis, mycoplasma pneumonias, chlamydial infections

Adverse Effects

Relatively few adverse effects are associated with the macrolides. The most frequent ones, which involve the direct effects of the drug on the GI tract, are often uncomfortable enough to limit the use of the drug. These include abdominal cramping, anorexia, diarrhea, vomiting, and pseudomembranous colitis. Other effects include neurological symptoms such as confusion, abnormal thinking, and uncontrollable emotions, which could be related to drug effects on the CNS membranes; hypersensitivity reactions ranging from rash to anaphylaxis; and superinfections related to the loss of normal flora.

Clinically Important Drug–Drug Interactions

Increased serum levels of digoxin occur when digoxin is taken concurrently with macrolides. Patients who receive both drugs should have their digoxin levels monitored and dosage adjusted during and after treatment with the macrolide.

In addition, when oral anticoagulants, theophyllines, carbamazepine, or corticosteroids are administered concurrently with macrolides, the effects of these drugs reportedly increase as a result of metabolic changes in the liver. Patients who take any of these combinations may require reduced dosage of the particular drug and careful monitoring.

When cycloserine is taken with macrolides, increased serum levels of cycloserine have occurred, with a resultant risk of renal toxicity. This combination should be avoided if at all possible.

Because the combination of macrolides and astemizole may lead to potentially fatal cardiac arrhythmias, this combination should also be avoided.

Clinically Important Drug–Food Interactions

Food in the stomach decreases the absorption of oral macrolides. Therefore, the antibiotic should be given on an empty stomach, 1 hour before or at least 2 to 3 hours after meals. A macrolide should be taken with a full, 8-oz glass of water.

Nursing Considerations for Patients Receiving Macrolides

Assessment: History and Examination

Screen for the following possible contraindications or precautions for use of the drug: known allergy to any macrolide (obtain specific information about the nature and occurrence of allergic reactions); history of liver disease that could interfere with metabolism of the drug; and current pregnancy or lactation status, because of potential adverse effects on the fetus or infant.

Physical assessment should be performed to establish baseline data for assessing the effectiveness of the drug and the occurrence of any adverse effects associated with drug therapy. Obtain specimens for culture and sensitivity testing from the site of infection. Examine the skin for any rash or lesions to provide a baseline for possible adverse effects. Monitor temperature to detect infection. Conduct assessment of orientation, affect, and reflexes to establish a baseline for any CNS effects of the drug. Assess liver and renal function test

values to determine the status of renal and liver functioning and to determine any needed alteration in dosage.

Nursing Diagnoses

The patient receiving a macrolide may have the following nursing diagnoses related to drug therapy:

- Acute Pain related to GI or CNS effects of the drug
- Risk for Infection related to potential for superinfections
- Deficient Knowledge regarding drug therapy

Implementation

- Check culture and sensitivity reports *to ensure that this is the drug of choice for this patient.*
- Monitor hepatic and renal function test values before therapy begins *to arrange to reduce dosage as needed.*
- Ensure that the patient receives the full course of the macrolide as prescribed *to eradicate the infection and to help prevent the emergence of resistant strains.*
- Monitor the site of infection and presenting signs and symptoms (eg, fever, lethargy, urinary tract signs and symptoms) throughout the course of drug therapy. *Failure of these signs and symptoms to resolve may indicate the need to reculture the site. Arrange to continue drug therapy for at least 2 days after all signs and symptoms resolve.*
- Provide small, frequent meals as tolerated *to ensure adequate nutrition with GI upset;* frequent mouth care and ice chips or sugarless candy to suck *to provide relief of discomfort if dry mouth is a problem;* and adequate fluids *to replace fluid lost with diarrhea.*
- Ensure ready access to bathroom facilities *to assist patients with problems associated with diarrhea.*
- Institute safety measures *to protect patient from injury if CNS effects occur.*
- Arrange for appropriate treatment of superinfections as needed *to decrease severity of infection and complications.*
- Ensure patient instruction about the appropriate dosage regimen and possible adverse effects *to enhance patient knowledge about drug therapy and to promote compliance.*

The patient should

Take safety precautions, including changing position slowly and avoiding driving and hazardous tasks, if CNS effects occur.

Try to drink a lot of fluids and to maintain nutrition (very important) even though nausea, vomiting, and diarrhea may occur.

Report difficulty breathing, severe headache, severe diarrhea, severe skin rash, and mouth or vaginal sores to a health care provider.

Evaluation

- Monitor patient response to the drug (resolution of bacterial infection).

- Monitor for adverse effects (orientation and affect, GI effects, superinfections).
- Evaluate the effectiveness of the teaching plan (patient can name the drug, dosage, possible adverse effects to expect, and specific measures to help avoid adverse effects.)
- Monitor the effectiveness of comfort and safety measures and compliance with the regimen.

LINCOSAMIDES

The lincosamides are similar to the macrolides but more toxic. The lincosamides react at almost the same site in bacterial protein synthesis and are effective against the same strains of bacteria (Figure 9–2).

Clindamycin (*Cleocin*) is reserved for severe infections caused by the same strains of bacteria that are susceptible to macrolides. The drug is rapidly absorbed from the GI tract or from IM injections. Clindamycin has a half-life of 2 to 3 hours; it is metabolized in the liver and excreted in the urine and feces. Caution needs to be used in patients with hepatic or renal impairment, which could interfere with the metabolism and excretion of the drug. The drug crosses the placenta and enters breast milk; it should be used during pregnancy and lactation only if the benefit clearly outweighs the risk to the fetus and neonate. GI reactions, which are often severe, limit the usefulness of clindamycin. Severe pseudomembranous colitis has occurred as a result of treatment. However, for a serious infection caused by a susceptible bacterium, clindamycin may be the drug of choice. It is available in a parenteral form as well as in topical and vaginal forms for the treatment of local infections.

Lincomycin (*Lincocin*) is indicated to treat severe infections when penicillin cannot be given and other, less toxic antibiotics, such as the macrolides, cannot be used. It is rapidly absorbed from the GI tract or from IM injections. Lincomycin is metabolized in the liver and excreted in the urine and feces. It has a half-life of 5 hours. Caution needs to be used in patients with hepatic or renal impairment, which could interfere with the metabolism and excretion of the drug. The drug crosses the placenta and enters breast milk; it should be used during pregnancy and lactation only if the benefit clearly outweighs the risk to the fetus or the neonate. Severe GI reactions, including fatal pseudomembranous colitis, have occurred. Some other toxic effects that limit the usefulness of this drug are pain, skin infections, and bone marrow depression. Nursing care of patients taking these drugs is the same as for those taking macrolides, with additional precautions that include careful monitoring of GI activity and fluid balance and stopping the drug at the first sign of severe or bloody diarrhea.

MONOBACTAM ANTIBIOTICS

The only monobactam antibiotic currently available for use is aztreonam (*Azactam*). Among the antibiotics, its structure is unique, and little cross-resistance occurs. Aztreonam is effective against gram-negative enterobacteria and has no effect on gram-positive or anaerobic bacteria. The drug is a safe alter-

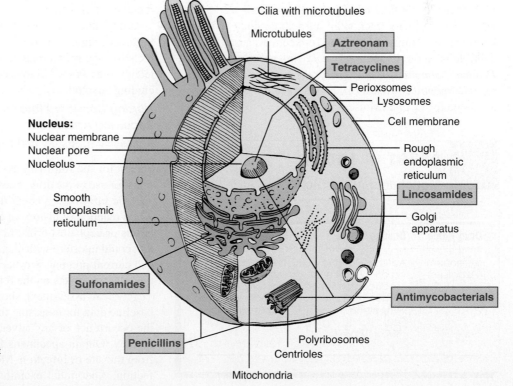

FIGURE 9–2. Sites of cellular action of lincosamides, aztreonam, penicillins, sulfonamides, tetracyclines, and antimycobacterial drugs. Lincosamides change protein function and prevent cell division or cause cell death. Aztreonam alters cell membranes to allow leakage of intracellular substances and causes cell death. Penicillins prevent bacteria from building their cells during division. Sulfonamides inhibit folic acid synthesis for RNA and DNA production. Tetracyclines inhibit protein synthesis and thus prevent reproduction. Antimycobacterial drugs affect myocbacteria in three ways. They (1) affect the mycotic coat of the bacteria, (2) alter DNA and RNA, and (3) prevent cell division.

DRUGS IN FOCUS
Lincosamides

Drug Name	Dosage/Route	Usual Indications
(P) clindamycin (*Cleocin*)	Adult: 150–300 mg PO q6h or 600–2700 mg/d in two to four equal doses; reduce dosage with renal impairment Pediatric: 8–25 mg/kg per day PO or 15–40 mg/kg per day IM or IV in three to four divided doses	Treatment of severe infections when penicillin or other less toxic antibiotics cannot be used
lincomycin (*Lincocin*)	Adult: 500 mg PO q6–8h, 600 mg IM q12–24h, or 600 mg to 1 g q8–12h; reduce dosage with renal impairment Pediatric: 30–60 mg/kg per day PO in three to four divided doses, 10 mg/kg IM q12–24h, or 10–20 mg/kg per day IV in divided doses	Treatment of severe infections when penicillin or other less toxic antibiotics cannot be used

native for treating infections caused by susceptible bacteria in patients who may be allergic to penicillins or cephalosporins. Aztreonam is absorbed well after IM injection, reaching peak effect levels in 1 to 1.5 hours. Its half-life is 1.5 to 2 hours, and it is excreted unchanged in the urine. It crosses the placenta and enters breast milk; it therefore should be used during pregnancy and lactation only if the benefit clearly outweighs the potential risk to the fetus and the neonate.

Therapeutic Actions and Indications

Aztreonam disrupts bacterial cell wall synthesis, which promotes leakage of cellular contents and cell death in susceptible bacteria (see Figure 9–2). The drug is indicated for the treatment of urinary tract, skin, intra-abdominal, and gynecological infections, as well as septicemia caused by susceptible bacteria, including *E. coli, Enterobacter, Serratia, Proteus, Salmonella, Providencia, Pseudomonas, Citrobacter, Haemophilus, Neisseria,* and *Klebsiella.* Aztreonam is available for IV and IM use only.

DRUGS IN FOCUS
Monobactam Antibiotic

Drug Name	Dosage/Route	Usual Indications
aztreonam (*Azactam*)	Adult: 500 mg to 1 g q8–12h IM or IV; reduce dosage in renal and hepatic impairment Pediatric: 30 mg/kg IM or IV q6–8h	Treatment of gram-negative onterobacterial infections, often as an alternative to penicillin

Contraindications and Cautions

Aztreonam is contraindicated with any known allergy to aztreonam. Caution should be used in patients with a history of acute allergic reaction to penicillins or cephalosporins because of the possibility of cross-reactivity; in those with renal or hepatic dysfunction that could interfere with the clearance and excretion of the drug; and in pregnant and lactating women, because of potential adverse effects on the neonate.

Adverse Effects

The adverse effects associated with the use of aztreonam are relatively mild. Local GI effects include nausea, GI upset, vomiting, and diarrhea. Hepatic enzyme elevations related to direct drug effects on the liver may also occur. Other effects include inflammation, phlebitis, and discomfort at injection sites as well as the potential for allergic response, including anaphylaxis.

Nursing Considerations for Patients Receiving Aztreonam
Assessment: History and Examination

Screen for the following possible contraindications or cautions for use of the drug: known allergy to aztreonam (obtain specific information about the nature and occurrence of allergic reactions); history of acute allergic reactions to penicillins or cephalosporins; history of liver or kidney disease that could interfere with clearance and excretion of the drug; and current pregnancy or lactation status, because of potential adverse effects on the fetus or infant.

Physical assessment should be performed to establish baseline data for assessing the effectiveness of the drug and the occurrence of any adverse effects associated with drug therapy. Obtain specimens for culture and sensitivity tests from the site of infection. Monitor temperature to detect infection. Abdominal examination should be performed and liver and kidney function tests should be done to determine any needed alteration in dosage.

Nursing Diagnoses

The patient receiving aztreonam may have the following nursing diagnoses related to drug therapy:

- Acute Pain related to GI and local effects of drug
- Deficient Knowledge regarding drug therapy
- Deficient Fluid Volume (diarrhea)

Implementation

- Check culture and sensitivity reports *to ensure that this is the drug of choice for this patient.*
- Monitor hepatic and renal function tests before therapy *to arrange to reduce dosage as needed.*
- Ensure that the patient receives the full course of aztreonam as prescribed *to eradicate the infection and to help prevent the emergence of resistant strains.*
- Monitor the site of infection and presenting signs and symptoms (eg, fever, lethargy) throughout the course of drug therapy. *Failure of drug therapy to resolve these signs and symptoms may indicate the need to reculture the site. Arrange to continue drug therapy for at least 2 days after the resolution of all signs and symptoms.*
- Provide small, frequent meals as tolerated, frequent mouth care, and ice chips or sugarless candy to suck if dry mouth is a problem *to relieve discomfort and ensure nutrition.*
- Provide adequate fluids *to replace fluid lost with diarrhea.*
- Ensure ready access to bathroom facilities *to assist patients with problems associated with diarrhea.*
- Ensure that the patient is instructed about the route of administration and possible side effects *to enhance patient knowledge about drug therapy and to promote compliance.* The drug can only be given IV or IM, so the patient will not be responsible for administering the drug.

The patient should:

Try to drink a lot of fluids and to maintain nutrition (very important), even though nausea, vomiting, and diarrhea may occur.

Report difficulty breathing, severe diarrhea, or mouth or vaginal sores to a health care provider.

Evaluation

- Monitor patient response to the drug (resolution of bacterial infection).
- Monitor for adverse effects (orientation and affect, GI effects, local inflammation).
- Evaluate the effectiveness of the teaching plan (patient can name the drug, dosage, possible adverse effects to expect, and specific measures to help avoid adverse effects).
- Monitor the effectiveness of comfort and safety measures and compliance with the regimen.

PENICILLINS AND PENICILLINASE-RESISTANT ANTIBIOTICS

Penicillin was the first antibiotic introduced for clinical use. Sir Alexander Fleming used *Penicillium* molds to produce the original penicillin in the 1920s. Subsequent versions of penicillin were developed to decrease the adverse effects of the drug and to modify it to act on resistant bacteria.

With the prolonged use of penicillin, more and more bacterial species have synthesized the enzyme penicillinase to counteract the effects of penicillin. Researchers have developed a group of drugs with a resistance to penicillinase, which allows them to remain effective against bacteria that are now resistant to the penicillins. The actual drug chosen depends on the sensitivity of the bacteria causing the infection, the desired and available routes, and the personal experience of the clinician with the particular agent. Culture and sensitivity tests should always be performed to ensure that the causative organism is sensitive to the penicillin selected for use. With the emergence of many resistant strains of bacteria, this has become increasingly important.

Therapeutic Actions and Indications

The penicillins and penicillinase-resistant antibiotics produce bactericidal effects by interfering with the ability of susceptible bacteria to build their cell walls when they are dividing (see Figure 9–2). These drugs prevent the bacteria from biosynthesizing the framework of the cell wall, and the bacteria with weakened cell walls swell and then burst from osmotic pressure within the cell. Because human cells do not use the biochemical process that the bacteria use to form the cell wall, this effect is a selective toxicity.

The penicillins are indicated for the treatment of streptococcal infections, including pharyngitis, tonsillitis, scarlet fever, and endocarditis; pneumococcal infections; staphylococcal infections; fusospirochetal infections; ratbite fever; diphtheria; anthrax; syphilis; and uncomplicated gonococcal infections. At high doses, these drugs are also used to treat meningococcal meningitis.

Pharmacokinetics

Most of the penicillins are rapidly absorbed from the GI tract, reaching peak levels in 1 hour. They are sensitive to the gastric acid levels in the stomach and should be taken on an empty stomach to ensure adequate absorption. Penicillins are excreted unchanged in the urine, making renal function an important factor in safe use of the drug. There are no adequate studies of use during pregnancy, so the drug should be used in pregnancy only if the benefit clearly outweighs the potential risk to the fetus. Penicillins enter breast milk and can cause diarrhea and adverse reactions in the baby. Use during lactation should be limited to situations in which the mother clearly would benefit from the drug.

Contraindications and Cautions

These drugs are contraindicated in patients with allergies to penicillin, cephalosporins, or other allergens. Penicillin sensitivity tests are available if the patient's history of allergy is

DRUGS IN FOCUS
Penicillins

Drug Name	Dosage/Route	Usual Indications
Penicillins		
penicillin G benzathine (*Bicillin, Permapen*)	Adult: 1.2–2.4 million units IM Pediatric: 900,000 to 1.2 million units IM as a single injection	Severe infections caused by sensitive organisms; treatment of syphilis and erysipeloid infections
penicillin G potassium (*Pfizerpen*)	Adult: 1–20 million U/d IM or IV, depending on condition Pediatric: 100,000 to 1 million U/d IM or IV	Treatment of severe infections; used for several days in some cases
penicillin G procaine (*Crysticillin-AS*)	Adult: 600,000 to 1.2 million U/d IM Pediatric: 50,000 U/kg per day IM	Treatment of moderately severe infections daily for 8–12 d
penicillin V (*Beepen-VK*)	Adult 250–500 mg q6–8h PO Pediatric: 15–62.5 mg/kg per day PO in divided doses q6–8h	Used for prophylaxis for bacterial endocarditis; Lyme disease, urinary tract infections (UTIs), and other susceptible infections
Extended-spectrum Penicillins		
ampicillin (*D-Amp, Omnipen*)	Adult: 250–500 mg IM or IV q6h, then 500 mg PO q6h when oral use is feasible Pediatric: 60 mg/kg per day IM or IV in four to six divided doses, then 250 mg PO q6h	Broad spectrum of activity; useful form if switch from parenteral to oral is anticipated; monitor for nephritis
P amoxicillin (*Amoxil, Trimox*)	Adult 250–500 mg PO q8h Pediatric: 20 mg/kg per day PO in divided doses q8h	Broad spectrum of uses for adults and children
carbenicillin (*Geocillin*)	Adult: 382–764 mg PO q.i.d. Pediatric: safety not established	Treatment of UTIs in adults; not used in children
mezlocillin (*Mezlin*)	Adult: 200–300 mg/kg per day IV or IM in four to six divided doses Pediatric: 50–75 mg/kg q8h IV or IM	Treatment of severe infections and broad range of susceptible infections; four to six injections per day may make this drug undesirable for some patients
piperacillin (*Pipracil*)	Adult: 3–4 g q4–6h IM or IV; reduce dosage with renal impairment Pediatric: 200–300 mg/kg per day IM or IV in four to six divided doses	Treatment of severe infections and for postoperative prophylaxis; need for four to six injections per day or IV infusion limits use in some patients
ticarcillin (*Ticar*)	Adult: 1 g IM or direct IV q6h; reduce dosage with renal impairment Pediatric: 50–100 mg/kg per day IM or direct IV q6–8h	Severe infections caused by susceptible bacteria
Penicillinase-resistant Antibiotics		
P cloxacillin (*Cloxapen, Tegapen*)	Adult: 250–500 mg PO q6h Pediatric: 50 mg/kg per day PO in divided doses q6h	Infections by penicillinase-producing staphylococci; must be taken around the clock for 10 d
dicloxacillin (*Dyapen, Dycill*)	Adult: 125 mg PO q6h Pediatric: 12.5 mg/kg per day PO in divided doses q6h	Infections by penicillinase-producing staphylococci; must be taken around the clock for 10 d
nafcillin (*Nafcil, Nallpen*)	Adult: 500–1000 mg IV q4h, 500 mg IM q6h, or 250–500 mg PO q4–6h Pediatric: 25 mg/kg IM b.i.d. or 25–50 mg/kg/day PO in four divided doses	Infections by penicillinase-producing staphylococci as well as group A hemolytic streptococci, plus *Streptococcus viridans*; drug of choice if switch to oral form is anticipated
oxacillin (*Bactocill, Prostaphilin*)	Adult: 500 mg PO q4–6h or 250–500 mg IM or IV q4–6h Pediatric: 50 mg/kg per day IM, IV or PO in equally divided doses q4–6h	Infections by penicillinase-producing staphylococci; streptococci; drug of choice if switch to oral form is anticipated

unclear and a penicillin is the drug of choice. Caution should be exercised in patients with renal disease (lowered doses are necessary because excretion is reduced), in those who are pregnant, and in lactating women (diarrhea and superinfections may occur in the infant).

Adverse Effects

The major adverse effects of penicillin therapy involve the GI tract. Common adverse effects include nausea, vomiting, diarrhea, abdominal pain, glossitis, stomatitis, gastritis, sore mouth, and furry tongue. These effects are primarily related to the loss of bacteria from the normal flora and the subsequent opportunistic infections that occur. Superinfections, including yeast infections, are also very common and are again associated with the loss of bacteria from the normal flora. Pain and inflammation at the injection site can occur with injectable forms of the drugs. Hypersensitivity reactions may include rash, fever, wheezing, and, with repeated exposure, anaphylaxis that can progress to anaphylactic shock and death.

Clinically Important Drug–Drug Interactions

If penicillins and penicillinase-resistant antibiotics are taken concurrently with tetracyclines, a decrease in the effectiveness of the penicillins results. This combination should be avoided if at all possible, or the penicillin dosages should be raised, which could increase the occurrence of adverse effects.

In addition, when the parenteral forms of penicillins and penicillinase-resistant drugs are administered in combination with any of the parenteral aminoglycosides, inactivation of the aminoglycosides occurs. These combinations should also be avoided.

Nursing Considerations for Patients Receiving Penicillins and Penicillinase-Resistant Antibiotics
Assessment: History and Examination

Screen for the following possible contraindications or cautions for use of the drug: known allergy to any cephalosporins, penicillins, or other allergens, because cross-sensitivity often occurs (obtain specific information about the nature and occurrence of allergic reactions); history of renal disease that could interfere with excretion of the drug; and current pregnancy or lactation status.

Physical assessment should be performed to establish baseline data for evaluating the effectiveness of the drug and the occurrence of any adverse effects associated with drug therapy. Perform culture and sensitivity tests at the site of infection. Examine the skin and mucous membranes for any rashes or lesions to provide a baseline for possible adverse effects. Note respiratory status to provide a baseline for the occurrence of hypersensitivity reactions. Examine the abdomen to monitor for adverse effects. Evaluate renal function test findings, including BUN and creatinine clearance, to assess the status of renal functioning and to determine any needed alteration in dosage. Examine injection sites to provide a baseline for determining adverse reactions or abscess formation.

Nursing Diagnoses

The patient receiving a penicillin may have the following nursing diagnoses related to drug therapy:

- Acute Pain related to GI effects of drug
- Imbalanced Nutrition: Less than Body Requirements related to multiple GI effects of the drug or to superinfections
- Deficient Knowledge regarding drug therapy

Implementation

- Check culture and sensitivity reports *to ensure that this is the drug of choice for this patient.*
- Monitor renal function tests before and periodically during therapy *to arrange for dosage reduction as needed.*
- Ensure that the patient receives the full course of the penicillin as prescribed, in doses around the clock, *to increase effectiveness.*
- Explain storage requirements for suspensions and the importance of completing the prescribed therapeutic course even if signs and symptoms have disappeared, *to increase the effectiveness of the drug and decrease the risk of developing resistant strains.*
- Monitor the site of infection and presenting signs and symptoms (eg, fever, lethargy) throughout the course of drug therapy. *Failure of these signs and symptoms to resolve may indicate the need to reculture the site. Arrange to continue drug therapy for at least 2 days after the resolution of all signs and symptoms.*
- Provide small, frequent meals as tolerated, ensure frequent mouth care, and offer ice chips or sugarless candy to suck if stomatitis and sore mouth are problems *to relieve discomfort and ensure nutrition.*
- Provide adequate fluids *to replace fluid lost with diarrhea.*
- Monitor the patient for any signs of superinfection and *arrange for treatment if superinfections occur.*
- Monitor injection sites regularly and *provide warm compresses and gentle massage to injection sites if painful or swollen.* If signs of phlebitis occur, remove the IV line and reinsert it in a different vein *to continue the drug regimen.*
- Be sure to instruct the patient regarding the appropriate dosage regimen and possible adverse effects *to enhance the patient's knowledge about drug therapy and promote compliance.*

The patient should

Try to drink a lot of fluids and to maintain nutrition (very important) even though nausea, vomiting, and diarrhea may occur.
Report difficulty breathing, severe headache, severe diarrhea, dizziness, weakness, mouth sores, and vaginal itching or sores to a health care provider.

See the accompanying Patient Teaching Checklist for penicillins.

PATIENT TEACHING CHECKLIST
Penicillins

Create customized patient teaching materials for a specific antibiotic, such as penicillin, from the CD-ROM. Patient teaching should stress the following points for drugs within this antibiotic class:

- The penicillins are used to help destroy specific bacteria that are causing infections in the body. They are effective against only certain bacteria; they are not effective against viruses (such as cold germs) or other bacteria. To clear up a bacterial infection, the penicillins must act on the bacteria over a period of time, so it is very important to complete the full course of this penicillin to avoid recurrence of the infection.
- The drug should be taken on an empty stomach with a full 8-oz glass of water—1 hour before meals or 2 to 3 hours after meals is best. Do not use fruit juice, soft drinks, or milk to take your drug, because these foods may interfere with its effectiveness. (This does not apply to bacampicillin, amoxicillin, or penicillin V.)
- Common effects of these drugs include stomach upset, diarrhea, changes in taste, and change in the color of the tongue. Small, frequent meals may help. It is important to try to maintain good nutrition. These effects should go away when the drug is stopped.
- Report any of the following to your health care provider: hives, rash, fever, difficulty breathing, severe diarrhea.
- Tell any doctor, nurse, or other health care provider that you are taking this drug.
- Keep this drug and all medications out of the reach of children.
- Do not share this drug with other people, and do not use this medication to self-treat other infections.
- It is very important that you complete the full course of your prescription, even if you feel better before you finish it.

This Teaching Checklist reflects general patient teaching guidelines. It is not meant to be a substitute for drug-specific teaching information, which is available in nursing drug guides.

Evaluation

- Monitor patient response to the drug (resolution of bacterial infection).
- Monitor for adverse effects (GI effects; local irritation, phlebitis at injection and IV sites; superinfections).
- Evaluate the effectiveness of the teaching plan (patient can name the drug, dosage, possible adverse effects to expect, and specific measures to help avoid adverse effects).
- Monitor the effectiveness of comfort and safety measures and compliance with the regimen (see Nursing Care Guide: Antibiotics/Penicillins).

SULFONAMIDES

The sulfonamides, or sulfa drugs, are drugs that inhibit folic acid synthesis. Folic acid is necessary for the synthesis of purine and pyrimidines, which are precursors of RNA and DNA. For cells to grow and reproduce, they require folic acid. Humans cannot synthesize folic acid and depend on the folate found in the diet to obtain this essential substance. Bacteria are impermeable to folic acid and must synthesize it inside the cell.

Because of the emergence of resistant bacterial strains and the development of newer antibiotics, the sulfa drugs are not used much any more. However, they remain an inexpensive and effective treatment for urinary tract infections and trachoma, especially in developing countries and when cost is an issue.

Sulfadiazine (generic) is an oral agent with broad use in infections caused by susceptible bacteria. It is slowly absorbed from the GI tract, reaching peak levels in 3 to 6 hours.

Sulfisoxazole (generic) is used for a broad spectrum of infections caused by susceptible bacteria. This drug is also recommended by the Centers for Disease Control and Prevention (CDC) for the treatment of sexually transmitted diseases and has the unlabeled use of prophylaxis for recurrent otitis media. It is rapidly absorbed from the GI tract, reaching peak levels in 2 hours. After being metabolized in the liver, it is excreted in the urine with a half-life of 4.5 to 7.8 hours.

Sulfasalazine (*Azulfidine*) is a sulfapyridine that is carried by aminosalicylic acids (aspirin) that release the aminosalicylic acid in the colon. Sulfasalazine is used to treat ulcerative colitis and Crohn's disease because of the direct anti-inflammatory effect of the aspirin. In a delayed-release form, this sulfa drug is also used to treat rheumatoid arthritis that does not respond to other treatments. It is rapidly absorbed from the GI tract, reaching peak levels in 2 to 6 hours. After being metabolized in the liver, it is excreted in the urine with a half-life of 5 to 10 hours.

Cotrimoxazole (*Septra, Bactrim*) is a combination drug that contains sulfamethoxazole and trimethoprim, another antibacterial drug. This combination has proved to be very effective in the treatment of otitis media, bronchitis, urinary tract infections, and pneumonitis caused by *Pneumocystis carinii,* which is a serious problem in patients with compromised immune systems (eg, those with AIDS). It is rapidly absorbed from the GI tract, reaching peak levels in 2 hours. After being metabolized in the liver, it is excreted in the urine with a half-life of 7 to 12 hours.

Therapeutic Actions and Indications

The sulfonamides competitively block para-aminobenzoic acid (PABA) to prevent the synthesis of folic acid in susceptible bacteria that synthesize their own folates for the production of RNA and DNA (see Figure 9–2). This includes gram-negative and gram-positive bacteria such as *C. trachomatis; Nocardia;* and some strains of *H. influenzae, E. coli,* and *P. mirabilis.* These drugs are used to treat trachoma (a leading cause of blindness), nocardiosis (which causes pneumonias as well as brain abscesses and inflammation), urinary tract infections, and sexually transmitted diseases.

NURSING CARE GUIDE

Antibiotics/Penicillins

Assessment	Nursing Diagnoses	Implementation	Evaluation
HISTORY Allergies to any of these drugs or other antibiotics; renal or liver dysfunction; pregnancy or lactation; other drugs administered	Acute Pain related to GI effects, superinfections	Check culture and sensitivity tests before giving drug.	Evaluate drug effects: resolution of bacterial infection.
	Deficient Knowledge regarding drug therapy	Monitor renal function and arrange to reduce dose as necessary.	Monitor for adverse effects: GI effects, superinfections, liver changes.
		Ensure that patient receives the full course of treatment; space dosage around the clock; administer oral drug on an empty stomach.	
	Imbalanced Nutrition: Less than Body Requirements, related to GI effects	Provide small, frequent meals and monitor nutritional status.	Monitor for drug–drug interactions as indicated for each drug.
		Monitor for superinfections and arrange treatment as indicated.	Evaluate effectiveness of patient teaching program.
		Provide support and reassurance for dealing with drug effects and discomfort.	Evaluate effectiveness of comfort and safety measures.
		Provide patient teaching regarding drug name, dosage, adverse effects, precautions, and warning signs to report.	
PHYSICAL EXAMINATION General: temperature, culture site of infection, affect Skin: color, lesions, texture Local: infection sites GI: abdominal, liver evaluation Hematologic: CBC and differential; renal and hepatic function test			

Pharmacokinetics

The sulfonamides are absorbed from the GI tract, metabolized in the liver, and excreted in the urine. The time to peak level and the half-life of the individual drug varies (described earlier). The sulfonamides are teratogenic; they are distributed into breast milk and should not be used during pregnancy or lactation.

Contraindications and Cautions

The sulfonamides are contraindicated with any known allergy to any sulfonamide, to sulfonylureas, or to thiazide diuretics, because cross-sensitivities occur; during pregnancy, because the drugs can cause birth defects as well as kernicterus; and during lactation, because of a risk of kernicterus, diarrhea, and rash in the infant. Caution should be used in patients with renal disease or a history of kidney stones because of the possibility of increased toxic effects of the drugs.

Adverse Effects

Adverse effects associated with sulfonamides include GI effects such as nausea, vomiting, diarrhea, abdominal pain, anorexia, stomatitis, and hepatic injury, which are all related to direct irritation of the GI tract and the death of normal bacteria. Renal effects are related to the filtration of the drug

DRUGS IN FOCUS
Sulfonamides

Drug Name	Dosage/Route	Usual Indications
sulfadiazine (generic)	Adult: 2–4 g PO loading dose, then 2–4 g/d PO in four to six divided doses Pediatric: 75 mg/kg PO, then 120–150 mg/kg per day PO in four to six divided doses	Treatment of a broad spectrum of infections
sulfisoxazole (generic)	Adult: 2–4 g PO loading dose, then 4–8 g/d PO in four to six divided doses Pediatric: 75 mg/kg PO, then 120–150 mg/kg per day PO in four to six divided doses	Treatment of a wide range of infections including various sexually transmitted diseases
Ⓟ sulfasalazine (*Azulfidine*)	Adult: 3–4 g/d PO in evenly divided doses, then 500 mg PO q.i.d. Pediatric: 40–60 mg/kg per day PO in divided doses, then 20–30 mg/kg per day PO in four equally divided doses	Treatment of ulcerative colitis and Crohn's disease
cotrimoxazole (*Septra, Bactrim*)	Adult: 2 tablets PO q12h; reduce dosage with renal impairment Pediatric: 8 mg/kg per day trimethoprim plus 40 mg sulfamethoxazole PO q12h	Treatment of otitis media, bronchitis, urinary tract infections, and pneumonitis caused by *Pneumocystis carinii*

in the glomerulus and include crystalluria, hematuria, and proteinuria, which can progress to a nephrotic syndrome and possible toxic nephrosis. CNS effects include headache, dizziness, vertigo, ataxia, convulsions, and depression (possibly related to drug effects on the nerves). Bone marrow depression may occur and is related to drug effects on the cells that turn over rapidly in the bone marrow.

Dermatological effects include photosensitivity and rash related to direct effects on the dermal cells. A wide range of hypersensitivity reactions may also occur.

Clinically Important Drug–Drug Interactions

If sulfonamides are taken with tolbutamide, tolazamide, glyburide, glipizide, acetohexamide, or chlorpropamide, the risk of hypoglycemia increases. If this combination is needed, the patient should be monitored and a dosage adjustment of the antidiabetic agent should be made. An increase in dosage will then be needed when sulfonamide therapy stops.

When sulfonamides are taken with cyclosporine, the risk of nephrotoxicity rises. If this combination is essential, the patient should be monitored closely and the sulfonamide stopped at any sign of renal dysfunction.

Nursing Considerations for Patients Receiving Sulfonamides

Assessment: History and Examination

Screen for the following possible contraindications or cautions for use of the drug: known allergy to any sulfon-

amide, sulfonylureas, or thiazide diuretic, because cross-sensitivity often results (obtain specific information about the nature and occurrence of allergic reactions); history of renal disease that could interfere with excretion of the drug and lead to increased toxicity; and current pregnancy or lactation status.

Physical assessment should be performed to establish baseline data for assessing the effectiveness of the drug and the occurrence of any adverse effects associated with drug therapy. Obtain specimens for culture and sensitivity tests at the site of infection. Examine skin and mucous membranes for any rash or lesions to provide a baseline for possible adverse effects. Note respiratory status to provide a baseline for the occurrence of hypersensitivity reactions. Conduct assessment of orientation, affect, and reflexes to monitor for adverse drug effects and examination of the abdomen to monitor for adverse effects. Monitor renal function test findings, including BUN and creatinine clearance, to evaluate the status of renal functioning and to determine any needed alteration in dosage. A complete blood count (CBC) also should be performed to establish a baseline to monitor for adverse effects.

Nursing Diagnoses

The patient receiving a sulfonamide may have the following nursing diagnoses related to drug therapy:

• Acute Pain related to GI, CNS, or skin effects of drug

- Disturbed Sensory Perception related to CNS effects
- Imbalanced Nutrition: Less than Body Requirements, related to multiple GI effects of the drug
- Deficient Knowledge regarding drug therapy

Implementation

- Check culture and sensitivity reports *to ensure that this is the drug of choice for this patient*, and repeat cultures if response is not as anticipated.
- Monitor renal function tests before and periodically during therapy *to arrange for a dosage reduction as necessary*.
- Ensure that the patient receives the full course of the sulfonamide as prescribed *to increase therapeutic effects and decrease the risk for development of resistant strains*.
- Administer the oral drug on an empty stomach 1 hour before or 2 hours after meals with a full glass of water *to promote adequate absorption of the drug*.
- Discontinue the drug immediately if hypersensitivity reactions occur *to prevent potentially fatal reactions*.
- Provide small, frequent meals and adequate fluids as tolerated; encourage frequent mouth care; and offer ice chips or sugarless candy to suck if stomatitis and sore mouth are problems *to relieve discomfort, ensure nutrition, and replace fluid lost with diarrhea*.
- Monitor CBC and urinalysis test results before and periodically during therapy *to check for adverse effects*.
- Be sure to instruct the patient about the appropriate dosage regimen, the proper way to take the drug (on an empty stomach with a full glass of water), and possible adverse effects, *to enhance patient knowledge about drug therapy and to promote compliance*.

The patient should

Avoid driving or operating dangerous machinery, because dizziness, lethargy, and ataxia may occur.
Try to drink a lot of fluids and to maintain nutrition (very important), even though nausea, vomiting, and diarrhea may occur.
Report any difficulty in breathing, rash, ringing in the ears, fever, sore throat, or blood in the urine to a health care provider.

Evaluation

- Monitor patient response to the drug (resolution of bacterial infection).
- Monitor for adverse effects (GI effects, CNS effects, rash, and crystalluria).
- Evaluate the effectiveness of the teaching plan (patient can name the drug, dosage, possible adverse effects to expect, and specific measures to help avoid adverse effects).
- Monitor the effectiveness of comfort and safety measures and compliance with the regimen.

TETRACYCLINES

The tetracyclines were developed as semisynthetic antibiotics based on the structure of a common soil mold. They work by inhibiting protein synthesis in susceptible bacteria. They are composed of four rings, which is how they got their name. Researchers have developed newer tetracyclines to increase absorption and tissue penetration. Widespread resistance to the tetracyclines has limited their use in recent years.

Tetracycline (*Sumycin, Panmycin,* and others) is available in oral and topical forms for treatment of a wide variety of infections, including acne vulgaris and minor skin infections caused by susceptible organisms. When penicillin is contraindicated, tetracycline is often used. Tetracycline is also available as an ophthalmic agent to treat superficial ocular lesions caused by susceptible microorganisms and as a prophylactic agent for ophthalmia neonatorum caused by *N. gonorrhoeae* and *C. trachomatis*.

Demeclocycline (*Declomycin*) is available in oral form for treating a wide variety of infections. Like tetracycline, it is also often used when penicillin is contraindicated.

Doxycycline (*Doryx, Doxy Caps,* and others) is available in oral and IV forms. Used for a wide variety of infections, this drug is recommended in the treatment of traveler's diarrhea and some sexually transmitted diseases.

Minocycline (*Minocin*) is also available in IV and oral forms. It is used to treat severe infections caused by susceptible bacteria. In addition, minocycline is the drug of choice in treating meningococcal carriers (not the disease itself) and various uncomplicated GU and gynecological infections.

Oxytetracycline (*Terramycin*) is available for oral, IM, and IV use. It is used to treat a wide variety of infections caused by susceptible bacteria and when penicillin is contraindicated. Oxytetracycline is also used as an adjunctive therapy in the treatment of acute intestinal amebiasis.

Therapeutic Actions and Indications

The tetracyclines inhibit protein synthesis in susceptible bacteria, leading to the inability of the bacteria to multiply (see Figure 9–2). Because the affected protein is similar to a protein found in human cells, these drugs can be toxic to humans at high concentrations. Tetracyclines, which are effective against a wide range of bacteria, are indicated for treatment of infections caused by rickettsiae, *M. pneumoniae, Borrelia recurrentis, H. influenzae, Haemophilus ducreyi, Pasteurella pestis, Pasteurella tularensis, Bartonella bacilliformis, Bacteroides* species, *Vibrio comma, Vibrio fetus, Brucella* species, *E. coli, E. aerogenes, Shigella* species, *Acinetobacter calcoaceticus, Klebsiella* species, *Diplococcus pneumoniae,* and *S. aureus;* against agents that cause psittacosis, ornithosis, lymphogranuloma venereum, and granuloma inguinale; when penicillin is contraindicated in susceptible infections; and for treatment of acne and uncomplicated GU infections caused by *C. trachomatis*. Some of the tetracyclines are also used as adjuncts in the treatment of certain protozoal infections.

DRUGS IN FOCUS
Tetracyclines

Drug Name	Dosage/Route	Usual Indications
demeclocycline (*Declomycin*)	Adult: 150 mg PO q.i.d. or 300 mg PO b.i.d. Pediatric (>8 y): 6–12 mg/kg per day PO in two to four divided doses	Treatment of a wide variety of infections when penicillin cannot be used
doxycycline (*Doryx, Doxy Caps*)	Adult: 200 mg/d IV in two infusions of 1–4 h each or 100–300 mg/d PO Pediatric (>8 y): 4.4 mg/kg per day IV in one or two transfusions or 4.4 mg/kg per day PO	Treatment of a wide variety of infections, including traveler's diarrhea and sexually transmitted diseases
minocycline (*Minocin*)	Adult: 200 mg IV, followed by 100 mg IV q12h, or 200 mg PO, then 100 mg PO q12h Pediatric (>8 y): 4 mg/kg IV, followed by 2 mg/kg IV or PO q12h	Treatment of meningococcal carriers and of various uncomplicated genitourinary and gynecological infections
oxytetracycline (*Terramycin*)	Adult: 250 mg q.d. IM, or 250–500 mg IV q12h, or 1–2 g/d PO in divided doses Pediatric (>8 y): 15–25 mg/kg per day IM or 12 mg/kg per day IV in divided doses or 25–50 mg/kg per day PO in two to four divided doses	Treatment of a variety of infections caused by susceptible bacteria when penicillin is contraindicated; adjunct therapy in the treatment of acute intestinal amebiasis
Ⓟ tetracycline (*Sumycin, Panmycin*)	Adult: 1–2 g/d PO in divided doses; topical applied generously to affected area Pediatric (>8 y): 25–50 mg/kg per day PO in four divided doses	Treatment of a wide variety of infections, including acne vulgaris and minor skin infections caused by susceptible organisms; as an ophthalmic agent to treat superficial ocular lesions caused by susceptible microorganisms; as a prophylactic agent for ophthalmia neonatorum caused by *Neisseria gonorrhoeae* and *Chlamydia trachomatis*

Pharmacokinetics

Tetracyclines are absorbed adequately, but not completely, from the GI tract. Their absorption is affected by food, iron, calcium, and other drugs in the stomach. Tetracyclines are concentrated in the liver and excreted unchanged in the urine, with half-lives ranging from 12 to 25 hours. These drugs cross the placenta and pass into breast milk. They should not be used in women who are pregnant or lactating, or in children younger than 8 years of age, because they can permanently discolor and damage enamel in developing teeth. They can also promote calcium complex formations in bone, which leads to decreased bone growth.

Contraindications and Cautions

Tetracyclines are contraindicated in patients with known allergy to tetracyclines or to tartrazine (ie, in specific oral preparations that contain tartrazine) and during pregnancy and lactation because of effects on the bones and teeth.

Tetracyclines should be used with caution in children younger than 8 years of age, because they can potentially damage the bones and teeth. They are also used with caution in patients with hepatic or renal dysfunction, because they are concentrated in the bile and excreted in the urine. The ophthalmic preparation is contraindicated in patients who have fungal, mycobacterial, or viral ocular infections, because the drug kills not only the undesired bacteria but also bacteria of the normal flora, which increases the risk for exacerbation of the ocular infection that is being treated.

Adverse Effects

The major adverse effects of tetracycline therapy involve direct irritation of the GI tract and include nausea, vomiting, diarrhea, abdominal pain, glossitis, and dysphagia. Fatal hepatotoxicity related to the drug's irritating effect on the liver has also been reported. Skeletal effects involve damage to the teeth and bones. Because tetracyclines have an affinity for teeth and bones, they accumulate there, weakening the structure and causing staining and pitting of teeth and bones. Dermatological effects include photosensitivity and rash. Superinfections, including yeast infections, occur when bacteria of the normal flora are destroyed. Local effects, such as pain and stinging with topical or ocular application, are fairly common. Less frequent are hematological effects, such as hemolytic anemia and bone marrow depression secondary to the effects on bone marrow cells that turn over rapidly. Hypersensitivity reactions reportedly range from urticaria to anaphylaxis and also include intracranial hypertension.

Clinically Important Drug–Drug Interactions

When penicillin G and tetracyclines are taken concurrently, the effectiveness of penicillin G decreases. If this combination is used, the dose of the penicillin should be increased.

When oral contraceptives are taken with tetracyclines, the effectiveness of the contraceptives decreases. Therefore, patients who take oral contraceptives should be advised to use an additional form of birth control while receiving the tetracycline.

When methoxyflurane is combined with tetracycline, the risk of nephrotoxicity increases. If at all possible, this combination should be avoided.

In addition, digoxin toxicity rises when tetracyclines are taken concurrently. Digoxin levels should be monitored and dosage adjusted appropriately during treatment and after tetracycline therapy is discontinued.

Finally, decreased absorption of tetracyclines results from oral combinations with calcium salts, magnesium salts, zinc salts, aluminum salts, bismuth salts, iron, urinary alkalinizers, and charcoal.

Clinically Important Drug–Food Interactions

Because oral tetracyclines are not absorbed effectively if taken with food or dairy products, tetracyclines should be given on an empty stomach 1 hour before or 2 to 3 hours after any meal or other medication.

Nursing Considerations for Patients Receiving Tetracyclines
Assessment: History and Examination

Screen for the following possible contraindications or cautions for use of the drug: known allergy to any tetracycline or to tartrazine in certain oral preparations, because cross-sensitivity often occurs (obtain specific information about the nature and occurrence of allergic reactions); any history of renal or hepatic disease that could interfere with metabolism and excretion of the drug and lead to increased toxicity; current pregnancy or lactation status; and age.

Physical examination should be performed to establish baseline data for assessing the effectiveness of the drug and the occurrence of any adverse effects associated with drug therapy. Perform culture and sensitivity tests at the site of infection. Conduct examination of the skin for any rash or lesions to provide a baseline for possible adverse effects. Note respiratory status to provide a baseline for the occurrence of hypersensitivity reactions. Evaluate renal and liver function test reports, including BUN and creatinine clearance, to assess the status of renal and liver functioning, which helps to determine any needed changes in dosage.

Nursing Diagnoses

The patient receiving a tetracycline may have the following nursing diagnoses related to drug therapy:

- Diarrhea related to drug effects
- Imbalanced Nutrition: Less than Body Requirements related to GI effects, alteration in taste, superinfections
- Impaired Skin Integrity related to rash and photosensitivity
- Deficient Knowledge regarding drug therapy

Implementation

- Check culture and sensitivity reports *to ensure that this is the drug of choice for this patient.* Arrange for repeated cultures if response is not as anticipated.
- Monitor renal and liver function test results before and periodically during therapy *to arrange for a dosage reduction as needed.*
- Ensure that the patient receives the full course of the tetracycline as prescribed. The oral drug should be taken on an empty stomach 1 hour before or 2 hours after meals with a full 8-oz glass of water. Concomitant use of antacids or salts should be avoided, because they interfere with drug absorption. *These precautions will increase drug effectiveness and decrease development of resistant strains of bacteria.*
- Discontinue the drug immediately if hypersensitivity reactions occur *to avoid the possibility of severe reactions.*
- Provide small, frequent meals as tolerated; frequent mouth care; and ice chips or sugarless candy to suck if stomatitis and sore mouth are problems *to relieve discomfort and ensure nutrition.* Also provide adequate fluids *to replace fluid lost with diarrhea.*
- Monitor for signs of superinfections *to arrange for treatment as appropriate.*
- Encourage the patient to apply sunscreen and wear clothing *to protect exposed skin from skin rashes and sunburn associated with photosensitivity reactions.*
- Be sure to instruct the patient about the appropriate dosage regimen, how to take the oral drug, and possible side effects *to enhance patient knowledge about drug therapy and to promote compliance.*

The patient should:

Try to drink a lot of fluids and maintain nutrition (very important) even though nausea, vomiting, and diarrhea may occur.

Use a barrier contraceptive method, because oral contraceptives may not be effective while a tetracycline is being used.

Know that superinfections may occur. Appropriate treatment can be arranged through the health care provider.

Use sunscreens and protective clothing if sensitivity to the sun occurs.

Know when to report dangerous adverse effects, such as difficulty breathing, rash, itching, watery diarrhea, cramps, or changes in color of urine or stool, to the health care provider.

Evaluation

- Monitor the patient's response to the drug (resolution of bacterial infection).

CASE STUDY

Antibiotics and Oral Contraceptives

THE SITUATION

In mid-January, G. S., a 27-year-old married graduate student, is seen at the student health clinic with a number of complaints, which are found to be caused by pregnancy. At the time of the visit, uterine size is consistent with a 12-week gestation.

G. S. tells you that she is surprised. She began graduate school with plans to start a family in 2 years after completion of her program, not during the program. She has organized her rigorous course work and her nonacademic activities so that almost every hour is scheduled. An interruption in her schedule is not expected or planned for. She has successfully used low-dose birth control pills for 4 years and denies any lapse in continuing this method of birth control.

In reviewing her health history, you learn that a few weeks into the fall semester she developed severe sinusitis. The student health records disclose that culture and sensitivity testing identified the infecting organism as a strain of *Klebsiella* sensitive to tetracycline. G. S. received treatment with a standard 5-day course of the antibiotic, after which the sinusitis resolved.

CRITICAL THINKING

What most likely led to this pregnancy?
How do tetracyclines and some other antibiotics and oral contraceptives interact? What are the possible ramifications of continuing to take oral contraceptives during a pregnancy?
What nursing interventions are appropriate at this time?
What options are available, and what plans for nursing interventions should be made at this first visit?

Think about the possibility of birth defects, about the stage in the patient's life, and the issues that G. S. is trying to cope with. Also think about the nature of her personality and the problems that she may face with an unplanned pregnancy and potential problems with the fetus.

DISCUSSION

Several antibiotics, including tetracycline, are known to lead to the failure of oral contraceptives as evidenced by breakthrough bleeding and unplanned pregnancy. Although the exact way in which these drugs interact is incompletely understood, it is thought that the antibiotics destroy certain bacteria in the normal flora of the GI tract. These bacteria are necessary for the breakdown and eventual absorption of the female hormones contained in the contraceptives.

The 5 days of antibiotic treatment together with the time necessary for rebuilding the normal flora was long enough for the hypothalamus to lose the negative feedback signal provided by the contraceptives that prevents ovulation and preparation of the uterus. Sensing the low hormone levels, the hypothalamus released gonadotropin-releasing hormone, which led to the release of follicle-stimulating hormone and luteinizing hormone, with subsequent ovulation.

G. S., a compulsively organized woman, may be overwhelmed by the emotional and physical stress of this unplanned pregnancy. She may investigate the possibility of birth defects caused by taking oral contraceptives during pregnancy and discover that cardiac and sexual organ and accessory organ deformities can occur. Because she may wish to undergo further studies to determine fetal abnormalities, she should be referred to an obstetrician and possibly to a genetic counselor.

G. S. will need a great deal of support and understanding during the next few days and weeks. Just having someone to talk to may be beneficial. She should receive help in understanding the reason for the birth control failure and should be encouraged to read all of the literature that comes with oral contraceptives as well as patient teaching information that should have been given out with the antibiotic. Whether she decides to terminate the pregnancy or carry it to term, she will need continued medical management and emotional support. All of the health care professionals who are involved with her care should use this as an example of the importance of clear, concise patient teaching in the administration of drug therapy.

- Monitor for adverse effects (GI effects, rash, and superinfections).
- Evaluate the effectiveness of the teaching plan (patient can name the drug, dosage, possible adverse effects to expect, and specific measures to help avoid adverse effects).
- Monitor the effectiveness of comfort and safety measures and compliance with the regimen.

For related data, see the accompanying case study, Antibiotics and Oral Contraception.

ANTIMYCOBACTERIAL ANTIBIOTICS

Mycobacteria, the group of bacteria that contain the pathogens that cause tuberculosis and leprosy, are classified on the basis of their ability to hold a stain even in the presence of a "destaining" agent such as acid. Because of this property, they are called "acid-fast" bacteria. The mycobacteria have an outer coat of mycolic acid that protects them from many disinfectants and allows them to survive for long periods in the environment. These slow-growing bacteria may need to be treated for several years before they can be eradicated.

Mycobacteria cause serious infectious diseases. The bacterium *Mycobacterium tuberculosis* causes tuberculosis, the leading cause of death from infectious disease in the world. For several years the disease was thought to be under control, but with the increasing number of people with compromised immune systems and the emergence of resistant bacterial strains, tuberculosis is once again on the rise.

Mycobacterium leprae causes leprosy, also known as

Hansen's disease, which is characterized by disfiguring skin lesions and destructive effects on the respiratory tract. Leprosy is also a worldwide health problem; it is infectious when the mycobacteria invade the skin or respiratory tract of susceptible individuals. *Mycobacterium avium-intracellulare,* which causes mycobacterium avium complex (MAC), is seen in patients with AIDS or in other patients who are severely immunocompromised. Rifabutin (*Mycobutin*), which was developed as an antituberculosis drug, is most effective against *M. avium-intracellulare.*

Antituberculosis Drugs

Tuberculosis can lead to serious damage in the lungs, the GU tract, bones, and the meninges. Because *M. tuberculosis* is so slow growing, the treatment must be continued for 6 months to 2 years. The first-line drugs for treating tuberculosis are as follows:

- Isoniazid [INH] (*Nydrazid*), which affects the mycolic acid coating of the bacterium
- Rifampin (*Rifadin, Rimactane*), which alters DNA and RNA activity in the bacterium
- Ethionamide (*Trecator SC*), which prevents cell division
- Rifapentine (*Priftin*), which alters DNA and RNA activity, causing cell death

These drugs are used in combinations of two or more agents until bacterial conversion occurs or maximum improvement is seen.

If the patient cannot take one or more of these drugs, or if the disease continues to progress because of the emergence of a resistant strain, the second-line drugs can be used:

- Ethambutol (*Myambutol*), which inhibits cellular metabolism
- Pyrazinamide (generic), which is both bactericidal and bacteriostatic

These drugs are used in combination with at least one other antituberculosis drug.

If therapeutic success is still not achieved, a third-line combination of two antituberculosis drugs can be tried:

- Capreomycin (*Capastat*), whose mechanism of action is not known
- Cycloserine (*Seromycin*), which inhibits cell wall synthesis and leads to cell death

Using the drugs in combination helps to decrease the emergence of resistant strains and to affect the bacteria at various phases during their long and slow life cycle.

Leprostatic Drugs

Antibiotics used to treat leprosy include dapsone and clofazimine.

Dapsone (generic) has been the mainstay of leprosy treatment for many years, although resistant strains are emerging. Similar to the sulfonamides, dapsone inhibits folate synthesis in susceptible bacteria. In addition to its use in leprosy, dapsone is used to treat *P. carinii* pneumonia in AIDS patients and for a variety of infections caused by susceptible bacteria, as well as for brown recluse spider bites.

Clofazimine (*Lamprene*), which binds to bacterial DNA sites and causes cell death, has been useful in the treatment of dapsone-resistant leprosy. The drug is used as part of initial leprosy treatment in combination with dapsone to prevent the development of resistant strains.

Recently, the hypnotic drug thalidomide (*Thalomid*) was approved in use for a condition that occurs after treatment for leprosy (Box 9–3).

Therapeutic Actions and Indications

Most of the antimycobacterial agents act on the DNA of the bacteria, leading to a lack of growth and eventually to bacterial death (see Figure 9–2). INH specifically affects the mycolic acid coat around the bacterium. Although many of the antimycobacterial agents are effective against other species of susceptible bacteria, their primary indications are in the treatment of tuberculosis or leprosy (as previously indicated). The antituberculosis drugs are always used in combination to affect the bacteria at various stages and to help to decrease the emergence of resistant strains.

Pharmacokinetics

The antimycobacterial agents are generally well absorbed from the GI tract, metabolized in the liver, and excreted in the urine. Caution should be used in patients with hepatic or renal dysfunction, which could interfere with the metabolism and excretion of the drugs. These drugs cross the placenta and enter breast milk; they should not be used during pregnancy and lactation unless the benefit to the mother clearly outweighs the potential risk to the neonate.

BOX 9-3

Thalidomide Approved for New Use

In the 1950s, the drug thalidomide became internationally known because it caused serious abnormalities (eg, lack of limbs, defective limbs) in the fetuses of many women who received the drug during pregnancy to help them sleep and to decrease stress. This tragedy led to the recall of thalidomide in the United States and the establishment of more stringent standards for drug testing and labeling.

In 1998, the U. S. Food and Drug Administration (FDA) approved the use of this controversial drug for the treatment of erythema nodosum leprosum, which is a painful inflammatory condition related to an immune reaction to dead bacteria that occurs after treatment for leprosy. To take thalidomide, a woman must have a negative pregnancy test, receive instruction in using birth control, and sign a release stating that she understands the risks associated with the drug. These limits on the use of a drug were the first such restrictions ever ordered by the FDA.

Thalidomide (*Thalomid*) is given in doses of 100 to 300 mg/d PO at bedtime for at least 2 wk, followed by tapered dosage in 50-mg increments over the next 2 to 4 wk.

DRUGS IN FOCUS
Antimycobacterial Drugs

Drug Name	Dosage/Route	Usual Indications
Antituberculosis Drugs		
capreomycin (*Capastat*)	Adult: 1 g/d IM for 60–120 d, followed by 1 g IM 2–3 times per wk for 18–24 mo; reduce dosage with renal impairment Pediatric: 15 mg/kg per day IM	Second-line drug for treatment of *Mycobacterium tuberculosis*
cycloserine (*Seromycin*)	Adult: 250 mg PO b.i.d. for 2 wk, then 500 mg to 1 g/d PO in divided doses Pediatric: safety not established	Second-line drug for treatment of *M. tuberculosis*
ethambutol (*Myambutol*)	Adult: 15 mg/kg per day PO as a single dose Pediatric: not recommended for children <13 y	Second-line drug for treatment of *M. tuberculosis*
ethionamide (*Trecator S.C.*)	Adult: 15–20 mg/kg per day PO in divided doses with pyridoxine Pediatric: 10–20 mg/kg per day PO individual doses with pyridoxine	First-line drug for treatment of *M. tuberculosis*
Ⓟ isoniazid (INH) (*Nydrazid*)	Adult: 5 mg/kg per day PO Pediatric: 10–20 mg/kg per day PO	First-line drug for treatment of *M. tuberculosis*
pyrazinamide (generic)	Adult and pediatric: 15–30 mg/g per day PO	Second-line drug for treatment of *M. tuberculosis*
rifabutin (*Mycobutin*)	Adult: 300 mg PO q.d. Pediatric: safety not established	Treatment of *Mycobacterium avium-intracellulare* (MAC) in patients with advanced HIV infection
rifampin (*Rifadin, Rimactane*)	Adult: 600 mg PO or IV as a single daily dose Pediatric: 10–20 mg/kg per day PO or IV	First-line drug for treatment of *M. tuberculosis*
rifapentine (*Priftin*)	Adult: 600 mg PO 2 times per week for 2 mo Pediatric: safety not established	First-line drug for treatment of *M. tuberculosis*
Leprostatic Drugs		
Ⓟ dapsone (generic)	Adult: 50–100 mg/d PO Pediatric: 1–2 mg/kg per day PO for 3 y	Treatment of leprosy, *Pneumocystis carinii* pneumonia in AIDS patients, a variety of infections caused by susceptible bacteria and brown recluse spider bites
clofazimine (*Lamprene*)	Adult: 100 mg/d PO for at least 2 y Pediatric: safety not established	Treatment of dapsone-resistant leprosy

Contraindications and Cautions

Antimycobacterial drugs are contraindicated for patients with any known allergy to these agents; in those with severe renal or hepatic failure that could interfere with the metabolism or excretion of the drug; in those with severe CNS dysfunction that could be exacerbated by the actions of the drugs; and in pregnancy because of possible adverse effects on the fetus. If an antituberculosis regimen is necessary during pregnancy, the combination of isoniazid, ethambutol, and rifampin is considered the safest.

Adverse Effects

CNS effects, such as neuritis, dizziness, headache, malaise, drowsiness, and hallucinations, are often reported and are related to direct effects of the drugs on neurons. These drugs also are irritating to the GI tract, causing nausea, vomiting, anorexia, stomach upset, and abdominal pain. Rifampin, rifabutin, and rifapentine cause discoloration of body fluids from urine to sweat and tears. Patients should be alerted that in many instances orange-tinged urine, sweat, and tears may stain clothing and permanently stain contact lenses. This can be frightening if the patient is not alerted to the possibility that it will happen. As with other antibiotics, there is always a possibility of hypersensitivity reactions and the patient should be monitored on a regular basis.

Clinically Important Drug–Drug Interactions

When rifampin and INH are used in combination, the possibility of toxic liver reactions increases. Patients should be monitored closely.

Increased metabolism and decreased drug effectiveness occur as a result of administration of quinidine, metoprolol, propranolol, corticosteroids, oral contraceptives, oral anticoagulants, oral antidiabetic agents, digoxin, theophylline, methadone, phenytoin, verapamil, cyclosporine, or ketoconazole in combination with rifampin or rifabutin. Patients who are taking these drug combinations should be monitored closely and dosage adjustments made as needed.

Nursing Considerations for Patients Receiving Antimycobacterial Antibiotics

Assessment: History and Examination

Screen for the following possible contraindications or cautions for use of the drug: known allergy to any antimycobacterial drug (obtain specific information about the nature and occurrence of allergic reactions); history of renal or hepatic disease that could interfere with metabolism and excretion of the drug and lead to toxicity; history of CNS dysfunction, including seizure disorders and neuritis, that could be exacerbated by adverse drug effects; and current pregnancy status.

Physical examination should be performed to establish baseline data for assessing the effectiveness of the drug and the occurrence of any adverse effects associated with drug therapy. Obtain specimens for culture and sensitivity testing to establish the sensitivity of the organism being treated. Examine skin for any rash or lesions to provide a baseline for possible adverse effects. Evaluate CNS for orientation, affect, and reflexes to establish a baseline and to monitor for adverse effects. Note respiratory status to provide a baseline for the occurrence of hypersensitivity reactions. Evaluate renal and liver function tests, including BUN and creatinine clearance, to assess the status of renal and liver functioning so as to determine any needed alteration in dosage.

Nursing Diagnoses

The patient receiving an antimycobacterial drug may have the following nursing diagnoses related to drug therapy:

- Imbalanced Nutrition: Less than Body Requirements, related to GI effects
- Disturbed Sensory Perception (Kinesthetic) related to CNS effects of the drug
- Acute Pain related to GI effects of drug
- Deficient Knowledge regarding drug therapy

Implementation

- Check culture and sensitivity reports *to ensure that this is the drug of choice for this patient,* and arrange repeated cultures if response is not as anticipated.
- Monitor renal and liver function test results before and periodically during therapy *to arrange for dosage reduction as needed.*
- Ensure that the patient receives the full course of the drugs *to improve effectiveness and decrease the risk of development of resistant bacterial strains.* These drugs are taken for years and often in combination. Periodic medical evaluation and reteaching are often essential to ensure compliance.
- Discontinue the drug immediately if hypersensitivity reactions occur, *to avert potentially serious reactions.*
- Encourage the patient to eat small, frequent meals as tolerated; perform frequent mouth care; and drink adequate fluids *to ensure adequate nutrition and hydration.* Monitor nutrition if GI effects become a problem.
- Ensure that the patient is instructed about the appropriate dosage regimen, use of drug combinations, and possible adverse effects *to enhance patient knowledge about drug therapy and to promote compliance.*

The patient should:

Try to drink a lot of fluids to maintain nutrition (very important) even though nausea, vomiting, and diarrhea may occur.

Use barrier contraceptives and understand that oral contraceptives may not be effective if antimycobacterial drugs are being used.

Understand that normally some of these drugs impart an orange stain to body fluids. If this occurs, the fluids may stain clothing and tears may stain contact lenses.

Report difficulty breathing, hallucinations, numbness and tingling, worsening of condition, fever and chills, or changes in color of urine or stool to a health care provider.

Evaluation

- Monitor patient response to the drug (resolution of mycobacterial infection).
- Monitor for adverse effects (GI effects, CNS changes, and hypersensitivity reactions).
- Evaluate the effectiveness of the teaching plan (patient can name the drug, dosage, possible adverse effects to expect, and specific measures to help avoid adverse effects).
- Monitor the effectiveness of comfort and safety measures and compliance with the regimen.

NEW CLASSES OF ANTIBIOTICS

Two new classes of antibiotics are described in Box 9–4 and Box 9–5.

BOX 9-4

Ketolide Approved for Treatment of Respiratory Infections

In June, 2001, the U.S. Food and Drug Administration approved the first of a new class of antibiotics, the ketolides. These antibiotics are effective against most respiratory infections and are given only once a day. Telithromycin (*Ketek*) is the first drug approved in this class. This drug is used to treat community-acquired pneumonia, acute bacterial exacerbations of chronic bronchitis, and acute bacterial sinusitis. It is given in one 800-mg oral dose each day.

BOX 9-5

New Carbepenem Antibiotic Available for Parenteral Use

In late 2001, ertapenem (*Invanz*), a methyl-carbepenem antibiotic, was approved for use in treating community-acquired pneumonias, complicated skin and skin structure infections, and complicated intra-abdominal and pelvic infections. The carbepenem inhibits the synthesis of the bacterial cell wall, causing death of the bacteria. Its effectiveness against a wide range of bacteria may help to slow the emergence of resistant strains previously sensitive only to well-established antibiotics and may also provide successful treatment of some infections that are resistant to regularly used antibiotics. *Invanz* is given as 1 g IV or IM for 3–14 d, depending on the infection. It is not approved for use in children younger than 18 years of age. It can cause allergic reactions in patients known to be allergic to penicillins or cephalosporins and is associated with gastrointestinal upset and possibly with pseudomembranous colitis. It is anticipated that other antibiotics in this class will be forthcoming if this drug proves successful.

◼▮▸◼ WEB LINKS

Health care providers, students, and patients may want to consult the following Internet resources:

Information on aminoglycosides:
  http://www.cop.ufl.edu
Information on cephalosporins:
  http://www.fhsu.edu/nursing
Information on penicillins:
  http://www.healthanswers.com
Information on tuberculosis:
  http://www.lupingroup.com
Information on resources for patients with tuberculosis:
  http://www.cpmc.columbia.edu/resources/tbcpp
Information on leprosy:
  http://www.christianity.com
Information on infectious diseases, disease prevention, recommendations for treatment, and treatment schedules (CDC):
  http://www.cdc.gov

CHAPTER SUMMARY

- Antibiotics work by disrupting protein or enzyme systems within a bacterium, causing cell death (bactericidal) or preventing multiplication (bacteriostatic).
- The proteins or enzyme systems affected by antibiotics are more likely to be found or used in bacteria than in human cells.
- The goal of antibiotic therapy is to reduce the number of invading bacteria so that the normal immune system can deal with the infection.

- The primary therapeutic use of each antibiotic is determined by the bacterial species that are sensitive to that drug, the clinical condition of the patient receiving the drug, and the benefit-to-risk ratio for the patient.
- The longer an antibiotic has been available, the more likely it is that mutant bacterial strains resistant to the mechanisms of antibiotic activity will have developed.
- The most common adverse effects of antibiotic therapy involve the GI tract (nausea, vomiting, diarrhea, anorexia, abdominal pain) and superinfections (invasion of the body by normally occurring microorganisms that are usually kept in check by the normal flora).
- To prevent or contain the growing threat of drug-resistant strains of bacteria, it is very important to use antibiotics cautiously, to complete the full course of an antibiotic prescription, and to avoid saving antibiotics for self-medication in the future. A patient and family teaching program should address these issues as well as the proper dosing procedure for the drug (even if the patient feels better) and the importance of keeping a record of any reactions to antibiotics.

Review Questions

1. A bacteriostatic substance is one that
   a. directly kills any bacteria it comes in contact with.
   b. directly kills any bacteria that are sensitive to the substance.
   c. prevents the growth of any bacteria.
   d. prevents the growth of specific bacteria that are sensitive to the substance.
2. Gram-negative bacteria
   a. are mostly found in the respiratory tract.
   b. are mostly associated with soft tissue infections.
   c. are mostly found in the GI and GU tracts.
   d. accept a positive stain when tested.
3. Antibiotics that are used together to increase their effectiveness and limit the associated adverse effects are said to be
   a. broad spectrum.
   b. synergistic.
   c. bacteriocidal.
   d. anaerobic.
4. An aminoglycoside antibiotic might be the drug of choice in treating
   a. serious infections caused by susceptible strains of gram-negative bacteria.
   b. otitis media in an infant.
   c. cystitis in a woman who is 4 months' pregnant.
   d. suspected pneumonia, before the culture results are available.
5. Which of the following is not a caution for the use of cephalosporins?
   a. allergy to penicillin
   b. renal failure
   c. allergy to aspirin
   d. concurrent treatment with aminoglycosides

6. The fluoroquinolones
   a. are found freely in nature.
   b. are associated with severe adverse reactions.
   c. are widely used to treat gram-positive infections.
   d. are broad-spectrum antibiotics with few associated adverse effects.

7. Cipro, a widely used antibiotic, is an example of
   a. a penicillin.
   b. a fluoroquinolone.
   c. an aminoglycoside.
   d. a macrolide antibiotic.

8. One commonly associated adverse effect related to fluoroquinolone use is
   a. increased salivation.
   b. constipation.
   c. photosensitivity.
   d. cough.

9. The goal of antibiotic therapy is
   a. to eradicate all bacteria from the system.
   b. to suppress resistant strains of bacteria.
   c. to reduce the number of invading bacteria so that the immune system can deal with the infection.
   d. to stop the drug as soon as the patient feels better.

10. The penicillins
    a. are bacteriostatic.
    b. are bactericidal, interfering with bacteria cell walls.
    c. are effective only if given intravenously.
    d. do not produce cross-sensitivity within their class.

11. Tetracycline use during pregnancy has been associated with
    a. gray baby syndrome.
    b. tooth and bone defects in the neonate.
    c. acne.
    d. excessive bleeding.

12. Patients receiving antibiotics do not usually need to receive teaching regarding
    a. completing the full course of drug therapy.
    b. the possibility of oral contraceptive failure.
    c. timing of the drug doses.
    d. the need for screening blood tests.

BIBLIOGRAPHY

Anonymous. The choice of antibacterial drugs. (1996). *Medical Letter on Drugs and Therapeutics, 38*, 971.

Bullock, B. L. (2000). *Focus on pathophysiology*. Philadelphia: Lippincott Williams & Wilkins.

Drug facts and comparisons. (2002). St. Louis: Facts and Comparisons.

Gilman, A., Hardman, J. G., & Limbird, L. E. (Eds.) (2002). *Goodman and Gilman's the pharmacological basis of therapeutics* (10th ed.). New York: McGraw-Hill.

Karch, A. M. (2002). *2003 Lippincott's nursing drug guide*. Philadelphia: Lippincott Williams & Wilkins.

Professional's guide to patient drug facts. (2002). St. Louis: Facts and Comparisons.

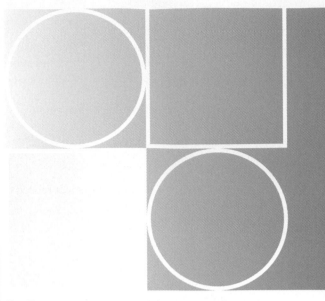

Antiviral Agents

Viruses cause a variety of conditions, ranging from warts, to the common cold and "flu," to diseases such as chickenpox and measles. A single virus particle is composed of a piece of DNA or RNA inside a protein coat. To carry on any metabolic processes, including replication, a virus must enter a cell. Once a virus has injected its DNA or RNA into its host cell, that cell is altered—that is, it is "programmed" to control the metabolic processes that the virus needs to survive. The virus, including the protein coat, replicates in the host cell (Figure 10–1). When the host cell can no longer carry out its own metabolic functions because of the viral invader, the host cell dies and releases the new viruses into the body to invade other cells.

Because viruses are contained inside human cells while they are in the body, it has proved difficult to develop effective drugs that destroy a virus without harming the human host. **Interferons** (see Chapter 15) are released by the host in response to viral invasion of a cell and prevent the replication of that particular virus. Some interferons that affect particular viruses are now available through genetic engineering programs. Other drugs that are used in treating viral infections have been effective against a limited number of viruses. Viruses that respond to some antiviral therapy include influenza A and some respiratory viruses, herpes viruses, cytomegalovirus (CMV), the human immunodeficiency virus (HIV) that causes acquired immunodeficiency syndrome (AIDS), and some viruses that cause warts and certain eye infections.

AGENTS FOR INFLUENZA A AND RESPIRATORY VIRUSES

Influenza A and other respiratory viruses, including influenza B and respiratory syncytial virus (RSV), invade the respiratory tract and cause the signs and symptoms of respiratory "flu."

Amantadine (*Symmetrel*) was first used to treat Parkinson's disease. However, patients who took amantadine did not get influenza during flu season. This drug is now used for both treatment and prevention of respiratory viral infections. It is slowly absorbed from the gastrointestinal (GI) tract, reaching peak levels in 4 hours. Excretion occurs unchanged through the urine, with a half-life of 15 hours. Because of its renal clearance, amantadine must be used at reduced doses and with caution in patients who have any renal impairment. Amantadine is embryotoxic in animals and crosses into breast milk; it should be used during pregnancy and lactation only if the benefits clearly outweigh the risks to the neonate.

Oseltamivir (*Tamiflu*) is effective in the treatment of uncomplicated influenza infections that have been symptomatic for less than 2 days. It is readily absorbed from the GI tract, extensively metabolized in the urine, and excreted in the urine with a half-life of 6 to 10 hours. The dosage should be reduced and the patient closely monitored if there is renal dysfunction. There are no adequate studies in pregnancy and lactation, so oseltamivir should be used during pregnancy and lactation only if the benefits clearly outweigh the risks to the neonate.

Ribavirin (*Virazole*) is effective against influenza A, RSV,

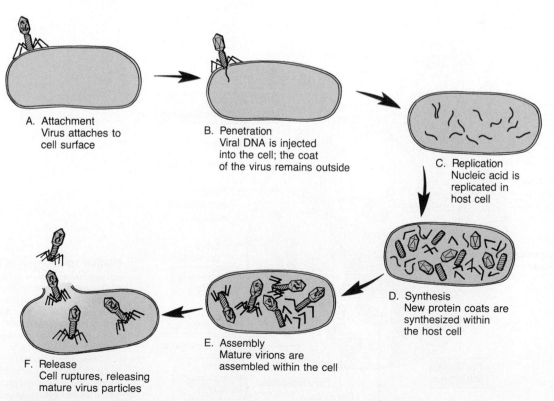

A. Attachment
Virus attaches to cell surface

B. Penetration
Viral DNA is injected into the cell; the coat of the virus remains outside

C. Replication
Nucleic acid is replicated in host cell

D. Synthesis
New protein coats are synthesized within the host cell

E. Assembly
Mature virions are assembled within the cell

F. Release
Cell ruptures, releasing mature virus particles

FIGURE 10–1. The stages in the replication cycle of a virus. (From Bullock, B. L. [2000]. *Focus on pathophysiology*. Philadelphia: Lippincott Williams & Wilkins.)

and herpes viruses. This agent has been used in the treatment of children with RSV and has been tested for use in several other viral conditions. It is available in a combination packet with interferon-alfa-2b as an oral drug, *Rebetron,* for the treatment of chronic hepatitis C in adults. Ribavirin is absorbed well through the respiratory tract and has a half-life of 9.5 hours. It is teratogenic and is rated pregnancy category X. Women of child-bearing age should be advised to use barrier contraceptives if they are taking this drug, although the drug is not normally indicated for use in adults.

Rimantadine (*Flumadine*), a synthetic agent, is used for the prevention and treatment of influenza A infections. It is absorbed from the GI tract with peak levels achieved in 6 hours. Rimantadine is extensively metabolized in the liver and excreted in the urine. Rimantadine is embryotoxic in animals and should be used during pregnancy only if the benefits clearly outweigh the risks. It should not be used by nursing mothers, because it crosses into breast milk and can cause toxic reactions in the neonate. Use in children should be limited to prevention of influenza A infections.

Zanamivir (*Relenza*) was approved in 1999 to treat uncomplicated influenza infections in adults and in children older than 12 years of age who have had symptoms for less than 2 days. This drug must be delivered by a *Diskhaler* device, which comes with every prescription of zanamivir. It is absorbed through the respiratory tract and excreted unchanged in the urine with a half-life of 2.5 to 5.1 hours. Because of the renal excretion, the drug should be used cau-

tiously in patients with any renal impairment. It should be used during pregnancy and lactation only if the benefits clearly outweigh the risks to the neonate.

Therapeutic Actions and Indications

Although the exact mechanism of action of drugs that combat respiratory viruses is not known, it is believed that these agents prevent shedding of the viral protein coat and entry of the virus into the cell (Figure 10–2). This action prevents viral replication, causing viral death. These antiviral drugs are indicated for prevention of influenza A infection, which is especially important in health care workers and other high-risk individuals, and for reducing the severity of infection if it occurs.

Contraindications and Cautions

Caution should be used when giving these antiviral agents to patients with a known allergy; to pregnant or lactating women; or to patients with renal or liver disease, which could alter metabolism and excretion of the drug.

Adverse Effects

Use of these antiviral agents is frequently associated with various adverse effects that may be related to possible effects on dopamine levels in the brain. These adverse effects include lightheadedness, dizziness, and insomnia; nausea; orthostatic hypotension; and urinary retention.

Clinically Important Drug–Drug Interactions

Patients who receive amantadine or rimantadine may experience increased atropine-like effects if either of these drugs is given with an anticholinergic drug.

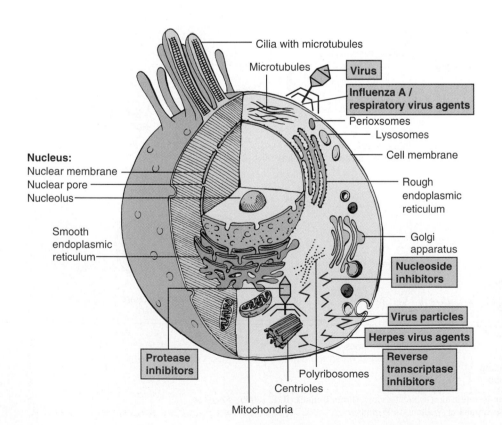

FIGURE 10–2. Agents for influenza A and respiratory viruses prevent shedding of the protein coat and entry of virus into the cell. Herpes virus agents alter viral DNA production. Agents that attempt to control HIV and AIDS work in the following ways: nucleosides interfere with HIV replication by blocking protein synthesis; reverse transcriptase inhibitors block the transfer of information that allows viral replication; protease inhibitors block protease within the virus, leading to immature, noninfective virus particles.

DRUG THERAPY ACROSS THE LIFESPAN

Antivirals

Children	Adults	Older Adults

Children are very sensitive to the effects of most antiviral drugs, and more severe reactions can be expected when these drugs are used in children.
 	
    Many of these drugs do not have proven safety and efficacy in children, and extreme caution should be used.
 	
    Most of the drugs for prevention and treatment of influenza virus infections can be used, in smaller doses, for children.
 	
    Acyclovir is the drug of choice for children with herpes virus or cytomegalovirus infections.
 	
    The drugs used in the treatment of AIDS are frequently used in children, even when no scientific data are available, because of the seriousness of the disease. Dosage should be lowered according to body weight, and children must be monitored very closely for adverse effects on kidneys, bone marrow, and liver.
	Adults need to know that these drugs are specific for the treatment of viral infections. The use of antibiotics to treat such infections can lead to the development of resistant strains and superinfections that can cause more problems.
	
	    Patients with HIV infection who are taking antiviral medications need to be taught that these drugs do not cure the disease, that opportunistic infections can still occur, and that precautions to prevent transmission of the disease need to be taken.
	
	    Pregnant women, for the most part, should not use these drugs unless the benefit clearly outweighs the potential risk to the fetus or neonate. Women of child-bearing age should be advised to use barrier contraceptives if any of these drugs are used. Zidovudine has been safely used in pregnant women.
	
	    The Centers for Disease Control and Prevention advises that women with HIV infection should not breast feed, to protect the neonate from the virus.
		Older patients may be more susceptible to the adverse effects associated with these drugs; they should be monitored closely.
		
		    Patients with hepatic dysfunction are at increased risk for worsening hepatic problems and toxic effects of those drugs that are metabolized in the liver. Drugs that are excreted unchanged in the urine can be especially toxic to patients who have renal dysfunction. If hepatic or renal dysfunction is expected (extreme age, alcohol abuse, use of other hepatotoxic or nephrotoxic drugs), the dosage may need to be lowered and the patient should be monitored more frequently.

DRUGS IN FOCUS

Influenza A and Respiratory Virus Drugs

Drug Name	Dosage/Route	Usual Indications
amantadine (*Symmetrel*)	Adult: 200 mg PO q.d. Pediatric (9–12 y): 100 mg PO b.i.d. Pediatric (1–9 y): 2–4 mg/lb PO q.d.	Treatment of Parkinson's disease; treatment and prevention of respiratory virus infections
oseltamivir (*Tamiflu*)	Adult: 75–150 mg PO b.i.d. for 5 d Pediatric (1–12 y): 30–75 mg b.i.d. PO for 5 days	Treatment of uncomplicated influenza
ribavirin (*Virazole*) (*Rebetron*)	Pediatric: 20 mg/mL in the reservoir for aerosol treatment over 12–18 h each day for 3–7 d Adult: 400 mg/d PO in AM with 600 mg/d PO in PM with 3 million IU interferon alfa-2b SC 3 times per week	Treatment of influenza A, respiratory syncytial virus, and herpes virus infections Treatment of chronic hepatitis C in patients who relapse after interferon-alfa therapy
rimantadine (*Flumadine*)	Adult: 100 mg PO b.i.d. Pediatric (<10 y): 5 mg/kg PO q.d.	Prevention and treatment of influenza A infections
zanamivir (*Relenza*)	Adult and children ≥7 y: Two inhalations, b.i.d. (12 h apart) for 5 d	Treatment of uncomplicated influenza infections

Nursing Considerations for Patients Receiving Influenza A and Respiratory Virus Drugs

Assessment: History and Physical Examination

Patients who receive respiratory antiviral agents should be assessed for the following conditions, which either are contraindications to the use of these drugs or necessitate precautionary measures: known history of allergy to antivirals; history of liver or renal dysfunction that might interfere with drug metabolism and excretion; and current pregnancy or lactation status.

Physical assessment should be performed to establish baseline data for evaluating the effectiveness of the drug and the occurrence of any adverse effects associated with drug therapy. Include screening for orientation and reflexes to evaluate any central nervous system (CNS) effects of the drug; vital signs (respiratory rate, adventitious sounds, temperature) to assess for signs and symptoms of the viral infection; blood pressure to monitor for orthostatic hypotension; urinary output to monitor genitourinary (GU) effects of the drug; and renal and hepatic function tests to determine baseline function of these organs.

Nursing Diagnoses

The patient receiving a respiratory antiviral drug may have the following nursing diagnoses related to drug therapy:

- Acute Pain related to GI, CNS, GU effects of drug
- Disturbed Sensory Perception (Kinesthetic) related to CNS effects of drug
- Deficient Knowledge regarding drug therapy

Implementation

- Start drug regimen as soon after exposure to the virus as possible *to achieve best effectiveness and decrease the risk of complications of viral infection.*
- Administer influenza A vaccine before the flu season begins if at all possible, *to prevent the disease and decrease the risk of complications.*
- Administer the full course of the drug *to obtain the full beneficial effects.*
- Provide safety provisions if CNS effects occur, *to protect the patient from injury.*
- Instruct the patient about the appropriate dosage scheduling regimen; safety precautions, including changing position slowly and avoiding driving and hazardous tasks, to take if CNS effects occur; and the need to report any difficulty walking or talking *to enhance patient knowledge about drug therapy and to promote compliance.*

Evaluation

- Monitor patient response to the drug (prevention of respiratory flu-like symptoms; alleviation of flu-like symptoms).
- Monitor for adverse effects (orientation and affect, blood pressure, urinary output).

- Evaluate the effectiveness of the teaching plan (patient can name the drug, dosage, possible adverse effects to watch for, and specific measures to help avoid adverse effects).
- Monitor the effectiveness of comfort and safety measures and compliance with the regimen.

AGENTS FOR HERPES AND CYTOMEGALOVIRUS

Herpes viruses account for a broad range of conditions, including cold sores, encephalitis, shingles, and genital infections. **Cytomegalovirus (CMV),** although slightly different from the herpes virus, can affect the eye, respiratory tract, and liver and reacts to many of the same drugs. A number of antiviral drugs are used to combat these infections.

Acyclovir (*Zovirax*) is specific for herpes virus infections. It is excreted unchanged in the urine and therefore must be used cautiously in the presence of renal impairment. Acyclovir crosses into breast milk and exposes the neonate to high levels of the drug, so extreme caution must be used during lactation.

Cidofovir (*Vistide*) is used to treat CMV retinitis in patients with AIDS only. It is associated with severe renal toxicity and granulocytopenia. Cidofovir is excreted unchanged in the urine and must be given with probenecid to increase renal clearance of the drug. The dosage must be decreased according to renal function and creatinine clearance. Use in children with AIDS should be very cautious because of potential carcinogenic effects and effects on fertility. If no other treatment option is available, monitor the child very closely.

Famciclovir (*Famvir*) is most effective in treating herpes infections. It is well absorbed from the GI tract, reaching peak levels in 2 to 3 hours. Famciclovir is metabolized in the liver and excreted in the urine and feces. Safety of use in children younger than 18 years of age has not been established.

Foscarnet (*Foscavir*) is available in intravenous (IV) form only. It can be highly toxic to the kidneys and is reserved for treatment of CMV retinitis in immunocompromised patients and for mucocutaneous acyclovir-resistant herpes simplex infections. About 90% of foscarnet is excreted unchanged in the urine, so it should be used cautiously and at reduced dosage in patients with renal impairment. Foscarnet has been shown to affect bone development and growth and should not be used in children unless the benefit clearly outweighs the risk and the child is monitored very closely.

Ganciclovir (*Cytovene*), which is available in IV and oral forms, is used for long-term treatment and prevention of CMV infections. Ganciclovir is primarily excreted unchanged in the feces with some urinary excretion. Ganciclovir is carcinogenic and should be used only with extreme caution in children.

Valacyclovir (*Valtrex*) is an oral agent used for the treatment of herpes zoster and recurrent genital herpes. It is rapidly absorbed from the GI tract and metabolized in the liver to acyclovir. Excretion occurs through the urine, so caution should be used in patients with renal impairment. Safety for use in children has not been established.

Valganciclovir (*Valcyte*), which is the oral prodrug of ganciclovir, is used for the treatment of CMV retinitis in AIDS patients. It is primarily excreted unchanged in the feces with some urinary excretion. Valganciclovir is also carcinogenic and should be used only with extreme caution in children.

Pharmacokinetics

Of the agents used in the treatment of herpes and CMV, Cidofovir (*Vistide*), has proved embryotoxic in animals. For many of the other agents, there have been no adequate studies during human pregnancy and lactation, but because of the toxicities of all of these drugs, they should be used only if the benefits clearly outweigh the potential risks to the neonate.

Therapeutic Actions and Indications

Drugs that combat herpes and CMV inhibit viral DNA replication by competing with viral substrates to form shorter, noneffective DNA chains (see Figure 10–2). This action prevents replication of the virus, but it has little effect on the host cells of humans, because their DNA uses different substrates. These antiviral agents are indicated for treatment of the DNA viruses herpes simplex, herpes zoster, and CMV. Research has shown that they are very effective in immunocompromised individuals such as patients with AIDS, those taking immunosuppressants, and those with multiple infections.

Contraindications and Cautions

Drugs indicated for the treatment of herpes and CMV should not be used during pregnancy or lactation or in patients with known allergies to antiviral agents; renal disease, which could interfere with excretion of the drug; or severe CNS disorders.

Adverse Effects

The adverse effects most commonly associated with these antivirals include nausea and vomiting, headache and depression, and rash and hair loss. Rash, inflammation, and burning often occur at sites of IV injection and topical application. Renal dysfunction and renal failure also have been reported.

Clinically Important Drug–Drug Interactions

The risk of nephrotoxicity increases when agents indicated for the treatment of herpes and CMV are used in combination with other nephrotoxic drugs.

The risk of drowsiness also rises when these antiviral agents are taken with zidovudine, an antiretroviral agent.

Nursing Considerations for Patients Receiving Agents for Herpes Virus and Cytomegalovirus
Assessment: History and Physical Assessment

Patients receiving DNA-active antiviral agents should be assessed for the following conditions, which are cautions or contraindications to use of these drugs: any history of allergy

---

DRUGS IN FOCUS
Agents for Herpes Virus and Cytomegalovirus (CMV)

Drug Name	Dosage/Route	Usual Indications
Ⓟ acyclovir (*Zovirax*)	Adult: 5–10 mg/kg q8h IV, IM, or SC, *or* 200 mg PO 5 times per day for 10 d and then 400 mg PO b.i.d. for 12 mo Pediatric: 250–500 mg/m² q8h IV, IM, or SC for 7–10 d, *or* 20 mg/kg q.i.d. PO for 5 d	Treatment of herpes virus infections
cidofovir (*Vistide*)	5 mg/kg IV (over 1 h) once weekly for 2 weeks, then every other week, with probenecid 2 g PO 3 h before and 1 g PO 2 h and 8 h after cidofovir infusion	Treatment of CMV retinitis in AIDS patients
famciclovir (*Famvir*)	Herpes zoster: 500 mg PO q8h for 7 d Genital herpes: 125 mg b.i.d. PO for 5 d	Treatment of herpes virus infections
foscarnet (*Foscavir*)	Adult: 40–60 mg/kg q8–12h IV given as a 2-h infusion Pediatric: safety and efficacy not established	Treatment of CMV and herpes simplex infections in immunocompromised patients
ganciclovir (*Cytovene*)	Adult: 5 m/kg q12h IV given over 1 h for 14–21 d, then over 1 h daily 7 d/wk or 6 mg/kg per day for 5 d/wk for prophylaxis	Long-term treatment and prevention of CMV infection
valacyclovir (*Valtrex*)	Herpes zoster: 1 g PO t.i.d. for 7 d Genital herpes: 500 mg b.i.d. PO for 5 d	Treatment of herpes virus infections
valganciclovir (*Valcyt*)	900 mg PO b.i.d. for 21 d, then 900 mg PO once a day for maintenance; reduce dosage with renal impairment	Treatment of CMV retinitis in AIDS patients

to antivirals; renal dysfunction that might interfere with the metabolism and excretion of the drug; severe CNS disorders that could be aggravated; and pregnancy or lactation.

Physical assessment should be performed to establish baseline data for assessing the effectiveness of the DNA-active antiviral drug and the occurrence of any adverse effects associated with drug therapy. Assess orientation and reflexes to evaluate any CNS effects of the drug. Examine skin (color, temperature, and lesions) to monitor the effectiveness of the drug. Evaluate renal function tests to determine baseline function of the kidneys.

Nursing Diagnoses

The patient receiving a DNA-active antiviral agent may have the following nursing diagnoses related to drug therapy:

- Acute Pain related to GI, CNS, local effects of drug
- Disturbed Sensory Perception (Kinesthetic) related to CNS effects of drug
- Deficient Knowledge regarding drug therapy

Implementation

- Ensure good hydration *to decrease the toxic effects on the kidneys.*
- Administer the drug as soon as possible after the diagnosis has been made *to improve effectiveness of the antiviral activity.*
- Ensure that the patient takes the complete course of the drug regimen *to improve effectiveness and decrease the risk of the emergence of resistant viruses.*
- Wear protective gloves when applying the drug topically *to decrease risk of exposure to the drug and inadvertent absorption.*
- Provide safety precautions if CNS effects occur (e.g., use of side rails, appropriate lighting, orientation, assistance) *to protect the patient from injury.*
- Warn the patient that GI upset, nausea, and vomiting can occur, *to prevent undue anxiety and increase awareness of the importance of nutrition.*
- Monitor renal function tests periodically during treatment *to detect and respond to renal toxicity as soon as possible.*
- Provide the patient with instructions about the drug *to enhance patient knowledge about drug therapy and to promote compliance.*

The patient should

Avoid sexual intercourse if genital herpes is being treated, because these drugs do not cure the disease.
Wear protective gloves when applying topical agents.
Avoid driving and hazardous tasks if dizziness or drowsiness occurs.

Evaluation

- Monitor patient response to the drug (alleviation of signs and symptoms of herpes or CMV infection).

- Monitor for adverse effects (orientation and affect, GI upset, and renal function).
- Evaluate the effectiveness of the teaching plan (patient can name the drug, dosage, possible adverse effects to watch for, and specific measures to help avoid adverse effects).
- Monitor the effectiveness of comfort and safety measures and compliance with the regimen.

AGENTS FOR HIV AND AIDS

The **human immunodeficiency virus (HIV)** attacks the **helper T cells** within the immune system. This virus enters the helper T cell and multiplies within the cell. When the cell ruptures, many new viruses are released to attack other helper T cells. The end result is that the immune system loses an important monitor that propels the immune reaction into full force when the body is invaded.

Loss of T-cell function causes **acquired immunodeficiency syndrome (AIDS)** or **AIDS-related complex (ARC),** diseases that are characterized by the emergence of a variety of opportunistic infections and cancers that occur when the immune system is depressed and unable to function properly. The HIV mutates over time, presenting a slightly different configuration with each new generation. Treatment of AIDS and ARC has been difficult for two reasons: (1) the length of time the virus can remain dormant within the T cells (i.e., months to years), and (2) the adverse effects of many potent drugs, which may include further depression of the immune system. At present, a combination of several different antiviral drugs is used to attack the virus at various points in its life cycle, so as to achieve maximum effectiveness with the least amount of toxicity. The types of antiviral agents that are used to treat HIV infections are the reverse transcriptase inhibitors, the protease inhibitors, and the nucleosides. These drugs are known as antiretroviral agents.

Reverse Transcriptase Inhibitors

The **reverse transcriptase inhibitors** bind directly to HIV reverse transcriptase, blocking both RNA- and DNA-dependent DNA polymerase activities. They prevent the transfer of information that would allow the virus to replicate and survive.

Delavirdine (*Rescriptor*) must be used in combination therapy regimens, because resistant strains develop rapidly when it is used alone. It is rapidly absorbed from the GI tract, with peak levels occurring within 1 hour. Delavirdine is extensively metabolized by the cytochrome P450 system in the liver and is excreted through the urine. Safety for use in children has not been established.

Efavirenz (*Sustiva*) is used in adults and children in combination with other antiretroviral agents. It is absorbed rapidly from the GI tract, reaching peak levels in 3 to 5 hours. Efavirenz is metabolized in the liver by the cytochrome P450 system and is excreted in the urine and feces with a half-life of 52 to 76 hours.

Nevirapine (*Viramune*) is recommended for use in adults

NURSING CHALLENGE
Public Education About AIDS

When AIDS was first diagnosed in the early 1980s, it was found in a certain population in New York City. The people in this group tended to be homosexuals, intravenous drug users, and debilitated persons with poor hygiene and nutrition habits. Originally, a number of health care practitioners thought that the disease was a syndrome of opportunistic infections that occurred in a population with repeated exposures to infections that naturally deplete the immune system. It was not until several years later that the human immunodeficiency virus (HIV) was identified. Since then, it has been discovered that HIV infection is rampant in many African countries. The infection also has spread throughout the United States in populations that are not homosexual or intravenous drug users and who have good nutrition and hygiene habits. As health care practitioners have learned, HIV is not particular about the body it invades. And once introduced into a body, it infects T cells and causes HIV infection.

When a patient is diagnosed with HIV infection, the nurse faces a tremendous challenge for patient education and support. The patient and any significant others should be counseled about the risks of transmission and reassured about ways in which the virus is not transmitted. They will need to learn about drug protocols, T-cell levels, adverse drug effects, and anticipated progress of the disease. They also will need consistent support and a telephone number to call with questions at any time. Many communities have AIDS support groups and other resources that can be very helpful; the nurse can direct the patient to these resources as appropriate.

The combinations of drugs that are being used today and the constant development of more drugs make the disease less of a death sentence than it was in the past. The result, however, is that many people must take a large number of pills each day, at tremendous cost and inconvenience. Many people today do live for long periods with HIV infection. An AIDS vaccine is currently being studied and offers hope for preventing this disease in the future.

Public education is key for promoting the acceptance and support of patients with HIV infection or AIDS, who need a great deal of support and assistance. Nurses can be role models for dealing with HIV patients and can provide informal public education whenever the opportunity presents.

and children. After rapid GI absorption, nevirapine is metabolized by the cytochrome P450 system in the liver. Excretion is through the urine with a half-life of 45 hours. Safety for use in children has not been established.

Pharmacokinetics
There are no adequate studies of reverse transcriptase inhibitors in pregnancy, so use should be limited to situations in which the benefits clearly outweigh any risks. It is suggested that women not breast feed if they are infected with HIV.

Protease Inhibitors

The **protease inhibitors** block protease activity within the HIV virus. Protease is essential for the maturation of infectious virus; without it, an HIV particle is immature and noninfective. The protease inhibitors that are available for use include the following.

Amprenavir (*Agenerase*) was approved in 1999 for the treatment of adults and children with HIV in combination with other antiretroviral agents. It is rapidly absorbed from the GI tract, reaching peak levels in 1 to 2 hours. After undergoing metabolism in the liver, amprenavir is excreted in the urine and feces with a half-life of 7.1 to 10.6 hours. Because of the extensive hepatic metabolism, caution must be used in any patient with hepatic dysfunction.

Indinavir (*Crixivan*) is available for treatment of adults with HIV. It is rapidly absorbed from the GI tract, reaching peak levels in 0.8 hours. Indinavir is metabolized in the liver by the cytochrome P450 system. It is excreted in the urine with a half-life of 1.8 hours. Patients with hepatic or renal impairment are at risk for increased toxic effects, and the dosage may need to be reduced. The safety of indinavir for use in children has not been established.

Lopinavir (*Kaletra*) is a fixed combination drug that combines lopinavir and ritonavir. The ritonavir inhibits the metabolism of lopinavir, leading to increased lopinavir serum levels and effectiveness. This drug is approved for use in adults and children in combination with other antiretroviral agents for the treatment of HIV infection. It is readily absorbed from the GI tract and undergoes extensive hepatic metabolism by the cytochrome P450 system. Lopinavir is excreted in urine and feces.

Nelfinavir (*Viracept*) must be given in combination with other drugs and can be used in the treatment of children with HIV. It is well absorbed from the GI tract, reaching peak levels in 2 to 4 hours. Nelfinavir is metabolized in the liver, and caution must be used in patients with any hepatic dysfunction. It is primarily excreted in the feces, with a half-life of 3.5 to 5 hours. Because there is little renal excretion, this is considered a good drug for patients with renal impairment.

Ritonavir (*Norvir*) can be used alone and is available for use in adults and children. It is rapidly absorbed from the GI tract, reaching peak levels in 2 to 4 hours. Ritonavir undergoes extensive metabolism in the liver and is excreted in feces and urine. Many potentially serious toxic effects can occur when ritonavir is taken with nonsedating antihistamines, sedative/hypnotics, or antiarrhythmics because of the activity of ritonavir in the liver. Patients with hepatic dysfunction are at increased risk for serious effects when taking ritonavir and require a reduced dosage and close monitoring.

Saquinavir (*Fortovase, Invirase*) is used in combination regimens for adults. This drug is slowly absorbed from the GI tract and is metabolized in the liver by the cytochrome P450 mediator, so it must be used cautiously in the presence of hepatic dysfunction. It is primarily excreted in the feces with a short half-life. It has not been shown to be teratogenic, but use during pregnancy should limited. Saquinavir crosses into breast milk, and women are advised not to breast feed while taking this drug. The safety for use in children younger than 16 years of age has not been established.

Pharmacokinetics

Of the protease inhibitors listed, saquinavir (*Fortovase, Invirase*) is the only agent that has not been shown to be teratogenic; however, as mentioned, its use during pregnancy should be limited. Saquinavir crosses into breast milk, and women are advised not to breast feed while taking this drug. For the other agents listed, there are no adequate studies in pregnancy, so use should be limited to situations in which the benefits clearly outweigh any risks. It is suggested that women not breast feed if they are infected with HIV.

Nucleosides

Nucleosides interfere with HIV replication by inhibiting cell protein synthesis, leading to viral death. The nucleosides include the following agents.

Abacavir (*Ziagen*) is used in combination therapy in adults and children. Serious to fatal hypersensitivity reactions have occurred with this drug, and it must be stopped immediately at any sign of a hypersensitivity reaction (fever, chills, rash, fatigue, GI upset, flu-like symptoms). Patients exhibiting any signs of hypersensitivity should be listed with the Abacavir Hypersensitivity Registry, a drug follow-up registry that is maintained by the drug company and reporting to the U. S. Food and Drug Administration. After rapid GI absorption, abacavir is metabolized in the liver and excreted in feces and urine.

Didanosine (*Videx*) is used to treat advanced infections in adults and children. It is rapidly destroyed in an acid environment and therefore must be taken in a buffered form. It reaches peak levels in 15 to 75 minutes. Didanosine undergoes intracellular metabolism with a half-life of 8 to 24 hours. Serious pancreatitis, hepatomegaly, and neurological problems have been reported with this drug, which is why its use should be limited to the treatment of advanced infections.

Lamivudine (*Epivir*) is recommended specifically for use with other antiretroviral agents; as an oral solution, *Epivir-HBV,* it is also recommended for the treatment of chronic hepatitis B. After rapid GI absorption, lamivudine is excreted primarily unchanged in the urine, with a half-life of 5 to 7 hours. Because excretion depends on renal function, dosage reduction is recommended in the presence of renal impairment.

Stavudine (*Zerit*) is recommended specifically for use with other antiretroviral agents. It is rapidly absorbed from the GI tract, reaching peak levels in 1 hour. Most of the drug is excreted unchanged in the urine, making it important to reduce dosage and monitor patients carefully in the presence of renal dysfunction.

Tenafovir (*Viread*) is a new drug that affects the virus at a slightly different point in replication—a nucleotide that becomes a nucleoside. It is used only in combination with other antiretroviral agents. It is rapidly absorbed from the GI tract, reaching peak levels in 45 to 75 minutes. Its metabolism is not known, but it is excreted in the urine. Severe hepatomegaly with steatosis has been reported with tenafovir, so it must be used with great caution in any patient with hepatic impairment or lactic acidosis. Patients also should be alerted that the drug may cause changes in body fat distribution, with loss of fat from arms, legs, and face and deposition of fat on the trunk, neck, and breasts.

Zalcitabine (*Hivid*) is used to treat advanced cases of HIV/AIDS in adults, as a monotherapy in adults who have become intolerant to zidovudine or who have progressive disease while taking zidovudine, and as combination therapy with zidovudine for the treatment of advanced HIV infection. After absorption from the GI tract, zalcitabine is excreted unchanged in the urine with a half-life of 2 hours. It is not advisable to use zalcitabine during pregnancy, and women of child-bearing age should use barrier contraceptives while taking this drug. Safety for use in children has not been established. Severe and even fatal adverse reactions, including neuropathies, lactic acidosis, pancreatitis, and hepatic toxicity, have occurred with this drug. Use should be limited to severe or recalcitrant cases.

Zidovudine [AZT] (*Retrovir*) was one of the first drugs found to be effective in the treatment of AIDS. It is used to treat symptomatic disease in adults and children and to prevent maternal transmission of HIV. It is rapidly absorbed from the GI tract, with peak levels occurring within 30 to 75 minutes. Zidovudine is metabolized in the liver and excreted in the urine, with a half-life of 1 hour. Severe bone marrow suppression has occurred with this drug, which must be used very cautiously in patients with compromised bone marrow function. Patients with marked renal or hepatic impairment may require lower doses because of the role of these organs in metabolism and excretion. Zidovudine has been used safely during pregnancy.

Box 10–1 discusses combination drugs used for the treatment of HIV infection.

Pharmacokinetics

Of the nucleosides mentioned, zidovudine is the only agent that has been proven to be safe when used during pregnancy. Of the other agents, there have been no adequate studies in pregnancy, so use should be limited to situations in which the benefits clearly outweigh any risks. It is suggested that women not breast feed if they are infected with HIV.

Therapeutic Actions and Indications

The antiviral agents used to treat HIV and AIDS operate at various points in the life cycle of the virus and result in its death or inactivation (see Figure 10–2). Use of these drugs in combination can affect more viral particles and reduce the number of mutant viruses that are formed and spread to noninfected cells. These antiviral agents are indicated for the treatment of patients with documented AIDS or ARC who have decreased numbers of T cells and evidence of increased opportunistic infections.

Contraindications and Cautions

Because these drugs are used in the treatment of a potentially fatal disease with no known cure, there are no true con-

BOX 10-1

Fixed Combination Drugs for Treatment of HIV Infection

Patients who are taking combination drug therapy for HIV infection may have to take a very large number of pills each day. Keeping track of these pills and swallowing such a large number each day can be an overwhelming task. In an effort to improve patient compliance and make it easier for some of these patients, some anti-HIV agents are now available in combination products.

Combivir is a combination of 150 mg lamivudine and 300 mg zidovudine. The patient takes one tablet, twice a day. Because this is a fixed combination drug, it is not the drug of choice for patients who require a dosage reduction owing to renal impairment or adverse effects that limit dose tolerance.

Trizivir combines 300 mg abacavir, 150 mg lamivudine, and 300 mg zidovudine. The patient takes one tablet, twice a day. Because this is a fixed combination drug, it is not the drug of choice for patients who require a dosage reduction owing to renal impairment or adverse effects that limit dose tolerance. Patients taking *Trizivir* should be warned at the time the prescription is filled about the potentially serious hypersensitivity reactions associated with abacavir and should be given a written list of warning signs to watch for.

CULTURAL CONSIDERATIONS

Alternative Therapies and Antiviral Drugs

An increasing number of people in our culture are using alternative therapies as part of their daily regimen. St. Jonh's wort is one of the more popular alternative therapies sold today. This herb has been used as an anti-inflammatory agent, as an antidepressant, as a diuretic, and as a treatment for gastritis and insomnia. Multimedia advertisements urge the use of St. John's wort to increase one's sense of well-being and to decrease depression "without the use of drugs." Many people with viral infections just do not feel well. They are tired, have muscle aches and pains, and feel feverish and low on energy. This herb seems to be a remedy aimed at these people. Unfortunately, St. John's wort has been shown to interact with many prescription drugs. When taken with St. John's wort, the protease inhibitors used in treating HIV were found to have decreased serum levels, leading to possible treatment failure. Because St. John's wort may induce the cytochrome P450 system in the liver, there is a possibility that it could increase the metabolism of many other antiviral drugs that are metabolized by that system and cause treatment failures with those drugs.

Patients may be reluctant to discuss their use of alternative therapies with the health care provider, because they want to maintain control over that aspect of their medical regimen or because they believe that the health care provider would not approve of the use of these therapies. It is important, when a patient is prescribed an antiviral agent, to ask specifically about the use of herbal or alternative medicines. Explain to the patient that antiviral drugs may interact with some herbal medicines and that it is important to try to avoid any adverse effects or drug failures.

traindications to their use. Zidovudine is the drug of choice during pregnancy to block maternal transmission of the virus. Caution should be used with known allergies to any of these drugs; with hepatic or renal dysfunction, which could lead to increased drug levels and toxicity; and with pregnancy or lactation, because of potential adverse effects on the neonate.

Adverse Effects

The adverse effects reported with the use of these drugs often are not distinguishable from the effects of the ongoing disease process. Adverse effects that are most often reported include the CNS effects of headache, dizziness, and myalgia; GI upset, including nausea, vomiting, and diarrhea; hepatic toxicity related to direct drug effects on the liver; fever and flu-like symptoms; rash (which is potentially fatal in some patients); and bone marrow depression, including agranulocytosis and anemia.

Clinically Important Drug–Drug Interactions

If nelfinavir is combined with astemizole, cisapride, rifampin, triazolam, or midazolam, severe toxic effects and life-threatening arrhythmias may occur. Such combinations should be avoided.

Indinavir and nevirapine interact to cause severe toxicity. If these two drugs are given in combination, the dosages should be adjusted and the patient should be monitored closely.

Tenafovir can cause large increases in the serum level of didanosine. If both of these drugs are given, tenafovir should be given 2 hours before or 1 hour after didanosine.

When oral contraceptives are taken in combination with several of the antiviral agents, episodes of ineffective contraception may occur. Affected patients should be advised to use barrier contraceptives.

Nursing Considerations for Patients Receiving Agents for HIV and AIDS

Assessment: History and Physical Assessment

Screen for the following conditions, which are cautions or contraindications to use of these drugs: any history of allergy to antivirals; renal or hepatic dysfunction that might interfere with the metabolism and excretion of the drug; and pregnancy or lactation.

Physical assessment should be performed to establish baseline data for assessing the effectiveness of the drug and the occurrence of any adverse effects associated with drug therapy. Perform assessment of orientation and reflex to evaluate any CNS effects of the drug. Examine the skin (color, temperature, and lesions) to monitor the effectiveness of the drug. Check temperature to monitor for infections. Evaluate hepatic and renal function tests to determine baseline function of the kidneys and liver. Check results of a complete blood count (CBC) with differential to monitor bone marrow activity and T-cell number to indicate effectiveness of the drugs.

DRUGS IN FOCUS
HIV and AIDS Drugs

Drug Name	Dosage/Route	Usual Indications
Reverse Transcriptase Inhibitors		
delaviridine (*Rescriptor*)	Adult: 400 mg PO t.i.d.	Part of combination therapy regimens for treatment of HIV in adults
efavirenz (*Sustiva*)	Adult: 600 mg PO q.d. Pediatric: dosage determined by age and weight	Treatment of adults and children with HIV in combination with other antiretroviral agents
℗ nevirapine (*Viramune*)	Adult: 200 mg PO q.d. for 14 d, then 200 mg PO b.i.d. Pediatric: 4 mg/kg PO for 14 days then 4–7 mg/kg PO b.i.d.	Treatment of adults or children with HIV in combination with other antiretroviral agents
Protease inhibitors		
amprenavir (*Agenerase*)	Adult: 1200 mg (8 tablets) PO b.i.d. Pediatric (13–16 y): adult dose Pediatric (4–12 y): 20 mg/kg PO b.i.d. (capsules) 22.5 mg/kg PO b.i.d (solution)	Treatment of adults and children with HIV, in combination with other antiretroviral agents
℗ indinavir (*Crixivan*)	Adult: 800 mg PO q8h	Treatment of adults with HIV
lopinavir (*Kaletra*)	Adult: 3 capsules or 5 mL PO b.i.d. Pediatric (6 mo to 12 y): 10–12 mg/kg PO b.i.d.	Treatment of adults and children with HIV, in combination with other antiretroviral agents
nelfinavir (*Viracept*)	Adult: 750 mg PO t.i.d. Pediatric (2–13 y): 20–30 mg/kg per dose PO t.i.d.	Combination therapy for the treatment of adults and children with HIV
ritonavir (*Norvir*)	Adult and Pediatric (> 2 y): 600 mg PO b.i.d.	Part of combination therapy for the treatment of adults and children with HIV
saquinavir (*Fortovase*) (*Invirase*)	*Fortovase*, Adult: Six 200-mg tablets PO t.i.d. *Invirase*, Adult: Three 200-mg tablets PO t.i.d.	Treatment of adults with HIV as part of combination therapy
Nucleosides		
abacavir (*Ziagen*)	Adult: 300 mg PO b.i.d. Pediatric: 8 mg/kg PO b.i.d.	Combination therapy for the treatment of adults and children with HIV
didanosine (*Videx*)	Adult: 250–400 mg PO q.d. *or* 125–200 mg PO b.i.d. Pediatric: 120 mg/m² PO b.i.d.	Treatment of advanced infections in adults and children with HIV
lamivudine (*Epivir*)	Adult: 150 mg PO b.i.d.; for chronic hepatitis B, 100 mg PO q.d. Pediatric (3 mo–16 y): 4 mg/kg PO b.i.d.	With other antiretroviral agents for the treatment of adults and children with HIV; as an oral solution for the treatment of chronic hepatitis B
stavudine (*Zerit*)	Adult (≥60 kg): 40 mg PO b.i.d. Adult (30–60 kg): 30 mg PO b.i.d. Pediatric (>30 kg): adult dosage Pediatric (<30 kg): 1 mg/kg per dose PO b.i.d.	Treatment of adults and children with HIV, in combination with other anti-retroviral agents
tenofovir (*Viread*)	Adult: 300 mg/d PO with food	Treatment of adults with HIV infection, in combination with other antiretroviral drugs
zalcitabine (*Hivid*)	Adult: 0.75 mg PO q8h	Treatment of advanced infections in adults with HIV
℗ zidovudine (AZT) (*Retrovir*)	Adult: 100 mg PO q4h Pediatric (3 mo to 12 y): 180 mg/m² PO q6h Maternal: 100 mg PO 5 times per day until start of labor, then 2 mg/kg IV over 1 h, and then 1 mg/kg per hour IV until clamping of the cord	Treatment of symptomatic HIV in adults and children; prevention of maternal transmission of HIV

Antiviral Agents for HIV and AIDS

THE SITUATION

H. P. is a 34-year-old attorney who was diagnosed with AIDS, having had a positive HIV test 3 years ago. Although his T-cell count had been stabilized with treatment with zidovudine, it recently dropped remarkably. He presents with numerous opportunistic infections and Kaposi's sarcoma. H. P. admits that he has been under tremendous stress at work and at home in the past few weeks. He begins a combination regimen of lamivudine, zidovudine, ritonavir, and zalcitabine.

CRITICAL THINKING

What are the important nursing implications in this case?
What role would stress play in the progress of this disease?
What specific issues should be discussed?
What other clinical implications should be considered?

DISCUSSION

Combination therapy with antivirals has been found to be effective in decreasing some of the morbidity and mortality associated with HIV and AIDS. However, this treatment does not cure the disease. H. P. needs to understand that opportunistic infections can still occur and that regular medical help should be sought. H. P. also needs to understand that these drugs do not decrease the risk of transmitting HIV by sexual contact or through blood contamination and should be encouraged to take appropriate precautions.

It is important to make a dosing schedule for H. P., or even to prepare a weekly drug box, to ensure that all of the medications are taken as indicated. H. P. should also receive interventions to help him decrease his stress, because activation of the sympathetic nervous system during periods of stress is known to depress the immune system. Further depression of his immune system could accelerate the development of opportunistic infections and decrease the effectiveness of his antiviral drugs. Measures that could be used to decrease stress should be discussed and tried with H. P.

Discussion of adverse effects that H. P. may experience is important. Gastrointestinal upset and discomfort may occur while he is taking all of these anti-HIV/AIDS medications. Small, frequent meals may help alleviate the discomfort. It is important that every effort be made to maintain H. P.'s nutritional state, and a nutritional consultation may be necessary if gastrointestinal effects are severe. H. P. also may experience dizziness, fatigue, and confusion, which could cause more problems for him at work and may necessitate changes in his workload. Because some of the prescribed drugs must be taken around the clock, provisions may be needed to allow H. P. to take his drugs on time throughout the day. For example, H. P. may need to wear an alarm wristwatch, establish planned breaks in his schedule at dosing times, or devise other ways to follow his drug regimen without interfering with his work schedule. The adverse effects and inconvenience of taking this many drugs may add to the stress that H. P. is experiencing. It is important that a health care provider work consistently with him to help him to manage his disease and treatment as effectively as possible.

Nursing Diagnoses

The patient receiving drugs for HIV and AIDS may have the following nursing diagnoses related to drug therapy:

- Acute Pain related to GI, CNS, dermatological effects of drug
- Disturbed Sensory Perception (Kinesthetic) related to CNS effects of drug
- Imbalanced Nutrition: Less than Body Requirements, related to GI effects of the drugs
- Deficient Knowledge regarding drug therapy

Implementation

- Monitor renal and hepatic function before and periodically during therapy *to detect renal or hepatic function changes and arrange to reduce dosage or provide treatment as needed*.
- Ensure that the patient takes the complete course of the drug regimen and takes all drugs included in a particular combination *to improve effectiveness of the drug and decrease the risk of emergence of resistant viral strains*.

- Administer drug around the clock, if indicated, *to provide the critical concentration needed for the drug to be effective*.
- Monitor nutritional status if GI effects are severe, and *take appropriate action to maintain nutrition*.
- Stop drug if severe rash occurs, especially if accompanied by blisters, fever, and so on, *to avert potentially serious reactions*.
- Provide safety precautions (e.g., the use of side rails, appropriate lighting, orientation, assistance) if CNS effects occur, *to protect patient from injury*.
- Teach the patient about the drugs prescribed, *to enhance patient knowledge about drug therapy and to promote compliance*. Include as a teaching point the fact that these drugs do not cure the disease and therefore appropriate precautions should still be taken to prevent transmission.

The patient should

Have regular medical care.
Have periodic blood tests, which are necessary to monitor the effectiveness and toxicity of the drug.
Realize that GI upset, nausea, and vomiting may occur but that efforts must be taken to maintain adequate nutrition.

Avoid driving and hazardous tasks if dizziness or drowsiness occurs.

Report extreme fatigue, severe headache, difficulty breathing, or severe rash to a health care provider.

See accompanying Patient Teaching Checklist for the antiviral agents used for HIV and AIDS.

Evaluation

• Monitor patient response to the drug (alleviation of signs and symptoms of AIDS or ARC and maintenance of T-cell levels).

PATIENT TEACHING CHECKLIST
Antiviral Agents for HIV and AIDS

Create customized patient teaching materials for a specific antiviral agent from the CD-ROM. Patient teaching should stress the following points for drugs within this class:

• An antiviral agent works in combination with other antivirals to stop the replication of HIV, to control AIDS, and to maintain the functioning of your immune system.
• These drugs are not a cure for HIV, AIDS, or AIDS-related complex (ARC). Opportunistic infections may occur, and regular medical follow-up should be sought to deal with the disease.
• These drugs do not reduce the risk of transmission of HIV to others by sexual contact or by blood contamination; use appropriate precautions.

Common effects of these drugs include the following:

• *Dizziness, weakness, and loss of feeling*—Change positions slowly. If you feel drowsy, avoid driving and dangerous activities.
• *Headache, fever, muscle aches*—Analgesics may be ordered to alleviate this discomfort. Consult with your health care provider.
• *Nausea, loss of appetite, change in taste*—Small, frequent meals may help. It is important to try to maintain good nutrition. Consult your health care provider if this becomes a severe problem.

Report any of the following to your health care provider: excessive fatigue, lethargy, severe headache, difficulty breathing, or skin rash.

Avoid over-the-counter medications. If you feel that you need one of these, check with your health care provider first.

Regular medical evaluations, including blood tests, are needed to monitor the effects of these drugs on your body and to adjust dosages as needed.

Tell any doctor, nurse, or other health care provider that you are taking these drugs.

Keep this drug and all medications out of the reach of children. Do not share these drugs with other people.

Note: This Teaching Checklist reflects general patient teaching guidelines. It is not meant to be a substitute for drug-specific teaching information, which is available in nursing drug guides.

• Monitor for adverse effects (orientation and affect, GI upset, renal and hepatic function, skin, levels of blood components).
• Evaluate the effectiveness of the teaching plan (patient can name the drug, dosage, possible adverse effects to watch for, and specific measures to help avoid adverse effects).
• Monitor the effectiveness of comfort and safety measures and compliance with the regimen (see Nursing Care Guide: Antiviral Agents for HIV/AIDS).

WEB LINKS

Health care providers and patients may want to consult the following Internet sources:

Information on AIDS and HIV research, treatments, and resources:
http://www.infoweb.org
Information on drug protocols and new HIV research:
http://www.cdc.gov
Information on AIDS:
http://www.critpath.org
Health information for professionals and consumers:
http://www.aegis.com

LOCALLY ACTIVE ANTIVIRAL AGENTS

Some antiviral agents are given locally to treat local viral infections. These agents include the following:

• Idoxuridine (*Herplex*), which is applied directly to the eye and is used to treat herpes simplex keratitis
• Imiquimod (*Aldara*), which is applied locally for the treatment of genital and perianal warts
• Fomivirsen (*Vitravene*), which is injected into the eye to treat CMV retinitis in patients with AIDS
• Ganciclovir (*Vitrasert*), which is implanted into the eye every 5 to 8 months for treatment of patients with CMV retinitis
• Penciclovir (*Denavir*), which is applied locally for the treatment of herpes labialis (cold sores) on the face and lips (not to be applied to mucous membranes)
• Trifluridine (*Viroptic*), which is applied locally to treat herpes simplex infections in the eye
• Vidarabine (*Vira-A*), which is used locally to treat herpes simplex infections of the eye that are not responsive to idoxuridine

Therapeutic Actions and Indications
These antiviral agents act on viruses by interfering with normal viral replication and metabolic processes. They are indicated for specific, local viral infections.

Contraindications and Cautions
Locally active antiviral drugs are not absorbed systemically, but caution should be used in patients with known allergic reactions to any topical drugs.

Adverse Effects
Because these drugs are not absorbed systemically, the adverse effects most commonly reported are local burning,

NURSING CARE GUIDE

Antiviral Agents for HIV/AIDS

Assessment	Nursing Diagnoses	Implementation	Evaluation
HISTORY Allergies to any of these drugs; bone marrow depression; renal or liver dysfunction; pregnancy and lactation	Acute Pain related to GI, skin, CNS effects	Monitor CBC and differential before and every 2 weeks during therapy.	Evaluate drug effects: relief of signs and symptoms of AIDS and ARC; stabilization of T-cell levels.
	Disturbed Sensory Perception (Kinesthetic) related to CNS effects	Provide comfort and implement safety measures: assistance, temperature control, lighting control, mouth care, back rubs.	Monitor for adverse effects: GI alterations, dizziness, confusion, headache, fever.
	Imbalanced Nutrition: More than Body Requirements related to GI effects	Provide small, frequent meals and monitor nutritional status.	Monitor for drug–drug interactions as indicated for each drug.
	Deficient Knowledge regarding drug therapy	Monitor for opportunistic infections and arrange treatment as indicated.	Evaluate effectiveness of patient teaching plan.
		Provide support and reassurance for dealing with drug effects and discomfort.	Evaluate effectiveness of comfort and safety measures.
		Provide patient teaching regarding drug name, dosage, adverse effects, warnings, precautions, and signs to report.	
PHYSICAL EXAMINATION Skin: color, lesions, texture CNS: affect, reflexes, *orientation* GI: abdominal and liver evaluation Hematological: CBC and differential; renal and hepatic function tests			

stinging, and discomfort. These effects usually occur at the time of administration and pass with time.

Nursing Considerations for Patients Receiving Locally Active Antiviral Agents
Assessment: History and Physical Assessment

Patients receiving locally active antiviral agents should be assessed for any history of allergy to antivirals.

Physical assessment should be performed to establish baseline data for evaluating the effectiveness of the drug and the occurrence of any adverse effects associated with drug therapy, including inflammation at the site of infection.

Nursing Diagnoses

The patient receiving locally active antiviral drugs may have the following nursing diagnoses related to drug therapy:

• Acute Pain related to local effects of drug
• Deficient Knowledge regarding drug therapy

Implementation

• Ensure proper administration of the drug *to improve effectiveness and decrease risk of adverse effects*.
• Stop the drug if severe local reaction occurs or if open lesions occur near the site of administration, *to prevent systemic absorption*.
• Teach the patient about the drug being used, *to enhance patient knowledge about drug therapy and to promote compliance*. Include as a teaching point the fact that these drugs do not cure the disease but should alleviate discomfort and prevent damage to healthy tissues. Encourage the patient to report severe local reaction or discomfort.

DRUGS IN FOCUS
Locally Active Antiviral Agents

Drug Name	Usual Indications
fomivirsen (*Vitravene*)	Ophthalmic injection to treat cytomegalovirus (CMV) retinitis in patients with AIDS
ganciclovir (*Vitrasert*)	Implanted for treatment of CMV in patients with AIDS
Ⓟ idoxuridine (*Herplex*)	Ophthalmic agent used to treat herpes simplex keratitis (drug of choice)
imiquimod (*Aldara*)	Local treatment of genital and perianal warts
penciclovir (*Denavir*)	Local treatment of herpes labialis (cold sores) on the face and lips
trifluridine (*Viroptic*)	Ophthalmic ointment to treat herpes simplex infections in the eye
vidarabine (*Vira-A*)	Ophthalmic agent to treat herpes simplex infections of the eye that are not responsive to idoxuridine

Evaluation

- Monitor patient response to the drug (alleviation of signs and symptoms of viral infection).
- Monitor for adverse effects (local irritation and discomfort).
- Evaluate the effectiveness of the teaching plan (patient can name the drug, the dosage, proper administration technique, and adverse effects to watch for and report to a health care provider).
- Monitor the effectiveness of comfort and safety measures and compliance with the regimen.

CHAPTER SUMMARY

- Viruses are particles of DNA or RNA surrounded by a protein coat that survive by injecting their own DNA or RNA into a healthy cell and taking over its functioning.
- Because viruses are contained within human cells, it has been difficult to develop drugs that are effective antivirals and yet do not destroy human cells. Antiviral agents are available that are effective against only a few types of viruses.
- Influenza A and respiratory viruses cause the signs and symptoms of the common cold or "flu." The drugs that are available to prevent the replication of these viruses are used for prophylaxis against these diseases during peak seasons.
- Herpes viruses and CMV are DNA viruses that cause a multitude of problems, including cold sores, encephalitis, infections of the eye and liver, and genital herpes.
- Helper T cells are essential for maintaining a vigilant, effective immune system. When these cells are decreased in

number or effectiveness, opportunistic infections occur. AIDS and ARC are syndromes of opportunistic infections that occur when the immune system is depressed.
- HIV, which specifically attacks helper T cells, may remain dormant in T cells for long periods and has been known to mutate easily.
- Antiviral agents that are effective against HIV and AIDS include reverse transcriptase inhibitors, protease inhibitors, and nucleosides, all of which affect the way the virus communicates, replicates, or matures within the cell. These drugs are known as antiretroviral agents. These drugs are given in combination to most effectively destroy the HIV virus and prevent mutation.
- Some antivirals are available only for the local treatment of viral infections, including warts and eye infections. These drugs are not absorbed systemically.

Review Questions

1. Viruses are known to cause
   a. tuberculosis.
   b. leprosy.
   c. the common cold.
   d. gonorrhea.
2. Virus infections have proved difficult to treat because
   a. viruses have a protein coat.
   b. viruses inject themselves into human cells to survive and to reproduce.
   c. viruses are bits of RNA or DNA.
   d. viruses easily resist drug therapy.
3. Naturally occurring substances that are released in the body in response to viral invasion are called
   a. antibodies.

b. immunoglobulins.
c. interferons.
d. interleukins.

4. Herpes viruses cause a broad range of conditions, but have not been identified as the causative agent in
   a. cold sores.
   b. shingles.
   c. genital infections.
   d. leprosy.

5. An important teaching point for the patient receiving an agent to treat herpes virus or CMV would be the following:
   a. stop taking the drug as soon as the lesions have disappeared.
   b. sexual intercourse is fine—as long as you are taking the drug, you are not contagious.
   c. drink plenty of fluids to decrease the drug's toxic effects on the kidneys.
   d. there are no associated GI adverse effects.

6. HIV (human immunodeficiency virus) attacks
   a. B clones.
   b. helper T cells.
   c. suppressor T cells.
   d. cytotoxic T cells.

7. The reasoning behind using combination therapy in the treating of HIV does not include which of the following:
   a. the virus can remain dormant within the T cell for a very long time.
   b. adverse effects of many of the drugs used to treat this virus include immune depression.
   c. the drugs are cheaper if used in combination.
   d. the virus slowly mutates with each generation.

8. Nursing interventions for the patient receiving antiviral drugs for the treatment of HIV probably would not include
   a. monitoring renal and hepatic function periodically during therapy.

b. administering the drugs around the clock to increase drug effectiveness.
c. encouraging the patient to avoid eating if GI upset is severe.
d. stopping the drugs and notifying the prescriber if severe rash occurs.

9. Locally active antiviral agents can be used to treat
   a. HIV infection.
   b. herpes simplex, keratitis, and warts.
   c. RSV.
   d. CMV systemic infections.

10. The clinical presentations of AIDS and ARC are related to
    a. direct virus attacks on specific cells.
    b. the appearance of opportunistic infections that occur when the immune system is depressed.
    c. activation of the immune system.
    d. dermatological deterioration secondary to the virus' entering skin cells.

BIBLIOGRAPHY

Bullock, B. L. (2000). *Focus on pathophysiology*. Philadelphia: Lippincott Williams & Wilkins.

Centers for Disease Control and Prevention. (1997). USPHS/IDSA guidelines for the prevention of opportunistic infections in persons infected with HIV. U. S. Department of Health and Human Services. *MMWR Morbidity and Mortality Weekly Report, 46*(No. RR 12).

Drug facts and comparisons. (2002). St. Louis: Facts and Comparisons.

Guberski, R. D. (1997). Treatment of AIDS in adults: An update. *American Journal for Nurse Practitioners, 1*(1), 22–26.

Gilman, A., Hardman, J. G., & Limbird, L. E. (Eds.) (2002). *Goodman and Gilman's the pharmacological basis of therapeutics* (10th ed.). New York: McGraw-Hill.

Karch, A. M. (2002). *2003 Lippincott's nursing drug guide*. Philadelphia: Lippincott Williams & Wilkins.

Professional's guide to patient drug facts. (2002). St. Louis: Facts and Comparisons.

11

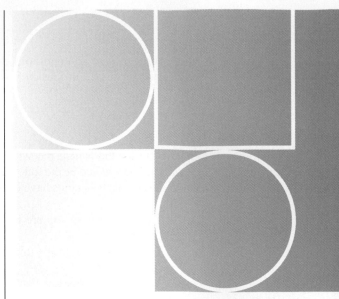

Key Terms
Candida
ergosterol
fungus
mycosis
tinea

Antifungal Agents

130

Systemic antifungals	terbinafine	haloprogin
amphotericin B	**Topical antifungals**	miconazole
P fluconazole	butenafine	naftifine
flucytosine	butoconazole	oxiconazole
griseofulvin	ciclopirox	terbinafine
itraconazole	**P** clotrimazole	tolnaftate
ketoconazole	econazole	undecyclenic acid
nystatin	gentian violet	

Fungal infections in humans range from conditions such as the annoying "athlete's foot" to potentially fatal systemic infections. An infection caused by a **fungus** is called a **mycosis.** Fungi differ from bacteria in that the fungus has a rigid cell wall that is made up of chitin and various polysaccharides and a cell membrane that contains **ergosterol.** The composition of the protective layers of the fungal cell makes the organism resistant to antibiotics. Conversely, because of their cellular makeup, bacteria are resistant to antifungal drugs.

The incidence of fungal infections has increased with the rising number of immunocompromised individuals—patients with acquired immunodeficiency syndrome (AIDS) and AIDS-related complex (ARC), those taking immunosuppressant drugs, those who have undergone transplantation surgery or cancer treatment, and members of the increasingly large elderly population, who are no longer able to protect themselves from the many fungi that are found throughout the environment. For example, *Candida,* a fungus that is normally found on mucous membranes, can cause yeast infections or "thrush" of the gastrointestinal (GI) tract and vagina in immunosuppressed patients.

SYSTEMIC ANTIFUNGALS

The drugs used to treat systemic fungal infections can be toxic to the host and are not used indiscriminately. It is important to get a culture of the fungus causing the infection to ensure that the right drug is being used, so that the patient is not put at additional risk from the toxic adverse effects associated with these drugs.

Amphotericin B (*Fungizone, Abelcet, Amphotec, AmBisome*), available in intravenous (IV) form, is a very potent drug with many unpleasant side effects that can cause renal failure. This drug is indicated for advanced and progressive systemic fungal infections, including aspergillosis, leishmaniasis, cryptococcosis, blastomycosis, moniliasis, coccidioidomycosis, histoplasmosis, and mucormycosis. Amphotericin B can also be used topically to treat resistant *Candida* infections. Because of the many adverse effects associated this agent, its use is reserved for progressive, potentially fatal infections. Amphotericin B is excreted in the urine, with an initial half-life of 24 hours and then a 15-day half-life. Its metabolism is not fully understood. Amphotericin B has been used successfully during pregnancy, but it should be used cautiously. It crosses into breast milk and should not be used during lactation because of the potential risk to the neonate.

Flucytosine (*Ancobon*), available in an oral form, is a less toxic drug that is used for the treatment of systemic infections caused by *Candida* or *Cryptococcus*. It is well absorbed from the GI tract, with peak levels occurring in 2 hours. Most of the drug is excreted unchanged in the urine, and a small amount in the feces, with a half-life of 2.4 to 4.8 hours. Because the drug is excreted primarily in the urine, extreme caution is needed in the presence of renal impair-

DRUG THERAPY ACROSS THE LIFESPAN

Antifungal Agents

Children	Adults	Older Adults
Children are very sensitive to the effects of most antifungal drugs, and more severe reactions can be expected when these drugs are used in children. Many of these drugs do not have proven safety and efficacy in children, and extreme caution should be exercized when using them. Fluconazole, ketoconazole, and griseofulvin have established pediatric doses and would be drugs of choice if appropriate for a particular infection. Topical agents should not be used over open or draining areas that would increase the risk of systemic absorption and toxicity. Occlusive dressings including tight diapers, should be avoided over the affected areas.	These drugs can be very toxic to the body, and their use should be reserved for situations in which the causative organism has been identified. Over-the-counter topical preparations are widely used, and patients should be cautioned to follow the instructions and to report continued problems to their health care provider. Pregnant and nursing women should not use these drugs unless the benefit clearly outweighs the potential risk to the fetus or neonate. Women of child-bearing age should be advised to use barrier contraceptives if any of these drugs are used. A severe fungal infection may threaten the life of the mother and/or fetus; in these situations, the potential risk of treatment should be carefully explained. Topical agents should not be used over open or draining areas that would increase the risk of systemic absorption.	Older patients may be more susceptible to the adverse effects associated with these drugs and should be monitored closely. Patients with hepatic dysfunction are at increased risk for worsening hepatic problems and toxic effects of many of these drugs (ketoconazole, itraconazole, griseofulvin). If hepatic dysfunction is expected (extreme age, alcohol abuse, use of other hepatotoxic drugs), the dosage may need to be lowered and the patient monitored more frequently. Other agents are associated with renal toxicity (flucytosine, fluconazole, griseofulvin) and should be used cautiously in the presence of renal impairment. Patients at risk for renal toxicity should be monitored carefully.

ment, since drug accumulation and toxicity can occur. Because of the potential for adverse reactions in the neonate, flucytosine should be used during pregnancy and lactation only if the benefits clearly outweigh the risks. Safety for use in children has not been established.

Griseofulvin (*Fulvicin, Grifulvin V, Grisactin, Gris-PEG*) is an oral drug that is used for the treatment of ringworm infections—tinea corporis, tinea pedis, tinea cruris, tinea barbae, tinea capitis, and tinea unguium. It is not effective against bacterial infections or for candidiasis. Griseofulvin can be very toxic and should only be used after the fungus responsible for an infection has been identified. It is absorbed from the GI tract, and peak levels are achieved within 4 hours. Griseofulvin is metabolized in the liver and excreted in the urine. It was shown to be fetotoxic in preclinical studies and should not be used during pregnancy. Women of child-bearing age who need this drug should be advised to use barrier contraceptives.

Nystatin (*Mycostatin, Nilstat, Nystex*) is used orally for the treatment of intestinal candidiasis. In addition, it is available in a number of topical preparations—oral suspension; troche; and vaginal suppository, cream, and ointment—for the treatment of local candidiasis, vaginal candidiasis, and cutaneous and mucocutaneous infections caused by *Candida* species. It is not absorbed from the GI tract and passes unchanged in the stool. It is not known whether nystatin crosses the placenta or enters breast milk, so it should not be used during pregnancy or lactation unless the benefits clearly outweigh the potential risks.

Another group of agents, called azoles, are newer drugs that are used to treat systemic fungal infections. Although they are less toxic than amphotericin B, they may also be less effective in very severe and progressive infections. The azoles include the following drugs.

- Ketoconazole (*Nizoral*) is used orally to treat many of the same mycoses as amphotericin B. It works by blocking the activity of a steroid in the fungal wall and has the side effect of blocking the activity of human steroids, including testosterone and cortisol. Because of this action, ketoconazole is not the drug of choice for patients with endocrine or fertility problems. It has been associated with severe hepatic toxicity and should be avoided in patients with hepatic dysfunction. It is absorbed rapidly from the GI tract, with peak levels occurring within 1 to 3 hours. It is extensively metabolized in the liver and excreted through the feces. It strongly inhibits the cytochrome P450 (CYP450) enzyme system in the liver and is associated with many drug–drug interactions. This agent is also used topically as a shampoo to reduce the scaling associated with dandruff and as a cream to treat topical mycoses.
- Fluconazole (*Diflucan*) is available in oral and IV preparations, so a patient who is seriously ill can be treated with the IV form and then switched to the oral form as his or her condition improves. Fluconazole, which is not associated with the endocrine problems seen with ketoconazole, is used to treat candidiasis, cryptococcal meningitis, and

other systemic fungal infections. This drug has been used successfully as a prophylactic agent for reducing the incidence of candidiasis in bone marrow transplant recipients. Peak levels after administration occur within 1 to 2 hours. Most of the drug is excreted unchanged in the urine, making use with renal dysfunction difficult. Fluconazole also strongly inhibits the CYP450 liver enzyme system and may be associated with drug–drug interactions.
- Itraconazole (*Sporanox*) is an oral agent used for the treatment of assorted systemic mycoses. This drug, which has been associated with hepatic failure, should not be used in patients with hepatic failure and should be used with caution in those with hepatic impairment. Itraconazole is slowly absorbed from the GI tract and is metabolized in the liver by the CYP450 system. It is excreted in the urine and feces.

Ketoconazole (*Nizoral*), fluconazole (*Diflucan*), and itraconazole (*Sporanox*) have all been shown to be teratogenic in animals and should not be used in pregnancy or lactation unless the benefits clearly outweigh the potential risks.

Terbinafine (*Lamisil*) is a similar drug which blocks the formation of ergosterol. It inhibits a CYP2D6 enzyme system, so it could be a better choice for patients who need to take drugs metabolized by the CYP450 system. Terbinafine is available as an oral drug for the treatment of onychomycosis of the toenail or fingernail. It is rapidly absorbed from the GI tract, extensively metabolized in the liver, and excreted in the urine.

Therapeutic Actions and Indications

All of the systemic antifungal drugs function to alter the cell permeability of the fungus, leading to cell death and prevention of replication (Figure 11–1). Some agents, including amphotericin B, nystatin, fluconazole, and itraconazole, bind to the ergosterol to open pores in the cell membrane. In contrast, ketoconazole and terbinafine impair the synthesis of ergosterol, allowing increased cell permeability and leakage of cellular components, leading to cell death. These agents are indicated for the treatment of systemic infections caused by susceptible fungi.

Contraindications and Cautions

Caution should be used when systemic antifungal agents are administered to anyone with a known allergy; during pregnancy and lactation (with the exception of terbinafine, use should be reserved for life-threatening infections); or to patients with renal or liver disease, which could either alter drug metabolism and excretion or worsen as a result of the actions of the drug.

Adverse Effects

Adverse effects frequently encountered with the use of systemic antifungal agents include central nervous system (CNS) effects such as headache, dizziness, fever, shaking, chills, and malaise. GI effects include nausea, vomiting, dyspepsia, and anorexia. Hepatic dysfunction, which is seen more often with itraconazole, is associated with the toxic effects of the drug on the liver. Dermatological effects, such as rash and pruritus as-

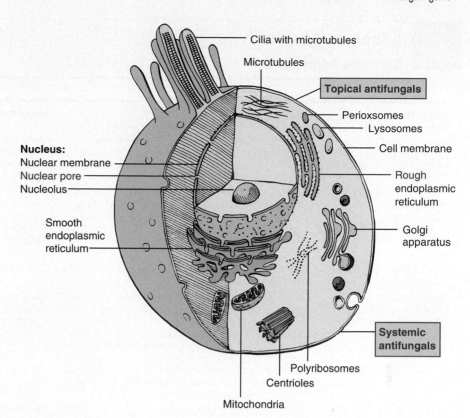

FIGURE 11–1. Sites of action of antifungal agents. Both systemic and topical antifungals alter fungal cell permeability, leading to prevention of replication and cell death.

sociated with local irritation, may occur. Renal dysfunction, which is more often seen with amphotericin B, is probably related to the drug effects on cell membranes.

Clinically Important Drug–Drug Interactions

Patients who receive amphotericin B should take neither other nephrotoxic drugs nor corticosteroids unless absolutely necessary, because of the increased risk of severe renal toxicity.

The azole family of antifungal drugs can cause increased serum levels of the following agents: cyclosporine, digoxin, oral hypoglycemics, warfarin, oral anticoagulants, and phenytoin. Toxicity may occur because the azoles inhibit the CYP450 liver enzyme system needed for metabolism of these drugs. If these combinations cannot be avoided, patients should be closely monitored and dosage adjustments made.

Because the azoles have also been associated with potentially severe cardiovascular events when taken with lovastatin, simvastatin, astemizole, cisapride, triazolam, and midazolam, use of these drugs in combination with azoles should be avoided.

Nursing Considerations for Patients Receiving Systemic Antifungals

Assessment: History and Physical Assessment

Screen for the following, which are cautions or contraindications for use of these drugs: history of allergy to antifungals; history of liver or renal dysfunction that might interfere with metabolism and excretion of the drug; and pregnancy or lactation.

Physical assessment should be performed to establish

baseline data for assessing the effectiveness of the drug and the occurrence of any adverse effects associated with drug therapy. Perform a culture of the infected area to make an accurate determination of the type and responsiveness of fungus. Assess orientation and reflexes to evaluate any CNS effects of the drug. Examine the skin for color and lesions to check for dermatological effects of the drug. Evaluate renal and hepatic function tests to determine baseline function of these organs, to assess possible toxicity during drug therapy.

Nursing Diagnoses

The patient receiving a systemic antifungal drug may have the following nursing diagnoses related to drug therapy:

• Acute Pain related to GI, CNS, local effects of drug
• Disturbed Sensory Perception (Kinesthetic) related to CNS effects
• Deficient Knowledge regarding drug therapy

Implementation

• Arrange for appropriate culture and sensitivity tests before beginning therapy *to ensure that the appropriate drug is being used.* However, in some cases, treatment can begin before test results are known because of the seriousness of the systemic infections.
• Administer the entire course of the drug *to get the full beneficial effects;* this may take as long as 6 months for some chronic infections.

DRUGS IN FOCUS
Systemic Antifungals

Drug Name	Dosage/Route	Usual Indications
amphotericin B (*Fungizone, Abelcet, Amphotec, AmBisone*)	0.25–1.5 mg/kg per day IV, based on the infection and its severity; also used topically	Treatment of aspergillosis, leishmaniasis, cryptococcosis, blastomycosis, moniliasis, coccidioidomycosis, histoplasmosis, and mucormycosis; topical treatment of resistant *Candida*
fluconazole (*Diflucan*)	Adult: 200–400 mg PO on day 1, followed by 100 mg PO q.d.; IV route can be used, but do not exceed 200 mg/h Pediatric: 3–6 mg/kg PO; do not exceed 12 mg/kg	Treatment of candidiasis, cryptococcal meningitis, other systemic fungal infections; prophylaxis for reducing the incidence of candidiasis in bone marrow transplant recipients
flucytosine (*Ancobon*)	50–150 mg/kg per day PO in divided doses at 6-h intervals	Treatment of candidiasis, cryptococcosis
griseofulvin (*Fulvicin, Grifulvin V, Grisactin, Gris-PEG*)	Tinea corporis, tinea cruris, and tinea capitis: Adult: 500 mg (microsize) or 330–375 mg (ultramicrosize) q.d. PO Tinea pedis and tinea unguium: Adult: 0.75–1 g (microsize) or 660–750 mg (ultramicrosize) q.d. PO Pediatric (> 2 y): 11 mg/kg per day (microsize) or 7.3 mg (ultramicrosize) PO q.d. (not recommended for children ≤ 2 y)	Treatment of tinea corporis, tinea pedis, tinea cruris, tinea barbae, tinea capitis, and tinea unguium
itraconazole (*Sporanox*)	Adult: 100–400 mg PO q.d. Pediatric: safety and efficacy not established	Treatment of blastomycosis, histoplasmosis, and aspergillosis
ketoconazole (*Nizoral*)	Adult: 200 mg PO q.d., up to 400 mg PO q.d. in severe cases Pediatric (≥2 y): 3.3–6.6 mg/kg per day PO Pediatric (<2 y): safety not established Topical: as a shampoo	Treatment of aspergillosis, leishmaniasis, cryptococcosis, blastomycosis, moniliasis, coccidioidomycosis, histoplasmosis, and mucormycosis; topical treatment of mycoses, to reduce the scaling of dandruff
nystatin (*Mycostatin, Nilstat, Nystex*)	500,000–1,000,000 units t.i.d. PO; continue for 48 h after resolution to prevent relapse; also used topically	Treatment of candidiasis
terbinafine (*Lamisil*)	250 mg/d PO for 6 wk (fingernail) or 12 wk (toenail)	Treatment of onychomycosis of the fingernail or toenail

- Monitor IV sites *to ensure that phlebitis does not occur.* Treat appropriately and restart IV at another site if phlebitis occurs.
- Monitor renal and hepatic function before and periodically during treatment and *arrange to stop drug if signs of organ failure occur.*
- Provide comfort and safety provisions if CNS effects occur (eg, siderails and assistance with ambulation for dizziness and weakness, analgesics for headache, antipyretics for fever and chills, temperature regulation for fever) *to protect the patient from injury.*
- Provide small, frequent, nutritious meals if GI upset is severe. Monitor nutritional status, and arrange a dietary consultation as needed *to ensure nutritional status.* GI upset may be decreased by taking an oral drug with food.
- Provide patient instruction *to enhance patient knowledge about drug therapy and to promote compliance.*

The patient should

Follow the appropriate dosage regimen.

Take safety precautions, including changing position slowly and avoiding driving and hazardous tasks, if CNS effects occur.

Take an oral drug with meals and try small, frequent meals if GI upset is a problem.

Report to a health care provider any of the following: sore throat, unusual bruising and bleeding, or yellowing of the eyes or skin, all of which could indicate hepatic toxicity; severe nausea and vomiting, which could interfere with nutritional state and slow recovery; and severe local irritation with local application, which could indicate a sensitivity reaction and worsening of the infection.

See the accompanying Patient Teaching Checklist for antifungal agents.

PATIENT TEACHING CHECKLIST
Antifungal Agents

Create customized patient teaching materials for a specific antifungal agent from the CD-ROM.
   Patient teaching should stress the following points for drugs within this class:

• An antifungal drug works to destroy the fungi that have invaded the body.
• Because of the way that antifungal drugs work, they may need to be taken over a long period of time.

   It is very important to take all of the prescribed medication.
   Common adverse effects of this drug include the following:

• *Headache and weakness*—Change positions slowly. An analgesic may be ordered to help alleviate the headache. If you feel drowsy, avoid driving or dangerous activities.
• *Stomach upset, nausea, and vomiting*—Small, frequent meals may help. Take the drug with food if appropriate, because this may decrease the gastrointestinal upset associated with these drugs. (*Note:* Ketoconazole must be taken on an empty stomach at least 2 hours before taking a meal, antacids, milk products, or any other drugs.) Try to maintain adequate nutrition.

   Report any of the following to your health care provider: severe vomiting, abdominal pain, fever or chills, yellowing of the skin or eyes, dark urine or pale stools, or skin rash.
   Avoid over-the-counter medications. If you feel that you need one of these, check with your health care provider first.
   Take the full course of your prescription. Never use this drug to self-treat any other infection or give it to any other person.
   Tell any doctor, nurse, or other health care provider that you are taking this drug.
   Keep this drug and all medications out of the reach of children.
   Note: This Teaching Checklist reflects general patient teaching guidelines. It is not meant to be a substitute for drug-specific teaching information, which is available in nursing drug guides.

Evaluation

• Monitor patient response to the drug (resolution of fungal infection).
• Monitor for adverse effects (orientation and affect, nutritional state, skin color and lesions, renal and hepatic function).
• Evaluate the effectiveness of the teaching plan (patient can name the drug, dosage, possible adverse effects to watch for, and specific measures to help avoid adverse effects).
• Monitor the effectiveness of comfort and safety measures and compliance with the regimen (see Nursing Care Guide: Antifungal Agents).

TOPICAL ANTIFUNGALS

Some antifungal drugs are available only in topical forms for treating a variety of mycoses of the skin and mucous membranes. Fungi that cause these infections are called *dermatophytes*. These diseases include a variety of tinea infections, which are often referred to as ringworm, although the causal organism is a fungus, not a worm. Types of **tinea** include athlete's foot (tinea pedis), jock itch (tinea cruris), and yeast infections of the mouth and vagina often caused by *Candida*. Because the antifungal drugs reserved for use as topical agents are often too toxic for systemic administration, care should always be taken when using them near open or draining wounds that might permit systemic absorption.

   Amphotericin B (*Fungizone*) is available as a cream, lotion, or ointment for the treatment of cutaneous and mucocutaneous infections caused by *Candida*.

   Gentian violet (generic), a very old agent, is of limited usefulness because it stains skin and clothing. In addition, it is very toxic when absorbed, so it cannot be used near active lesions.

   Butenafine (*Mentax*), which is applied only once a day for 4 weeks, is used for tinea infections.

   Butoconazole (*Femstat 3*), an over-the-counter (OTC) cream, is used in the treatment of vaginal *Candida* infections.

   Ciclopirox (*Loprox, Penlac Nail Lacquer*) is available as a cream or lotion for topical tinea infections and as a solution used specifically for fungal infections of the toenails and fingernails caused by *Trichophyton rubrum*.

   Clotrimazole (*Lotrimin, Mycelex*), another OTC preparation, is used for treating oral and vaginal *Candida* infections and as a cream or lotion for treating tinea infections.

   Econazole (*Spectazole*) is used to treat tinea infections. This drug can cause intense, local burning and irritation, and it should be discontinued if these conditions become severe.

   Haloprogin (*Halotex*) is a prescription cream or solution used for the treatment of athlete's foot, jock itch, and ringworm infections.

   Miconazole *(Monistat, Fungoid, Lotrimin,* and others) is available as an OTC product in several topical forms (vaginal suppository, cream, powder, and spray) for treatment of local, topical mycoses, including bladder and vaginal infections and athlete's foot.

   Naftifine (*Naftin*) is a very powerful local antifungal agent that should not be used for longer than 4 weeks.

   Oxiconazole (*Oxistat*) can be used for up to 1 month and is applied once daily or twice daily as needed.

   Terbinafine (*Lamisil*) can be used for 1 to 4 weeks and is applied twice daily. This drug should be stopped when the fungal condition appears to be improved or if local irritation and pain become too great.

   Tolnaftate (*Tinactin, Aftate*), an OTC drug, is very effective in the treatment of athlete's foot.

   Undecyclenic acid (*Cruex, Desenex, Pedi-Dri, Fungoid AF*) is an OTC product that is recommended for athlete's foot, jock itch, diaper rash, and burning and chafing in the groin area.

NURSING CARE GUIDE

Antifungal Agents

Assessment	Nursing Diagnoses	Implementation	Evaluation
HISTORY Allergies to any of these drugs, renal or liver dysfunction, pregnancy and lactation	Acute Pain related to GI, local, CNS effects	Culture infection before beginning therapy.	Evaluate drug effects: relief of signs and symptoms of fungal infection.
	Disturbed Sensory Perception (Kinesthetic) related to CNS effects	Provide comfort and implement safety measures: assistance and siderails, temperature control, lighting control, mouth care, skin care.	Monitor for adverse effects: GI alterations, dizziness, confusion, headache, fever, renal or hepatic dysfunction, local pain, discomfort.
	Imbalanced Nutrition: Less than Body Requirements, related to GI effects	Provide small, frequent meals and monitor nutritional status.	Monitor for drug–drug interactions as indicated for each drug.
	Deficient Knowledge regarding drug therapy	Provide support and reassurance for dealing with drug effects and discomfort.	Evaluate effectiveness of patient teaching program.
		Provide patient teaching regarding drug name, dosage, adverse effects, precautions, and warning signs to report.	Evaluate effectiveness of comfort and safety measures.
PHYSICAL EXAMINATION Local: culture of infected site Skin: color, lesions, texture GU: urinary output GI: abdominal, liver evaluation Hematological: renal and hepatic function tests			

■□●■ WEB LINKS
Health care providers and patients may want to consult the following Internet sources:

Information on drug protocols, fungal research:
  http://www.cdc.gov
Information about athlete's foot infections:
  http://www.athletesfoot.com
Health information for professionals and consumers:
  http://www.critpath.org/aric/dirt/05-06

Therapeutic Actions and Indications
The topical antifungal drugs work to alter the cell permeability of the fungus, causing prevention of replication and fungal death (see Figure 11–1). They are indicated only for local treatment of mycoses, including tinea infections. Because these agents are very toxic, they are not intended for systemic use, and they are not indicated for use near open lesions or wounds because of the increased risk of systemic absorption.

Contraindications and Cautions
Because these drugs are not absorbed systemically, contraindications are limited to known allergy to any of these drugs.

Adverse Effects
When these drugs are applied locally as a cream, lotion, or spray, local effects include irritation, burning, rash, and swelling. When they are taken as a suppository or troche, adverse effects include nausea, vomiting, and hepatic dysfunction (related to absorption of some of the drug by the GI tract) or urinary frequency, burning, and change in sexual activity (related to local absorption in the vagina).

Clinically Important Drug–Drug Interactions

Because these drugs are not generally absorbed systemically, there are no reported drug–drug interactions.

Nursing Considerations for Patients Receiving Topical Antifungals

Assessment: History and Physical Assessment

Patients who receive a topical antifungal agent should be assessed for any known allergy to any topical antifungal agent.

Physical assessment should be performed to establish baseline data for assessment of the effectiveness of the drug and the occurrence of any adverse effects associated with drug therapy. Perform culture and sensitivity testing of the affected area to determine the causative fungus and appropriate medication. Conduct local evaluation (eg, color, temperature, lesions) to monitor the effectiveness of the drug and to monitor for local adverse effects of the drug.

Nursing Diagnoses

The patient receiving a topical antifungal drug may have the following nursing diagnoses related to drug therapy:

- Acute Pain related to local effects of drug
- Deficient Knowledge regarding drug therapy

Implementation

- Culture the affected area before beginning therapy *to identify the causative fungus.*

DRUGS IN FOCUS
Topical Antifungals

Drug Name	Usual Indications
amphotericin B (*Fungizone*)	Treatment of cutaneous and mucocutaneous *Candida* infections
gentian violet (generic)	Treatment of topical mycosis
butenafine (*Mentax*)	Treatment of tinea infections
butoconazole (*Femstat 3*)	Available over the counter (OTC) for treatment of vaginal *Candida* infections
ciclopirox (*Loprox, Penlac, Nail Lacquer*)	Treatment of topical tinea infections; as solution for treatment of toenail and fingernail tinea infections
(P) clotrimazole (*Lotrimin, Mycelex*)	Available OTC for treatment of oral and vaginal *Candida* infections; tinea infections
econazole (*Spectazole*)	Treatment of tinea infections
haloprogin (*Halotex*)	Treatment of athlete's foot, jock itch and ringworm infections
miconazole (*Monistat, Fungoid, Lotrimin*)	Treatment of local, topical mycoses, including bladder and vaginal infections and athlete's foot
naftifine (*Naftin*)	Short-term (up to 4 wk) treatment of severe topical mycosis
oxiconazole (*Oxistat*)	Short-term (up to 4 wk) treatment of topical mycosis
terbinafine (*Lamisil*)	Short-term (1–4 wk) treatment of topical mycosis
tolnaftate (*Tinactin, Aftate*)	Available OTC for treatment of athlete's foot
undecyclenic acid (*Cruex, Desenex, Pedi-Dri, Fungoid AF*)	Available OTC for treatment of athlete's foot, jock itch, diaper rash, burning and chafing in the groin area

Dosage/Route for all antifungals: Apply topically to affected area once or twice a day.

C A S E   S T U D Y

Poor Nutrition and Opportunistic Infections

THE SITUATION

P. P., a 19-year-old woman and aspiring model, complains of abdominal pain, difficulty swallowing, and a very sore throat. The strict diets she has followed for long periods have sometimes amounted to a starvation regimen. In the past 18 months, she has received treatment for a variety of bacterial infections (eg, pneumonia, cystitis) with a series of antibiotics.

P. P. appears to be a very thin, extremely pale young woman who looks older than her stated age. Her mouth is moist, and small, white colonies that extend down the pharynx cover the mucosa. A vaginal examination reveals similar colonies. Cultures are performed, and it is determined that she has mucocutaneous candidiasis. She is prescribed ketoconazole (*Nizoral*) and asked to return in 10 days for follow-up.

CRITICAL THINKING

What are the effects of taking a variety of antibiotics on the normal flora? *Think about the possible cause of the mycosis.*

What happens to the immune system and to the skin and mucous membranes when a person's nutritional status becomes insufficient?

How is P. P.'s chosen profession affecting her health? What are the possible ramifications of suggesting that P. P. change her profession or her lifestyle?

What are the important nursing implications for P. P.?

Think about how the nurse can work with P. P. to ensure some compliance with therapy and a return to a healthy state.

DISCUSSION

Because of P. P.'s appearance, a complete physical examination should be performed before drug therapy is initiated. It is necessary to know baseline functioning in order to evaluate any underlying problems that may exist. Poor nutrition and total starvation result in characteristic deficiencies that predispose individuals to opportunistic infections and prevent their bodies from protecting themselves adequately through inflammatory and immune responses. In this case, the fact that liver changes often occur with poor nutrition is particularly important; such hepatic dysfunction may cause deficient drug metabolism and lead to toxicity.

An intensive program of teaching and support should be started for P. P., who should have an opportunity to vent her feelings and fears. She needs help accepting her diagnosis and adapting to the drug therapy and nutritional changes that are necessary for the effective treatment of this infection. She should understand the possible causes of her infection (poor nutrition and the loss of normal flora secondary to antibiotic therapy); the specifics of her drug therapy, including timing and administration; and adverse effects and warning signs that should be reported. P. P. should be monitored closely for adverse effects and should return for follow-up regularly while taking the ketoconazole. Nutritional counseling or referral to a dietitian for thorough nutritional teaching may prove beneficial.

The actual resolution of the fungal infection may occur only after a combination of prolonged drug and nutritional therapy. Because the required therapy will affect P. P.'s lifestyle tremendously, she will need a great deal of support and encouragement to make the necessary changes and to maintain compliance. A health care provider, such as a nurse whom P. P. trusts and with whom she can regularly discuss her concerns, may be an essential element in helping eradicate the fungal infection.

- Ensure that the patient takes the complete course of the drug regimen *to achieve maximal results.*
- Ensure that the patient is using the correct method of administration depending on the route *to improve effectiveness and decrease risk of adverse effects:*

  Troches should be dissolved slowly in the mouth.
  Vaginal suppositories, creams, and tablets should be inserted high into the vagina with the patient remaining recumbent for at least 10 to 15 minutes after insertion.
  Topical creams and lotions should be rubbed into the affected area after it has been cleansed with soap and water.

- Stop the drug if a severe rash occurs, especially if it is accompanied by blisters or if local irritation and pain are very severe. *This development may indicate a sensitivity to the drug or worsening of the condition being treated.*
- Provide patient instruction *to enhance patient knowledge about drug therapy and to promote compliance.*

  The patient should

Know the correct method of drug administration.
Know the length of time necessary to treat the infection adequately.
Use clean, dry socks when treating athlete's foot, to help eradicate the infection.
Avoid occlusive dressings because of the risk of increasing systemic absorption. Drugs should not be placed near open wounds or active lesions, because these agents are not intended to be absorbed systemically.

Report severe local irritation, burning, or worsening of the infection to a health care provider (refer to the Patient Teaching Checklist: Antifungal Agents).

Evaluation

- Monitor patient response to the drug (alleviation of signs and symptoms of the fungal infection).
- Monitor for adverse effects: rash, local irritation, and burning.
- Evaluate the effectiveness of the teaching plan (patient can name the drug, dosage, possible adverse effects to watch for, and specific measures to help avoid adverse effects).
- Monitor the effectiveness of comfort and safety measures and compliance with the regimen (refer to the Nursing Care Guide: Antifungal Agents).

CHAPTER SUMMARY

- A fungus is a cellular organism with a hard cell wall that contains chitin and polysaccharides and a cell membrane that contains ergosterols.
- Any infection with a fungus is called a mycosis. Systemic fungal infections, which can be life-threatening, are increasing with the rise in the number of immunocompromised patients.
- Systemic antifungals alter the cell permeability, leading to leakage of cellular components. This causes prevention of cell replication and cell death.
- Because systemic antifungals can be very toxic, patients should be monitored closely while receiving them. Adverse effects may include hepatic and renal failure.
- Local fungal infections include vaginal and oral yeast infections (*Candida*) and a variety of tinea infections, including athlete's foot and jock itch.
- Topical antifungals are agents that are too toxic to be used systemically but are effective in the treatment of local fungal infections.
- Proper administration of topical antifungals improves their effectiveness. They should not be used near open wounds or lesions.
- Topical antifungals can cause serious local irritation, burning, and pain. The drug should be stopped if these conditions occur.

Review Questions

1. A fungus is resistant to antibiotics because
   a. a fungus cell wall contains many protective layers including folic acid and vitamin B.
   b. a fungus cell wall contains many protective layers including chitin and ergosterol.
   c. a fungus does not reproduce by cell division.
   d. antibiotics affect only bacterial cell walls.
2. All systemic antifungal drugs function to
   a. break apart the fungus nucleus.
   b. interfere with fungus DNA production.
   c. alter cell permeability of the fungus, leading to cell death.
   d. prevent the fungus from absorbing needed nutrients.
3. Amphotericin B is associated with potentially serious nephrotoxicity and should not be given concurrently with
   a. digoxin.
   b. oral anticoagulants.
   c. phenytoin.
   d. corticosteroids.
4. Fungi that cause infections of the skin and mucous membranes are called
   a. mycoses.
   b. meningeal fungi.
   c. dermatophytes.
   d. worms.
5. Tinea infections include all of the following except
   a. athlete's foot.
   b. Rocky Mountain spotted fever.
   c. jock itch.
   d. vaginal yeast infections.
6. Vaginal yeast infections often respond very well to
   a. tolnaftate.
   b. butenafine.
   c. clotrimazole.
   d. naftifine.
7. Care must be taken when using topical antifungal agents to prevent systemic absorption because
   a. the fungus is only on the surface.
   b. these drugs are too toxic to be given systemically.
   c. absorption would prevent drug effectiveness.
   d. these drugs can cause serious local burning and pain.

BIBLIOGRAPHY

Bullock, B. L. (2000). *Focus on pathophysiology*. Philadelphia: Lippincott Williams & Wilkins.

Drug facts and comparisons. (2002). St. Louis: Facts and Comparisons.

Gilman, A., Hardman, J. G., & Limbird, L. E. (Eds.) (2002). *Goodman and Gilman's the pharmacological basis of therapeutics* (10th ed.). New York: McGraw-Hill.

Karch, A. M. (2002). *2003 Lippincott's nursing drug guide*. Philadelphia: Lippincott Williams & Wilkins.

Lewis, R. E., & Klepser, M. E. (1999). The changing face of nosocomial candidemia: Epidemiology, resistance and drug therapy. *American Journal of Health-System Pharmacy, 56*, 525–536.

Professional's guide to patient drug facts. (2002). St. Louis: Facts and Comparisons.

C H A P T E R

12

Antiprotozoal Agents

140

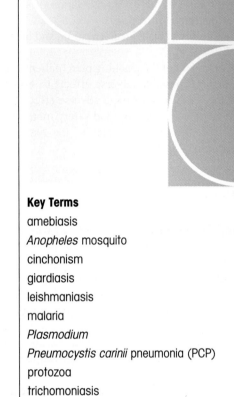

Key Terms
amebiasis
Anopheles mosquito
cinchonism
giardiasis
leishmaniasis
malaria
Plasmodium
Pneumocystis carinii pneumonia (PCP)
protozoa
trichomoniasis
trophozoite
trypanosomiasis

Antimalarials
Ⓟ chloroquine
halofantrine
hydroxychloroquine
mefloquine
primaquine

pyrimethamine
quinine
Other antiprotozoals
atovaquone
Ⓟ metronidazole
pentamidine

Infections caused by **protozoa** are very common in several parts of the world. In tropical areas, where these types of illnesses are most prevalent, many people suffer multiple infestations at the same time. These infections are relatively rare in the United States, but with people traveling throughout the world in increasing numbers, it is not unusual to find an individual who returns home from a trip to Africa, Asia, or South America with fully developed protozoal infections. Protozoa thrive in tropical climates, but they may also survive and reproduce in any area where people live in very crowded and unsanitary conditions. This chapter focuses on protozoal infections that are caused by insect bites (malaria, trypanosomiasis, and leishmaniasis) and on those that result from ingestion or contact with the causal organism (amebiasis, giardiasis, and trichomoniasis).

MALARIA

Malaria is a parasitic disease that has killed hundreds of millions of people and even changed the course of history. The courses of several African battles and the building of the Panama Canal were altered by outbreaks of malaria. Even with the introduction of drugs for the treatment of this disease, it remains endemic in many parts of the world. Malaria is spread via the bite of an **Anopheles mosquito,** which har-bors the protozoal parasite and carries it to humans. This is the only known method of disease transmission.

Four protozoal parasites, all in the genus **Plasmodium,** have been identified as causes of malaria:

• *Plasmodium falciparum* is considered to be the most dangerous type of protozoan. Infection with this protozoan results in an acute, rapidly fulminating disease with high fever, severe hypotension, swelling and reddening of the limbs, loss of red blood cells, and even death.
• *Plasmodium vivax* causes a milder form of the disease, which seldom results in death.
• *Plasmodium malariae* is endemic in many tropical countries and causes very mild signs and symptoms in the population. It can cause more acute disease in travelers to endemic areas.
• *Plasmodium ovale,* which is rarely seen, seems to be in the process of being eradicated.

Part of the problem with malaria control is that the female mosquito, which is responsible for transmitting the disease, has developed a resistance to the insecticides designed to eradicate the mosquito. Widespread efforts at mosquito control were successful for a long period, with fewer cases of malaria seen each year. Because the insecticide-resistant mosquitoes continue to flourish, however, the incidence of malaria is again increasing. In addition, the protozoa that cause malaria have developed strains resistant to the usual

DRUG THERAPY ACROSS THE LIFESPAN

Antiprotozoal Agents

Children	Adults	Older Adults
Children are very sensitive to the effects of most antiprotozoal drugs, and more severe reactions can be expected when these drugs are used in children. Many of these drugs do not have proven safety and efficacy in children, and extreme caution should be used. The dangers of infection resulting from travel to areas endemic with many of these diseases are often much more severe than the potential risks associated with cautious use of these drugs. If a child needs to travel to an area with endemic protozoal infections, the CDC or local health department should be consulted about the safest possible preventative measures.	Adults should be well advised about the need for prophylaxis against various protozoal infections and the need for immediate treatment if the disease is contracted. It is very helpful to mark calendars as reminders of the days before, during, and after exposure on which the drugs should be taken. Pregnant and nursing women should not use these drugs unless the benefit clearly outweighs the potential risk to the fetus or neonate. Women of child-bearing age should be advised to use barrier contraceptives if any of these drugs are used. A pregnant woman traveling to an area endemic with protozoal infections should be advised of the serious risks to the fetus associated with both preventive therapy and treatment of acute attacks, as well as the risks associated with contracting the disease.	Older patients may be more susceptible to the adverse effects associated with these drugs. They should be monitored closely. Patients with hepatic dysfunction are at increased risk for worsening hepatic problems and toxic effects of many of these drugs. If hepatic dysfunction is expected (extreme age, alcohol abuse, use of other hepatotoxic drugs), the dosage may need to be lowered and the patient monitored more frequently.

antimalarial drugs. This combination of factors has led to a worldwide public health challenge.

Life Cycle of *Plasmodium*

The parasites that cause human malaria spend part of their life in the *Anopheles* mosquito and part in the human host (Figure 12–1). When a mosquito bites a human who is infected with malaria, it sucks blood infested with gametocytes, which are male and female forms of the plasmodium. These gametocytes mate in the stomach of the mosquito and produce a zygote that goes through several phases before forming sporozoites (spore animals) that make their way to the mosquito's salivary glands.

The next person who is bitten by that mosquito is injected with thousands of sporozoites. These animals travel through the bloodstream, where they quickly become lodged in the human liver and other tissues and invade the cells.

Inside human cells, the organisms undergo asexual cell division and reproduction. Over the next 7 to 10 days, these primary tissue schizonts grow and multiply within their invaded cells (as trophozoites). Merozoites are formed from the primary schizonts and then burst from invaded cells when they rupture because of overexpansion. These merozoites enter the circulation and invade red blood cells, in which they continue to divide until the blood cells also burst, sending more merozoites into the circulation to invade yet more red blood cells.

FIGURE 12–1. Types of antimalarial drugs in relation to the stages in the life cycle of *Plasmodium*.

Eventually, there are a large number of merozoites in the body as well as many ruptured and invaded red blood cells. At this point, the acute malarial attack occurs. The rupture of the red blood cells causes chills and fever related to the pyrogenic effects of the protozoa and the toxic effects of the red blood cell components on the system. This cycle of chills and fever usually occurs about every 72 hours.

With *P. vivax* and *P. malariae* malaria, this cycle may continue for a long period. Many of the tissue schizonts lay dormant until they eventually find their way to the liver, where they multiply and then invade more red blood cells, again causing the acute cycle. This may occur for years in an untreated patient.

With *P. falciparum* malaria, there are no extrahepatic sites for the schizonts. If the patient survives an acute attack, no prolonged periods of relapse occur. The first attack of this type of malaria can destroy so many red blood cells that the patient's capillaries become clogged and the circulation to vital organs is interrupted, leading to death.

Antimalarials

Antimalarial drugs are usually given in combination form to attack the plasmodium at various stages of its life cycle. Using this approach, it is possible to prevent the acute malarial reaction in individuals who have been infected by the parasite.

Quinine (generic), the first drug found to be effective in the treatment of malaria, is now reserved for treatment of chloroquine-resistant infections in combination with other agents. Quinine affects the DNA synthesis of the plasmodium, leading to an inability to reproduce effectively. The drug may lead to severe diarrhea and a condition called **cinchonism** (nausea, vomiting, tinnitus, and vertigo), which makes it less desirable than newer, less toxic drugs. Quinine is readily absorbed from the top of the small intestine, with peak serum levels occurring within 1 to 3 hours. It is metabolized in the liver, with a half-life of 4 to 5 hours, and is excreted in the urine. Quinine is toxic to the fetus and is classified as pregnancy category X. Barrier contraceptive use should be advised for women of child-bearing age who need to take quinine.

Chloroquine (*Aralen*) is currently the mainstay of antimalarial therapy. This drug enters human red blood cells and changes the metabolic pathways necessary for the reproduction of the plasmodium. In addition, this agent is directly toxic to parasites that absorb it; it is acidic and it decreases the ability of the parasite to synthesize DNA, leading to a blockage of reproduction. Chloroquine sometimes has serious adverse effects such as hepatic toxicity, permanent eye damage, and blindness. Chloroquine is readily absorbed from the GI tract, with peak serum levels occurring in 1 to 6 hours. It is concentrated in the liver, spleen, kidney, and brain and is excreted very slowly in the urine, primarily as unchanged drug. Use during pregnancy and lactation should be restricted to situations in which the benefit clearly outweighs the potential risk to the neonate.

Hydroxychloroquine (*Plaquenil*) inhibits parasite reproduction, and, by blocking the synthesis of protein production, it can cause the death of the plasmodium. This drug is used in combination therapy, usually with primaquine, for greatest effectiveness. Hydroxychloroquine is readily absorbed from the GI tract, with peak serum levels occurring in 1 to 6 hours. It is excreted slowly in the urine, primarily as unchanged drug. Use during pregnancy and lactation should be restricted to situations where the benefit clearly outweighs the potential risk to the neonate.

Mefloquine (*Lariam*) increases the acidity of plasmodial food vacuoles, causing cell rupture and death. In combination therapy, mefloquine is used in malarial prevention as well as treatment. Mefloquine is a mixture of molecules that are absorbed, metabolized, and excreted at different rates. The terminal half-life is 13 to 24 days. Metabolism occurs in the liver, and caution should be used in patients with hepatic dysfunction. Pregnancy should be avoided during and for 2 months after completion of therapy. Mefloquine is teratogenic in preclinical studies. Mefloquine crosses into breast milk and can be very toxic to the baby. Breast feeding should be discontinued if this drug is essential for therapy.

Primaquine (generic), another very old drug for treating malaria, similar to quinine, disrupts the mitochondria of the plasmodium. It also causes death of gametocytes and exoerythrocytic forms and prevents other forms from reproducing. Because of this action, it is especially useful in preventing relapses of *P. vivax* and *P. malariae* infections. Primaquine is readily absorbed and metabolized in the liver. Excretion occurs primarily in the urine. Safety for use during pregnancy has not been established.

Pyrimethamine (*Daraprim*) is used in combination with agents that act more rapidly to suppress malaria by blocking the use of folic acid in protein synthesis by the plasmodium, eventually leading to inability to reproduce and cell death. Pyrimethamine is readily absorbed from the GI tract, with peak levels occurring within 2 to 6 hours. It is metabolized in the liver and has a half-life of 4 days. It usually maintains suppressive concentrations in the body for about 2 weeks. As with other antiprotozoals, pyrimethamine should not be used during pregnancy or lactation unless the benefit clearly outweighs the potential risk to the fetus.

Halofantrine (*Halfan*), the newest antimalarial agent, is effective in the erythrocyte stage of the disease and causes the death of the plasmodium. Apparently, it has no effect on the sporozoite or gametocyte phases or on the hepatic stage of the disease, so it is most effective when used in combination with other antimalarials. Halofantrine is readily absorbed from the GI tract, with peak levels occurring in 5 to 7 hours. It is metabolized in the liver and has a long termination half-life of 6 to 10 days. Excretion occurs primarily in the feces. Halofantrine has caused fetal abnormalities in rabbits and should be avoided during pregnancy and lactation because of the potential risks to the neonate. Halofantrine prolongs the QTc interval (a syndrome associated with syncope, ventricular arrhythmias, and sudden death) and should not be used in patients with known cardiac conduction abnormalities or combined with other drugs that prolong the QTc interval. A baseline electrocardiogram (ECG) should be obtained before treatment with this drug is started.

Combination drugs for malaria prevention and treatment are discussed in Box 12–1.

Therapeutic Actions and Indications
Research has demonstrated that the antimalarial agents are effective in interrupting plasmodial reproduction of protein synthesis in the red blood cell stage of the life cycle as well as in the hepatic and gametocyte stages in some cases (Figure 12–2). Chemotherapeutic agents, which do not appear to affect the sporozoites, are used for prophylaxis and treatment of acute attacks of malaria caused by susceptible strains of *Plasmodium*.

Contraindications/Cautions
Contraindications to the use of antimalarials are the presence of known allergy to any of these drugs; liver disease or alcoholism, both because of the parasitic invasion of the liver and because of the need for the hepatic metabolism to avoid reaching toxic levels; and lactation, because the drugs can enter breast milk and could be toxic to the infant. Caution should be used in patients with retinal disease or damage, because many of these drugs can affect vision and the retina and the likelihood of problems increases if the retina is already damaged; with psoriasis or porphyria, because of skin damage; with damage to mucous membranes, which can occur as a result of the effects of the drug on proteins and protein synthesis; or with prolonged QTc intervals, if using halofantrine.

Adverse Effects
A number of adverse effects are encountered with the use of these antimalarial agents. Headache, dizziness, fever, shaking, chills, and malaise are associated with central nervous system (CNS) effects of the drugs and immune reaction to the release of the mitozoites. Nausea, vomiting, dyspepsia, and anorexia are associated with direct drug effects on the gastrointestinal (GI) tract and effects on CNS control of vomiting related to cell death and protein changes. Hepatic dysfunction is associated with the toxic effects of the drug on the liver and the effects of the disease on the liver. Dermatological effects include rash, pruritus, and loss of hair associated with changes in protein synthesis. Visual changes, including possible blindness related to retinal damage from the drug, and ototoxicity related to additional nerve damage may occur. Cinchonism (nausea, vomiting, tinnitus, and vertigo) is more commonly seen with high levels of quinine and is related to drug effects in the CNS. This effect can be seen with any quinine-related drug if toxic levels occur.

BOX 12-1
Combination Drugs Used For Malaria Prevention and Treatment

Two fixed combination drugs are available for use in the prevention and treatment of malaria. Combining two different preparations in one drug may increase compliance by reducing the number of pills a patient has to take, and it conforms to the treatment protocol of taking drugs that effect the protozoa at different stages on their life cycle.

Fansidar is a combination of sulfadoxine and pyrimethamine. It is indicated for the treatment of *Plasmodium falciparum* malaria when chloroquine resistance is suspected. It is used for prophylaxis of malaria when travelers are going to areas in which chloroquine-resistant strains are known to be endemic. *Fansidar* is contraindicated in pregnancy, and women should be advised to use barrier contraceptives while taking it. Both of the constituent drugs cross into breast milk and can cause serious reactions in the neonate.

Usual dosage, acute attack

Adult: 2–3 tablets PO as a single dose
Pediatric (9–14 y): 2 tablets PO as a single dose
Pediatric (4–8 y): 1 tablet PO as a single dose
Pediatric (<4 y): ½ tablet PO as a single dose

Usual dosage, prevention

Adult: 1 tablet PO every week or 2 tablets every other week
Pediatric (9–14 y): ¾ tablet PO every week or 1½ tablets every other week
Pediatric (4–8 y): ½ tablet PO every week or 1 tablet every other week
Pediatric (<4 y): ¼ tablet PO every week or ½ tablet every other week

Preventive therapy should begin 1–2 d before exposure and should continue throughout and 4–6 wk after leaving the area.

Malarone and *Malarone Pediatric* combine atovaquone and proguanil. They are indicated for the prevention of *P. falciparum* malaria when chlorquine resistance has been reported. It is used for the treatment of uncomplicated *P. falciparum* malaria when chloroquine, halofantrine, mefloquine, and amodiaquine have not proved successful, most likely because of resistance. This combination should be used in pregnancy and lactation only if the benefit clearly outweighs the potential risk to the neonate.

Usual dosage, acute attack:

Adult: 4 tablets PO as a single daily dose for 3 consecutive days
Pediatric (11–20 kg): 1 adult tablet PO q.d. for 3 consecutive days
Pediatric (21–30 kg): 2 adult tablets PO q.d. as a single daily dose for 3 consecutive days
Pediatric (31–40 kg): 3 adult tablets PO q.d. as a single daily dose for 3 consecutive days
Pediatric (>40 kg): 4 adult tablets PO q.d. as a single daily dose for 3 consecutive days

Prevention

Adult: 1 tablet PO q.d.
Pediatric (11–20 kg): 1 pediatric tablet PO q.d.
Pediatric (21–30 kg): 2 pediatric tablets PO q.d.
Pediatric (31–40 kg): 3 pediatric tablets PO q.d.
Pediatric (>40 kg): 1 adult tablet PO q.d.
Prevention should start 1–2 d before exposure and continue throughout and 7 d after leaving the area.

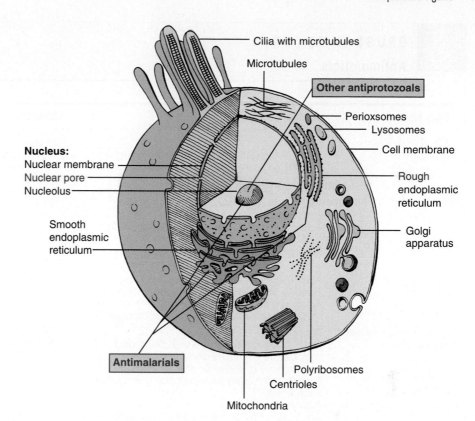

FIGURE 12-2. Sites of action of antimalarials and other antiprotozoals. Antimalarials block protein synthesis and cause cell death. Other antiprotozoals block DNA synthesis, prevent cell reproduction, and lead to cell death.

Clinically Important Drug–Drug Interactions

The patient who is receiving combinations of the quinine derivatives and quinine is at increased risk for cardiac toxicity and convulsions and should be checked very closely. Drug levels should be monitored and dosage adjustments made as needed.

Patients taking halofantrine are at increased risk for serious cardiac arrhythmias and even death if they are taking other drugs that prolong the QTc interval.

Nursing Considerations for Patients Receiving Antimalarial Agents

Assessment: History and Physical Assessment

Screen for the following: history of allergy to any of the antimalarials; liver dysfunction or alcoholism that might interfere with the metabolism and excretion of the drug; porphyria or psoriasis, which could be exacerbated by the drug effects; retinal disease that could increase the visual disturbances associated with these drugs; prolonged QTc interval, which could increase the risk for cardiac arrhythmias if taking halofantrine; pregnancy and lactation, because these drugs could affect the fetus and could enter the breast milk and be toxic to the infant.

Physical assessment should be performed to establish baseline data for assessment of the effectiveness of the drug and the occurrence of any adverse effects associated with drug therapy. Assess CNS (reflexes and muscle strength). Perform retinal examination and auditory and ophthalmic screening to detect cautions for drug use and to evaluate changes that occur as a result of drug therapy. Perform liver evaluation and obtain liver function tests to determine ap-

propriateness of therapy and to monitor for toxicity. Perform blood culture to determine which *Plasmodium* species is causing the disease. Conduct examination of the skin (lesions, color, temperature, and texture) to monitor for adverse effects. Obtain a baseline ECG if halofantrine is being used.

Nursing Diagnoses

The patient receiving an antimalarial drug may have the following nursing diagnoses related to drug therapy:

- Acute Pain related to GI, CNS, skin effects of drug
- Disturbed Sensory Perception (Kinesthetic, Visual) related to CNS effects
- Deficient Knowledge regarding drug therapy

Implementation

- Arrange for appropriate culture and sensitivity tests before beginning therapy *to ensure proper drug for susceptible Plasmodium species.* Treatment may begin before tests results are known.
- Administer the complete course of the drug *to get the full beneficial effects.* Mark a calendar for prophylactic doses. Use combination therapy as indicated.
- Monitor hepatic function and ophthalmologic examination before and periodically during treatment to effectively arrange to stop the drug if signs of failure or deteriorating vision occur.
- Provide comfort and safety measures if CNS effects occur

DRUGS IN FOCUS
Antimalarials

Drug Name	Dosage/Route	Usual Indications
Ⓟ chloroquine (*Aralen*)	*Suppression:* Adult: 300 mg PO every week beginning 1–2 wk before exposure and continuing for 4 wk after leaving endemic area Pediatric: 5 mg/kg per week PO, using same schedule as for an adult *Acute attacks:* Adult: 600 mg PO followed by 300 mg PO in 6 h; then 300 mg PO on days 2 and 3 Pediatric: 10 mg/kg PO, followed by 5 mg/kg PO in 6 h and on days 2 and 3.	Prevention and treatment of *Plasmodium* malaria; treatment of extraintestinal amebiasis
halofantrine (*Halfan*)	Adult, never previously exposed: 500 mg PO q6h for three doses, then repeat in 7 days Adult, semi-immune: use for only one course Pediatric: safety and efficacy not established	Treatment of *Plasmodium* malaria in combination with other drugs
hydroxychloroquine (*Plaquenil*)	*Suppression:* Adult: 310 mg PO every week, beginning 1–2 wk before exposure and continuing for 4 wk after leaving endemic area Pediatric: 5 mg/kg per week, following adult schedule *Acute attack:* Adult: 620 mg PO, followed by 310 mg PO in 6 h and on days 2 and 3 Pediatric: 10 mg/kg PO, followed by 5 mg/kg PO in 6 h and on days 2 and 3	Treatment of *Plasmodium* malaria in combination with other drugs, particularly primaquine
mefloquine (*Lariam*)	*Treatment:* Adult: 1250 mg PO as a single dose *Prevention:* Adult: 250 mg PO once weekly for 4 wk, then 250 mg PO every other week, starting 1 wk before travel and continuing for 4 wk after leaving area Pediatric: 15–19 kg, ¼ tablet; 20–30 kg, ½ tablet; 31–45 mg, ¾ tablet; >45 kg, 1 tablet. Take once a week, starting 1 wk before travel and continuing until 4 wk after leaving area	Prevention and treatment of *Plasmodium* malaria in combination with other drugs
primaquine (generic)	Adult: 26.3 mg/d PO for 14 d Pediatric: 0.5 mg/kg per day PO for 14 d Begin therapy during last 2 wk of (or after) therapy with chloroquine or other drugs	Prevention of relapses of *P. vivax* and *P. malariae* infections; radical cure of *P. vivax* malaria
pyrimethamine (*Daraprim*)	*Prevention:* Adult: 25 mg PO every week Pediatric (>10 y): same as adult Pediatric (4–10 y): 12.5 mg PO every week Pediatric (<4 y): 6.25 mg PO every week *Toxoplasmosis:* Adult: 50–75 mg PO qd with 1–4 g of a sulfonamide, for 4–5 wk Pediatric: 1 mg/kg per day PO, divided into two equal doses, for 2–4 d; then cut dose in half and continue for 1 mo	Prevention of *Plasmodium* malaria, in combination with other agents to suppress transmission; treatment of toxoplasmosis
quinine (generic)	Adult: 260–650 mg PO t.i.d. for 6–12 d Pediatric: 10 mg/kg PO q8h for 5–7 d	Treatment of chloroquine-resistant *Plasmodium* infections

(eg, siderails and assistance with ambulation if dizziness and weakness are present) *to prevent patient injury.* Provide oral hygiene and ready access to bathroom facilities as needed *to cope with GI effects.*

• Provide small, frequent, nutritious meals if GI upset is severe *to ensure adequate nutrition.* Monitor nutritional status and arrange a dietary consultation as needed. Taking the drug with food may also decrease GI upset.

- Ensure that the patient is instructed concerning the appropriate dosage regimen *to enhance patient knowledge about drug therapy and to promote compliance.*

   The patient should

Take safety precautions, including changing position slowly and avoiding driving and hazardous tasks, if CNS effects occur.

Take the drug with meals and try small, frequent meals if GI upset is a problem.

Report blurring of vision, which could indicate retinal damage; loss of hearing or ringing in the ears, which could indicate CNS toxicity; and fever or worsening of condition, which could indicate a resistant strain or noneffective therapy.

Evaluation

- Monitor patient response to the drug (resolution of malaria or prevention of malaria).
- Monitor for adverse effects (orientation and affect, nutritional state, skin color and lesions, hepatic function, and visual and auditory changes).
- Evaluate the effectiveness of the teaching plan (patient can name the drug, dosage, possible adverse effects to watch for, and specific measures to help avoid adverse effects).
- Monitor the effectiveness of comfort and safety measures and compliance with the regimen.

◻◼◉◼ WEB LINKS

Health care providers and patients may want to consult the following Internet sources:

Information on malaria, including information for travelers:
   http://www.cdc.gov/travel/malinfo.htm
Information on malaria incidence, treatment, prevention, and support:
   http://www.hawaii.gov/doh/resource/comm_dis/cddmalar. htm
Information on trypanosomiasis:
   http://www.thirdworldtraveler.com/Disease/sleeping_ sickness.html
Information about giardiasis—support, treatment, prevention, teaching:
   http://www.vdh.state.va.us/epi/giarf.htm
Information about amebiasis prevention, incidence, and treatments:
   http://www.aomc.org/ComDiseases/Amebiasis.html

OTHER PROTOZOAL INFECTIONS

Other protozoal infections that are encountered in clinical practice include amebiasis, leishmaniasis, trypanosomiasis, trichomoniasis, and giardiasis. These infections, which are caused by single-celled protozoa, are usually associated with

CULTURAL CONSIDERATIONS
Potential for Hemolytic Crisis

Patients with glucose-6-phosphate dehydrogenase (G6PD) deficiency—which is more likely to occur in Greeks, Italians, and other people of Mediterranean descent—may experience a hemolytic crisis if taking the antimalarial agents chloroquine, primaquine, or quinine. Patients of Greek, Italian, or Mediterranean ancestry should be questioned about any history of potential G6PD deficiency. If no history is known, the patient should be tested before any of these drugs are prescribed. If testing is not possible and the drugs are needed, the patient should be monitored very closely and informed about the potential need for hospitalization and emergency services.

unsanitary, crowded conditions and use of poor hygienic practices. Patients traveling to some other countries may encounter these infections, which also appear increasingly in the United States.

Amebiasis

Amebiasis, an intestinal infection caused by *Entamoeba histolytica,* is often known as amebic dysentery. *E. histolytica* has a two-stage life cycle (Figure 12–3). The organism exists in two stages: (1) a cystic, dormant stage, in which the protozoan can live for long periods outside the body or in the human intestine, and (2) a **trophozoite** stage in the ideal environment—the human large intestine.

   The disease is transmitted while the protozoan is in the cystic stage in fecal matter, from which it can enter water and the ground. It can be passed to other humans who drink this water or eat food that has been grown in this ground. The cysts are swallowed and pass, unaffected by gastric acid, into the intestine. Some of these cysts are passed in fecal matter, and some of them become trophozoites that grow and reproduce. The trophozoites migrate into the mucosa of the colon, where they penetrate into the intestinal wall, forming erosions. These forms of *Entamoeba* release a chemical that dissolves mucosal cells, and eventually they eat away tissue until they reach the vascular system, which carries them throughout the body. The trophozoites lodge in the liver, lungs, heart, brain, and so on.

   Early signs of amebiasis include mild to fulminate diarrhea. In the worst cases, if the protozoan is able to invade extraintestinal tissue, it can dissolve the tissue and eventually cause the death of the host. Some individuals can become carriers of the disease without having any overt signs or symptoms. These people seem to be resistant to the intestinal invasion but pass the cysts on in the stool.

Leishmaniasis

Leishmaniasis is a disease caused by a protozoan that is passed from sand flies to humans. The sand fly injects an asexual form of this flagellated protozoan, called a promastigote,

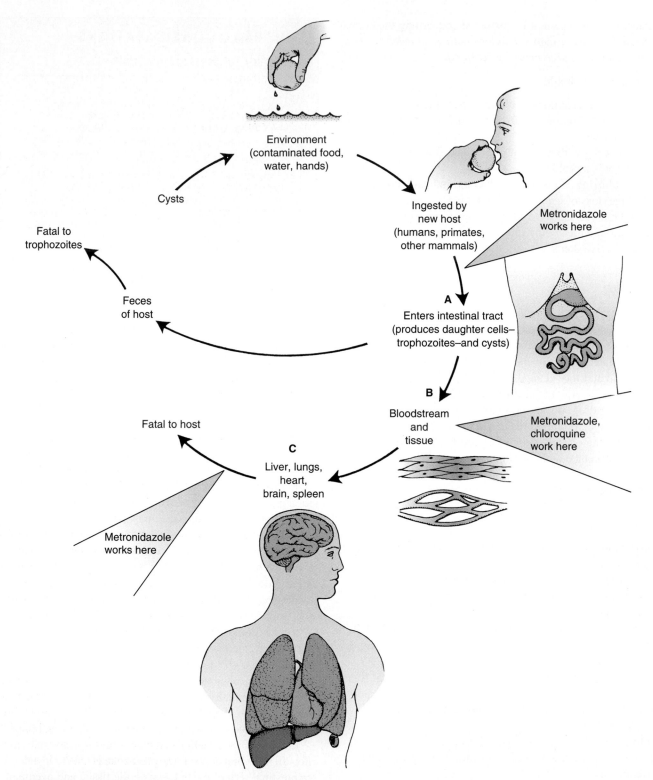

FIGURE 12-3. Life cycle of *Entamoeba histolytica* and the sites of action of metronidazole and chloroquine, which are used to treat amebiasis.

into the body of a human, where it is rapidly attacked and digested by human macrophages. Inside the macrophages, the promastigote divides, developing many new forms called amastigotes, which keep dividing and eventually kill the macrophage, releasing the amastigotes into the system to be devoured by more macrophages. Thus, a cyclic pattern of infection is established. These amastigotes can cause serious lesions in the skin, the viscera, or the mucous membranes of the host.

Trypanosomiasis

Trypanosomiasis is caused by infection with *Trypanosoma*. Two parasitic protozoal species cause very serious and often fatal diseases in humans.

NURSING CHALLENGE
World Travel and the Spread of Pathogens

Nowadays, people are traveling to more exotic areas of the world than ever before. Because of this, people are being exposed to more pathogens than ever before, and they also are potentially spreading pathogens to different areas of the world. Pathogens that are endemic in one area of the world, causing mild disease, can be quite devastating in a population that has not previously been exposed to that pathogen.

World health agencies and governments have established guidelines for prophylaxis and treatment of such diseases for travelers. People who are planning to travel out of the country should contact their local Health Department or the Centers for Disease Control and Prevention (CDC; website available at http://www.cdc/gov/travel) for the latest information on what prophylactic measures are required in the area they plan to visit and to learn about potential health hazards in that area. The information is updated frequently and should be consulted regularly.

Patients who have been traveling to other areas of the world and who present with any illness should be questioned about where they traveled, what precautions (including prophylactic measures) were taken, and when they first experienced any signs or symptoms of illness. The CDC can be consulted about diagnosis and treatment guidelines for any tropical disease that is unfamiliar to a health care provider, as well as what precautions should be used in caring for such patients.

African sleeping sickness, which is caused by *Trypanosoma brucei gambiense,* is transmitted by the tsetse fly. After the pathogenic organism has lived and grown in human blood, it eventually invades the CNS, leading to an acute inflammation that results in lethargy, prolonged sleep, and even death.

Chagas' disease, which is caused by *Trypanosoma cruzi,* is almost endemic in many South American countries. This protozoan results in a severe cardiomyopathy that accounts for numerous deaths and disabilities in certain regions.

Trichomoniasis
Trichomoniasis, which is caused by another flagellated protozoan, *Trichomonas vaginalis,* is a common cause of vaginitis. This infection is usually spread during sexual intercourse by men who have no signs and symptoms of infection. In women, this protozoan causes reddened, inflamed vaginal mucosa, itching, burning, and a yellowish-green discharge.

Giardiasis
Giardiasis, which is caused by *Giardia lamblia,* is the most commonly diagnosed intestinal parasite in the United States. This protozoan forms cysts, which survive outside the body and allow transmission through contaminated water or food, and trophozoites, which break out of the cysts in the upper small intestine and eventually cause signs and symptoms of disease. Diarrhea, rotten egg–smelling stool, and pale and mucous-filled stool are commonly seen. Some patients ex-perience epigastric distress, weight loss, and malnourishment as a result of the invasion of the mucosa.

Pneumocystis carinii Pneumonia
Pneumocystis carinii is an endemic protozoan that does not usually cause illness in humans. When an individual's immune system becomes suppressed, because of acquired immunodeficiency syndrome (AIDS) or AIDS-related complex (ARC), the use of immunosuppressant drugs, or advanced age, this parasite is able to invade the lungs, leading to severe inflammation and the condition known as **Pneumocystis carinii pneumonia (PCP).** This disease is the most common opportunistic infection in patients with AIDS.

Other Antiprotozoal Agents

Drugs that are available specifically for the treatment of these various protozoan infections include many of the malarial drugs; chloroquine is effective against extraintestinal amebiasis and pyrimethamine is also effective in treating toxoplasmosis. Other drugs, including some tetracyclines and aminoglycosides, are used for treating these conditions at various stages of the disease. Other antiprotozoals include the following agents.

- Atovaquone (*Mepron*), which is especially active against PCP, is slowly absorbed and is highly protein bound in circulation. It is excreted slowly through the feces, with a half-life of 67 to 76 hours. Use during pregnancy and lactation should be limited to those situations in which the benefit to the mother clearly outweighs the potential risks to the fetus. The safety and efficacy of atovaquone in children has not been established.
- Metronidazole (*Flagyl, MetroGel, Noritate*), which is used to treat amebiasis, trichomoniasis, and giardiasis, is well absorbed orally, reaching peak levels in 1 to 2 hours. It is metabolized in the liver with a half-life of 8 to 15 hours. Excretion occurs primarily through the urine. Metronidazole rapidly crosses the placenta and enters fetal circulation. It passes into breast milk. Use during pregnancy and lactation should be restricted to those situations when the benefit clearly outweighs the risk to the neonate. Safety and efficacy in children has not been established.
- Pentamidine (*Pentam 300, NebuPent*) is used as an inhalation agent and a systemic agent in the treatment of PCP and as a systemic drug in the treatment of trypanosomiasis and leishmaniasis. Pentamidine is readily absorbed through the lungs. Excretion occurs in the urine, with traces found in the urine for up to 6 weeks. The safety and efficacy of pentamidine during pregnancy and lactation, and for children, have not been established.

Therapeutic Actions and Indications
These antiprotozoal agents act to inhibit DNA synthesis in susceptible protozoa, leading to the inability to reproduce and subsequent cell death (see Figure 12–2). These drugs are indicated for the treatment of infections caused by susceptible protozoa.

Contraindications and Cautions
Contraindications include the presence of any known allergy or hypersensitivity to any of these drugs and pregnancy, be-

CASE STUDY

Coping With Amebiasis

PRESENTATION

J. C., a 20-year-old male college student, reported to the university health center complaining of severe diarrhea, abdominal pain, and, most recently, blood in his stool. He had a mild fever and appeared to be dehydrated and very tired. The young man, who denied travel outside the country, reported eating most of his meals at the local beer joint, where he worked in the kitchen each night making pizza.

A stool sample for ova and parasites (O&P) was obtained, and a diagnosis of amebiasis was made. J. C. was prescribed metronidazole. A public health referral was sent to find the source of the infection, which was the kitchen of the beer joint where J. C. worked. The kitchen was shut down until all the food, utensils, and environment passed state health inspection. Although a potential epidemic was averted (only three other cases of amebiasis were reported), the action of the public health officials added a new stress to this student's life, because he was unemployed for several months.

CRITICAL THINKING

What are the important nursing implications for J. C.? *Think about the usual nutritional state of a college student who eats most of his meals in a pizza place.*

What are the implications for recovery when a patient is malnourished and then has a disease that causes severe diarrhea, dehydration, and potential malnourishment? *Consider how difficult it will be for J. C. to be a full-time student while trying to cope with the signs and symptoms of his disease as well as the adverse effects associated with his drug therapy and the need to maintain adequate nutrition to allow some healing and recovery.*

What potential problems could the added stress of being out of work have for J.C.? *Consider the physiological impact of stress as well as the psychological problems of trying to cope with one more stressor.*

DISCUSSION

J. C. needed a great deal of reassurance and an explanation of his disease. He learned that oral hygiene and small, frequent meals would help alleviate some of his discomfort until the metronidazole could control the amebiasis and that good hygiene and strict hand washing when the disease is active would help to prevent transmission. He was advised to watch for the occurrence of specific adverse drug effects such as a possible severe reaction to alcohol (he was advised to avoid alcoholic beverages while taking this drug); gastrointestinal upset and a strange metallic taste (the importance of good nutrition to promote healing of the gastrointestinal tract was stressed); dizziness or lightheadedness; and superinfections.

J. C. was scheduled for a follow-up examination for stool O&P and nutritional status. Metronidazole was continued until the stool sample came back negative. He needed and received a great deal of support and encouragement, because he was far from home and the disease and the drug effects were sometimes difficult to cope with.

The effects of stress—decreasing blood flow to the gastrointestinal tract, for example—can make it more difficult for patients such as J. C. to recover from this disease. Support and encouragement can be major factors in their eventual recovery. J. C. was given a telephone number to call if he needed information or support and a complete set of written instructions regarding the disease and the drug therapy.

---

cause drug effects on developing fetal DNA and proteins can cause fetal abnormalities and even death. Caution should be used in the presence of CNS disease because of possible exacerbation when the drug affects the CNS; hepatic disease, because of possible exacerbation when hepatic drug effects occur; candidiasis, because of the risk of superinfections; and lactation, because these drugs may pass into breast milk and could have severe adverse effects on the infant.

Adverse Effects

Adverse effects that can be seen with these antiprotozoal agents include such CNS effects as headache, dizziness, ataxia, loss of coordination, and peripheral neuropathy related to drug effects on the neurons. GI effects include nausea, vomiting, diarrhea, unpleasant taste, cramps, and changes in liver function. Superinfections also can occur when the normal flora is disrupted.

Nursing Considerations for Patients Receiving Antiprotozoal Agents

Assessment: History and Physical Assessment

Screen for the following conditions: history of allergy to any of the antiprotozoals; liver dysfunction that might interfere with metabolism and excretion of the drug or be exacerbated by the drug; pregnancy, which is a contraindication, and lactation, because these drugs could enter the breast milk and be toxic to the infant; CNS disease that could be exacerbated by the drug; and candidiasis that could become severe as a result of the effects of these drugs on the normal flora.

Physical assessment should be performed to establish baseline data for determination of the effectiveness of the drug and the occurrence of any adverse effects associated with drug therapy. Conduct an examination of the CNS to check reflexes and of muscle strength to detect cautions for drug use and to evalu-

DRUGS IN FOCUS
Antiprotozoal Agents

Drug Name	Dosage/Route	Usual Indications
atovaquone (*Mepron*)	*Prevention:* Adult and Pediatric >13 y: 1500 mg PO q.d. *Treatment:* Adult and Pediatric >13 y: 750 mg PO b.i.d. with meals, for 12 d	Prevention and treatment of *Pneumocystis carinii* pneumonia
Ⓟ metronidazole (*Flagyl, MetroGel, Noritate*)	*Amebiasis:* Adult: 750 mg PO t.i.d. for 5–10 d Pediatric: 35–50 mg/kg per day PO in three divided doses for 10 d *Trichomoniasis:* Adult: 2 g PO as one dose, or divided into two doses given on the same day or 250 mg PO t.i.d. for 7 d Pediatric: 5 mg/kg per dose PO t.i.d. for 7 d	Treatment of amebiasis, trichomoniasis, giardiasis
pentamidine (*Pentam 300, Nebupent*)	Inhalation: 300 mg once every 4 wk Injection: 4 mg/kg per day IM or IV for 14 d	As inhalation treatment of PCP; as a systemic agent in the treatment of trypanosomiasis and leishmaniasis

ate changes that occur as a result of drug therapy. Evaluate liver and liver function tests to determine appropriateness of therapy and to monitor for toxicity. Obtain cultures to determine the exact protozoal species causing the disease. Examine the skin and mucous membranes to check for lesions, color, temperature, and texture, to monitor for adverse effects and superinfections.

Nursing Diagnoses

The patient receiving an antiprotozoal drug may have the following nursing diagnoses related to drug therapy:

• Acute Pain related to GI, CNS effects of drug
• Imbalanced Nutrition: Less than Body Requirements, related to severe GI effects of drug
• Disturbed Sensory Perception (Kinesthetic, Visual) related to CNS effects
• Deficient Knowledge regarding drug therapy

Implementation

• Arrange for appropriate culture and sensitivity tests before beginning therapy *to ensure proper drug for susceptible organisms.* Treatment may begin before tests results are known.
• Administer the complete course of the drug *to get the full beneficial effects.* Use combination therapy as indicated.
• Monitor hepatic function before and periodically during treatment *to arrange to effectively stop the drug if signs of failure or worsening liver function occur.*
• Provide comfort and safety measures if CNS effects occur, such as siderails and assistance with ambulation if dizzi-

ness and weakness are present, *to prevent injury to the patient.* Provide oral hygiene and ready access to bathroom facilities as needed *to cope with GI effects.*
• Arrange for treatment of superinfections as appropriate *to prevent severe infections.*
• Provide small, frequent, nutritious meals if GI upset is severe, *to ensure proper nutrition.* Monitor nutritional status and arrange a dietary consultation as needed. Taking the drug with food may also decrease GI upset.
• Ensure that the patient is instructed about the appropriate dosage regimen *to enhance patient knowledge about drug therapy and to promote compliance.*

The patient should

Take safety precautions, including changing position slowly and avoiding driving and hazardous tasks, if CNS effects occur.
Take the drug with meals and try small, frequent meals if GI upset is a problem.
Report severe GI problems and interference with nutrition; fever and chills, which may indicate the presence of a superinfection; and dizziness, unusual fatigue, or weakness, which may indicate CNS effects

See accompanying Patient Teaching Checklist on antiprotozoal agents.

Evaluation

• Monitor patient response to the drug (resolution of infection and negative cultures for parasite).
• Monitor for adverse effects (orientation and affect, nutri-

PATIENT TEACHING CHECKLIST

Antiprotozoal Agents

Create customized patient teaching materials for a specific antiprotozoal agent from the CD-ROM. Patient teaching should stress the following points for drugs within this class:

- An antiprotozoal drug acts to destroy certain protozoa that have invaded your body. Because it affects specific phases of the protozoal life cycle, it must be taken over a period of time to be effective. It is very important to take all the drug that has been ordered for you.
- This drug frequently causes stomach upset. If it causes you to have nausea, heartburn, or vomiting, take the drug with meals or a light snack.

Common effects of this drug include the following:

- *Nausea, vomiting, and loss of appetite*—Take the drug with food and have small, frequent meals.
- *Superinfections of the mouth, vagina, and skin*—These go away when the course of the drug has been completed. If they become uncomfortable, notify your health care provider for an appropriate solution.
- *Dry mouth, strange metallic taste (metronidazole)*—Frequent mouth care and sucking sugarless lozenges may help. This effect will also go away when the course of the drug is finished.
- *Intolerance to alcohol (nausea, vomiting, flushing, headache, and stomach pain)*—Avoid alcoholic beverages or products containing alcohol while taking this drug.

Report any of the following to your health care provider: sore throat, fever, or chills; skin rash or redness; severe gastrointestinal upset; and unusual fatigue, clumsiness, or weakness.

Take the full course of your prescription. Never use this drug to self-treat any other infection or give it to any other person.

Tell any doctor, nurse, or other health care provider that you are taking this drug.

Keep this drug and all medications out of the reach of children.

Note: This Teaching Checklist reflects general patient teaching guidelines. It is not meant to be a substitute for drug-specific teaching information, which is available in nursing drug guides.

tional state, skin color and lesions, hepatic function, and occurrence of superinfections).
- Evaluate the effectiveness of the teaching plan (patient can name the drug, dosage, possible adverse effects to watch for, and specific measures to help avoid adverse effects).
- Monitor the effectiveness of comfort and safety measures and compliance with the regimen (see Nursing Care Guide: Antiprotozoal Agents).

CHAPTER SUMMARY

- A protozoan is a parasitic cellular organism. Its life cycle includes a parasitic phase inside human tissues or cells.

- Malaria, which occurs in many tropical parts of the world, has been spreading in recent years because of resistance to insecticides occurring in the *Anopheles* mosquito.
- Malaria is caused by *Plasmodium* protozoa, which must go through a cycle in the *Anopheles* mosquito before being passed to humans by the mosquito bite. Once inside a human, the protozoa invade red blood cells.
- The characteristic cyclic chills and fever of malaria occur when red blood cells burst, releasing more protozoa into the bloodstream.
- Malaria is treated with a combination of drugs that attack the protozoan at various stages in its life cycle.
- Amebiasis is caused by the protozoan *Entamoeba histolytica,* which invades human intestinal tissue after being passed to humans through unsanitary food or water.
- Leishmaniasis, a protozoan-caused disease, can result in serious lesions in the mucosa, viscera, and skin.
- Trypanosomiasis, which is caused by infection with a *Trypanosoma* parasite, may assume two forms. African sleeping sickness leads to inflammation of the CNS, and Chagas' disease results in serious cardiomyopathy.
- Trichomoniasis is caused by *Trichomonas vaginalis*. This common cause of vaginitis results in no signs or symptoms in men but serious vaginal inflammation in women.
- Giardiasis, which is caused by *Giardia lamblia,* is the most commonly diagnosed intestinal parasite in the United States. This disease may lead to serious malnutrition when the pathogen invades intestinal mucosa.
- *Pneumocystis carinii* is an endemic protozoan that does not usually cause illness in humans unless they become immunosuppressed. *P. carinii* pneumonia (PCP) is the most common opportunistic infection seen in AIDS patients.
- Patients receiving antiprotozoal agents should be monitored regularly to detect any serious adverse effects, including loss of vision, liver toxicity, and so on.

Review Questions

1. Of the following protozoal infections, the one that is not caused by insect bites is
   a. malaria.
   b. trypanosomiasis.
   c. leishmaniasis.
   d. giardiasis.
2. Malaria is caused by the *Plasmodium* protozoan, which depends on
   a. a snail to act as intermediary in the life cycle of the protozoan.
   b. a mosquito and a red blood cell for maturation.
   c. a human liver cell for cell division and reproduction.
   d. stagnant water for maturation.
3. Drugs used to treat malaria are given in combination because
   a. they are less toxic that way.
   b. they are absorbed better if taken together.
   c. mosquitos are less likely to bite a person who is taking combination drugs.

NURSING CARE GUIDE

Antiprotozoal Agents

Assessment	Nursing Diagnoses	Implementation	Evaluation
HISTORY Allergies to any of these drugs, renal or liver dysfunction, pregnancy and lactation	Acute Pain related to GI, super-infection effects	Culture infection before beginning therapy.	Evaluate drug effects: resolution of protozoal infection.
	Disturbed Sensory Perception (Kinesthetic, Visual) related to CNS effects	Provide comfort and safety measures: oral hygiene, safety precautions, treatment of superinfections, maintenance of nutrition.	Monitor for adverse effects: GI alterations, dizziness, confusion, CNS changes, vision loss, renal, hepatic function, superinfections.
	Imbalanced Nutrition: Less than Body Requirements, related to GI effects	Provide small, frequent meals and monitor nutritional status.	Monitor for drug–drug interactions as indicated for each drug.
	Deficient Knowledge regarding drug therapy	Provide support and reassurance for dealing with drug effects and discomfort.	Evaluate effectiveness of patient teaching program.
		Provide patient teaching regarding drug name, dosage, adverse effects, precautions, and warning signs to report and hygiene measures to observe.	Evaluate effectiveness of comfort and safety measures.
PHYSICAL EXAMINATION Local: culture of infection CNS: orientation, affect, vision, reflexes Skin: color, lesions, texture Respiratory: respiration rate, adventitious sounds GI: abdominal, liver evaluation Hematologic: renal and hepatic function tests			

d. the drugs can then affect the protozoan at various stages of the life cycle.
4. A patient traveling to an area of the world where malaria is known to be endemic should
   a. avoid drinking the water.
   b. begin prophylactic antimalarial therapy before traveling and continue it through the visit and for 2 to 3 weeks after the visit.
   c. take a supply of antimalarial drugs in case he or she gets a mosquito bite.
   d. begin prophylactic antimalarial therapy 2 weeks before traveling and stop the drugs on arrival at the destination.
5. Amebiasis or amebic dysentery
   a. is seen only in Third World countries.
   b. is caused by a protozoan that enters the body through an insect bite.
   c. is caused by a protozoan that can enter the body in the cyst stage in water or food, usually under unsanitary conditions.
   d. usually has no signs and symptoms.
6. Giardiasis is the most common intestinal parasite seen in the United States, and it
   a. does not respond to drug therapy.
   b. can invade the liver and cause death.
   c. is seen only in areas with no sanitation.
   d. is associated with rotten egg–smelling stool, diarrhea, and mucous-filled stool.
7. PCP (*Pneumocystis carinii* pneumonia) is not
   a. an endemic protozoan found in the human respiratory system.
   b. responsive to inhaled pentamidine.
   c. an opportunistic bacterial infection.

    d. frequently associated with immune suppression and AIDS.

8. Trypanosomiasis may assume two different forms:
    a. African sleeping sickness and Chagas' disease.
    b. elephantiasis and malaria.
    c. dysentery and African sleeping sickness.
    d. malaria and Chagas' disease.

9. A patient receiving halofantrine antimalarial treatment should be assessed routinely for
    a. ECG changes.
    b. renal function changes.
    c. changes in vision or hearing.
    d. bone marrow suppression.

BIBLIOGRAPHY

Andrews, M., & Boyle, J. (1999). *Transcultural concepts in nursing care*. Philadelphia: Lippincott Williams & Wilkins.

Bullock, B. L. (2000). *Focus on pathophysiology*. Philadelphia: Lippincott Williams & Wilkins.

Drug facts and comparisons. (2002). St. Louis: Facts and Comparisons.

Gilman, A., Hardman, J. G., & Limbird, L. E. (Eds.) (2002). *Goodman and Gilman's the pharmacological basis of therapeutics* (10th ed.). New York: McGraw-Hill.

Karch, A. M. (2002). *2003 Lippincott's nursing drug guide*. Philadelphia: Lippincott Williams & Wilkins.

Professional's guide to patient drug facts. (2002). St. Louis: Facts and Comparisons.

13

Anthelmintic Agents

155

albendazole

ivermectin

P mebendazole

praziquantel

pyrantel

thiabendazole

About 1 billion people have worms in their gastrointestinal (GI) tract or other tissues, which makes helminthic infections among the most common of all diseases. These infestations are very common in tropical areas, but they are also often found in other regions, including countries such as the United States and Canada. With so many people traveling to many parts of the world, it is not uncommon for a traveler to pick up a helminthic infection in another country and inadvertently bring it home, where the worms are able to infect other individuals. The **helminths** that most commonly infect humans are of two types: the **nematodes** or **roundworms,** and the platyhelminths or flatworms.

INTESTINE-INVADING WORMS

Many of the worms that infect humans live only in the intestinal tract. Proper diagnosis of a helminthic infection requires a stool examination for ova (eggs) and parasites. Treatment of a helminthic infection entails the use of an anthelmintic drug. Another important part of therapy for helminthic infections involves the prevention of reinfection or spread of an existing infection. Measures such as thorough hand washing after use of the toilet; frequent laundering of bed linens and underwear in very hot, chlorine-treated water; disinfection of toilets and bathroom areas after each use; and good personal hygiene to wash away ova are important to the effectiveness of drug therapy and prevention of the spread of the disease.

Nematodes

Nematodes, or roundworms, include the commonly encountered **pinworms, whipworms, threadworms,** *Ascaris,* and hookworms. These worms cause diseases that range from mild to potentially deadly.

Pinworms

Pinworms, which stay in the intestine, cause little discomfort except for perianal itching or occasionally vaginal itching. Infection with pinworms is the most common helminthic infection among school-age children.

Whipworms

Whipworms attach themselves to the wall of the colon; when large numbers of them are in the intestine, they cause colic and bloody diarrhea. In severe cases, whipworm infestation may result in prolapse of the intestinal wall and anemia related to blood loss.

Threadworms

Threadworms are more pervasive than most of the other helminths. After burrowing into the wall of the small intestine, female worms lay eggs, which hatch into larvae that invade many body tissues, including the lungs, liver, and heart. In very severe cases, death may occur from pneumonia or from lung or liver abscesses that result from larval invasion.

NURSING CHALLENGE
Pinworm Infections

Infestation with worms can be a frightening and traumatic experience for most people. Seeing the worm can be an especially difficult experience. Some worm infestations are not that uncommon in this country, especially infestation with pinworms.

Pinworms can spread very rapidly among children in schools, summer camps, and other institutions. Once the infestation starts, careful hygiene measures and drug therapy are required to eradicate the disease. After the diagnosis has been made and appropriate drug therapy started, proper hygiene measures are essential. Some suggested hygiene measures that might help to control the infection include the following:

• Keep the child's nails cut short and hands well scrubbed, because reinfection results from the worm's eggs being carried back to the mouth after becoming lodged under the fingernails when the child scratches the pruritic perianal area.
• Give the child a shower in the morning to wash away any ova deposited in the anal area during the night.
• Change and launder undergarments, bed linens, and pajamas every day.
• Disinfect toilet seats daily and the floors of bathrooms and bedrooms periodically.
• Encourage the child to wash hands vigorously after using the toilet.

In some areas of the country, parents are asked to check for worm ova by pressing sticky tape against the anal area in the morning before bathing. The sticky tape is then pressed against a slide that can be taken or sent to a clinical laboratory for evaluation. It may take 5 to 6 weeks to get a clear reading with this method of testing. Some health care providers believe that the psychological trauma involved in doing this type of follow-up, especially with a school-age child, makes this task too onerous to ask parents to do. Instead, many believe that the ease of treating this relatively harmless disease makes it more prudent to continue to treat as prescribed and to forgo the follow-up testing.

It is important to reassure patients and families that these types of infections do not necessarily reflect negatively on their hygiene or lifestyle. It takes a coordinated effort among medical personnel, families, and patients to get control of a pinworm infestation.

Ascaris

Worldwide, *Ascaris* infection is the most prevalent helminthic infection. It may occur wherever sanitation is poor. Although many individuals have no idea that they have this infestation unless they see a worm in their stool, others become quite ill.

Initially, the individual ingests fertilized roundworm eggs, which hatch in the small intestine and then make their way to the lungs, where they may cause cough, fever, and other signs of a pulmonary infiltrate. The larvae then migrate back to the intestine, where they grow to adult size (ie, about as long and as big around as an earthworm) and can cause abdominal distention and pain. In the most severe cases, intestinal obstruction by masses of worms can occur.

Hookworms

Hookworms attach themselves to the small intestine of infected individuals and suck blood from the walls of the intestine. This damages the intestinal wall and can cause severe anemia with lethargy, weakness, and fatigue. Malabsorption problems may occur as the small intestinal mucosa is altered. Treatment for anemia and fluid and electrolyte disturbances is an important part of the therapy for this infection.

Platyhelminths: Cestodes

The platyhelminths (flatworms) include the **cestodes** (tapeworms) that live in the human intestine and the flukes (schistosomes) that invade other tissues as part of their life cycle. Cestodes are segmented flatworms with a head, or scolex, and a variable number of segments that grow from the head; they sometimes form worms that are several yards long. Persons with a tapeworm may experience some abdominal discomfort and distention as well as weight loss, because the worm eats ingested nutrients. Many infected patients require a great deal of psychological support when they excrete parts of the tapeworm or when the worm comes out the mouth or nose, which may occur occasionally.

TISSUE-INVADING WORM INFECTIONS

Some of the worms that invade the body exist outside the intestinal tract and can seriously damage the tissues they invade. Because of their location within healthy tissue, they can also be more difficult to treat.

Trichinosis

Trichinosis is the disease caused by ingestion of the encysted larvae of the roundworm, *Trichinella spiralis,* in undercooked pork. The larvae of this worm, which is deposited in the intestinal mucosa, pass into the bloodstream and are carried throughout the body. They can penetrate skeletal muscle and can cause an inflammatory reaction in cardiac muscle and in the brain. Fatal pneumonia, heart failure, and encephalitis may occur.

The best treatment for trichinosis is prevention. Because the larvae are ingested by humans in undercooked pork, freezing pork meat, monitoring the food eaten by pigs, and instructing people in the proper cooking of pork can be most beneficial.

Filariasis

Filariasis refers to infection of the blood and tissues of healthy individuals by worm embryos, which are injected by biting insects. These thread-like embryos, or filariae, can overwhelm the lymphatic system and cause massive inflammatory reactions. This may lead to severe swelling of the hands, feet, legs, arms, scrotum, or breast—a condition called elephantiasis.

Schistosomiasis

Schistosomiasis (Figure 13–1) is an infection by a fluke that is carried by a snail. This disease is a common problem in parts of Africa, Asia, and certain South American and Caribbean countries that have climates and snails conducive to the life cycle of *Schistosoma.*

A description of the life cycle of *Schistosoma* follows. The eggs, which are excreted in the urine and feces of infected individuals, hatch in freshwater into a form that infects a certain snail. Larvae, known as cercariae, develop in the snail, which sheds the cercariae back into the freshwater pond or lake. People become infected when they come in contact with the infested water. The larvae attach to the skin and quickly burrow into the bloodstream and lymphatics. After they move into the lungs, and later the liver, they mature into adult worms that mate and migrate to the intestines and urinary bladder. The female worms then lay large numbers of eggs, which are expelled in the feces and urine, and the cycle begins again.

Signs and symptoms of infection with this helminth may include a pruritic rash where the larva attaches to the skin, which is often called swimmer's itch. About 1 or 2 months later, affected individuals may experience several weeks of fever, chills, headache, and other symptoms. Chronic or severe infestation may lead to abdominal pain and diarrhea as well as blockage of blood flow to areas of the liver, lungs, and central nervous system (CNS). These blockages can lead to liver and spleen enlargement as well as signs of CNS and cardiac ischemia.

ANTHELMINTICS

The anthelmintic drugs act on metabolic pathways that are present in the invading worm but absent or significantly different in the human host. Mebendazole (*Vermox*), probably the most commonly used of all of the anthelmintics, is effective against pinworms, roundworms, whipworms, and hookworms. It is available in the form of a chewable tablet, and a typical 3-day course can be repeated in 3 weeks if needed. Because very little of the mebendazole is absorbed systemically, it has few adverse effects. The drug is not metabolized in the body, and most of it is excreted unchanged in the feces, though a small amount may be excreted in the urine. It should not be used during pregnancy, because teratogenic effects do occur in rats and there is a risk of possible fetal harm. Other anthelmintics cross into breast milk and can cause harm to the neonate, and it is not known whether mebendazole passes into breast milk; therefore, lactating women should be advised to select another way to feed the baby.

Pyrantel (*Antiminth, Pin-Rid, Pin-X, Reese's Pinworm*) is an oral drug that is effective against pinworms and roundworms. Because this agent is given as a single dose, it may be preferred for patients who could have trouble remembering to take medications or following drug regimens. Pyrantel is poorly absorbed, and most of the drug is excreted unchanged

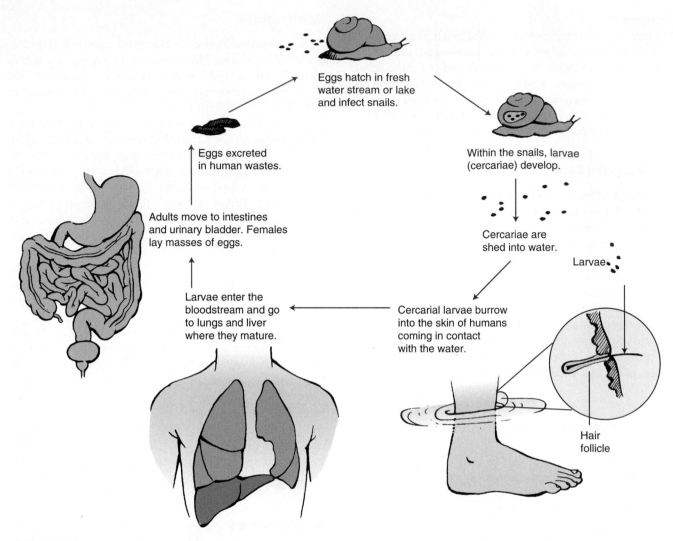

FIGURE 13-1. Life cycle of *Schistosoma*.

in the feces, although a small amount may be found in the urine. It is not recommended for use during pregnancy or lactation, and safety has not been established for children younger than 2 years of age. Adverse effects associated with pyrantel include possible uncomfortable GI side effects and diarrhea.

Thiabendazole (*Mintezol*) may also be used in the treatment of roundworm, hookworm, and whipworm infections. However, it is not the drug of choice if one of the other drugs can be used, because it is not as effective as other agents and can cause more uncomfortable adverse effects. Nevertheless, thiabendazole is the drug of choice for treatment of threadworm infections, and it can be used to alleviate the signs and symptoms of invasive trichinosis. It is readily absorbed from the GI tract, reaching peak levels in 1 to 2 hours. It is completely metabolized in the liver and primarily excreted in the urine. There are no established studies regarding use during pregnancy or lactation, so it is recommended that the drug not be used, unless the benefit clearly outweighs potential risk.

Albendazole (*Albenza*) is effective against active lesions caused by pork tapeworm and cystic disease of the liver, lungs, and peritoneum caused by dog tapeworm. A very powerful drug, albendazole has serious adverse effects, including renal failure and bone marrow depression. It should be used only after the causative worm has been identified. It is poorly absorbed from the GI tract, reaching peak plasma levels in about 5 hours. It is metabolized in the liver and primarily excreted in urine. Albendazole has been shown to be teratogenic in animal studies and should not be used during pregnancy or lactation. Women of child-bearing age should be advised to use barrier contraceptives while taking this drug.

Ivermectin (*Stromectol*) is effective against the nematode that causes onchocerciasis, or river blindness, which is found in tropical areas of Africa, Mexico, and South America. The drug is also used to treat threadworm disease or strongyloidiasis. It is readily absorbed from the GI tract and reaches peak plasma levels in 4 hours. It is completely metabolized in the liver with a half-life of 16 hours; excretion is through the feces. Ivermectin should never be taken during pregnancy, be-

DRUG THERAPY ACROSS THE LIFESPAN

Anthelmintic Agents

Children	Adults	Older Adults
Culture of the suspected worm is important before beginning any drug therapy. The more toxic drugs—albendazole, ivermectin and praziquantel—should be avoided in children. The most commonly used anthelmintic, mebendazole, comes in a chewable tablet that is convenient for use in children. Nutritional status and hydration are major concerns with children taking these drugs who develop serious gastrointestinal effects.	Adults may be somewhat repulsed by the idea that they have a worm infestation, and they may be reluctant to discuss the needed lifestyle adjustments and treatment plans. Pregnant and nursing women should not use these drugs unless the benefit clearly outweighs the potential risk to the fetus or neonate. If a severe helminth infestation threatens the mother, some of the drugs can be used as long as the mother is informed of the potential risk.	Older patients may be more susceptible to the central nervous system and gastrointestinal effects of some of these drugs. Dosage adjustment is needed for these agents. Monitor hydration and nutritional status carefully.

cause it can cause serious fetal harm. Women of child-bearing age should be advised to use barrier contraceptives while taking this drug. Ivermectin crosses into breast milk; the risk of toxic reactions in the neonate should be considered, and the drug should be used with caution during lactation.

Praziquantel (*Biltricide*) is very effective in the treatment of a wide number of schistosomes or flukes. This drug, which is taken in a series of three doses at 4- to 6-hour intervals, has relatively few adverse effects. The drug is rapidly absorbed

CULTURAL CONSIDERATIONS

Travelers and Helminths

People who come from or travel to areas of the world where schistosomiasis is endemic should always be assessed for the possibility of infection with such a disease when seen for health care. Areas of the world in which this disease is endemic are mainly tropical settings, such as Puerto Rico, islands of the West Indies, Africa, parts of South America, the Philippines, China, Japan, and Southeast Asia. People traveling to these areas should be warned about wading, swimming, or bathing in freshwater streams, ponds, or lakes. For example, swimming in the Nile River is a popular attraction on Egyptian vacation tours; however, this activity may result in a lasting (unhappy) memory when the traveler returns home and is diagnosed with schistosomiasis. The nurse can suggest to patients who are planning a visit to one of these areas that they contact the Centers for Disease Control and Prevention (CDC) for health and safety guidelines, as well as signs and symptoms to watch for after returning home. The CDC can be reached on the World Wide Web at http://www.cdc.gov/travel.

from the GI tract and reaches peak plasma levels within 1 to 3 hours. It is metabolized in the liver with a half-life of 0.8 to 1.5 hours. Excretion of praziquantel occurs primarily through the urine. There are no adequate studies regarding the use of this drug during pregnancy, and it should be used cautiously. Praziquantel crosses into breast milk and should not be used during lactation; in addition, the baby should not be nursed for 72 hours after treatment is finished.

Therapeutic Actions and Indications

Anthelmintic agents are indicated for the treatment of infections by certain susceptible worms and are not interchangeable. Anthelmintics interfere with metabolic processes in particular worms, as noted previously (Figure 13–2).

Contraindications and Cautions

Contraindications to the use of anthelmintic drugs include the presence of known allergy to any of these drugs; lactation, because the drugs can enter breast milk and could be toxic to the infant; and pregnancy (in most cases), because of reported associated fetal abnormalities or death. Caution should be used in the presence of renal or hepatic disease that interferes with the metabolism or excretion of drugs that are absorbed systemically and in cases of severe diarrhea and malnourishment, which could alter the effects of the drug on the intestine and any pre-existing helminths.

Adverse Effects

Adverse effects frequently encountered with the use of these anthelmintic agents are related to their absorption or direct action in the intestine. Mebendazole and pyrantel are not generally absorbed systemically and may cause abdominal discomfort, diarrhea, or pain. Anthelmintics that are absorbed systemically may cause the following effects: headache and dizziness; fever, shaking, chills, and malaise, asso-

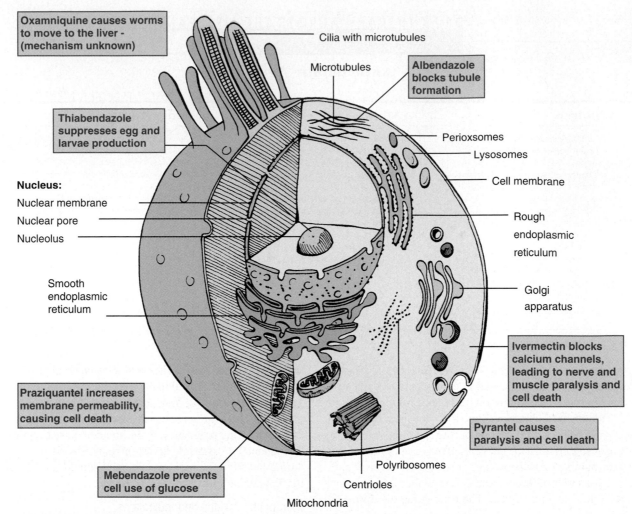

Oxamniquine causes worms to move to the liver - (mechanism unknown)

Cilia with microtubules

Microtubules

Albendazole blocks tubule formation

Thiabendazole suppresses egg and larvae production

Perioxsomes

Lysosomes

Cell membrane

Nucleus:

Nuclear membrane

Nuclear pore

Nucleolus

Rough endoplasmic reticulum

Smooth endoplasmic reticulum

Golgi apparatus

Ivermectin blocks calcium channels, leading to nerve and muscle paralysis and cell death

Praziquantel increases membrane permeability, causing cell death

Pyrantel causes paralysis and cell death

Mebendazole prevents cell use of glucose

Polyribosomes

Centrioles

Mitochondria

FIGURE 13–2. General structure of a cell, showing the sites of action of the anthelmintic agents. Mebendazole interferes with the ability to use glucose, leading to an inability to reproduce and cell death. Albendazole blocks tubule formation, resulting in cell death. Ivermectin blocks calcium channels, leading to nerve and muscle paralysis and cell death. Pyrantel is a neuromuscular polarizing agent that causes paralysis and cell death. Thiabendazole both suppresses egg and larva production and blocks a helminth-specific enzyme that promotes the development of eggs and larvae. Praziquantel increases membrane permeability, leading to a loss of intracellular calcium and muscular paralysis; it may also result in disintegration of the integument.

ciated with an immune reaction to the death of the worms; rash; pruritus; and loss of hair.

Changes in protein synthesis by the liver to Stevens–Johnson syndrome is associated with thiabendazole use and can be fatal. Also, renal failure and severe bone marrow depression are associated with albendazole, which is toxic to some human tissues. Patients taking this drug should be monitored carefully.

Clinically Important Drug–Drug Interactions

Combinations of theophylline and thiabendazole may lead to increased theophylline levels, and patients who take both of these drugs may require frequent monitoring and dosage reduction.

The effects of albendazole, which are already severe, may increase if the drug is combined with dexamethasone, prazi-

quantel, or cimetidine. These combinations should be avoided if at all possible; if they are necessary, patients should be monitored closely for occurrence of adverse effects.

Nursing Considerations for Patients Receiving Anthelmintics

Assessment: History and Physical Assessment

Screen for the following: history of allergy to any of the anthelmintics; hepatic or renal dysfunction that might interfere with the metabolism and excretion of the drug; pregnancy, which is a contraindication to the use of some of these agents because of reported effects on the fetus; and lactation, because these drugs could enter the breast milk and be toxic to the infant.

Physical assessment should be performed to establish

DRUGS IN FOCUS
Anthelmintics

Drug Name	Dosage/Route	Usual Indications
albendazole (*Albenza*)	*Hydatid disease:* ≥60 kg: 400 mg b.i.d. PO ≤60 kg: 15 mg/kg per day PO in divided doses, b.i.d., on a 28-d cycle followed by 14 d rest, for a total of three cycles *Neurocysticercosis:* ≥60 kg: 400 mg b.i.d. PO ≤60 kg: 15/mg/kg per day PO in divided doses, b.i.d., for 8–30 days of treatment	Treatment of active lesions caused by pork tapeworm and cystic disease of the liver, lungs, and peritoneum caused by dog tapeworm
ivermectin (*Stromectol*)	150–200 μg/kg PO as a single dose	Treatment of threadworm disease or strongyloidiasis; onchocerciasis or river blindness
Ⓟ mebendazole (*Vermox*)	100 mg PO morning and evening on three consecutive days *Enterobiasis:* 100 mg PO as a single dose	Treatment of diseases caused by pinworms, roundworms, whipworms, and hookworms
praziquantel (*Biltricide*)	30 doses of 20–25 mg/kg PO as a 1-day treatment	Treatment of a wide number of shistosomes or flukes
pyrantel (*Antiminth, Pin-Rid, Reese's Pinworm, Pin-X*)	11 mg/kg PO as a single dose; maximum dose, 1 g	Treatment of diseases caused by pinworms and roundworms
thiabendazole (*Mintezol*)	<150 lb: 10 mg/lb per dose PO, 2 doses/day ≥150 lb: 1.5 g/dose PO, 2 doses/day	Treatment of diseases caused by round- worms, hookworms, and whipworms

baseline data for determining the effectiveness of the drug and the occurrence of any adverse effects associated with drug therapy. Obtain a culture of stool for ova and parasites to determine the infecting worm and establish appropriate treatment. Examine reflexes and muscle strength to evaluate changes that occur as a result of drug therapy. Conduct hepatic evaluation, including liver function tests, and also renal function tests to determine appropriateness of therapy and to monitor for toxicity. Examine skin (lesions, color, temperature, and texture), to monitor for adverse effects, and abdomen, to evaluate any changes from baseline related to the infection and to monitor for improvement and the possibility of adverse effects.

Nursing Diagnoses

The patient receiving an anthelmintic drug may have the following nursing diagnoses related to drug therapy:

- Acute Pain related to GI, CNS, skin effects of drug
- Disturbed Personal Identity related to diagnosis and treatment
- Deficient Knowledge regarding drug therapy

Implementation

- Arrange for appropriate culture and sensitivity tests before beginning therapy *to ensure that the appropriate drug is being used.*
- Administer the complete course of the drug *to obtain the full beneficial effects.* Ensure that chewable tablets are chewed. The drug may be taken with food if necessary, but high-fat meals might interfere with drug effectiveness and should be avoided.
- Monitor hepatic and renal function before and periodically during treatment *to arrange to stop administration of albendazole if signs of failure occur.*
- Provide comfort and safety measures if CNS effects occur (eg, siderails and assistance with ambulation in the presence of dizziness and weakness), *to protect patient from injury.* Provide oral hygiene and ready access to bathroom facilities as needed *to cope with GI effects.*
- Provide small, frequent, nutritious meals if GI upset is severe *to ensure adequate nutrition.* Monitor nutritional status and arrange a dietary consultation as needed. Taking the drug with food may also decrease GI upset.

CASE STUDY

Anthelmintics

THE SITUATION

V. Y., a 33-year-old Vietnamese man, underwent a complete physical examination in preparation for a training job in custodial work at a local hospital. He was a refugee who had come to the United States 6 months ago as part of a church-sponsored resettlement program. In the course of the examination, it was found that he had a history of chronic diarrhea, hepatomegaly, pulmonary rales, and splenomegaly. Further tests indicated that he had chronic schistosomiasis. Because of V. Y.'s limited use of the English language, he was hospitalized so that his disease, which was unfamiliar to most of the associated health care providers, could be monitored. He was treated with praziquantel.

CRITICAL THINKING

What are the important nursing implications for V. Y.? *Think about the serious limitations that are placed on medical care, particularly patient teaching, when the patient and the health care workers do not speak the same language.*

What innovative techniques could be used to teach this patient about the disease, the drugs, and the hygiene measures that are important for him to follow?

Are the other patients or workers in the hospital exposed to any health risks? What sort of educational program should be developed to teach them about this disease and to allay any fears or anxieties they may have?

What special interventions are needed to explain the drug therapy and any adverse effects or warning signs that V. Y. should be watching for?

DISCUSSION

A language barrier can be a real handicap in the health care system. In many cases, pictures can assist communication. For example, the need for nutritious food is conveyed by using appropriate pictures of foods that should be eaten. Frequent reinforcement is necessary, because the patient has no way of letting you know that he really understands the message that you are trying to convey. The patient is prepared for discharge through careful patient teaching that may involve pictures, calendars, and clocks so that he is given every opportunity to comply with his medical regimen.

In addition, the nursing staff should contact the local health department to determine whether the local sewer system can properly handle contaminated wastes. In this case, the staff learned from the Centers for Disease Control and Prevention that the snail intermediate host does not live in this country, so the hazards posed by this waste are small and normal disposal of the wastes should be appropriate.

V. Y. should also be observed for signs of adverse effects, although praziquantel is a relatively mild drug. Drug fever, abdominal pain, or dizziness may occur. If dizziness occurs, safety precautions, such as assistance with ambulation, use of side rails, and adequate lighting, need to be taken without alarming the patient.

• Ensure that the patient is instructed about the appropriate dosage regimen and other measures *to enhance patient knowledge about drug therapy and to promote compliance.*

The patient should

Take safety precautions, including changing position slowly and avoiding driving and hazardous tasks, if CNS effects occur.

Take the drug with meals and try small, frequent meals if GI upset is a problem.

Note the importance of strict hand washing and hygiene measures, including daily laundering of underwear and bed linens, daily disinfection of toilet facilities, and periodic disinfection of bathroom floors.

Report fever, severe diarrhea, or aggravation of condition, which could indicate a resistant strain or noneffective therapy, to a health care provider

See the accompanying Patient Teaching Checklist for anthelmintic agents.

Evaluation

• Monitor patient response to the drug (resolution of helminth infestation and improvement in signs and symptoms).

• Monitor for adverse effects (orientation and effect, nutritional state, skin color and lesions, hepatic and renal function, and abdominal discomfort and pain).

• Evaluate the effectiveness of the teaching plan (patient can name the drug, dosage, possible adverse effects to watch for, and specific measures to help avoid adverse effects).

• Monitor the effectiveness of comfort and safety measures and compliance with the regimen (see Nursing Care Guide: Anthelmintic Agents).

◻◼◉◼ WEB LINKS

Health care providers and patients may want to consult the following Internet sources:

Information on preventing and dealing with pinworm infections:
http://www.rockwoodclinic.com/abc.htm

PATIENT TEACHING CHECKLIST
Anthelmintic Agents

Create customized patient teaching materials for a specific anthelmintic agent from the CD-ROM. Patient teaching should stress the following points for drugs within this class:

• An anthelmintic destroys certain helminths, or worms, that have invaded your body.
• It is important that you take the full course of the drug to ensure that all of the worms, in all phases of their life cycle, have disappeared from your body.
• You may take this drug with meals or with a light snack to help decrease any stomach upset that you may experience. If you have chewable tablets, be sure to chew them before swallowing. If you have regular tablets, swallow them whole and avoid holding them in your mouth for any length of time, because a very unpleasant taste may occur.

Common effects of this drug include

• *Nausea, vomiting, and loss of appetite*—Take the drug with food, and eat small, frequent meals.
• *Dizziness and drowsiness*—If this occurs, avoid driving a car or operating dangerous machinery. Change positions slowly to avoid falling or injury.
• Report any of the following conditions to your health care provider: fever, chills, rash, headache, weakness, or tremors.
• Take all the drug that has been prescribed. Never use this drug to self-treat any other infection or give it to any other person.
• Tell any doctor, nurse, or other health care provider that you are taking this drug.
• Keep this drug and all medications out of the reach of children.

For intestinal worm infections, some measures that help prevent worm reinfection or spread to other family members include the following:

• Vigorous hand washing with soap after use of toilet facilities.
• Showering in the morning to wash away any ova deposited in the anal area during the night.
• Changing and laundering undergarments, bed linens, and pajamas daily.
• Disinfecting toilets and toilet seats daily and bathroom and bedroom floors periodically.
Note: This Teaching Checklist reflects general patient teaching guidelines. It is not meant to be a substitute for drug-specific teaching information, which is available in nursing drug guides.

Information on schistosomiasis—incidence, precautions, treatments:
  http://www.who.int/ctd/schisto/index.html
Information about other intestinal parasites:
  http://www.cdfound.to.it
Information for travelers about potential helminth infestations, precautions, treatments, warning signs:
  http://www.cdc.gov/travel

CHAPTER SUMMARY

• Helminths are worms that cause disease by invading the human body. Helminths that affect humans include nematodes (round-shaped worms) such as pinworms, hookworms, threadworms, whipworms, and roundworms.
• Pinworms are the most frequent cause of helminth infection in the United States, and roundworms called *Ascaris* are the most frequent cause of helminth infections throughout the world.
• Platyhelminths (flatworms) include tapeworms and flukes.
• Some helminths invade body tissues and can seriously damage lymphatic tissue, lungs, CNS, heart, liver, and so on. These include trichinosis-causing tapeworms, which are found in undercooked pork; filariae, which occur when thread-like worm embryos clog up vascular spaces; and schistosomiasis-causing flukes, which can invade the liver, lungs, CNS, and other tissues. Schistosomiasis is a common problem in many tropical areas where the snail that is necessary in the life cycle of the fluke lives.
• Anthelmintic drugs affect metabolic processes that are either different in worms than in human hosts or are not found in humans. These agents all cause death of the worm by interfering with normal functioning.
• Prevention is a very important part of the treatment of helminths. Thorough hand washing; laundering of bed linens, pajamas, and underwear to destroy ova that are shed during the night; and disinfection of toilet facilities at least daily and of bathroom floors periodically help stop the spread of these diseases. In addition, proper sanitation and hygiene in food preparation and storage is essential for reducing the incidence of these infestations.
• Patient teaching is important for decreasing the stress and anxiety that may occur when individuals are diagnosed with a worm infestation.

Review Questions

1. Effective treatment of pinworm infections would involve all of the following except
   a. keeping nails cut short and hands well scrubbed.
   b. laundering undergarments, bed linens, and pajamas every day.
   c. boiling all drinking water.
   d. disinfecting toilet seats and bathroom floors daily.
2. *Ascaris* infections are the most prevalent worldwide helminthic infections and may cause
   a. cough, fever, and signs of pulmonary infestation.
   b. cardiac arrhythmias.
   c. seizures and disorientation.
   d. bloody diarrhea.
3. Schistosomiasis is an infection caused by
   a. a protozoan carried by a mosquito.
   b. improperly cooked pork.
   c. a fluke carried by a snail.
   d. eating food contaminated by fecal material.

NURSING CARE GUIDE

Anthelmintic Agents

Assessment	Nursing Diagnoses	Implementation	Evaluation
HISTORY Allergies to any of these drugs, renal or liver dysfunction, pregnancy or lactation	Acute Pain related to GI, CNS effects Disturbed Personal Identity related to diagnosis and treatment Deficient Knowledge regarding drug therapy	Culture for ova and parasites before beginning therapy. Provide comfort and safety measures: antipruritics for anal rash; small, frequent meals; safety precautions; hygiene measures; maintenance of nutrition. Monitor nutritional status as needed. Provide support and reassurance to deal with drug effects, discomfort, and diagnosis. Provide patient teaching regarding drug name, dosage regimen, adverse effects and precautions to report, and hygiene measures to observe.	Evaluate drug effects: resolution of helminth infection. Monitor for adverse effects: GI alterations, CNS changes, dizziness and confusion, renal and hepatic function. Monitor for drug–drug interactions as indicated for each drug. Evaluate effectiveness of patient teaching program. Evaluate effectiveness of comfort and safety measures.
PHYSICAL EXAMINATION Local: culture of infection CNS: orientation, affect Skin: color, lesions, texture GI: abdominal and liver evaluation, including hepatic function tests GU: renal function tests			

4. A patient has traveled to Egypt and come home with schistosomiasis. The family is very concerned about spreading the disease. Important teaching information that could help the family would include which of the following:
a. strict hand washing will stop the spread of the disease.
b. isolating the patient will be necessary to stop the spread of the disease.
c. carefully cooking all of the patient's food will help to stop the spread of the disease.
d. the snail that is needed for the life cycle of this worm does not live in this climate and the disease cannot be spread without the snail.

5. Mebendazole is the most commonly used anthelmintic. It is effective against
a. pinworms, roundworms, whipworms, and hookworms.
b. trichinosis and flukes.
c. pork tapeworm and threadworms.
d. all stages of schistosomal infections.

6. Patient teaching regarding the use of anthelmintics should include counseling about
a. the use of oral contraceptives.
b. the importance of maintaining nutrition during therapy.
c. the use of oral anticoagulants.
d. cardiac drug effects.

7. Patients may experience anxiety about the diagnosis and treatment of helminthic infections. Teaching may help to alleviate this anxiety and should include all except which of the following:
a. what they may experience if the worms are passed from the body.
b. the prevalence of such infections worldwide, assuring them that it is not a personal problem.
c. measures to prevent reinfection and the spread of the infection.
d. criticism of their personal hygiene practices.

BIBLIOGRAPHY

Andrews, M., & Boyle, J. (1999). *Transcultural concepts in nursing care*. Philadelphia: Lippincott Williams & Wilkins.

Bullock, B. L. (2000). *Focus on pathophysiology*. Philadelphia: Lippincott Williams & Wilkins.

Gilman, A., Hardman, J. G., & Limbird, L. E. (Eds.) (2002). *Goodman and Gilman's the pharmacological basis of therapeutics* (10th ed.). New York: McGraw-Hill.

Karch, A. M. (2002). *2003 Lippincott's nursing drug guide*. Philadelphia: Lippincott Williams & Wilkins.

Drug facts and comparison. (2002.) St. Louis: Facts and Comparisons.

Professional's guide to patient drug facts. (2002). St. Louis: Facts and Comparisons.

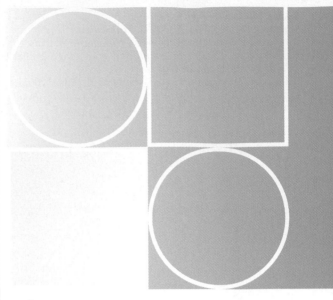

CHAPTER 14

Antineoplastic Agents

166

Key Terms

alopecia
anaplasia
antineoplastic drug
autonomy
bone marrow suppression
carcinoma
metastasis
neoplasm
sarcoma

Alkylating Agents
busulfan
carboplatin
carmustine
🅟 chlorambucil
cisplatin
cyclophosphamide
ifosfamide
lomustine
mechlorethamine
melphalan
streptozocin
thiotepa

Antimetabolites
capecitabine
cladribine
cytarabine
floxuridine
fludarabine
fluorouracil
mercaptopurine
🅟 methotrexate
pentostatin
thioguanine
Antineoplastic Antibiotics
bleomycin

dactinomycin
daunorubicin
🅟 doxorubicin
idarubicin
mitomycin
mitoxantrone
plicamycin
valrubicin
Mitotic Inhibitors
docetaxel
etoposide
paclitaxel
teniposide

vinblastine
🅟 vincristine
vinorelbine
Hormones and Hormone Modulators
anastrazole
bicalutamide
diethylstilbestrol
estramustine
flutamide
goserelin
letrozole
leuprolide

nilutamide
🅟 tamoxifen
testolactone
toremifene
Miscellaneous Antineoplastic Agents
altretamine
asparaginase
dacarbazine
gemcitabine
hydroxyurea
irinotecan

mitotane
pegaspargase
porfimer
procarbazine
topotecan
tretinoin
Antineoplastic Adjunctive Therapy
amifostine
dexrazoxane
leucovorin
mesna

One branch of chemotherapy involves drugs developed to act on and kill or alter human cells—the **antineoplastic drugs,** which are designed to fight **neoplasms,** or cancers. When chemotherapy is mentioned, most people think of cancer treatment. Antineoplastic drugs alter human cells in a variety of ways, and they are intended to have a greater impact on the abnormal cells that make up the neoplasm or cancer than on normal cells. This area of pharmacology, which has grown tremendously in recent years, now includes many drugs that act on or are part of the immune system; these substances fight the cancerous cells using components of the immune system instead of destroying cells directly (see Chapter 15). This chapter discusses the classic antineoplastic approach and those drugs that are used in cancer chemotherapy.

NEOPLASMS

Cancer is a disease that can strike a person at any age. It remains second only to coronary disease as the leading cause of death in the United States. Treatment of cancer can be a long and debilitating experience that leads to many disabilities in adults.

All cancers start with a single cell that is genetically different from the other cells in the surrounding tissue. This cell divides, passing along its abnormalities to daughter cells, eventually producing a tumor or neoplasm that has characteristics quite different from the original tissue (Figure 14–1). The cancerous cells exhibit **anaplasia,** a loss of cellular differentiation and organization, which leads to a loss of their ability to function normally. They also exhibit **autonomy,** growing without the usual homeostatic restrictions that regulate cell growth and control, which allows the cells to form a tumor.

Over time, these neoplastic cells grow uncontrollably, invading and damaging healthy tissue in the area and even undergoing **metastasis,** or traveling from the place of origin to develop new tumors in other areas of the body where conditions are favorable for cell growth (Figure 14–2). The abnormal cells release enzymes that generate blood vessels in the area to supply both oxygen and nutrients to the cells, thus contributing to their growth. Overall, the cancerous cells rob the host cells of energy and nutrients and block normal lymph and vascular vessels as the result of pressure and intrusion on normal cells, leading to a loss of normal cellular function.

The body's immune system can damage or destroy some neoplastic cells. T cells, which recognize the abnormal cells and destroy them; antibodies, which form in response to parts of the abnormal cell protein; interferons; and tissue necrosis factor (TNF) all play a role in the body's attempt to eliminate the abnormal cells before they become uncontrollable and threaten the life of the host. Once the neoplasm has grown and enlarged, it may overwhelm the immune system, which is no longer able to manage the problem.

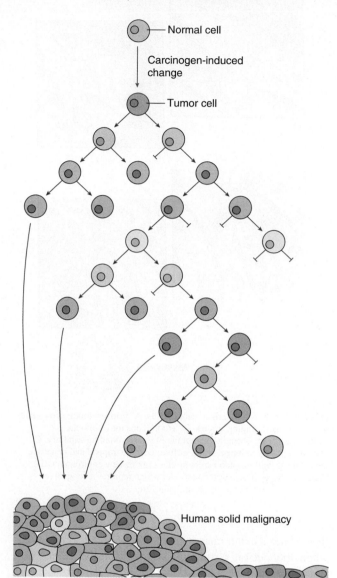

FIGURE 14-1. Tumor development from one cell, with somatic mutations occurring during cell division as the tumor grows.

Causes of Cancer

What causes the cells to mutate and become genetically different is not clearly understood. In some cases, a genetic predisposition to such a mutation can be found. Breast cancer, for example, seems to have a definite genetic link. In other cases, viral infection, constant irritation and cell turnover, and even stress have been blamed for the ensuing cancer. Stress reactions suppress the activities of the immune system (see Chapter 29), so if a cell is mutating while a person is under prolonged stress, research indicates that

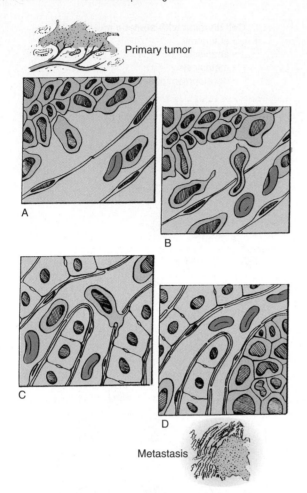

Primary tumor

A

B

C

D

Metastasis

FIGURE 14-2. Metastasis of cancer cells. A: Primary tumor grows and invades the surrounding tissues. B: Tumor cells move into the endothelium and basement membrane of the surrounding capillary. C: Shed tumor cells in lungs, brain, or liver become trapped and penetrate the capillary wall to establish themselves in this new environment. D: Cancer cells proliferate at the new site, which requires a conducive environment with blood supply and nutrition.

the cell has a better chance of growing into a neoplasm than when the person's immune system is fully active. Pipe smokers are at increased risk for development of tongue and mouth cancers because the heat and chemicals in the pipe are constantly destroying normal cells, which must be replaced rapidly, increasing the chances for development of a mutant cell. People living in areas with carcinogenic or cancer-causing chemicals in the air, water, or even the ground are at increased risk of developing mutant cells as a reaction to these toxic chemicals. Cancer clusters are often identified in such high-risk areas. Most likely, a mosaic of factors coming together in one person lead to development of the neoplasm.

Types of Cancer

Cancers can be divided into two groups: (1) solid tumors, and (2) hematological malignancies such as the leukemias and lymphomas, which occur in the blood-forming organs.

Solid tumors may originate in any body organ and may be further divided into **carcinomas,** or tumors that originate in epithelial cells, and **sarcomas,** or tumors that originate in the mesenchyma and are made up of embryonic connective tissue cells. Examples of carcinomas include granular cell tumors of the breast, bronchogenic tumors arising in cells lining the bronchial tubes, and squamous and basal tumors of the skin. Sarcomas include osteogenic tumors, which form in the primitive cells of the bone, and rhabdomyosarcomas, which occur in striated muscles.

ANTINEOPLASTIC DRUGS

Antineoplastic drugs can work by affecting cell survival or by boosting the immune system in its efforts to combat the abnormal cells. Chapter 17 discusses the immune agents that are used to combat cancer. This chapter focuses on those drugs that affect cell survival. The antineoplastic drugs that are commonly used today include the alkylating agents, antimetabolites, antineoplastic antibiotics, mitotic inhibitors, hormones and hormone modulators, and a group of antineoplastic agents that cannot be classified elsewhere.

As discussed in Chapter 7, all cells progress through a cell cycle. Different types of cells progress at different rates (see Figure 7–6 in Chapter 7). Rapidly multiplying cells, or cells that replace themselves quickly, include those that line the gastrointestinal (GI) tract and those in hair follicles, skin, and bone marrow. These cells complete the cell cycle every few days. Cells that proceed very slowly through the cell cycle include those in the breasts, testicles, and ovaries. Some cells take weeks, months, or even years to complete the cycle.

Cancer cells tend to move through the cell cycle at about the same rate as their cells of origin, and malignant cells that remain in a dormant phase for long periods are difficult to destroy. These cells can emerge long after cancer treatment has finished—after weeks, months, or years—to begin their division and growth cycle all over again. For this reason, antineoplastic agents are often given in sequence over periods of time, in the hope that the drugs will affect the cancer cells as they emerge from dormancy or move into a new phase of the cell cycle.

The adverse effects of cancer chemotherapy are often unpleasant and debilitating, and it is essential that patients understand the importance of returning every few weeks to go through the chemotherapy, with its adverse effects, over and over again. Most cancer patients are not considered to be "cured" until they have been cancer-free for a period of 5 years because of the possibility of cancer cells emerging from dormancy and causing new tumors or problems. No cells have yet been identified that can remain dormant for longer than 5 years, so the chances of the emergence of one after that time are very slim.

The goal of cancer therapy, much like that of anti-infective therapy, is to limit the offending cells enough so that the immune system can control them and without causing too much toxicity to the host. However, this is a particularly difficult task when using antineoplastic drugs, because these agents are not specific to mutant cells but affect normal human cells, too. In most cases, antineoplastic drugs primarily affect rapidly multiplying human cells, which have many cells in many phases of the cell cycle (eg, those in the hair follicles, GI tract, bone marrow). (See Box 14–1 for a discussion of a recently approved abnormal cell–specific antineoplastic agent.) Some of these drugs also influence fertility as a result of toxic effects on ova and sperm production. In addition, these agents are usually selective for rapidly growing cells, so they are dangerous during pregnancy. Because of the possible occurrence of serious fetal effects, pregnancy is a contraindication to the use of antineoplastic drugs.

Cancer treatment is aimed at destroying cancer cells through several methods, including surgery to remove them, stimulation of the immune system to destroy them, radiation therapy to destroy them, and drug therapy to kill them during various phases of the cell cycle. To do this effectively, and without too much damage to the host, combination therapy is often most successful. Surgery, followed by radiation or chemotherapy or both, is very effective with some cancers. A collection of chemotherapeutic agents that work at different phases of the cell cycle is frequently most effective in treating many cancers.

Many antineoplastic drugs often cause another adverse effect, cancer itself, because they cause cell death, leading to the need for cell growth and the increased risk of mutant cell development. In addition, they jeopardize the immune system by causing **bone marrow suppression,** inhibiting the blood-forming components of the bone marrow and interfering with the body's normal protective actions against abnormal cells. Other specific adverse effects may occur with particular drugs. The patient's hematological profile must always be assessed for toxic effects.

A cancerous mass may be so large that no therapy can arrest its growth without killing the host. In such cases, cancer chemotherapeutic agents are used as palliative therapy to shrink the size of the tumor and alleviate some of the signs and symptoms of the cancer, decreasing pain and increasing function. Here the goal of drug therapy is not to cure the disease but to try to improve the patient's quality of life in a situation in which there is no cure.

Some emerging antineoplastic agents are discussed in Box 14–2.

ALKYLATING AGENTS

The alkylating agents produce their cytotoxic effects by reacting chemically with portions of the RNA, DNA, or other cellular proteins, and they are most potent when they bind with cellular DNA. The oldest drugs in this class are the nitrogen mustards, and modifications of the structure of these drugs have led to the development of the nitrosoureas. Be-

BOX 14-1
Abnormal Cell–Specific Antineoplastic Agent

Imatinib mesylate (*Gleevec*) was approved in 2001 for the treatment of adults with chronic myeloid leukemia (CML) who are in blast crisis, accelerated phase, or chronic phase after failure with interferon-alpha therapy. This oral antineoplastic drug is a protein tyrosine kinase inhibitor that selectively inhibits the Bcr-Abl tyrosine kinase created by the Philadelphia chromosome abnormality in CML; this inhibits proliferation and induces apoptosis in the Bcr-Abl–positive cell lines as well as fresh leukemic cells, leading to an inhibition of tumor growth in CML patients in blast crisis. Because of its specific effects on these tumor cells, it is not associated with adverse effects on normal human cells. The adverse effects associated with this drug include GI upset, muscle cramps, fluid retention, and skin rash. The bone marrow suppression, alopecia, and severe GI effects associated with more traditional antineoplastic therapy do not occur. Imatinib is slowly absorbed from the GI tract, reaching peak levels in 2 to 4 hours. It is extensively metabolized in the liver, with a half-life of 18 and then 40 hours. Caution should be used with known hepatic dysfunction and when using drugs affected by the cytochrome P450 enzyme system. St. John's wort decreases the effectiveness of this drug and should be avoided. This drug crosses the placenta and is in pregnancy category D. Women of child-bearing age should be advised to use barrier contraceptives while taking this drug. It can enter breast milk, and it should be used during lactation only if the benefits to the mother clearly outweigh the risks to the fetus. Dosage recommendations for adults are as follows:

Chronic phase CML:
400 mg/d PO as a once-a-day dose; increase to 600 mg/d may be considered if response is not satisfactory and patient can tolerate the drug

Accelerated phase or blast crisis CML:
600 mg/d PO as a single dose; increase to 400 mg PO bid may be considered if response is not satisfactory and patient can tolerate the drug

CML patients who have been switched to this drug after traditional chemotherapy have been amazed at how good they feel and how much they have recovered. Long-term effects are not yet known because the drug is new. It is being researched for possible use in other cancers. The down side to this drug is the cost. It is estimated that 1 year of treatment with the drug (which needs to be taken continually) costs the patient between $30,000 and $35,000. Novartis, the drug company that manufactures *Gleevec,* has set up a patient assistance program with a sliding-scale price reduction based on income. They do not want patients to have to pay more than 20% of their annual income for the drug. Patients prescribed this drug may need support and assistance in obtaining financial help.

cause alkylating agents can affect cells even in the resting phase, these drugs are said to be non–cell cycle-specific (Figure 14–3). They are most useful in the treatment of slow-growing cancers, which have many cells in the resting phase.

Therapeutic Actions and Indications

The alkylating agents work by disrupting cellular mechanisms that affect DNA, causing cell death. They are effective against various lymphomas; leukemias; myelomas; some ovarian, testicular, and breast cancers; and some pancreatic cancers. The table on page 172 lists the various alkylating agents, their indications and dosages, and specific information about each drug. These agents are not used interchangeably.

Pharmacokinetics

The alkylating agents vary in their degree of absorption, and little is known about their distribution in the tissues. They are metabolized and sometimes activated in the liver, with many of these agents using the cytochrome P450 systems, and they are excreted in the urine, so caution must be used in patients with hepatic or renal dysfunction. Their use during pregnancy and lactation is contraindicated because of the potential harm to the neonate.

Contraindications and Cautions

Caution should be used when giving alkylating agents to any individual with a known allergy to any of the alkylating agents; during pregnancy or lactation, when these drugs are contraindicated because of potential severe effects on the neonate; with bone marrow suppression, which is often the index for redosing and dosing levels; or with suppressed renal or hepatic function, which may interfere with metabolism or excretion of these drugs and often indicates a need to change the dosage.

Adverse Effects

Adverse effects frequently encountered with the use of these alkylating agents are listed here; Table 14–1 indicates the most common adverse effects for each agent. Amifostine (*Ethyol*) and mesna (*Mesnex*) are cytoprotective (cell-protecting) drugs that may be given to limit certain effects of cisplatin and ifosfamide, respectively (Box 14–3).

DRUG THERAPY ACROSS THE LIFESPAN

Antineoplastic Agents

Children	Adults	Older Adults
Antineoplastic protocols have been developed for the treatment of most pediatric cancers. Combination therapy is stressed to eliminate as many of the mutant cells as possible. Dosage and timing of these combinations is crucial. Double checking of dosage, including recalculating desired dose and verifying the drug amount with another nurse, is good practice when giving these toxic drugs to children. Children need to monitored closely for hydration and nutritional status. The nutritional needs of a child are greater than those of an adult, and this needs to be considered when formulating a care plan. Children need support and comfort and also need to be allowed to explore and learn like any other children. Body image problems, lack of energy and the need to protect the child from exposure to infection can isolate a child receiving antineoplastic agents. The total care plan of the child needs to include social, emotional, and intellectual stimulation. Monitor bone marrow activity very carefully, and adjust the dosage accordingly.	The adult receiving antineoplastic drugs is confronted with many dilemmas that the nurse needs to address. Changes in body image are common with loss of hair, skin changes, gastrointestinal complaints, and weight loss. Fear of the diagnosis and the treatment is also common with these patients. Networking support systems and providing teaching, reassurance, and comfort can have a tremendous impact on the success of the drug therapy. Pregnant and nursing women should not receive these drugs, which are toxic to the developing cells of the fetus. Pregnant women who are diagnosed with cancer are in a difficult situation: the drug therapy can have serious adverse effects on the fetus, and not using the drug therapy can be detrimental to the mother. Education, support, and referrals to appropriate specialists are important. Nursing women should find another method of feeding the baby, to prevent the adverse effects to the fetus that occur when these drugs cross into breast milk. Use of barrier contraceptives is urged when these drugs are being used by women of child-bearing age.	Older adults may be more susceptible to the CNS and gastrointestinal effects of some of these drugs. Older patients should be monitored for hydration and nutritional status regularly. Safety precautions should be instituted if CNS effects occur, including increased lighting, assistance with ambulation, and use of supports. Many older patients have decreased renal and/or hepatic function. Many of these drugs depend on the liver and kidney for metabolism and excretion. Renal and liver function tests should be done before (baseline) and periodically during the use of these drugs, and dosage should be adjusted accordingly. Protecting these patients from exposure to infection and injury is a very important aspect of their nursing care. Older patients are naturally somewhat immunosuppressed because of age, and giving drugs that further depress the immune system can lead to infections that are serious and difficult to treat. Monitor blood counts carefully, and arrange for rest or reduced dosage as indicated.

BOX 14-2
New Drugs in the Battle Against Cancer

Arsenic trioxide (*Trisenox*), known as a poison in forensic medicine, has been approved for the induction and remission of promyelocytic leukemia (PML) in patients whose disease is refractory to conventional therapy and whose leukemia is characterized by t(15:17) translocation of PML/RAR-alpha gene expression. It is given intravenously at a rate of 0.15 mg/kg per day until bone marrow remission occurs and then 0.15 mg/kg per day starting 3 to 6 weeks after induction. The patient needs to be screened carefully for toxic reactions.

Other drugs are under development that target specific areas of the human genome. In the future, antineoplastic drugs may be able to target abnormal cells and not affect the healthy cells. This could relieve the suffering of many patients undergoing cancer chemotherapy.

Hematological effects include bone marrow suppression, with leukopenia, thrombocytopenia, anemia, and pancytopenia, secondary to the effects of the drugs on the rapidly multiplying cells of the bone marrow. GI effects include nausea, vomiting, anorexia, diarrhea, and mucous membrane deterioration, all of which are related to the drugs' effects on the rapidly multiplying cells of the GI tract. Hepatic toxicity and renal toxicity may occur, depending on the exact mechanism of action. **Alopecia,** or hair loss, related to effects on the hair follicles, may also occur.

Clinically Important Drug–Drug Interactions
Alkylating agents that are known to cause hepatic or renal toxicity should be used cautiously with any other drugs that have similar effects. In addition, drugs that are toxic to the liver may adversely affect drugs that are metabolized in the liver or that act in the liver (eg, oral anticoagulants). Specific drug–drug interactions for each agent should be checked in your nursing drug guide.

Nursing Considerations for Patients Receiving Alkylating Agents
Assessment: History and Examination

Screen for the following, which will alert you to specific cautions or contraindications to the use of the drug: history of allergy to any of the alkylating agents; bone marrow suppression; renal or hepatic dysfunction; and pregnancy or lactation.

Physical assessment should be performed to establish

FIGURE 14-3. Sites of action of non–cell cycle-specific antineoplastic agents. Hormone modulators react with specific receptor sites to block cell growth and activity. Docetaxel and paclitaxel inhibit microtubular reorganization. Cladribine and hydroxyurea block DNA synthesis; dacarbazine blocks DNA and RNA synthesis; irinotecan disrupts DNA strands; procarbazine inhibits DNA, RNA, and protein synthesis.

DRUGS IN FOCUS
Alkylating Agents

Drug Name	Dosage/Route	Usual Indications
busulfan (*Myleran*)	Induction: 4–8 mg PO q.d. Maintenance: 1–3 mg PO q.d.	Treatment of chronic myelogenous leukemia; not effective in blastic phase or without the Philadelphia chromosome **Special considerations:** Dosing monitored by effects on bone marrow; always push fluids to decrease toxic renal effects; alopecia is common
carboplatin (*Paraplatin*)	360 mg/m^2 IV on day 1 every 4 wk; reduce dosage as needed based on blood counts and with renal impairment	Palliative treatment of returning ovarian cancer after prior chemotherapy; may be useful in several other cancers **Special considerations:** Dosage and timing determined by bone marrow response; alopecia is common
carmustine (*BiCNU, Gliadel*)	150–200 mg/m^2 IV every 6 wk as a single dose or divided daily injections	Treatment of brain tumors, Hodgkin's disease, and multiple myelomas; available in implantable wafer form for treatment of glioblastoma **Special considerations:** Dosage determined by bone marrow toxicity, usually not repeated for 6 wk; often used in combination therapy
Ⓟ chlorambucil (*Leukeran*)	0.1–0.2 mg/kg per day PO for 3–6 wk; *or* 0.4 mg/kg PO every 2 wk with maintenance dose of 0.03–0.1 mg/kg per day PO	Treatment of lymphomas and leukemias including Hodgkin's disease; being considered for the treatment of rheumatoid arthritis and other conditions **Special considerations:** Toxic to liver and bone marrow; dosing based on bone marrow response
cisplatin (*Platinol-AQ*)	20–50 mg/m^2/d IV, once every 3 wk used in combination with other antineoplastic agents	Combination therapy for metastatic testicular or ovarian tumors, advanced bladder cancers **Special considerations:** Neurotoxic, nephrotoxic, and can cause serious hypersensitivity reactions
cyclophosphamide (*Cytoxan, Neosar*)	Induction: 40–50 m/kg IV over 2–5 d, *or* 1–5 mg/kg per day PO Maintenace: 1–5 mg/kg per day PO, *or* 10–15 mg/kg IV q7–10d	Treatment of lymphoma, myelomas, leukemias, and other cancers in combination with other drugs **Special considerations:** Hemorrhagic cystitis is a potentially fatal side effect; alopecia is common
ifosfamide (*Ifex*)	1.2 g/m^2 per day IV for 5 consecutive days; repeat every 3 wk	Combination therapy as a third-line agent in treating germ cell testicular cancers; being tested for treatment of other cancers **Special considerations:** Alopecia is common
lomustine (*CeeNu*)	130 mg/m^2 PO as a single dose every 6 wk; adjust dosage based on blood counts	Palliative combination therapy for Hodgkin's disease and primary and metastatic brain tumors **Special considerations:** Immune suppression and gastrointestinal effects are common
mechlorethamine (*Mustargen*)	0.4 mg/kg IV for each course; usually repeated every 3–6 wk	Nitrogen mustard; palliative treatment in Hodgkin's disease, leukemia, bronchial carcinoma, other cancers; injected for treatment of effusions secondary to cancer metastases **Special considerations:** Gastrointestinal toxicity, bone marrow suppression, and impaired fertility are common
melphalan (*Alkeran*)	Multiple myeloma: 6 mg/d PO for 2–3 wk, then a rest period Ovarian cancer: 0.2 mg/kg per day PO for 5 d; repeat course every 4–5 wk	Nitrogen mustard; palliative treatment for multiple myeloma, ovarian cancers **Special considerations:** Oral route is preferred; pulmonary fibrosis, bone marrow suppression, and alopecia are common

DRUGS IN FOCUS (CONTINUED)

Alkylating Agents

Drug Name	Dosage/Route	Usual Indications
streptozocin (*Zanosar*)	500 mg/m^2 IV for 5 consecutive days, usually given every week	Treatment of metastatic islet cell carcinoma of the pancreas **Special considerations:** Gastrointestinal and renal toxicity are common; causes infertility; wear rubber gloves to avoid drug contact with the skin—if contact occurs, wash with soap and water
thiotepa (*Thioplex*)	0.3–0.4 mg/kg IV at 4-wk intervals	Treatment of adenocarcinoma of the breast and uterus and papillary carcinoma of the bladder; available intrathecally to treat effusion **Special considerations:** Infertility, rash, gastrointestinal toxicity, dizziness, headache, and bone marrow suppression are common

baseline data for determining the effectiveness of the drug and the occurrence of any adverse effects associated with drug therapy. Include screening for orientation and reflexes to evaluate any central nervous system (CNS) effects; respiratory rate and adventitious sounds to monitor the disease and to evaluate for respiratory or hypersensitivity effects; pulse, rhythm, and auscultation to monitor for systemic or cardiovascular effects; and bowel sounds and mucous membrane status to monitor for GI effects. Evaluate the complete blood count (CBC) with differential and renal and liver function tests to monitor for dosage adjustment as needed and to evaluate toxic drug effects.

BOX 14-3

Drugs that Protect Cells from Alkylating Agents

Amifostine (*Ethyol*) is a cytoprotective (cell-protecting) drug that preserves healthy cells from the toxic effects of cisplatin. It is thought to react to the specific acidity and vascularity of nontumor cells to protect them, and it may also act as a scavenger of free radicals released by cells that have been exposed to cisplatin. Amifostine is given at a dose of 910 mg/m^2 q.i.d. as a 15-min IV infusion starting within 30 min after starting cisplatin therapy; timing is very important to its effectiveness. Now approved for use to prevent the renal toxicity associated with the use of cisplatin in patients with advanced ovarian cancer, amifostine is under investigation as an agent to protect lung fibroblasts from the effects of paclitaxel. Because amifostine is associated with severe nausea and vomiting, concurrent administration of an antiemetic is recommended. It also can cause hypotension, and patients should be monitored closely for this condition.

Mesna (*Mesnex*) is a cytoprotective agent that is used to reduce the incidence of hemorrhagic cystitis caused by ifosfamide or cyclophosphamide. Mesna, which is known to react chemically with urotoxic metabolites of ifosfamide, is given intravenously at the time of the ifosfamide injection at a dose that is 20% of the ifosfamide dose, and is repeated 4 hours and 8 hours afterward. Because mesna has been associated with nausea and vomiting, an antiemetic may be useful.

Nursing Diagnoses

The patient receiving an alkylating agent may have the following nursing diagnoses related to drug therapy:

- Acute Pain related to GI, CNS, skin effects of drug
- Disturbed Body Image related to alopecia, skin effects, impaired fertility
- Fear, Anxiety related to diagnosis and treatment
- Deficient Knowledge regarding drug therapy

Implementation

- Arrange for blood tests before, periodically during, and for at least 3 weeks after therapy *to monitor bone marrow function. Discontinue the drug or reduce the dose as needed.*
- Administer medication according to scheduled protocol and in combination with other drugs as indicated *to improve effectiveness.*
- Ensure that the patient is well hydrated *to decrease risk of renal toxicity.*
- Provide small, frequent meals, frequent mouth care, and dietary consultation as appropriate *to maintain nutrition when GI effects are severe.* Antiemetics may be helpful in some cases.

- Arrange for proper head covering at extremes of temperature if alopecia occurs; a wig, scarf, or hat is *important for maintaining body temperature*. If alopecia is an anticipated effect of drug therapy, advise the patient to obtain a wig or head covering before the condition occurs *to promote self-esteem and a positive body image*.
- Provide patient teaching *to enhance patient knowledge about drug therapy and to promote compliance* regarding

The appropriate dosage regimen, including dates to return for further doses.

The importance of covering the head at extremes of temperature.

The need to try to maintain nutrition if GI effects are severe.

The need to plan appropriate rest periods, because fatigue and weakness are common effects of the drugs.

The possibility of impaired fertility; the patient may wish to consult a health care provider.

The importance of not taking the drugs during pregnancy and of using barrier contraceptives.

See the accompanying Patient Teaching Checklist for antineoplastic agents.

Evaluation

- Monitor patient response to the drug (alleviation of cancer being treated, palliation of signs and symptoms of cancer).
- Monitor for adverse effects (bone marrow suppression, GI toxicity, neurotoxicity, alopecia, renal or hepatic dysfunction).
- Evaluate the effectiveness of the teaching plan (patient can name the drug, dosage, possible adverse effects to watch for, and specific measures to help avoid adverse effects). (See Nursing Care Guide: Antineoplastic Agents.)

PATIENT TEACHING CHECKLIST
Antineoplastic Agents

Create customized patient teaching materials for a specific antineoplastic agent from the CD-ROM. Patient teaching should stress the following points for drugs within this class:

- Antineoplastic agents work to destroy cells at various phases of their life cycle. These drugs are prescribed to kill cancer cells that are growing in the body. Because these drugs also affect normal cells, they sometimes cause many adverse effects.

    Common adverse effects of this drug include

- *Nausea and vomiting*—Antiemetic drugs and sedatives may help. Your health care provider will be with you to help if these effects occur.
- *Loss of appetite*—It is very important to keep up your strength. Tell people if there is something that you would be interested in eating—anything that appeals to you. Alert someone if you feel hungry, regardless of the time of day.
- *Loss of hair*—Your hair will grow back, although its color or consistency may be different from what it was originally. It may help to purchase a wig before you lose your hair so that you can match appearance if you would like to. Hats and scarves may also be worn. It is very important to keep your head covered in extremes of temperature and to protect yourself from sun, heat, and cold. Because much of the body's heat can be lost through the head, not protecting yourself could cause serious problems.
- *Mouth sores*—Frequent mouth care is very helpful. Try to avoid very hot or spicy foods.
- *Fatigue, malaise*—Frequent rest periods and careful planning of your day's activities can be very helpful.
- *Bleeding*—You may bruise more easily than you normally do, and your gums may bleed while you are brushing your teeth. Special care should be taken when

shaving or brushing your teeth. Avoid activities that might cause an injury, and avoid medications that contain aspirin.
- *Susceptibility to infection*—Avoid people with infections or colds, and avoid crowded, public places. In some cases, the people who are caring for you may wear gowns and masks to protect you from their germs.

    Report any of the following to your health care provider: bruising and bleeding, fever, chills, sore throat, difficulty breathing, flank pain, and swelling in your ankles or fingers.

    Take the full course of your prescription. It is very important to take the complete regimen that has been ordered for you. Cancer cells grow at different rates, and they go through rest periods during which they are not susceptible to the drugs. The disease must be attacked over time to eradicate the problem.

    Tell any doctor, nurse, or other health care provider that you are taking this drug.

    Try to maintain a balanced diet while you are taking this drug. Drink 10 to 12 glasses of water each day during the drug therapy.

    Use a barrier contraceptive while you are taking this drug. These drugs can cause serious effects to a developing fetus, and precautions must be taken to avoid pregnancy. If you think that you are pregnant, consult your health care provider immediately.

    You need to have periodic blood tests and examinations while you are taking this drug. These tests help guard against serious adverse effects and may be needed to determine the next dose of your drug.

This Teaching Checklist reflects general patient teaching guidelines. It is not meant to be a substitute for drug-specific teaching information, which is available in nursing drug guides.

NURSING CARE GUIDE

Antineoplastic Agents

Assessment	Nursing Diagnoses	Implementation	Evaluation
HISTORY	Acute Pain related to GI, CNS, skin effects	Ensure safe administration of the drug.	Evaluate drug effects: resolution of cancer.
Allergies to any of these drugs, renal or hepatic dysfunction, pregnancy or lactation, bone marrow suppression, GI ulceration	Imbalanced Nutrition: Less than Body Requirements related to GI effects	Provide comfort and safety measures: mouth and skin care, rest periods, safety precautions, antiemetics as needed, maintenance of nutrition, head covering.	Monitor for adverse effects: GI toxicity, bone marrow suppression, CNS changes, renal and hepatic damage, alopecia, extravasation of drug.
	Disturbed Body Image related to diagnosis, therapy, adverse effects	Provide support and reassurance to deal with drug effects, discomfort, and diagnosis.	Monitor for drug–drug interactions as indicated for each drug.
	Deficient Knowledge regarding drug therapy	Provide patient teaching regarding drug name, dosage, adverse effects, precautions to take, signs and symptoms to report, and comfort measures to observe.	Evaluate effectiveness of patient teaching program.
			Evaluate effectiveness of comfort and safety measures.
PHYSICAL EXAMINATION			
Local: evaluation of injection site			
CNS: orientation, affect, reflexes			
Skin: color, lesions, texture			
GI: abdominal, liver evaluation			
Laboratory tests: CBC with differential; renal and hepatic function tests			

ANTIMETABOLITES

Antimetabolites are drugs that have chemical structures similar to those of various natural metabolites that are necessary for the growth and division of rapidly growing neoplastic cells and normal cells. Antimetabolites replace those needed metabolites and thereby prevent normal cellular function. The use of these drugs has been somewhat limited because of the ability of neoplastic cells to develop resistance to these agents rather rapidly. For this reason, these drugs are usually administered as part of a combination therapy.

Therapeutic Actions and Indications

The antimetabolites inhibit DNA production in cells that depend on certain natural metabolites to produce their DNA. Many of these agents inhibit thymidylate synthetase, DNA polymerase, or folic acid reductase, all of which are needed for

DNA synthesis. They are considered to be S phase–specific in the cell cycle. They are most effective in rapidly dividing cells, in which they prevent cell replication, leading to cell death (Figure 14–4). The antimetabolites are indicated for the treatment of various leukemias, including some GI and basal cell cancers. The table on page 177 lists the antimetabolites, their indications, and specific information about each drug. Methotrexate is also indicated for the treatment of rheumatoid arthritis and psoriasis.

Pharmacokinetics

Methotrexate is absorbed well from the GI tract and is excreted unchanged in the urine. Patients with renal impairment may require reduced dosage and increased monitoring when taking methotrexate. Methotrexate readily crosses the blood–brain barrier. Cytarabine, floxuridine, and fluorouracil are not absorbed well from the GI tract and need to be ad-

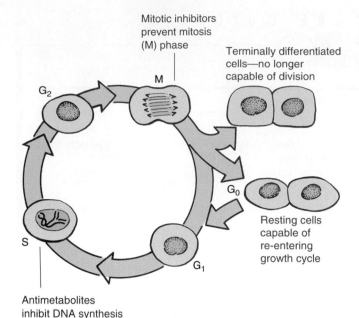

Mitotic inhibitors
prevent mitosis
(M) phase

Terminally differentiated
cells—no longer
capable of division

Resting cells
capable of
re-entering
growth cycle

Antimetabolites
inhibit DNA synthesis
(S) phase

FIGURE 14–4. Sites of action of cell cycle–specific antineoplastic agents.

ministered by a different route. They are metabolized in the liver and excreted in the urine, making it important to monitor patients with hepatic or renal impairment who are receiving these drugs. Mercaptopurine and thioguanine are absorbed slowly from the GI tract and are metabolized in the liver and excreted in the urine. All of these agents are contraindicated during pregnancy and lactation because of the potential risk to the neonate.

Contraindications and Cautions

Caution should be used when administering antimetabolites to any individual with a known allergy to any of the antimetabolites; during pregnancy and lactation, when these drugs are contraindicated because of potential severe effects on the neonate; with bone marrow suppression, which is often the index for redosing and dosing levels; with renal or hepatic dysfunction, which might interfere with the metabolism or excretion of these drugs and often indicates a need to change the dosage; and with known GI ulcerations or ulcerative diseases that might be exacerbated by the effects of these drugs.

Adverse Effects

Adverse effects frequently encountered with the use of the antimetabolites are listed here. To counteract the effects of treatment with one antimetabolite, methotrexate, the drug leucovorin is sometimes given (Box 14–4).

Hematological effects include bone marrow suppression, with leukopenia, thrombocytopenia, anemia, and pancytopenia, secondary to the effects of the drugs on the rapidly multiplying cells of the bone marrow. Toxic GI effects include nausea, vomiting, anorexia, diarrhea, and mucous membrane deterioration, all of which are related to drug effects on the rapidly multiplying cells of the GI tract. CNS

effects include headache, drowsiness, aphasia, fatigue, malaise, and dizziness. Patients should be advised to take precautions if these conditions occur. As with alkylating agents, effects of the antimetabolites may include possible hepatic toxicity or renal toxicity depending on the exact mechanism of action. Alopecia may also occur.

Clinically Important Drug–Drug Interactions

Antimetabolites that are known to cause hepatic or renal toxicity should be used with care with any other drugs known to have the same effect. In addition, drugs that are toxic to the liver may adversely affect drugs that are metabolized in the liver or that act in the liver (eg, oral anticoagulants). Specific drug–drug interactions for each agent should be checked in your nursing drug guide.

Nursing Considerations for Patients Receiving Antimetabolites

Assessment: History and Examination

Screen for the following, which will alert you to cautions and contraindications for the use of the drug: history of allergy to the specific antimetabolite; bone marrow suppression; renal or hepatic dysfunction; pregnancy or lactation; and GI ulcerative disease.

Physical assessment should be performed to establish baseline data for determining the effectiveness of the drug and the occurrence of any adverse effects associated with drug therapy. Include screening for orientation and reflexes to evaluate any CNS effects; respiratory rate and adventitious sounds to monitor the disease and to evaluate for respiratory or hypersensitivity effects; pulse, rhythm, and cardiac auscultation to monitor for systemic or cardiovascular effects; and bowel sounds and mucous membrane status to monitor for GI effects. Evaluate the CBC with differential and renal and liver function tests to monitor for dosage adjustment as needed and to evaluate toxic drug effects.

Nursing Diagnoses

The patient receiving an antimetabolite may have the following nursing diagnoses related to drug therapy:

- Acute Pain related to GI, CNS, skin effects of drug
- Disturbed Body Image related to alopecia, skin effects, impaired fertility
- Fear, Anxiety related to diagnosis and treatment
- Deficient Knowledge regarding drug therapy

Implementation

- Arrange for blood tests to monitor bone marrow function before, periodically during, and for at least 3 weeks after therapy *to arrange to discontinue the drug or reduce the dose as needed.*
- Administer medication according to scheduled protocol and in combination with other drugs as indicated *to improve effectiveness of drug therapy.*

DRUGS IN FOCUS
Antimetabolites

Drug Name	Dosage/Route	Usual Indications
capecitabine (*Xeloda*)	2500 mg/m²/d PO in two divided doses for 2 wk, then 1 wk rest, for 3 cycles	Treatment of metastatic breast cancer with resistance to paclitaxel or anthracylcines; treatment of metastatic colorectal cancer as first-line therapy **Special considerations:** Severe diarrhea can occur—monitor hydration and nutrition; monitor for bone marrow suppression
cladribine (*Leustatin*)	0.09 mg/kg per day IV for 7 consecutive days	Treatment of active hairy cell leukemia **Special considerations:** Severe bone marrow depression can occur—monitor patient closely and reduce dosage as needed; fever is common, especially early in treatment
cytarabine (*Ara-C, Cytosar-U*)	200 mg/m² per day by continuous IV infusion for 5 d, repeat every 2 wk	Treatment of meningeal and myolocytic leukemias; used in combination with other agents **Special considerations:** GI toxicity and cytarabine syndrome (fever, myalgia, bone pain, chest pain, rash, conjunctivitis, and malaise) are common—this syndrome sometimes responds to corticosteroids; alopecia may occur
floxuridine (*FUDR*)	0.1–0.6 mg/kg per day via intra-arterial line	Palliative management of GI adenocarcinoma metastatic to the liver in patients who are not candidates for surgery **Special considerations:** Administer by intra-arterial line only; bone suppression, GI toxicity, neurotoxicity, and alopecia are common
fludarabine (*Fludara*)	25 mg/m² per day IV for 5 d; repeat every 28 d	Treatment of chronic lymphocytic leukemia (CLL); unresponsive B cell CLL with no progress with at least one other treatment **Special considerations:** CNS toxicity can be severe; GI toxicity, respiratory complications, renal failure, and a tumor lysis syndrome are common
fluorouracil (*Adrucil, Efudex, Fluoroplex*)	12 mg/kg per day IV on days 1–4, then 6 mg/kg IV on days 6, 8, 10, and 12	Palliative treatment of various GI cancers; topical treatment of basal cell carcinoma and actinic and solar keratoses **Special considerations:** GI toxicity, bone marrow suppression, alopecia, and skin rash are common; avoid occlusive dressings with topical forms; wash hands thoroughly after coming in contact with drug
mercaptopurine (*Purinethol*)	2.5 mg/kg per day PO for 4 wk; then re-evaluate	Remission induction and maintenance therapy in acute leukemias **Special considerations:** Bone marrow toxicity and GI toxicity are common; hyperuricemia is a true concern—ensure that the patient is well hydrated during therapy
Ⓟ methotrexate (*Folex, Rheumatrex*)	Dosage varies with route and disease being treated; 15–30 mg PO or IM is common	Treatment of leukemias, psoriasis, and rheumatoid arthritis **Special considerations:** Hypersensitivity reactions can be severe; liver toxicity and GI complications are common; monitor for bone marrow suppression and increased susceptibility to infections; dose pack available for the oral treatment of psoriasis and rheumatoid arthritis

Drugs in Focus continues on page 178

DRUGS IN FOCUS (CONTINUED)
Antimetabolites

Drug Name	Dosage/Route	Usual Indications
pentostatin (*Nipent*)	4 mg/m² IV every other week	Hairy cell leukemia in adults if refractory to interferon-alpha therapy **Special considerations:** Associated with severe renal, hepatic, CNS, and pulmonary toxicities—monitor patient closely and reduce dosage accordingly; 3–6 mo of interferon-alpha therapy should be tried before using pentostatin
thioguanine (generic)	2 mg/kg per day PO for 4 wk; then dosage may be increased if tolerated well	Remission induction and maintenance of acute leukemias alone or as part of combination therapy **Special considerations:** Bone marrow suppression, GI toxicity, miscarriage, and birth defects have been reported; monitor bone marrow status to determine dosage and redosing; ensure that the patient is well hydrated during therapy to minimize hyperuricemia—patient may respond to allopurinol and urine alkalinization

- Ensure that the patient is well hydrated *to decrease risk of renal toxicity.*
- Provide small, frequent meals; frequent mouth care; and dietary consultation as appropriate *to maintain nutrition when GI effects are severe.* Antiemetics may be helpful in some cases.
- Arrange for proper head covering at extremes of temperature if alopecia occurs; a wig, scarf, or hat is *important for maintaining body temperature.* If alopecia is an anticipated effect of drug therapy, advise the patient to obtain a wig or head covering before the condition occurs *to promote self-esteem and a positive body image.*

BOX 14-4
A Drug That Protects Against an Antimetabolite

Leucovorin (*Wellcovorin*) is an active form of folic acid that is used to "rescue" normal cells from the adverse effects of methotrexate therapy in the treatment of osteosarcoma. This drug is also used to treat folic acid deficiency conditions such as sprue, nutritional deficiency, pregnancy, and lactation. Leucovorin is given orally or intravenously at the time of methotrexate therapy and for the next 72 h at a dose of 12–15 g/m² PO or IV followed by 10 mg/m² PO q6h for 72 h. Use of this drug has been associated with pain at the injection site.

- Provide patient teaching *to enhance patient knowledge about drug therapy and to promote compliance regarding*
  The appropriate dosage regimen, including dates to return for further doses.
  The need to try to maintain nutrition if GI effects are severe.
  The importance of covering the head at extremes of temperature if alopecia is anticipated.
  The need to plan appropriate rest periods because fatigue and weakness are common effects of the drugs.
  Possible dizziness, headache, and drowsiness; if these occur, the patient should avoid driving or using dangerous equipment.
  The possibility of impaired fertility; the patient may wish to consult a health care provider.
  The importance of not taking the drugs during pregnancy and using barrier contraceptives.

  Refer to the Patient Teaching Checklist for Antineoplastic Agents.

Evaluation

- Monitor patient response to the drug (alleviation of cancer being treated, palliation of signs and symptoms of cancer, palliation of rheumatoid arthritis or psoriasis).
- Monitor for adverse effects (bone marrow suppression, GI toxicity, neurotoxicity, alopecia, renal or hepatic dysfunction).
- Evaluate the effectiveness of the teaching plan (patient can

NURSING CHALLENGE

Antiemetics and Cancer Chemotherapy

Antineoplastic drugs can directly stimulate the chemoreceptor trigger zone (CTZ) in the medulla to induce nausea and vomiting. These drugs also cause cell death, which releases many toxins into the system—and which in turn stimulate the CTZ. Because patients expect nausea and vomiting with the administration of antineoplastic agents, the higher cortical centers of the brain can stimulate the CTZ to induce vomiting just at the thought of the chemotherapy.

A variety of antiemetic agents have been used in the course of antineoplastic therapy. Sometimes a combination of drugs is most helpful. It should also be remembered that an accepting environment, plenty of comfort measures (eg, environmental control, mouth care, ice chips), and support for the patient can help decrease the discomfort associated with the emetic effects of these drugs. Antihistamines to decrease secretions and corticosteroids to relieve inflammation are useful as adjunctive therapies.

Drugs that are known to help in treating antineoplastic chemotherapy–induced nausea and vomiting include the following:

• Dronabinol (*Marinol*) is a synthetic derivative of delta-9-tetrahydrocannabinol, the active ingredient in marijuana; this is not usually a first-line drug because of associated CNS effects. The usual dosage is 5 mg/m^2 PO 1–3 h before chemotherapy and repeated q2–4h after chemotherapy.
• Ondansetron (*Zofran*) and granisetron (*Kytril*) block serotonin receptors in the CTZ and are among the most effective antiemetics, especially if combined with a corticosteriod such as dexamethasone. The usual dosage is three 0.15-mg/kg doses IV or 8 mg PO t.i.d. starting 30 min before chemotherapy (ondansetron) or 10 µg/kg IV or 1 mg PO b.i.d. (granisetron).
• Two benzodiazepines, alprazolam (*Xanax*), 0.5 mg PO t.i.d., and lorazepam (*Ativan*), 2–6 mg/d PO, seem to be effective in directly blocking the CTZ to relieve nausea and vomiting caused by cancer. chemotherapy; they are especially effective when combined with a corticosteroid.
• Haloperidol (*Haldol*), 0.5–2.0 mg PO t.i.d. or 2–25 mg IM or IV, is a dopaminergic blocker that also is believed to have direct CTZ effects.
• Metoclopramide (*Reglan*), 2 mg/kg IV over at least 30 min, calms the activity of the GI tract; it is especially effective if combined with a corticosteroid, an antihistamine, and a centrally acting blocker such as haloperidol or lorazepam.
• Prochlorperazine (*Compazine*), 5–10 mg PO t.i.d. to q.i.d. or 5–10 mg IM, is a phenothiazine that has been found to have strong antiemetic action in the CNS; it can be given by a variety of routes.

Nausea and vomiting are unavoidable aspects of many chemotherapeutic regimens. However, treating the patient as the chemotherapy begins, using combination regimens, and providing plenty of supportive and comforting nursing care can help to alleviate some of the distress associated with these adverse effects.

name the drug, dosage, possible adverse effects to watch for, and specific measures to help avoid adverse effects).
• Monitor the effectiveness of comfort and safety measures and compliance with the regimen (refer to Nursing Care Guide: Antineoplastic Agents.)

ANTINEOPLASTIC ANTIBIOTICS

Antineoplastic antibiotics are selective not only for bacterial cells; they are also toxic to human cells. Because these drugs tend to be more toxic to cells that are multiplying rapidly, they are useful in the treatment of certain cancers. These cell cycle–specific drugs interfere with cellular DNA, disrupting it and causing cell death (see Figure 14–4). Some antineoplastic antibiotics break up DNA links, and others prevent DNA synthesis. Like other antineoplastics, the main adverse effects of these drugs are seen in cells that multiply rapidly: cells in the bone marrow, GI tract, and skin.

Therapeutic Actions and Indications
The antineoplastic antibiotics are cytotoxic and interfere with DNA synthesis by inserting themselves between base pairs in the DNA chain and causing a mutant DNA molecule, leading to cell death. The table on pages 180 and 181 lists the various antineoplastic antibiotics, their indications, and specific information about each drug. Their potentially serious adverse effects may limit their usefulness in patients with pre-existing diseases and in those who are debilitated and therefore more susceptible to these effects.

Pharmacokinetics
The antineoplastic antibiotics are not absorbed well from the GI tract and are given IV or injected into specific sites. They are metabolized in the liver and excreted in the urine at various rates. Many of them have very long half-lives (45 hours for idarubicin, more than 5 days for mitoxantrone). Daunorubicin and doxorubicin do not cross the blood–brain barrier, but they are widely distributed in the body and are taken up by the heart, lungs, kidneys, and spleen. All of these agents are contraindicated for use during pregnancy and lactation because of the potential risk to the neonate.

Contraindications and Cautions
Caution should be used when giving antineoplastic antibiotics to an individual with a known allergy to the antibiotic or related antibiotics and during pregnancy and lactation. Care should also be taken in patients with the following conditions: bone marrow suppression, which is often the index for redosing and dosing levels; suppressed renal or hepatic function, which might interfere with the metabolism or excretion of these drugs and often indicates a need to change the dosage; known GI ulcerations or ulcerative diseases, which may be exacerbated by the effects of these drugs; pulmonary problems with bleomycin or mitomycin, cardiac problems with idarubicin or mitoxantrone, and bleeding disorders with plicamycin, which are specifically toxic to these systems.

DRUGS IN FOCUS
Antineoplastic Antibiotics

Drug Name	Dosage/Route	Usual Indications
bleomycin (*Blenoxane*)	0.25–0.5 units/kg IM, IV, or SC once or twice weekly	Palliative treatment of squamous cell carcinomas, testicular cancers, and lymphomas; used to treat malignant pleural effusion **Special considerations:** GI toxicity, severe skin reactions, and hypersensitivity reactions may occur; pulmonary fibrosis can be a serious problem—baseline and periodic chest radiographs and pulmonary function tests are necessary.
dactinomycin (*Cosmegen*)	Adult: 0.5 mg/d IV for up to 5 d Pediatric: 0.015 mg/kg per day IV for up to 5 d or a total dose of 2.5 mg/m^2/wk	Part of combination drug regimen in the treatment of a variety of sarcomas and carcinomas; potentiates the effects of radiation therapy **Special considerations:** Bone marrow suppression and GI toxicity, which may be severe, limit the dose; effects may not appear for 1 to 2 wk; local extravasation can cause necrosis and should be treated with injectable corticosteroids, ice to the area, and restarting of the IV line in a different vein
daunorubicin (*DaunoXome*)	40 mg/m^2 IV, infused over 1 h; repeat every 2 wk	First-line treatment of advanced HIV infection and associated Kaposi's sarcoma **Special considerations:** Complete alopecia is common, and GI toxicity and bone marrow suppression may also occur; severe necrosis may occur at sites of local extravasation—immediate treatment with corticosteroids, normal saline, and ice may help; if ulcerations occur, a plastic surgeon should be called
ⓟ doxorubicin (*Adriamycin*)	60–75 mg/m^2 as a single IV dose; repeat every 21 d	Treatment of a number of leukemias and cancers; used to induce regression; available in a liposomal form for treatment of AIDs-associated Kaposi's sarcoma **Special considerations:** Complete alopecia is common; GI toxicity and bone suppression may occur; severe necrosis may occur at sites of local extravasation—immediate treatment with corticosteroids, normal saline and ice may help; if ulcerations occur, a plastic surgeon should be called; toxicity is dose related—an accurate record of each dose received is important in determining dosage. Severe pulmonary toxicity, alopecia, and injection site and GI toxicity occur.
idarubicin (*Idamycin*)	12 mg/m^2 per day IV for 3 d with cytarabine	Combination therapy for treatment of acute myeloid leukemia in adults **Special considerations:** May cause severe bone marrow suppression, which regulates dosage; associated with cardiac toxicity, which can be severe; GI toxicity and local necrosis with extravasation are also common; severe necrosis may occur at sites of local extravasation—immediate treatment with corticosteroids, normal saline, and ice may help; if ulcerations occur, a plastic surgeon should be called; it is essential to monitor heart and bone marrow function to protect the patient from potentially fatal adverse effects
mitomycin (*Mutamycin*)	20 mg/m^2 IV as a single dose at 6–8 wk intervals	Treatment of disseminated adenocarcinoma of the stomach and pancreas **Special considerations:** Severe pulmonary toxicity, alopecia, and injection site and GI toxicity occur

DRUGS IN FOCUS (CONTINUED)
Antineoplastic Antibiotics

Drug Name	Dosage/Route	Usual Indications
mitoxantrone (*Novantrone*)	12 mg/m^2 per day IV for 1–3 d Multiple sclerosis: 12 mg/m^2 IV as a short infusion every 3 mo	Part of combination therapy in the treatment of adult leukemias; treatment of bone pain in advanced prostatic cancer; reduction of neurological disability and frequency of relapses in chronic, progressive, relapsing multiple sclerosis **Special considerations:** Severe bone marrow suppression may occur and limits dosage; alopecia, GI toxicity, and congestive heart failure often occur; avoid direct skin contact with the drug—use gloves and goggles; monitor bone marrow activity and cardiac activity to adjust dosage or discontinue drug as needed
plicamycin (*Mithracin*)	25–30 μg/kg per day IV for 8–10 d	Treatment of malignant testicular tumor not amenable to surgery or radiation therapy; treatment of hypercalcemia and hypercalciuria not responsive to other treatments in patients with advanced neoplasms **Special considerations:** GI toxicity, local cellulitis, fever, and pain are common; hemorrhagic syndrome with epistaxis to severe bleeding and death has occurred; monitor bleeding times and adjust dosage as needed; monitor injection sites for cellulitis and arrange appropriate treatment
valrubicin (*valstar*)	800 mg intravesically once a week for 6 weeks	Intravesical therapy for carcinoma in situ of the bladder if refractory to bacille Calmette-Guérin (BCG) therapy **Special considerations:** Use goggles and gloves when handling, avoid contact with eyes; severe bladder spasms have occurred, use caution with history of irritable bowel syndrome, do not clamp bladder catheter in place

Adverse Effects

Adverse effects frequently encountered with the use of these antibiotics include bone marrow suppression, with leukopenia, thrombocytopenia, anemia, and pancytopenia, secondary to the effects of the drugs on the rapidly multiplying cells of the bone marrow. Toxic GI effects include nausea, vomiting, anorexia, diarrhea, and mucous membrane deterioration, all of which are related to drug effects on the rapidly multiplying cells of the GI tract. As with the alkylating agents and antimetabolites, effects of antineoplastic antibiotics may include renal or hepatic toxicity, depending on the exact mechanism of action. Alopecia may also occur. Specific drugs are toxic to the heart and lungs; Box 14–5 discusses a cardioprotective drug that interferes with the effects of doxorubicin. Plicamycin has been associated with a hemorrhagic syndrome (see Table 14–3).

Clinically Important Drug–Drug Interactions

Antimetabolites that are known to cause hepatic or renal toxicity should be used with care with any other drugs known to

have the same effect. Drugs that result in toxicity to the heart or lungs should be used with caution with any other drugs that produce that particular toxicity. Specific drug–drug interactions for each agent are listed in your nursing drug guide.

Nursing Considerations for Patients Receiving Antineoplastic Antibiotic Agents
Assessment: History and Examination

Screen for the following, which could be cautions or contraindications to the use of the drug: history of allergy to the antibiotic in use; bone marrow suppression; renal or hepatic dysfunction; respiratory or cardiac disease; pregnancy or lactation; and GI ulcerative disease.

Physical assessment should be performed to establish baseline data for determining the effectiveness of the drug and the occurrence of any adverse effects associated with drug therapy. Include screening for orientation and reflexes to evaluate any CNS effects; respiratory rate and adventitious sounds to monitor the disease and evaluate for respiratory or hypersensitivity effects; pulse, rhythm, cardiac aus-

CASE STUDY

Antineoplastic Therapy and Breast Cancer

THE SITUATION

A 34-year-old white woman, B. P., is a school teacher with two young daughters. She noticed a slightly painful lump under her arm when showering. About 2 weeks later, she found a mass in her right breast. Initial patient assessment found that she had no other underlying medical problems, had no allergies, and took no medications. Her family history was most indicative: many of the women in her family—her mother, two grandmothers, three aunts, two older sisters, and one younger sister—died of breast cancer when they were in their early 30s. All data from the initial examination, including an evaluation of the lump in the upper outer quadrant of her breast and the presence of a fixed axillary node, were recorded as baseline data for further drug therapy and treatment. B. P. underwent a radical mastectomy with biopsy report for grade IV infiltrating ductal carcinoma (28 of 35 lymph nodes were positive for tumor) and then radiation therapy. Then she began a 1-year course of cytoxan, methotrexate, and fluorouracil (CMF).

CRITICAL THINKING

What are the important nursing implications for B.P.? *Think about the outlook for B.P., based on her biopsy results and her family history.*

What are the effects of high levels of stress on the immune system and the body's ability to fight cancer?

What impact will this disease have on B. P.'s job and her family? *Think about the adverse drug effects that can be anticipated.* How can good patient teaching help B. P. to anticipate and cope with these many changes and unpleasant effects?

What future concerns should be addressed or at least approached at this point in the treatment of B. P's disease? What are the implications for her two daughters? How may a coordinated health team work to help the daughters cope with their mother's disease as well as the prospects for their future?

DISCUSSION

The extent of B. P.'s disease, as evidenced by the biopsy results, does not signify a very hopeful prognosis. In this case, the overall nursing care plan should take into account not only the acute needs related to surgery and drug therapy but also future needs related to potential debilitation and even the prospect of death. Immediate needs include comfort and teaching measures to help B. P. deal with the mastectomy and recovery from the surgery. She should be given an opportunity to vent her feelings and thoughts in a protected environment. Efforts should be made to help her to organize her life and plans around her radiation therapy and chemotherapy.

The adverse effects associated with the antineoplastic agents she will be given should be explained and possible ways to cope should be discussed. These effects include the following:

Alopecia—B. P. should be reassured that her hair will grow back, but she will need to cover her head in extremes of temperature. Purchasing a wig before the hair loss begins may be a good alternative to trying to remember later what her hair was like.

Nausea and vomiting—These effects will most often occur immediately after the drugs are given. Antiemetics may be ordered, but they are frequently not very effective.

Bone marrow suppression—This will make B. P. more susceptible to disease, which could be a problem for a teacher and a mother with young children. Ways to avoid contact and infection as well as warning signs to report immediately should be discussed.

Mouth sores—Stomatitis and mucositis are common problems. Frequent mouth care is important. The patient should be encouraged to maintain fluid intake and nutrition.

Because the antineoplastic therapy will be a long-term regimen, it might help to prepare a calendar of drug dates for use in planning other activities and events. All of B. P.'s treatment should be incorporated into a team approach that helps B. P. and her family deal with the impact of this disease and its therapy, as well as with the potential risk to her daughters. B. P.'s daughters are in a very-high-risk group for this disease, so the importance of frequent examinations as they grow up needs to be stressed. In some areas of the country, health care providers are encouraging prophylactic mastectomies for women in this very-high-risk group.

---

cultation, and baseline electrocardiogram to monitor for systemic or cardiovascular effects; and bowel sounds and mucous membrane status to monitor for GI effects. Evaluate the CBC with differential and renal and liver function tests to monitor for dosage adjustment as needed and to evaluate toxic drug effects. Clotting times should be obtained for patients receiving plicamycin.

Nursing Diagnoses

The patient receiving an antineoplastic antibiotic may have the following nursing diagnoses related to drug therapy:

- Acute Pain related to GI, CNS, local effects of drug
- Disturbed Body Image related to alopecia, skin effects
- Fear, Anxiety related to diagnosis and treatment
- Deficient Knowledge regarding drug therapy

Implementation

- Arrange for blood tests to monitor bone marrow function before, periodically during, and for at least 3 weeks after therapy *to arrange to discontinue the drug or reduce the dose as needed.* Monitor cardiac and respiratory function as well as clotting times as appropriate for the drug being

BOX 14-5
A Cardioprotective Antineoplastic Drug

Dexrazoxane (*Zinecard*), a powerful intracellular chelating agent, is a cardioprotective drug that interferes with the cardiotoxic effects of doxorubicin. The associated adverse effects are difficult to differentiate from those attributable to doxorubicin. This agent is approved for use to prevent the cardiomyopathy associated with doxorubicin in doses greater than 300 mg/m^2 in women with metastatic breast cancer. Dexrazoxane is given intravenously in a dosage proportional to (10 times greater than) the doxorubicin dose 30 minutes before the doxorubicin is administered.

used *to arrange to discontinue the drug or reduce the dose as needed.*
- Administer medication according to scheduled protocol and in combination with other drugs as indicated *to improve effectiveness of drug therapy.*
- Ensure that the patient is well hydrated *to decrease risk of renal toxicity.*
- Provide small, frequent meals; frequent mouth care; and dietary consultation as appropriate *to maintain nutrition when GI effects are severe.* Antiemetics may be helpful in some cases.
- Arrange for proper head covering at extremes of temperature if alopecia occurs; a wig, scarf, or hat is *important for maintaining body temperature.* If alopecia is an anticipated effect of drug therapy, advise the patient to obtain a wig or head covering before the condition occurs *to promote self-esteem and a positive body image.*
- Provide patient teaching *to enhance patient knowledge about drug therapy and to promote compliance* regarding

The appropriate dosage regimen, including dates to return for further doses.
The need to try to maintain nutrition if GI effects are severe.
The importance of covering the head at extremes of temperature if alopecia is anticipated.
The need to plan appropriate rest periods because fatigue and weakness are common effects of the drugs.
Possible dizziness, headache, and drowsiness; if these occur, the patient should avoid driving or using dangerous equipment.
The possibility of impaired fertility; the patient may wish to consult a health care provider.
The importance of not taking the drugs during pregnancy and of using barrier contraceptives.

Refer to the Patient Teaching Checklist for Antineoplastic Agents

Evaluation
- Monitor patient response to the drug (alleviation of cancer being treated and palliation of signs and symptoms of cancer).

- Monitor for adverse effects (bone marrow suppression, GI toxicity, neurotoxicity, alopecia, renal or hepatic dysfunction, and cardiac or respiratory dysfunction).
- Evaluate the effectiveness of the teaching plan (patient can name the drug, dosage, possible adverse effects to watch for, and specific measures to help avoid adverse effects). (Refer to Nursing Care Guide: Antineoplastic Agents.)

WEB LINKS
Health care providers and patients may want to consult the following Internet sources:

Information on cancer, including research, protocols, and new information, maintained by the National Cancer Institute of the National Institutes of Health:
http://cancer.gov/cancer_information
Information on cancer care and general patient education:
http://cancerguide.org
Information on numerous cancer connections, support groups, treatment, resources:
http://www.cancer.org
Information about on-line resources related to all types of cancer:
http://www.acor.org
Information about the Oncology Nurses Society:
http://www.ons.org

MITOTIC INHIBITORS

Mitotic inhibitors are drugs that kill cells as the process of mitosis begins (see Figure 14–4). These cell-cycle-specific agents inhibit DNA synthesis. Like other antineoplastics, the main adverse effects with the mitotic inhibitors occur with cells that rapidly multiply: those in the bone marrow, GI tract, and skin.

Therapeutic Actions and Indications
The mitotic inhibitors interfere with the ability of a cell to divide, block, or alter DNA synthesis, thus causing cell death. They work in the M phase of the cell cycle. These drugs are used for the treatment of a variety of tumors and leukemias. The table on page 184 lists the mitotic inhibitors, their indications, and specific information about each drug. These drugs are not interchangeable, and each has a specific use.

Pharmacokinetics
Generally, these drugs are not well absorbed from the GI tract and are given intravenously. They are metabolized in the liver and excreted primarily in the feces, making them safer for use in patients with renal impairment than the antineoplastics that are cleared through the urine. They should not be used during pregnancy or lactation because of the potential risk to the neonate.

Contraindications and Cautions
Caution should be used when giving these drugs to anyone with a known allergy to the drug or related drugs and during

DRUGS IN FOCUS
Mitotic Inhibitors

Drug Name	Dosage/Route	Usual Indications
docetaxel (*Taxotere*)	60–100 mg/m^2 IV over 1 h every 3 wk	Treatment of breast cancer and non–small cell lung cancer **Special considerations:** Monitor patient closely—deaths have occurred during use; severe fluid retention can occur—premedicate with corticosteroids and monitor for weight gain; skin rash and nail disorders are usually reversible; monitor patients closely during use
etoposide (*Toposar, VePesid*)	35–100 mg/m^2 per day IV for 4–5 d	Treatment of testicular cancers refractory to other agents **Special considerations:** Fatigue, GI toxicity, bone marrow depression and alopecia are common side effects; avoid direct skin contact with the drug, use protective clothing and goggles; monitor bone marrow function to adjust dosage; rapid fall in blood pressure can occur during IV infusion—monitor patient carefully
paclitaxel (*Taxol, Onxol*)	135–175 mg/m^2 per day IV over 3 h every 3 weeks	Treatment of advanced ovarian cancer, breast cancer, non–small cell lung cancer, and AIDS-related Kaposi's sarcoma **Special considerations:** Anaphylaxis and severe hypersensitivity reactions have occurred—monitor very closely during administration; also monitor for bone marrow suppression; cardiovascular toxicity and neuropathies have occurred
teniposide (*Vumon*)	165–250 mg/m^2 IV weekly in combination with other drugs	In combination with other drugs for induction therapy in childhood acute lymphoblastic leukemia **Special considerations:** GI toxicity, CNS effects, bone marrow suppression, and alopecia are common effects; avoid direct skin contact with the drug—use protective clothing and goggles; monitor bone marrow function to adjust dosage; rapid fall in blood pressure can occur during IV infusion—monitor patient carefully
vinblastine (*Velban*)	Adult: 3.7 mg/m^2 IV once weekly Pediatric: 2 mg/m^2 IV once weekly Dosage may then be increased based on leukocyte count and patient response	Palliative treatment of various lymphomas and sarcomas; advanced Hodgkin's disease; alone or as part of combination therapy for the treatment of advanced testicular germ cell cancers **Special considerations:** GI toxicity, CNS effects, and total loss of hair are common; antiemetics may help; avoid contact with drug, and monitor injection sites for reactions
vincristine (*Oncovin, Vincasar*)	Adult: 1.4 mg/m^2 IV at weekly intervals Pediatric: 1.5–2 mg/m^2 IV once weekly	Treatment of acute leukemia, various lymphomas, and sarcomas **Special considerations:** Extensive CNS effects are common, GI toxicity, local irritation at injection IV site, and hair loss commonly occur; syndrome of inappropriate secretion of antidiuretic hormone (SIADH) has been reported—monitor urine output and arrange for fluid restriction and diuretics as needed.
vinorelbine (*Navelbine*)	30 mg/m^2 IV once weekly, based on granulocyte count	First-line treatment of unresectable advanced small cell lung cancer; stage IV non–small cell lung cancer and stage III non–small cell lung cancer with cisplatin **Special considerations:** GI and CNS toxicity are common; total loss of hair, local reaction at injection site, and bone marrow depression also occur; prepare a calendar with return dates for the series of injections; avoid extravasation but arrange for hyaluronidase infusion if it occurs; antiemetics may be helpful

pregnancy and lactation. Care should also be taken in patients with the following conditions: bone marrow suppression, which is often the index for redosing and dosing levels; renal or hepatic dysfunction, which could interfere with the metabolism or excretion of these drugs and often indicates a need to change the dosage; and known GI ulcerations or ulcerative diseases, which may be exacerbated by the effects of these drugs.

Adverse Effects

Adverse effects frequently encountered with the use of mitotic inhibitors include bone marrow suppression, with leukopenia, thrombocytopenia, anemia, and pancytopenia, secondary to the effects of the drugs on the rapidly multiplying cells of the bone marrow. GI effects include nausea, vomiting, anorexia, diarrhea, and mucous membrane deterioration. As with the other antineoplastic agents, effects of the mitotic inhibitors may include possible hepatic or renal toxicity, depending on the exact mechanism of action. Alopecia may also occur. These drugs also cause necrosis and cellulitis if extravasation occurs, so injection sites should be regularly monitored and appropriate action taken as needed (Box 14–6).

Clinically Important Drug–Drug Interactions

Mitotic inhibitors that are known to be toxic to the liver or the CNS should be used with care with any other drugs known to have the same adverse effect. Specific drug–drug interactions for each agent are listed in your nursing drug guide.

Nursing Considerations for Patients Receiving Mitotic Inhibitors

Assessment: History and Examination

Screen for the following, which could be cautions or contraindications to the use of the drug: history of allergy to the drug used (or related drugs); bone marrow suppression; renal or hepatic dysfunction; pregnancy or lactation; and GI ulcerative disease.

Physical assessment should be performed to establish baseline data for determining the effectiveness of the drug and the occurrence of any adverse effects associated with drug therapy. Include screening for orientation and reflexes to evaluate any CNS effects; skin, to evaluate for lesions, as well as hair and hair distribution, to monitor for adverse effects; respiratory rate and adventitious sounds to monitor the disease and to evaluate for respiratory or hypersensitivity effects; and bowel sounds and mucous membrane status to monitor for GI effects. Evaluate the CBC with differential and renal and liver function tests to monitor for dosage adjustment as needed and to evaluate toxic drug effects. Regular evaluation of injection sites should be performed to check for signs of extravasation or inflammation.

Nursing Diagnoses

The patient receiving a mitotic inhibitor may have the following nursing diagnoses related to drug therapy:

- Acute Pain related to GI, CNS, local effects of drug
- Disturbed Body Image related to alopecia, skin effects

BOX 14-6
Treating Extravasation

When an IV antineoplastic drug extravasates, or infiltrates into the surrounding tissue, serious tissue damage can occur. These drugs are toxic to cells, and the resulting tissue injury can result in severe pain, scarring, nerve and muscle damage, infection, and in very severe cases even amputation of the limb.

Prevention is the best way to deal with extravasation. Interventions that can help to prevent extravasation include the following: use a distal vein, avoiding small veins on the wrist or digits; never use an existing line unless it is clearly open and running well; start the infusion with plain 5% dextrose in water (D5W) and monitor for any sign of extravasation; check the site frequently and ask the patient to report any discomfort in the area; if at all possible, do not use an infusion pump to administer one of these drugs, because it will continue to deliver the drug under pressure and can cause a severe extravasation.

If extravasation occurs, there are specific antidotes to use with some antineoplastic drugs. The antidote is usually administered through the IV line to allow it to infiltrate the same tissue, but if the line has been pulled, a tuberculin syringe can be used to inject the antidote subcutaneously into the tissue surrounding the infiltrated area.

Drug	Antidote and Suggested Dosage
etoposide teniposide vinblastine vincristine	hyaluronidase (Wydase), 0.2 mL SC; then apply heat to disperse drug and alleviate pain
daunorubicin doxorubicin vinblastine vincristine	8.4% sodium bicarbonate, 5 mL; flood area with normal saline, apply cold compress; local infiltration with corticosteroids may also be ordered at 25 to 50 mg/mL of extravasate; if ulceration occurs, a plastic surgery consultation should be obtained
mechlorethamine	isotonic sodium thiosulfate (1/6 M), 10 mL infused immediately, then apply an ice compress for 6 to 12 h
dactinomycin	50 mg ascorbic acid injection; flush area with normal saline and apply cold compresses; consider use of an injectable corticosteroid if reaction is severe

- Fear, Anxiety related to diagnosis and treatment
- Deficient Knowledge regarding drug therapy

Implementation

- Arrange for blood tests to monitor bone marrow function before, periodically during, and for at least 3 weeks after therapy *to arrange to discontinue the drug or reduce the dose as needed.*

- Avoid direct skin or eye contact with the drug. *Wear protective clothing and goggles while preparing and administering the drug to prevent toxic reaction to the drug.*
- Administer medication according to scheduled protocol and in combination with other drugs as indicated *to improve effectiveness of drug therapy.*
- Ensure that the patient is well hydrated *to decrease risk of renal toxicity.*
- Monitor injection sites *to arrange appropriate treatment for extravasation, local inflammation, or cellulitis.*
- Provide small, frequent meals; frequent mouth care; and dietary consultation as appropriate *to maintain nutrition if GI effects are severe.* Antiemetics may be helpful in some cases.
- Arrange for proper head covering at extremes of temperature if alopecia or epilation occurs; a wig, scarf, or hat is *important for maintaining body temperature.* If alopecia is an anticipated effect of drug therapy, advise the patient to obtain a wig or head covering before the condition occurs *to promote self-esteem and a positive body image.*
- Provide patient teaching to enhance patient knowledge about drug therapy and *to promote compliance regarding*

The appropriate dosage regimen, including dates to return for further doses.
The need to try to maintain nutrition if GI effects are severe.
The importance of covering the head at extremes of temperature if alopecia is anticipated.
The need to plan appropriate rest periods because fatigue and weakness are common effects of the drugs.
Possible dizziness, headache, and drowsiness; if these occur, the patient should avoid driving or using dangerous equipment.
The possibility of impaired fertility; the patient may wish to consult a health care provider.
The importance of not taking the drugs during pregnancy and using barrier contraceptive.

Refer to the Patient Teaching Checklist on antineoplastic agents.

Evaluation

- Monitor patient response to the drug (alleviation of cancer being treated and palliation of signs and symptoms of cancer).
- Monitor for adverse effects (bone marrow suppression, GI toxicity, neurotoxicity, alopecia, renal or hepatic dysfunction, and local reactions at the injection site).
- Evaluate the effectiveness of the teaching plan (patient can name the drug, dosage, possible adverse effects to watch for, and specific measures to help avoid adverse effects). (Refer to Nursing Care Guide: Antineoplastic Agents.)

HORMONES AND HORMONE MODULATORS

Some cancers, particularly those involving the breast tissue, ovaries, and uterus, are sensitive to estrogen stimulation. Estrogen receptor sites on the tumor react with circulating estrogen, and this reaction stimulates the tumor cells to grow and divide. Several antineoplastic agents are used to block or interfere with these receptor sites so as to prevent growth of the cancer and in some situations to actually cause cell death. Some hormones are used to block the release of gonadotropic hormones in breast or prostate cancer if the tumors are responsive to gonadotropic hormones. Others may block androgen receptor sites directly and are useful in the treatment of advanced prostate cancers.

Therapeutic Actions and Indications
The hormones and hormone modulators used as antineoplastics are receptor site–specific or hormone-specific to block the stimulation of growing cancer cells that are sensitive to the presence of that hormone (see Figure 14–3). These drugs are indicated for the treatment of breast cancer in postmenopausal women or in other women without ovarian function, and some are indicated for the treatment of prostatic cancers that are sensitive to hormone manipulation. The table on pages 187–189 lists the hormones and hormone modulators, their uses, and specific information about each drug.

Pharmacokinetics
These drugs are readily absorbed from the GI tract, metabolized in the liver, and excreted in the urine. Caution must be used with any patient who has hepatic or renal impairment. These drugs cross the placenta and enter into breast milk and are contraindicated during pregnancy and lactation because of toxic effects on the neonate.

Contraindications and Cautions
Caution should be used when giving hormones and hormone modulators to anyone with a known allergy to any of these drugs; during pregnancy, when blocking of estrogen effects or any gonadotropic effects can lead to fetal death and serious problems for the mother; and during lactation. Care should also be taken in patients with bone marrow suppression, which is often the index for redosing and dosing levels, and in those with renal or hepatic dysfunction, which could interfere with the metabolism or excretion of these drugs and often indicates a need to change the dosage. Hypercalcemia is a contraindication to the use of toremifene, which is known to increase calcium levels.

Adverse Effects
Adverse effects frequently encountered with the use of these drugs involve the effects that are seen when estrogen is blocked or inhibited. Menopause-associated effects include hot flashes, vaginal spotting, vaginal dryness, moodiness, and depression. Other effects include bone marrow suppression and GI toxicity, including hepatic dysfunction. Hypercalcemia is also encountered as the calcium is pulled out of the bones without estrogen activity to promote calcium deposition.

Clinically Important Drug–Drug Interactions
If hormones and hormone modulators are taken with oral anticoagulants, there is often an increased risk of bleeding. Care should also be taken with any drugs that might increase serum lipid levels.

DRUGS IN FOCUS
Hormones and Hormone Modulators

Drug Name	Dosage/Route	Usual Indications
anastrazole (*Arimidex*)	1 mg PO q.d.	Treatment of advanced breast cancer in post-menopausal women after tamoxifen therapy **Actions:** Antiestrogen drug; blocks estradiol production without effects on adrenal hormones **Special considerations:** GI effects, signs and symptoms of menopause—hot flashes, mood swings, edema, vaginal dryness and itching—as well as bone pain and back pain, treatable with analgesics, may occur; monitor lipid concentrations in patients at risk for high cholesterol level
bicalutamide (*Casodex*)	50 mg PO q.d.	In combination with a leutinizing hormone for the treatment of advanced prostate cancer **Actions:** Antiandrogen drug that competitively binds androgen receptor sites **Special considerations:** Gynecomastia and breast tenderness occur in 33% of patients; GI complaints are common. Pregnancy category X.
estramustine (*Emcyt*)	10–16 mg/kg per day PO in three to four divided doses for 30–90 d, then reevaluate	Palliative for treatment of metastatic and progressive prostate cancer **Actions:** Binds to estrogen steroid receptors, causing cell death **Special considerations:** GI toxicity, rash, bone marrow depression, breast tenderness, and cardiovascular toxicity are common adverse effects; 30–90 d of therapy may be required before effects are seen; monitor cardiovascular, liver, and bone marrow function throughout therapy
flutamide (*Eulexin*)	250 mg PO t.i.d. given 8 h apart	With a luteinizing hormone for treatment of locally confined and metastatic prostate cancer **Actions:** Antiestrogenic drug, inhibits androgen uptake and binding on target cells **Special considerations:** May cause liver toxicity, so liver function should be monitored regularly; associated with impaired fertility and cancer development; urine may become greenish; protect patient from exposure to the sun—photosensitivity is common
goserelin (*Zoladex*)	3.6–10.8 mg implant, SC, every 28 d to 12 wk	Treatment of advanced prostatic and breast cancers **Actions:** Synthetic luteinizing hormone that inhibits pituitary release of gonadotropic hormones **Special considerations:** 3.6-mg dose is effective in decreasing the signs and symptoms of endometriosis; associated with hypercalcemia and bone density loss—monitor serum calcium levels regularly; impairs fertility and is carcinogenic; monitor male patients for possible ureteral obstruction, especially during the first month

Drugs in Focus continues on page 188

DRUGS IN FOCUS (CONTINUED)
Hormones and Hormone Modulators

Drug Name	Dosage/Route	Usual Indications
letrozole (*Femara*)	2.5 mg PO q.d.	Treatment of advanced breast cancer in post-menopausal women with disease after antiestrogen therapy **Actions:** Prevents the conversion of precursors to estrogens in all tissues **Special considerations:** GI toxicity, bone marrow depression, alopecia, hot flashes, and CNS depression are common effects; discontinue drug at any sign that the cancer is progressing
leuprolide (*Lupron*)	3.7–30 mg by injection, implant, or depot	Treatment of advanced prostate cancer; also used to treat precocious puberty and endometriosis **Actions:** A natural leuteinizing hormone that blocks the release of gonadotropic hormones **Special considerations:** Monitor cancer patient's prostate-specific antigen levels periodically; monitor bone density and serum calcium levels; warn patient that he may have difficulty voiding the first few weeks and may experience bone pain, hot flashes, and pain at injection site
nilutamide (*Nilandron*)	300 mg PO q.d. for 30 d, then 150 mg PO q.d.	With surgical castration for treatment of metastatic prostate cancer **Actions:** Antiestrogenic drug, inhibits androgen uptake and binding on target cells **Special considerations:** May cause liver toxicity and liver function test results should be monitored regularly; associated with interstitial pneumonitis—baseline and periodic chest radiographs should be obtained, and discontinue drug at first sign of dyspnea
tamoxifen (*Nolvadex*)	20–40 mg PO q.d.	In combination therapy with surgery to treat breast cancer; treatment of advanced breast cancer in men and women; first drug approved for the prevention of breast cancer in women at high risk for breast cancer **Actions:** Antiestrogen, competes with estrogen for receptor sites in target tissues **Special considerations:** Signs and symptoms of menopause are common effects; CNS depression, bone marrow depression, and GI toxicity are also common; can change visual acuity and cause corneal opacities and retinopathy—pretherapy and periodic ophthalmic examinations are indicated
testolactone (*Teslac*)	250 mg PO q.i.d.	Treatment of breast cancer in postmenopausal women and in premenopausal women in whom ovarian function has been terminated **Actions:** Synthetic androgen; antineoplastic effects in postmenopausal women with breast cancer are not clearly understood—thought to act via competitive reaction for estrogen receptor sites **Special considerations:** GI effects and hypercalcemia are common reactions; virilization—hirsutism, deepening of voice, clitoral enlargement, facial hair growth, altered libido—is often an unacceptable reaction that limits drug use in some women; monitoring of serum calcium is important during the course of the therapy; a class III controlled substance

DRUGS IN FOCUS (CONTINUED)
Hormones and Hormone Modulators

Drug Name	Dosage/Route	Usual Indications
toremifene (*Fareston*)	60 mg PO q.d.	Treatment of advanced breast cancer in women with estrogen receptor–positive disease **Actions:** Binds to estrogen receptors and prevents growth of breast cancer cells **Special considerations:** Signs and symptoms of menopause are common effects; CNS depression and GI toxicity are also common

Nursing Considerations for Patients Receiving Hormones and Hormone Modulators

Assessment: History and Examination

Screen for the following, which could be cautions or contraindications to the use of the drug: history of allergy to the drug in use or any related drugs; bone marrow suppression; renal or hepatic dysfunction; pregnancy or lactation; hypercalcemia; and hypercholesterolemia.

Physical assessment should be performed to establish baseline data for determining the effectiveness of the drug and the occurrence of any adverse effects associated with drug therapy. Include screening for orientation and reflexes to evaluate any CNS effects; skin, to evaluate for lesions; hair and hair distribution to monitor for adverse drug effects; blood pressure, pulse, and perfusion to evaluate the status of the cardiovascular system and monitor for adverse drug effects; and bowel sounds and mucous membrane status to monitor for GI effects. Evaluate the CBC with differential, serum calcium levels, and renal and liver function tests to monitor for dosage adjustment as needed and to evaluate toxic drug effects.

Nursing Diagnoses

The patient receiving a hormone or hormone modulator may have the following nursing diagnoses related to drug therapy:

- Acute Pain related to GI, CNS, menopausal effects of drug
- Disturbed Body Image related to antiestrogen effects, virilization
- Fear, Anxiety related to diagnosis and treatment
- Deficient Knowledge regarding drug therapy

Implementation

- Arrange for blood tests to monitor bone marrow function before and periodically during therapy *to discontinue the drug or reduce the dose as needed.*

- Provide small, frequent meals; frequent mouth care; and dietary consultation as appropriate *to maintain nutrition when GI effects are severe.*
- Provide comfort measures *to help the patient cope with menopausal signs and symptoms* such as hygiene measures, temperature control, and stress reduction. Reduce the dosage if these effects become severe or intolerable.
- Advise the patient of the need to use barrier contraceptive measures while taking these drugs *to avert serious fetal harm which could result.*
- Provide patient teaching *to enhance patient knowledge about drug therapy and to promote compliance* regarding

The appropriate dosage regimen, including dates to return for further doses.
Maintenance of nutrition even if GI effects are severe.
Not taking these drugs during pregnancy and using barrier contraceptives.
Staying in a cool environment.
Practicing good hygiene and skin care and using stress reduction to cope with menopausal effects.

Refer to the Patient Teaching Checklist for Antineoplastic Agents.

Evaluation

- Monitor patient response to the drug (alleviation of cancer being treated and palliation of signs and symptoms of cancer being treated).
- Monitor for adverse effects (bone marrow suppression, GI toxicity, menopausal signs and symptoms, hypercalcemia, and cardiovascular effects).
- Evaluate the effectiveness of the teaching plan (patient can name the drug, dosage, possible adverse effects to watch for, and specific measures to help avoid adverse effects). (Refer to Nursing Care Guide: Antineoplastic Agents.)

MISCELLANEOUS ANTINEOPLASTIC AGENTS

Many other agents that do not fit into one of the previously discussed groups are used as antineoplastics to cause cell death. These drugs are used for treating a wide variety of cancers. The table on pages 190–192 lists the unclassified antineoplastic drugs, their indications, and anticipated adverse effects. Specific information about each drug may be obtained in your nursing drug guide. (See Figure 14–3 for sites of action of the miscellaneous antineoplastic agents.)

DRUGS IN FOCUS
Miscellaneous Antineoplastics

Drug Name	Dosage/Route	Usual Indications
altretamine (*Hexalen*)	260 mg/m² per day PO for 14–21 d in a 28-d cycle	Single agent used in the palliative treatment of persistent or recurrent ovarian cancer **Actions:** Cytotoxic; mechanism of action unknown **Special considerations:** Severe bone marrow depression and peripheral sensory neuropathy as well as severe GI toxicity can limit the use of this drug; a 14-d rest may alleviate the side effects sufficiently to allow redosing
asparaginase (*Elspar*)	1000–6000 U/m² IM or IV and specific days as part of a specific combination regimen	As part of combination therapy to induce remission in children with acute lymphocytic leukemia **Actions:** An enzyme that hydrolyzes the amino acid asparagine, which is needed by malignant cells for protein synthesis; inhibits cell proliferation; most effective in G_1 phase of the cell cycle **Special considerations:** Can cause severe bone marrow depression, renal toxicity, and fatal hyperthermia; hypersensitivity reactions to this drug are common, and patients should be tested and desensitized, if necessary, before using the drug
dacarbazine (*DTIC-Dome*)	2–4.5 mg/kg per day IV for 10 d, repeat at 4-wk intervals; *or* 150–250 mg/m² per day IV for 5 d in combination with other drugs	Treatment of metastatic malignant melanoma and as second-line therapy in combination with other drugs for the treatment of Hodgkin's disease **Actions:** Inhibits DNA and RNA synthesis, causing cell death; cell-cycle nonspecific **Special considerations:** Bone marrow depression, GI toxicity and severe photosensitivity are common effects; extravasation can cause tissue necrosis or cellulitis—use extreme care and monitor injection sites regularly
gemcitabine (*Gemzar*)	1000 mg/m² IV over 30 min, once a week for 7 wk	First-line treatment of locally advanced or metastatic adenocarcinoma of the pancreas in patients who have received fluorouracil (5-FU) **Actions:** S-phase cell-cycle specific; causes cell death by disrupting DNA and RNA synthesis **Special considerations:** Can cause severe bone marrow depression, GI toxicity, pain, and alopecia
hydroxyurea (*Hydrea*)	20–30 mg/kg PO q.d.	Inhibits enzymes essential for the synthesis of DNA, causing cell death **Actions:** Treatment of melanoma, ovarian cancer, chronic myelocytic leukemia; in combination therapy for primary squamous cell cancers of the head and neck; also used in the treatment of sickle cell anemia **Special considerations:** Can cause bone marrow depression, headache, rash, GI toxicity, and renal dysfunction; encourage patient to drink 10–12 glasses of water each day while taking this drug

DRUGS IN FOCUS (CONTINUED)
Miscellaneous Antineoplastics

Drug Name	Dosage/Route	Usual Indications
irinotecan (*Camptosar*)	125 mg/m^2 IV over 90 min, once a week for 4 wk, followed by a 2-wk rest; repeat every 6 wk	Treatment of metastatic colon or rectal cancer after treatment with 5-FU **Actions:** Disrupts DNA strands during DNA synthesis, causing cell death **Special considerations:** Can cause severe bone marrow depression, which regulates dose of the drug; causes GI toxicity, dyspnea, and alopecia
mitotane (*Lysodren*)	2–6 mg PO in divided doses t.i.d. to q.i.d. to a maximum of 9–10 g/d	Treatment of inoperable adrenocortical carcinoma **Actions:** Cytotoxic to corticosteroid-forming cells of the adrenal gland **Special considerations:** Can cause GI toxicity, CNS toxicity with vision and behavioral changes, adrenal insufficiency; monitor for adrenal insufficiency and arrange for replacement therapy as indicated
pegasparagase (*Oncaspar*)	2500 IU/m^2 IM or IV q14 d	Treatment of acute lymphocytic leukemia in patients who are hypersensitive to asparaginase **Actions:** An enzyme that hydrolyzes the amino acid asparagine, which is needed by malignant cells for protein synthesis; inhibits cell proliferation; most effective in G$_1$ phase of the cell cycle **Special considerations:** Can cause potentially fatal hyperthermia, bone marrow depression, renal toxicity, and pancreatitis, monitor patient regularly, and arrange decreased dosage as appropriate if toxic effects occur
porfimer (*Photofrin*)	2 mg/kg IV over 3–5 min; may repeat in 40–50 h and again in 96–120 h	Photosensitizing agent that is used with laser light to decrease tumor size in patients with obstructive esophageal cancers not responsive to laser treatment alone **Special considerations:** Has been associated with pleural effusion and fistula; associated with GI and cardiac toxicity; must given in conjunction with scheduled laser treatment, with at least 30 d between treatments; protect patient from exposure to light with protective clothing for 30 d after treatment (sunscreens are not effective); avoid direct contact with the drug—protective clothing and goggles are suggested
procarbazine (*Matulane*)	Adult: 2–6 mg/kg per day PO; base the dose on bone marrow response Pediatric: 50 mg/m^2 per day, adjust based on bone marrow response	Used in combination therapy for treatment of stage III and IV Hodgkin's disease **Actions:** Inhibits DNA, RNA, and protein synthesis, leading to cell death **Special considerations:** Bone marrow toxicity; GI toxicity and skin lesions also limit use in some patients; severity of adverse effects regulates the dose of the drug
topotecan (*Hycamtin*)	1.5 mg/m^2 per day IV for 5 d; as part of a 2 d course; minimum of 4 courses	Treatment of patients with metastatic ovarian cancer after failure of other agents **Actions:** Damages DNA strand, causing cell death during cell division **Special considerations:** Can cause severe bone marrow depression, which regulates the dose of the drug; total alopecia, GI toxicity, and CNS effects may also limit the use of the drug; analgesics may be helpful

Drugs in Focus continues on page 192

DRUGS IN FOCUS (CONTINUED)
Miscellaneous Antineoplastics

Drug Name	Dosage/Route	Usual Indications
tretinoin (*Vesanoid*)	45 mg/m^2 per day PO for 30 d	Used to induce remission in acute promyelocytic leukemia (APL); can cause severe respiratory and cardiac toxicity, including myocardial infarction and cardiac arrest **Actions:** Promotes cell differentiation and the repopulation of the bone marrow with normal cells in patients with APL **Special considerations:** GI toxicity, pseudotumor cerebri (papilledema, headache, nausea, vomiting, visual changes), skin rash, and fragility may limit use in some patients; discontinue drug at first sign of toxic effects; use for induction of remission only—then other chemotherapeutic agents should be used

CHAPTER SUMMARY

- Cancers arise from a single abnormal cell that multiplies and grows.
- Cancers can manifest as diseases of the blood and lymph tissue or as growth of tumors arising from epithelial cells (carcinomas) or from mesenchymal cells and connective tissue (sarcomas).
- Cancer cells lose their normal function (anaplasia), develop characteristics that allow them to grow in an uninhibited way (autonomy), and have the ability to travel to other sites in the body that are conducive to their growth (metastasis).
- Antineoplastic drugs affect both normal cells and cancer cells by disrupting cell function and division at various points in the cell cycle.
- Cancer drugs are usually most effective against cells that multiply rapidly (ie, proceed through the cell cycle quickly). These cells include most neoplasms, bone marrow cells, cells in the GI tract, and cells in the skin or hair follicles.
- The goal of cancer chemotherapy is to decrease the size of the neoplasm so that the human immune system can deal with it.
- Antineoplastic drugs are often given in combination so that they can affect cells in various stages of the cell cycle, including cells that are emerging from rest or moving to a phase of the cycle that is disrupted by these drugs.
- Adverse effects associated with antineoplastic therapy include effects caused by damage to the rapidly multiplying cells, such as bone marrow suppression, which may limit the drug use; GI toxicity, with nausea, vomiting, mouth sores, and diarrhea; and alopecia, or hair loss.
- Chemotherapeutic agents should not be used during pregnancy or lactation because they may result in potentially serious adverse effects on the rapidly multiplying cells of the neonate.

CULTURAL CONSIDERATIONS
Alternative Therapies and Cancer

The diagnosis of cancer and the sometimes devastating effects of cancer treatment often drive patients to seek out alternative therapies, either as adjuncts to traditional cancer therapy or sometimes instead of traditional therapy. Because Asian-Americans and Pacific islanders often see drug therapy and other cancer therapies as part of the yin/yang belief system, they may turn to a variety of herbal therapies to balance their systems.

The nurse should be aware of some potential interactions that may occur when alternative therapies are used:

- *Echinacea*—may be hepatotoxic; increases the risk of hepatotoxicity when taken with antineoplastics that are hepatotoxic
- Ginkgo—inhibits blood clotting, which can cause problems after surgery or with bleeding neoplasms
- *Saw palmetto*—may increase the effects of various estrogen hormones and hormone modulators; advise patients taking such drugs to avoid this herb
- St. John's wort—can greatly increase photosensitivity, which can cause problems with patients who have received radiation therapy or are taking drugs that cause other dermatological effects

If a patient has an unexpected reaction to a drug being used, ask about the use of alternative therapies. Many of these agents are untested, and interactions and adverse effects are not well documented.

Review Questions

1. Many properties of neoplastic cells are different than those of normal cells, with the exception of

a. anaplasia.
b. metastasis.
c. miosis.
d. autonomy.

2. Carcinomas are tumors that
   a. originate in the mesenchyma and are made up of embryonic connective tissue cells.
   b. originate in the bone marrow and affect the blood.
   c. originate in the striated muscle.
   d. originate in epithelial cells.

3. The goal of traditional antineoplastic drug therapy is to
   a. reduce the size of the mass of abnormal cells so that the immune system can take care of destroying them.
   b. eradicate all of the abnormal cells that have developed.
   c. destroy all cells of the originating type.
   d. stimulate the immune system to destroy the neoplastic cells.

4. Cancer can be a difficult disease to treat because
   a. cells no longer progress through the normal cell cycle.
   b. cells can develop resistance to drug therapy.
   c. cells can remain in the dormant state for long periods and emerge months to years later.
   d. the exact cause of cancer is not known.

5. Antineoplastic drugs destroy human cells. They are most likely to cause cell death among healthy cells that
   a. have poor cell membranes.
   b. are rapidly turning over and progress through their cell cycle rapidly.
   c. are in dormant tissues.
   d. are across the blood–brain barrier.

6. Cancer treatment usually occurs in several different treatment phases. A common determinant of the appropriateness of another round of chemotherapy is
   a. hair loss.
   b. bone marrow function.
   c. anorexia.
   d. heart rate.

7. Patient teaching can be very important in helping the patient receiving cancer chemotherapy and should stress all of the following except
   a. the importance of keeping the head covered at extremes of temperature.
   b. the need to use barrier contraceptives because of the risk of serious fetal effects.
   c. avoiding exposure to infection or to injury because the ability to heal or to fight infection is impaired.
   d. the importance of avoiding food if nausea or vomiting is a problem.

8. Chemotherapeutic agents should not be used during pregnancy
   a. because the tendency to cause nausea and vomiting will be increased.
   b. because of potentially serious adverse effects on the rapidly multiplying cells of the fetus.
   c. because bone marrow toxicity could alter hormone levels.
   d. because patients may be weakened by the drug regimen.

9. Hair loss, or alopecia, is an adverse effect of many antineoplastic agents. Patient teaching points would not include
   a. warnings that this will occur.
   b. encouraging the patient to arrange for appropriate head covering at extremes of temperature.
   c. advising the patient to lie with the legs elevated and head low to promote circulation and prevent hair loss.
   d. encouragement to arrange for a wig or other head covering before the hair loss occurs.

10. Most cancer drugs are most effective against
    a. slowly growing cells.
    b. cells in the dormant phase of the cell cycle.
    c. cells that multiply rapidly and go through the cell cycle quickly.
    d. cells that have moved from their normal site in the body.

BIBLIOGRAPHY

Bullock, B. L. (2000). *Focus on pathophysiology*. Philadelphia: Lippincott Williams & Wilkins.

Gilman, A., Hardman, J. G., & Limbird, L. E. (Eds.) (2002). *Goodman and Gilman's the pharmacological basis of therapeutics* (10th ed.). New York: McGraw-Hill.

Grochow, L. B., & Ames, M. M. (1998). *A clinician's guide to chemotherapy pharmacokinetics and pharmacodynamics*. Baltimore: Williams & Wilkins.

Karch, A. M. (2002). *2003 Lippincott's nursing drug guide*. Philadelphia: Lippincott Williams & Wilkins.

Drug facts and comparisons. (2002). St. Louis. Facts and Comparisons.

Navarro, T. M. (1998) Chemotherapy extravasation. *American Journal of Nursing, 98*(11), 38.

Professional's guide to patient drug facts. (2001). St. Louis: Facts and Comparisons.

PART

III

Drugs Acting on
the Immune
System

Introduction to the Immune Response and Inflammation

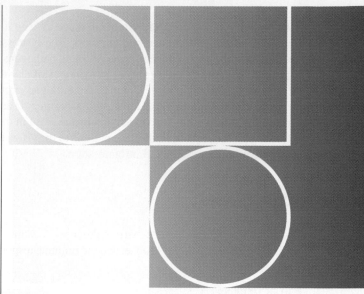

197

The body has many defense systems in place to keep it intact and to protect it from external stressors. These stressors can include bacteria, viruses, other foreign pathogens or nonself-cells, trauma, and exposure to extremes of environmental conditions. The same defense systems that protect the body also help to repair it after cellular trauma or damage. Understanding the basic mechanisms involved in these defense systems helps to explain the actions of the drugs that affect the immune system and inflammation.

BODY DEFENSES

The body's defenses include barrier defenses, cellular defenses, the inflammatory response, and the immune response.

Barrier Defenses

Certain anatomical barriers exist to prevent the entry of foreign pathogens and to serve as important lines of defense in protecting the body.

Skin

The skin is the first line of defense. The skin acts as a physical barrier to protect the internal tissues and organs of the body. Glands in the skin secrete chemicals that destroy or repel many pathogens. The skin sloughs off daily, making it difficult for any pathogen to colonize on the skin. Finally, an array of normal flora bacteria live on the skin and destroy many disease-causing pathogens.

Mucous Membranes

Mucous membranes line the areas of the body that are exposed to external influences but do not have the benefit of skin protection. These body areas include the respiratory tract, which is exposed to air; the gastrointestinal (GI) tract, which is exposed to anything ingested by mouth; and the genitourinary (GU) tract, which is exposed to many pathogens from the rectal area. Like the skin, the mucous membrane is a physical barrier to invasion. It also secretes a sticky mucus, which traps invaders and inactivates them for later destruction and removal by the body. The mucus works much like flypaper at trapping flies.

In the respiratory tract, the mucous membrane is lined with tiny, hair-like processes called *cilia*. The cilia sweep any captured pathogens or foreign materials upward toward the mouth, either to be swallowed or to cause irritation to the area and be removed by a cough or a sneeze.

In the GI tract, the mucous membrane serves as a protective coating, preventing erosion of GI cells by the acidic environment of the stomach, the digestive enzymes of the small intestine, and the waste products that accumulate in the large intestine. The mucous membrane also secretes mucus that serves as a lubricant throughout the GI tract to facilitate movement of the food bolus and of waste products.

In the GU tract, the mucous membrane provides direct protection against injury and trauma and traps any pathogens in the area for destruction by the body.

Gastric Acid

The stomach secretes acid in response to many stimuli. The acidity of the stomach not only aids digestion but also destroys many would-be pathogens that are either ingested or swallowed after removal from the respiratory tract.

Major Histocompatibility Complex

The body's last barrier defense is the ability to distinguish between self-cells and foreign cells. All of the cells and tissues of each person are marked for identification as part of that individual's genetic code. No two people have exactly the same code. In humans, the genetic identification code is carried on a chromosome and is called the major histocompatibility complex (MHC). The MHC produces several proteins called histocompatibility antigens, or human leukocyte antigens (HLAs), that are found on the cell membrane and allow the body to recognize cells as being self-cells. Cells that do not have these proteins are identified as foreign and are destroyed by the body.

Cellular Defenses

Any foreign pathogen that manages to get past the barrier defenses will encounter the human immune system, or mononuclear phagocyte system (MPS). Previously called the reticuloendothelial system, the MPS is composed of the thymus gland, the lymphatic tissue, leukocytes, lymphocytes, and numerous chemical mediators.

Myelocytes

Stem cells in the bone marrow produce two types of white blood cells or **leukocytes:** lymphocytes and myelocytes. The **lymphocytes** are the key components of the immune system and consist of T cells, B cells, and natural killer cells (see later discussion of the immune response). The myelocytes can develop into a number of different cell types that are important in both the basic inflammatory response and the immune response. Myelocytes include neutrophils, basophils, eosinophils, and monocytes or macrophages (Figure 15–1).

Neutrophils

Neutrophils are polymorphonuclear leukocytes that are capable of diapedesis (moving outside of the bloodstream) and **phagocytosis** (engulfing and digesting foreign material). When the body is injured or invaded by a pathogen, neutrophils are rapidly produced and move to the site of the insult to attack the foreign substance. Because neutrophils are able to engulf and digest foreign material, they are called **phagocytes.** Phagocytes are able to identify nonself-cells by use of the MHC, and they can engulf these cells or mark them for destruction by cytotoxic T cells.

Basophils

Basophils are myelocytic leukocytes that are not capable of phagocytosis. They are full of chemical substances that are im-

FIGURE 15-1. Types of white blood cells, or leukocytes, produced by the body.

FIGURE 15-2. Appearance of various types of leukocytes. (Bullock, B. L. [2000]. *Focus on pathophysiology.* Philadelphia: Lippincott Williams & Wilkins.)

portant for initiating and maintaining an immune or inflammatory response. These substances include histamine, heparin, and other chemicals used in the inflammatory response.

Eosinophils

Eosinophils are circulating myelocytic leukocytes whose exact function is not understood. They are often found at the site of allergic reactions and may be responsible for removing the proteins and active components of the immune reaction from the site of an allergic response.

Monocytes/Macrophages

Monocytes or mononuclear phagocytes are also called **macrophages.** They are mature leukocytes that are capable of phagocytizing an **antigen** (foreign protein). They also can process antigens and present them to active lymphocytes for destruction. Macrophages can be circulating phagocytes, or they can be fixed in specific tissues, such as the Kupffer cells in the liver, the cells in the alveoli of the respiratory tract, and the microglia in the central nervous system (CNS), GI, circulatory, and lymph tissues. These cells are active phagocytes and can release chemicals that are necessary to elicit a strong inflammatory reaction. Macrophages help remove foreign material from the body, including pathogens, debris from dead cells, and necrotic tissue from injury sites, so that the body can heal. These cells respond to chemical mediators (released by other cells that are active in the inflammatory and immune responses) to increase the intensity of a response and to facilitate the body's reaction (Figure 15-2).

Mast Cells

Mast cells are fixed basophils that do not circulate; they are found in the respiratory and GI tracts and in the skin. They release many of the chemical mediators of the inflammatory and immune responses when they are stimulated by local irritation.

Tissue and Gland Connections

Lymphoid tissues that play an important part in the cellular defense system include the following: lymph nodes, spleen, thymus gland (a bipolar gland located in the middle of the chest, which becomes smaller with age), bone marrow, and lymphoid tissue throughout the respiratory and GI tracts. The bone marrow and the thymus gland are important for creation of the cellular components of the MPS and also have a role in their differentiation and regulation. The lymph nodes and lymphoid tissue store concentrated populations of leukocytes and lymphocytes in positions that facilitate their surveillance for and destruction of foreign proteins. Other cells travel through the cardiovascular and lymph systems to search for foreign proteins or to reach the sites of injury or pathogen invasion.

The Inflammatory Response

The inflammatory response is the local reaction of the body to invasion or injury. Any insult to the body that injures cells or tissues sets into action a series of events and chemical reactions.

Cell injury causes the activation of a chemical in the plasma called factor XII or **Hageman factor.** Hageman factor is responsible for activating at least three systems in the body: the **kinin system,** which is discussed here; the clotting cascade, which starts blood clotting; and the plasminogen system, which starts the dissolution of blood clots. The last two systems are discussed in Part VII of this book, Drugs Acting on the Cardiovascular System.

Hageman factor activates kallikrein, a substance found in the local tissues, which causes the precursor substance kininogen to be converted to bradykinin and other kinins. Bradykinin was the first kinin identified and remains the one that is best understood. Bradykinin causes local vasodilation to bring more blood to the injured area and to allow white blood cells to escape into the tissues. It also stimulates nerve endings to cause pain, which alerts the body to the injury.

Bradykinin also causes the release of **arachidonic acid** from the cell membrane. Arachidonic acid is known to cause the release of other substances called *autocoids.* These substances act like local hormones—they are released from cells, cause an effect in the immediate area, and then are broken down. These autocoids include the following:

- Prostaglandins, some of which augment the inflammatory reaction and some of which block it
- Leukotrienes, some of which can cause vasodilation and increased capillary permeability and some of which can block the reactions
- Thromboxanes, which cause local vasoconstriction and facilitate platelet aggregation and blood coagulation

While this series of Hageman factor–initiated events is proceeding, another locally mediated response is occurring. Injury to a cell membrane causes the local release of histamine. Histamine causes vasodilation, which brings more blood and blood components to the area; changes capillary permeability, making it easier for neutrophils and blood chemicals to leave the bloodstream and enter the injured area; and stimulates pain perception. These activities bring neutrophils to the area to engulf and get rid of the invader, or to remove the cell that has been injured.

Some leukotrienes activated by arachidonic acid have a property called **chemotaxis.** Chemotaxis is the ability to attract neutrophils and to stimulate them and other macrophages in the area to be very aggressive. As the neutrophils become active and other chemicals are released into the area, they can injure or destroy local cells. The destruction of a cell results in the release of various lysosomal enzymes from the cell. These enzymes lyse or destroy cell membranes and cellular proteins. They are an important part of biological recycling and the breakdown of once-living tissues after death. In the case of an inflammatory reaction, they can cause local cellular breakdown and further inflammation, which can develop into a vicious cycle leading to cell death.

Many inflammatory diseases, such as rheumatoid arthritis and systemic lupus erythematosus, are examples of these uncontrolled cycles. The prostaglandins and leukotrienes are important to the inflammatory response because they act to moderate the reaction, thus preventing this destructive cycle from happening on a regular basis. Many of the drugs used to affect the inflammatory and immune systems modify or interfere with these inflammatory reactions.

Clinical Presentation

Activation of the inflammatory response produces a characteristic clinical picture. The Latin words **calor** (heat), **tumor** (swelling), **rubor** (redness), and **dolor** (pain) describe a typical inflammatory reaction. Calor, or heat, occurs because of the increased blood flow to the area. Tumor, or swelling, occurs because of the fluid that leaks into the tissues as a result of the change in capillary permeability. Rubor, or redness, is related again to the increase in blood flow caused by the vasodilation. Dolor, or pain, comes from the activation of pain fibers by histamine and the kinin system. These signs and symptoms occur anytime a cell is injured (Figure 15–3).

For example, if you scratch the top of your hand and wait for about a minute, the direct line of the scratch will be red

(rubor) and raised (tumor). If you feel it gently, it will be warmer than the surrounding area (calor). You should also experience a burning sensation or discomfort at the site of the scratch (dolor). Invasion of the lungs by bacteria can produce pneumonia. If the lungs could be examined closely, they would also show the signs and symptoms of inflammation. They would be very red from increased blood flow; fluid would start to leak out of the capillaries (often this can be heard as rales); the patient would complain of chest discomfort; and the increased blood flow to the area of infection would make it appear hot or very active on a scan. No matter what the cause of the insult, the body's local response is the same.

Once the inflammatory response is underway and neutrophils become active, engulfing and digesting injured cells or the invader, they release a chemical that is a natural **pyrogen,** or fever-causing substance. This pyrogen resets specific neurons in the hypothalamus to maintain a higher body temperature, seen clinically as a fever. The higher temperature acts as a catalyst to many of the body's chemical reactions, making the inflammatory and immune responses more effective. Treating fevers remains a controversial subject, because lowering a fever decreases the efficiency of the immune and inflammatory responses.

The leukotrienes (activated through the kinin system) affect the brain to induce slow-wave sleep, which is thought to be important for saving energy to fight the invader. They also cause myalgia and arthralgia (muscle and joint pain)—common signs and symptoms of various inflammatory diseases—which also cause reduced activity and save energy. All of these chemical responses make up the total clinical picture of an inflammatory reaction.

The Immune Response

More specific invasion can stimulate a more specific response through the immune system. The lymphocytes produced in the bone marrow by the stem cells can develop into T lymphocytes (so named because they migrate from the bone marrow to the thymus gland for activation and maturation) or B lymphocytes (so named because they are activated in the bursa of Fabricius in the chicken, although the specific point of activation in humans has not been identified). Other identified lymphocytes include natural killer cells and lymphokine-activated killer cells. These cells are aggressive against neoplastic or cancer cells and promote rapid cellular death. They do not seem to be programmed for specific identification of cells. Research in the area of lymphocyte identification is relatively new and continues to grow. There may be other lymphocytes with particular roles in the immune response that have not yet been identified.

T Cells

T cells are programmed in the thymus gland and provide what is called cell-mediated immunity (Figure 15–4). T cells develop into at least three different cell types.

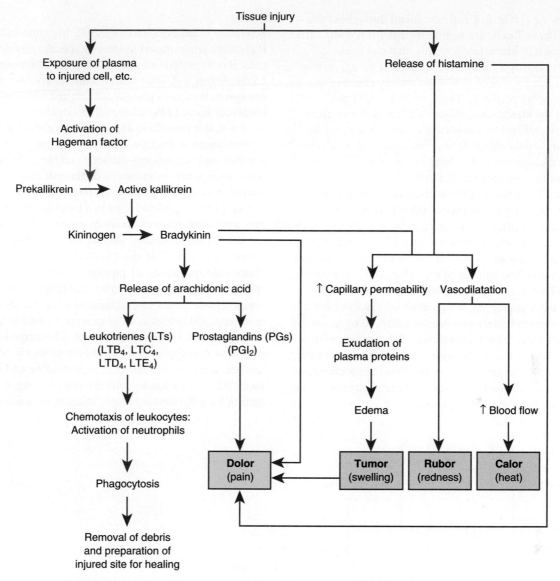

FIGURE 15–3. The inflammatory response in relation to the four cardinal signs of inflammation.

FIGURE 15–4. The cell-mediated immune response. Activation of a T cell by a "nonself—cell" results in responses that destroy the foreign cell.

1. *Effector or cytotoxic T cells* are found throughout the body. These T cells are aggressive against nonself-cells, releasing cytokines, or chemicals, that can either directly destroy a foreign cell or mark it for aggressive destruction by phagocytes in the area by eliciting an inflammatory response. These nonself-cells have membrane identifying antigens that are different from those established by the person's MHC. They may be the body's own cells that have been invaded by a virus, which changes the cell membrane; neoplastic cancer cells; or transplanted foreign cells.

2. *Helper T cells* respond to the chemical indicators of immune activity and stimulate other lymphocytes, including B cells, to be more aggressive and responsive.

3. *Suppressor T cells* respond to rising levels of chemicals associated with an immune response to suppress or slow the reaction. The balance of the helper and suppressor T cells allows for a rapid response to body injury or invasion by pathogens, which may destroy foreign antigens immediately and then be followed by a slowing reaction if the invasion continues. This slowing allows the body to conserve energy and the components of the immune and inflammatory reaction that are needed for basic protection and to prevent cellular destruction from a continued inflammatory reaction.

B Cells

B cells are found throughout the MPS in groups called clones. B cells are programmed to identify specific proteins, or antigens. B cells provide what is called *humoral immunity* (Figure 15–5). When a B cell reacts with its specific antigen, it changes to become a plasma cell. Plasma cells produce **antibodies,** or immunoglobulins, which circulate in the body and react with this specific antigen when it is encountered. This is a direct chemical reaction. When the antigen and antibody react, they form an antigen–antibody complex. This new structure reveals a new receptor site on the antibody that activates a series of plasma proteins in the body called **complement.**

Complement proteins react in a cascade fashion to form a ring around the antigen–antibody complex. The complement can destroy the antigen by altering the membrane to allow an osmotic inflow of fluid that bursts the cell. They also induce chemotaxis (attraction of phagocytic cells to the area), increase the activity of phagocytes, and release histamine. Histamine release causes vasodilation, which increases blood flow to the area and brings in all of the components of the inflammatory reaction to destroy the antigen. The antigen–antibody–complement complex precipitates out of the circulatory system and deposits in various sites, including end arteries in joints, the eye, the kidney, and the skin. The signs and symptoms of the inflammatory response can be seen where the anti-

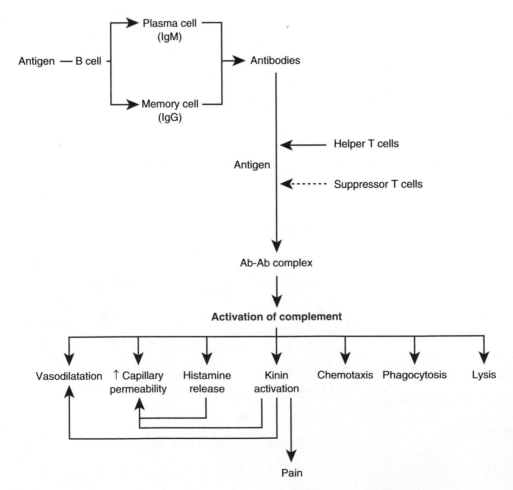

FIGURE 15–5. The humoral immune response.

gen–antibody complexes are deposited. Chicken pox eruptions are an example of an antigen–antibody–complement complex that deposits in the skin and causes a local inflammatory reaction.

The initial formation of antibodies, or primary response, takes several days. Once activated, the B cells form memory cells that will produce antibodies for immediate release in the future if the antigen is encountered. The antibodies are released in the form of immunoglobulins. Five different types of immunoglobulins have been identified. The first one that is released is called immunoglobulin M (IgM), and it contains the antibodies produced at the first exposure to the antigen. IgG, another form of immunoglobulin, contains antibodies made by the memory cells that circulate and enter the tissue; most of the immunoglobulin found in the serum is IgG. IgA is found in tears, saliva, sweat, mucus, and bile. It is secreted by plasma cells in the GI and respiratory tracts and in epithelial cells. These antibodies react with specific pathogens that are encountered in exposed areas of the body. IgE is present in small amounts and seems to be related to allergic responses and to the activation of mast cells. IgD is another identified immunoglobulin whose role has not been determined.

This process of antibody formation, called *acquired* or *active immunity,* is a lifelong reaction. For example, a person exposed to chicken pox will have a mild respiratory reaction when the virus (varicella) first enters the respiratory tract. There will then be a 2- to 3-week incubation period as the body is forming IgM antibodies and preparing to attack any chicken pox virus that appears. The chicken pox virus enters a cell and multiplies. The cell eventually ruptures and ejects more viruses into the system. When this happens, the body is ready to respond with the immediate release of antibodies and a full-scale antigen–antibody response is seen throughout the body. Fever, myalgia, arthralgia, and skin lesions are all part of the immune response to the virus. Once all of the invading chicken pox viruses have been destroyed, or have entered the CNS to safely hibernate away from the antibodies, the clinical signs and symptoms resolve. (Varicella can enter the CNS and stay dormant for many years. The antibodies are not able to cross into the CNS, and the virus remains unaffected while it stays there.)

The B memory cells will continue to make a supply of immunoglobulin, IgG, for use with any future exposure to the chicken pox virus. That exposure usually does not evolve into a clinical case because the viruses are destroyed immediately on entering the body and do not have a chance to multiply. Older patients with weakened immune systems, people who are immunosuppressed, and individuals who have depleted their immune system fighting an infection are at risk for development of shingles if they had chicken pox earlier in their lives. The dormant virus, which has aged and changed somewhat, is able to leave the CNS along a nerve root because the immunosuppressed body is slow to respond. The antibodies do eventually respond to the varicella, and the signs and symptoms of shingles occur as the virus is attacked along the nerve root. Figure 15–6 outlines this entire process.

B clones cluster in areas where they are most likely to encounter the specific antigen that they have been programmed to recognize. For example, pathogens or antigens that are introduced into the body via the respiratory tract will meet up with the B cells in the tonsils and upper respiratory tract; antigens that enter the body through the GI tract will meet their B cells situated in the esophagus and GI tract. Theorists believe that the B cells are programmed genetically and are formed by the time of birth. Clones of B cells contain similar cells. The introduction of an antigen to which there are no preprogrammed B cells could result in widespread disease, because the body would have no way of responding. A big concern of space travel has always been the introduction of a completely new antigen to the earth; for this reason, long periods of decontamination have been used after rocks or debris are brought back to earth. Germ warfare research is ongoing in some countries to develop an antigen that has not been seen before and to which people would have no response.

Other Mediators

Several other factors also play an important role in the immune reaction. **Interferons** are chemicals that are secreted by cells that have been invaded by viruses and possibly by other stimuli. The interferons prevent viral replication and also suppress malignant cell replication and tumor growth.

Interleukins are chemicals secreted by active leukocytes to influence other leukocytes. Interleukin 1 (IL-1) stimulates T and B cells to initiate an immune response. IL-2 is released from active T cells to stimulate production of more T cells and to increase the activity of B cells, cytotoxic cells, and natural killer cells. Interleukins also cause fever, arthralgia, myalgia, and slow-wave sleep induction—all things that help the body to conserve energy for use in fighting off the invader. Several other factors released by lymphocytes and basophils have been identified. These include interleukins such as B-cell growth factor, macrophage-activating factor, macrophage-inhibiting factor, platelet-activating factor, eosinophil chemotactic factor, and neutrophil chemotactic factor. The thymus gland also releases a number of hormones that aid in the maturation of T cells and that circulate in the body to stimulate and communicate with T cells. Thymosin, a thymus hormone that has been replicated, is important in the maturation of T cells and cell-mediated immunity. Research is ongoing on the use of thymosin in certain leukemias and melanomas to stimulate the immune response.

Tumor necrosis factor (TNF), a cytokine, is a chemical released by macrophages that inhibits tumor growth and can actually cause tumor regression. It also works with other chemicals to make the inflammatory and immune responses more aggressive and efficient. Research is ongoing to determine the therapeutic effectiveness of TNF. TNF receptor sites are now available for injection into patients with acute rheumatoid arthritis. These receptor sites react with TNF released by the macrophages in this inflammatory disease. All of these chemicals act as communication factors within the immune system, allowing the coordination of the immune response.

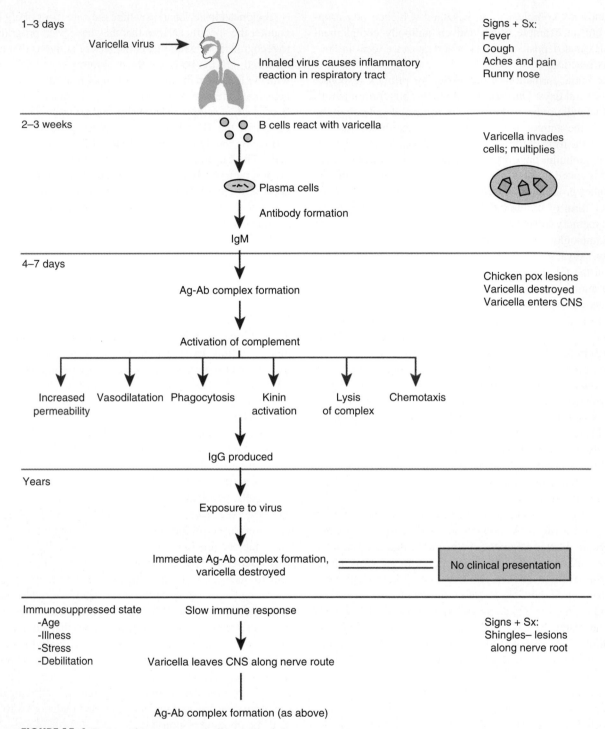

FIGURE 15-6. Process of response to varicella exposure in humans.

Interrelationship of the Immune and Inflammatory Responses

The immune and inflammatory responses work together to protect the body and to maintain a level of homeostasis within the body. Helper T cells stimulate the activity of B cells and effector T cells. Suppressor T cells monitor the chemical activity in the body and act to suppress B-cell and T-cell activity when the foreign antigen is under control. Both B cells and T cells ultimately depend on an effective in-

flammatory reaction to achieve the end goal of destruction of the foreign protein or cell (Figure 15–7).

PATHOPHYSIOLOGY INVOLVING THE IMMUNE SYSTEM

Several conditions can arise that cause problems involving the immune system. These conditions, many of which are treated by drugs that stimulate or suppress the immune sys-

FIGURE 15–7. Interrelationship of immune and inflammatory reactions.

tem, include neoplasm, viral invasion, autoimmune disease, and transplant rejection.

Neoplasms

Neoplasms occur when mutant cells escape the normal surveillance of the immune system and begin to grow and multiply. This can happen in many ways. For example, aging causes a decreased efficiency of the immune system, allowing some cells to escape. Location of the mutant cells can present a problem for getting lymphocytes to an area to respond. Mutant cells in breast tissue, for example, are not well perfused with blood and may escape detection until they are quite abundant. "Sneaking through" of a cell can occur. Sometimes cells are able to avoid detection by the T cells until the growing mass of cells is so large that the immune system cannot deal with it. Tumors can produce blocking antibodies that cover the antigen receptor sites on the tumor and prevent recognition by cytotoxic T cells. A weakly antigenic tumor may develop; such a tumor elicits a mild response from the immune system and somehow tricks the T cells into allowing it to survive.

Viral Invasion of Cells

Viruses are parasites that can survive only by invading a host cell that provides the nourishment necessary for viral repli-

cation. Invasion of a cell alters the cell membrane and the antigenic presentation of the cell (the MHC). This change can activate cellular immunity, or it can be so subtle that the immune system's response to the cell is mild or absent. In some cases the response activates a cellular immune reaction to normal cells similar to the one that was invaded. This is one theory for the development of autoimmune disease.

Autoimmune Disease

Autoimmune disease occurs when the body responds to specific self-antigens to produce antibodies or cell-mediated immune responses against its own cells. The actual cause of autoimmune disease is not known, but theories speculate that (1) it could be a result of response to a cell that was invaded by a virus, leading to antibody production to similar cells; (2) production of autoantibodies is a normal process that goes on all the time, and in a state of immunosuppression the suppressor T cells do not suppress autoantibody production; or (3) there is a genetic predisposition to develop autoantibodies.

Transplant Rejection

With the growing field of organ transplantation, more is being learned about the reaction to foreign cells that are introduced into the body. Effort is always made to match a donor's HLA molecules as closely as possible to those of the recipient for histocompatibility. The more closely the foreign cells can be matched, the less aggressive will be the immune reaction to the donated tissue. Self-transplantation, or autotransplantation, results in no immune response. All other transplants produce an immune reaction. The effector T cells are activated by the presence of the foreign cells, and cytokines are released to stimulate an immune and inflammatory reaction and to destroy the foreign cells.

◻◼●◼ WEB LINKS

Health care providers and patients may want to consult the following Internet sources:

Detailed review of the immune system:
  http://www.keratin.com/am/amindex.shtml
Fun travel through the virtual immune system:
  http://www.thebody.com/step/immune.html

CHAPTER SUMMARY

- The body has several defense mechanisms in place to protect it from injury or foreign invasion: the skin, mucous membranes, normal flora, gastric acid, and the inflammatory and immune responses.
- The inflammatory response is a general response to any cell injury.
- The inflammatory response involves activation of Hageman factor to stimulate the kinin system and release of histamine from injured cells to generate local inflammatory responses.
- The response to the inflammatory stimuli involves local vasodilation, increased capillary permeability, and the stimulation of pain fibers. These reactions alert the person to the injury and bring an increased blood flow to the area.
- The clinical presentation of an inflammatory reaction is heat, redness, swelling, and pain (ie, calor, rubor, tumor, and dolor).
- The immune response provides a specific reaction to foreign cells or proteins.
- Several types of T cells exist: effector or cytotoxic T cells, helper T cells, and suppressor T cells. Effector or cytotoxic T cells immediately destroy foreign cells. Helper T cells stimulate the immune and inflammatory reactions. Suppressor T cells dampen the immune and inflammatory responses to conserve energy and prevent cellular damage.
- B cells are programmed to recognize specific proteins or foreign antigens. Once in contact with that protein, the B cell produces antibodies (immunoglobulins) that react directly with the protein.
- Reaction of an antibody with the specific receptor site on the protein activates the complement cascade of proteins and lyses the associated protein or precipitates an aggressive inflammatory reaction around it.
- Other chemicals are involved in communication among

parts of the immune system and in local response to invasion. Any of these chemicals has the potential to alter the immune response.
- The T cells, B cells, and inflammatory reaction work together to protect the body from invasion, limit the response to that invasion, and return the body to a state of homeostasis.
- Patient problems that occur within the immune system include the development of neoplasms, viral invasions of cells that trigger immune responses, autoimmune diseases, and rejections of transplanted organs.

Review Questions

1. Antibodies
   a. are carbohydrates.
   b. are secreted by activated T cells.
   c. are not found in circulating gamma globulins.
   d. are effective only against specific antigens.
2. B and T cells are similar in that they both
   a. secrete antibodies.
   b. play important roles in the immune response.
   c. are activated in the thymus gland.
   d. release cytotoxins to destroy cells.
3. Which of the following is not a cytokine?
   a. interleukin 2.
   b. antibody.
   c. tumor necrosis factor.
   d. interferon.
4. As part of the nonspecific defense against infection
   a. blood flow and vascular permeability to proteins increases throughout the circulatory system.
   b. particles in the respiratory tract are engulfed by phagocytes.
   c. B cells are released from the bone marrow.
   d. neutrophils release lysosomes, heparin and kininogen into the extracellular fluid.
5. B cells respond to an initial antigen challenge by
   a. reducing in size.
   b. immediately producing antigen-specific antibodies.
   c. producing a large number of cells that are unlike the original B cell.
   d. producing new cells that become plasma cells and memory cells.
6. All of the following statements about neutrophils are true, except
   a. they possess the property of phagocytosis.
   b. when activated they release a pyrogen that causes fever.
   c. when the body is injured, they are produced rapidly and in large numbers.
   d. they are not capable of movement outside the circulatory system.
7. The inflammatory response is activated whenever cell injury occurs. It involves all of the following except
   a. activation of Hageman factor.
   b. vasodilation in the area of the injury.

c. generalized edema and tumor development.

d. changes in capillary permeability to allow proteins to leak out of the capillaries.

8. Treating fevers remains a controversial subject because

a. fevers make people feel ill.

b. higher temperatures act as catalysts to many of the body's chemical reactions, so the inflammatory and immune responses are more effective.

c. higher temperatures can suppress the body's normal metabolism.

d. higher temperatures can alter the body's hormone levels, particularly progesterone.

9. T cells are programmed in the thymus gland and can become any of the following except

a. cytotoxic T cells.

b. helper T cells.

c. suppressor T cells.

d. antibody-secreting T cells.

10. Interleukins are

a. chemicals released when a virus enters a cell.

b. chemicals secreted by activated leukocytes to influence other leukocytes.

c. part of the kinin system.

d. activated by arachidonic acid.

BIBLIOGRAPHY

Bullock, B. L. (2000). *Focus on pathophysiology*. Philadelphia: Lippincott Williams & Wilkins.

Ganong, W. (1999). *Review of medical physiology* (18th ed.). Norwalk, CT: Appleton & Lange.

Guyton, A., & Hall, J. (1999). *Textbook of medical physiology*. Philadelphia: W. B. Saunders.

Gilman, A., Hardman, J. G., & Limbird, L. E. (Eds.) (2002). *Goodman and Gilman's the pharmacological basis of therapeutics* (10th ed.). New York: McGraw-Hill.

Karch, A. M. (2002). *2003 Lippincott's nursing drug guide*. Philadelphia: Lippincott Williams & Wilkins.

Peakman, M., & Vergani, D. (1997). *Basic and clinical immunology*. New York: Churchill-Livingstone.

Stites, D. P., Terr, A. I., & Parslow, T. G. (Eds.). (1997). *Medical immunology* (9th ed.). Stamford, CT: Appleton & Lange.

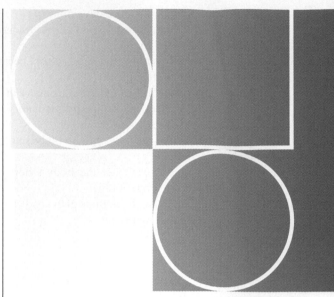

CHAPTER 16

Anti-inflammatory Agents

Key Terms

analgesic

anti-inflammatory

antipyretic

chrysotherapy

nonsteroidal anti-inflammatory drugs (NSAIDs)

salicylates

Salicylates

- Ⓟ aspirin
- balsalazide
- choline magnesium trisalicylate
- choline salicylate
- mesalamine
- olsalazine
- salsalate
- sodium thiosalicylate

Nonsteroidal Anti-inflammatory Drugs

- celecoxib
- diclofenac
- diflunisal
- etodolac

- fenoprofen
- flurbiprofen
- Ⓟ ibuprofen
- indomethacin
- ketoprofen
- ketorolac
- meclofenamate
- mefenamic acid
- nabumetone
- naproxen
- oxaprozin
- piroxicam
- rofecoxib
- sulindac

- tolmetin
- valdecoxib

Other Related Drugs

- Ⓟ acetaminophen
- anakinra
- auranofin
- Ⓟ aurothioglucose
- etanercept
- gold sodium thiomalate
- hylan G-F 20
- leflunomide
- penicillamine
- sodium hyaluronate

The inflammatory response is designed to protect the body from injury and pathogens. It employs a variety of potent chemical mediators to produce the reaction that helps to destroy pathogens and promote healing. As the body reacts to these chemicals, it produces some signs and symptoms of disease, such as swelling, pain, fever, aches, and pains. Occasionally, the inflammatory response becomes a chronic condition and can actually result in body damage, leading to increased inflammatory reactions. Anti-inflammatory agents generally block or alter the chemical reactions associated with the inflammatory response to stop one or more of the signs and symptoms of inflammation.

ANTI-INFLAMMATORY AGENTS

Several different types of drugs are used as anti-inflammatory agents. Corticosteroids (discussed in Chapter 36) are used systemically to block the inflammatory and immune systems. Blocking these important protective processes may produce many adverse effects, including decreased resistance to infection and neoplasms. Corticosteroids also are used topically to produce a local anti-inflammatory effect without as many adverse effects. Antihistamines (discussed in Chapter 54) are used to block the release of histamine in the initiation of the inflammatory response. In this chapter, discussion of anti-inflammatory agents focuses on salicylates, nonsteroidal anti-inflammatory drugs, and other related drugs.

Salicylates are popular anti-inflammatory agents, not only because of their ability to block the inflammatory response, but also because of their **antipyretic** (fever-blocking) and **analgesic** (pain-blocking) properties. They are generally available without prescription and are relatively nontoxic when used as directed.

Nonsteroidal anti-inflammatory drugs (NSAIDs) are some of the most widely used drugs in the United States. They provide strong anti-inflammatory and analgesic effects yet do not have the adverse effects that are associated with the corticosteroids.

Acetaminophen also is a widely used agent. It has antipyretic and analgesic properties but does not have the anti-inflammatory effects of the salicylates or the NSAIDs.

Because many of these anti-inflammatory drugs are available over the counter (OTC), there is a potential for abuse and overdosing. In addition, patients may take these drugs and block the signs and symptoms of a present illness, thus causing the potential for misdiagnosis of a problem. Patients also may combine these drugs and unknowingly produce toxic levels. All of these drugs have adverse effects that can be dangerous if toxic levels are reached.

SALICYLATES

Salicylates are some of the oldest anti-inflammatory drugs used. They were extracted from willow bark, poplar trees, and other plants by ancient peoples to treat fever, pain, and what we now call inflammation. The synthetic salicylates include the following drugs

Aspirin (*Bayer, Empirin,* and others) is one of the most widely used drugs for treating inflammatory conditions; it is available OTC.

Balsalazide (*Colazal*) is a new drug that is delivered intact to the colon, where it delivers a local anti-inflammatory effect for patients with ulcerative colitis.

Choline magnesium trisalicylate (*Trilisate*) is used for mild pain and fevers and to treat arthritis.

Choline salicylate (*Arthropan*) is used to treat mild pain and fevers as well as arthritis; it is available only as an OTC drug.

Mesalamine (*Pentasa* and others) is a unique compound that releases aspirin in the large intestine for a direct anti-inflammatory effect in ulcerative colitis or other conditions involving inflammation of the large intestine.

Olsalazine (*Dipentum*) is a drug that is converted to mesalamine in the colon and has the same direct anti-inflammatory effects.

Salsalate (*Argesic* and others) is used to treat pain, fever, and inflammation.

Sodium thiosalicylate (*Rexolate*) is used mainly for episodes of acute gout and muscular pain, and to treat rheumatic fever.

A person who does not respond to one salicylate may respond to a different one.

Therapeutic Actions and Indications

Salicylates inhibit the synthesis of prostaglandin, an important mediator of the inflammatory reaction (Figure 16–1). The antipyretic effect of salicylates may be related to blocking of a prostaglandin mediator of pyrogens (chemicals that cause an increase in body temperature and that are released by active white blood cells) at the thermoregulatory center of the hypothalamus. At low levels, aspirin also affects platelet aggregation by inhibiting the synthesis of thromboxane A, a potent vasoconstrictor that normally increases platelet aggregation and blood clot formation. At higher levels, aspirin inhibits the synthesis of prostacyclin, a vasodilator that inhibits platelet aggregation.

Salicylates are indicated for the treatment of mild to moderate pain, fever, and numerous inflammatory conditions, including rheumatoid arthritis and osteoarthritis. Aspirin at low doses is indicated for the prevention of transient ischemic attack (TIA) and stroke in men with a history of emboli. It also is indicated to reduce the risk of death and myocardial infarction (MI) in patients with a history of MI or unstable angina.

Pharmacokinetics

Salicylates are readily absorbed directly from the stomach, reaching peak levels within 5 to 30 minutes. They are metabolized in the liver and excreted in the urine, with a half-life of 15 minutes to 12 hours, depending on the salicylate involved. Salicylates cross the placenta and enter breast milk; they are not indicated for use during pregnancy or lac-

DRUG THERAPY ACROSS THE LIFESPAN

Anti-inflammatory Agents

Children	Adults	Older Adults
Children are more susceptible to the GI and CNS effects of these drugs. Care must be taken to make sure that the child receives the correct dose of any anti-inflammatory agent. This can be a problem because many of these drugs are available in OTC pain, cold, flu, and combination products. Parents need to be taught to read the label to find out the ingredients and the dosage they are giving the child.	Adults need to be cautioned about the presence of these drugs in many OTC products and taught to be aware of exactly what they are taking to avoid serious toxic effects. They should also be cautioned to report OTC drug use to their health care provider when they are receiving any other prescription drug, to avoid possible drug–drug interactions and the masking of signs and symptoms of disease.	Older patients may be more susceptible to the CNS and GI effects of some of these drugs. Dosage adjustment is not needed for many of these agents.
Acetaminophen is probably the most used anti-inflammatory drug for children. Care must be taken to avoid overdosage, which can cause severe hepatotoxicity.	Pregnant and nursing women should not use these drugs unless the benefit clearly outweighs the potential risk to the fetus or neonate. The salicylates, NSAIDs, and gold products have been found to have potentially severe adverse effects on the neonate and possibly the mother. Acetaminophen can be used cautiously if a pain preparation or antipyretic are needed. Nondrug measures should be taken when at all possible to decrease the potential risk. These women also need to be urged to avoid OTC drugs unless they are suggested by their health care providers.	Geriatric warnings have been associated with naproxen, ketorolac, and ketoprofen because of reports of increased toxicity when they are used by older patients. These NSAIDs should be avoided if possible.
Aspirin and choline magnesium trisalicylate are the only salicylates recommended for children. They should not be used when any risk of Reyes' syndrome exists.		Gold salts, used to treat arthritis, which is more common in older patients, are particularly toxic for geriatric patients. Accumulations in tissues can lead to increased renal, GI, and even liver problems. If gold is used in this group, the dosage should be reduced and the patient monitored very closely for toxic effects.
Ibuprofen, naproxen, tolmetin, and, in some cases, indomethacin are the NSAIDs approved for use in children.		
Children with arthritis may receive treatment with gold salts or etanercept; they must be monitored very closely for toxic effects.		

tation because of the potential adverse effects on the neonate and associated bleeding risks for the mother.

Contraindications and Cautions

The use of salicylates is contraindicated in the presence of known allergy to salicylates, other NSAIDs (more common with a history of nasal polyps, asthma, or chronic urticaria), or tartrazine (a dye that has a cross-sensitivity with aspirin); bleeding abnormalities (because of the changes in platelet aggregation associated with these drugs); impaired renal function (because the drug is excreted in the urine); chicken pox or influenza (risk of Reye's syndrome in children and teenagers); surgery or other invasive procedures scheduled within 1 week (because of the risk of increased bleeding); and pregnancy or lactation.

Adverse Effects

The adverse effects associated with use of salicylates may be the result of direct drug effects on the stomach (nausea, dyspepsia, heartburn, epigastric discomfort) and on clotting systems (blood loss, bleeding abnormalities). Salicylism can occur with high levels of aspirin; dizziness, ringing in the ears, difficulty hearing, nausea, vomiting, diarrhea, mental confu-

sion, and lassitude can occur. Acute salicylate toxicity may occur at doses of 20 to 25 g in adults or 4 g in children. Signs of salicylate toxicity include respiratory alkalosis; hyperpnea; tachypnea; hemorrhage; excitement; confusion; pulmonary edema; convulsions; tetany; metabolic acidosis; fever; coma; and cardiovascular, renal, and respiratory collapse.

Clinically Important Drug–Drug Interactions

The salicylates interact with many other drugs, primarily because of alterations in absorption, effects on the liver, or extension of the therapeutic effects of the salicylate or the interacting drug (or both). The list of interacting drugs in each drug monograph in a nursing drug guide should be consulted and the prescriber consulted before adding or removing a salicylate from any drug regimen.

Nursing Considerations for Patients Receiving Salicylates

Assessment: History and Examination

Screen for any of the following, which could be contraindications or cautions for the use of the drug: known allergies to any salicylates, NSAIDs, or tartrazine; renal disease; bleeding disorders; chicken pox; influenza; and pregnancy or lactation.

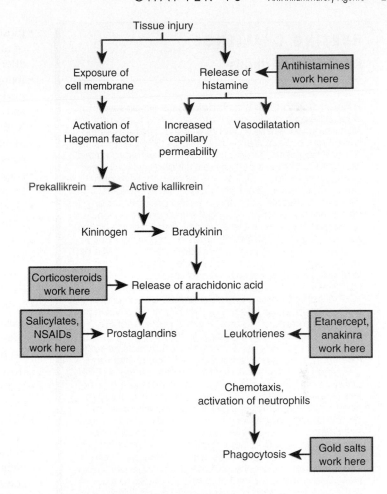

FIGURE 16-1. Sites of action of anti-inflammatory agents.

Include screening for baseline status before beginning therapy and for any potential adverse effects: the presence of any skin lesions; temperature; orientation, reflexes, eighth cranial nerve function, and affect; pulse, blood pressure, perfusion; respirations, adventitious sounds; liver evaluation; bowel sounds; and complete blood count (CBC), liver and renal function tests, urinalysis, stool guaiac, and clotting times.

Nursing Diagnoses

The patient receiving salicylates may have the following nursing diagnoses related to drug therapy:

- Acute Pain related to central nervous system (CNS) and gastrointestinal (GI) effects
- Ineffective Breathing Pattern if toxic effects occur
- Disturbed Sensory Perception (Auditory, Kinesthetic) if toxic effects occur
- Deficient Knowledge regarding drug therapy

Implementation

- Administer with food if GI upset is severe; provide small, frequent meals *to alleviate GI effects.*
- Administer drug as indicated; monitor dosage *to avoid toxic levels.*
- Monitor for severe reactions *to avoid problems and pro-*

vide emergency procedures (gastric lavage, induction of vomiting, charcoal) if they occur.
- Arrange for supportive care and comfort measures (rest, environmental control) *to decrease body temperature or to alleviate inflammation.*
- Ensure that the patient is well hydrated during therapy *to decrease the risk of toxicity.*
- Provide thorough patient teaching, including measures to avoid adverse effects and warning signs of problems as well as proper administration, *to increase knowledge about drug therapy and to increase compliance with drug regimen.*
- Offer support and encouragement *to deal with the drug regimen.*

Evaluation

- Monitor patient response to the drug (improvement in condition being treated, relief of signs and symptoms of inflammation).
- Monitor for adverse effects (GI upset, CNS changes, bleeding).
- Evaluate effectiveness of teaching plan (patient can name drug, dosage, adverse effects to watch for, specific measures to avoid adverse effects).
- Monitor effectiveness of comfort measures and compliance with the drug regimen.

212   PART III   Drugs Acting on the Immune System

NURSING CHALLENGE
Rheumatoid Arthritis

Rheumatoid arthritis is a chronic, systemic disease that affects people of all ages. It is considered to be an autoimmune disease. Patients with rheumatoid arthritis have high levels of rheumatoid factor (RF), an antibody to immunoglobulin G (IgG). RF interacts with circulating IgG to form immune complexes, which tend to deposit in the synovial fluid of joints as well as in the eye and other small vessels. The formation of the immune complex activates complement and precipitates an inflammatory reaction. During the immune reaction, lysosomal enzymes are released that destroy the tissues surrounding the joint. This destruction of normal tissue causes a further inflammatory reaction, and a cycle of destruction and inflammation ensues. Over time, the joint becomes severely damaged and the synovial space fills with scar tissue.

The patient with rheumatoid arthritis is in chronic pain, related to the release of the chemicals involved in the inflammatory process and the pressure of the swelling tissues in the joint capsule. At this time there is no cure for rheumatoid arthritis. Treatment is aimed at relieving the signs and symptoms of inflammation and delaying the progressive damage to the joints. The patient with this disease will progressively lose the use of the joint, which affects mobility as well as the ability to carry on the activities of daily living. Depression is not an uncommon side effect to this disease.

Specific nursing interventions can help to alleviate some of the signs and symptoms of rheumatoid arthritis and help the patient to cope with the disease. These interventions include physical therapy; range-of-motion exercises; application of hot and cold packs to the joints; weight-bearing exercises; spacing activities throughout the day to make the most of energy and movement reserves; and assistance devices for normal daily activities (eg, big handles on utensils and pens to help patients do things for themselves when they cannot grasp small handles). Thorough teaching about drug regimens can also help prevent adverse effects and increase compliance.

Patients may have to progress through a series of drugs as various agents lose their effectiveness. Aspirin, NSAIDs, gold therapy, and more potent antiarthritis drugs may all be used at one time or another. The patient with rheumatoid arthritis will profit from a relationship with a consistent, reliable health care provider who listens, offers support, and has knowledge of new drugs and treatments to improve the quality of life. Many community support and information groups are available as resources to patients—and to health care providers who work with these patients. For a listing of available resources in your area, contact the Arthritis Foundation: http://www.arthritis.org.

NONSTEROIDAL ANTI-INFLAMMATORY DRUGS

The NSAIDs are a relatively new drug class that has become one of the most commonly used types in the United States. This group of drugs includes the following agents.

Propionic Acids
- Fenoprofen (*Nalfon*) is used to treat pain and manage arthritis.
- Flurbiprofen (*Ansaid*) is used for long-term management of arthritis and as a topical preparation for managing pain after eye surgery.
- Ibuprofen (*Motrin, Advil,* and others) is used as an OTC pain medication and for long-term management of arthritis pain and dysmenorrhea; it is the most widely used of the NSAIDs.
- Ketoprofen (*Orudis*) is available for short-term management of pain and as a topical agent to relieve ocular itching caused by seasonal rhinitis.
- Naproxen (*Naprosyn*) is available for OTC pain relief and to treat arthritis and dysmenorrhea.
- Oxaprozin (*Daypro*) is very successfully used to manage arthritis.

Acetic Acids
- Diclofenac (*Voltaren*) is used to treat acute and long-term pain associated with inflammatory conditions.
- Etodolac (*Lodine*) is widely used for arthritis pain.
- Indomethacin (*Indocin*) is available in oral, topical, and rectal preparations for the relief of moderate to severe pain associated with inflammatory conditions and in intravenous form to promote closure of the patent ductus arteriosus in premature infants.
- Ketorolac (*Toradol*) is used for short-term management of pain and topically to relieve ocular itching.
- Nabumetone (*Relafen*) is used to treat acute and chronic arthritis pain.
- Sulindac (*Clinoril*) is used for long- and short-term treatment of the signs and symptoms of various inflammatory conditions.
- Tolmetin (*Tolectin*) is used to treat acute attacks of rheumatoid arthritis and juvenile arthritis.

Fenamates
- Meclofenamate (generic) is used to treat dysmenorrhea, mild pain, and arthritis.
- Mefenamic acid (*Ponstel*) is used only for short-term treatment of pain.
- Piroxicam (*Feldene*) is used to treat acute and chronic arthritis.
- Diflunisal (*Dolobid*) is used for moderate pain and for the treatment of arthritis.

Cyclooxygenase-2 Inhibitors
- Celecoxib (*Celebrex*) is used for the acute and long-term treatment of arthritis, particularly in patients who cannot tolerate the GI effects of other NSAIDs; for acute pain in adults; and for primary dysmenorrhea.
- Rofecoxib (*Vioxx*) used for the relief of the signs and symptoms of osteoarthritis, acute pain in adults, and the treatment of primary dysmenorrhea, particularly in patients who cannot tolerate the GI effects of other NSAIDs.
- Valdecoxib (*Bextra*) is used as a once-a-day treatment for osteoarthritis, treatment of adult rheumatoid arthritis, and primary dysmenorrhea.

The choice of NSAID depends on personal experience and the patient's response to the drug. A patient may have little response to one NSAID and a huge response to another.

DRUGS IN FOCUS
Salicylates

Drug Name	Dosage/Route	Usual Indications
(P) aspirin (*Bayer, Empirin,* others)	Adult: 325–650 mg PO or PR q4h Myocardial infarction (MI): 300–325 mg PO Pediatric: 65–100 mg/kg per day PO or PR in four to six divided doses; if <2 y of age, consult with prescriber	Treatment of fever, pain, inflammatory conditions; at low dose to prevent the risk of death and MI in patients with history of MI, prevention of transient ischemic attacks in men
balsalazide (*Colazal*)	Three 750-mg capsules PO t.i.d. for 8 wk	Treatment of mildly to moderately acute ulcerative colitis in adults
choline magnesium trisalicylate (*Trilisate*)	Adult: 1.5–3 g/d PO in two to three divided doses Pediatric: 50 mg/kg per day PO in two divided doses	Relief of mild pain, fevers; treatment of arthritis
choline salicylate (*Arthropan*)	Adult and children >12 y: 870 mg PO q3–4h	Relief of mild pain, fevers; treatment of arthritis
mesalamine (*Pentasa,* others)	800 mg PO t.i.d. for 6 wk; or 4 g/60 mL rectal suspension q.d. at bedtime *or* 500 mg suppository PR, retained for 1–3 h b.i.d.	Treatment of ulcerative colitis and other inflammatory bowel disease in adults
olsalazine (*Dipentum*)	1 g/d PO in two divided doses	Treatment of ulcerative colitis and other inflammatory bowel disease in adults
salsalate (*Argesic,* others)	3000 mg/d PO in divided doses	Treatment of pain, fever, inflammation in adults
sodium thiosalicylate (*Rexolate*)	50–150 mg IM q3–6h	Relief of gout, muscular pain; treatment of rheumatic fever in adults

It may take several trials to determine the drug of choice for any particular patient.

Therapeutic Actions and Indications

The anti-inflammatory, analgesic, and antipyretic effects of the NSAIDs are largely related to inhibition of prostaglandin synthesis (see Figure 16–1). The NSAIDs block two enzymes, known as cyclooxygenase-1 (COX-1) and cyclooxygenase-2 (COX-2). COX-1 is present in all tissues and seems to be involved in many body functions, including blood clotting, protecting the stomach lining, and maintaining sodium and water balance in the kidney. COX-1 turns arachidonic acid into prostaglandins as needed in a variety of tissues. COX-2 is active at sites of trauma or injury when more prostaglandins are needed, but it does not seem to be involved in the other tissue functions. By interfering with this part of the inflammatory reaction, NSAIDs block inflammation before all of the signs and symptoms can develop. Most NSAIDs also block various other functions of the prostaglandins, including protection of the stomach lining, regulation of blood clotting, and water and salt balance in the kidney. The newer COX-2 inhibitors are thought to act only at sites of trauma and injury to more specifically block the inflammatory reaction.

The adverse effects associated with most NSAIDs are related to blocking of both of these enzymes and changes in the functions that they influence—GI integrity, blood clotting, and sodium and water balance. The COX-2 inhibitors are designed to affect only the activity of COX-2, the enzyme that becomes active in response to trauma and injury. They do not interfere with COX-1, which is needed for normal functioning of these systems. Consequently, these drugs should not have the associated adverse effects seen when both COX-1 and COX-2 are inhibited. These drugs are relatively new; with experience, it has been shown that the COX-2 inhibitors still have some effect on these other functions, and patients should still be evaluated for GI effects, changes in bleeding time, and water retention.

The NSAIDs are indicated for relief of the signs and symptoms of rheumatoid arthritis and osteoarthritis; for relief of mild to moderate pain; for treatment of primary dysmenorrhea; and for fever reduction.

Pharmacodynamics

The NSAIDs are rapidly absorbed from the GI tract, reaching peak levels in 1 to 3 hours. They are metabolized in the liver and excreted in the urine. NSAIDs cross the placenta

DRUGS IN FOCUS
Nonsteroidal Anti-inflammatory Drugs

Drug Name	Dosage/Route	Usual Indications
celecoxib (*Celebrex*)	100–200 mg PO b.i.d.	Treatment of acute and chronic arthritis in adults; acute pain; primary dysmenorrhea
diclofenac (*Voltaren*) (*Cataflam*)	150–200 mg/d PO 25–50 mg b.i.d to q.i.d. PO	Treatment of acute and chronic pain associated with inflammatory conditions in adults
diflunisal (*Dolobid*)	500–1000 mg/d PO q12h	Treatment of moderate pain, arthritis in adults
etodolac (*Lodine*)	800–1200 mg/d PO in divided doses	Treatment of arthritis pain in adults
fenoprofen (*Nalfon*)	200–600 mg PO t.i.d.	Treatment of pain, arthritis in adults
flurbiprofen (*Ansaid*)	200–300 mg PO in divided doses; ophthalmic solution 1 gtt q 30 min beginning 2 h after surgery	Long-term management of arthritis; topically to manage pain after eye surgery in adults
ⓟ ibuprofen (*Motrin, Advil,* others)	Adult: 400–800 mg PO t.i.d. to q.i.d. Pediatric: 30–70 mg/kg per day PO in three to four divided doses for arthritis, or 5–10 mg/kg PO q6–8h for fever	Treatment of pain, arthritis, dysmenorrhea
indomethacin (*Indocin*)	Adult: 75–150 mg/d PO in three to four divided doses Pediatric >2 y: in special circumstances, 2 mg/kg per day PO in divided doses	Relief of moderate to severe pain in PO, topical, and PR forms; closure of patent ductus arteriosus in premature infants (given IV)
ketoprofen (*Orudis*)	25–75 mg PO t.i.d. to q.i.d.; reduce dosage with hepatic or renal impairment	Short-term management of pain; topically to relieve ocular itching
ketorolac (*Toradol*)	10 mg PO q4–6h, *or* 30–60 mg IM, switching to oral form as soon as possible, *or* 30 mg IV as a single dose Ophthalmic: 1 gtt to affected eye q.i.d. Reduce dosage with renal impairment and in patients >65 y	Short-term management of pain in adults; topically to relieve ocular itching
meclofenamate (generic)	200–400 mg/d PO in divided doses	Treatment of dysmenorrhea, mild pain, arthritis in adults
mefenamic acid (*Ponstel*)	500 mg PO, then 250 mg PO q6h as needed	Short-term treatment of pain in adults and children >14 y.
nabumetone (*Relafen*)	1000 mg/d PO as a single dose	Treatment of acute and chronic arthritis pain in adults
naproxen (*Naprosyn*)	Adult: 250–500 mg PO b.i.d.; do not give >200 mg q12h for geriatric patients Pediatric: 10 mg/kg per day PO in two divided doses for juvenile arthritis; do not give OTC versions to children <12 y without consulting health care provider	Treatment of pain, arthritis, dysmenorrhea
oxaprozin (*Daypro*)	1200 mg PO q.d.	Treatment of arthritis in adults
piroxicam (*Feldene*)	20 mg PO q.d. as a single dose	Treatment of acute and chronic arthritis in adults
rofecoxib (*Vioxx*)	12.5 mg PO q.d.; 50 mg PO q.d. for pain and primary dysmenorrhea for no longer than 5 d	Treatment of osteoarthritis, acute pain and primary dysmenorrhea in adults
sulindac (*Clinoril*)	150–200 mg PO b.i.d.	Treatment of various inflammatory conditions in adults
tolmetin (*Tolectin*)	Adult: 400 mg PO t.i.d. Pediatric: 20 mg/kg per day PO in three to four divided doses	Treatment of acute flares of rheumatoid and juvenile arthritis
Valdecoxib (*Bextra*)	Adult: 10 mg/d PO	Treatment of osteoarthritis; rheumatoid arthritis; primary dysmenorrhea

and cross into breast milk. Therefore, they are not recommended during pregnancy and lactation because of the potential adverse effects on the neonate.

Contraindications and Cautions

The NSAIDs are contraindicated in the presence of allergy to any NSAID or salicylate, and celecoxib is also contraindicated in the presence of allergy to sulfonamides. Additional contraindications are cardiovascular dysfunction or hypertension, because of the varying effects of the prostaglandins; peptic ulcer or known GI bleeding, because of the potential to exacerbate the GI bleeding; and pregnancy or lactation. Caution should be used with renal or hepatic dysfunction, which could alter the metabolism and excretion of these drugs, and with any other known allergies, which indicate increased sensitivity.

Adverse Effects

Patients receiving NSAIDs often experience nausea, dyspepsia, GI pain, constipation, diarrhea, or flatulence caused by direct GI effects of the drug. The potential for GI bleeding is often a cause of discontinuation of the drug. Headache, dizziness, somnolence, and fatigue also occur frequently and could be related to prostaglandin activity in the CNS. Bleeding, platelet inhibition, and even bone marrow depression have been reported with chronic use and are probably related to blocking of prostaglandin activity. Rash and mouth sores may occur, and anaphylactoid reactions ranging to fatal anaphylactic shock have been reported in cases of severe hypersensitivity.

Clinically Important Drug–Drug Interactions

There is often a decreased diuretic effect when these drugs are taken with loop diuretics; there is a potential for decreased antihypertensive effect of β-blockers if these drugs are combined; and there have been reports of lithium toxicity, especially when combined with ibuprofen. Patients who receive these combinations should be monitored closely and appropriate dosage adjustments should be made by the prescriber.

Nursing Considerations for Patients Receiving NSAIDs

Assessment: History and Examination

Screen for any of the following, which could be contraindications or cautions for the use of the drug: known allergies to any salicylates, NSAIDs, or tartrazine; pregnancy or lactation; hepatic or renal disease; cardiovascular dysfunction; hypertension; and GI bleeding or peptic ulcer.

Include screening for baseline status before beginning therapy and for any potential adverse effects: presence of any skin lesions; temperature; orientation, reflexes, and affect; pulse, blood pressure, perfusion; respirations, adventitious sounds; liver evaluation; bowel sounds; and CBC, liver and renal function tests, urinalysis, stool guaiac, and serum electrolytes.

Nursing Diagnoses, Implementation, and Evaluation

Refer to the nursing consideration sections for the salicylates. (See the accompanying Patient Teaching Checklist for NSAIDs and the Nursing Care Guide: NSAIDs.)

PATIENT TEACHING CHECKLIST

NSAIDs

Create customized patient teaching materials for a specific NSAID form your CD-ROM. Patient teaching should stress the following points for drugs within this class:

- Nonsteroidal anti-inflammatory drugs, or NSAIDs, work in the body to decrease inflammation and to relieve the signs and symptoms of inflammation, such as pain, swelling, heat, tenderness, and redness.

Some of the following adverse effects may occur:

- *Nausea, vomiting, abdominal discomfort*—Taking the drug with food or eating small, frequent meals may help. If these effects persist, consult with your health care provider.
- *Diarrhea, constipation*—These effects may decrease over time; ensure ready access to bathroom facilities and consult with your health care provider for possible treatment.
- *Drowsiness, dizziness, blurred vision*—Avoid driving or performing tasks that require alertness if you experience any of these problems.
- *Headache*—If this becomes a problem, consult with your health care provider. Do not self-treat with aspirin or other analgesics.
- Tell any health care provider who is taking care of you that you are taking this drug.
- Avoid the use of over-the-counter preparations while you are taking this drug. If you feel that you need one of these drugs, consult with your health care provider for the most appropriate choice.
- Report any of the following to your health care provider: sore throat, fever, rash, itching, weight gain or swelling in the ankles or fingers, changes in vision, black or tarry stools.
- Keep this drug and all medications out of the reach of children.

This Teaching Checklist reflects general patient teaching guidelines. It is not meant to be a substitute for drug-specific teaching information, which is available in nursing drug guides.

▢▣◗◖ WEB LINKS

Health care providers and patients may want to consult the following Internet sources for additional information:

Information on arthritis—disease, treatments, research:
  http://www.arthritis.org
Guide to finding additional information, support groups:
  http://www.interaccess.com/ihpnet/health.html
Information on drug research and development, warnings, information:
  http://www.fda.gov

OTHER RELATED DRUGS

Other drugs that are used to treat inflammatory conditions include acetaminophen (*Tylenol*), gold compounds, and other antiarthritic drugs. Acetaminophen is used to treat moderate to mild pain and fever and often is used in place of

NURSING CARE GUIDE

NSAIDs

Assessment	Nursing Diagnoses	Implementation	Evaluation
HISTORY Allergies to any NSAID or aspirin, sulfonamides (COX-2 inhibitors), pregnancy, lactation; renal or hepatic impairment; ulcerative GI disease, peptic ulcer, hearing impairment, blood dyscrasias	Acute Pain related to GI effects, headache Disturbed Sensory Perception related to CNS effects (Auditory, Kinesthetic) Ineffective Gas Exchange secondary to hypersensitivity reactions Deficient Knowledge deficit regarding drug therapy	Ensure proper administration of the drug. Administer with food if GI upset occurs. Provide supportive and comfort measures to deal with adverse effects: small, frequent meals, safety measures if CNS effects occur, measures for headache, bowel training as needed. Provide life support and emergency measures in cases of hypersensitivity. Provide patient teaching regarding drug name, dosage, side effects, precautions, and warnings to report.	Evaluate drug effects: decrease in signs and symptoms of inflammation. Monitor for adverse effects: CNS changes, rash, GI upset, congestive heart failure, liver dysfunction, asthma, anaphylaxis. Monitor for drug–drug interactions as indicated for each drug. Evaluate effectiveness of patient teaching program. Evaluate effectiveness of comfort/safety measures. Evaluate effectiveness of life support and emergency measures if appropriate.
PHYSICAL EXAMINATION Neurological: orientation, reflexes, affect Skin: color, lesions CV: P, cardiac auscultation, BP, perfusion GI: liver evaluation, bowel sounds Lab tests: CBC, liver and renal function tests			

the NSAIDs or salicylates. The gold compounds are used to prevent and suppress arthritis in selected patients with rheumatoid arthritis. The other antiarthritic drugs are specifically used to block the inflammatory process and tissue damage associated with rheumatoid arthritis.

Acetaminophen

Therapeutic Actions and Indications

Acetaminophen acts directly on the thermoregulatory cells in the hypothalamus to cause sweating and vasodilation; this in turn causes the release of heat and lowers fever. The mechanism of action related to the analgesic effects of acetaminophen has not been identified.

Acetaminophen is indicated for the treatment of pain and fever associated with a variety of conditions, including influenza; for the prophylaxis of children receiving diphtheria–pertussis–tetanus (DPT) immunizations (aspirin may mask Reye's syndrome in children); and for the relief of musculoskeletal pain associated with arthritis.

Pharmacokinetics

Acetaminophen is rapidly absorbed from the GI tract, reaching peak levels in 0.5 to 2 hours. It is extensively metabolized in the liver and excreted in the urine, with a half-life of about 2 hours. Caution should be used in patients with hepatic or renal impairment, which could interfere with metabolism and excretion of the drug, leading to toxic levels. Acetaminophen crosses the placenta and enters breast milk; it should be used cautiously during pregnancy or lactation because of the potential adverse effects on the fetus.

Contraindications and Cautions

Acetaminophen is contraindicated in the presence of allergy to acetaminophen. It should be used cautiously in pregnancy or lactation and in hepatic dysfunction or chronic alcoholism (because of associated toxic effects on the liver).

Adverse Effects

Adverse effects associated with acetaminophen use include headache, hemolytic anemia, renal dysfunction, skin rash, and fever. Hepatotoxicity is a potentially fatal adverse effect that is usually associated with chronic use and overdose and is related to direct toxic effects on the liver.

Clinically Important Drug–Drug Interactions
There is an increased risk of bleeding with oral anticoagulants because of effects on the liver; of toxicity with chronic ethanol ingestion because of toxic effects on the liver; and of hepatotoxicity with barbiturates, carbamazepine, hydantoins, rifampin, or sulfinpyrazone. These combinations should be avoided, but if they must be used, appropriate dosage adjustment should be made and the patient should be monitored closely.

Gold Compounds

Some patients with rheumatic inflammatory conditions do not respond to the usual anti-inflammatory therapies and their conditions worsen despite weeks or months of standard pharmacological treatment. Some of these patients respond to treatment with gold salts, also known as chrysotherapy. The gold salts that are currently available for use include auranofin (*Ridaura*), an oral agent used for long-term therapy; aurothioglucose (*Solganal*), an injected drug that is recommended for treatment early in the disease, before too much tissue damage has been done; and gold sodium thiomalate (*Aurolate*), an injected drug much like aurothioglucose.

Therapeutic Actions and Indications
Gold salts are absorbed by macrophages, which results in inhibition of phagocytosis (see Figure 16–1). Because phagocytosis is blocked, the release of lysosomal enzymes is inhibited and tissue destruction is decreased. This action allows gold salts to suppress and prevent some arthritis and synovitis. Gold salts are indicated to treat selected cases of rheumatoid and juvenile rheumatoid arthritis in patients whose disease has been unresponsive to standard therapy. These drugs do not repair damage; they prevent further damage and so are most effective if used early in the disease.

Pharmacokinetics
The gold salts are absorbed at varying rates depending on their route of administration. They are widely distributed throughout the body but seem to concentrate in the hypothalamo-pituitary-adrenocortical (HPA) system and in the adrenal and renal cortices. The gold salts are excreted in urine and feces. These drugs cross the placenta and cross into breast milk. They have been shown to be teratogenic in animal studies and should not be used during pregnancy or lactation. Barrier contraceptives should be recommended to women of childbearing age, and another method of feeding the baby should be used if gold therapy is needed in a lactating woman.

Contraindications and Cautions
Gold salts can be quite toxic and are contraindicated in the presence of any known allergy to gold, severe diabetes, congestive heart failure, severe debilitation, renal or hepatic impairment, hypertension, blood dyscrasias, recent radiation treatment, history of toxic levels of heavy metals, and pregnancy or lactation.

Adverse Effects
A variety of adverse effects are common with the use of gold salts and are probably related to their deposition in the tissues and effects at that local level: stomatitis, glossitis, gingivitis, pharyngitis, laryngitis, colitis, diarrhea, and other GI inflammation; gold bronchitis and interstitial pneumonitis; bone marrow depression; vaginitis, nephrotic syndrome; dermatitis, pruritus, exfoliative dermatitis; and allergic reactions ranging from flushing, fainting, and dizziness to anaphylactic shock.

Clinically Important Drug–Drug Interactions
These drugs should not be combined with penicillamine, antimalarials, cytotoxic drugs, or immunosuppressive agents other than low-dose corticosteroids because of the potential for severe toxicity.

Other Antiarthritis Drugs

Six other drugs have become available to relieve the pain and suffering of patients with acute rheumatoid arthritis that is no longer responsive to conventional therapy: etanercept (*Enbrel*), leflunomide (*Arava*), penicillamine (*Depen*), hylan G-F 20 (*Synvisc*), sodium hyaluronate (*Hyalgan*), and anakinra (*Kineret*).

Therapeutic Actions and Indications
Etanercept (*Enbrel*) contains genetically engineered tumor necrosis factor (TNF) receptors derived from Chinese hamster ovary cells. These receptors react with free-floating TNF released by active leukocytes in autoimmune inflammatory disease to prevent the damage caused by TNF. Etanercept is indicated for subcutaneous use to reduce the signs and symptoms of active rheumatoid arthritis and prevent

CULTURAL CONSIDERATIONS
Sensitivity to Anti-inflammatory Drugs

African Americans have a documented decreased sensitivity to the pain-relieving effects of many of the anti-inflammatory drugs. They do, however, have an increased risk of developing gastrointestinal adverse effects to these drugs, including acetaminophen. This should be taken into consideration when using these drugs as analgesics. Increased dosages may be needed to achieve a pain-blocking effect, but the increased dosage will put these patients at an even greater risk for development of the adverse GI effects associated with these drugs. These patients should be monitored closely, and efforts should be made to decrease pain using nondrug measures such as positioning, environmental control, physical therapy, warm soaks, and so on. If African American patients are prescribed anti-inflammatory drugs, they should be educated about the signs and symptoms of gastrointestinal bleeding and what to report. They also should be monitored regularly for any adverse reactions to these drugs.

damage in the early stages of the disease. A warning has been issued stating that the drug has been associated with the development of serious CNS problems, including multiple sclerosis. It can also cause severe myelosuppression and increased risk of infections and cancer development. Patients who use this drug need to be monitored very closely.

Leflunomide (*Arava*) directly inhibits an enzyme, dihydroorotate dehydrogenase (DHODH), which is active in the autoimmune process that leads to rheumatoid arthritis, preventing the signs and symptoms of inflammation and blocking the structural damage this inflammation can cause. Leflunomide is indicated for the treatment of active rheumatoid arthritis to relieve symptoms and to slow the progression of the disease. It has been associated with severe hepatic toxicity. and the patient's liver function needs to be monitored closely.

Penicillamine (*Depen*) lowers the immunoglobulin M (IgM) rheumatoid factor levels in patients with acute rheumatoid arthritis, relieving the signs and symptoms of inflammation. It may take 2 to 3 months of therapy before a response is noted.

Hylan G-F 20 (*Synvisc*) and sodium hyaluronate (*Hyalgan*) are hyaluronic acid derivatives that have elastic and viscous properties. These drugs are injected directly into the joints of patients with severe rheumatoid arthritis of the knee. They seem to cushion and lubricate the joint and relieve the pain associated with degenerative arthritis.

Anakinra (*Kineret*) is the newest of the antiarthritis drugs. This drug is an interleukin-1 receptor antagonist. It blocks the increased interleukin-1, which is responsible for the degradation of cartilage in rheumatoid arthritis. This drug must be given each day by subcutaneous injection.

Contraindications and Cautions

These drugs are contraindicated in the presence of allergy to the drugs or to the animal products from which they were derived (Chinese hamster products in etanercept; chicken products in hylan G-F 20 and sodium hyaluronate); pregnancy or lactation, because of the potential for adverse effects on the neonate; acute infection, because of the blocking of normal inflammatory pathways; and liver or renal impairment, which could be exacerbated by these drugs.

Adverse Effects

A variety of adverse effects are common with the use of these drugs, including local irritation at injection sites (anakinra, etanercept, hylan G-F 20, and sodium hyaluronate), pain with injection, and increased risk of infection. Leflunomide is associated with potentially fatal hepatic toxicity and rashes. Penicillamine is associated with a potentially fatal myasthenic syndrome, bone marrow depression, and assorted hypersensitivity reactions. Etanercept is associated with severe bone marrow suppression as well as serious CNS disorders, including multiple sclerosis.

Clinically Important Drug–Drug Interactions

Hylan G-F 20 and sodium hyaluronate should not be injected at the same time as local anesthetics.

Because leflunomide can cause severe liver dysfunction if combined with other hepatotoxic drugs, this combination should be avoided.

There is decreased absorption of penicillamine if taken with iron salts or antacids; if these are given together, they should be separated by at least 2 hours.

Anakinra and etanercept should not be used together because of an increased risk of serious infections.

Nursing Considerations for Patients Receiving Other Related Drugs

Nursing considerations for patients receiving the drugs listed in this section are similar to those for patients receiving other anti-inflammatory drugs. Details related to each individual drug can be found in the specific drug monograph in your nursing drug guide.

CHAPTER SUMMARY

- The inflammatory response, which is important for protecting the body from injury and invasion, produces many of the signs and symptoms associated with disease, including fever, aches and pains, and lethargy.
- Chronic or excessive activity by the inflammatory response can lead to the release of lysosomal enzymes and tissue destruction.
- Anti-inflammatory drugs block various chemicals associated with the inflammatory reaction. Anti-inflammatory drugs also may have antipyretic (fever-blocking) and analgesic (pain-blocking) activities.
- Salicylates block prostaglandin activity. NSAIDs block prostaglandin synthesis. Acetaminophen causes vasodilation and heat release, lowering fever and working to relieve pain. Gold salts prevent macrophage phagocytosis, lysosomal release, and tissue damage. Etanercept contains TNF receptors to deactivate TNF and slow progression of autoimmune diseases. Leflunomide deactivates an enzyme active in autoimmune disease. Penicillamine is a chelating agent that lowers levels of IgM rheumatoid factor in acute rheumatoid arthritis. Hylan G-F 20 and hyaluronate are viscous and elastic hyaluronic acid derivatives that lubricate arthritic knees and stop some of the pain of inflammation. Anakinra is an interleukin-1 receptor antagonist that blocks the degradation of cartilage in rheumatoid arthritis.
- Salicylates can cause acidosis and eighth cranial nerve damage. NSAIDs are most associated with GI irritation and bleeding. Acetaminophen can cause serious liver toxicity. The gold salts cause many systemic inflammatory reactions. Other antiarthritis drugs are associated with local injection site irritation and increased susceptibility to infection. Leflunomide is associated with severe hepatic toxicity.
- Many anti-inflammatory drugs are available OTC, and care must be taken to prevent abuse or overuse of these drugs. Many combination products contain the same ingredients, and overdose can easily occur.

DRUGS IN FOCUS
Anti-inflammatory and Antiarthritis Agents

Drug Name	Dosage/Route	Usual Indications
(P) acetaminophen (*Tylenol*)	Adult: 1000 mg PO t.i.d. to q.i.d. *or* 325–650 mg PR q4–6h Pediatric: adjust dosage based on age	Relief of pain and fever in a variety of situations
anakinra (*Kineret*)	Adult: 100 mg/d SC	Reduction of signs and symptoms of rheumatoid arthritis in patients ≥18 y if one or more other arthritis agents have failed
auranofin (*Ridaura*)	Adult: 6 mg/d PO; monitor geriatric patients carefully Pediatric: 0.1–0.15 mg mg/kg per day PO	Long-term therapy for rheumatic disorders
(P) aurothioglucose (*Solganal*)	Adult: 10 mg IM, then 2 doses of 25 mg IM, then 2 doses of 50 mg IM; then 50 mg IM every 3–4 wk; monitor geriatric patients carefully Pediatric: one-quarter the adult dose	Injected drug for early treatment of rheumatic disorders
etanercept (*Enbrel*)	Adult: 25 mg SC two times per week Pediatric 4–17 y: 0.4 mg/kg SC two times per week with 72–96 h between doses; not recommended for patients <4 y	Reduction of signs and symptoms of severe rheumatoid arthritis in patients whose disease is unresponsive to other therapy; prevention of damage early in the disease
gold sodium thiomalate (*Aurolate*)	Adult: 10 mg IM, then 25 mg IM every other week; use caution in geriatric patients Pediatric: 10 mg IM, then 1 mg/kg IM every other week	Injected drug for early treatment of rheumatic disorders
hylan G-F 20 (*Synvisc*)	2 mL once a week for 3 wk injected into the affected knee	Relief of pain in the knees of arthritis patients whose disease is unresponsive to conventional treatment
leflunomide (*Arava*)	100 mg PO q.d. for 3 d, then 20 mg PO q.d.	Treatment of active rheumatoid arthritis, to relieve signs and symptoms and to slow progression of disease in adults
penicillamine (*Depen*)	125–250 mg PO q.d.	Treatment of severe, active rheumatoid arthritis in adults whose disease is unresponsive to conventional therapy
sodium hyaluronate (*Hyalgan*)	2 mg once a week for 5 wk injected into the affected knee	Relief of pain in the knees of arthritis patients whose disease is unresponsive to conventional treatment

Review Questions

1. An analgesic is a drug that
   a. reduces fever.
   b. reduces swelling.
   c. reduces redness.
   d. reduces pain.
2. An antipyretic is a drug that can
   a. block pain.
   b. block swelling.
   c. block fever.
   d. block inflammation.
3. Salicylates are very popular anti-inflammatory agents for all of the following reasons, except
   a. they have antipyretic properties.
   b. they have analgesic properties.
   c. they are available without a prescription.
   d. they must be given parenterally.

4. The NSAIDs affect the COX-1 and COX-2 enzymes. By blocking COX-2 enzymes, the NSAIDs block inflammation and the signs and symptoms of inflammation at the site of injury or trauma. By blocking COX-1 enzymes, these drugs block
   a. fever regulation.
   b. prostaglandins that protect the stomach lining.
   c. swelling in the periphery.
   d. liver function.
5. Your patient has been receiving ibuprofen for many years to relieve the pain of osteoarthritis. Assessment of the patient should include
   a. Electrocardiogram.
   b. CBC with differential.
   c. respiratory auscultation.
   d. renal evaluation.
6. Patients taking NSAIDs should be taught to avoid the use

CASE STUDY

Aspirin and Rheumatoid Arthritis

THE SITUATION

G. T. is an 82-year-old man on a fixed income with a 14-year history of rheumatoid arthritis. He is seen in the clinic for evaluation of his arthritis and to address his complaint that the drugs are not doing any good. On examination, it is found that G. T.'s range of motion, physical examination of joints, and overall presentation has not changed since his last visit. G. T. states that he had been taking aspirin, as prescribed, for his arthritis. But he read that aspirin can cause severe stomach problems, so he had switched to *Ecotrin* (an aspirin and antacid combination). This drug was much more expensive than he could handle on his fixed income, so he had started taking the drug only once every 3 days.

CRITICAL THINKING

Think about the pathophysiology of rheumatoid arthritis and how the drugs ordered act on the inflammatory process. How can the nurse best explain the disease and the drug regimen to this patient?

What could be contributing to G.T.'s perception that his condition has worsened?

What nursing interventions would be appropriate to help G. T. cope with his disease and his need for medication?

DISCUSSION

G. T. should be offered encouragement and support to deal with his progressive disease and the drug regimen required. The fact that his physical status has not changed but he perceives that the disease is worse may reflect other underlying problems that are making it more difficult

for him to cope with chronic pain and limitations. The nurse should explore his social situation, any changes in his living situation, and support services. An examination should be done to determine whether other physical problems have emerged that could be adding to his sense that things are getting worse. The actions of aspirin on the arthritic process should be reviewed in basic terms, with emphasis on the importance of preventing further damage and maintaining high enough levels of aspirin to control the arthritis signs and symptoms. Pictures of the process involved in rheumatoid arthritis may help—the simpler the better in most cases.

G. T. also should be taught that all aspirin is the same, so it is acceptable to buy the cheapest generic aspirin. He can check the expiration date to make sure that the drug is fresh and still therapeutic and check that it does not smell like vinegar. Express that the expensive combination product that G. T. has been using has not been proven to be any more effective at helping arthritis or at decreasing adverse effects than generic aspirin.

If G. T. has been having gastrointestinal complaints with the aspirin, he can be encouraged to take the drug with food and to have small, frequent meals to keep stomach acid levels at a more steady state. If G. T. has not been having any gastrointestinal complaints, he should be asked to report any immediately. The importance of the placebo effect cannot be overlooked with this patient. Many patients actually state that they feel better when they are using well-recognized, brand-name products. With support and encouragement, G. T. can be helped to follow his prescribed drug regimen and delay further damage from his arthritis.

---

of OTC medications without checking with their prescriber because

a. many of the OTC preparations contain NSAIDs and inadvertent toxicity could occur.

b. no one should take more than one type of pain reliever at a time.

c. increased GI upset could occur.

d. there is a risk of Reye's syndrome.

7. Treatment of severe rheumatoid arthritis could include use of any of the following except

a. etanercept—tumor necrosis factor.

b. gold therapy.

c. hylan G-F 20—hylans with elastic properties.

d. ketoprofen.

8. Chronic or excessive activity by the inflammatory response can lead to

a. loss of white blood cells.

b. coagulation problems.

c. release of lysosomal enzymes and tissue destruction.

d. adrenal suppression.

9. Oxaprozin (*Daypro*) would not be the drug of choice for the treatment of arthritis in a patient with

a. headaches.

b. dysmenorrhea.

c. active peptic ulcer disease.

d. chronic obstructive pulmonary disease.

10. A patient with rheumatoid arthritis who is on a fixed income and is being treated with aspirin should be advised

a. to use only brand-name aspirin.

b. to use only enteric-coated aspirin.

c. to use generic aspirin, checking the expiration date before use.

d. to switch to one of the NSAIDs.

BIBLIOGRAPHY

Agrawal, N. M., & Aziz, K. (1998). Prevention of gastrointestinal complications with nonsteroidal antiinflammatory drugs. *Journal of Rheumatology Supplement, 51,* 17–20.

Bullock, B. L. (2000). *Focus on pathophysiology.* Philadelphia: Lippincott Williams & Wilkins.

Cash, J. M., & Wilder, R. L. (1995). Refractory rheumatoid arthritis: Therapeutic options. *Rheumatic Diseases Clinics North America, 21*(1), 1–18.

Gilman, A., Hardman, J. G., & Limbird, L. E. (Eds.) (2002). *Goodman and Gilman's the pharmacological basis of therapeutics* (10th ed.). New York: McGraw-Hill.

Karch, A. M. (2002). *2003 Lippincott's nursing drug guide*. Philadelphia: Lippincott Williams & Wilkins.

Lancaster, C. (1995). Effective nonsteroidal antiinflammatory drugs devoid of gastrointestinal side effects: Do they really exist? *Digestive Diseases and Sciences, 13*(Suppl 1), 40–47.

Drug facts and comparisons. (2002). St. Louis: Facts & Comparisons.

The medical letter on drugs and therapeutics. (2002). New Rochelle, NY: Medical Letter.

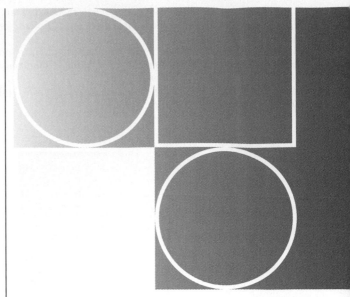

CHAPTER

17

Key Terms
immune stimulant
immune suppressant
monoclonal antibodies
recombinant DNA technology

Immune Modulators

222

As the name implies, immune modulators are used to modify the actions of the immune system. **Immune stimulants** are used to energize the immune system when it is exhausted from fighting prolonged invasion or needs help fighting a specific pathogen or cancer cell. **Immune suppressants** are used to block the normal effects of the immune system in cases of organ transplantation (in which nonself-cells are transplanted into the body and destroyed by the immune reaction) and in autoimmune disorders (in which the body's defenses recognize self-cells as foreign and work to destroy them).

The knowledge base about the actions and components of the immune system is growing and changing daily. As new discoveries are made and interactions understood, new applications will be found for modulating the immune system in a variety of disorders.

IMMUNE STIMULANTS

Immune stimulants include the interferons, which are naturally released from human cells in response to viral invasion; the interleukins, synthetic compounds much like the interleukins that communicate between lymphocytes, which stimulate cellular immunity and inhibit tumor growth; and a T- and B-cell modulator called levamisole (*Ergamisol*), which restores immune function and also stimulates immune system activity (Figure 17–1).

Interferons

Interferons are naturally produced and released by human cells that have been invaded by viruses. They may also be released from cells in response to other stimuli. A number of interferons are available for use today. Several are produced by **recombinant DNA technology,** including interferon alfa-2a (*Roferon-A*), interferon alfa-2b (*Intron-A*), interferon alfacon-1 (*Infergen*), interferon alfa-n1 lymphoblastoid (*Wellferon*), peginterferon alfa-2b (*Peg-Intron*), and interferon beta-1b (*Betaseron*). Interferon alfa-n3 (*Alferon N*) is produced by harvesting human leukocytes and is injected directly into warts, a viral infection. Interferon beta-1a (*Avonex*) is produced from Chinese hamster ovary cells. Interferon gamma-1b (*Actimmune*) is produced by *Escherichia coli* bacteria. The interferon of choice depends on the condition being treated.

Therapeutic Actions and Indications

Interferons act to prevent virus particles from replicating inside other cells. They also stimulate interferon receptor sites on noninvaded cells to produce antiviral proteins, which prevent viruses from entering the cell. In addition, interferons have been found to inhibit tumor growth and replication.

DRUG THERAPY ACROSS THE LIFESPAN

Immune Modulators

Children	Adults	Older Adults
Most of the drugs that affect the immune system are not recommended for use in children or have not been tested in children. The exceptions—interferon alfa-2b, azathioprine, cyclosporine, tacrolimus, and palivizumab—should be used cautiously, monitoring the child frequently for infection, GI, renal, hematological, or CNS effects. The immune suppressants (azathioprine, cyclosporine, and tacrolimus) are usually needed in higher doses for children than for adults to achieve the same therapeutic effect. Protecting the child from infection and injury is a very important part of the care of a child taking an immune modulator. This can be a great challenge with an active child.	Both the adult patient who is receiving a parenteral immune modulator and a significant other should learn the proper technique for injection, disposal of needles, and special storage precautions for the drug. It is important to stress ways to avoid exposure to infection and injury to prevent further complications. The patient should be encouraged to seek regular follow-up and medical care. Immune modulators are contraindicated during pregnancy and lactation because of the potential for adverse effects on the fetus and complications for the mother. Women of child-bearing age should be advised to use barrier contraceptives while taking these drugs and, if breast feeding, should be counseled to find another method of feeding the baby. Some of these drugs impair fertility, and the patient should be advised of this fact before taking the drug.	Older patients may be more susceptible to the effects of the immune modulators, partly because the aging immune system is less efficient and less responsive. These patients need to be monitored closely for infection, GI, renal, hepatic, and CNS effects. Baseline renal and liver function tests can help to determine whether a decreased dosage will be needed before beginning therapy. Because these patients are more susceptible to infection, they need to receive extensive teaching about ways to avoid infection and injury.

FIGURE 17–1. Sites of action of the immune modulators.

Interestingly, interferon gamma-1b also acts like an interleukin, stimulating phagocytes to be more aggressive.

Interferons are indicated for treating selected leukemias (alfa-2a, alfa-2b); multiple sclerosis (beta-1a, beta-1b); intralesional treatment of warts (alfa-n3, alfa-2b); chronic hepatitis B or non-A/non-B/C hepatitis (alfa-2b); chronic hepatitis C (alfa-n-1 lymphoblastoid, alfacon-1, peginterferon); acquired immunodeficiency syndrome (AIDS)–related Kaposi's sarcoma (alfa-2a, alfa-2b, and unlabeled uses for several other interferons); and severe infections caused by chronic granulomatous disease (gamma-1b). Most of the interferons are being tested for the treatment of various cancers and AIDS-related problems.

Contraindications and Cautions

The use of interferons is contraindicated in the presence of known allergy to any interferon or product components and during pregnancy and lactation because of the potential risk to the neonate. Caution should be used in the presence of known cardiac disease, because hypertension and arrhythmias have been reported with the use of these drugs; with myelosuppression, because these drugs may further suppress the bone marrow; and with central nervous system (CNS) dysfunction of any kind, because of the potentials for CNS depression and personality changes that have been reported.

Pharmacokinetics

The interferons are generally well absorbed after subcutaneous or intramuscular injection. They are broken down in the tissues and seem to be excreted primarily through the kidneys. Many of them are teratogenic in animals and therefore should not be used during pregnancy. Use of barrier contraceptives is advised for women of child-bearing age. It is not known whether these drugs cross into breast milk, but because of the potential adverse effects on the baby, it is advised that the drugs not be used during lactation unless the benefits to the mother clearly outweigh any risks to the baby.

Adverse Effects

The adverse effects associated with the use of interferons are related to the immune or inflammatory reaction that is being stimulated (eg, lethargy, myalgia, arthralgia, anorexia, nausea). Other commonly seen adverse effects include headache, dizziness, bone marrow depression, depression and suicidal ideation, photosensitivity, and liver impairment.

Interleukins

Interleukins are chemicals produced by T cells to communicate between leukocytes. Two interleukin-2 preparations are available for use. Interleukin-2 stimulates cellular immunity by increasing the activity of natural killer cells, platelets, and

DRUGS IN FOCUS
Interferons

Drug Name	Dosage/Route	Usual Indications
interferon alfa-2a (*Roferon-A*)	*Leukemia:* 3 million IU/d SC or IM for 16–24 wk *Kaposi's sarcoma:* 36 million IU/d SC or IM for 10–12 wk	Treatment of leukemias, Kaposi's sarcoma in adults
Ⓟ interferon alfa-2b (*Intron-A*)	Adult: dosage varies widely based on indication Pediatric: for hepatitis B, adjust adult dosage to weight	Treatment of leukemias, Kaposi's sarcoma, warts, hepatitis B, malignant melanoma
interferon alfacon-1 (*Infergen*)	9 μg SC as a single dose three times per week for 24 wk	Treatment of chronic hepatitis C in adults
interferon alfa-n1 lymphoblastoid (*Wellferon*)	3 million IU SC or IM three times per week for 48 wk	Treatment of chronic hepatitis C in adults
interferon alfa-n3 (*Alferon N*)	250,000 IU intralesionally two times per week for 8 wk	Intralesional treatment of warts; AIDS-related complex, AIDS orphan drug indication
interferon beta-1a (*Avonex*)	30 μg IM once a week	Treatment of multiple sclerosis in adults
interferon beta-1b (*Betaseron*)	0.25 mg SC every other day; discontinue if disease is unremitting >6 mo	Treatment of multiple sclerosis in adults
interferon gamma-1b (*Actimmune*)	50 μg/m² SC three times per week	Treatment of serious, chronic granulomatous disease in adults
peginterferon alfa-2b (*Peg-Intron*)	1 μg/kg SC once a week for 1 yr	Treatment of chronic hepatitis C in adults

cytokines. Aldesleukin (*Proleukin*) is a human interleukin produced by recombinant DNA technology using *E. coli* bacteria. Oprelvekin (*Neumega*) is a newer agent, released in 1998, that is also produced by DNA technology.

Therapeutic Actions and Indications
Natural interleukin-2 is produced by helper T cells to activate cellular immunity and inhibit tumor growth by increasing lymphocyte numbers and their activity. When interleukins are administered, there are increases in the number of natural killer cells and lymphocytes, in cytokine activity, and in the number of circulating platelets. Interleukins are indicated for the treatment of specific renal carcinomas (aldesleukin, which is also being investigated for use in the treatment of AIDS and AIDS related disorders) and for the prevention of severe thrombocytopenia (an abnormal decrease in the number of platelets) after myelosuppressive chemotherapy in select patients (oprelvekin).

Pharmacokinetics
The interleukins are rapidly distributed after injection and are primarily cleared from the body by the kidney. They were shown to be embryocidal and teratogenic in animal studies and should not be used during pregnancy. Use of barrier contraceptives is recommended for women of childbearing age who require one of these drugs. It is not clear whether the drugs cross into breast milk, but it is recom-

mended that they not be used during lactation and that another method of feeding the baby be chosen because of the potential for adverse effects in the baby.

Contraindications and Cautions
Interleukins are contraindicated in the presence of any allergy to an interleukin or *E. coli*–produced product and during pregnancy and lactation. Caution should be used with renal, liver, or cardiovascular impairment because of the adverse effects of the drugs.

Adverse Effects
The adverse effects associated with the interleukins can be attributed to their effect on the body during inflammation (eg, lethargy, myalgia, arthralgia, fatigue, fever). Respiratory difficulties, CNS changes, and cardiac arrhythmias also have been reported, and the patient should be monitored for these effects and the drug stopped if they do occur.

T- and B-cell Modulator
The drug levamisole (*Ergamisol*) is an immune stimulant that restores suppressed immune function in certain situations.

Therapeutic Actions and Indications
Levamisole stimulates B cells, which in turn stimulate antibody formation, enhance T cell activity, and increase the ac-

DRUGS IN FOCUS

Interleukins

Drug Name	Dosage/Route	Usual Indications
℗ aldesleukin (*Proleukin*)	Two 5-d cycles of 600,000 IU/kg IV q8h given over 15 min	Treatment of specific renal carcinomas in adults
oprelvelkin (*Neumega*)	50 µg/kg per day SC starting 1 d after chemotherapy and continuing for 14–21 d	Prevention of severe thrombocytopenia after myelosuppressive chemotherapy

tivity of both monocytes and macrophages. Levamisole is indicated for the treatment of Dukes stage C colon cancer after surgical resection and in conjunction with fluorouracil therapy. With further research, the indications may be expanded to include other carcinomas.

Pharmacokinetics

Levamisole is readily absorbed from the gastrointestinal (GI) tract, reaching peak levels in 1.5 to 2 hours. It is extensively metabolized in the liver and excreted in the urine, with a half life of 16 hours. Levamisole was embryotoxic in animal studies and should not be used during pregnancy. Women of child-bearing age should be advised to use barrier contraceptives. It is not known whether levamisole crosses into breast milk, but because of the potentially severe adverse effects it could have on a neonate, it is recommended that the drug not be used during lactation.

Contraindications and Cautions

Levamisole is contraindicated in the presence of any known allergy to levamisole or its components, and in pregnancy and lactation because of possible adverse effects to the neonate.

Adverse Effects

The most common adverse effects seen with levamisole are related to immune stimulation (so-called flu-like effects: fatigue, lethargy, myalgia, arthralgia, fever). Other adverse effects that have been reported include GI upset, nausea, taste perversions, and diarrhea; dizziness, headache, and depression; bone marrow depression; dermatitis; and hair loss.

Clinically Important Drug–Drug Interactions

There is a possibility of a disulfiram-type reaction if this drug is combined with alcohol. Patients should be cautioned to avoid this combination. There also is a possibility of increased phenytoin levels and toxicity if levamisole is combined with phenytoin. If such a combination cannot be avoided, phenytoin levels should be monitored and appropriate dosage reductions made.

Nursing Considerations for Patients Receiving Immune Stimulants

Assessment: History and Examination

Screen for any of the following conditions, which would contraindicate or require cautious use of the drug: known allergies to any of these drugs or their components; pregnancy or lactation; hepatic, renal, or cardiac disease; bone marrow depression; and CNS disorders, including seizures.

Include screening for baseline status before beginning therapy and for any potential adverse effects: presence of any skin lesions; weight; temperature; orientation, reflexes; pulse, blood pressure, electrocardiogram (ECG), heart rhythm; liver evaluation; complete blood count (CBC), liver and renal function tests; and assessment of condition being treated.

DRUGS IN FOCUS

T- and B-Cell Modulator

Drug Name	Dosage/Route	Usual Indications
℗ levamisole (*Ergamisol*)	50 mg PO q8h given with fluorouracil	Treatment of Dukes stage C colon cancer after resection in adults

Nursing Diagnoses

The patient receiving immune stimulants may have the following nursing diagnoses related to drug therapy:

- Acute Pain related to CNS, GI, and flu-like effects
- Imbalanced Nutrition: Less than Body Requirements, related to flu-like effects
- Anxiety related to diagnosis and drug therapy
- Deficient Knowledge regarding drug therapy

Implementation

- Arrange for laboratory tests before and periodically during therapy, including CBC and differential, *to monitor for drug effects and adverse effects.*
- Administer drug as indicated; instruct the patient and a significant other if injections are required, *to ensure that the drug will be given even if the patient is not able to administer it.*
- Monitor for severe reactions and *arrange to discontinue drug immediately if they occur.*
- Arrange for supportive care and comfort measures for flu-like symptoms (eg, rest, environmental control, acetaminophen) *to help the patient cope with the drug effects.* Ensure that the patient is well hydrated during therapy *to prevent severe adverse effects.*
- Instruct female patients in the use of barrier contraceptives *to avoid pregnancy during therapy, because of the potential for adverse effects on the fetus.*
- Provide thorough patient teaching, including measures to avoid adverse effects, warning signs of problems, and proper administration, *to increase knowledge about drug therapy and to increase compliance with the drug regimen.*
- Offer support and encouragement *to deal with the diagnosis and the drug regimen.*

Evaluation

- Monitor patient response to the drug (improvement in condition being treated).
- Monitor for adverse effects (flu-like symptoms, GI upset, CNS changes, bone marrow depression).
- Evaluate the effectiveness of the teaching plan (patient can name drug, dosage, adverse effects to watch for, specific measures to avoid adverse effects).
- Monitor the effectiveness of comfort measures and compliance to the regimen.

IMMUNE SUPPRESSANTS

Immune suppressants often are used in conjunction with corticosteroids, which block the inflammatory reaction and decrease initial damage to cells. They are especially beneficial in cases of organ transplantation and in the treatment of autoimmune diseases. The immune suppressants include T-and B-cell suppressors and **monoclonal antibodies**—antibodies produced by a single clone of B cells that react with specific antigens.

T- and B-cell Suppressors

There are several T- and B-cell immune suppressors available for use. Only one, cyclosporine (*Sandimmune, Neoral*), is used to suppress rejection in a variety of transplantation scenarios. It also is the most commonly used immune suppressant. *Neoral* is also used to treat rheumatoid arthritis and psoriasis. It is well absorbed from the GI tract, reaching peak levels in 1 to 2 hours. Cyclosporine is extensively metabolized in the liver by the cytochrome P450 system and is primarily excreted in the bile. The half-life of the drug is about 19 hours for *Sandimmune* and 8.4 hours for *Neoral*. Cyclosporine was embryotoxic in animal studies and crosses into breast milk. The drug should not be used during pregnancy or lactation, and women of child-bearing age should be advised to use barrier contraceptives.

Azathioprine (*Imuran*) is used specifically to prevent rejection in renal homotransplants and to treat rheumatoid arthritis (an autoimmune disorder) in selected patients. It is rapidly absorbed from the GI tract, reaching peak levels in 1 to 2 hours. This drug is catabolized in the liver and on red blood cells. It was highly teratogenic in animal studies and crosses into breast milk. Because of the potential effects on the neonate, the drug should not be used during pregnancy or lactation, and women of child-bearing age should be advised to use barrier contraceptives.

Glatiramer acetate (*Copaxone*) is used specifically to reduce the number of relapses in multiple sclerosis, which is thought to be related to an autoimmune reaction. Little is known about the pharmacokinetics of this drug. Some of it is immediately hydrolyzed on injection, some enters the lymph system, and some may actually reach the systemic circulation. Because it is not known whether this drug crosses the placenta or crosses into breast milk, use during pregnancy and lactation should be reserved for those situations in which the benefit to the mother clearly outweighs the potential risk to the neonate.

Mycophenolate (*CellCept*) is an oral drug that is used with cyclosporine and corticosteroids to prevent organ rejection after renal or heart transplantation. It is readily absorbed and immediately metabolized to its active metabolite. Most of the metabolized drug is then excreted in the urine. Caution should be used if serious renal impairment exists, and the dosage should be lowered. Mycophenolate was teratogenic in animal studies, and women of child-bearing age should be advised to use barrier contraceptives whenever this drug is used. It is not known whether mycophenolate crosses into human breast milk, but because of the potential for adverse effects in the baby, it should not be used during lactation.

Sirolimus (*Rapamune*) is used to prevent organ rejection in patients receiving renal transplants and should be used with cyclosporine and corticosteroids. It is being studied for use in the treatment of psoriasis. Sirolimus is rapidly absorbed from the GI tract, reaching peak levels in 1 hour. It is extensively metabolized in the liver, partly by the cytochrome P450 system. Reduced dosage may be needed if hepatic impairment is present. The drug is then excreted primarily in the feces. Sirolimus was embryotoxic in animal studies and should not be used during pregnancy unless the benefit to the mother clearly outweighs the potential risks to the fetus. It is not known whether sirolimus crosses into breast milk, but because of the potential for serious adverse effects in the baby, the drug should not be used during lactation.

Tacrolimus (*Prograf*) is used to prevent liver transplant rejection. This drug is rapidly absorbed from the GI tract, reaching peak levels in 1.5 to 3.5 hours. It is extensively metabolized in the liver by the cytochrome P450 system and is excreted in the urine. Lower doses of the drug may be needed in the presence of hepatic or renal impairment, which would interfere with the metabolism and excretion of the drug. Tacrolimus crosses the placenta and has been associated with hyperkalemia and renal dysfunction in the fetus. Avoid use in pregnancy unless the benefit to the mother clearly outweighs the risk to the fetus. It crosses into breast milk and is contraindicated during lactation because of the potential for serious adverse effects on the baby.

Ongoing drug studies continue to explore unlabeled uses of many of these agents to prevent other transplant rejections.

Therapeutic Actions and Indications

The exact mechanism of action of the T- and B-cell suppressors is not clearly understood. It has been shown that they do block antibody production by B cells, inhibit suppressor and helper T cells, and modify the release of interleukins and of T-cell growth factor (see Figure 17–1).

The T- and B-cell suppressors are indicated for the prevention and treatment of specific transplant rejections. Azathioprine has also been approved for the treatment of rheumatoid arthritis. Many of the T- and B-cell suppressors are used to treat a variety of autoimmune disorders and other transplant rejections as unlabeled uses for the drugs.

Contraindications and Cautions

The use of T- and B-cell suppressors is contraindicated in the presence of any known allergy to the drug or its components, and during pregnancy and lactation because of the potential adverse effects on the neonate. Caution should be used with renal or hepatic impairment, which could interfere with the metabolism or excretion of the drug, and in the presence of known neoplasms, which potentially could spread with immune system suppression.

Adverse Effects

Patients receiving these drugs are at increased risk for infection and for the development of neoplasms because of the blockage of the immune system. Other potentially danger-

CASE STUDY

Holistic Care for a Transplantation Patient

After waiting on a transplant list for 4 years, T. B. received a human heart transplant to replace his heart, which had been severely damaged by cardiomyopathy. Before getting the transplant, T. B. was bedridden, on oxygen, and near death. The transplant has given T. B. a "new lease on life," and he is determined to do everything possible to stay healthy and improve his activity and lifestyle. Currently, he is being maintained on cyclosporine, mycophenolate, and steroids.

CRITICAL THINKING

What important teaching facts would help T. B. to achieve his goal? *Think about the psychological impact of the heart transplant and the "new lease on life."*
What activity, dietary, and supportive guidelines should be outlined for T. B?
What impact will T. B.'s drug regimen have on his plans?
How can all of the aspects of his condition and medical care be coordinated to give T. B. the best possible advantages for the future?

DISCUSSION

T. B.'s medical regimen will include a very complicated combination of rehabilitation, nutrition, drug therapy, and prevention. T. B. should know the risks of transplant rejection and the measures that will be used to prevent it. He also should know the names of his medications and when to take them, the signs and symptoms of rejection to watch for, and what to do if they occur. T. B. must understand the need to prevent exposure to infections and the precautions required, such as avoiding crowded areas and people with known diseases, avoiding injury, and taking steps to maintain cleanliness and avoid infection if an injury occurs.

The medications that T. B. is taking may cause him to experience flu-like symptoms, which can be quite unpleasant. A restful, quiet environment may help to decrease his stress. Acetaminophen may be ordered to help alleviate the fever, aches, and pains.

T. B. also may experience gastrointestinal upset, nausea, and vomiting related to drug effects. A nutritional consultation may be requested to help T. B. maintain a good nutritional state. Frequent mouth care and small, frequent meals may help. Proper nutrition will help T. B. to recover, heal, and maintain his health.

T. B.'s primary health care provider will need to work with the transplantation surgeon, rehabilitation team, nutritionist, and cardiologist to coordinate a total program that will help T. B. to avoid problems and make the most of his transplanted heart.

ous adverse effects include hepatotoxicity, renal toxicity, renal dysfunction, and pulmonary edema. Patients may experience headache, tremors, secondary infections such as acne, GI upset, diarrhea, and hypertension.

Clinically Important Drug–Drug Interactions

There is an increased risk of toxicity if these drugs are combined with other drugs that are hepatotoxic or nephrotoxic. Extreme care should be used if such combinations are necessary. Other reported drug–drug interactions are drug-specific (see your nursing drug guide).

Monoclonal Antibodies

Antibodies that attach to specific receptor sites are being developed to respond to very specific situations. In 1998 alone, six new monoclonal antibodies were marketed, exemplifying the rapid pace with which these agents are being developed and approved for clinical use.

Therapeutic Actions and Indications

Muromonab-CD3 (*Orthoclone OKT3*), the first monoclonal antibody approved for use, is a T cell–specific antibody that is available as an intravenous (IV) agent. It reacts as an antibody to human T cells, disabling the T cells and acting as an immune suppressor (see Figure 17–1). Muromonab is indicated for the treatment of acute allograft rejection in patients undergoing renal transplantation. It also is indicated for the treatment of steroid-resistant acute allograft rejection in those receiving heart or liver transplants.

Alemtuzumab (*Campath*) is a monoclonal antibody that is specific for lymphocyte receptor sites; it is used for the treatment of B-cell chronic lymphocytic leukemia in patients who have been treated with alkylating agents and have failed fludarabine therapy.

Basiliximab (*Simulect*) and daclizumab (*Zenapax*) are monoclonal antibodies to interleukin-2 receptor sites on activated T lymphocytes; they react with those sites and block

---

DRUGS IN FOCUS
T- and B-Cell Suppressors

Drug Name	Dosage/Route	Usual Indications
azathioprine (*Imuran*)	Adult: 3–5 mg/kg/d PO for prevention of rejection; maintenance: 1–3 mg/kg per day PO Rheumatoid arthritis: 1–2.5 mg/kg per day PO Reduce dosage with renal impairment Pediatric: 3–5 mg/kg per day IV or PO to prevent rejection; maintenance: 1–3 mg/kg per day PO	Prevention of rejection in renal homotransplants; treatment of rheumatoid arthritis
Ⓟ cyclosporine (*Sandimmune*) (*Neoral*)	15 mg/kg PO as a single oral dose 4–12 h before transplantation, then 5–10 mg/kg per day PO Pediatric: larger doses may be needed to achieve therapeutic levels 9–15 mg/kg PO as a single oral dose 4–12 h before transplantation, then 5–10 mg/kg per day PO—titrate down Rheumatoid arthritis: 2.5 mg/kg per day PO in two divided doses Psoriasis: 2.5 mg/kg PO b.i.d.	Suppression of rejection in a variety of transplant situations; rheumatoid arthritis, psoriasis (*Neoral*)
glatiramer acetate (*Copaxone*)	20 mg/d SC	Reduction of the number of relapses in multiple sclerosis in adults
mycophenolate (*CellCept*)	1–1.5 mg PO b.i.d.; may be started IV during transplantation, with switch to oral route as soon as possible 6 mg PO as soon after transplant as possible; then 2 mg per day PO	Prevention of rejection after renal or heart transplantation in adults
sirolimus (*Rapamune*)	Children <13 yr: 3 mg/m² PO loading dose, then 1 mg/m² per day PO	Prevention of rejection after renal transplantation
tacrolimus (*Prograf*)	0.15–0.3 mg/kg per day PO in two divided doses; may begin as continuous IV infusion of 0.05–0.1 mg/kg per day, with switch to oral form as soon as possible Pediatric: may require higher doses to achieve therapeutic levels	Prevention of rejection after liver transplantation

cellular response to allograft transplants. They are approved for use in preventing renal transplant rejection.

Ibritumomab (*Zevalin*) is an antibody to specific sites on activated B lymphocytes. It is used for the treatment of follicular B-cell non-Hodgkin's lymphoma in patients no longer responding to rituximab. Ibritumomab is used in combination with radiation therapy.

Infliximab (*Remicade*) is a monoclonal antibody to tumor necrosis factor. It is used to decrease the signs and symptoms of Crohn's disease in patients who do not respond to conventional therapy. It also is approved for use with methotrexate in the treatment of progressing moderate to severe rheumatoid arthritis.

Omalizumab (*Xolair*) is a monoclonal antibody used for the treatment of asthma with a strong allergic component, and for patients with seasonal rhinitis that is not well controlled with traditional medications. It is an antibody to immunoglobulin E, an important factor in allergic reactions.

Palivizumab (*Synagis*) is a monoclonal antibody to the antigenic site on respiratory syncytial virus (RSV); it inactivates that virus. It is used to prevent RSV disease in high-risk children.

Rituximab (*Rituxan*) is a monoclonal antibody to specific sites on activated B lymphocytes; it is used in the treatment of follicular B-cell non-Hodgkin's lymphoma.

Trastuzumab (*Herceptin*) is a monoclonal antibody that reacts with human epidermal growth factor receptor 2 (HER2), a genetic defect that is seen in certain metastatic breast cancers. It is used in the treatment of metastatic breast cancer in tumors that overexpress HER2.

Pharmacokinetics

The monoclonal antibodies must be injected. They are processed by the body like other antibodies. It is not known whether they cross the placenta or enter breast milk, but because of the potential for adverse effects, they should not be used during pregnancy or lactation unless the benefit clearly outweighs the potential risk to the fetus.

Contraindications and Cautions

Monoclonal antibodies are contraindicated in the presence of any known allergy to the drug or to murine products, and in the presence of fluid overload. They should be used cautiously with fever (treat the fever before beginning therapy), previous administration of the monoclonal antibody (serious hypersensitivity reactions can occur with repeat administration), and pregnancy or lactation.

Adverse Effects

The most serious adverse effects associated with the use of monoclonal antibodies are acute pulmonary edema (dyspnea, chest pain, wheezing), which is associated with severe fluid retention, and cytokine release syndrome (flu-like symptoms than can progress to third-spacing of fluids and shock). Other adverse effects that can be anticipated include fever, chills, malaise, myalgia, nausea, diarrhea, vomiting, and increased susceptibility to infection.

Clinically Important Drug–Drug Interactions

Use caution and arrange to reduce the dosage if a monoclonal antibody is combined with any other immunosuppressant drug, because severe immune suppression with increased infections and neoplasms can occur.

Nursing Considerations for Patients Receiving Immune Suppressants

Assessment: History and Examination

Screen for the following, which could be contraindications or cautions to use of the drug: any known allergies to any of these drugs or their components; pregnancy or lactation; renal or hepatic impairment; and history of neoplasm.

Include screening for baseline status before beginning therapy and for any potential adverse effects: presence of any skin lesions; weight; temperature; orientation, reflexes; pulse, blood pressure, ECG; liver evaluation; CBC, liver, and renal function tests; and assessment of condition being treated.

Nursing Diagnoses

The patient receiving immune suppressants may have the following nursing diagnoses related to drug therapy:

- Acute Pain related to CNS, GI, and flu-like effects
- Risk for Infection related to immune suppression
- Imbalanced Nutrition: Less than Body Requirements, related to nausea and vomiting
- Deficient Knowledge regarding drug therapy

Implementation

- Arrange for laboratory tests before and periodically during therapy, including CBC, differential, and liver and renal function tests, *to monitor for drug effects and adverse effects.*
- Administer the drug as indicated; instruct the patient and a significant other if injections are required, *to ensure proper administration of the drug.*
- Protect the patient from exposure to infections and maintain strict aseptic technique for any invasive procedures *to prevent infections during immunosuppression.*
- Arrange for supportive care and comfort measures for flu-like symptoms (rest, environmental control, acetaminophen) *to decrease patient discomfort and increase compliance.*
- Monitor nutritional status during therapy; provide small, frequent meals, mouth care, and nutritional consultation as necessary *to ensure adequate nutrition.*
- Instruct female patients in the use of barrier contraceptives *to avoid pregnancy during therapy, because of the risk of adverse effects to the fetus.*
- Provide thorough patient teaching, including measures to avoid adverse effects, warning signs of problems, and proper administration *to increase knowledge about drug therapy and to increase compliance with drug regimen* (see Patient Teaching Checklist: Immune Suppressants).

DRUGS IN FOCUS
Monoclonal Antibodies

Drug Name	Dosage/Route	Usual Indications
alemtuzumab (*Campath*)	3 mg/d IV as a 2-h infusion; increase slowly to maintenance dose of 30 mg/d IV three times per week for up to 12 wk.	Treatment of B-cell chronic lymphocytic leukemia in patients who have been treated with alkylating agents and have failed fludarabine therapy
basiliximab (*Simulect*)	20 mg IV twice—first dose within 24 h of transplantation then at 4 d	Prevention of renal transplant rejection
daclizumab (*Zenapax*)	1 mg/kg IV for 5 doses, the first within 24 h of transplantation, and the last within 14 d after transplantation	Prevention of renal transplant rejection
ibritumomab (*Zevalin*)	2 mg antibody labeled with 0.3 or 0.4 mCi/kg yttrium-90 IV	Treatment of B-cell non-Hodgkin's lymphoma in conjunction with rituxivmab
infliximab (*Remicade*)	5 mg/kg IV over 2 h; may be repeated at 2 wk and 6 wk	To decrease the signs and symptoms of Crohn's disease in patients who do not respond to other therapy
Ⓟ muromonab-CD3 (*Orthoklone OKT3*)	5 mg/d IV for 10–14 d infused as an IV bolus over <1 min	Prevention of renal transplant rejection; treatment of steroid-resistant rejection of heart and liver transplants in adults
omaluzimab (*Xolair*)	0.15 mg/kg per day SC	Treatment of asthma with a very strong allergic component and seasonal allergic rhinitis not well controlled with traditional medications
palivizumab (*Syangis*)	15 mg/kg IM as a single dose at the start of RSV season	Prevention of serious respiratory syncytial virus (RSV) infection in high-risk children
rituximab (*Rituxan*)	375 mg/m² IV once weekly for 4 doses	Treatment of relapsed follicular B-cell non-Hodgkin's lymphoma
trastuzumab (*Herceptin*)	4 mg/kg IV over 90 min, then 2 mg/kg IV once a week over at least 30 min	Treatment of metastatic breast cancer with tumors that overexpress human epidermal growth factor receptor 2 (HER2)

GENDER CONSIDERATIONS
Immune Modulators and Pregnancy

Generally, immune modulators are contraindicated for use during pregnancy and lactation, largely because these drugs have been associated with fetal abnormalities, increased maternal and fetal infections, and suppressed immune responses in nursing babies. Female patients should be informed of the risk of using these drugs during pregnancy and receive counseling in the use of barrier contraceptives. (The use of barrier contraceptives is advised because the effects of oral contraceptives may be altered by liver changes or by changes in the body's immune response, potentially resulting in unexpected pregnancy.)

If a patient taking immune modulators becomes pregnant or decides that she wants to become pregnant, she should discuss this with her health care provider and review the risks associated with use of the drug or drugs being taken. The monoclonal antibodies should be used with caution during pregnancy and lactation. Because long-term studies of most of these drugs are not yet available, it may be prudent to advise patients taking these drugs to avoid pregnancy if possible.

• Offer support and encouragement *to help the patient deal with the diagnosis and the drug regimen.*

Evaluation

• Monitor patient response to the drug (prevention of transplant rejection; improvement in autoimmune disease or cancer; prevention of RSV disease; improvement in signs and symptoms of Crohn's disease or rheumatoid arthritis).
• Monitor for adverse effects (flu-like symptoms, GI upset, increased infections, neoplasms, fluid overload).
• Evaluate the effectiveness of the teaching plan (patient can name drug, dosage, adverse effects to watch for, specific measures to avoid adverse effects).
• Monitor the effectiveness of comfort measures and compliance to the regimen (see Nursing Care Guide: Immune Suppressants).

▢◼◗◼ WEB LINKS

Health care providers and patients may want to consult the following Internet sources:

PATIENT TEACHING CHECKLIST
Immune Suppressants

Create customized patient teaching materials for a specific immune suppressant from the CD-ROM. Patient teaching should stress the following points for drugs within this class:

• An immune suppressant is given to depress your body's immune system and prevent rejection of your transplanted tissue.
• You should never stop taking your drug without consulting your health care provider. If your prescription is low or you are unable to take the medication for *any* reason, notify your health care provider.

Some of the following adverse effects may occur:

• *Nausea, vomiting*—Taking the drug with food and eating small, frequent meals may help.
• *Diarrhea*—This may not decrease; ensure ready access to bathroom facilities.
• *Flu-like symptoms*—Rest and a cool, peaceful environment may help; acetaminophen may be ordered to help relieve this discomfort.
• *Skin rash, mouth sores*—Frequent skin and mouth care may ease these effects.
• You will have an increased susceptibility to infection because your body's normal defenses will be decreased. You should avoid crowded places and people with known infections. If you notice any signs of illness or infection, notify your health care provider immediately.
• This drug should not be taken during pregnancy. Use of a barrier contraceptive is recommended. If you wish to become pregnant, or find that you are pregnant, consult with your health care provider immediately.
• Tell any doctor, nurse, or other health care provider that you are taking this drug.
• You will need to have periodic blood tests and perhaps biopsies while you are being treated with this drug.
• Report any of the following to your health care provider: unusual bleeding or bruising; fever, sore throat, mouth sores; fatigue; any sign of infection; injury.
• Keep this drug out of the reach of children. Do not give this medication to anyone else or take any similar medication that has not been prescribed for you.

This Teaching Checklist reflects general patient teaching guidelines. It is not meant to be a substitute for drug-specific teaching information, which is available in nursing drug guides.

Information on cancers (including leukemias and Kaposi's sarcoma) and treatments:
http://www.oncolink.upenn.edu
Information on multiple sclerosis (updates, treatments, contact groups):
http://www.nmss.org
Information on drug research and development, new approvals, alerts, and warnings:
http://www.fda.gov

CHAPTER SUMMARY

• Immune stimulants boost the immune system when it is exhausted from fighting off prolonged invasion or needs help fighting a specific pathogen or cancer cell.
• Immune suppressants are used to depress the immune system when needed to prevent transplant rejection or severe tissue damage associated with autoimmune disease.
• Interferons are naturally released from cells in the response to viral invasion; they are used to treat various cancers and warts.
• Interleukins stimulate cellular immunity and inhibit tumor growth; they are used to treat very specific cancers.
• Adverse effects seen with immune stimulants are related to the immune response (flu-like symptoms including fever, myalgia, lethargy, arthralgia, and fatigue).
• Immune suppressants are used in a variety of specific transplantation situations. Research is ongoing to extend the use of various immune suppressants to other situations, including various autoimmune disorders.
• Increased susceptibility to infection and increased risk of neoplasm are potentially dangerous effects associated with the use of immune suppressants. Patients need to be protected from infection, injury, and invasive procedures.

Review Questions

1. Immune suppressants are used in all of the following except
   a. treatment of transplant rejection.
   b. treatment of autoimmune disease.
   c. reduction of the number of relapses in multiple sclerosis.
   d. treatment of aggressive cancers.
2. Interferon alfa-n3 (*Alferon N*) would be the drug of choice for
   a. treatment of leukemias.
   b. treatment of multiple sclerosis.
   c. intralesional treatment of warts.
   d. treatment of Kaposi's sarcoma.
3. Patient teaching of a patient receiving an interferon would include
   a. proper use of oral contraceptives.
   b. use of aspirin to control adverse effects.
   c. importance of exercise and cardiovascular workouts.
   d. proper methods for drawing up and injecting the drug.
4. Patients who are receiving an immune stimulant may experience any of the clinical signs of immune response activity, including
   a. flu-like symptoms (arthralgia, myalgia, fatigue, anorexia).
   b. diarrhea.
   c. constipation.
   d. headache.
5. Organ transplants are often rejected by the body because the T cells recognize the transplanted cells as foreign and try to destroy them. Treatment with an immune suppressant would
   a. activate antibody production.
   b. stimulate interleukin release.

NURSING CARE GUIDE

Immune Suppressants

Assessment	Nursing Diagnoses	Implementation	Evaluation
HISTORY Allergies to any immune suppressant, pregnancy, lactation, renal or hepatic impairment, history of neoplasm	Acute Pain related to CNS, GI, flu-like symptoms Risk for Infection, related to immune suppression Imbalanced Nutrition: Less than Body Requirements, related to GI effects Deficient Knowledge regarding drug therapy	Arrange for laboratory tests before and periodically during therapy. Administer drug as indicated. Protect patient from exposure to infection. Provide supportive and comfort measures to deal with adverse effects. Monitor nutritional status and intervene as needed. Provide patient teaching regarding drug name, dosage, adverse effects and precautions, warning signs to report.	Evaluate drug effects: prevention of transplant rejection; improvement of autoimmune disease. Monitor for adverse effects: infection, flu-like symptoms, GI upset, fluid overload, neoplasm. Monitor for drug–drug interactions as indicated for each drug. Evaluate effectiveness of patient teaching program. Evaluate effectiveness of comfort and safety measures.
PHYSICAL EXAMINATION Neurological: orientation, reflexes, affect General: temperature, weight CV: pulse, cardiac auscultation, BP, edema, ECG GI: liver evaluation Lab tests: CBC, liver and renal function tests, condition being treated			

   c. stimulate thymus secretions.

   d. block the inflammatory reaction and initial damage to the transplanted cells.

6. Anticipated adverse effects that occur when the immune system is suppressed include all of the following except

   a. development of cancers.

   b. increased risk of infection.

   c. cardiac standstill.

   d. development of secondary infections.

7. A patient taking cyclosporine to prevent rejection of a renal transplant would not be instructed to

   a. use barrier contraceptives to avoid pregnancy.

   b. use acetaminophen, rest, and a cool environment to cope with the flu-like illness that may occur.

   c. take the drug with food and eat small, frequent meals to avoid GI problems.

   d. stop taking the drug if GI upset or fever occurs.

8. Monoclonal antibodies are available for use in treating

   a. warts.

   b. herpes zoster.

   c. metastatic breast cancers with tumors that overexpress HER2.

   d. Kaposi's sarcoma.

BIBLIOGRAPHY

Bullock, B. L. (2000). *Focus on pathophysiology.* Philadelphia: Lippincott Williams & Wilkins.

Gilman, A., Hardman, J. G., & Limbird, L. E. (Eds.) (2002). *Goodman and Gilman's the pharmacological basis of therapeutics* (10th ed.). New York: McGraw-Hill.

Karch, A. M. (2002). *2003 Lippincott's nursing drug guide.* Philadelphia: Lippincott Williams & Wilkins.

Drug facts and comparisons. (2002). St. Louis: Facts & Comparisons.

The medical letter on drugs and therapeutics. (2002). New Rochelle, NY: Medical Letter.

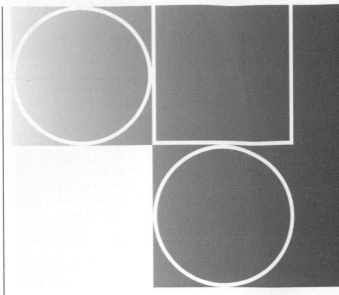

CHAPTER

18

Vaccines and Sera

234

Key Terms

active immunity
antitoxins
immune sera
immunization
passive immunity
serum sickness
vaccine

Immune Sera

cytomegalovirus immune globulin

hepatitis B immune globulin

Ⓟ immune globulin intramuscular

immune globulin intravenous

lymphocyte immune globulin

rabies immune globulin

respiratory syncytial virus immune
  globulin

RHO immune globulin

RHO immune globulin, microdose

tetanus immune globulin

varicella zoster immune globulin

Antitoxins and Antivenins

Ⓟ antivenin

Black Widow spider antivenin

crotalidae polyvalent immune fab

Vaccines, immune sera, and antitoxins are usually referred to as *biologicals*. They are used to stimulate the production of antibodies, to provide preformed antibodies to facilitate an immune reaction, or to react specifically with the toxins produced by an invading pathogen. Prudent, prophylactic medical care requires the routine administration of certain vaccines to prevent diseases before they occur.

IMMUNITY

Immunity is a state of relative resistance to a disease that develops after exposure to the specific disease-causing agent. People are not born with immunity to diseases, so they must acquire immunity by stimulating B-cell clones to form plasma cells, and then antibodies.

Active immunity occurs when the body recognizes a foreign protein and begins producing antibodies to react with that specific protein or antigen. After plasma cells are formed to produce antibodies, specific memory cells that produce the same antibodies are created. If the specific foreign protein is introduced into the body again, these memory cells react immediately to release antibodies. This type of immunity is thought to be lifelong.

Passive immunity occurs when preformed antibodies are injected into the system and react with a specific antigen. These antibodies come from animals that have been infected with the disease or from humans who have had the disease and have developed antibodies. The circulating antibodies act the same as those produced from plasma cells, recognizing the foreign protein and attaching to it, rendering it harmless. Unlike active immunity, passive immunity is limited. It lasts only as long as the circulating antibodies last, because the body does not produce its own antibodies. In some cases, the host human produces antibodies to the circulating injected antibodies. This results in **serum sickness,** a massive immune reaction. Signs and symptoms of serum sickness include fever, arthritis, flank pain, myalgia, and arthralgia.

IMMUNIZATION

Immunization is the process of artificially stimulating active immunity by exposing the body to weakened or less toxic proteins associated with specific disease-causing organisms. The goal is to cause an immune response without having the patient suffer the full course of a disease. Children routinely are immunized against many infections that were once quite devastating (Figure 18–1). For example, smallpox was one of the first diseases against which children were immunized. Today, it has virtually been wiped out in the world. Diphtheria, pertussis, tetanus, haemophilus B, hepatitis B, hepatitis A, chickenpox, polio, measles, mumps, and rubella are all standard childhood immunizations today. The use of vaccines is not without controversy. Severe reactions, although rare, have occurred. The central reporting of adverse effects or suspected adverse effects may help to clarify concerns about reactions to immunizations (Box 18–1). Adults may also require immunizations in certain situations: exposure, travel to an area endemic in a disease they have not had and have not been immunized against, occupations that are considered high risk (see Figure 18–1). People who receive allergy shots to help them cope with the signs and symptoms of allergic reactions are receiving antigenic proteins that stimulate antibody production to prevent the allergic response (Box 18–2).

VACCINES

The word **vaccine** comes from the Latin word for smallpox, *vaccinia*. Vaccines are immunizations containing weakened or altered protein antigens that stimulate formation of antibodies against a specific disease (Figure 18–2). They are used to promote active immunity.

Box 18–3 discusses vaccines and the use of biological weapons.

Vaccines can be made from chemically inactivated microorganisms or from live, weakened viruses or bacteria. Toxoids are vaccines that are made from the toxins produced by the microorganism. The toxins are altered so that they are no longer poisonous but still have the recognizable protein antigen that will stimulate antibody production.

The particular vaccine that is used depends on the possible exposure a person will have to a particular disease and the age of the patient. Some vaccines are used only in children, and some cannot be used in infants. Some vaccines require booster doses—doses that are given a few months after the initial dose to further stimulate antibody production. In many cases, antibody titers (levels of the antibody in the

Recommended Immunization Schedule, Pediatric

Vaccine	Birth	2 mo	4 mo	6 mo	12 mo	15 mo	18 mo	24 mo	4–6 y	11–12 y	14–16 y
Hepatitis B		X	X		X					0	
Hepatitis B*	X	X		X							
DPT		X	X	X			X		X		
Tetanus Booster										X	X
H. influenzae b		X	X	X	X						
Poliovirus (IPV)		X	X			X			X		
Measles, mumps, rubella					X				X	0	
Varicella						X				0	
Hepatitis A‡									X		

0—suggested timing of immunization if recommended immunizations have been missed, or given early.
* Infants born to HBsAg-positive mothers.
‡Recommended in selected areas only, check with your local Health Department.
Suggested by the Center for Disease Control (CDC) and the American Academy of Pediatrics, January, 2000

Recommendations for Adult Immunizations

Adults often need immunizations because of exposure or being in an immune-compromised state. As with children, these vaccines should not be given to patients with any previous anaphylactic reaction to any vaccine or in the presence of moderate or severe infections. these vaccines can be given with other vaccines, but separate injection sites should be used.

Vaccine/route	Recommendation	Schedule	Schedule for Those Fallen Behind
Influenza IM	All people ≥65 yr; people with chronic medical conditions; all health care workers; pregnant women who will be in 2nd or 3rd trimester during the flu season; anyone wishing to avoid the flu	October–November; any time during the flu season.	May be given any time during the flu season.
Pneumococcal IM or SC	All people >65 yr; people with chronic medical conditions; people in immune-suppressed or debilitated states	Given once as a one-time dose. May be repeated in 5 y for people in the highest risk group, or if first dose was given <65 y.	
Hepatitis B IM	High-risk adults; all adolescents	Three-dose series. Must be 4 wk between doses #1 and #2, and 8 wk between doses #2 and #3. (4 mo between dose#1 and dose #3.)	If series is delayed, do not start over. Continue series from where it was left off.
Hepatitis A IM	Adults who travel outside the United States; people with chronic liver disease, hepatitis C; IV drug users; food handlers

In many areas of the country, prevaccination titers may remove the need for this vaccine. | Two-dose series. At least 6 mo between dose #1 and dose #2. | If dose #2 is delayed, do not repeat dose #1; give dose #2 when possible. |
| Td IM | After a primary series, a booster dose every 10 years; may give a booster after 5 yrs. For wound management. | Booster every 10 yr; make sure the patient has received the 3-dose primary series. | If no primary series has been given, give dose #2 four wk after dose #1; give dose #3 6–12 mo after dose #2. |
| MMR SC | Adults born in 1957 or later and> 18n yr should receive one dose of MMR.

High-risk adults, including health care workers, college students, and international travelers should receive a second dose.

Adults born after 1957 or with a positive titer are considered immune and do not need the vaccine.

Should be spaced 4 wk apart from varicella vaccine. | Dose #2, if recommended, is given no sooner than 4 wk after dose#1. | Dose #2 may be given as early as 4 wk after dose #1 if needed. |
| Varicella SC | All susceptible adults should be vaccinated, including people living in institutional settings and non-pregnant women of childbearing age.

Reliable proof of having had chicken pox, or positive titers can be an assumption of immunity.

Should be given 4 wk apart from MMR. Should not be given to immune-compromised people. | Two-dose series. Dose #2 should be given 4–8 wk after dose #1. | Give dose #2 no sooner than 4 wk after dose #1. |
| Polio (IPV) IM or SC | Not recommended for adults >18 yr. Adults traveling to endemic areas with reported outbreaks may receive one booster dose. | | |

Adapted from the Center for Disease Control (CDC) and the Advisory Committee on Immunization Practices (ACIP). October 2001.

FIGURE 18-1. Recommended immunization schedules for adults and children. (From Karch, A. M. [2002]. *2003 Lippincott's nursing drug guide*. Philadelphia: Lippincott Williams & Wilkins.)

BOX 18-1

MMR Vaccine Links to Autism

In 2001, the U.S. Food and Drug Administration (FDA) began conducting a study to investigate published reports linking the use of measles–mumps–rubella (MMR) vaccine with the development of autism. In reviewing the case reports, there was no clear association between receiving the vaccine and developing signs of autism. Timing of the vaccination and the onset of symptoms was unclear. The media, however, continue to pursue this possible connection, raising concerns for parents about the use of vaccines in children. The FDA study will use a questionnaire to gather information about the symptoms reported and the temporal relationship between onset of these symptoms and the vaccination. A second aspect of the study will look at the specific Vaccine Adverse Event Reporting System (VAERS) reports in an effort to find out exactly how the reporter came to think that autism was related to the vaccination. The information obtained from these surveys will be used to determine a need for further research and to update and clarify educational efforts for parents.

Along the same lines, the National Institutes of Health (NIH) and the Centers for Disease Control and Prevention (CDC) have been cosponsoring a study to look at the temporal association between MMR vaccinations and the onset of autism, looking at early-onset versus regressive autism. A second phase of this study will try to duplicate earlier reports of persistent measles infections in children with documented autism versus healthy controls. It is hoped that this type of scientific study will provide more data for a possible link between the measles virus and autism. Early indications of study results seemed to point to an immune system alteration in some children with autism, but no correlation between vaccines and autism can be seen in further reports. There was an increase in febrile seizures in children with vaccines, but no link to autism related to seizures has been found.

BOX 18-2

Use of Allergenic Extracts

Many people receive "allergy shots" or injections of allergenic extracts. These extracts contain various antigens based on specific standardizations. The exact action of these extract is not completely understood, but it has been shown that after injection specific immunoglobulin G (IgG) antibodies appear in the serum. These antibodies compete with IgE for the receptor site on a specific antigen which is the cause of the allergy. (IgE is the immune globulin that is associated with allergic reactions; these antibodies react with mast cells, causing the release of histamine and other inflammatory chemicals when they have combined with the antigen). After repeated exposure to the antigens, the levels of IgG antibodies increase and the circulating levels of IgE seem to decrease, leading to less allergic response. It may take 4 to 6 months of subcutaneous injections of the allergenic extract every 3 to 14 days to achieve relief from the symptoms of the allergic reaction. The IgG levels remain high for weeks or sometimes months, but the individual response varies widely. Many people are maintained with a weekly injection once the desired response has been achieved.

serum) can be used to evaluate a person's response to an immunization and determine the need for a booster dose.

Therapeutic Actions and Indications

Vaccines stimulate active immunity in people who are at high risk for development of a particular disease. The vaccine needed for a patient depends on the exposure that person will have to the pathogen. Exposure is usually determined by where the person lives, travel plans, and work or family environment exposures. Vaccines are thought to provide lifelong immunity to the disease against which the patient is being immunized.

Contraindications and Cautions

The use of vaccines is contraindicated in the presence of immune deficiency (the vaccine could cause disease, and the body would not be able to respond as anticipated if in an immunodeficient state); during pregnancy (because of potential effects on the fetus and on the success of the pregnancy); with known allergies to any of the components of the vac-

cine (refer to each individual vaccine for specifics); or in patients who are receiving immune globulin or who have received blood or blood products within the last 3 months (a serious immune reaction could occur).

Caution should be used any time a vaccine is given to a child with a history of febrile convulsions or cerebral injury, or in any condition in which a potential fever would be dangerous. Caution also should be used in the presence of any acute infection.

Adverse Effects

Adverse effects of vaccines are associated with the immune or inflammatory reaction that is being stimulated: moderate fever, rash, malaise, chills, fretfulness, drowsiness, anorexia, vomiting, and irritability. Pain, redness, swelling, and even nodule formation at the injection site are also common. In rare instances, severe hypersensitivity reactions have been reported.

Nursing Considerations for Patients Receiving Vaccines

Assessment: History and Examination

Screen for any of the following, which could be contraindications or cautions for use of the drug: known allergies to any vaccines or to the components of the one being used; pregnancy; recent administration of immune globulin or blood products; immune deficiency; and acute infection.

Include screening for baseline status before beginning therapy and for any potential adverse effects: presence of any skin lesions; temperature; affect; range of motion; pulse, blood pressure, perfusion; respirations and adventitious sounds.

DRUG THERAPY ACROSS THE LIFESPAN

Biologicals

Children	Adults	Older Adults
Routine immunizations for children has become a standard of care in this country. Parents should receive written records of immunizations given to their children to assure continuity of care. The parent should be asked to report adverse reactions to any immunization. Sensitive children may receive divided doses of their immunizations to help prevent adverse reactions. Simple comfort measures—warm soaks at the injection site, acetaminophen to reduce fever or aches and pains, comfort from parents or caregivers—will help the child deal with the immunization experience. Parent education is a very important aspect of the immunization procedure. Parents may need reassurance and educational materials when concerns about the safety of immunizations arise.	There are a number of reasons why adults should receive certain immunizations. For example, adults who are traveling to areas with high risk for particular diseases—and who may not have previously been exposed to those diseases—are advised to be immunized. In addition, adults with chronic diseases are advised to be immunized yearly with an influenza vaccine, and once with a pneumococcal pneumonia vaccine. These vaccines provide some protection against diseases that can prove dangerous for people with chronic lung, cardiovascular, or endocrine disorders. The influenza vaccine changes yearly, depending on predictions of which flu strain might be emergent in that year. The pneumonia vaccine contains 23 strains and is believed to offer lifetime protection. Tetanus shots also are recommended for adults every 10 years, or with any injury that potentially could precipitate a tetanus infection.	Older patients are at greater risk for severe illness from influenza and pneumococcal infections. The yearly flu shot and the pneumococcal vaccine should be stressed for this group. A tetanus booster every 10 years will also help to protect older adults from exposure to that illness. Ask the patient about any adverse reaction to previous tetanus boosters, and weigh the risk against the possible exposure to tetanus. If an older patient is traveling to an area where a particular disease is endemic and the risk of exposure is great, the Centers for Disease Control and Prevention should be contacted to determine whether the appropriate vaccine is acceptable for use in the older patient.

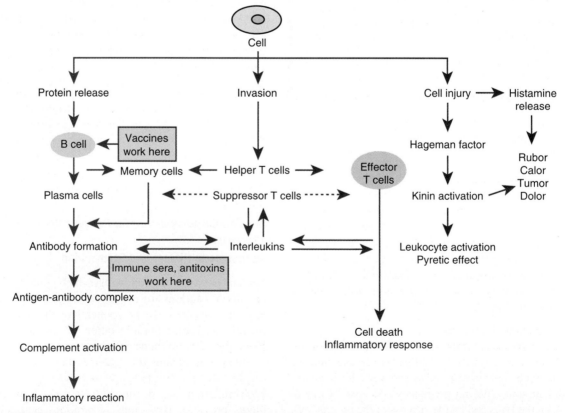

FIGURE 18–2. Sites of action of vaccines, immune sera, and antitoxins.

BOX 18-3
Vaccines and Biological Weapons

The events of September 11, 2001, and the subsequent war on terrorism have heightened awareness of several diseases that might be in development as biological weapons. Anthrax, plague, tularemia, smallpox, botulism, and a variety of viral hemorrhagic fevers are all considered to be likely weapons if biological warfare became a reality.

ANTHRAX
A vaccine is available in the United States made from inactivated cell-free filtrate of an avirulent strain of the anthrax bacillus. It is available only for military use. Active production had stopped in 1998, but production and supply issues were made high priorities. Ciprofloxacin, and, in sensitive cases, doxycycline and penicillins are effective in treating postexposure cases. The vaccine is given and repeated in 2 and 4 weeks, along with the appropriate antibiotic, to patients who have been exposed.

PLAGUE
Plague is easily spread from person to person and without treatment can progress rapidly to respiratory failure and death. There is currently no vaccine for plague; a whole-cell vaccine that was used for many years is no longer available. Research is ongoing using a pneumonic plague vaccine that has successfully protected animals. Several drugs have been found to be life-saving with plague—streptomycin, doxycycline, ciprofloxacin, and chloramphenicol.

SMALLPOX
Smallpox was considered eradicated since no new cases had been seen in 20 years. Smallpox is highly transmissable and has a 30% mortality rate in unvaccinated people. Immunization against smallpox ended in the 1970s. There is no commercially available vaccine, but some stockpiled supplies do exist. It is currently thought that the vaccine is no longer effective after 20 years, though there is no definite evidence that previously vaccinated people have no protection. After exposure, vaccination can prevent the disease if it is given within the first 3 to 4 days; if it has been 7 days or longer since exposure, the vaccine and a vaccinia immune globulin should be used, if any are available. So far no drugs are thought to be effective in treating smallpox. Early studies have, however, shown cidofovir to be effective in vitro.

TULAREMIA
Tularemia in an aerosolized form can cause systemic and respiratory illness with a 35% mortality rate. It is not passed from person to person. There is no vaccine available, but doxycycline and ciprofloxacin can be used after exposure, and gentamicin has been shown to be effective after symptoms appear.

BOTULISM
Botulism, produced by *Clostridium botulinum,* can be aerosolized or used to contaminate food. The toxin it produces causes cranial nerve palsies that can result in muscle paralysis and respiratory failure. A botulinum toxoid is available through the Centers for Disease Control

BOX 18-3
Vaccines and Biological Weapons (CONTINUED)

and Prevention for the military and high-risk workers. Antitoxin is also available for patients with specific exposures, and research is ongoing with an equine antitoxin effective against all seven serotypes of botulism that is thought to cause fewer hypersensitivity reactions than what is currently available.

VIRAL HEMORRHAGIC FEVER
Lassa, Marburg, Junin, and Ebola viruses cause hemorrhagic fevers with mortality rates as high as 90%. No vaccines are currently available for these agents, although the United States Army has had success with a vaccine for Junin. Ribavirin has been effective in some cases of Lassa fever and has been effective orally for postexposure prophylaxis. It is being studied for effectiveness with these other viruses. Currently there is no established treatment, and this area is one of the highest priorities for combating possible biological warfare.

CULTURAL CONSIDERATIONS
Pediatric Immunization

It is a well-documented concept that by preventing potentially devastating diseases, society not only can prevent unneeded suffering and even death but also can save valuable citizens for the future. Pediatric immunization has helped to greatly decrease the incidence of most childhood diseases and has prevented the complications associated with many of these diseases. In the United States, routine immunization is considered standard medical practice.

Ensuring that every child has the opportunity to receive the recommended immunizations has become a political as well as a social issue. The cost of preventing a disease that most people have never even seen may be difficult to justify to families who have trouble putting food on the table. Widespread campaigns to provide free immunizations and health screening to all children have tried to address this problem but have not been totally successful.

In addition, periodic reports of severe or even fatal reactions to standard immunizations alarm many parents about the risks of immunizations. These parents need facts as well as reassurance about modern efforts to prevent and screen for these reactions.

Public education efforts should be directed at providing parents with information about pediatric immunization, and encouraging them to act on that information. Nurses are often in the ideal position to provide this information, during prenatal visits, while screening for other problems, or even standing in line at a grocery store. It is important for nurses to be well versed on the need for standard immunizations and screening to prevent severe reactions. The Centers for Disease Control and Prevention (http://www.cdc.gov) offers current information and updates for health care providers.

DRUGS IN FOCUS
Vaccines

Drug Name	Dosage/Route	Usual Indications
Bacterial Vaccines		
BCG (*TICE BCG*)	0.2–0.3 mL percutaneously	Prevention of tuberculosis with high risk of exposure
cholera vaccine (generic)	0.2–0.5 mL IM with a 0.5-mL booster after 10 y	Immunization against cholera for areas high in cholera
P haemophilus B conjugated vaccine and hepatitis B surface antigen (*ActHIB, Comvax, HibTITER, Liquid PedvaxHIB*)	Three 0.5-mL IM injections at 2, 4, and 6 mo with 0.5 mL booster at 15–18 mo	Immunization of children against *haemophilus B* and hepatitis B infections
meningococcal polysaccharide vaccine (*Menomune-A/C/Y/W-135*)	0.5 mL SC	Immunization against meningococcal infections in endemic areas
pneumococcal vaccine, polyvalent (*Pneumovax 23, Pnu-Imune 23*)	0.5 mL SC or IM, not recommended for children <2 y of age	Immunization against pneumococcal infections
pneumococcal 7-valent conjugate vaccine (*Prevnar*)	7–11 mo: three 0.5-mg IM doses at least 4 wk apart and the last one at >1 y 12–23 mo: two 0.5-mg IM doses 2 mo apart 24 mo–9 y: one 0.5-mg IM dose	Prevention of invasive pneumococcal disease in infants and children
typhoid vaccine	Two doses of 0.5 mL SC at intervals >4 wk with booster given every 3 y, *or*	Immunization against typhoid fever
Vivotif Berna Typhim VI	One capsule PO on days 1, 3, 5, and 7	
Toxoids		
diphtheria and tetanus toxoids, combined, adsorbed (*DT, Td*)	Two IM injections of 0.5 mL at intervals of 4–8 wk, with booster of 0.5 mL in 6–12 mo and every 10 years	Immunization of adults and children >7 y of age against diphtheria and tetanus
P diphtheria and tetanus toxoids and acellular pertussis vaccine, absorbed (*DTaP*)	0.5 mL IM at 18 mo, at least 6 mo after DTwP as the fourth dose; then 0.5 mL IM at 4–6 y	Immunization of children against diphtheria, tetanus, and pertussis as the fourth and fifth doses of the immunization series
Viral Vaccines		
hepatitis A vaccine, inactivated (*Havrix, Vaqta*)	Adult: 1 mL IM with a booster dose in 6–12 mo Pediatric: 0.5 mL IM with a repeat dose in 6–12 mo	Immunization of adults and children against hepatitis A infection
hepatitis A vaccine, inactivated, with hepatitis B recombinant vaccine (*Twinrix*)	1 mL IM followed by booster doses at 1 mo and 6 mo	Immunization against hepatitis A and hepatitis B infections in people ≥18 y of age
hepatitis B vaccine (*Energix-B, Recombivax-HB*)	0.5–1 mL IM followed by 0.5–1 mL IM at 1 mo and 6 mo	Immunization against hepatitis B infections in susceptible people and in infants born to mothers with hepatitis B
influenza virus vaccine (*Fluzone, Flu-Shield, Fluvirin, Fluogen*)	Adult: 0.5 mL IM Pediatric: 0.25–0.5 mL IM repeated in 4 wk	Prophylaxis in adults and children at high risk for complications of influenza infections
Japanese encephalitis vaccine (*JE-VAX*)	1 mL SC on days 0, 7, and 30	Immunization of persons >1 y of age who reside in or will travel to endemic areas
measles virus vaccine (*Attenuvax*)	0.5 mL SC	Immunization against measles

DRUGS IN FOCUS (CONTINUED)
Vaccines

Drug Name	Dosage/Route	Usual Indications
P measles, mumps, rubella vaccine (*MMR-II*)	0.5 mL SC	Immunization against measles, mumps, and rubella in adults and children >15 mo of age
measles and rubella virus vaccine, live (*M-R-Vax II*)	0.5 mg SC	Immunization against measles and rubella in children ≥15 mo of age
mumps virus vaccine (*Mumpsvax*)	0.5 mL SC	Immunization against mumps in persons >12 mo of age
poliovirus vaccine, live, oral, trivalent (*Orimune*)	0.5 mL PO at 2, 4, and 18 mo Older children: 0.5 mL PO, two doses 8 wk apart and a third dose 6–12 mo later	Immunization against polio infections in children through 18 y of age; not recommended for adults
poliovirus vaccine, inactivated (*IPOL*)	0.5 mL SC at 2, 4, and 12–15 mo; booster when starting school Adult: 0.5 mL SC, two doses at intervals of 1–2 mo, with a third dose 6–12 mo later	Immunization against polio infections in adults and children who cannot take oral polio vaccine
rabies vaccine (*Imovax Rabies, RabAvert*)	Pre-exposure: 1 mL IM on days 0, 7, 21, and 28 Postexposure: 1 mL IM on days 0, 3, 7, 21, and 28	Pre-exposure immunization against rabies for high-risk people; postexposure antirabies regimen with rabies immune globulin
rubella virus vaccine (*Meruvax II*)	One dose SC (>1000 times the median tissue culture infective dose ($TCID_{50}$))	Immunization against rubella in adults and children >12 mo of age
rubella and mumps vaccine, live (*Biavax II*)	0.5 mg SC	Immunization against rubella and mumps in children > 12 mo, preferably at 15 mo
varicella virus vaccine (*Varivax*)	0.5 mL SC, followed by 0.5 mL SC 4–8 wk later Children 1–12 y: 0.5 mL SC	Immunization against chickenpox infections in adults and children ≥12 mo of age
yellow fever vaccine (*YF-Vax*)	0.5 mL SC, booster every 10 yr	Immunization of travelers to areas where yellow fever is endemic

Nursing Diagnoses

The patient receiving a vaccine may have the following nursing diagnoses related to drug therapy:

• Acute Pain related to injection, GI, and flu-like effects
• Ineffective Tissue Perfusion if severe reaction occurs
• Deficient Knowledge regarding drug therapy

Implementation

• Do not use to treat acute infection; *a vaccine is only used to prevent infection with future exposures.*
• Do not administer if the patient exhibits signs of acute infection or immune deficiency, *because the vaccine can cause a mild infection and can exacerbate acute infections.*
• Do not administer if the patient has received blood, blood products, or immune globulin within the past 3 months, *because a severe immune reaction could occur.*
• Arrange for proper preparation and administration of the vaccine; check on each injection, timing and dosage, *be-*

cause dosage, preparation, and timing vary with individual vaccines.
• Maintain emergency equipment on standby, including epinephrine, *in case of severe hypersensitivity reaction.*
• Arrange for supportive care and comfort measures for flu-like symptoms (rest, environmental control, acetaminophen) and for injection discomfort (local heat application, anti-inflammatories, resting arm) *to promote patient comfort.*
• Be aware that children should not receive aspirin to treat the discomforts associated with the immunization. *Aspirin can mask warning signs of Reye's syndrome, a potentially serious disease.*
• Provide thorough patient teaching, including measures to avoid adverse effects; warning signs of problems; and the need to keep a written record of immunizations, *to increase knowledge about drug therapy and to increase compliance with drug regimen.* (See Patient Teaching Checklist: Vaccines.)
• Provide a written record of the immunization, including the need to return for booster immunizations and timing of the

PATIENT TEACHING CHECKLIST
Vaccines

Create customized patient teaching materials for a specific vaccine from the CD-ROM. Patient teaching should stress the following points for drugs within this class:

• This immunization helps your body to develop antibodies to protect you against _____ if you should be exposed to the disease.
• The injection site might be sore and painful. Heat applied to the area may help this discomfort and speed your recovery.
• Adverse effects that you might experience include fever, muscle aches, joint aches, fatigue, and malaise. Aspirin or acetaminophen may help these discomforts; check with your health care provider for the best choice for you. Children should not be given aspirin because it could prevent the recognition of a disease called Reye's syndrome. Rest, small meals, and a quiet environment may also help you to feel better.
• The adverse effects should pass within 2 to 3 days. If they become unduly uncomfortable or persist longer than a few days, notify your health care provider.
• Booster immunizations are required for many, but not all immunizations. You should receive a booster immunization in _____ months (if appropriate).

This Teaching Checklist reflects general patient teaching guidelines. It is not meant to be a substitute for drug-specific teaching information, which is available in nursing drug guides.

boosters, if necessary, *to increase patient compliance to medical regimens.*

Evaluation

• Monitor patient response to the drug (prevention of disease, appropriate antibody titer levels).
• Monitor for adverse effects (flu-like symptoms; GI upset; local pain, swelling, nodule formation at injection site).
• Evaluate the effectiveness of the teaching plan (patient can name drug, dosage, adverse effects to watch for, has written record of immunizations).
• Monitor the effectiveness of comfort measures and compliance to the regimen. (See Nursing Care Guide: Vaccines.)

▮▮◀▮ WEB LINKS
Patients traveling to various parts of the world can obtain information on vaccines that are needed and food and travel precautions online at:

http://www.travelhealth.com

IMMUNE SERA AND ANTITOXINS

As explained earlier, passive immunity can be achieved by providing preformed antibodies to a specific antigen. These antibodies are found in immune sera, which may contain antibodies to toxins, venins, bacteria, viruses, or even red blood cell antigenic factors. The term **immune sera** is usually used to refer to sera that contain antibodies to specific bacteria or viruses. The terms **antitoxin** and antivenin are used to refer to immune sera that has antibodies to very specific toxins that might be released by invading pathogens or to venom that might be injected through spider or snake bites.

Therapeutic Actions and Indications

Immune sera are used to provide passive immunity to a specific antigen or disease. They also may be used as prophylaxis against specific diseases after exposure in patients who are immunosuppressed. In addition, immune sera may be used to lessen the severity of a disease after known or suspected exposure (see Figure 18–2 for sites of action of immune sera and antitoxins).

Contraindications and Cautions

Immune sera are contraindicated in the presence of a history of severe reaction to any immune sera or to products similar to the components of the sera. They should be used with caution during pregnancy (because of potential risk to the fetus); with coagulation defects or thrombocytopenia; or with a known history of previous exposure to the immune sera (because increased risk of hypersensitivity reaction occurs with each use).

Adverse Effects

Adverse effects can be attributed either to the effect of immune sera on the immune system (rash, nausea, vomiting, chills, fever) or to allergic reactions (chest tightness, falling blood pressure, difficulty breathing). Local reactions are very common (swelling, tenderness, pain, muscle stiffness at the injection site).

Nursing Considerations for Patients Receiving Immune Sera or Antitoxins
Assessment: History and Examination

Screen for the following, which could be contraindications or cautions to the use of the drug: any known allergies to any of these drugs or their components; pregnancy; previous exposure to the serum being used; thrombocytopenia, coagulation disorders; and immunization history.

Include screening for baseline status before beginning therapy and for any potential adverse effects: presence of any skin lesions; temperature; orientation, reflexes; pulse, blood pressure, respirations, and adventitious sounds.

Nursing Diagnoses

The patient receiving immune sera may have the following nursing diagnoses related to drug therapy:

• Acute Pain related to local, GI, and flu-like effects
• Ineffective Tissue Perfusion related to possible severe reactions
• Deficient Knowledge regarding drug therapy

NURSING CARE GUIDE

Vaccines

Assessment	Nursing Diagnoses	Implementation	Evaluation
HISTORY Allergies to the serum base, pregnancy, lactation, acute infection, immunosuppression	Acute Pain related to infection, flu-like symptoms Ineffective Tissue Perfusion if severe reaction occurs Deficient Knowledge regarding drug therapy	Ensure proper preparation and administration of vaccine within appropriate time frame. Provide supportive and comfort measures to deal with adverse effects: anti-inflammatory/antipyretic, local heat application, small meals, rest, quiet environment. Provide patient teaching regarding drug name, dosage, adverse effects and precautions, warning signs to report. Provide emergency life support if needed for acute reaction.	Evaluate drug effects: serum titers reflecting immunization (if appropriate). Monitor for adverse effects: pain, flu-like symptoms, local discomfort. Monitor for drug–drug interactions as indicated for each drug. Evaluate effectiveness of patient teaching program. Evaluate effectiveness of comfort and safety measures. Evaluate effectiveness of emergency measures if needed.
PHYSICAL EXAMINATION General: temperature CV: pulse, cardiac auscultation, BP, edema, perfusion Respiratory: respirations, adventitious sounds Skin: lesions Joints: range of motion			

Implementation

- Do not administer to any patient with a history of severe reaction to immune globulins or to the components of the drug being used, *because severe immune reactions can occur.*
- Administer the drug as indicated. *Preparation varies with each product; always check manufacturer's guidelines.*
- Monitor for severe reactions and *have emergency equipment ready.*
- Arrange for supportive care and comfort measures for flu-like symptoms (rest, environmental control, acetaminophen) and for the local reaction (heat to injection site, anti-inflammatories) *to promote patient comfort.*
- Provide thorough patient teaching, including measures to avoid adverse effects and warning signs of problems *to improve patient compliance.*
- Provide a written record of immune sera use and encourage the patient or family to keep that information *to ensure proper medical treatment and to avert future reactions.*

Evaluation

- Monitor the patient's response to the drug (improvement in disease signs and symptoms, prevention of severe disease).
- Monitor for adverse effects (flu-like symptoms, GI upset, local inflammation and pain).
- Evaluate the effectiveness of the teaching plan (patient can name drug, dosage, adverse effects to watch for, specific measures to avoid adverse effects, need to retain written record of injection).
- Monitor the effectiveness of comfort measures and compliance to the regimen.

CHAPTER SUMMARY

- Immunity is a state of relative resistance to a disease that develops only after exposure to the specific disease-causing agent.
- Active immunity occurs when a person's body is stimu-

DRUGS IN FOCUS
Immune Sera

Drug Name	Dosage/Route	Usual Indications
cytomegalovirus immune globulin (*CytoGam*)	15 mg/kg IV over 30 min increased to 30 mg/kg IV over 30 min, then 60 mg/kg IV to a max of 150 mg/kg; infuse at 72 h, at 2 wk, and then at 4, 6, 8, 12, and 16 wk after transplantation	Attenuation of primary cytomegalovirus disease after renal transplantation
hepatitis B immune globulin (*Nabi-HB*)	0.06 mL/kg IM, repeated at 3 mo and 6 mo	Postexposure prophylaxis against hepatitis B
P immune globulin, intramuscular (*BayGam*, others)	Dosage varies with exposure; check manufacturer's instructions	Prophylaxis after exposure to hepatitis A, measles, varicella, or rubella
immune globulin, intravenous (*Gamimune, Gammagard*)	Dosage varies with indication and preparation; always check manufacturer's instructions	Prophylaxis after exposure to hepatitis A, measles, varicella, or rubella; bone marrow and other transplants; Kawasaki's disease; chronic lymphocytic leukemia; treatment of patients with immunoglobulin deficiency
lymphocyte immune globulin (*Atgam*)	Adult: 10–30 mg/kg per day IV Pediatric: 5–25 mg/kg per day IV Aplastic anemia: 10–20 mg/kg per day IV for 8–14 d	Management of allograft rejection in renal transplantation; treatment of aplastic anemia
rabies immune globulin (*BayRab, Imogam*)	20 IU/kg IM	Protection against rabies in nonimmunized patients exposed to rabies
respiratory syncytial virus immune globulin (*RespiGAM*)	1.5 mL/kg per hour for 15 min; then 3 mL/kg per hour for 15 min, then 6 mL/kg per hour to a total monthly infusion of 750 mg/kg	Prevention of respiratory syncytial virus infection in children <24 mo of age with bronchopulmonary dysplasia or premature birth
RHO immune globulin (*BayRab-D, RhoGAM*)	1 vial IM within 72 h after delivery	Prevention of sensitization to the Rh factor
RHO immune globulin, microdose (*BayRho-D Mini-Dose, MICRhoGAM*)	1 vial IV within 72 h after delivery	Prevention of sensitization to the Rh factor
tetanus immune globulin (*Bay Tet*)	250 units IM	Passive immunization against tetanus at time of injury
varicella zoster immune globulin (*Varicella Zoster Immune Globulin*)	125 units/10 kg IM, to a maximum of 625 units	Passive immunization against varicella zoster in immunosuppressed patients exposed to disease

Antitoxins and Antivenins

Drug Name	Dosage/Route	Usual Indications
P antivenin (generic)	20–40 mL IV, up to 100–150 mL in severe cases	Neutralizes the venom of various snakes
Black Widow spider antivenin (*Antivenin*)	25 mL IM or IV in 10–50 mL saline over 15 min	Treatment of symptoms of Black Widow spider bites
crotalidae polyvalent immune fab (*CroFab*)	Four to six vials IV given diluted over 60 min	Treatment of rattlesnake bites

lated to make antibodies against specific proteins; memory cells then release antibodies immediately if that protein enters the body again.

- Passive immunity occurs when a person is given preformed antibodies to a specific protein. This offers immediate protection from exposure to the protein, but the protection is limited to the life of the circulating antibodies.
- Immunizations are given to stimulate active immunity in a person who is at high risk for exposure to specific diseases. Immunizations are a standard part of preventive medicine.
- Vaccines contain weakened or partial proteins from specific antigens that stimulate the production of antibodies to that protein, thus providing active immunity.
- Immune sera provide preformed antibodies to specific proteins for people who have been exposed to them or are at high risk for exposure.

CASE STUDY

Educating a Parent About Vaccines

THE SITUATION

S. D. is a 25-year-old, first-time mother who has brought her 2-month-old daughter to the well baby clinic for a routine evaluation. The baby is found to be healthy, growing well, and within normal parameters for her age. At the end of the visit, the nurse prepares to give the baby the first of her routine immunizations. S. D. became concerned and expresses fears about paralysis and infant deaths associated with immunizations.

CRITICAL THINKING

What information should S. D. be given about immunizations?

What nursing interventions would be appropriate at this time? *Think of ways to explain the importance of immunizations to S. D. while supporting her concerns for the welfare of her baby.*

How can this experience be incorporated into a teaching plan for S. D. and her baby?

DISCUSSION

S. D. should be reassured before the baby is immunized. The nurse can tell her that in the past, paralysis and infant deaths were reported, but that efforts continue to make the vaccines pure. Careful monitoring of the child and the child's response to each immunization can help avoid such problems. Reassure S. D. that the immunizations will prevent her daughter from contracting many, sometimes deadly, diseases. Praise S. D.'s efforts for researching information that might affect her baby and for asking questions that could have an impact on her child and her understanding of her care.

The recommended schedule of immunizations should be given to S. D. so that she is aware of what is planned and how the various vaccines are spaced and combined. She should be encouraged to monitor the baby after each injection for fever, chills, and flu-like reactions. When she gets home, she can medicate the baby with acetaminophen to avert many of these symptoms before they happen. (S. D. should be advised not to give the baby aspirin, which could cover up Reye's syndrome, a potentially serious disorder.) S. D. also should be told that the injection site might be sore, swollen, and red, but that this will pass in a couple of days. S. D. can ease the baby's discomfort by applying warm soaks to the area for about 10 to 15 minutes every 2 hours.

S. D. should be encouraged to write down all of the immunizations that the baby has had and to keep this information handy for easy reference. She should also be encouraged to record any adverse effects that occur after each immunization. If reactions are uncomfortable, it is possible to split doses of future immunizations.

The nurse should give S. D. a chance to vent her concerns and fears. First-time parents may be more anxious than experienced ones when dealing with issues involving a new baby. To alleviate S. D.'s anxiety, the nurse should provide a telephone number that S. D. can call if the baby seems to be having a severe reaction or if S. D. wants to discuss any questions or concerns. She should feel that support is available for any concern that she may have. Because this interaction is likely to form the basis for future interactions with S. D., it is important to establish a sense of respect and trust.

- Serum sickness, a massive immune reaction, occurs more frequently with immune sera than with vaccines. Patients need to be monitored for any history of hypersensitivity reactions, and emergency equipment should be available.
- Patients should be advised to keep a written record of all immunizations or immune sera used. Booster doses may be needed to further stimulate antibody production.

Review Questions

1. Vaccines are used to stimulate
   a. passive immunity to a foreign protein.
   b. active immunity to a foreign protein.
   c. serum sickness.
   d. a mild disease in healthy people.
2. A public education campaign to stress the importance of childhood immunizations would include all of the following except
   a. prevention of potentially devastating diseases outweighs the discomfort and risks of immunization.
   b. routine immunization is standard practice in the United States.
   c. the practice of routine immunizations has virtually wiped out many previously deadly or debilitating diseases.
   d. the risk of severe adverse reactions is on the increase and is not being addressed.
3. Common adverse effects associated with routine immunizations would not include
   a. difficulty breathing.
   b. fever and rash.
   c. drowsiness and fretfulness.
   d. pain, redness, swelling, and nodule formation at the site of injection.
4. A child would not be a candidate for routine immunization at his 18-month well-baby visit if
   a. he cried at his last immunization.
   b. he developed a fever or rash after his last immunization.
   c. he currently has a fever and symptoms of a cold.
   d. he is allergic to aspirin.

5. A 6-month-old child would not be a candidate for
   a. DTaP.
   b. *H. influenza* B.
   c. poliovirus.
   d. chickenpox vaccine.
6. Every fall, older adults and people who are at high risk for complications of influenza should receive a flu vaccine. This is repeated every year because
   a. the immunity wears off after a year.
   b. the strains of virus predicted to cause the flu change every year.
   c. a booster shot will activate the immune system.
   d. older people do not produce good antibodies.
7. Tetanus booster shots should routinely be given
   a. only with exposure to anaerobic bacteria.
   b. every 2 years.
   c. every 5 years.
   d. every 10 years.
8. A nurse suffers a needle stick after injecting a patient with suspected hepatitis B. The nurse should
   a. have repeated titers to determine whether she was exposed to hepatitis B and, if she was, have hepatitis immune globulin.
   b. immediately receive hepatitis immune globulin and begin hepatitis B vaccines if she has not already received it.
   c. start antibiotic therapy immediately.
   d. go on sick leave until all screening tests are negative.
9. A patient is to receive immune globulin after exposure to hepatitis A. The patient has a previous history of allergies to various drugs. Before giving the immune globulin, the nurse should
   a. make sure that emergency equipment is readily available in case of a massive immune reaction.
   b. premedicate the patient with aspirin.
   c. make sure all of the patient's vaccinations are up to date.
   d. make sure the patient has a ride home.

BIBLIOGRAPHY

AMA drug evaluations. (2002). Chicago: American Medical Association.

Bullock, B. L. (2000). *Focus on pathophysiology.* Philadelphia: Lippincott Williams & Wilkins.

Gilman, A., Hardman, J. G., & Limbird, L. E. (Eds.) (2002). *Goodman and Gilman's the pharmacological basis of therapeutics* (10th ed.). New York: McGraw-Hill.

Karch, A. M. (2002). *2003 Lippincott's nursing drug guide.* Philadelphia: Lippincott Williams & Wilkins.

Drug facts and comparisons. (2002). St. Louis: Facts & Comparisons.

The medical letter on drugs and therapeutics. (2002). New Rochelle, NY: Medical Letter.

PART

IV

Drugs Acting on
the Central and
Peripheral
Nervous Systems

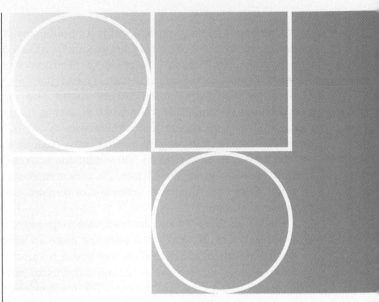

Introduction to Nerves and the Nervous System

Key Terms

action potential

afferent

axon

dendrite

depolarization

effector

efferent

engram

forebrain

hindbrain

limbic system

midbrain

neuron

neurotransmitter

repolarization

Schwann cell

soma

synapse

The nervous system is responsible for controlling the functions of the human body, analyzing incoming stimuli, and integrating internal and external responses. The nervous system is composed of the central nervous system (the brain and spinal cord) and the peripheral nervous system. The peripheral nervous system (PNS) is composed of sensory receptors that bring information into the central nervous system (CNS) and motor nerves that carry information away from the CNS to facilitate response to stimuli. The autonomic nervous system, which is discussed in Chapter 29, uses components of the CNS and PNS to regulate automatic or unconscious responses to stimuli.

The structural unit of the nervous system is the nerve cell, or neuron. The billions of nerve cells that make up the nervous system are organized to allow movement; realization of various sensations; response to internal and external stimuli; and learning, thinking, and emotion. The mechanisms that are involved in all of these processes are not clearly understood. The actions of drugs that are used to affect the functioning of the nerves and the responses that these drugs cause throughout the nervous system provide some of the current theories about the workings of the nervous system.

PHYSIOLOGY OF THE NERVOUS SYSTEM

The nervous system operates through the use of electrical impulses and chemical messengers to transmit information throughout the body and to respond to internal and external stimuli. The properties and function of the neuron provide the basis for all nervous system function.

Neurons

As noted previously, the **neuron** is the structural unit of the nervous system. The human body contains about 14 billion neurons. About 10 billion of these are located in the brain, and the remainder make up the spinal cord and PNS.

Neurons have several distinctive cellular features. Each neuron is made up of a cell body, or **soma,** which contains the cell nucleus, cytoplasm, and various granules and other particles (Figure 19–1). Short, branch-like projections that cover most of the surface of a neuron are known as **dendrites.** These structures, which provide increased surface area for the neuron, bring information into the neuron from other neurons.

One end of the nerve body extends into a long process that does not branch out until the very end of the process. This elongated process is called the nerve **axon,** and it emerges from the soma at the axon hillock (see Figure 19–1). The axon of a nerve can be extremely tiny, or it can extend for several feet. The axon carries information from a nerve to be transmitted to **effector** cells—cells in a muscle, a gland, or another nerve. This transmission occurs at the

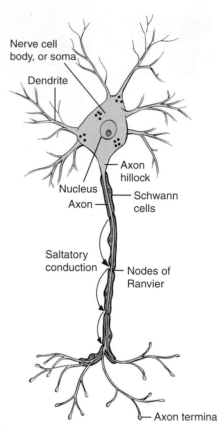

FIGURE 19-1. The neuron, functional unit of the nervous system.

end of the axon, where the axon branches out in what is called the axon terminal.

The axons of many nerves are packed closely together in the nervous system and look like cable or fiber tracts. **Afferent** fibers are nerve axons that run from peripheral receptors into the CNS. In contrast, **efferent** fibers are nerve axons that carry nerve impulses from the CNS to the periphery to stimulate muscles or glands. (An easy way to remember the difference between afferent and efferent is to recall that *e*fferent fibers *e*xit from the CNS.)

It is currently thought that neurons are unable to reproduce; so, if nerves are destroyed, they are lost. If dendrites and axons are lost, nerves regenerate those structures. For this regeneration to occur, the soma and the axon hillock must remain intact. For a clinical example, consider a person who has closed a car door on his or her finger. Sensation and movement may be lost or limited for a certain period, but because the nerve bodies for most of the nerves in the hand are located in ganglia (groups of nerve bodies) in the wrist, they are able to regenerate the damaged axon or dendrites. Over time, sensation and full movement should return.

Research on possible ways to stimulate the reproduction of nerves is under way. Although scientists have used nerve growth factor with fetal cell implants to stimulate some nerve growth, it is currently assumed that nerves are unable to reproduce.

Action Potential

Nerves send messages by conducting electrical impulses called **action potentials.** Nerve membranes, which are capable of conducting action potentials along the entire membrane, send messages to nearby neurons or to effector cells that may be located inches to feet away via this electrical communication system. Like all cell membranes, nerve membranes have various channels or pores that control the movement of substances into and out of the cell. Some of these channels allow the movement of sodium, potassium, and calcium. When cells are at rest, their membranes are impermeable to sodium. However, the membranes are permeable to potassium ions.

The sodium–potassium pump that is active in the membranes of neurons is responsible for this property of the membrane. This system pumps sodium ions out of the cell and potassium ions into the cell. At rest, more sodium ions are outside the cell membrane and more potassium ions are inside. Electrically, the inside of the cell is relatively negative compared with the outside of the membrane, which establishes an electrical potential along the nerve membrane. When nerves are at rest, this is referred to as the resting membrane potential of the nerve.

Stimulation of a neuron causes **depolarization** of the nerve, which means that the sodium channels open in response to the stimulus, and sodium ions rush into the cell, following the established concentration gradient. If an electrical monitoring device is attached to the nerve at this point, a positive rush of ions is recorded. The electrical charge on the inside of the membrane changes from relatively negative to relatively positive. This sudden reversal of membrane potential, called the action potential (Figure 19–2), lasts less than a microsecond. Using the sodium–potassium pump, the cell then returns that section of membrane to the resting membrane potential, a process called **repolarization.** The action potential generated at one point along a nerve membrane stimulates the generation of an action potential in adjacent portions of the cell membrane, and the stimulus travels the length of the cell membrane.

Nerves can respond to stimuli several hundred times per second, but for a given stimulus to cause an action potential, it must have sufficient strength and must occur when the nerve membrane is able to respond—that is, when it has repolarized. A nerve cannot be stimulated again while it is depolarized. The balance of sodium and potassium across the cell membrane must be reestablished.

Nerves require energy (ie, oxygen and glucose) and the correct balance of the electrolytes sodium and potassium to maintain normal action potentials and transmit information into and out of the nervous system. If an individual has anoxia or hypoglycemia, the nerves might not be able to maintain the sodium—potassium pump, and he or she may become severely irritable or too stable (not responsive to stimuli).

Long nerves are myelinated: they have a myelin sheath that speeds electrical conduction and protects the nerves from the fatigue that results from frequent formation of ac-

FIGURE 19-2. The action potential. **A:** A segment of an axon showing that, at rest, the inside of the membrane is relatively negatively charged and the outside is positively charged. A pair of electrodes placed as shown would record a potential difference of about −70 mV; this is the resting membrane potential. **B:** An action potential of about 1 msec that, as shown, would be recorded if the axon shown in **A** were brought to threshold. At the peak of the action potential, the charge on the membrane reverses polarity.

tion potentials. Even though many of the tightly packed nerves in the brain do not need to travel far to stimulate another nerve, they are myelinated. The effect of this myelination is not understood.

Myelinated nerves have **Schwann cells,** which are very resistant to electrical stimulation (Figure 19–3), located at specific intervals along the axons. The Schwann cells wrap themselves around the axon in jelly-roll fashion. Between the Schwann cells are areas of uncovered nerve membrane called the nodes of Ranvier. So-called "leaping" nerve conduction occurs along these exposed nerve fibers. An action potential excites one section of nerve membrane, and the electrical impulse then "skips" from one node to the next, generating an action potential. Because the membrane is forming fewer action potentials, the speed of conduction is much faster and the nerve is protected from exhaustion or using up energy to form multiple action potentials. This

FIGURE 19-3. Formation of a myelin sheath in a peripheral axon. Successive wrappings of the Schwann cell membranes form the sheath, with most of the Schwann cell cytoplasm left outside the myelin. Therefore, the neurilemmal sheath of Schwann cells is outside the myelin sheath.

node-to-node mode of conduction is termed *saltatory* or *leaping transmission.*

If the Schwann cells become enlarged or swollen and block the nodes of Ranvier, conduction does not occur because the electrical impulse has a limited firing range. A stimulus may simply be "lost" along the nerve, as in the neuromuscular disease multiple sclerosis. Believed to be an autoimmune disorder that attacks Schwann cells and leads to swelling and scarring of these cells, this disease is characterized by a progressive loss of nerve response and muscle function.

Nerve Synapse

When the electrical action potential reaches the end of an axon, the electrical impulse comes to a halt. At this point the stimulus no longer travels at the speed of electricity. The transmission of information between two nerves and between a nerve and a gland or muscle is chemical. Nerves communicate with other nerves or effectors at the nerve **synapse** (Figure 19–4). The synapse is made up of a presynaptic nerve, the synaptic cleft, and the postsynaptic effector cell. The nerve axon, called the presynaptic nerve, releases a chemical called a **neurotransmitter** into the synaptic cleft, and the neurotransmitter reacts with a very specific receptor site on the postsynaptic cell to cause a reaction.

Neurotransmitters

Neurotransmitters stimulate postsynaptic cells either by exciting or by inhibiting them. The reaction that occurs when a neurotransmitter stimulates a receptor site depends on the specific neurotransmitter that it releases and the receptor site it activates. A nerve may produce only one type of neurotransmitter, using building blocks such as tyrosine or choline from the extracellular fluid, often absorbed from dietary sources. The neurotransmitter, packaged into vesicles, moves to the terminal membrane of the axon, and when the nerve is stimulated the vesicles contract and push the neurotransmitter into the synaptic cleft. The calcium channels in the nerve membrane are open during the action potential, and the presence of calcium causes the contraction. When the cell repolarizes, calcium leaves the cell, and the contraction stops. Once released into the synaptic cleft, the neurotransmitter reacts with very specific receptor sites to cause a reaction.

To return the effector cell to a resting state so that it can be stimulated again, if needed, neurotransmitters must be inactivated. Neurotransmitters may be either reabsorbed by the presynaptic nerve in a process called reuptake (ie, a recycling effort by the nerve to reuse the materials and save resources) or broken down by enzymes in the area (eg, monoamine oxidase breaks down the neurotransmitter norepinephrine; the enzyme acetylcholinesterase breaks down the neurotransmitter acetylcholine). Several neurotransmitters have been identified. As research continues, other neurotransmitters may be discovered, and the actions of known neurotransmitters will be better understood.

The following are selected neurotransmitters:

- *Acetylcholine,* which communicates between nerves and muscles, is also important as the preganglionic neurotrans-

FIGURE 19–4. The sequence of events in synaptic transmission: (1) synthesis of the neurotransmitter; (2) uptake of the neurotransmitter into storage vesicles; (3) release of the neurotransmitter by an action potential in the presynaptic nerve; (4) diffusion of the neurotransmitter across the synaptic cleft; (5) combination of the neurotransmitter with a receptor; (6) a sequence of events leading to activation of second messengers within the postsynaptic nerve; (7) change in permeability of the postsynaptic membrane to one or more ions, causing (8a) an inhibitory postsynaptic potential or (8b) an excitatory postsynaptic potential. Characteristic responses of the postsynaptic cell are as follows: (9a) the gland secretes hormones; (9b) the muscle cells have an action potential; and (10) the muscle contracts. The action of the neurotransmitter is terminated by one or more of the following processes: (A) inactivation by an enzyme; (B) diffusion out of the synaptic cleft and removal by the vascular system; and (C) reuptake into the presynaptic nerve followed by storage in a synaptic vesicle or deactivation by an enzyme.

mitter throughout the autonomic nervous system and as the postganglionic neurotransmitter in the parasympathetic nervous system and in several pathways in the brain.

• *Norepinephrine* and *epinephrine* are catecholamines, which are released by nerves in the sympathetic branch of the autonomic nervous system. These neurotransmitters also occur in high levels in particular areas of the brain such as the limbic system.

• *Dopamine,* which is found in high concentrations in certain areas of the brain, is involved in the coordination of impulses and responses, both motor and intellectual.

• *Gamma-aminobutyric acid* (GABA), which is found in the brain, inhibits nerve activity and is important in preventing overexcitability or stimulation such as seizure activity.

• *Serotonin,* which is also found in the limbic system, is important in arousal and sleep as well as in preventing depression and promoting motivation.

Many of the drugs that affect the nervous system involve altering the activity of the nerve synapse. These drugs have several functions, including blocking the reuptake of neurotransmitters so that they are present in the synapse in greater quantities and cause more stimulation of receptor sites; blocking receptor sites so that the neurotransmitter cannot stimulate the receptor site; blocking the enzymes that break down neurotransmitters to cause an increase in neurotransmitter concentration in the synapse; stimulating specific receptor sites when the neurotransmitter is not available; and causing the presynaptic nerve to release greater amounts of the neurotransmitter.

WEB LINKS

To explore the virtual nervous system, visit this Internet site:

http://www.InnerBody.com

CENTRAL NERVOUS SYSTEM

The CNS consists of the brain and the spinal cord, the two parts of the body that contain the vast majority of nerves. The bones of the vertebrae protect the spinal cord, and the bones of the skull, which are corrugated much like an egg carton and designed to absorb impact, protect the brain (Figure 19–5). In addition, the meninges, which are membranes that cover the nerves in the brain and spine, furnish further protection.

The blood–brain barrier, a functioning boundary, also plays a defensive role. It keeps toxins, proteins, and other large structures out of the brain and prevents their contact with the sensitive and fragile neurons. The blood–brain barrier represents a therapeutic challenge to drug treatment of brain-related disorders, because a large percentage of drugs are carried bound to plasma proteins and are unable to cross into the brain. When a patient is suffering from a brain infection, antibiotics cannot cross into the brain until the infection is so severe that the blood–brain barrier can no longer function.

The brain has a unique blood supply to protect the neurons from lack of oxygen and glucose. Two arteries, the carotids, branch off the aortic arch and go up into each side of the brain at the front of the head, and two other arteries, the vertebrals, enter the back of the brain to become the basilar arteries. These arteries all deliver blood to a common vessel at the bottom of the brain called the circle of Willis, which distributes the blood to the brain as it is needed (Figure 19–6). The role of the circle of Willis becomes apparent when an individual has an occluded carotid artery. Although the passage of blood through one of the carotid arteries may be negligible, the areas of the brain on that side will still have

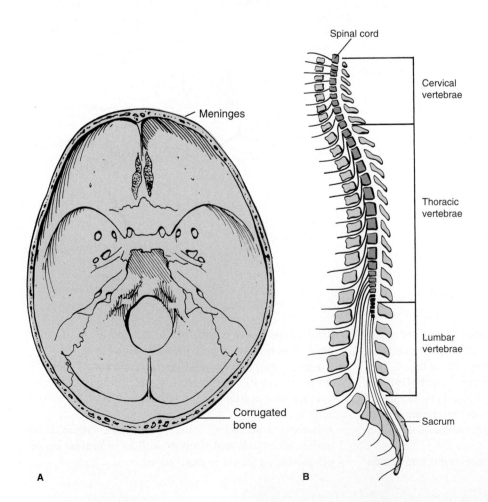

A

B

FIGURE 19-5. Bony and membranous protection of the brain (**A**) and the spine (**B**).

FIGURE 19-6. The protective blood supply of the brain: the carotid, vertebral, and basilar arteries join to form the circle of Willis. (From Bullock, B. L. [2000]. Focus on pathophysiology. Philadelphia: Lippincott Williams & Wilkins.)

a full blood supply because of the blood sent to those areas via the circle of Willis.

Anatomy of the Brain

The brain has three major divisions: the hindbrain, the midbrain, and the forebrain (Figure 19–7).

The **hindbrain,** which runs from the top of the spinal cord into the midbrain, is the most primitive area of the brain and contains the brainstem, where the pons and medulla oblongata are located. These areas of the brain control basic, vital functions such as the respiratory centers, which control breathing; the cardiovascular centers, which regulate blood pressure; the chemoreceptor trigger zone and emetic zone, which control vomiting; the swallowing center, which coordinates the complex swallowing reflex; and the reticular activating system (RAS), which controls arousal and awareness of stimuli and contains the sleep center. The RAS filters the billions of incoming messages, selecting only the most significant for response. When levels of serotonin become high in the RAS, the system shuts down, and sleep occurs. The medulla absorbs serotonin from the RAS, when the levels are low enough, consciousness or arousal results.

The cranial nerves (see Figure 19–7), which also emerge from the hindbrain, involve *specific* senses (sight, smell, hearing, balance, taste) and some muscle activity of the head and neck (eg, chewing, eye movement). The cerebellum, a part of the brain that looks like a skein of yarn and lies behind the other parts of the hindbrain, coordinates the motor function that regulates posture, balance, and voluntary muscle activity.

The **midbrain** contains the thalamus, the hypothalamus, and the limbic system (see Figure 19–7). The thalamus sends direct information into the cerebrum to transfer sensations such as cold, heat, pain, touch, and muscle sense. The hypo-

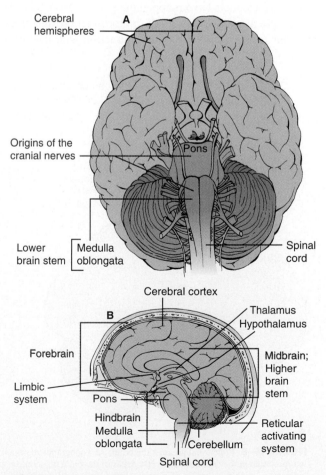

FIGURE 19-7. Anatomy of the brain. **A:** A view of the underside of the brain. **B:** The medial or midsagittal view of the brain.

thalamus, which is poorly protected by the blood–brain barrier, acts as a major sensor for activities in the body. Areas of the hypothalamus are responsible for temperature control, water balance, appetite, and fluid balance. In addition, the hypothalamus plays a central role in the endocrine system and in the autonomic nervous system.

The **limbic system** is an area of the brain that contains high levels of three neurotransmitters: epinephrine, norepinephrine, and serotonin. Stimulation of this area, which appears to be responsible for the expression of emotions, may lead to anger, pleasure, motivation, stress, and so on. This part of the brain seems to be largely responsible for the human aspect of brain function. Drug therapy aimed at alleviating emotional disorders such as depression and anxiety often involves attempting to alter the levels of epinephrine, norepinephrine, and serotonin.

The **forebrain** is made up of two cerebral hemispheres joined together by an area called the corpus callosum. These two hemispheres contain the sensory neurons, which receive nerve impulses, and the motor neurons, which send them. They also contain areas that coordinate speech and communication and seem to be the area where learning takes place (see Figures 19–7 and 19–8).

Different areas of the brain appear to be responsible for receiving and sending information to specific areas of the body. When the brain is viewed at autopsy, it looks homogenous, but scientists have mapped the general areas that are responsible for sensory response, motor function, and other functions (see Figure 19–8). In conjunction with the cere-

bellum, groups of ganglia or nerve cell bodies called the basal ganglia, located at the bottom of the brain, make up the extrapyramidal motor system. This system coordinates motor activity for unconscious activities such as posture and gait.

Anatomy of the Spinal Cord

The spinal cord is made up of 31 pairs of spinal nerves. Each spinal nerve has two components or roots. These mixed nerve parts include a sensory fiber (called the dorsal root) and a motor fiber (called the ventral root). The spinal sensory fibers bring information into the CNS from the periphery. The motor fibers cause movement or reaction.

Functions of the Central Nervous System

The brain is responsible for coordinating reactions to the constantly changing external and internal environment. In all animals, the function of this organ is essentially the same. The human component involving emotions, learning, and conscious response takes the human nervous system beyond a simple reflex system and complicates the responses seen to any stimulus.

Sensory Functions

Millions of sensory impulses are constantly streaming into the CNS from peripheral receptors. Many of these impulses go directly to specific areas of the brain designated to deal with in-

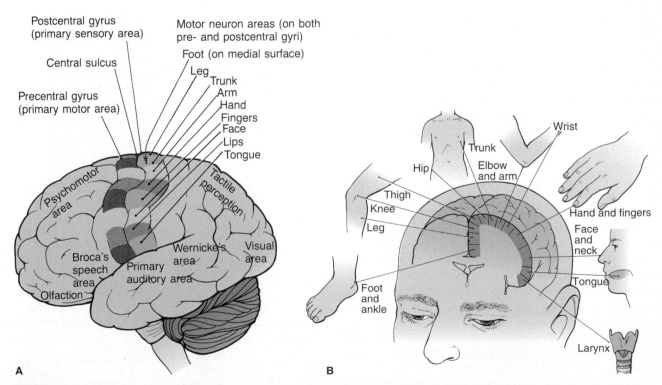

FIGURE 19–8. Functional areas of the brain. **A:** Topographical organization of functions of control and interpretation in the cerebral cortex. **B:** Areas of the brain that control specific areas of the body. Size indicates relative distribution of control. (From Bullock, B. L. [2000]. Focus on pathophysiology. Philadelphia: Lippincott Williams & Wilkins.)

put from particular areas of the body or from the senses. The responses that occur as a result of these stimuli can be altered by efferent neurons that respond to emotions through the limbic system, to learned responses stored in the cerebral cortex, or to autonomic input mediated through the hypothalamus.

The intricacies of the human brain can change the response to a sensation depending on the situation. People may react differently to the same stimulus. For example, if an individual drops a can on his or her foot, the physiologic response is one of pain and a stimulation of the sympathetic branch of the autonomic nervous system. If the person is alone or in a very comfortable environment (e.g., fixing dinner at home), he or she may scream, swear, or jump around. But if that person is in the company of other people (e.g., a cooking teacher working with a class), he or she may be much more dignified and quiet.

Motor Functions

The sensory nerves that enter the brain react with related motor nerves to cause a reaction mediated by muscles or glands. The motor impulses that leave the cortex are further regulated or coordinated by the pyramidal system, which coordinates voluntary movement, and the extrapyramidal system, which coordinates unconscious motor activity that regulates control of position and posture. For example, some drugs may interfere with the extrapyramidal system and cause tremors, shuffling gait, and lack of posture and position stability. Motor fibers from the cortex cross to the other side of the spinal cord before emerging to interact with peripheral effectors. In this way, motor stimuli coming from the right side of the brain affect motor activity on the left side of the body. For example, an area of the left cortex may send an impulse down to the spinal cord that reacts with an interneuron, crosses to the other side of the spinal cord, and causes a finger on the right hand to twitch.

Intellectual and Emotional Functions

The way that the cerebral cortex uses sensory information is not clearly understood, but research has demonstrated that the two hemispheres of the brain process information in different ways. The right side of the brain is the more artistic side, concerned with forms and shapes, and the left side is more analytical, concerned with names, numbers, and processes. Why the two hemispheres are different and how they develop differently is not known.

When learning takes place, distinct layers of the cerebral cortex are affected, and an actual membrane change occurs in a neuron to store information in the brain permanently. Learning begins as an electrical circuit called an **engram,** a reverberating circuit of action potentials that eventually becomes a long-term, permanent memory in the presence of the proper neurotransmitters and hormones. Scientists do not understand how this happens, but it is known that the nerve requires oxygen, glucose, and sleep to process an engram into a permanent memory. The engram is responsible for short-term memory. When patients have a decreased blood supply to the brain, short-term memory may be lost, and they are not able to remember new things. Because they are un-

able to remember new things, the brain falls back on long-term, permanent memory for daily functioning. For example, a patient may be introduced to a nurse and have no recollection of the nurse 2 hours later, and yet be able to recall the events of several years ago vividly.

Several substances appear to affect learning. Antidiuretic hormone, which is released during reactions to stress, increases learning. In situations in which a person is trying to learn, it may help to feel slightly stressed. Too much stress prevents learning, however. A patient who is a little nervous about upcoming surgery seems to display a better mastery of facts about the surgery and postoperative procedures than either one who is very stressed and scared or one who appears to show no interest or concern. Oxytocin also seems to increase actual learning. Because childbirth is the only known time that oxytocin levels increase, the significance of this is not understood. Nurses who work with maternity patients should know that women in labor will very likely remember the smallest details about the whole experience and should use whatever opportunity is made available to do teaching.

In addition, the limbic system appears to play an important role in how a person learns and reacts to stimuli. The emotions associated with a memory as well as with the present have an impact on stimulus response. The placebo effect (a documented effect of the mind on drug therapy: if a person perceives that a drug will be effective, it is much more likely to actually be effective), which uses the actions of the cerebrum and the limbic system, can have a tremendous impact on drug response. Events that are perceived as stressful by some patients may be seen as positive by other patients.

CLINICAL SIGNIFICANCE OF DRUGS THAT ACT ON THE NERVOUS SYSTEM

The features of the human nervous system, including the complexities of the human brain, sometimes make it difficult to predict the exact reaction of a particular patient to a given drug. When a drug is used to affect the nervous system, the occurrence of many systemic effects is always a possibility, because the nervous system affects the entire body. The chapters in this section address the individual classes of drugs used to treat disorders of the nervous system, including their adverse effects. An understanding of the actions of specific drugs makes it easier to anticipate what therapeutic and adverse effects might occur. In addition, nurses should also consider all of the learned, cultural, and emotional aspects of the patient's situation in an attempt to provide optimal therapeutic benefit and minimal adverse effects.

CHAPTER SUMMARY

- The nervous system, which consists of the CNS and the PNS, is responsible for control of the human body, analysis of stimuli coming into the system, and integration of internal and external responses to stimuli.

- The neuron, the functional unit of the nervous system, consists of a cell body or soma, dendrites that bring information to the nerve, and an axon that takes information away from the nerve.
- Although nerves do not reproduce, they can regenerate injured parts if the soma and axon hillock remain intact.
- Efferent nerves are nerves that take information out of the CNS to effector sites; afferent nerves are sensory nerves that take information into the CNS.
- Nerves transmit information by way of electrical charges called action potentials. An action potential is a sudden change in membrane charge from negative to positive. It is caused when stimulation of a nerve opens sodium channels and allows positive sodium ions to flow into the cell.
- The flow of sodium ions into a nerve results in depolarization of the nerve membrane. Immediately, repolarization occurs: the sodium—potassium pump in the cell membrane pumps out sodium and potassium ions and leaves the inside of the membrane relatively negative to the outside.
- When the transmission of action potentials reaches the axon terminal, it causes the release of chemicals called neurotransmitters, which cross the synaptic cleft to stimulate an effector cell, which can be another nerve, a muscle, or a gland.
- A neurotransmitter must be produced by a nerve (each nerve can produce only one kind); it must be released into the synapse when the nerve is stimulated; it must react with a very specific receptor site to cause a reaction; and it must be immediately broken down or removed from the synapse so that the cell can be ready to be stimulated again.
- Much of the drug therapy in the nervous system involves receptor sites and the release or reuptake and breakdown of neurotransmitters.
- The CNS consists of the brain and spinal cord, which are protected by bone and meninges. To ensure blood flow to the brain if a vessel should become damaged, the brain also has a protective blood supply moderated by the circle of Willis.
- The hindbrain, the most primitive area of the brain, contains the centers that control basic, vital functions. The pons, the medulla, and the reticular activating system (RAS), which regulates arousal and awareness, are all located in the hindbrain. The cerebellum, which helps coordinate motor activity, is found at the back of the hindbrain.
- The midbrain consists of the hypothalamus, the thalamus, and the limbic system. The limbic system is responsible for the expression of emotion, and the thalamus and hypothalamus coordinate internal and external responses and direct information into the cerebral cortex.
- The cerebral cortex consists of two hemispheres, which regulate the communication between sensory and motor neurons and are the sites of thinking and learning.
- The mechanisms of learning and processing learned information are not understood. Emotion-related factors influence the human brain, which handles stimuli and responses in complex ways.
- Much remains to be learned about the human brain and how drugs influence it. The actions of many drugs that have known effects on human behavior are not understood.

Review Questions

1. The reasons that the brain must have a constant blood supply do not include which of the following?
   a. Energy is needed to maintain nerve membranes and cannot be produced without oxygen.
   b. Carbon dioxide must constantly be removed to maintain the proper pH.
   c. Little glucose is stored in nerve cells.
   d. The brain needs a constant supply of insulin and thyroid hormone.
2. The cerebellum
   a. initiates voluntary muscle movement.
   b. helps regulate the tone of skeletal muscles.
   c. if destroyed, would result in the loss of all voluntary skeletal activity.
   d. contains the centers responsible for the regulation of body temperature.
3. At those regions of the nerve membrane where myelin is present, there is
   a. low resistance to electrical current.
   b. high resistance to electrical current.
   c. high conductance of electrical current.
   d. energy loss for the cell.
4. The nerve synapse
   a. is not resistant to electrical current.
   b. cannot become exhausted.
   c. has a synaptic cleft.
   d. transfers information at the speed of electricity.
5. The blood–brain barrier can be described by all but which of the following?
   a. It is produced by the cells that make up the meninges.
   b. It is regulated by the microglia in the CNS.
   c. It is weaker in certain parts of the brain.
   d. It is uniform in its permeability throughout the CNS.
6. Which of the following could result in the initiation of an action potential?
   a. depolarizing the membrane.
   b. decreasing the extracellular potassium concentration.
   c. increasing the activity of the sodium–potassium active transport system.
   d. stimulating the nerve with a threshold electrical stimulus during the absolute refractory period of the membrane.
7. Neurotransmitters are
   a. produced in the muscle to communicate with nerves.
   b. the chemicals used to stimulate or suppress effectors at the nerve synapse.
   c. usually found in the diet.
   d. nonspecific in their action on various nerves.
8. The limbic system is an area of the brain that
   a. is responsible for coordination of movement.
   b. is responsible for the special senses.
   c. is responsible for the expression of emotions.
   d. controls sleep.

9. The most primitive area of the brain, the brainstem, contains areas responsible for
   a. vomiting, swallowing, respiration, arousal, and sleep.
   b. learning.
   c. motivation and memory.
   d. taste, sight, hearing, and balance.

10. A clinical indication of poor blood supply to the brain, particularly to the higher levels where learning takes place, would be
   a. loss of long-term memory.
   b. loss of short-term memory.
   c. living in the past.
   d. insomnia.

BIBLIOGRAPHY

Bullock, B. L. (2000). *Focus on pathophysiology*. Philadelphia: Lippincott Williams & Wilkins.

Fox, S. (1991). *Perspectives on human biology*. Dubuque, IA: Wm. C. Brown Publishers.

Ganong, W. (1999). *Review of medical physiology* (19th ed.). Norwalk, CT: Appleton & Lange.

Guyton, A. & Hall, J. (2000). *Textbook of medical physiology*. Philadelphia: W. B. Saunders.

Gilman, A., Hardman, J. G., & Limbird, L. E. (Eds.) (2002). *Goodman and Gilman's the pharmacological basis of therapeutics* (10th ed.). New York: McGraw-Hill.

CHAPTER

20

Anxiolytic and Hypnotic Agents

Key Terms
anxiety
anxiolytic
barbiturate
benzodiazepine
hypnosis
hypnotic
sedation
sedative

260

Benzodiazepines
alprazolam
chlordiazepoxide
clonazepam
clorazepate
 diazepam
estazolam
flurazepam
halazepam
lorazepam
oxazepam

quazepam
temazepam
triazolam
Barbiturates
amobarbital
aprobarbital
butabarbital
mephobarbital
pentobarbital
 phenobarbital
secobarbital

Other Anxiolytic and Hypnotic Drugs
buspirone
chloral hydrate
diphenhydramine
ethchlorvynol
glutethimide
paraldehyde
promethazine
zaleplon
zolpidem

The drugs discussed in this chapter are used to alter an individual's responses to the environment. They have been called **anxiolytics,** because they can prevent feelings of tension or fear; **sedatives,** because they can calm patients and make them unaware of their environment; **hypnotics,** because they can cause sleep; and minor tranquilizers, because they can produce a state of tranquility in anxious patients. In the past, a given drug would be used at different dosages to yield each of these effects. Further research into how the brain reacts to outside stimuli has resulted in the increased availability of specific agents that produce particular goals and avoid unwanted adverse effects.

STATES AFFECTED BY ANXIOLYTIC AND HYPNOTIC DRUGS

Anxiety

Anxiety is a feeling of tension, nervousness, apprehension, or fear that usually involves unpleasant reactions to a stimulus, whether actual or unknown. Anxiety is often accompanied by signs and symptoms of the sympathetic stress reaction (see Chapter 29), which may include sweating, fast heart rate, rapid breathing, and elevated blood pressure. Mild anxiety, a not uncommon reaction, may serve as a stimulus or motivator in some situations. A person who feels anxious about being alone in a poorly lit parking lot at night may be motivated to take extra safety precautions. When anxiety becomes overwhelming or severe, it can interfere with the activities of daily living and lead to medical problems related to chronic stimulation of the sympathetic nervous system. A severely anxious person may, for example, be afraid to leave the house or to interact with other people. In these cases, treatment is warranted. Anxiolytic drugs are drugs that are used to lyse or break the feeling of anxiety.

Sedation

The loss of awareness and reaction to environmental stimuli is termed **sedation.** This condition may be desirable in patients who are restless, nervous, irritable, or overreacting to stimuli. Although sedation is anxiolytic, it may frequently lead to drowsiness. For example, sedative-induced drowsiness is a concern for outpatients who need to be alert and responsive in their normal lives. On the other hand, this tiredness may be desirable for patients who are about to undergo surgery or other procedures and who are receiving medical support. The choice of an anxiolytic drug depends on the situation in which it will be used, keeping the related adverse effects in mind.

Hypnosis

Extreme sedation results in further central nervous system (CNS) depression and sleep, or **hypnosis.** Hypnotics are used to help people fall asleep by causing sedation. Drugs that are effective hypnotics act on the reticular activating system (RAS) and block the brain's response to incoming stimuli. Hypnosis, therefore, is the extreme state of sedation, in which the person no longer senses or reacts to incoming stimuli.

BENZODIAZEPINES

Benzodiazepines, the most frequently used anxiolytic drugs, prevent anxiety without causing much associated sedation. In addition, they are less likely to cause physical dependence than many of the older sedatives/hypnotics that are used to relieve anxiety. Table 20–1 lists the currently available benzodiazepines, including common indications and specific information about each drug.

Therapeutic Actions and Indications
The benzodiazepines act in the limbic system and the RAS to make γ-aminobutyric acid (GABA) more effective, causing interference with neuron firing (Figure 20–1). This leads to an anxiolytic effect at doses lower than those required to induce sedation and hypnosis. The exact mechanism of action is not clearly understood.

The benzodiazepines are indicated for the treatment of the following conditions: anxiety disorders, alcohol withdrawal, hyperexcitability and agitation, and preoperative relief of anxiety and tension to aid in balanced anesthesia.

Pharmocokinetics
The benzodiazepines are well absorbed from the gastrointestinal (GI) tract with peak levels achieved in 30 minutes to 2 hours. They are lipid soluble and well distributed throughout the body, crossing the placenta and entering breast milk. The benzodiazepines are metabolized extensively in the liver. Patients with liver disease must receive a smaller dose and be monitored closely. Excretion is primarily through the urine.

Contraindications and Cautions
Contraindications to benzodiazepines include the presence of allergy to any benzodiazepine; psychosis, which could be exacerbated by sedation; and acute narrow-angle glaucoma, shock, coma, or acute alcoholic intoxication, all of which could be exacerbated by the depressant effects of these drugs.

In addition, these sedatives/hypnotics are contraindicated in pregnancy, because a predictable syndrome of cleft lip or palate, inguinal hernia, cardiac defects, microcephaly, or pyloric stenosis occurs when they are taken in the first trimester. Neonatal withdrawal syndrome may also result. Lactation is also a contraindication, because of potential adverse effects on the neonate (eg, sedation).

Caution should be used in elderly or debilitated patients, because of the possibility of unpredictable reactions, and in cases of renal or hepatic dysfunction, which may alter the metabolism and excretion of these drugs, resulting in direct toxicity. Dosage adjustments usually are needed for such patients.

DRUG THERAPY ACROSS THE LIFESPAN

Anxiolytic and Hypnotic Agents

Children	Adults	Older Adults
Use of anxiolytic and hypnotic drugs with children is challenging. The response of the child to the drug may be unpredictable; inappropriate aggressiveness, crying, irritability, and tearfulness are common. Of the benzodiazepines, only chlordiazepoxide, clonazepam, clorazepate, and diazepam have established pediatric dosages. Some of the others are used in pediatric settings and dosage may be calculated using age and weight. The barbiturates, being older drugs, have established pediatric dosages. These drugs must be used with caution because of the often unexpected responses. Children must be monitored very closely for CNS depression and excitability. Chloral hydrate and paraldehyde are approved for use in children. The potential for adverse effects and the unpleasant taste and odor of paraldehyde make them less desirable as sleep agents. The antihistamines diphenhydramine and promethazine are more popular for use in helping to calm children and to induce rest and sleep. Care must be taken to assess for possible dried secretions and effects on breathing. Dosage must be calculated carefully.	Adults using these drugs for the treatment of insomnia need to be cautioned that they are for short-term use only. The reason for the insomnia should be sought (eg, medical, hormonal, or anxiety problems). Other methods for helping to induce sleep—established routines, quiet activities before bed, a backrub or warm bath—should be encouraged before drugs are prescribed. Adults receiving anxiolytics also may need referrals for counseling and diagnosis of possible causes. Liver function should be evaluated before and periodically during therapy. These drugs are contraindicated during pregnancy and lactation because of the potential for adverse effects on the fetus and possible sedation of the baby. The antihistamines, which have not been associated with congenital malformations, may be the safest to use, with caution, if an anxiolytic or hypnotic drug must be used.	Older patients may be more susceptible to the adverse effects of these drugs, from unanticipated CNS effects to increased sedation, dizziness, and even hallucinations. Dosages of all of these drugs should be reduced and the patient should be monitored very closely for toxic effects and to provide safety measures if CNS effects do occur. Baseline liver and renal function tests should be performed, and these values should be monitored periodically for any changes that would indicate a need to decrease dosage further or to stop the drug. Nondrug measures to reduce anxiety and to help induce sleep are important with older patients. The patient should be screened for physical problems, neurological deterioration, or depression, which could contribute to the insomnia or anxiety.

DRUGS IN FOCUS

Benzodiazepines

Drug Name	Dosage/Route	Usual Indications
alprazolam (*Xanax*)	0.25–0.5 mg PO t.i.d. up to 1–10 mg/d PO have been used; reduce dosage with older patients	Anxiety; panic attacks **Onset:** 30 min **Duration:** 4–6 hr **Special considerations:** Taper after long-term therapy
chlordiazepoxide (*Librium*)	Adult: 5–25 mg PO t.i.d. to q.i.d.; or 50–100 mg IV or IM; may be repeated; reduce dosage with older patients. Pediatric > 6 y: 5 mg PO b.i.d. to q.i.d.; 25–50 mg IV or IM	Anxiety; alcohol withdrawal; preoperative anxiolytic **Onset:** 10–15 min **Duration:** 2–3 d **Special considerations:** Monitor injection sites
clonazepam (*Klonopin*)	Adult: 1.5 mg/d PO in divided doses; up to 20 mg/d Pediatric: 0.01–0.03 mg/kg per day PO in two to three divided doses, up to 0.1–0.3 mg/kg per day	Seizures; panic attacks; restless leg syndrome; neuralgias; acute manic episodes **Onset:** varies **Duration:** weeks

DRUGS IN FOCUS (CONTINUED)

Benzodiazepines

Drug Name	Dosage/Route	Usual Indications
clorazepate (*Tranxene*)	Adult: 15–60 mg/d in divided doses; 7.5–15 mg/d PO for elderly patients Pediatric: 7.5 mg PO b.i.d. as adjunct therapy for epilepsy	Anxiety; alcohol withdrawal; adjunctive therapy for partial seizures **Onset:** rapid **Duration:** days **Special considerations:** Taper dosage
P diazepam (*Valium*)	Adult: 2–10 mg PO b.i.d. to q.i.d.; or 0.2 mg/kg PR; or 2–30 mg IM b.i.d. or IV; 2–2.5 mg PO b.i.d. for elderly patients Pediatric: 1–2.5 mg PO t.i.d. to q.i.d.; 0.3–0.5 mg/kg PR; or 1–3 mg IM or IV	Anxiety; alcohol withdrawal; muscle relaxant; antiepileptic; antitetanus; preoperative anxiolytic **Onset:** 5–60 min **Duration:** 3 h **Special considerations:** Monitor injection sites; drug of choice if route change is anticipated; taper after long-term therapy
estazolam (*ProSom*)	1 mg PO h.s.; start with 0.5 mg for elderly or debilitated patient	Hypnotic; treatment of insomnia **Onset:** 45–60 min **Duration:** 2 h **Special considerations:** Monitor liver and renal function as well as complete blood count (CBC) if used long-term
flurazepam (*Dalmane*)	30 mg PO h.s.; 15 mg PO h.s. for elderly	Hypnotic; treatment of insomnia **Onset:** varies **Duration:** 30–60 min **Special considerations:** Monitor liver and renal function as well as CBC if used for long-term therapy
halazepam (*Paxipam*)	20–40 mg PO t.i.d. to q.i.d.; 20 mg PO q.d. or b.i.d. for elderly patients	Treatment of anxiety disorders **Onset:** slow **Duration:** 12–14 h
lorazepam (*Ativan*)	2–6 mg/d PO in divided doses; or 0.05 mg/kg IM; or 0.044 mg/kg IV	Anxiety, preanesthesia anxiolytic **Onset:** 1–30 min **Duration:** 12–24 h **Special considerations:** Monitor injection sites; reduce dosage of narcotics given with this drug
oxazepam (*Serax*)	10–15 mg PO t.i.d. to q.i.d.	Anxiety; alcohol withdrawal **Onset:** slow **Duration:** 2–4 h **Special considerations:** Preferred for use in elderly patients
quazepam (*Doral*)	15 mg PO h.s.	Hypnotic; treatment of insomnia **Onset:** varies **Duration:** 4–6 h **Special considerations:** Monitor liver and renal function, CBC if used for long-term therapy; taper after long-term therapy
temazepam (*Restoril*)	15–30 mg PO h.s.	Hypnotic; treatment of insomnia **Onset:** varies **Duration:** 4–6 h **Special considerations:** Taper after long-term therapy
triazolam (*Halcion*)	0.125–0.5 mg PO h.s.	Hypnotic; treatment of insomnia **Onset:** varies **Duration:** 2–4 h **Special considerations:** Monitor liver and renal function, CBC if used for long-term therapy; taper after long-term therapy

*Onset of action and duration are important in selecting the correct drug for a particular use.

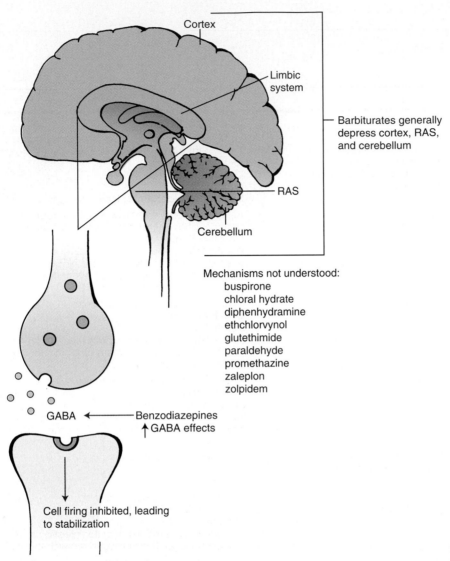

Mechanisms not understood:
buspirone
chloral hydrate
diphenhydramine
ethchlorvynol
glutethimide
paraldehyde
promethazine
zaleplon
zolpidem

FIGURE 20-1. Sites of action of the benzodiazepines and barbiturates.

Adverse Effects

The adverse effects of benzodiazepines are associated with the impact of these drugs on the central and peripheral nervous systems. Nervous system effects include sedation, drowsiness, depression, lethargy, blurred vision, headaches, apathy, light-headedness, and confusion. In addition, mild paradoxical excitatory reactions may occur during the first 2 weeks of therapy.

Several other kinds of adverse effects may occur. GI conditions such as dry mouth, constipation, nausea, vomiting, and elevated liver enzymes may result. Cardiovascular problems may include hypotension, hypertension, arrhythmias, palpitations, and respiratory difficulties. Hematological conditions such as blood dyscrasias and anemia are possible. Genitourinary (GU) effects include urinary retention and hesitancy, loss of libido, and changes in sexual functioning. Because phlebitis, local reactions, and thrombosis may occur at local injection sites, such sites should be monitored.

Abrupt cessation of these drugs may lead to a withdrawal syndrome characterized by nausea, headache, vertigo, malaise, and nightmares.

Clinically Important Drug–Drug Interactions

The risk of CNS depression increases if benzodiazepines are taken with alcohol or other CNS depressants, so such combinations should be avoided.

In addition, the therapeutic effects of benzodiazepines increase if they are taken with cimetidine, oral contraceptives, or disulfiram. If any of these drugs are used with benzodiazepines, patients should be monitored and the appropriate dosage adjustments made.

Finally, the impact of benzodiazepines may be decreased if they are given with theophyllines or ranitidine. If either of these drugs is used, dosage adjustment may be necessary.

Nursing Considerations for Patients Receiving Benzodiazepines

Assessment: History and Examination

Screen for the following conditions, which could be contraindications or cautions to the use of the drug: any known allergies to benzodiazepines; impaired liver or kidney function, which could alter the metabolism and excretion of a

CASE STUDY

Benzodiazepines

THE SITUATION

P. P., a 43-year-old mother of three teenage sons, comes to the outpatient department for a routine physical examination. Results are unremarkable except for blood pressure of 145/90 mm Hg, a pulse of 98 beats/min, and apparent tension—she is jittery, avoids eye contact, and sometimes has teary eyes. She says that she is having some difficulty dealing with "life in general."

P. P. then describes her problems. Her sons present many stresses, and her husband is busy with job-related concerns, has little time to deal with home problems, and is demanding when at home. In addition, she is entering early menopause and having trouble coping with the idea of menopause as well as with some of the symptoms. Overall, she feels that she has no outlet for her anger, tension, or stress.

A health care provider, who reassures P. P. that this problem is common in women of her age, prescribes the benzodiazepine diazepam (*Valium*) to help her deal with her anxiety.

CRITICAL THINKING

What sort of crisis intervention would be most appropriate for P. P.?
What nursing interventions should be done at this point?
What nondrug interventions might be helpful?
What other support systems could be used to help P. P. deal with all that is going on in her life?
Think about the overwhelming problems that P. P. has to deal with on a day-to-day basis and how the anxiolytic effects of diazepam might change her approach to these problems. Could they actually get worse?
Develop a care plan for the long-term care of P. P.

DISCUSSION

Anxiolytics are useful for controlling the unpleasant signs and symptoms of anxiety. The benzodiazepine prescribed for P. P. may provide some immediate relief, enabling her to survive the "crisis" period and plan changes in her "life in general." However, the associated drowsiness and sedation may make coping with the problems in her life even more difficult. She should be taught the adverse effects of diazepam, the warning signs to look for, and the health problems to report.

Follow-up evaluation should be scheduled. Further meetings with the same health care provider are important for the long-term solution to P. P.'s anxiety. Her need for the drug therapy should be re-evaluated once she is able to discover other support systems and develop other ways of coping. Although anxiolytics may be beneficial initially, they do not solve the problems that are causing the anxiety in the first place. In this case, the causes for the anxiety are specific, and the anxiolytic should be considered only as an aid in getting over a crisis period.

Unlike P. P., many patients in severe crisis do not consciously identify the many causes of stress, or stressors. However, P. P. has identified a list of factors that make her life stressful. This facilitates the development of strategies for helping her to cope with her stressors. She may use the following support systems to find ways of coping:

Referral to a counselor, involving the entire family in identification of problems and ways of dealing with them.
Community supports—clergy, support groups.
Support groups for women in various stages of life (e.g., entering menopause, mothers of children who are becoming teenagers). Just having the opportunity to discuss problems and explore ways of dealing with them helps many people.
Hormone replacement therapy to ease her way through menopause. Additional benefits include decreased risk of both heart disease and osteoporosis. Controlling some of the irritating signs and symptoms of menopause may alleviate some of the stress.

---

particular drug; any condition that might be exacerbated by the depressant effects of the drugs (eg, glaucoma, coma, psychoses, shock, acute alcohol intoxication); and pregnancy and lactation.

Include screening for baseline status before beginning therapy to check for occurrence of any potential adverse effects. Assess for the following: temperature and weight; skin color and lesions; affect, orientation, reflexes, and vision; pulse, blood pressure, and perfusion; respiratory rate, adventitious sounds, and presence of chronic pulmonary disease; and bowel sounds on abdominal examination. Laboratory tests should include renal and liver function tests and complete blood count (CBC).

Nursing Diagnoses

The patient receiving a benzodiazepine may have the following nursing diagnoses related to drug therapy:

- Disturbed Thought Processes and Disturbed Sensory Perception (Visual, Kinesthetic) related to CNS effects
- Risk for Injury related to CNS effects
- Disturbed Sleep Pattern related to CNS effects
- Deficient Knowledge regarding drug therapy

Implementation

- Do not administer intra-arterially, *because serious arteriospasm and gangrene could occur.* Monitor injection sites carefully for local reactions *to institute treatment as soon as possible.*
- Do not mix intravenous (IV) drugs in solution with any other drugs *to avoid potential drug–drug interactions.*
- Give parenteral forms only if oral forms are not feasible or available, and switch to oral forms, *which are safer and less likely to cause adverse effects,* as soon as possible.

- Give IV drugs slowly, *because these agents have been associated with hypotension, bradycardia, and cardiac arrest.*
- Arrange to reduce the dosage of narcotic analgesics in patients receiving a benzodiazepine *to decrease potentiated effects and sedation.*
- Maintain patients who receive parenteral benzodiazepines in bed for a period of at least 3 hours. Do not permit ambulatory patients to operate a motor vehicle after an injection, *to ensure patient safety.*
- Monitor hepatic and renal function as well as CBC during long-term therapy *to detect dysfunction and to arrange to taper and discontinue drug if dysfunction occurs.*
- Taper dosage gradually after long-term therapy, especially in epileptic patients. *Acute withdrawal could precipitate seizures in these patients. It may also cause withdrawal syndrome.*
- Provide comfort measures *to help patients tolerate drug effects,* such as having them void before dosing, instituting a bowel program as needed, giving food with the drug if GI upset is severe, environmental control (lighting, temperature, stimulation), safety precautions (use of siderails, assistance with ambulation), orientation.
- Provide thorough patient teaching, including drug name, prescribed dosage, measures for avoidance of adverse effects, and warning signs that may indicate possible problems. Instruct patients about the need for periodic monitoring and evaluation *to enhance patient knowledge about drug therapy and to promote compliance.* (See Patient Teaching Checklist: Benzodiazepines.)
- Offer support and encouragement *to help the patient cope with the diagnosis and the drug regimen.*
- If necessary, use flumazenil (Box 20–1), the benzodiazepine antidote, *for treatment of overdose.*

Evaluation

- Monitor patient response to the drug (alleviation of signs and symptoms of anxiety; sleep; sedation).
- Monitor for adverse effects (sedation, hypotension, cardiac arrhythmias, hepatic or renal dysfunction, blood dyscrasias).
- Evaluate effectiveness of teaching plan (patient can give the drug name, dosage, possible adverse effects to watch for, specific measures to help avoid adverse effects, and the importance of continued follow-up).
- Monitor effectiveness of comfort measures and compliance with regimen (see Nursing Care Guide: Benzodiazepines).

BARBITURATES

The **barbiturates** were once the sedative/hypnotic drugs of choice. Not only is the likelihood of sedation and other adverse effects greater with these drugs than with newer sedative/hypnotic drugs, but the risk of addiction and dependence is also greater. For these reasons, newer anxiolytic drugs have replaced the barbiturates in most instances. Table 20–2 lists the currently available barbiturates, including common indications, and specific information about each drug.

PATIENT TEACHING CHECKLIST
Benzodiazepines

Create customized patient teaching materials for a specific benzodiazepine from the CD-ROM. Patient teaching should stress the following points for drugs within this class:

- Benzodiazepines are used to relieve tension or nervousness. Although the exact way that these drugs work is not completely understood, this group of drugs relaxes muscle spasms, relieves insomnia, and may help manage convulsive disorders.

    Common effects of these drugs include the following:

- *Dizziness, drowsiness, nervousness, and insomnia—* Avoid driving or performing hazardous or delicate tasks that require concentration if these effects occur.
- *Nausea, vomiting, and weight loss—*Small, frequent meals may help to relieve the nausea. Monitor your weight loss and, if it becomes severe, consult your health care provider. Do not take this drug with antacids.
- *Constipation or diarrhea—*These reactions often pass with time. If they do not, consult with your health care provider for appropriate therapy.
- *Vision changes, slurred speech, and unsteadiness—* These effects also may pass with time. Take extra care in your activities for the first few days. If these reactions do not go away after 3 to 4 days, consult your health care provider.

    Report any of the following conditions to your health care provider: rash, fever, sore throat, insomnia, depression, clumsiness, or nervousness.

    If you are discontinuing this drug, tell your health care provider about the following conditions: trembling, muscle cramps, sweating, irritability, confusion, or seizures.

    Tell any doctor, nurse, or other health care provider that you are taking this drug.

    Keep this drug and all medications out of the reach of children.

    Avoid the use of over-the-counter (OTC) medications while you are taking this drug. If you feel that you need one of these OTC preparations, consult with your health care provider about the best choice. Many OTC drugs can interfere with your benzodiazepine.

    Avoid alcohol while you are taking this drug. The alcohol–benzodiazepine combination can cause serious problems.

    If you have been taking this drug for a prolonged period, do not stop taking it suddenly. Your body will need time to adjust to the loss of the drug, and the dosage will need to be reduced gradually to prevent the development of serious problems.
This Teaching Checklist reflects general patient teaching guidelines. It is not meant to be a substitute for drug-specific teaching information, which is available in nursing drug guides.

Therapeutic Actions and Indications
The barbiturates are general CNS depressants that inhibit neuronal impulse conduction in the ascending RAS, depress the cerebral cortex, alter cerebellar function, and depress motor output (see Figure 20–1). Thus, they can cause seda-

BOX 20-1
A Benzodiazepine Antidote

Flumazenil (*Romazicon*), a benzodiazepine antidote, acts by inhibiting the effects of the benzodiazepines at the γ-aminobutyric acid (GABA) receptors. It is used for three purposes: to treat benzodiazepine overdose, to reverse the sedation caused by benzodiazepines that are used as adjuncts for general anesthesia, and to reverse sedation produced for diagnostic tests or other medical procedures.

Flumazenil, which is available for IV use only, is injected into the tubing of a running IV. The drug has a rapid onset of action that peaks 5 to 10 minutes after administration. It is metabolized in the liver. Because this drug has a half-life of about 1 hour, it may be necessary to repeat injections of flumazenil if a long-acting benzodiazepine was used.

Patients who receive flumazenil should be monitored continually, and life-support equipment should be readily available. If the patient has been taking a benzodiazepine for a long period, administration of flumazenil may precipitate a rapid withdrawal syndrome that necessitates supportive measures. Headache, dizziness, vertigo, nausea, and vomiting may be associated with use of fumazenil.

tion, hypnosis, anesthesia, and, in extreme cases, coma. In general, barbiturates are indicated for relief of the signs and symptoms of anxiety, sedation, insomnia, preanesthesia, and seizures. Parenteral forms, which reach peak levels faster and have a faster onset of action, may be used for treatment of acute manic reactions and many forms of seizures (see Chapter 23).

Pharmacokinetics
The barbiturates are absorbed well, reaching peak levels in 20 to 60 minutes. They are metabolized in the liver to varying degrees, depending on the drug, and excreted in the urine. The longer-acting barbiturates tend to be metabolized slower and excreted to a greater degree unchanged in the urine. The barbiturates are known to induce liver enzyme systems, increasing the metabolism of the barbiturate broken down by that system as well as that of any other drug that may be metabolized by that enzyme system. Patients with hepatic or renal dysfunction require lower doses of the drug to avoid toxic effects and should be monitored closely. Barbiturates are lipid soluble; they readily cross the placenta and enter breast milk.

Contraindications and Cautions
Contraindications to barbiturates are the presence of allergy to any barbiturate and a previous history of addiction to sedative/hypnotic drugs, because the barbiturates are more addicting than many other anxiolytics. Other contraindications are latent or manifest porphyria, which may be exacerbated; marked hepatic impairment or nephritis, which may alter the metabolism and excretion of these drugs; and respiratory distress or severe respiratory dysfunction, which could be exacerbated by the CNS depression caused by these

drugs. Pregnancy is a contraindication because of potential adverse effects on the fetus; congenital abnormalities have been reported with barbiturate use.

Caution should be used in patients with acute or chronic pain, because barbiturates can cause paradoxical excitement, masking other symptoms; with seizure disorders, because abrupt withdrawal of a barbiturate can precipitate status epilepticus; and with chronic hepatic, cardiac, or respiratory diseases, which could be exacerbated by the depressive effects of these drugs. Care should be taken with lactating women because of the potential for adverse effects on the infant.

Adverse Effects
As previously stated, the adverse effects caused by barbiturates are more severe than those associated with other, newer sedatives/hypnotics. For this reason, barbiturates are no longer considered the mainstay for the treatment of anxiety. In addition, the development of physical tolerance and psychological dependence is more likely with the barbiturates than with other anxiolytics.

The most common adverse effects are related to general CNS depression. CNS effects may include drowsiness, somnolence, lethargy, ataxia, vertigo, a feeling of a "hangover," thinking abnormalities, paradoxical excitement, anxiety, and hallucinations. GI signs and symptoms such as nausea, vomiting, constipation, diarrhea, and epigastric pain may occur. Associated cardiovascular effects may include bradycardia, hypotension (particularly with IV administration), and syncope. Serious hypoventilation may occur, and respiratory depression and laryngospasm may also result, particularly with IV administration. Hypersensitivity reactions, including rash, serum sickness, and Stevens–Johnson syndrome, which is sometimes fatal, may also occur.

Clinically Important Drug–Drug Interactions
Increased CNS depression results if these agents are taken with other CNS depressants, including alcohol, antihistamines, and other tranquilizers. If other CNS depressants are used, dosage adjustments are necessary.

There often is an altered response to phenytoin if it is combined with barbiturates. Evaluate the patient frequently if this combination cannot be avoided.

If barbiturates are combined with monoamine oxidase (MAO) inhibitors, increased serum levels and effects occur. If the older sedatives/hypnotics are combined with MAO inhibitors, patients should be monitored closely and necessary dosage adjustments made.

In addition, because of an enzyme induction effect of barbiturates in the liver, the following drugs may not be as effective as desired: oral anticoagulants, digoxin, tricyclic antidepressants (TCAs), corticosteroids, oral contraceptives, estrogens, acetaminophen, metronidazole, phenmetrazine, carbamazepine, β-blockers, griseofulvin, phenylbutazones, theophyllines, quinidine, and doxycycline. If these agents are given in combination with barbiturates, patients should be monitored closely; frequent dosage adjustments may be necessary to achieve the desired therapeutic effect.

NURSING CARE GUIDE

Benzodiazepines

Assessment	Nursing Diagnoses	Implementation	Evaluation
HISTORY Allergies to any of these drugs; renal or hepatic dysfunction; pregnancy, lactation; glaucoma; coma; shock; acute alcohol intoxication	Disturbed Thought Processes and Disturbed Sensory Perception (Visual, Kinesthetic) related to CNS effects Risk for Injury related to CNS effects Disturbed Sleep patterns related to CNS effects Deficient Knowledge regarding drug therapy	Do not administer intra-arterially; monitor injection sites Provide comfort and safety measures: small meals; in bed for 3 h after parenteral use; siderails; drug with food if GI upset occurs; bowel program as needed; taper dosage after long-term use; reduce dosage if given with narcotics; lower dose with renal or hepatic impairment. Give IV drugs slowly. Provide support and reassurance to deal with drug effects. Provide patient teaching regarding drug, dosage, adverse effects, what to report, safety precautions.	Evaluate drug effects: Relief of signs and symptoms of anxiety, sedation, sleep. Monitor for adverse effects: sedation, dizziness, insomnia, blood dyscrasias; GI upset; hepatic or renal dysfunction; cardiovascular effects. Monitor for drug–drug interactions as indicated for each drug. Evaluate effectiveness of patient teaching program. Evaluate effectiveness of comfort and safety measures.
PHYSICAL EXAMINATION Cardiovascular: blood pressure, pulse, perfusion CNS: orientation, affect, reflexes, vision Skin: color, lesions, texture Respiratory: respiration, adventitious sounds GI: abdominal examination, bowel sounds Laboratory tests: liver and renal function tests, CBC			

Nursing Considerations for Patients Receiving Barbiturates

Assessment: History and Examination

Screen for the following, which could be contraindications or cautions for the use of the drug: any known allergies to barbiturates or a history of addiction to sedative/hypnotic drugs; impaired hepatic or renal function that could alter the metabolism and excretion of the drug; cardiac dysfunction or respiratory dysfunction; seizure disorders; acute or chronic pain disorders; and pregnancy or lactation.

Include screening for baseline status before beginning therapy and for the occurrence of any potential adverse effects. Assess the following: temperature and weight; blood pressure and pulse, including perfusion; skin color and lesions; affect, orientation, and reflexes; respiratory rate and adventitious sounds; and bowel sounds.

Nursing Diagnoses

The patient receiving a barbiturate may have the following nursing diagnoses related to drug therapy:

- Disturbed Thought Processes and Disturbed Sensory Perception (Visual, Auditory, Kinesthetic, Tactile) related to CNS effects
- Risk for Injury related to CNS effects
- Impaired Gas Exchange related to respiratory depression
- Deficient Knowledge regarding drug therapy

DRUGS IN FOCUS
Barbiturates Used as Anxiolytics/hypnotics*

Drug Name	Dosage/Route	Usual Indications
amobarbital (*Amytal sodium*)	Adult: 65–500 mg IM or IV; reduce dosage with older patients Pediatric: 65–500 mg IM or IV; monitor very closely	Sedative/hypnotic; convulsions; manic reactions **Onset:** 15–60 min **Duration:** 3–8 h **Special considerations:** Monitor carefully if administered by IV
butabarbital (*Butisol*)	Adult: 15–30 mg PO t.i.d. to q.i.d; 50–100 mg PO h.s. for sedation; reduce dosage in elderly Pediatric: 7.5–30 mg PO based on age and weight	Short-term sedative/hypnotic **Onset:** 45–60 min **Duration:** 6–8 h **Special considerations:** Taper gradually after long-term use; use caution in children, may produce aggressiveness, excitability
mephobarbital (*Mebaral*)	Adult: 32–100 mg PO t.i.d. to q.i.d.; 400–600 mg/d PO for seizures; reduce dosage in elderly patients Pediatric: 16–32 mg PO t.i.d. to q.i.d.; 16–64 mg PO t.i.d. to q.i.d. for seizures	Anxiolytic; antiepileptic **Onset:** 30–60 min **Duration:** 10–16 h **Special considerations:** Taper gradually after long-term use; use caution in children, may produce aggressiveness, excitability
pentobarbital (*Nembutal*)	Adult: 20 mg PO t.i.d. to q.i.d.; 100 mg h.s. for insomnia; 120–200 mg PR; 150–200 mg IM or 100 mg IV; reduce dosage in elderly patients Pediatric: 2–6 mg/kg per day; adjust dosage based on age and weight	Sedative/hypnotic; preanesthetic **Onset:** 10–15 min **Duration:** 2–4 h **Special considerations:** Taper gradually after long-term use; give IV slowly; monitor injection sites
℗ phenobarbital (*Luminal*)	Adult: 30–120 mg/d PO, IM, or IV; reduce dosage in elderly patients Pediatric: 1–3 mg/kg IV or IM	Sedative/hypnotic; control of seizures; preanesthetic **Onset:** 10–60 min **Duration:** 4–16 h **Special considerations:** Taper gradually after long-term use; give IV slowly; monitor injection sites
secobarbital (*Seconal*)	Adult: 100–300 mg PO; reduce dosage in elderly patients Pediatric: 2–6 mg/kg PO	Preanesthetic sedation; convulsive seizures of tetanus **Onset:** rapid **Duration:** 1–4 h **Special considerations:** Taper gradually after long-term use

*Onset of action and duration are important in selecting the correct drug for a particular use.

Implementation

- Do not administer these drugs intra-arterially, *because serious arteriospasm and gangrene could occur. Monitor injection sites carefully for local reactions.*
- Do not mix IV drugs in solution with any other drugs, *to avoid potential drug–drug interactions.*
- Give parenteral forms only if oral forms are not feasible or available, and switch to oral forms as soon as possible *to avoid serious reactions or adverse effects.*
- Give IV medications slowly, *because rapid administration may cause cardiac problems.*
- Provide standby life-support facilities *in case of severe respiratory depression or hypersensitivity reactions.*
- Taper dosage gradually after long-term therapy, especially

in patients with epilepsy. *Acute withdrawal may precipitate seizures or cause withdrawal syndrome in these patients.*
- Provide comfort measures *to help patients tolerate drug effects,* including small, frequent meals; access to bathroom facilities; bowel program as needed; consuming food with the drug if GI upset is severe; and environmental control, safety precautions, orientation, and appropriate skin care as needed.
- Provide thorough patient teaching, including drug name, prescribed dosage, measures for avoidance of adverse effects, and warning signs that may indicate possible problems. Instruct patients about the need for periodic monitoring and evaluation *to enhance patient knowledge about drug therapy and to promote compliance.*
- Offer support and encouragement *to help the patient cope with the diagnosis and the drug regimen.*

CULTURAL CONSIDERATIONS
Effects of Delayed Metabolism of Benzodiazepines

Special care should be taken when anxiolytic or hypnotic drugs are given to African Americans. About 15% to 20% of African Americans are genetically predisposed to delayed metabolism of benzodiazepines. As a result, they may develop high serum levels of these drugs, with increased sedation and an increased incidence of adverse effects. If an anxiolytic or hypnotic agent is the drug of choice for an African American individual, the smallest possible dose should be used, and the patient should be monitored very closely during the first week of treatment. Dosage adjustments are necessary to achieve the most effective dose with the fewest adverse effects.

Evaluation

- Monitor patient response to the drug (alleviation of signs and symptoms of anxiety, sleep, sedation, reduction in seizure activity).
- Monitor for adverse effects (sedation, hypotension, cardiac arrhythmias, hepatic or renal dysfunction, skin reactions, dependence).
- Evaluate effectiveness of teaching plan (patient can give the drug name, dosage, possible adverse effects to watch for, specific measures to help avoid adverse effects, and the importance of continued follow-up).
- Monitor effectiveness of comfort measures and compliance with regimen.

■□●■ WEB LINKS
Health care providers and patients may want to consult the following Internet sources:

Information on anxiety and anxiety-related disorders:
  http://www.anxiety.cmhc.com
Information on research, treatment, and support groups related to anxiety and anxiety-related disorders:
  http://www.adaa.org
Information on education programs related to anxiety and anxiety-related disorders:
  http://www.nimh.nih.gov
Patient-oriented and professional information on issues related to mental health:
  http://mhsource.com

OTHER ANXIOLYTIC AND HYPNOTIC DRUGS

There are other drugs used to treat anxiety or to produce hypnosis that do not fall into either the benzodiazepine or the barbiturate group. See Table 20–3 for a summary of the other anxiolytic/hypnotic drugs. Such medications include the following:

- Paraldehyde (*Paral*), a very old drug, is still used orally and rectally to sedate patients with delirium tremens or psychiatric conditions characterized by extreme excitement. It is rapidly absorbed and metabolized in the liver. Excretion of paraldehyde can occur unchanged through the lungs, or the metabolites can be found in the urine. Paraldehyde has a distinctive odor. It cannot be stored in plastic containers or dispensed with a plastic spoon or syringe.
- Chloral hydrate (*Aquachloral*) is frequently used to produce nocturnal sedation or preoperative sedation. Its mechanism of action is unknown. It is rapidly absorbed from the GI tract and metabolized in the liver and kidney for excretion in the bile and urine.
- Ethchlorvynol (*Placidyl*), glutethimide (generic), zaleplon (*Sonata*), and zolpidem (*Ambien*), all of which cause sedation, are used for the short-term treatment of insomnia. They are all metabolized in the liver and excreted in the urine. Caution should be used in patients with hepatic or renal impairment. Elderly patients are especially sensitive to these drugs; they should receive a lower dose and should be monitored carefully.
- Antihistamines (promethazine [*Phenergan*], diphenhydramine [*Benadryl*]) can be very sedating in some people. They are used as preoperative medications and postoperatively to decrease the need for narcotics. Patients need to be monitored for thickened respiratory secretions and breathing difficulties, a problem that can cause concern after anesthesia.
- Buspirone (*BuSpar*), a newer antianxiety agent, has no sedative, anticonvulsant, or muscle-relaxant properties, and its mechanism of action is unknown. However, it reduces the signs and symptoms of anxiety without many of the CNS effects and severe adverse effects associated with other anxiolytic drugs. It is rapidly absorbed from the GI tract, metabolized in the liver, and excreted in urine. Caution should be used in patients with hepatic or renal impairment and in elderly patients.

CHAPTER SUMMARY

- Anxiety is a feeling of tension, nervousness, apprehension, or fear. It is usually an unpleasant reaction to an actual or an unknown stimulus. In extreme cases, anxiety may produce physiological manifestations and may interfere with life.
- Anxiolytics, or minor tranquilizers, are drugs used to treat anxiety by depressing the CNS. When given at higher doses, these drugs may be sedatives or hypnotics.
- Sedatives block the awareness of and reaction to environmental stimuli, resulting in associated CNS depression that may cause drowsiness, lethargy, and other effects. This action can be beneficial when a patient is very excited or afraid.
- Hypnotics further depress the CNS, particularly the RAS, to cause an inhibition of neuronal arousal and sleep induction.
- Benzodiazepines are a group of drugs used as anxiolytics. They react with GABA inhibitory sites to depress the CNS. They can cause drowsiness, lethargy, and other CNS effects.

DRUGS IN FOCUS
Other Anxiolytic/Hypnotic Drugs

Drug Name	Usual Indications
buspirone (BuSpar)	Oral drug anxiety disorders; unlabeled use; signs and symptoms of premenstrual syndrome **Special considerations:** May cause dry mouth, headache
chloral hydrate (Aquachloral)	Administered PO or PR for nocturnal sedation, preoperative sedation **Special considerations:** Withdraw gradually over 2 wk in patients maintained for weeks or months
diphenhydramine (Benadryl)	Oral, IM, or IV for sleep aid, motion sickness, allergic rhinitis **Special considerations:** Antihistamine, drying effects common
ethchlorvynol (Placidyl)	Oral drug for short-term treatment of insomnia (up to 1 wk) **Special considerations:** Dispense least amount possible to depressed and/or suicidal patients; withdraw gradually if used for prolonged period
glutethimide (generic)	Oral drug for short-term treatment of insomnia (up to 1 wk) **Special considerations:** Dispense least amount possible to depressed and/or suicidal patients; withdraw gradually if used for prolonged period
paraldehyde (Paral)	Given PO or PR for sedation in acute psychiatric excitement and acute alcoholic withdrawal **Special considerations:** Dilute before use; use food to improve taste; avoid contact with plastic; keep away from heat or flame; discard any unused portion
promethazine (Phenergan)	Oral, IM, or IV use to decrease the need for postoperative pain relief and for preoperative sedation **Special considerations:** An antihistamine; monitor injection sites carefully
zaleplon (Sonata)	Oral drug for the short-term treatment of insomnia **Special considerations:** Must reman in bed for 4 h after taking drug
zolpidem (Ambien)	Oral drug for short-term treatment of insomnia **Special considerations:** Dispense least amount possible to depressed and/or suicidal patients; withdraw gradually if used for prolonged period

- Barbiturates are an older class of drugs used as anxiolytics, sedatives, and hypnotics. Because they are associated with potentially serious adverse effects and interact with many other drugs, they are less desirable than the benzodiazepines or other anxiolytics.

- Buspirone, a newer anxiolytic drug, does not cause sedation or muscle relaxation. Because of the absence of CNS effects, it is much preferred in certain circumstances (eg, when a person must drive, go to work, or maintain alertness).

Review Questions

1. Drugs that are used to alter a patient's response to the environment are called
   a. hypnotics.
   b. sedatives.
   c. antiepileptics.
   d. anxiolytics.

2. A patient who is experiencing anxiety would probably not present with
   a. rapid breathing.
   b. rapid heart rate.
   c. fear and apprehension.
   d. constricted pupils.

3. The benzodiazepines are the most frequently used anxiolytic drugs because

   a. they are anxiolytic at doses much lower than those needed for sedation or hypnosis.
   b. they can also be stimulating.
   c. they are more likely to cause physical dependence than older anxiolytic drugs.
   d. they do not affect any neurotransmitters.

4. Your patient has a long history of anxiety and has always responded well to diazepam. She has just learned that she is pregnant and feels very anxious. She would like a prescription for diazepam to get her through her early anxiety. In explaining why this is not recommended, the rationale would include all but which of the following?
   a. These drugs are known to cause a predictable syndrome of birth defects including cleft lip and pyloric stenosis.
   b. The baby born to a mother taking benzodiazepines may progress through a neonatal withdrawal syndrome.
   c. Cardiac defects and small brain development may occur it this drug is taken in the first trimester
   d. These drugs almost always cause loss of the pregnancy.

5. Barbiturates cause liver enzyme induction, which could lead to
   a. rapid metabolism and loss of effectiveness of other drugs metabolized by those enzymes.
   b. increased bile production.

  c. CNS depression.

  d. the need to periodically lower the barbiturate dose to avoid toxicity.

6. Anxiolytic drugs that are recommended for short-term treatment of insomnia do not include

  a. zolpidem.

  b. chloral hydrate.

  c. buspirone.

  d. glutethimide.

7. Anxiolytic drugs block the awareness of and reaction to the environment. This effect would not be beneficial

  a. to relieve extreme fear.

  b. to moderate anxiety related to unknown causes.

  c. in treating a patient who must drive a vehicle for a living.

  d. in treating a patient who is experiencing a stress reaction.

8. Mr. Jones is the chief executive officer of a large company and has been experiencing acute anxiety attacks. His physical examination was normal and he was diagnosed with anxiety. Considering his occupation and his need to be alert and present to large groups on a regular basis, the following anxiolytic would be a drug of choice for Mr. Jones:

  a. phenobarbital.

  b. diazepam.

  c. clorazepate.

  d. buspirone.

9. The benzodiazepines react with

  a. GABA receptor sites in the RAS to cause inhibition of neural arousal.

  b. norepinephrine receptor sites in the sympathetic nervous system.

  c. acetylcholine receptor sites in the parasympathetic nervous system.

  d. monoamine oxidase to increase norepinephrine breakdown.

BIBLIOGRAPHY

Bailey, K. (1998). *Psychotropic drug facts*. Philadelphia: Lippincott-Raven.

Bullock, B. L. (2000). *Focus on pathophysiology*. Philadelphia: Lippincott Williams & Wilkins.

Gilman, A., Hardman, J. G., & Limbird, L. E. (Eds.) (2002). *Goodman and Gilman's the pharmacological basis of therapeutics* (10th ed.). New York: McGraw-Hill.

Karch, A. M. (2002). *2003 Lippincott's nursing drug guide*. Philadelphia: Lippincott Williams & Wilkins.

Drug facts and comparisons. (2002). St. Louis: Facts and Comparisons.

Professional's guide to patient drug facts. (2002). St. Louis: Facts and Comparisons.

C H A P T E R

21

Antidepressant Agents

Key Terms
affect
biogenic amine
depression
monoamine oxidase (MAO) inhibitor
selective serotonin reuptake inhibitor (SSRI)
tricyclic antidepressant (TCA)
tyramine

273

When you ask people how they feel, they may say "pretty good" or "not so great." People's responses are usually appropriate to what is happening in their lives, and they describe themselves as being in a good mood or a bad mood. Some days are better than others.

Affect is a term that is used to refer to people's feelings in response to their environment, whether positive and pleasant or negative and unpleasant. All people experience different affective states at various times in their lives. These states of mind, which change in particular situations, usually do not last very long and do not often involve extremes of happiness or depression. If a person's mood goes far beyond the usual, normal "ups and downs," he or she is said to have an affective disorder.

DEPRESSION AND ANTIDEPRESSANTS

Depression, a very common affective disorder, strikes millions of people every year. In depression, feelings of sadness are much more severe and long-lasting than the suspected precipitating event, and the mood of affected individuals is much more intense. The depression may not even be traceable to a specific event or stressor (ie, there are no external causes). Patients who are depressed may have little energy, sleep disturbances, a lack of appetite, limited libido, and inability to perform activities of daily living. They may describe overwhelming feelings of sadness, despair, hopelessness, and disorganization.

In many cases, the depression is never diagnosed, and the patient is treated for physical manifestations of the underlying disease, such as fatigue, malaise, obesity, anorexia, or alcoholism and drug dependence. Clinical depression is an actual disorder that can interfere with a person's family life, job, and social interactions. Left untreated, it can produce multiple physical problems that can lead to further depression or, in extreme cases, even suicide.

Biogenic Amine Theory of Depression

Research on development of the drugs known to be effective in relieving depression led to formulation of the current hypothesis regarding the cause of depression. Scientists have theorized that depression results from a deficiency of norepinephrine (NE), dopamine, or serotonin (5HT), which are all **biogenic amines,** in key areas of the brain. Both NE and 5HT are released throughout the brain by neurons that react with multiple receptors to regulate arousal, alertness, attention, moods, appetite, and sensory processing. Deficiencies of these neurotransmitters may develop for three known reasons. First, monoamine oxidase (MAO) may break them down to be recycled or restored in the neuron. Second, rapid fire of the neurons may lead to their depletion. Third, the number or sensitivity of postsynaptic receptors may increase, thus depleting neurotransmitter levels.

Depression may also occur as a result of other, yet unknown causes. This condition may be a syndrome that reflects either activity or lack of activity in a number of sites in the brain including the arousal center (reticular activating system, or RAS), the limbic system, and basal ganglia.

Drug Therapy

Today, the use of agents that alter the concentration of neurotransmitters in the brain is the most effective means of treating depression with drugs. The antidepressant drugs used today counteract the effects of neurotransmitter deficiencies in three ways. First, they may inhibit the effects of MAO, leading to increased NE or 5HT in the synaptic cleft. Second, they may block reuptake by the releasing nerve, leading to increased neurotransmitter levels in the synaptic cleft. Third, they may regulate receptor sites and breakdown of neurotransmitters, leading to an accumulation of neurotransmitter in the synaptic cleft.

Antidepressants may be classified into three groups: the **tricyclic antidepressants** (TCAs), the **MAO inhibitors,** and the **selective serotonin reuptake inhibitors** (SSRIs). Other drugs that are used as antidepressants similarly increase the synaptic cleft concentrations of these neurotransmitters (Figure 21–1).

Tricyclic Antidepressants

The TCAs, including the amines, secondary amines, and tetracyclics, all reduce the reuptake of 5HT and NE into nerves. Because all TCAs are similarly effective, the choice of TCA depends on individual response to the drug and tolerance of adverse effects. A patient who does not respond to one TCA may respond to another drug from this class. Table 21–1 lists the currently available TCAs, including the specific type and the occurrence of sedation and other adverse effects.

Therapeutic Actions and Indications

The TCAs inhibit presynaptic reuptake of the neurotransmitters NE and 5HT, which leads to an accumulation of these neurotransmitters in the synaptic cleft and increased stimulation of the postsynaptic receptors. The exact mechanism of action in decreasing depression is not known, but is thought to be related to the accumulation of NE and 5HT in certain areas of the brain.

TCAs are indicated for the relief of symptoms of depression. The sedative effects of these drugs may make them more effective in patients whose depression is characterized by anxiety and sleep disturbances. They are effective for treating enuresis in children older than 6 years. Some of these drugs are being investigated for the treatment of chronic, intractable pain. In addition, the TCAs are anticholinergic. Clomipramine is now also approved for use in the treatment of obsessive–compulsive disorders (OCDs).

Pharmacokinetics

The TCAs are well absorbed from the gastrointestinal (GI) tract, reaching peak levels in 2 to 4 hours. They are highly

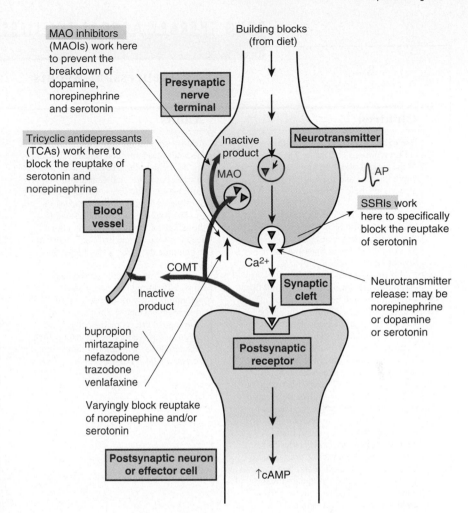

MAO inhibitors (MAOIs) work here to prevent the breakdown of dopamine, norepinephrine and serotonin

Tricyclic antidepressants (TCAs) work here to block the reuptake of serotonin and norepinephrine

Building blocks (from diet)

Presynaptic nerve terminal

Inactive product

MAO

Neurotransmitter

AP

Blood vessel

SSRIs work here to specifically block the reuptake of serotonin

COMT

Ca²⁺

Inactive product

Synaptic cleft

Neurotransmitter release: may be norepinephrine or dopamine or serotonin

bupropion
mitrazapine
nefazodone
trazodone
venlafaxine

Postsynaptic receptor

Varyingly block reuptake of norepinephine and/or serotonin

Postsynaptic neuron or effector cell

↑cAMP

FIGURE 21–1. Sites of action for the antidepressants: monoamine oxidase (MAO) inhibitors, tricyclic antidepressants, selective serotonin reuptake inhibitors (SSRIs), and other agents. cAMP, cyclic adenosine monophosphate; COMT, catecholamine-O-methyl transferase.

bound to plasma proteins and are lipid soluble; this allows them to be distributed widely in the tissues, including the brain. TCAs are metabolized in the liver and excreted in the urine, with relatively long half-lives ranging from 8 to 46 hours. Patients with liver impairment need a lower dose of the drug to avoid toxic levels. The TCAs cross the placenta and enter breast milk. They should not be used during pregnancy or lactation unless the benefit to the mother clearly outweighs the potential risk to the neonate.

Contraindications and Cautions

One contraindication to the use of TCAs is the presence of allergy to any of the drugs in this class. Other contraindications include recent myocardial infarction, because of the potential occurrence of reinfarction or extension of the infarct with the cardiac effects of the drug; myelography within the previous 24 hours or in the next 48 hours; and concurrent use of an MAO inhibitor, because of the potential for serious adverse effects or toxic reactions. In addition, pregnancy and lactation are contraindications because of the potential for adverse effects in the fetus and neonate.

Caution should be used with TCAs in patients with pre-existing cardiovascular (CV) disorders, because of the cardiac stimulatory effects of the drug, and with any condition that would be exacerbated by the anticholinergic effects, such as angle-closure glaucoma, urinary retention, prostate hypertrophy, or GI or genitourinary (GU) surgery. Care should also be taken with psychiatric patients, who may exhibit a worsening of psychoses or paranoia, and with manic–depressive patients, who may shift to a manic stage. In addition, caution is necessary in patients with a history of seizures, because the seizure threshold may be decreased secondary to stimulation of the receptor sites, and in elderly patients. The presence of hepatic or renal disease, which could interfere with metabolism and excretion of these drugs and lead to toxic levels, also necessitates caution.

Adverse Effects

The adverse effects of TCAs are associated with the effects of the drugs on the central nervous system (CNS) and on the peripheral nervous system. Sedation, sleep disturbances, fatigue, hallucinations, disorientation, visual disturbances, difficulty in concentrating, weakness, ataxia, and tremors may occur.

Use of TCAs may lead to GI anticholinergic effects such as dry mouth, constipation, nausea, vomiting, anorexia, increased salivation, cramps, and diarrhea. Resultant GU effects may include urinary retention and hesitancy, loss of li-

DRUG THERAPY ACROSS THE LIFESPAN

Antidepressant Agents

Children	Adults	Older Adults
Use of antidepressant drugs with children poses a challenge. The response of the child to the drug may be unpredictable, and the long-term effects of many of these agents are not clearly understood. Monoamine oxidase (MAO) inhibitors should be avoided in children if at all possible because of the potential for drug–food interactions and the serious adverse effects. Of the tricyclic drugs (TCAs), clomipramine, imipramine, nortriptyline, and trimipramine have established pediatric dosages. Children should be monitored closely for adverse effects, and dosage changes should be made as needed. The selective serotonin reuptake inhibitors (SSRIs) can cause serious adverse effects in children. Fluvoxamine and sertraline have established pediatric dosage guidelines for the treatment of obsessive–compulsive disorders. Fluoxetine is widely used to treat depression in adolescents, and a 2000 survey of off-label uses of drugs showed that it was being used in children as young as 6 months. Dosage regimens must be established according to the child's age and weight, and a child receiving an antidepressant should be monitored very carefully. Underlying medical reasons for the depression should be ruled out before antidepressant therapy is begun.	Adults using these drugs should have medical causes for their depression ruled out before therapy is begun. Thyroid disease, hormonal imbalance, and cardiovascular disorders can all lead to the signs and symptoms of depression. The patient needs to understand that the effects of drug therapy may not be seen for 4 weeks and that it is important to continue the therapy for at least that long. These drugs should be used very cautiously during pregnancy and lactation because of the potential for adverse effects on the fetus and possible neurological effects on the baby. Use should be reserved for situations in which the benefits to the mother far outweigh the potential risks to the neonate.	Older patients may be more susceptible to the adverse effects of these drugs, from unanticipated central nervous system (CNS) effects to increased sedation, dizziness, and even hallucinations. Dosages of all of these drugs need to be reduced and the patient monitored very closely for toxic effects. Safety measures should be provided if CNS effects do occur. Patients with hepatic or renal impairment should be monitored very closely while taking these drugs. Decreased dosages may be needed. Because many older patients also have renal or hepatic impairment, they need to be screened carefully.

bido, and changes in sexual functioning. CV effects such as orthostatic hypotension, hypertension, arrhythmias, myocardial infarction, angina, palpitations, and stroke may also pose problems. Miscellaneous reported effects include alopecia, weight gain or loss, flushing, chills, and nasal congestion.

These adverse effects may be intolerable to some patients, who then stop taking the particular TCA. Abrupt cessation of all TCAs causes a withdrawal syndrome characterized by nausea, headache, vertigo, malaise, and nightmares.

Clinically Important Drug–Drug Interactions
If TCAs are given with cimetidine, fluoxetine, or ranitidine, an increase in TCA levels results, with an increase in both therapeutic and adverse effects, especially anticholinergic conditions. Patients should be monitored closely, and appropriate dosage reductions should be made.

Other drug combinations may also pose problems. The combination of TCAs and oral anticoagulants leads to higher serum levels of the anticoagulants and increased risk of bleed-

ing. Blood tests should be done frequently, and appropriate dosage adjustments in the oral anticoagulant should be made.

If TCAs are combined with sympathomimetics or clonidine, the risk of arrhythmias and hypertension is increased. This combination should be avoided, especially in patients with underlying CV disease.

The combination of TCAs with MAO inhibitors leads to a risk of severe hyperpyretic crisis with severe convulsions, hypertensive episodes, and death. This combination should be avoided. Although TCAs and MAO inhibitors have been used together in selected patients who do not respond to a single agent, the risk of severe adverse effects is very high.

Nursing Considerations for Patients Receiving Tricyclic Antidepressants
Assessment: History and Examination

Screen for the following, which could be contraindications or cautions for the use of the drug: any known allergies to these drugs; impaired liver or kidney function that could al-

TABLE 21-1	The Tricyclic Antidepressants, Indicating Side Effects Most Frequently Associated with Each Drug

| Drug Name | Type | Common Side Effects | | | | Usual Dosage |
		Sedation	Anticholinergic	Hypotension	Cardiovascular	
amitriptyline (*Elavil*)	Amine	++++	++++	++++	++	75–150 mg/d PO
amoxapine (*Asendin*)	Amine	+	+	++	++	50–100 mg PO b.i.d.–t.i.d.
clomipramine (*Anafranil*)	Amine	+++	+++	+++	+++	Adult: 25–50 mg PO q.i.d. Pediatric: 25 mg PO q.i.d. to a maximum of 3 mg/kg per day
desipramine (*Norpramin*)	Secondary amine	+	+	++	++	100–200 mg/d PO
doxepin (*Sinequan*)	Amine	+++	+++	++	++	25–50 mg PO t.i.d.
ⓟ imipramine (*Tofranil*)	Amine	++	++	+++	++	Adult: 50–200 mg/d PO Pediatric: 30–40 mg/d PO Enuresis: 25 mg/d 1 h before bed
maprotiline (*Ludiomil*)	Tetracyclic	++	+	++	++	75–150 mg/d PO; reduce dosage in elderly patients
nortriptyline (*Aventyl, Pamelor*)	Secondary amine	+	+	+	+	Adult: 25–50 mg PO t.i.d.–q.i.d. Pediatric: 30–50 mg/d PO in divided doses Geriatric: 30–50 mg/d PO in divided doses
protriptyline (*Vivactil*)	Secondary amine	+	+++	+	+	15–40 mg/d PO in three or four divided doses; 5 mg PO t.i.d. for elderly patients
trimipramine (*Surmontil*)	Amine	+++	++	++	++	Adult: 75–150 mg/d PO Pediatric: 50 mg/d PO Geriatric: 50–100 mg/d PO

++++ = marked effects; +++ = moderate effects; ++ = mild effects; + = negligible effects.

ter metabolism and excretion of the drug; glaucoma, benign prostatic hypertrophy, cardiac dysfunction, GI obstruction, surgery, or recent myocardial infarction, all of which could be exacerbated by the effects of the drug; and pregnancy or lactation. Find out whether the patient has a history of seizure disorders, or a history of psychiatric problems or myelography within the past 24 hours or in the next 48 hours, or is taking an MAO inhibitor.

Include screening for baseline status before beginning therapy and for any potential adverse effects. Assess the following: temperature and weight; skin color and lesions; affect, orientation, and reflexes; vision; blood pressure, including orthostatic blood pressure; pulse and perfusion; respiratory rate and adventitious sounds; and bowel sounds on abdominal examination. Obtain an electrocardiogram as well as renal and liver function tests.

Nursing Diagnoses

The patient receiving a TCA may have the following nursing diagnoses related to drug therapy:

- Acute Pain related to anticholinergic effects, headache, CNS effects
- Decreased Cardiac Output related to CV effects
- Disturbed Thought Processes and Disturbed Sensory Perception (Visual, Auditory, Kinesthetic, Tactile, or Olfactory) related to CNS effects
- Risk for Injury related to CNS effects
- Deficient Knowledge regarding drug therapy

Implementation

- Limit drug access if the patient is suicidal, *because of the potential for overdose.*
- Maintain initial dosage for 4 to 8 weeks *to evaluate the therapeutic effect.*
- Give parenteral forms of the drug only if oral forms are not feasible or available; switch to an oral form, *which is less toxic and associated with fewer adverse effects,* as soon as possible.
- Give the major portion of the dose at bedtime if drowsiness and anticholinergic effects are severe, *to decrease the risk*

of patient injury. Elderly patients may not be able to tolerate larger doses.

- Reduce the dosage if minor adverse effects occur, and discontinue the drug slowly if major or potentially life-threatening adverse effects occur, *to ensure patient safety.*
- Provide comfort measures *to help the patient tolerate drug effects.* These measures may include voiding before dosing, instituting a bowel program as needed, taking food with the drug if GI upset is severe, and environmental control (lighting, temperature, stimuli).
- Provide thorough patient teaching, including drug name, prescribed dosage, measures for avoidance of adverse effects, and warning signs that may indicate possible problems. Instruct patients about the need for periodic monitoring and evaluation *to enhance patient knowledge about drug therapy and to promote compliance.*
- Offer support and encouragement *to help patients cope with the diagnosis and the drug regimen.*

Evaluation

- Monitor patient response to the drug (alleviation of signs and symptoms of depression).
- Monitor for adverse effects (sedation, anticholinergic effects, hypotension, cardiac arrhythmias).
- Evaluate effectiveness of teaching plan (patient can give the drug name, dosage, possible adverse effects to watch for, specific measures to help avoid adverse effects, and importance of continued follow-up).
- Monitor the effectiveness of comfort measures and compliance with the regimen.

MONOAMINE OXIDASE INHIBITORS

At one time, MAO inhibitors were used more often, but now they are used rarely because they require a specific dietary regimen to prevent toxicity. Safer drugs that are usually just as effective have replaced them. Agents still in use include the following:

- Isocarboxazid (*Marplan*), which once became unavailable because it was infrequently used, reappeared in 1998 when researchers found that some patients who did not respond to the newer, safer antidepressants could respond to this drug.
- Phenelzine (*Nardil*) is also reserved for patients who do not respond to other antidepressants or who cannot take other antidepressants for some reason.
- Tranylcypromine (*Parnate*) is used for adult outpatients with reactive depression. This agent is also associated with potentially fatal drug–food interactions.

The choice of an MAO inhibitor depends on the prescriber's experience and individual response. A patient who does not respond to one MAO inhibitor may respond to another.

Therapeutic Actions and Indications

The MAO inhibitors irreversibly inhibit MAO, an enzyme found in nerves and other tissues (including the liver) that breaks down the biogenic amines NE, dopamine, and 5HT. This allows these amines to accumulate in the synaptic cleft and in neuronal storage vesicles, causing increased stimulation of the postsynaptic receptors and, it is thought, relief of depression.

The MAO inhibitors are generally indicated for treatment of the signs and symptoms of depression in patients who cannot tolerate or do not respond to other, safer antidepressants.

Pharmacokinetics

The MAO inhibitors are well absorbed from the GI tract, reaching peak levels in 2 to 3 hours. They are metabolized in the liver primarily by acetylation and are excreted in the urine. Patients with liver or renal impairment and those known as "slow acetlyators" may require lowered doses to avoid exaggerated effects of the drugs. The MAO inhibitors cross the placenta and enter breast milk. Avoid use during pregnancy and lactation unless the benefit to the mother clearly outweighs the potential risk to the neonate.

Contraindications and Cautions

Contraindications to the use of MAO inhibitors include allergy to any of these antidepressants; pheochromocytoma, because the sudden increases in NE levels could result in severe hypertension and CV emergencies; CV disease, including hypertension, coronary artery disease, angina, and congestive heart failure, which could be exacerbated by increased NE levels; and known abnormal CNS vessels or defects, because the potential increase in blood pressure and vasoconstriction associated with higher NE levels could precipitate a stroke. A history of headaches may also be a contraindication.

Other contraindications include renal or hepatic impairment, which could alter the metabolism and excretion of these drugs and lead to toxic levels, and myelography within the past 24 hours or in the next 48 hours, because of the risk of severe reaction to the dye used in myelography.

In addition, caution should be used with psychiatric patients, who could be overstimulated or shift to a manic phase as a result of the stimulation associated with MAO inhibitors, and in patients with seizure disorders or hyperthyroidism, both of which could be exacerbated by the stimulation of these drugs. Care should also be taken with patients who are soon to undergo elective surgery, because of the potential for unexpected effects with NE accumulation during the stress reaction, and with female patients who are pregnant or breast feeding, because of potential adverse effects on the fetus and neonate.

Adverse Effects

The MAO inhibitors are associated with more adverse effects, more of which are fatal, than most other antidepressants. The effects relate to the accumulation of NE in the synaptic cleft. Dizziness, excitement, nervousness, mania, hyperreflexia, tremors, confusion, insomnia, agitation, and blurred vision may occur.

MAO inhibitors can cause liver toxicity. Other GI effects can include nausea, vomiting, diarrhea or constipation, anorexia, weight gain, dry mouth, and abdominal pain. Urinary retention, dysuria, incontinence, and changes in sexual function may also occur. CV effects can include orthostatic hypotension, arrhythmias, palpitations, angina, and the potentially fatal hypertensive crisis. This last condition is characterized by occipital headache, palpitations, neck stiffness, nausea, vomiting, sweating, dilated pupils, photophobia, tachycardia, and chest pain. It may progress to intracranial bleeding and fatal stroke.

Clinically Important Drug–Drug Interactions

Drug interactions of MAO inhibitors with other antidepressants include hypertensive crisis, coma, and severe convulsions with TCAs, and a potentially life-threatening serotonin syndrome with SSRIs. A period of 6 weeks should elapse after stopping an SSRI before beginning an MAO inhibitor.

If MAO inhibitors are given with other sympathomimetic drugs (eg, methyldopa, guanethidine), sympathomimetic effects increase. Combinations with insulin or oral antidiabetic agents result in additive hypoglycemic effects. Patients who receive these combinations must be monitored closely, and appropriate dosage adjustments should be made.

Clinically Important Drug–Food Interactions

Tyramine and other pressor amines that are found in food, which are normally broken down by MAO enzymes in the GI tract, may be absorbed in high concentrations in the presence of MAO inhibitors, resulting in increased blood pressure. The hypertensive crisis is often associated with eating foods that contain tyramine. In addition, tyramine causes the release of stored NE from nerve terminals, which further contributes to high blood pressure. Patients who take MAO inhibitors should avoid the tyramine-containing foods listed in Table 21–2.

Nursing Considerations for Patients Receiving Monoamine Oxidase Inhibitors

Assessment: History and Examination

Screen for the following, which could be contraindications or cautions for use of the drug: any known allergies to these drugs; impaired liver or kidney function that could alter the metabolism and excretion of the drug; cardiac dysfunction; GI or GU obstruction; surgery, including elective surgery; seizure disorders; psychiatric conditions; and occurrence of myelography within the past 24 hours or in the next 48 hours. Find out whether female patients are pregnant or breast feeding.

Include screening for baseline status before beginning therapy and for any potential adverse effects. Assess the following: temperature and weight; skin color and lesions; affect, orientation, and reflexes; vision; blood pressure, including orthostatic blood pressure; pulse and perfusion; respiratory rate and adventitious sounds; and bowel sounds on abdominal examination. Obtain an electrocardiogram and renal and liver function tests.

Nursing Diagnoses

The patient receiving an MAO inhibitor may have the following nursing diagnoses related to drug therapy:

- Acute Pain related to sympathomimetic effects, headache, CNS effects
- Decreased Cardiac Output related to CV effects
- Disturbed Thought Processes and Disturbed Sensory Perception (Visual, Kinesthetic) related to CNS effects
- Risk for Injury related to CNS effects
- Deficient Knowledge regarding drug therapy

Implementation

- Limit drug access to potentially suicidal patients *to decrease the risk of overdose.*
- Monitor the patient for 2 to 4 weeks *to ascertain onset of full therapeutic effect.*
- Monitor blood pressure and orthostatic blood pressure carefully *to arrange for a slower increase in dosage as needed for patients who show a tendency toward hypotension.*
- Monitor liver function before and periodically during therapy and *arrange to discontinue the drug at the first sign of liver toxicity.*
- Discontinue the drug and monitor the patient carefully at any complaint of severe headache *to decrease the risk of severe hypertension and cerebrovascular effects.*

TABLE 21-2 | Tyramine-Containing Foods

Foods High in Tyramine	Foods With Moderate Amounts of Tyramine	Foods With Low Amounts of Tyramine
Aged cheeses: cheddar cheese, bleu cheese, Swiss cheese, Camembert	Meat extracts: consommé, bouillon	Distilled liquors: vodka, gin, Scotch, rye
Aged or fermented meats, fish or poultry: chicken paté, beef liver paté, caviar	Pasteurized light and pale beer	Cheeses: American, mozzarella, cottage cheese, cream cheese
Brewer's yeast	Avocados	Chocolate
Fava beans		Fruits: figs, raisins, grapes, pineapple, oranges
Red wines: Chianti, burgundy, sherry, vermouth		Sour cream
Smoked or pickled meats, fish or poultry: herring, sausage, corned beef, salami, pepperoni		Soy sauce
		Yogurt

DRUGS IN FOCUS
Monoamine Oxidase Inhibitors

Drug Name	Dosage/Route	Usual Indications
isocarboxazid (Marplan)	10 mg PO b.i.d., may reach a maximum of 40 mg/d	Depression not responsive to other agents
℗ phenelzine (Nardil)	15 mg PO t.i.d.	Depression not responsive to other agents
tranylcypromine (Parnate)	30 mg/d PO in divided doses	Adult reactive depression

- Have phentolamine or another adrenergic blocker on standby *as treatment in case of hypertensive crisis.*
- Provide comfort measures *to help the patient tolerate drug effects.* These include voiding before dosing, instituting a bowel program as needed, taking food with the drug if GI upset is severe, and environmental control (lighting, temperature, decreased stimulation).
- Provide a list of potential drug–food interactions that can cause severe toxicity *to decrease the risk of a serious drug–food interaction.* Provide a diet that is low in tyramine-containing foods.
- Provide thorough patient teaching, including drug name, prescribed dosage, measures for avoidance of adverse effects, and warning signs that may indicate possible problems. Instruct patients about the need for periodic monitoring and evaluation *to enhance patient knowledge about drug therapy and to promote compliance.*
- Offer support and encouragement *to help patients cope with the disease and the drug regimen.*

Evaluation

- Monitor patient response to the drug (alleviation of signs and symptoms of depression).
- Monitor for adverse effects (sedation, sympathomimetic effects, hypotension, cardiac arrhythmias, GI disturbances, hypertensive crisis).
- Evaluate the effectiveness of the teaching plan (patient can give the drug name, dosage, possible adverse effects to watch for, specific measures to help avoid adverse effects, importance of continued follow-up, and importance of avoiding foods high in tyramine).
- Monitor the effectiveness of comfort measures and compliance with the regimen.

SELECTIVE SEROTONIN REUPTAKE INHIBITORS

SSRIs, the newest group of antidepressant drugs, specifically block the reuptake of 5HT, with little to no known effect on

NE. Because SSRIs do not have the many adverse effects associated with TCAs and MAO inhibitors, they are a better choice for many patients. SSRIs include the following agents:

- Fluoxetine (*Prozac*), the first SSRI, has been successfully used to treat depression, OCDs, bulimia, and premenstrual dysphoric disorder (PMDD). It is being investigated for use in the treatment of other psychiatric disorders, including depression in children, panic disorders, migraine headaches, narcolepsy, bipolar disorder, and attention deficit disorders.
- Fluvoxamine (*Luvox*), which is under investigation for the treatment of depression, anxiety, posttraumatic stress disorder, PMDD, and autism, is now indicated only for the treatment of OCDS.
- Paroxetine (*Paxil*) is indicated for the treatment of depression, panic disorders, posttraumatic stress reaction, social anxiety disorders, and OCDs. It is being investigated for the treatment of PMDD, chronic headache, premature ejaculation, bipolar depression, fibromyalgia syndrome, and diabetic neuropathy.
- Sertraline (*Zoloft*) is used to treat depression and OCDs, posttraumatic stress disorders, and panic disorders. It is being studied for use in the treatment of PMDD and social phobias.
- Citalopram (*Celexa*), the newest SSRI, is indicated only for the treatment of depression, but has been used to treat alcoholism, panic disorder, PMDD, and social phobias.

With the SSRIs, a period of up to 4 weeks is necessary for realization of the full therapeutic effect. Patients may respond well to one SSRI and yet show little or no response to another one. The choice of drug depends on the indications and individual response.

Therapeutic Actions and Indications

As previously stated, SSRIs more specifically block the reuptake of 5HT, with little known effect on NE. This action increases the levels of 5HT in the synaptic cleft and may contribute to the antidepressant and other effects attributed to these drugs.

SSRIs are indicated for the treatment of depression, OCDs, panic attacks, bulimia, PMDD, posttraumatic stress disorders, social phobias, and social anxiety disorders. Ongoing investigations are focusing on the use of these antidepressant drugs in the treatment of other psychiatric disorders.

Pharmacokinetics

The SSRIs are well absorbed from the GI tract, metabolized in the liver, and excreted in the urine and feces. The half-life varies widely with the drug being used. The SSRIs have been associated with congenital abnormalities in animal studies and should be used during pregnancy only if the benefits to the mother clearly outweigh the potential risks to the fetus. The SSRIs enter breast milk and can cause adverse effects in the baby, so a different method of feeding the baby should be selected if an SSRI is required by the mother.

Contraindications and Cautions

The SSRIs are contraindicated in the presence of allergy to any of these drugs and during pregnancy and lactation because of the potential for serious adverse effects on the neonate.

Caution should be used in patients with impaired renal or hepatic function that could alter the metabolism and excretion of the drug, leading to toxic effects, or with diabetes, which could be exacerbated by the stimulating effects of these drugs.

Adverse Effects

The adverse effects associated with SSRIs, which are related to the effects of increased 5HT levels, include CNS effects such as headache, drowsiness, dizziness, insomnia, anxiety, tremor, agitation, and seizures. GI effects such as nausea, vomiting, diarrhea, dry mouth, anorexia, constipation, and changes in taste often occur, as do GU effects including painful menstruation, cystitis, sexual dysfunction, urgency, and impotence. Respiratory changes may include cough, dyspnea, upper respiratory infections, and pharyngitis. Other reported effects are sweating, rash, fever, and pruritus.

Clinically Important Drug–Drug Interactions

Because of the risk of serotonin syndrome if SSRIs are used with MAO inhibitors, this combination should be avoided and at least 2 to 4 weeks should be allowed between the two types of drugs if switching from one to the other. In addition, the use of SSRIs with TCAs results in increased therapeutic and toxic effects. If these combinations are used, patients should be monitored closely, and appropriate dosage adjustments should be made.

Nursing Considerations for Patients Receiving Selective Serotonin Reuptake Inhibitors

Assessment: History And Examination

Screen for the following conditions, which could be contraindications or cautions for use of the drug: any known allergies to SSRIs; impaired liver or kidney function, which could alter metabolism and excretion of the drug; and diabetes mellitus. Find out whether female patients are pregnant or breast feeding.

Include screening for baseline status before beginning therapy and for any potential adverse effects. Assess for the fol-

CULTURAL CONSIDERATIONS
The Popularity of Prozac

A rise in the diagnosis of depression began in the 1990s, with that decade's fast-paced lifestyle, high-stress jobs, explosion of information availability, and rapid change. Many people who have high expectations of both themselves and others are overworked and overstimulated to a point at which they become clinically depressed.

There is now a selection of relatively safe and nontoxic drugs that can be used to treat depression—the selective serotonin reuptake inhibitors (SSRIs). For several years, the SSRIs remained in the top-selling category of prescription drugs. Fluoxetine (*Prozac*), in particular, has been the subject of numerous talk shows, books, and movies. In many ways, *Prozac* was the "in" drug of the 1990s. This societal phenomenon put pressure on health care providers to prescribe a drug even if it was not appropriate to a given patient's situation. In some instances, patients just wanted the drug that helped their friend. They may not have been willing to listen to their health care provider or to take the time to be properly diagnosed; they just wanted an SSRI. *Prozac* is not the solution to everyone's problem, and it is often difficult to explain this fact to a patient. It also may be hard to get the patient to understand that this drug is not a quick fix; it takes 4 to 6 weeks to achieve full therapeutic effectiveness. Fortunately, the SSRIs have the least adverse effects of the antidepressants, and such fads usually pass in a few years.

It is important to remember the powerful effects of the media on health care–seeking behavior. As more and more drugs are advertised in magazines and on television, patients are becoming aware of options and "cures" that they might like to try. Patient education is a tricky yet important part of any health care intervention and an extremely important aspect of health care in our society.

lowing: temperature and weight; skin color and lesions; affect, orientation, and reflexes; vision; blood pressure and pulse; respiratory rate and adventitious sounds; and bowel sounds on abdominal examination. Obtain renal and liver function tests.

Nursing Diagnoses

The patient receiving an SSRI may have the following nursing diagnoses related to drug therapy:

- Acute Pain related to GI, GU, CNS effects
- Disturbed Thought Processes and Disturbed Sensory Perception (Kinesthetic, Tactile) related to CNS effects
- Imbalanced Nutrition related to GI effects
- Deficient Knowledge regarding drug therapy

Implementation

- Arrange for lower dosage in elderly patients and in those with renal or hepatic impairment *because of the potential for severe adverse effects.*

DRUGS IN FOCUS
Selective Serotonin Reuptake Inhibitors

Drug Name	Dosage/Route	Usual Indications
citalopram (*Celexa*)	20 mg PO b.i.d.; up to 40 mg/d may be needed	Treatment of depression in adults
fluoxetine (*Prozac, Sarafem*)	20 mg PO in the AM; do not exceed 80 mg/d; reduce dosage with hepatic impairment; also available in a 90-mg, once-a-week formulation	Treatment of depression, bulimia, obsessive-compulsive disorders (OCDs) in adults, premenstrual dysphoric disorder
fluvoxamine (*Luvox*)	Adult: 50 mg PO at bedtime up to a maximum of 300 mg/d; reduce dosage with hepatic impairment Pediatric (8–17 y): 25 mg PO at bedtime; do not exceed 200 mg/d	Treatment of OCDs
paroxetine (*Paxil*)	10–20 mg/d PO; do not exceed 60 mg/d; reduce dosage in the presence of hepatic or renal dysfunction and in older adults	Treatment of depression, OCDs, panic disorders in adults, posttraumatic stress disorders
sertraline (*Zoloft*)	Adult: 25–50 mg/d PO; reduce dosage with hepatic dysfunction Pediatric: 25–50 mg/d PO based on age and severity of obsessive–compulsive disorder	Treatment of depression, OCDs, posttraumatic stress disorder

- Monitor patient for up to 4 weeks *to ascertain onset of full therapeutic effect before adjusting dosage.*
- Establish suicide precautions for severely depressed patients, and limit the quantity of the drug dispensed, *to decrease the risk of overdose.*
- Administer the drug once a day in the morning *to achieve optimal therapeutic effects.* If the dosage is increased or if the patient is having severe GI effects, the dosage can be divided.
- Suggest that patients use barrier contraceptives *to prevent pregnancy while taking this drug, because serious fetal abnormalities can occur.*
- Provide comfort measures *to help patients tolerate drug effects.* These may include voiding before dosing, instituting a bowel program as needed, taking food with the drug if GI upset is severe, or environmental control (lighting, temperature, stimuli).
- Provide thorough patient teaching, including the drug name, prescribed dosage, measures for avoidance of adverse effects, and warning signs that may indicate possible problems. Instruct patients about the need for periodic monitoring and evaluation *to enhance patient knowledge about drug therapy and to promote compliance.* (See Patient Teaching Checklist: Selective Serotonin Reuptake Inhibitors).
- Offer support and encouragement *to help patients cope with the disease and the drug regimen.*

Evaluation

- Monitor patient response to the drug (alleviation of signs and symptoms of depression, OCD, bulimia, panic disorder).

PATIENT TEACHING CHECKLIST
Selective Serotonin Reuptake Inhibitors (SSRIs)

Create customized patient teaching materials for a specific SSRI from the CD-ROM. Patient teaching should stress the following points for drugs within this class:

- SSRIs change the concentration of serotonin in specific areas of the brain. This increase in serotonin levels is believed to relieve depression.
- The drug should be taken once a day in the morning. If your dosage has been increased or you are having stomach upset, the dose may be divided.
- It may take up to 4 weeks before you feel the full effects of this drug. Continue to take the drug every day during that time so that the concentration of the drug in your body eventually reaches effective levels.

Common side effects of these drugs include the following:

- *Dizziness, drowsiness, nervousness, and insomnia*—If these effects occur, avoid driving or performing hazardous or delicate tasks that require concentration.
- *Nausea, vomiting, and weight loss*—Small, frequent meals may help. Monitor your weight loss; if it becomes excessive, consult your health care provider.
- *Sexual dysfunction and flu-like symptoms*—These effects may be temporary. Consult with your health care provider if these conditions become bothersome.

Report any of the following conditions to your health care provider: rash, mania, seizures, and severe weight loss.

Tell any doctor, nurse, or other health care provider that you are taking this drug.

Keep this drug and all medications out of the reach of children.

PATIENT TEACHING CHECKLIST
(CONTINUED)

Selective Serotonin Reuptake Inhibitors (SSRIs)

Do not take this drug during pregnancy because severe fetal abnormalities could occur. The use of barrier contraceptives is recommended while you are taking this drug. If you think that you are pregnant, or would like to become pregnant, consult with your health care provider.

This Teaching Checklist reflects general patient teaching guidelines. It is not meant to be a substitute for drug-specific teaching information, which is available in nursing drug guides.

- Monitor for adverse effects (sedation, dizziness, GI upset, respiratory dysfunction, GU problems, skin rash).
- Evaluate effectiveness of teaching plan (patient can give the drug name, dosage, possible adverse effects to watch for, specific measures to help avoid adverse effects, importance of continued follow-up, and importance of avoiding pregnancy).
- Monitor the effectiveness of comfort measures and compliance with the regimen (see Nursing Care Guide: Selective Serotonin Reuptake Inhibitors).

OTHER ANTIDEPRESSANTS

Some other effective antidepressants do not fit into any of the three groups that have been discussed in this chapter. These drugs have varying effects on NE, 5HT, and dopamine. Al-

NURSING CARE GUIDE

Selective Serotonin Reuptake Inhibitors (SSRIs)

Assessment	Nursing Diagnoses	Implementation	Evaluation
HISTORY Allergies to any of these drugs; renal or hepatic dysfunction; pregnancy or lactation; diabetes	Acute Pain related to GI, GU, CNS effects Disturbed Thought Processes related to CNS effects Imbalanced Nutrition related to GI effects Deficient Knowledge regarding drug therapy	Administer drug in morning; divide doses if high or GI upset. Provide comfort, safety measures: small meals; void before dosing; side rails; pain medication as needed; suggest barrier contraceptive; limit dosage with potentially suicidal patients; lower dose with renal or hepatic impairment. Provide support and reassurance to deal with drug effects (4-wk delay in full effectiveness). Provide patient teaching regarding drug, dosage, adverse effects, conditions to report, need to use barrier contraceptives.	Evaluate drug effects: relief of signs and symptoms of depression, obsessive–compulsive disorder, panic disorders. Monitor for adverse effects: sedation, dizziness, insomnia; respiratory dysfunction; GI upset; GU problems; skin rash. Monitor for drug–drug interactions as indicated for each drug. Evaluate effectiveness of patient teaching program. Evaluate effectiveness of comfort and safety measures.
PHYSICAL EXAMINATION Cardiovascular: BP, P CNS: orientation, affect, reflexes, vision Skin: color, lesions; texture Respiratory: respiration, adventitious sounds GI: abdominal examination, bowel sounds Laboratory tests: hepatic and renal function tests			

though it is not known how their actions are related to clinical efficacy, these agents may be most effective in treating depression in patients who do not respond to other antidepressants. They may even be used before MAO inhibitors or TCAs, which have many more adverse effects. Other antidepressants include the following:

- Bupropion (*Wellbutrin, Zyban*), which weakly blocks reuptake of NE, 5HT, and dopamine, is effective in the treatment of depression. At lower doses, this drug is effective in smoking cessation. It is well absorbed from the GI tract, metabolized in the liver, and excreted in the urine. There are no adequate studies done in pregnancy, and the drug should be used during pregnancy only if the benefits to the mother clearly outweigh the potential risks to the fetus. Bupropion does enter breast milk and should not be used by nursing mothers. The drug is available in a sustained-release formulation, which some patients find to be more convenient.
- Mirtazapine (*Remeron*) is used to treat depression. How its many anticholinergic effects relate to its antidepressive effects is not known. It is rapidly absorbed from the GI tract, extensively metabolized in the liver, and excreted in the urine. Mirtazapine has a half-life of 20 to 40 hours. Little is known about its effects in pregnancy and lactation, and it should be used during those times only if the benefit to the mother clearly outweighs the potential risk to the neonate.
- Nefazodone (*Serzone*), which is given twice daily, is effective in the treatment of some cases of depression. It has a short half-life of 2 to 4 hours. It is well absorbed from the GI tract, metabolized in the liver, and excreted in the urine. Little is known about its effects in pregnancy and lactation, and it should be used during those times only if the benefit to the mother clearly outweighs the potential risk to the neonate.

- Trazodone (*Desyrel*), which blocks 5HT and some 5HT precursor reuptake, is effective in some forms of depression but has many CNS effects associated with its use. It is readily absorbed from the GI tract, extensively metabolized in the liver, and excreted in urine and feces. Trazodone caused fetal abnormalities in animal studies and crosses into breast milk. It should be used during pregnancy and lactation only if the benefits to the mother clearly outweigh the potential risks to the fetus.
- Venlafaxine (*Effexor*) has fewer adverse CNS effects and is known to mildly block reuptake of NE, 5HT, and dopamine. It is very effective in treating some cases of depression, and its popularity has increased with the introduction of an extended-release form that does away with the multiple daily doses that are required with the regular form. Venlafaxine is readily absorbed from the GI tract, extensively metabolized in the liver, and excreted in urine. Adequate studies have not been done in pregnancy and lactation, and it should be used during those times only if the benefit to the mother clearly outweighs the potential risk to the neonate.

▭▭◉● WEB LINKS

Health care providers and patients may want to consult the following Internet sources:

Information on depression including diagnosis, research, treatment: http://www.depression.com

Information on depression, signs and symptoms, community resources, support groups: http://www.depressionalliance.org

Information on women and depression: http://www.nimh.nih.gov/publicat/depressionmenu.cfm

---

DRUGS IN FOCUS
Other Antidepressants

Drug Name	Dosage/Route	Usual Indications
℗ bupropion (*Wellbutrin, Wellbutrin SR, Zyban*)	300 mg/d PO given in three doses; or 150 mg PO b.i.d. in sustained-release form; 150–300 mg/d PO for smoking cessation for 7–12 wk	Treatment of depression in adults, smoking cessation
mirtazapine (*Remeron*)	15 mg/d PO; which may be increased to a maximum of 45 mg/d; reduce dosage in older adults and with renal or hepatic dysfunction	Treatment of depression in adults
nefazodone (*Serzone*)	100 mg PO b.i.d., up to a maximum of 600 mg/d; reduce dosage in older adults	Treatment of depression in adults
trazodone (*Desyrel*)	150 mg/d PO in divided doses; up to 600 mg/d	Treatment of depression in adults
venlafaxine (*Effexor, Effexor XR*)	75 mg/d PO in divided doses, up to 225 mg/d; 75 mg/d PO in sustained-release formulation, up to a maximum of 225 mg/d; reduce dosage with hepatic or renal impairment	Treatment of depression in adults

Information on education programs related to depression, stress, drug therapy, and so forth for patients and health professionals:
http://teachhealth.com

Patient-oriented and professional information on issues related to mental health:
http://nimh.nih.gov

CHAPTER SUMMARY

- *Affect* is a term that refers to the feelings that people experience when they respond emotionally.
- Depression is an affective disorder characterized by overwhelming sadness, despair, and hopelessness that is inappropriate with respect to the event or events that precipitated the depression. Depression is a very common problem; it is associated with many physical manifestations and is often misdiagnosed. It could be that depression is caused by a series of events that are not yet understood.

- The biogenic amine theory states that depression is caused by a deficiency of the biogenic amines—norepinephrine (NE), serotonin (5HT), and dopamine—in certain key areas of the brain.
- Antidepressant drugs—TCAs, MAO inhibitors, and SSRIs—increase the concentrations of the biogenic amines in the brain.
- Selection of an antidepressant depends on individual drug response and tolerance of associated adverse effects. The adverse effects of TCAs are sedating and anticholinergic; those of MAO inhibitors are CNS related and sympathomimetic. The adverse effects of SSRIs are fewer, but they do cause CNS changes.
- Other antidepressants with unknown mechanisms of action are also effective in treating depression.

Review Questions

1. Depression is a very common affective disorder that strikes many people. People with depression would not exhibit

C A S E   S T U D Y

Use of Selective Serotonin Reuptake Inhibitors

THE SITUATION
D. J., a 46-year-old married woman, complains of weight gain, malaise, fatigue, sleeping during the day, loss of interest in daily activities, and bouts of crying for no apparent reason. On examination, she weighs 8 pounds more than the standard weight for her height; all other findings are within normal limits. In conversation with a nurse, D. J. says that in the past 10 months, several events have occurred. She lost both her parents, her only child graduated from high school and went off to college, her nephew died of renal failure, her one sister received a diagnosis of metastatic breast cancer, and she herself lost her job as a day care provider when the client family moved out of town. In addition, a veterinarian diagnosed the family cat of 17 years with terminal leukemia. D. J. is prescribed fluoxetine (*Prozac*) and is given an appointment for a visit with a counselor.

CRITICAL THINKING
What nursing interventions are appropriate at this time? What sort of crisis intervention would be most appropriate? *Balance the benefits of pointing out all of the losses and points of grief that you detect in D. J.'s story with the risks of upsetting her strained coping mechanisms.* What can D. J. expect to experience as a result of the SSRI therapy? How can you help D. J. cope during the lengthy period it takes to reach therapeutic effects? What other future interventions should be planned with D. J.?

DISCUSSION
Many patients in severe crisis do not consciously identify the many things that are causing them stress. They have developed coping mechanisms to help them survive and cope with their day-to-day activities. However, D. J. seems to have reached her limit, and she exhibits many of the signs and symptoms of depression.

It is hoped that the fluoxetine, an SSRI, will enable D. J. to regain her ability to cope and her normal affect. The drug should give her brain a chance to reach a new biochemical balance. Before she begins taking the fluoxetine, she should receive a written sheet listing the pertinent drug information, adverse effects to watch for, warning signs to report, and a telephone number to call in case she has questions later or just needs to talk. The written information is especially important, because she may not remember drug-related discussions or instructions clearly.

Once the SSRI reaches therapeutic levels, which can take as long as 4 weeks, D. J. may start to feel like her "old self" and may be strong enough to finally begin dealing with all her grief. She may recover from her need for the SSRI over time and the medication can then be withdrawn.

Because it takes up to 4 weeks for the fluoxetine to produce its full therapeutic effect, the referral of D. J. to a counselor may be the best way to ensure that she can talk to someone who has the time to listen and to help her face her losses and resolve any problems she may be experiencing. If a counselor is not available, it is important to establish a trusting relationship and to give D. J. the time that she needs to work out some of her feelings. It might be possible to refer D. J. to community support groups for dealing with loss and grieving. She also might be able to consult with an employment agency regarding other positions as a day care provider that might fit her needs.

a. lack of energy.
b. hyperactivity.
c. sleep disturbances.
d. libido problems.

2. The biogenic amine theory of depression states that depression is a result of
   a. an unpleasant childhood.
   b. GABA inhibition.
   c. deficiency of NE, dopamine, or 5HT in key areas of the brain.
   d. blockages within the limbic system which controls emotions and affect.

3. A list of effective antidepressants would not include
   a. tetracyclic drugs.
   b. cholinergics.
   c. SSRIs.
   d. MAO inhibitors.

4. The tricyclic antidepressants (TCAs) are associated with many anticholinergic adverse effects. These could include
   a. increased libido and increased appetite.
   b. polyuria and polydipsia.
   c. urinary retention, arrhythmias and constipation.
   d. hearing changes, cataracts and nightmares.

5. Adverse effects may limit the usefulness of TCAs with some patients. Nursing interventions that could alleviate some of the unpleasant aspects of these adverse effects include
   a. always administering the drug when the patient has an empty stomach.
   b. reminding the patient not to void before taking the drug.
   c. increasing the dosage to override the adverse effects.
   d. taking the major portion of the dose at bedtime to avoid experiencing drowsiness and the unpleasant anticholinergic effects.

6. Monoamine oxidase (MAO) inhibitors are reserved for use in cases in which there has been no response to other agents, because
   a. MAO inhibitors can cause hair loss.
   b. MAO inhibitors are associated with potentially serious drug–food interactions.
   c. MAO inhibitors are mostly recommended for use in surgical patients.
   d. MAO inhibitors are more expensive than other agents.

7. Your patient is being treated for depression and is started on *Prozac* (fluoxetine). She calls you 10 days after the drug has started to report that nothing has changed and she wants to try a different drug. You should
   a. try sertraline (*Zoloft*), because some patients respond to one SSRI and not another.
   b. ask her to try a few days without the drug to see whether there is any difference.
   c. add an MAO inhibitor to her drug regimen to get an increased antidepressant effect.
   d. encourage her to keep taking the drug as prescribed because it usually takes up to 4 weeks to see the full antidepressant effect.

8. The drug of choice for a patient with a documented obsessive–compulsive disorder, who is also suffering from depression and occasional panic disorder, would be
   a. *Celexa.*
   b. *Paxil.*
   c. *Luvox.*
   d. *Prozac.*

9. Venlafaxine (*Effexor*) is a relatively new antidepressant that might be very effective for use in patients who
   a. have proven to be responsive to other antidepressants.
   b. can tolerate multiple side effects.
   c. are reliable at taking multiple daily dosings.
   d. have not responded to other antidepressants and would benefit from once-a-day dosing.

10. Depression is an affective disorder that is
    a. always precipitated by a specific event.
    b. most common in patients with head injuries.
    c. characterized by overwhelming sadness, despair, and hopelessness.
    d. very evident and easy to diagnose in the clinical setting.

BIBLIOGRAPHY

Bailey, K. (1998). *Psychotropic drug facts*. Philadelphia: Lippincott-Raven.

Bullock, B. L. (2000). *Focus of pathophysiology*. Philadelphia: Lippincott Williams & Wilkins.

Drug facts and comparisons. (2002). St. Louis: Facts and Comparisons.

Gilman, A., Hardman, J. G., & Limbird, L. E. (Eds.) (2002). *Goodman and Gilman's the pharmacological basis of therapeutics* (10th ed.). New York: McGraw-Hill.

Karch, A. M. (2002). *2003 Lippincott's nursing drug guide*. Philadelphia: Lippincott Williams & Wilkins.

Professional's guide to patient drug facts. (2002). St. Louis: Facts and Comparisons.

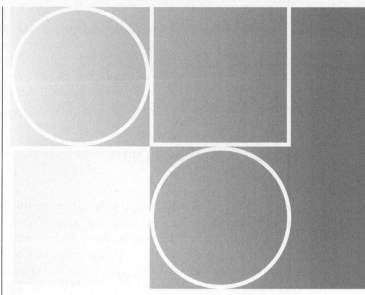

CHAPTER 22

Psychotherapeutic Agents

287

Key Terms

antipsychotic
attention-deficit disorder
major tranquilizer
mania
narcolepsy
neuroleptic
schizophrenia

Antipsychotic/Neuroleptic Drugs

Typical Antipsychotics

🅟 chlorpromazine
fluphenazine
haloperidol
loxapine
mesoridazine
molindone
perphenazine
pimozide
prochlorperazine
thioridazine
thiothixene

trifluoperazine
triflupromazine

Atypical Antipsychotics

🅟 clozapine
olanzapine
quetiapine
risperidone
ziprasidone

Antimanic Drug

lithium

Central Nervous System Stimulants

dexmethylphenidate
dextroamphetamine

🅟 methylphenidate
modafinil
pemoline

The drugs discussed in this chapter are used to treat psychoses—perceptual and behavioral disorders. These psychotherapeutic drugs are targeted at thought processes rather than affective states. Although these drugs do not cure any of these disorders, they do help patients function in a more acceptable manner and carry on activities of daily living.

MENTAL DISORDERS AND THEIR CLASSIFICATION

Mental disorders are now thought to be caused by some inherent dysfunction within the brain that leads to abnormal thought processes and responses. Most theories attribute these disorders to some sort of chemical imbalance in specific areas within the brain. Diagnosis of a mental disorder is often based on distinguishing characteristics described in the *Diagnostic and Statistical Manual of Mental Disorders,* 4th edition, text revision (DSM-IV-TR). Because no diagnostic laboratory tests are available, patient assessment and response must be carefully evaluated to determine the basis of a particular problem. Selected disorders are discussed here.

Schizophrenia, the most common type of psychosis, can be very debilitating and prevents affected individuals from functioning in society. Characteristics of schizophrenia include hallucinations, paranoia, delusions, speech abnormalities, and affective problems. This disorder, which seems to have a very strong genetic association, may reflect a fundamental biochemical abnormality.

Mania, with its associated bipolar illness (i.e., manic-depressive illness), is characterized by periods of extreme overactivity and excitement. Bipolar illness involves extremes of depression followed by hyperactivity and excitement. This condition may reflect a biochemical imbalance followed by overcompensation on the part of neurons and their inability to re-establish stability.

Narcolepsy is characterized by daytime sleepiness and sudden periods of loss of wakefulness. This disorder may reflect problems with stimulation of the brain by the reticular activating system (RAS) or problems with response to that stimulation.

DRUG THERAPY ACROSS THE LIFESPAN

Psychotherapeutic Agents

Children	Adults	Older Adults
Many of these agents are used in children, often in combination with other central nervous system (CNS) drugs in an attempt to control symptoms and behavior. Long-term effects of many of these agents are not known, and parents should be informed of this fact. Of the antipsychotics, chlorpromazine, haloperidol, pimozide, prochlorperazine, thioridazine, trifluoperazine, and triflupromazine are the only ones with established pediatric regimens. The dose is often higher than that required for adults. The child should be monitored carefully for adverse effects and developmental progress. Lithium does not have a recommended pediatric dose, and the drug should not ordinarily be used in children. If it is used, the dosage should be carefully calculated from the child's age and weight, and the child should be monitored very closely for renal, CNS, cardiovascular, and endocrine function. The CNS stimulants are often used in children to manage various attention-deficit disorders. Caution should be used with extended-release preparations, because they differ markedly in timing and effectiveness. The child should be assessed carefully and challenged periodically for the necessity of continuing the drug.	Adults using these drugs should be under regular care and should be monitored regularly for adverse effects. The QTc interval should be evaluated before thioridazine, ziprasidone, or mesoridazine is prescribed and periodically during use. Patients receiving lithium should be encouraged to maintain hydration and salt intake. They need to understand the importance of periodic monitoring of serum lithium levels. These drugs should be used very cautiously during pregnancy and lactation because of the potential for adverse effects on the neonate. A woman maintained on one of these drugs needs to be counseled about the risk to the fetus versus the risk of returning symptoms if the drug is stopped. Use should be reserved for situations in which the benefits to the mother far outweigh the potential risks to the neonate. Women of child-bearing age who need to take lithium should be advised to use barrier contraceptives while taking the drug because of the potential for serious congenital abnormalities.	Older patients may be more susceptible to the adverse effects of these drugs. Dosages of all of these drugs need to be reduced and patients monitored very closely for toxic effects and to provide safety measures if CNS effects do occur. Patients with renal impairment should be monitored very closely while taking lithium. Decreased dosages may be needed. Because many older patients may also have renal impairment, they need to be screened carefully. They should be urged to maintain hydration and salt intake, which can be a challenge with some older patients. Prolongation of the QTc interval, associated with use of thioridazine, ziprasidone, or mesoridazine, may be a concern in elderly patients with coronary disease. Careful screening and monitoring should be done if these drugs are needed for such patients.

Attention-deficit disorders involve a variety of conditions characterized by an inability to concentrate on one activity for longer than a few minutes and a state of hyperkinesis. These conditions are usually diagnosed in school-aged children but can occur in adults.

ANTIPSYCHOTIC/NEUROLEPTIC DRUGS

The **antipsychotic** drugs, which are essentially dopamine receptor blockers, are used to treat disorders that involve thought processes. Because of their associated neurological adverse effects, these medications are also called **neuroleptic** agents. At one time, these drugs were known as **major tranquilizers.** However, that name is no longer used because the primary action of these drugs is not sedation but a change in neuron stimulation and response (Figure 22–1).

Table 22–1 lists the antipsychotics in use today and gives information about their relative potencies and associated adverse effects. Any of these drugs may be effective in a particular patient; the selection of a specific drug depends on the desired potency and patient tolerance of the associated adverse effects. A patient who does not respond to one drug may react successfully to another agent. To determine the best therapeutic regimen for a particular patient, it may be necessary to try more than one drug.

Antipsychotics can be classified as either typical or atypical. The classic, typical antipsychotics are primarily dopamine receptor blockers that cause several adverse effects associated with dopamine blockade, including hypotension, anticholinergic effects, and extrapyramidal effects. Newer, atypical antipsychotics block both dopamine receptors and serotonin receptors. This dual action may help alleviate some of the unpleasant neurological effects and depression associated with the typical antipsychotics.

Therapeutic Actions and Indications

It is not understood which of the several actions of antipsychotics corrects the manifestations of schizophrenia. The typical antipsychotic drugs block dopamine receptors, preventing the stimulation of the postsynaptic neurons by dopamine. They also depress the RAS, limiting the stimuli coming into the brain, and they have anticholinergic, antihistamine, and α-adrenergic blocking effects, all related to the blocking of the dopamine receptor sites. Atypical antipsychotics block both dopamine and serotonin receptors.

The antipsychotics are indicated for schizophrenia and for manifestations of other psychotic disorders including hyperactivity, combative behavior, agitation in the elderly, and severe behavioral problems in children (short-term control).

Pharmacokinetics

The antipsychotics are erratically absorbed from the gastrointestinal (GI) tract, depending on the drug and the preparation of the drug. Intramuscular doses provide four to five times the active dose as oral doses, requiring caution if switching between routes. The antipsychotics are widely distributed in the tissues and are often stored in the tissues, being released for up to 6 months after the drug is stopped. They are metabolized in the liver and excreted through the bile and urine. Children tend to metabolize these drugs faster than adults, and elderly patients tend to metabolize them more slowly. The antipsychotics cross the placenta and enter breast milk. They should not be used during pregnancy or lactation unless the benefit to the mother clearly outweighs the potential risk to the neonate.

Contraindications and Cautions

Antipsychotic drugs are contraindicated in the presence of underlying diseases that could be exacerbated by the dopamine-blocking effects of these drugs. They are also contraindicated in the following conditions, which can be exacerbated by the drugs: central nervous system (CNS) depression, circulatory collapse, Parkinson's disease, coronary disease, severe hypotension, bone marrow suppression, and blood dyscrasias. Prolongation of the QTc interval is a contraindication to the use of mesoridazine, thioridazine, and zaprisidone, all of which can further prolong the QTc interval, leading to increased risk of serious cardiac arrhythmias.

Caution should be used in the presence of medical conditions that could be exacerbated by the anticholinergic effects of the drugs, such as glaucoma, peptic ulcer, and uri-

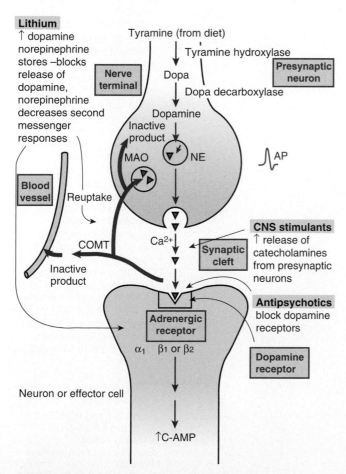

FIGURE 22-1. Sites of action of the drugs used to treat mental disorders: antipsychotics, central nervous system stimulants, lithium.

TABLE 22-1 | Antipsychotics/Neuroleptics, Indicating Side Effects Most Frequently Associated With Each Drug

Drug Name	Potency	Common Side Effects				Usual Dosage
		Sedation	Anticholinergic	Hypotension	Extrapyramidal	
TYPICAL ANTIPSYCHOTICS						
chlorpromazine (*Thorazine*)	Low	++++	+++	+++	++	Adult: 25 mg IM for acute episode, may be re-peated; switch to 25–50 mg PO t.i.d. Pediatric: 0.5–1 mg/kg q4–8h PO, IM, or PR
fluphenazine (*Moditen, Prolixin*)	High	+	+	+	++++	Adult: 0.5–10 mg/d PO in divided doses; 1.25–10 mg/d IM in divided doses Geriatric: 1–2.5 mg/d PO, adjust dose based on response
haloperidol (*Haldol*)	High	+	+/−	+	++++	Adult: 0.5–2 mg PO b.i.d.-t.i.d. or 2–5 mg IM, may be repeated in 1 h, 4–8 h more common Geriatric: reduce dosage Pediatric: (3–12 y): 0.5 mg/d PO; 0.05–0.075 mg/kg per day PO for Tourette's syndrome and behavioral syndromes
loxapine (*Loxitane*)	Medium	+++	++	++	+++	Adult: 60–100 mg/d PO; 12.5–50 mg IM or IV for acute states
mesoridazine (*Serentil*)	Low	++++	++	++	+	Adult: 25–50 mg PO t.i.d.; monitor QTc intervals
molindone (*Moban*)	Medium	+	++	+/−	+	Adult: initially 50–75 mg/d PO, maintenance at 5–25 mg PO t.i.d. to q.i.d.
perphenazine (*Trilafon*)	Medium	++	+	++	+++	Adult: 4–8 mg PO t.i.d. or 5 mg IM q6h; switch to oral as soon as possible Geriatric: one-half to one-third of adult dose
pimozide (*Orap*)	High	+	+	++	+++	Adult: 1–2 mg/d PO in divided doses Pediatric (>12 y): 0.05 mg/kg PO h.s.; do not exceed 10 mg/d
prochlorperazine (*Compazine*)	Low	+	++	+	+++	Adult: 5–10 mg PO t.i.d.–q.i.d.; 10–20 mg IM for acute states Geriatric: reduce dosage Pediatric: 2.5 mg PO t.i.d.; 0.03 mg/kg IM for acute states; 20–25 mg/d PR
thioridazine (*Mellaril*)	Low	++++	+++	+++	+	Adult: 50–100 mg PO t.i.d., monitor QTc intervals Pediatric: up to 3 mg/kg per day PO
thiothixene (*Navane*)	High	+	+	+	++++	Adult: 2 mg PO t.i.d.; up to a maximum 60 mg/d in severe cases
trifluoperazine (*Stelazine*)	High	+	+	+	++++	Adult: 2–5 mg PO b.i.d.; 1–2 mg IM q4–6h in severe cases Geriatric: reduce dosage Pediatric (6–12 y): 1 mg PO q.d. or b.i.d.: 1 mg IM q.d. or b.i.d. for severe cases

TABLE 22-1 Antipsychotics/Neuroleptics, Indicating Side Effects Most Frequently Associated With Each Drug (continued)

Drug Name	Potency	Common Side Effects				Usual Dosage
		Sedation	Anticholinergic	Hypotension	Extrapyramidal	
triflupromazine (*Vesprin*)	Low	+	++	+	+++	Adult: 60 mg IM, up to 150 mg/d Pediatric: 0.2–0.25 mg/kg IM to a maximum 10 mg/d; do not give to children <2.5 y
ATYPICAL ANTIPSYCHOTICS						
clozapine (*Clozaril*)	Low	++++	++	+++	+/−	Adult: initially 25 mg PO q.d.–b.i.d.; up to 500 mg/d; available only through the *Clozaril* Patient Management System, which monitors WBC and compliance issues, only 1-week supply given at a time.
olanzapine (*Zyprexa Zydis*)	High	++++	++	+++	+	Adult: 5–10 mg/d PO, up to 20 mg/d PO for bipolar mania; available in disintegrating tablets, which can be taken without swallowing (Zyprexa Zydis)
quetiapine (*Seroquel*)	Medium	++++	++	++	+/−	Adult: initially 25 mg PO b.i.d., up to 300–400 mg/d Geriatric: hepatic impairment or hypotensives; reduce dosage and titrate very slowly
risperidone (*Risperdal*)	High	+++	+	++	++	Adult: 1 mg PO b.i.d. up to 8 mg/d Geriatric, renal impairment, hypotension: 0.5 mg PO b.i.d. initially, titrate slowly
ziprasidone (*Geodon*)	Medium	+++	++	+	+	Adult: 20–80 mg PO b.i.d.; monitor QTc intervals

Each + indicates increased incidence of that adverse effect.

nary or intestinal obstruction. In addition, care should be taken in patients with seizure disorders, because the threshold for seizures could be lowered; in those with thyrotoxicosis, because of the possibility of severe neurosensitivity; and in active alcoholism, because of potentiation of the CNS depression.

Other situations that warrant caution include myelography within the last 24 hours or scheduled within the next 48 hours, because severe neuron reaction to the dye can occur, and pregnancy or lactation, because of the potential of adverse effects on the fetus or neonate. Because children are more apt to develop dystonia from the drugs, which could confuse the diagnosis of Reye's syndrome, caution should be used with children younger than 12 years of age who have a CNS infection or chicken pox. The use of antipsychotics may result in bone marrow suppression, leading to blood dyscrasias, so care should be taken with patients who are immunosuppressed and those who have cancer.

Adverse Effects

The adverse effects associated with the antipsychotic drugs are related to their dopamine-blocking, anticholinergic, antihistamine, and α-adrenergic activities. The most common CNS effects are sedation, weakness, tremor, drowsiness, and extrapyramidal effects—pseudoparkinsonism, dystonia, akathisia, tardive dyskinesia, and potentially irreversible neuroleptic malignant syndrome (Figure 22–2). Anticholinergic effects include dry mouth, nasal congestion, flushing, constipation, urinary retention, sexual impotence, glaucoma, blurred vision, and photophobia. Cardiovascular (CV) effects, which are probably related to the dopamine-blocking effects, include hypotension, orthostatic hypotension, cardiac arrhythmias, congestive heart failure, and pulmonary edema. Several of these agents (thioridazine, mesoridazine, zaprisidone) are associated with prolongation of the QTc interval, which could lead to serious or even fatal cardiac arrhythmias. Patients receiving these drugs should have a baseline and periodic electrocardiogram (ECG) during therapy.

A. Dystonia—spasms of the tongue, neck, back, and legs. Spasms may cause unnatural positioning of the neck, abnormal eye movements, excessive salivation.

B. Akathisia—continuous restlessness, inability to sit still. Constant moving, foot tapping, hand movements may be seen.

C. Pseudoparkinsonism—muscle tremors, cogwheel rigidity, drooling, shuffling gait, slow movements.

D. Tardive dyskinesia—abnormal muscle movements such as lip smacking, tongue darting, chewing movements, slow and aimless arm and leg movements.

FIGURE 22–2. Common neurologic effects of antipsychotic drugs.

Respiratory effects such as laryngospasm, dyspnea, and bronchospasm may also occur. The phenothiazines (chlorpromazine, fluphenazine, prochlorperazine, promethazine, and thioridazine) often turn the urine pink to reddish-brown as a result of their excretion. Although this effect may cause great patient concern, it has no clinical significance. In addition, bone marrow suppression is a possibility with some antipsychotic agents.

Clinically Important Drug–Drug Interactions

Because the combination of antipsychotics with β-blockers may lead to an increase in the effect of both drugs, this combination should be avoided if possible.

Antipsychotic–alcohol combinations result in an increased risk of CNS depression, and antipsychotic–anticholinergic combinations lead to increased anticholinergic effects, so dosage adjustments are necessary. Patients who take either of

these combinations should be monitored closely for adverse effects, and supportive measures should be provided.

Patients should not take mesoridazine, thioridazine, or zaprisidone with any other drug that is associated with prolongation of the QTc interval.

Nursing Considerations for Patients Receiving Antipsychotic/Neuroleptic Drugs

Assessment: History and Examination

Screen for the following conditions, which could be contraindications or cautions for the use of the drug: any known allergies to these drugs, severe CNS depression, circulatory collapse, coronary disease including prolonged QTc interval, brain damage, severe hypotension, glaucoma, respiratory depression, urinary or intestinal obstruction, thyrotoxicosis, seizure disorder, bone marrow suppression, pregnancy or lactation, and myelography within the past 24 hours or sched-

CASE STUDY

Chronic Schizophrenia and Long-Term Therapy With Phenothiazines

THE SITUATION

B. A., a 36-year-old, single, professional woman, was diagnosed with chronic schizophrenia when she was a senior in high school. Her condition has been well controlled with phenothiazines, and she is able to maintain steady employment, live in her own home, and carry on a fairly active social life. At her last evaluation, she appeared to be developing bone marrow suppression and her physician decided to try to taper the drug. As the dosage was being lowered, B. A. became withdrawn and listless, missed several days of work, and canceled most of her social engagements. Afraid of interacting with people, she stayed in bed most of the time. She reported having thoughts of death and paranoid ideation about her neighbors that she was beginning to think might be true.

CRITICAL THINKING

What nursing interventions are appropriate at this time?
What supportive measures might be useful to help B. A. cope with this crisis and allow her to function normally again?
What happens to brain chemistry after long-term therapy with phenothiazines?
What drug options should be tried?
Are there any other options that might be useful?

DISCUSSION

Schizophrenia is not a disorder that can be resolved with proper counseling. B. A., an educated woman with a long history of taking phenothiazines, realizes the necessity of drug therapy to correct the chemical imbalance in her brain. She may need an antipsychotic with a high potency to return her to the level of functioning she had reached before experiencing this setback. Her knowledge of her individual responses can be used to help select an appropriate drug and dosage. Her experiences may also facilitate her care planning and new drug regimen.

B. A. will need support to cope with problems at work from her inability to go in to work, to cope with feelings about not meeting her social obligations, and to find the motivation to get up and become active again. She might do well with behavior modification techniques that give her some control over her activities and allow her to use her knowledge and experience with her own situation to her advantage in forming a new medical regimen. She may need support in explaining her problem to her employer and her social contacts in ways that will avoid the prejudice associated with mental illness and will allow her every opportunity to return to her regular routine as soon as she can.

Because it may take several months to find the drug or drugs that will bring B. A. back to a point of stabilization, it is important to have a consistent, reliable health care team in place to support her through this stabilization period. She should have a reliable contact person to call when she has questions and when she needs support.

---

uled in the next 48 hours. In children younger than 12 years of age, screen for CNS infections.

Include screening for baseline status before beginning therapy and for any potential adverse effects. Assess the following: temperature; skin color and lesions; CNS orientation, affect, reflexes, and bilateral grip strength; bowel sounds and reported output; pulse, auscultation, and blood pressure, including orthostatic blood pressure; respiration rate and adventitious sounds; and urinary output. Obtain liver and renal function tests, thyroid function tests, ECG if appropriate, and complete blood count (CBC).

Nursing Diagnoses

The patient receiving antipsychotics may have the following nursing diagnoses related to drug therapy:

- Impaired Physical Mobility related to extrapyramidal effects
- Decreased Cardiac Output related to hypotensive effects
- Risk for Injury related to CNS effects and sedation
- Impaired Urinary Elimination related to anticholinergic effects
- Deficient Knowledge regarding drug therapy

Implementation

- Do not allow the patient to crush or chew sustained-release capsules, *which will decrease their absorption and effectiveness.*
- If the patient receives parenteral forms, keep the patient recumbent for 30 minutes *to reduce the risk of orthostatic hypotension.*
- Consider warning the patient or the patient's guardians about the risk of development of tardive dyskinesias with continued use *so they are prepared for that neurological change.*
- Monitor CBC *to arrange to discontinue the drug at signs of bone marrow suppression.*
- Arrange for gradual dose reduction after long-term use. *Abrupt withdrawal has been associated with gastritis, nausea, vomiting, dizziness, arrhythmias, and insomnia.*
- Provide positioning of legs and arms *to decrease the discomfort of dyskinesias.*
- Provide sugarless candy and ice chips *to increase secretions* and frequent mouth care *to prevent dry mouth from becoming a problem.*
- Encourage the patient to void before taking a dose *if urinary hesitancy or retention is a problem.*

- Provide safety measures such as side rails and assistance with ambulation if CNS effects or orthostatic hypotension occurs, *to prevent patient injury.*
- Provide for vision examinations *to determine ocular changes and arrange appropriate dosage change.*
- Provide thorough patient teaching, including drug name, prescribed dosage, measures for avoidance of adverse effects, warning signs that may indicate possible problems, and the need for monitoring and evaluation *to enhance patient knowledge about drug therapy and to promote compliance.* (See Patient Teaching Checklist: Antipsychotic/ Neuroleptic Drugs). Warn patients that urine may have a pink to reddish-brown color.
- Offer support and encouragement *to help patients cope with their drug regimen.*

Evaluation

- Monitor patient response to the drug (decrease in signs and symptoms of psychotic disorder).
- Monitor for adverse effects (sedation, anticholinergic effects, hypotension, extrapyramidal effects, bone marrow suppression).
- Evaluate effectiveness of teaching plan (patient can give the drug name and dosage, possible adverse effects to watch for, specific measures to prevent adverse effects, and warning signs to report).
- Monitor the effectiveness of comfort measures and compliance with the regimen (see Nursing Care Guide: Antipsychotic/Neuroleptic Drugs).

ANTIMANIC DRUG

Mania, the opposite of depression, occurs in individuals with bipolar disorder, who experience a period of depression followed by a period of mania. The cause of mania is not understood, but it is thought to be an overstimulation of certain neurons in the brain. The mainstay for treatment of mania is lithium.

Lithium salts (*Lithane, Lithotabs*) are taken orally for the management of manic episodes and prevention of future episodes. These very toxic drugs can cause severe CNS, renal, and pulmonary problems that may lead to death. Despite the potential for serious adverse effects, lithium is used with caution, because it is consistently effective in the treatment of mania. The therapeutically effective serum level is 0.6 to 1.2 mEq/L.

Therapeutic Actions and Indications

Lithium functions in several ways. It alters sodium transport in nerve and muscle cells; inhibits the release of norepinephrine and dopamine, but not serotonin, from stimulated neurons; increases the intraneuronal stores of norepinephrine and dopamine slightly; and decreases intraneuronal content of second messengers. This last mode of action may allow it to selectively modulate the responsiveness of hyper-

PATIENT TEACHING CHECKLIST

Antipsychotic/Neurologic Drugs

Create customized patient teaching materials for a specific antipsychotic/neurologic drug from the CD-ROM. Patient teaching should stress the following points for drugs within this class:

- Antipsychotic/neuroleptic drugs affect the activities of certain chemicals in your brain and are used to treat certain mental disorders.
- Drugs in this group should be taken exactly as prescribed.
- Because these drugs affect many body systems, it is important that you undergo medical evaluation regularly.

Common effects of these drugs include

- *Dizziness, drowsiness, and fainting*—Avoid driving or performing hazardous tasks or delicate tasks that require concentration if these occur. Change position slowly. The dizziness usually passes after 1 to 2 weeks of drug use.
- *Pink or reddish urine (with phenothiazines)*—These drugs sometimes cause the urine to change color. Do not be alarmed by this change; it does not mean that your urine contains blood.
- *Sensitivity to light*—Bright light might hurt your eyes and sunlight might burn your skin more easily. Wear sunglasses and protective clothing when you must be out in the sun.
- *Constipation*—Consult with your health care provider if this becomes a problem.

Report any of the following conditions to your health care provider: sore throat, fever, rash, tremors, weakness, and vision changes.

Tell any doctor, nurse, or other health care provider that you are taking this drug.

Keep this drug and all medications out of the reach of children.

Avoid the use of alcohol or other depressants while you are taking this drug. You also may want to limit your use of caffeine if you have increased tension or insomnia.

Avoid the use of over-the-counter drugs while you are on this drug. Many of them contain ingredients that could interfere with the effectiveness of your drug. If you feel that you need one of these preparations, consult with your health care provider about the most appropriate choice.

Take this drug exactly as prescribed. If you run out of medicine or find that you cannot take your drug for any reason, consult your health care provider. After this drug has been used for a period of time, additional adverse effects may occur if it is suddenly stopped. This drug will need to be tapered over time.

This Teaching Checklist reflects general patient guidelines. It is not meant to be a substitute for drug-specific teaching information, which is available in nursing drug guides.

active neurons that might contribute to the manic state. Although the biochemical actions of lithium are known, the exact mechanism of action in decreasing the manifestations of mania are not understood.

NURSING CARE GUIDE

Antipsychotic/Neuroleptic Drugs

Assessment	Nursing Diagnoses	Implementation	Evaluation
HISTORY Allergies to any of these drugs; CNS depression; CV disease; pregnancy or lactation; myelography; glaucoma; hypotension; thyrotoxicosis; seizures; CNS infections in children <12 y.	Impaired physical mobility related to extrapyramidal effects Risk for Injury related to CNS effects Decreased Cardiac Output related to CV effects Impaired Urinary Elimination related to anticholinergic effects Deficient Knowledge regarding drug therapy	Give drug in evening; do not allow patient to chew or crush sustained release capsules. Provide comfort and safety measures: void before dosing; side rails; sugarless lozenges; mouth care; safety measures if CNS effects occur; positioning to relieve dyskinesia discomfort; taper dose after long-term therapy. Provide support and reassurance to help patient cope with drug effects. Provide patient teaching regarding drug, dosage, adverse effects, conditions to report, precautions.	Evaluate drug effects: relief of signs and symptoms of psychotic disorders. Monitor for adverse effects: sedation, dizziness, insomnia; anticholinergic effects; extrapyramidal effects; bone marrow depression; skin rash. Monitor for drug–drug interactions as indicated for each drug. Evaluate effectiveness of patient teaching program. Evaluate effectiveness of comfort and safety measures.
PHYSICAL EXAMINATION CV: BP, P, orthostatic BP CNS: orientation, affect, reflexes, vision Skin: color, lesions, texture Respiratory: respiration, adventitious sounds GI: abdominal examination, bowel sounds Laboratory tests: thyroid, liver and renal function tests, CBC			

Lithium is indicated for the treatment of manic episodes of manic-depressive or bipolar illness and for maintenance therapy to prevent or diminish the frequency and intensity of future manic episodes. This agent is currently being investigated for the improvement of neutrophil counts in patients with cancer chemotherapy–induced neutropenia and as prophylaxis of cluster headaches and migraine headaches.

Pharmacokinetics

Lithium is readily absorbed from the GI tract, reaching peak levels in 30 minutes to 3 hours. It follows the same distribution pattern in the body as water. It slowly crosses the blood–brain barrier. Lithium is excreted from the kidney, although about 80% is reabsorbed. During periods of sodium depletion or dehydration, the kidney reabsorbs more lithium into the serum, often leading to toxic levels. Therefore, patients must be encouraged to maintain hydration while taking this drug. Lithium crosses the placenta and has been associated with congenital abnormalities. Women of childbearing age should be advised to use birth control while taking this drug. It also enters breast milk and can cause toxic effects in the baby. Breast feeding should be discontinued while using lithium.

Contraindications and Cautions

Lithium is contraindicated in the presence of hypersensitivity to lithium or tartrazine (found in *Lithane*). In addition, it is contraindicated in the following conditions: significant renal or cardiac disease that could be exacerbated by the toxic effects of the drug; a history of leukemia; metabolic disorders, including sodium depletion; dehydration; and diuretic use, because lithium depletes sodium reabsorption and severe hyponatremia may occur. (Hyponatremia leads to lithium retention and toxicity.) Pregnancy and lactation are also contraindications because of the potential for adverse effects on the fetus and neonate.

Caution should be used in any condition that could alter sodium levels, such as protracted diarrhea or excessive sweating; with suicidal or impulsive patients; and in patients who have infection with fever, which could be exacerbated by the toxic effects of the drug.

Adverse Effects

The adverse effects associated with lithium are directly related to serum levels of the drug.

- Serum levels of less than 1.5 mEq/L: CNS problems, including lethargy, slurred speech, muscle weakness, and fine tremor; polyuria, which relates to renal toxicity; and beginning of gastric toxicity, with nausea, vomiting, and diarrhea.
- Serum levels of 1.5 to 2 mEq/L: intensification of all of the above reactions, with ECG changes.
- Serum levels of 2 to 2.5 mEq/L: possible progression of CNS effects to ataxia, clonic movements, hyperreflexia, and seizures; possible CV effects such as severe ECG changes and hypotension; large output of dilute urine secondary to renal toxicity; fatalities secondary to pulmonary toxicity.
- Serum levels greater than 2.5 mEq/L: complex multiorgan toxicity, with a significant risk of death.

Clinically Important Drug–Drug Interactions

Some drug–drug combinations should be avoided. A lithium-haloperidol combination may result in an encephalopathic syndrome, consisting of weakness, lethargy, confusion, tremors, extrapyramidal symptoms, leukocytosis, and irreversible brain damage.

If lithium is given with carbamazepine increased CNS toxicity may occur, and a lithium–iodide salt combination results in an increased risk of hypothyroidism. Patients who receive either of these combinations should be monitored carefully. In addition, a thiazide diuretic–lithium combination increases the risk of lithium toxicity because of the loss of sodium and increased retention of lithium. If this combination is used, the dosage of lithium should be decreased and the patient should be monitored closely.

In the following instances, the serum lithium level should be monitored closely and appropriate dosage adjustments made. With the combination of lithium and some urine-alkalinizing drugs, including antacids and tromethamine, there is a possibility of decreased effectiveness of lithium. If lithium is combined with indomethacin or with some nonsteroidal anti-inflammatory drugs, higher plasma levels of lithium occur.

Nursing Considerations for Patients Receiving an Antimanic Drug

Assessment: History and Examination

Screen for the following conditions, which could be contraindications or cautions for the use of the drug: any known allergies to lithium or tartrazine; renal or CV disease; dehydration; sodium depletion, use of diuretics, protracted sweating, or diarrhea; suicidal or impulsive patients with severe depression; pregnancy or lactation; and infection with fever.

Include screening for baseline status before beginning therapy and for any potential adverse effects. Assess the following: temperature; skin color and lesions; CNS orientation, affect, and reflexes; bowel sounds and reported output; pulse, auscultation, and blood pressure, including orthostatic blood pressure; respiration rate and adventitious sounds; and urinary output. Obtain liver and renal function tests, thyroid function tests, CBC, and baseline ECG, and obtain serum lithium levels as appropriate.

Nursing Diagnoses

The patient receiving lithium may have the following nursing diagnoses related to drug therapy:

- Acute Pain related to GI, CNS, vision effects
- Risk for Injury related to CNS effects
- Impaired Urinary Elimination related to renal toxic effects
- Disturbed Thought Processes related to CNS effects
- Deficient Knowledge regarding drug therapy

Implementation

- Give the drug cautiously, with daily monitoring of serum lithium levels, to patients with significant renal or CV disease, dehydration, or debilitation, as well as those taking

DRUGS IN FOCUS
Antimanic Drug

Drug Name	Dosage/Route	Usual Indications
Lithium (*Lithane, Lithotabs*)	600 mg PO t.i.d. for acute episodes; 300 mg PO t.i.d.–q.i.d. for maintenance; reduce dosage with elderly patients	Treatment of manic episodes of manic-depressive illness; maintenance therapy to prevent or diminish the frequency and intensity of future manic episodes. Not recommended for children <12 y old.

diuretics, *to monitor for toxic levels and to arrange for appropriate dosage adjustment.*

- Give the drug with food or milk *to alleviate GI irritation if GI upset is severe.*
- Arrange to decrease dose after acute manic episodes. *Lithium tolerance is greatest during acute episodes and decreases when the acute episode is over.*
- Ensure that the patient maintains adequate intake of salt and fluid *to decrease toxicity.*
- Monitor the patient's clinical status closely, especially during the initial stages of therapy, *to provide appropriate supportive management as needed.*
- Arrange for small frequent meals, sugarless lozenges to suck, and frequent mouth care, *to increase secretions and decrease discomfort as needed.*
- Provide safety measures such as side rails and assistance with ambulation if CNS effects occur, *to prevent patient injury.*
- Provide thorough patient teaching, including drug name, prescribed dosage, measures for avoidance of adverse effects, warning signs that may indicate possible problems, and the need to avoid pregnancy while taking lithium, *to enhance patient knowledge about drug therapy and to promote compliance.*
- Offer support and encouragement *to help the patient cope with the drug regimen.*

Evaluation

- Monitor patient response to the drug (decreased manifestations and frequency of manic episodes).
- Monitor for adverse effects (CV toxicity, renal toxicity, GI upset, respiratory complications).
- Evaluate the effectiveness of the teaching plan (patient can give the drug name and dosage and describe the possible adverse effects to watch for, specific measures to help avoid adverse effects, warning signs to report, and the need to avoid pregnancy).
- Monitor the effectiveness of comfort measures and compliance with the regimen.

CENTRAL NERVOUS SYSTEM STIMULANTS

CNS stimulants are used clinically to treat both attention-deficit disorders and narcolepsy. Paradoxically, these drugs calm hyperkinetic children and help them focus on one activity for a longer period. They also redirect and excite the arousal stimuli from the RAS (Figure 22–3; see Figure 22–1).

The CNS stimulants that are used to treat attention-deficit disorder and narcolepsy include the following drugs.

- Methylphenidate (*Ritalin, Concerta*) is a very commonly used drug for the treatment of attention-deficit disorders and other behavioral syndromes associated with hyperactivity, as well as narcolepsy. It is now available in various forms allowing for once-, twice-, or three-times a day dosing.
- Dexmethylphenidate (*Focalin*), approved in late 2001, is an isomer of methylphenidate and is used in lower doses than methylphenidate. It is approved only for treatment of attention-deficit hyperactivity disorder in patients 6 years of age and older.
- Dextroamphetamine (*Dexedrine*), an oral drug, is also used as short-term adjunctive therapy for exogenous obesity.
- Modafinil (*Provigil*), a newer drug, is approved only for use in treating narcolepsy. It is not associated with many of the systemic stimulatory effects of some of the other CNS stimulants.
- Pemoline (*Cylert*), is approved only for use in attention-deficit disorders and other behavioral syndromes associated with hyperactivity. It is not associated with many of the systemic stimulatory effects of amphetamine-type stimulatory drugs.

Therapeutic Actions and Indications

The CNS stimulants act as cortical and RAS stimulants, possibly by increasing the release of catecholamines from presynaptic neurons, leading to an increase in stimulation of the postsynaptic neurons. The paradoxical effect of calming hyperexcitability through CNS stimulation seen in attention-deficit syndrome is believed to be related to increased stimulation of an immature RAS, which leads to the ability to be more selective in response to incoming stimuli.

The CNS stimulants are indicated for the treatment of attention-deficit syndromes, including behavioral syndromes characterized by hyperactivity and distractibility, as well as narcolepsy.

Pharmacokinetics

These drugs are rapidly absorbed from the GI tract, reaching peak levels in 2 to 4 hours. They are metabolized in the liver and excreted in the urine, with half-lives ranging from 2 to 15 hours, depending on the drug. Safety for use during preg-

FIGURE 22–3. Site of action of the central nervous system (CNS) stimulants in the reticular activating system (RAS).

CULTURAL CONSIDERATIONS
Antipsychotic Drugs

The ways in which patients in certain cultural groups respond to antipsychotic drugs—either physiologically or emotionally—may vary. Therefore, when a pharmacological regimen is incorporated into overall patient care, health care providers must consider and respect an individual patient's cultural beliefs and needs.

• African Americans respond more rapidly to antipsychotic medications and have a greater risk for development of disfiguring adverse effects, such as tardive dyskinesia. Consequently, these patients should be started off at the lowest possible dose and monitored closely. African Americans also display a higher red blood cell plasma lithium ratio than Caucasians do, and they report more adverse effects from lithium therapy. These patients should be monitored closely because they have a higher potential for lithium toxicity at standard therapeutic ranges.

• Patients in Asian countries, such as India, Turkey, Malaysia, China, Japan, and Indonesia, receive lower doses of neuroleptics and lithium to achieve the same therapeutic response as seen in patients in the United States. This may be related to these individuals' lower body mass as well as metabolic differences, and it may have implications for dosing protocols for patients in these ethnic groups who undergo therapy in the United States.

• Arab American patients metabolize antipsychotic medications more slowly than Asian Americans do and may require lower doses to achieve the same therapeutic effects as in Caucasians.

• Individuals in some cultures use herbs and other folk remedies, and the use of herbs may interfere with the metabolism of Western medications. The nurse should carefully assess for herbal use and be aware of potential interactions.

nancy and lactation has not been established; during those periods, these drugs should be used only if the benefit to the mother clearly outweighs the potential risk to the neonate.

Contraindications and Cautions

The CNS stimulants are contraindicated in the presence of known allergy to the drug. Other contraindications include the following conditions: marked anxiety, agitation, or tension and severe fatigue or glaucoma, which could be exacerbated by the CNS stimulation caused by these drugs; cardiac disease, which could be aggravated by the stimulatory effects of these drugs; and pregnancy and lactation, because of the potential for adverse effects on the fetus and neonate.

Caution should be used in the presence of a history of seizures, which could be potentiated by the CNS stimulation; with a history of drug dependence, including alcoholism, because these drugs may result in physical and psychological dependence; and with hypertension, which could be exacerbated by the stimulatory effects of these drugs.

Adverse Effects

The adverse effects associated with these drugs are related to the CNS stimulation they cause. CNS effects can include nervousness, insomnia, dizziness, headache, blurred vision, and difficulty with accommodation. GI effects such as anorexia, nausea, and weight loss may occur. CV effects can include hypertension, arrhythmias, and angina. Skin rashes are a common reaction to some of these drugs. Physical and psychological dependence may also develop. Because CNS stimulants have this effect, the drugs are controlled substances.

Clinically Important Drug–Drug Interactions

The combination of a CNS stimulant with a monoamine oxidase (MAO) inhibitor leads to an increased risk of adverse effects and increased toxicity and should be avoided if possible. Likewise, the combination of a CNS stimulant with guanethidine, which results in a decrease in antihypertensive effects, should be avoided.

In addition, the combination of CNS stimulants with tricyclic antidepressants or phenytoin leads to a risk of increased drug levels. Patients who receive such a combination should be monitored for toxicity.

Nursing Considerations for Patients Receiving Central Nervous System Stimulants
Assessment: History and Examination

Screen for the following conditions, which could be contraindications or cautions for the use of the drug: any known allergies to the drug; glaucoma, anxiety, tension, fatigue, or seizure disorder; cardiac disease and hypertension; pregnancy or lactation; a history of leukemia; and history of drug dependency, including alcoholism.

Include screening for baseline status before beginning therapy and for any potential adverse effects. Assess the following: temperature; skin color and lesions; CNS orientation, affect, and reflexes; ophthalmic examination; bowel sounds and reported output; pulse, auscultation, and blood pressure, including orthostatic blood pressure; respiration rate and adventitious sounds; and urinary output. Obtain a CBC.

Nursing Diagnoses

The patient receiving CNS stimulants may have the following nursing diagnoses related to drug therapy:

• Disturbed Thought Processes related to CNS effects of the drug
• Decreased Cardiac Output related to CV effects of the drug
• Risk for Injury related to CNS and visual effects of the drug
• Deficient Knowledge regarding drug therapy

Implementation

• Ensure proper diagnosis of behavioral syndromes and narcolepsy, *because these drugs should not be used until underlying medical causes of the problem are ruled out.*
• Arrange to interrupt the drug periodically in children who are

DRUGS IN FOCUS
Central Nervous System Stimulants

Drug Name	Dosage/Route	Usual Indications
dexmethylphenidate (*Focalin*)	2.5–5 mg PO b.i.d.; do not exceed 10 mg PO b.i.d.	Treatment of attention-deficit hyperactivity disorder in patients age ≥6 y
dextroamphetamine (*Dexedrine*)	Narcolepsy: 5–60 mg/d PO in divided doses Attention-deficit disorders: 2.5–5 mg per day PO taken in the morning Obesity: 5–30 mg/d PO (not recommended for children <12 y)	Narcolepsy, attention-deficit disorders, behavioral syndromes, exogenous obesity
methylphenidate (*Ritalin, Concerta, Metadate CD*)	Adult: 10–60 mg/d PO in divided doses depending on preparation Pediatric: 5 mg PO b.i.d.; increase gradually, do not exceed 60 mg/d	Narcolepsy, attention-deficit disorders, behavioral syndromes
modafinil (*Provigil*)	200 mg/d PO as a single dose; reduce dosage with hepatic impairment and in the elderly	Narcolepsy in adults
pemoline (*Cylert*)	37.5–75 mg/d PO in the morning	Attention-deficit disorders, behavioral syndromes in children

receiving the drug for behavioral syndromes, *to determine whether symptoms recur and therapy should be continued.*

- Arrange to dispense the least amount of drug possible, *to minimize the risk of overdose and abuse.*
- Administer the drug before 6 PM, *to reduce the incidence of insomnia.*
- Monitor weight, CBC, and ECG *to ensure early detection of adverse effects and proper interventions.*
- Consult with the school nurse or counselor *to ensure comprehensive care of school-aged children receiving CNS stimulants.*
- Provide safety measures such as siderails and assistance with ambulation if CNS effects occur, *to prevent patient injury.*
- Provide thorough patient teaching, including drug name, prescribed dosage, measures for avoidance of adverse effects, warning signs that may indicate possible problems, and the need for monitoring and evaluation, *to enhance patient knowledge about drug therapy and to promote compliance.* Offer support and encouragement *to help the patient cope with the drug regimen.*

Evaluation

- Monitor patient response to the drug (decrease in manifestations of behavioral syndromes, decrease in daytime sleep and narcolepsy).
- Monitor for adverse effects (CNS stimulation, CV effects, rash, physical or psychological dependence, GI dysfunction).
- Evaluate the effectiveness of the teaching plan (patient can give the drug name and dosage, name possible adverse effects to watch for and specific measures to help avoid adverse effects, and describe the need for follow-up and evaluation).

- Monitor the effectiveness of comfort measures and compliance with the regimen.

WEB LINKS

Health care providers and patients may want to consult the following Internet sources:

Information on sleep disorders research and treatment:
http://www.uic.edu/depts/cnr
Information on education programs, research, and other information related to mental illness:
http://www.cmhc.com
Information on mental health resources, support groups, and related information:
http://www.mhsource.com
Information on mental health–related issues in the child and adolescent:
http://www.aacp.org
Information about specific diagnoses, treatment, and support groups:
http://www.adhdnews.com
http://mentalhelp.net

CHAPTER SUMMARY

- Mental disorders are disorders of thought processes that may be caused by some inherent dysfunction within the brain. Psychoses are thought disorders.
- Schizophrenia, the most common psychosis, is characterized by delusions, hallucinations, and inappropriate responses to stimuli.

NURSING CHALLENGE
School Nursing and *Ritalin* Administration

In the past several years, the number of school children receiving diagnoses of attention-deficit disorder or minimal brain dysfunction and being prescribed methylphenidate (*Ritalin*) has increased dramatically. Because this drug needs to be given two or three times each day, it has become the responsibility of the school nurse to dispense the drug during the day. Some school nurses reportedly spend between 50% and 70% of their time administering these drugs and completing the necessary paperwork. In 2000–2001, several long-acting formulations of methylphenidate became available. *Concerta*, available in an extended-release tablet in 18- and 36-mg strengths, is now also available in a 54-mg strength. This form is suggested for every-12-hours dosing. *Metadate CD* is approved as a 20-mg extended-release capsule that is suggested as a once-daily treatment for children with attention deficit disorder. *Ritalin SR* is another extended-release formulation that is designed to be given every 8 hours. These extended-release forms are not interchangeable, and the instructions that come with the drug that is prescribed should be checked carefully. The advantage of these extended-release forms is expected to be a decrease in the number of students who must see the nurse for medication during the school day and, perhaps, a decrease in the stigma that may be associated with needing this drug.

The school nurse has additional responsibilities besides administering the drug. The school nurse is responsible for assessing children's response to the drug and for coordinating the teacher's and health care providers' input into each individual case, including the incidence of adverse effects and the appropriateness of the drug therapy. The nurse should

• Ensure that the proper diagnosis is made before supporting the use of the drug.
• Constantly evaluate and work with the primary health care provider to regularly challenge children without the drug to see whether the drug is doing what is expected or whether the child is maturing and no longer needs the drug therapy.

The school nurse needs to be prepared to be an advocate for the best therapeutic intervention for a particular child. Because long-term methylphenidate therapy is associated with many adverse effects, use of the drug should not be taken lightly.

• Lithium, a membrane stabilizer, is the only effective anti-manic drug. Because it is a very toxic salt, serum levels must be carefully monitored to prevent severe toxicity.
• CNS stimulants, which stimulate cortical levels and the RAS to increase RAS activity, are used to treat attention-deficit disorders and narcolepsy. These drugs improve concentration and the ability to filter and focus incoming stimuli.

Review Questions

1. Mental disorders are now thought to be caused by some inherent dysfunction within the brain that leads to abnormal thought processes and responses and include
   a. depression.
   b. anxiety.
   c. seizures.
   d. schizophrenia.
2. Antipsychotic drugs are basically
   a. serotonin reuptake inhibitors.
   b. norepinephrine blockers.
   c. dopamine receptor blockers.
   d. acetylcholine stimulators.
3. Adverse effects associated with antipsychotics drugs are related to the drugs' effects on receptor sites and can include
   a. insomnia, hypertension.
   b. dry mouth, hypotension, glaucoma.
   c. diarrhea, excessive urination.
   d. increased sexual drive, improved concentration.
4. Dyskinesias are a common side effect of antipsychotic drugs. Nursing interventions for the patient receiving antipsychotic drugs should include all of the following except
   a. positioning to decrease discomfort of dyskinesias.
   b. safety measures to prevent injury.
   c. encouraging the patient to chew tablets to prevent choking.
   d. careful teaching to alert the patient and family about this adverse effect.
5. Lithium toxicity can be dangerous. Patient assessment to evaluate for appropriate lithium levels would look for:
   a. serum lithium levels greater than 3 mEq/L.
   b. serum lithium levels greater than 4 mEq/L.
   c. serum lithium levels less than 1.5 mEq/L.
   d. undetectable serum lithium levels.
6. Your patient, a 6-year-old boy, is being started on *Ritalin* (methylphenidate) to control an attention-deficit disorder. Family teaching should include which of the following:
   a. This drug can be shared with other family members who might seem to need it.
   b. This drug may cause insomnia, weight loss, and GI upset.
   c. Do not alert the school nurse to the fact that this drug is being taken, because the child could have problems later on.
   d. This drug should not be stopped for any reason for several years.

• Mania is a state of hyperexcitability, one extreme of bipolar disorder.
• An attention-deficit disorder is a behavioral syndrome characterized by hyperactivity and a short attention span.
• Narcolepsy is a disorder characterized by daytime sleepiness and sudden loss of wakefulness.
• Antipsychotics are dopamine-receptor blockers that are effective in helping people with mental disorders to organize thought patterns and respond appropriately to stimuli.
• Antipsychotics can cause hypotension, anticholinergic effects, sedation, and extrapyramidal effects including parkinsonism, ataxia, and tremors.

7. Antipsychotic drugs are also known as neuroleptic drugs because
   a. they cause numerous neurological effects.
   b. they frequently cause epilepsy.
   c. they are also minor tranquilizers.
   d. they are the only drugs known to directly affect nerves.
8. Attention-deficit disorders (the inability to concentrate or focus on an activity) and narcolepsy (sudden episodes of sleep) are both most effectively treated with the use of
   a. neuroinhibitors.
   b. dopamine receptor blockers.
   c. major tranquilizers.
   d. CNS stimulants.
9. Haloperidol (*Haldol*) is a potent antipsychotic that is associated with
   a. severe extrapyramidal effects.
   b. severe sedation.
   c. severe hypotension.
   d. severe anticholinergic effects.

10. A severe adverse reaction that can include permanent brain damage may occur if lithium is combined with
    a. acetaminophen.
    b. haloperidol.
    c. thiazide diuretics.
    d. antacids.

BIBLIOGRAPHY

Bailey, K. (1998). *Psychotropic drug facts*. Philadelphia: Lippincott-Raven.

Bullock, B. L. (2000). *Focus on pathophysiology*. Philadelphia: Lippincott Williams & Wilkins.

Drug facts and comparisons. (2002). St. Louis: Facts and Comparisons.

Gilman, A., Hardman, J. G., & Limbird, L. E. (Eds.) (2002). *Goodman and Gilman's the pharmacological basis of therapeutics* (10th ed.). New York: McGraw-Hill.

Karch, A. M. (2002). *2003 Lippincott's nursing drug guide*. Philadelphia: Lippincott Williams & Wilkins.

Professional's guide to patient drug facts. (2002). St. Louis: Facts and Comparisons.

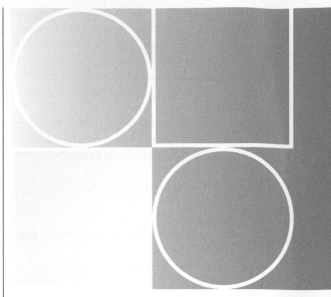

CHAPTER

23

Antiepileptic Agents

302

Key Terms

absence seizure

antiepileptic

convulsion

epilepsy

focal seizure

generalized seizure

grand mal seizure

petit mal seizure

seizure

status epilepticus

tonic–clonic seizure

Drugs for Treating Tonic–Clonic (Grand Mal) Seizures

Hydantoins

ethotoin

fosphenytoin

mephenytoin

🅟 phenytoin

Barbiturates and Barbiturate-Like Drugs

mephobarbital

🅟 phenobarbital

primidone

Benzodiazepines

clonazepam

🅟 diazepam

Drugs for Treating Absence (Petit Mal) Seizures

Succinimides

🅟 ethosuximide

methsuximide

phensuximide

Other Drugs for Absence (Petit Mal) Seizures

acetazolamide

🅟 valproic acid

zonisamide

Drugs for Treating Partial (Focal) Seizures

🅟 carbamazepine

clorazepate

felbamate

gabapentin

lamotrigine

levetiracetam

oxcarbazepine

tiagabine

topiramate

Epilepsy, the most prevalent of the neurological disorders, is not a single disease but a collection of different syndromes. All of these conditions are characterized by the same feature: sudden discharge of excessive electrical energy from nerve cells located within the brain, which leads to a **seizure.** In some cases, this release stimulates motor nerves, resulting in **convulsions,** with tonic–clonic muscle contractions that have the potential to cause injury, tics, or spasms. Other discharges may stimulate autonomic or sensory nerves and cause very different effects such as a barely perceptible, temporary lapse in consciousness or a sympathetic reaction.

The treatment of epilepsy varies widely, depending on the exact problem and its manifestations. The drugs that are used to manage epilepsy are called **antiepileptics.** These agents are sometimes referred to as anticonvulsants, but because not all types of epilepsy involve convulsions, this term is not generally applicable. The drug of choice for any given situation depends on the type of epilepsy and patient tolerance for associated adverse effects (Table 23–1).

NATURE OF EPILEPSY

The form that a particular seizure takes depends on the location of the cells that initiate the electrical discharge and the neural pathways that are stimulated by the initial volley of electrical impulses. For the most part, epilepsy seems to be caused by abnormal neurons that are very sensitive to stimulation or overrespond for some reason. They do not appear to be different from other neurons in any other way. Seizures caused by these abnormal cells are called primary seizures because no underlying cause can be identified. In some cases, however, outside factors—head injury, drug overdose, environmental exposure, and so on—may precipitate seizures. Such seizures are often referred to as secondary seizures.

Classification of Seizures

Correct diagnosis of seizure type is very important for determining the correct medication to prevent future seizures while causing the fewest problems and adverse effects. Seizures may be grouped into two main types, and they are further classified within these two categories.

Generalized Seizures
Generalized seizures begin in one area of the brain and rapidly spread throughout both hemispheres of the brain. Patients who have a generalized seizure usually experience a loss of consciousness resulting from this massive electrical activity throughout the brain. Generalized seizures are further classified into the following five types:

1. **Tonic–clonic seizures,** formerly known as **grand mal seizures,** involve dramatic tonic–clonic muscle contractions, loss of consciousness, and a recovery period characterized by confusion and exhaustion.
2. **Absence seizures,** formerly known as **petit mal seizures,** involve abrupt, brief (3- to 5-second) periods of loss of

TABLE 23-1 | Drugs Used to Treat Seizures and the Type of Seizures That They Treat

	Type of Seizure						
Drug	Grand Mal	Petit Mal	Myoclonic	Febrile	Status Epilepticus	Simple Focal	Complex Focal
Mephobarbital	O	O	—	—	—	—	—
Phenobarbital	O	—	—	X	O	O	—
Primidone	O	—	—	O	—	O	O
Clonazepam	—	O	X	—	—	—	—
Diazepam	O	—	—	—	X	—	—
Ethotoin	X	—	—	—	—	—	—
Fosphenytoin	—	—	—	—	X	—	—
Mephenytoin	O	—	O	—	—	O	O
Phenytoin	X	—	—	—	X	X	X
Ethosuximide	—	X	—	—	—	—	—
Methosuximide	—	O	—	—	—	—	—
Phenosuximide	—	O	—	—	—	—	—
Acetazolamide	O	—	—	—	—	—	—
Valproic acid	—	O	X	—	—	—	O
Zonisamide	—	O	—	—	—	—	—
Carbamazepine	X	—	—	—	—	X	X
Clorazepate	—	—	—	—	—	O	O
Felbamate	—	—	—	—	—	O	O
Gabapentin	—	—	—	—	—	O	O
Lamotrigine	—	—	—	—	—	O	O
Levetiracetam	—	—	—	—	—	O	O
Oxcarbazepine	—	—	—	—	—	O	O
Tiagabine	—	O	—	—	—	O	O
Topiramate	—	—	—	—	—	O	O

X, primary treatment, a drug of choice; O, adjunctive therapy or used when unresponsive to other treatments; —, not a use.

consciousness. Absence seizures occur commonly in children and frequently disappear at puberty.

3. Myoclonic seizures involve short, sporadic periods of muscle contractions that last for several minutes. They are relatively rare and are often secondary seizures.
4. Febrile seizures are related to very high fevers and usually involve convulsions. Febrile seizures most frequently occur in children; they are usually self-limited and do not reappear.
5. **Status epilepticus,** potentially the most dangerous of seizure conditions, is a state in which seizures rapidly recur again and again.

Partial Seizures

Partial seizures, also called **focal seizures,** involve one area of the brain and do not spread throughout the entire organ. The presenting symptoms depend on exactly where the excessive electrical discharge is occurring in the brain. Partial seizures can be further classified as follows:

1. Simple partial seizures occur in a single area of the brain and may involve a single muscle movement or sensory alteration.
2. Complex partial seizures involve complex sensory changes such as hallucinations, mental distortion, changes in personality, loss of consciousness, and loss of social inhibitions. Motor changes may include involuntary urination, chewing motions, diarrhea, and so on. The onset of complex partial seizures usually occurs by the late teens.

DRUGS FOR TREATING TONIC–CLONIC (GRAND MAL) SEIZURES

Various drugs are used to treat tonic–clonic (grand mal) seizures. Drugs that are used to treat generalized seizures stabilize the nerve membranes by blocking channels in the

DRUG THERAPY ACROSS THE LIFESPAN

Antiepiletic Agents

Children	Adults	Older Adults
Antiepileptic drugs can have an impact on a child's learning and social development. Children may also be more sensitive to the sedating effects of some of these drugs. Children should be monitored very closely and often require a switch to a different agent or dosage adjustments based on their response. Newborns (1 to 10 days of age) respond best to intramuscular phenobarbital if an antiepileptic is needed. Older children (2 months to 6 years of age) absorb and metabolize many of these drugs more quickly than adults do and require a larger dosage per kilogram to maintain therapeutic levels. Careful calculation of drug dosage using both weight and age are important in helping the child to receive the best therapeutic effect with the least toxicity. After the age of 10 to 14 years, many of these drugs can be given in the standard adult dose. Parents of children receiving these drugs should receive consistent support and education about the seizure disorder and the medications being used to treat it. Many communities have local support groups that can offer lots of educational materials and support programs. It is a very frightening experience to watch your child have a tonic–clonic seizure, and parents should be supported with this in mind.	Adults using these drugs should be under regular care and should be monitored regularly for adverse effects. They should be encouraged to carry or wear a Medic-Alert identification to alert emergency personnel that antiepileptic drugs are being taken. Adults also need education and support to deal with the old stigma of seizures as well as the lifestyle changes and drug effects that they may need to cope with. Most of these drugs have been associated with fetal abnormalities in animal studies. Some of them are clearly associated with predictable congenital effects in humans. Women of child-bearing age should be encouraged to use contraceptives while taking these drugs. If a pregnancy does occur, or if a woman taking one of these drugs desires to become pregnant, the importance of the drug to the mother should be weighed against the potential risk to the fetus. Stopping an antiepileptic can precipitate seizures that could cause anoxia and its related problems for the mother and the baby. Women who are nursing should be encouraged to find another way of feeding the baby to avoid the sedating and central nervous system effects that the drugs can have on the infant.	Older patients may be more susceptible to the adverse effects of these drugs. Dosages of all of these drugs may need to be reduced, and the patient should be monitored very closely for toxic effects and to provide safety measures if central nervous system effects do occur. Patients with renal or hepatic impairment should be monitored very closely. Baseline renal and liver function tests should be done and dosages adjusted as appropriate. Serum levels of the drug should be monitored closely in such cases to prevent serious adverse effects. The older patient should also be encouraged to wear or carry a Medic-Alert identification in case there is an emergency and the patient is not able to communicate information about the drug or disorder.

cell membrane or altering receptor sites. Because they work generally on the central nervous system (CNS), sedation and other CNS effects often result. In particular, the drugs that are indicated for tonic–clonic seizures (the hydantoins, the barbiturates, and the barbiturate-like drugs) affect the entire brain and reduce the chance of sudden electrical outburst. Associated adverse effects are often related to total brain stabilization (Figure 23–1).

Hydantoins

The hydantoins stabilize nerve membranes and limit the spread of excitability from the initiating focus (see Figure 23–1). Because hydantoins are generally less sedating than many other antiepileptics, they may be the drugs of choice for patients who are not willing to tolerate sedation and drowsiness. They do have significant adverse effects (eg, severe liver toxicity). In many situations, less toxic drugs (eg, the benzodiazepines) have replaced them.

The hydantoins include the following agents:

- Phenytoin (*Dilantin*), the prototype hydantoin, is used in the treatment of tonic–clonic seizures and status epilepticus as well as in the prevention and treatment of seizures after neurosurgery. It is available in oral and parenteral forms. It is well absorbed from the gastrointestinal (GI) tract, metabolized in the liver, and excreted in the urine. Patients with hepatic impairment are at risk for increased toxicity from the drug. Therapeutic serum levels ranges from 10 to 20 μg/mL.
- Ethotoin (*Peganone*) is used to control tonic–clonic and myoclonic seizures. It is also well absorbed from the GI tract, metabolized in the liver, and excreted in the urine. The therapeutic serum levels of ethotoin are from 15 to 50 μg/mL.
- Fosphenytoin (*Cerebyx*) is used for short-term control of status epilepticus and to prevent seizures after neurosurgery. It is given intramuscularly or intravenously. Fosphenytoin is metabolized in the liver and excreted in the urine. The ther-

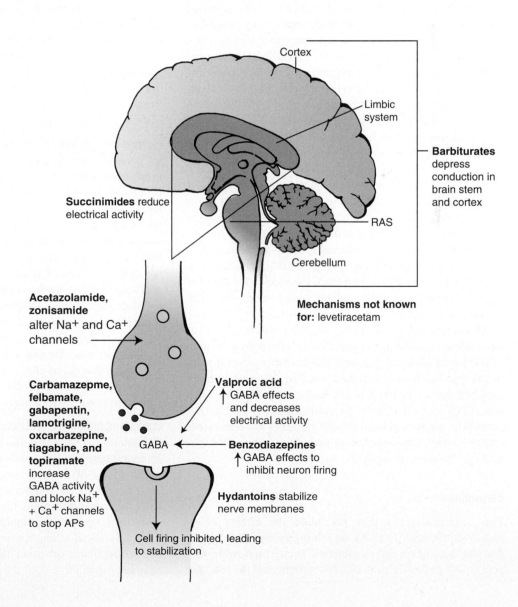

FIGURE 23–1. Sites of action of drugs used to treat various types of epilepsy. APs, action potentials; GABA, γ-aminobutyric acid; RAS, reticular activating system.

apeutic phenytoin serum levels peak about 10 to 20 minutes after the infusion, and the patient must be monitored closely for cardiovascular reactions during this period. Patients with hepatic and/or renal impairment are at increased risk for toxic effects because of alterations in metabolism and excretion of the drug. Such patients should be monitored closely, and the dosage should be reduced accordingly.

- Mephenytoin (*Mesantoin*) is used for the treatment of tonic–clonic, myoclonic, and partial (focal) seizures in patients who do not respond to less toxic antiepileptic agents. This drug has been associated with severe hepatic toxicity, bone marrow suppression, and often unacceptable dermatological reactions. Mephenytoin is well absorbed from the GI tract and metabolized in the liver with bile secretion. The therapeutic serum level has not been established. Patients with hepatic impairment should be monitored very closely.

Barbiturates and Barbiturate-Like Drugs

Phenobarbital (*Solfoton, Luminal*), which is available in oral and parenteral forms, is used for the emergency control of status epilepticus and acute seizures associated with eclampsia, tetanus, and other conditions. In addition, it is used orally for the long-term management of tonic–clonic and cortical focal seizures and can be very effective in the treatment of simple partial seizures. It is well absorbed from the GI tract, metabolized in the liver, and excreted in the urine. This drug has very low lipid solubility, giving it a slow onset and a very long duration of activity. The therapeutic serum level is 15 to 40 μg/mL.

Primidone (*Mysoline*), which is structurally very similar to phenobarbital, is an alternative choice in the treatment of tonic–clonic or partial seizures. It tends to have a longer half-life than phenobarbital and is available only in an oral form. Primidone may be combined with other agents to treat seizures that cannot be controlled by any other antiepileptic. It is well absorbed from the GI tract, metabolized in the liver to phenobarbital metabolites, and excreted in the urine. The therapeutic serum levels are 5 to 12 μg/mL.

Mephobarbital (*Mebaral*) is used for the treatment of tonic–clonic and absence seizures and is also used as an anxiolytic/hypnotic agent. It is well absorbed from the GI tract, metabolized in the liver, and excreted in the urine. It has a long half-life of 11 to 67 hours. It is commonly associated with CNS and GI effects. Its cardiovascular effects (hypotension, bradycardia, circulatory collapse) and respiratory effects (apnea, hypoventilation) make it less desirable than many of the other antiepileptic agents.

Benzodiazepines

The benzodiazepines may potentiate the effects of γ-aminobutyric acid (GABA), an inhibitory neurotransmitter that stabilizes nerve cell membranes. These drugs, which appear to act primarily in the limbic system and the reticular

activating system (RAS), also cause muscle relaxation and relieve anxiety without affecting cortical functioning substantially. In general, these drugs have limited toxicity and are well tolerated by most people. (See Chapter 20 for use of benzodiazepines as sedatives and anxiolytics.) The benzodiazepines described here are used as antiepileptics.

Diazepam (*Valium*), the prototype benzodiazepine, is useful in relieving tension, anxiety, and muscle spasm. Available in oral, rectal, and parenteral forms, it is used to treat severe convulsions and status epilepticus, alcohol withdrawal, and treatment of tetanus; is given to relieve preoperative anxiety; and is being studied for use in the treatment of panic attacks. Diazepam is not used for long-term management of epilepsy. Diazepam is well absorbed from the GI tract, metabolized in the liver, and excreted in the urine. It has a long half-life of 20 to 50 hours.

Clonazepam (*Klonopin*) is used for the treatment of absence (petit mal) seizures and myoclonic seizures. Patients who do not respond to succinimides may respond to this drug. Clonazepam may lose its effectiveness within 3 months (affected patients may respond to dosage adjustment). Clonazepam is being studied for use in the treatment of panic attacks, restless leg movements during sleep, hyperkinetic dysarthria, acute manic episodes, multifocal tic disorders, neuralgias, and as an adjunct in the treatment of schizophrenia. It is well absorbed from the GI tract, metabolized in the liver, and excreted in the urine. Clonazepam also has a long half-life of 18 to 50 hours.

Therapeutic Actions and Indications

In general, the hydantoins, barbiturates, and benzodiazepines all stabilize nerve membranes throughout the CNS to decrease excitability and hyperexcitability to stimulation. By decreasing conduction through nerve pathways, they reduce the tonic–clonic, muscular, and emotional responses to stimulation. Both hydantoins and barbiturates stabilize the nerve membrane directly by influencing ionic channels in the cell membrane. Specifically, phenobarbital depresses conduction in the lower brainstem and the cerebral cortex and depresses motor conduction. Benzodiazepines decrease excitability and conduction (see Figure 23–1).

Several drugs in these three groups are indicated for tonic–clonic seizures and status epilepticus, for prevention of seizures that occur after neurosurgery, and for adjunctive therapy for other seizure disorders or sedation and muscle relaxation (varies with drug).

Contraindications and Cautions

Hydantoins, barbiturates, and benzodiazepines are generally contraindicated in the presence of allergy to any of these drugs. Many of these agents are associated with specific birth defects and should not be used in pregnancy unless the risk of seizures outweighs the potential risk to the fetus. In such cases, the mother should be informed of the potential risks. The risk of taking a woman with a seizure disorder off of an antiepileptic drug that has stabilized her condition may be greater than the risk of the drug to the fetus. Discontinuing the drug could result in status epilepticus, which has a high risk of hypoxia for the mother and the fetus. Research has not been able to show the effects of even a minor seizure during pregnancy on the fetus, making it important to prevent seizures during pregnancy if at all possible. Women of child-bearing age should be urged to use barrier contraceptives while taking these drugs. If a pregnancy does occur, the woman should receive educational materials and counseling. Other contraindications include lactation, because these drugs cross into breast milk and may cause adverse effects on the neonate, and coma, depression, or psychoses that could be exacerbated by the generalized CNS depression.

Caution should be used with elderly or debilitated patients who may respond adversely to the CNS depression and with those patients who have impaired renal or liver function that may interfere with drug metabolism and excretion.

Adverse Effects

The most common adverse effects associated with drugs in all three groups—hydantoins, barbiturates, and benzodiazepines—relate to CNS depression and its effects on body function: depression, confusion, drowsiness, lethargy, fatigue, constipation, dry mouth, anorexia, cardiac arrhythmias and changes in blood pressure, urinary retention, and loss of libido.

Specific adverse effects with the hydantoins include severe liver toxicity, bone marrow suppression, gingival hyperplasia, and potentially serious dermatological reactions (eg, hirsutism, coarsening of facial skin), all of which are directly related to cellular toxicity.

In addition, benzodiazepines and phenobarbital may be associated with physical dependence and withdrawal syndrome. Phenobarbital has also been linked to severe dermatological reactions and the development of drug tolerance related to changes in drug metabolism over time.

Clinically Important Drug–Drug Interactions

Because the risk of CNS depression is increased when any of the drugs in these three groups are taken with alcohol, patients should be advised not to drink alcohol while they are taking these agents. In addition, the individual drugs are associated with a wide variety of drug–drug interactions. Therefore, a drug reference should be reviewed carefully before any drug is added or withdrawn from a therapeutic regimen that involves any of these agents.

Nursing Considerations for Patients Receiving Hydantoins

See Chapter 20 for nursing considerations for patients receiving barbiturates or benzodiazepines.

Assessment: History and Examination

Screen for the following conditions, which may be cautions or contraindications to the use of the drug: any known allergies to these drugs; cardiac arrhythmias, hypotension, diabetes, coma, psychoses; pregnancy and lactation; and renal

or hepatic dysfunction. Obtain a description of seizures, including onset, aura, duration, and recovery.

Include screening for baseline status before beginning therapy and for any potential adverse effects. Assess the following: skin color and lesions; temperature; CNS orientation, affect, reflexes, and bilateral grip strength; bowel sounds and reported output; pulse, auscultation, and blood pressure; urinary output; and electroencephalogram (EEG) if appropriate. Assess liver and renal function tests.

Nursing Diagnoses

The patient receiving hydantoins may have the following nursing diagnoses related to drug therapy:

- Acute Pain related to GI, CNS, genitourinary effects
- Disturbed Thought Processes related to CNS effects
- Risk for Injury related to CNS effects
- Impaired Skin Integrity related to dermatological effects
- Deficient Knowledge regarding drug therapy

Implementation

- Discontinue the drug at any sign of hypersensitivity reaction, liver dysfunction, or severe skin rash, *to limit reaction and prevent potentially serious reactions.*
- Administer the drug with food *to alleviate GI irritation if GI upset is a problem.*
- Monitor for adverse effects and provide appropriate supportive care as needed, *to help the patient cope with these effects.*
- Monitor for drug–drug interactions to arrange *to adjust dosages appropriately if any drug is added or withdrawn from the drug regimen.*
- Arrange for counseling for women of child-bearing age who are taking these drugs. *Because these drugs have the potential to cause serious damage to the fetus, women should understand the risk of birth defects and use barrier contraceptives to avoid pregnancy.*
- Provide thorough patient teaching, including drug name and prescribed dosage, as well as measures for avoidance of adverse effects, warning signs that may indicate possible problems, and the need for monitoring and evaluation, *to enhance patient knowledge about drug therapy and to promote compliance.* (See Patient Teaching Checklist: Antiepileptic Agents).
- Suggest the wearing or carrying of a Medic-Alert bracelet *to alert emergency workers and health care providers about the use of an antiepileptic drug.*
- Offer support and encouragement *to help the patient cope with the drug regimen.*

Evaluation

- Monitor patient response to the drug (decrease in incidence or absence of seizures; serum drug levels within the therapeutic range).

DRUGS IN FOCUS
Drugs for Treating Tonic–Clonic (Grand Mal) Seizures

Drug Name	Dosage/Route	Usual Indications
Hydantoins		
ethotoin (*Peganone*)	Adult: 2–3 g/d PO Pediatric: 500 mg to 1 g per day PO; consider age and weight	Tonic–clonic (grand mal) and psychomotor seizures
fosphenytoin (*Cerebyx*)	Adult: loading dose 15–20 mg phenytoin equivalent (PE) per kilogram IV given as 100–150 mg PE per minute; maintenance, 4–6 mg PE per kilogram per day; reduce dosage with renal or hepatic impairment	Short-term control of status epilepticus, prevention of seizures after neurosurgery
mephenytoin (*Mesantoin*)	Adult: 200–600 mg/d PO Pediatric: 100–400 mg/d PO	Tonic–clonic (grand mal), psychomotor, and partial (focal) seizures
℗ phenytoin (*Dilantin*)	Adult: 100 mg PO t.i.d., up to 300–400 mg/d; 10–15 mg/kg IV Pediatric: 5–8 mg/kg per day PO; 5–10 mg/kg IV in divided doses	Tonic–clonic (grand mal) seizures, status epilepticus prevention, and treatment of seizures after neuro-surgery
Barbiturates and Barbiturate-like Drugs		
mephobarbital (*Mebaral*)	Adult: 400–600 mg/d PO; decrease dosage and monitor elderly patients and debilitated patients closely Pediatric (≤5 y): 16–32 mg PO t.i.d.–q.i.d. Pediatric (>5 y): 32–64 mg PO t.i.d.–q.i.d.	Sedative/hypnotic, tonic–clonic (grand mal) and absence (petit mal) seizures
phenobarbital (*Solfoton, Luminal*)	Adult: 60–100 mg/d PO; 200–320 mg IM or IV for acute episodes, may be repeated in 6 h; reduce dosage with elderly and with renal or hepatic impairment Pediatric: 3–6 mg/kg per day PO; 4–6 mg/kg per day IM or IV; 15–20 mg/kg IV over 10–15 min for status epilepticus	Sedative hypnotic, tonic–clonic (grand mal) seizures, status epilepticus, cortical focal seizures, simple partial seizures
primidone (*Mysoline*)	Adult: 250 mg PO t.i.d.–q.i.d. Pediatric (>8 y): 250 mg PO t.i.d.–q.i.d. Pediatric (<8 y): 125–250 mg PO t.i.d.	Tonic–clonic (grand mal), partial, and refractory seizures
Benzodiazepines		
clonazepam (*Klonopin*)	Adult: initially 1.5 mg/d PO in three divided doses, up to a maximum 20 mg/d Pediatric (<10 y): 0.01–0.03 mg/kg per day PO initially, then up to 0.1–0.2 mg/kg per day PO	Absence (petit mal) and myoclonic seizures
℗ diazepam (*Valium*)	Adult: 2–10 mg PO b.i.d.–q.i.d.; or 0.2 mg/kg PR, may repeat in 4–12 h; 2–20 mg IM or IV Geriatric or debilitated patients: 2–2.5 mg PO q.d.–b.i.d. or 2–5 mg IM or IV Pediatric: 1–2.5 mg PO t.i.d.–q.i.d.; or 0.3–0.5 mg/kg PR with a repeat in 4–12 h if needed; 0.25 mg/kg IV over 3 min, may repeat in 15–30 min for up to three doses	Relieving tension, anxiety; muscle spasm; short-term treatment of severe convulsions, status epilepticus

- Monitor for adverse effects (CNS changes, GI depression, urinary retention, arrhythmias, blood pressure changes, liver toxicity, bone marrow suppression, severe dermatological reactions).
- Evaluate effectiveness of teaching plan (patient can give the drug name and dosage and name possible adverse effects to

watch for, and specific measures to prevent adverse effects; patient is aware of the risk of birth defects and the need to carry information about the diagnosis and use of this drug).
- Monitor the effectiveness of comfort measures and compliance with the regimen (see Nursing Care Guide: Antiepileptic Agents [Hydantoins]).

PATIENT TEACHING CHECKLIST
Antiepileptic Agents

Create customized patient teaching materials for a specific antiepileptic agent from the CD-ROM. Patient teaching should stress the following points for drugs within this class:

• Antiepileptic agents are used to stabilize abnormal cells in the brain that have been firing excessively and causing seizures.
• The timing of these doses is very important. To be effective, this drug must be taken regularly.
• Do not stop taking this drug suddenly. If for any reason you are unable to continue taking the drug, notify your health care provider at once. This drug must be slowly withdrawn when it is discontinued.

Common effects of these drugs include

• *Fatigue, weakness, and drowsiness*—Try to space activities evenly throughout the day and allow rest periods to avoid these effects. Take safety precautions and avoid driving or operating dangerous machinery if these conditions occur.
• *Headaches and difficulty sleeping*—These usually disappear as your body adjusts to the drug. If they persist and become too uncomfortable, consult with your health care provider.
• *Gastrointestinal upset, loss of appetite, and diarrhea or constipation*—Taking the drug with food or eating small, frequent meals may help alleviate this problem.

Report any of the following conditions to your health care provider: skin rash, severe nausea and vomiting, impaired coordination, yellowing of the eyes or skin, fever, sore throat, personality changes, and unusual bleeding or bruising.

It is advisable to wear or carry a Medic-Alert warning so that any person who takes care of you in an emergency will know that you are taking this drug.

Tell any doctor, nurse, or other health care provider that you are taking this drug.

Keep this drug and all medications out of the reach of children.

Do not take any other drug, including over-the-counter medications and alcohol, without consulting with your health care provider. Many of these preparations interact with the drug and could cause adverse effects.

If you become pregnant or decide to become pregnant while you are taking this drug, it is important that you discuss the implications with your health care provider. Use of barrier contraceptives is recommended to avoid pregnancy.

Report and record any seizure activity that you have while you are taking this drug.

Take this drug exactly as prescribed. Regular medical follow-up, which may include blood tests, will be necessary to evaluate the effects of this drug on your body.

This Teaching Checklist reflects general patient teaching guidelines. It is not meant to be a substitute for drug-specific teaching information, which is available in nursing drug guides.

DRUGS FOR TREATING ABSENCE (PETIT MAL) SEIZURES

Absence or petit mal seizures involve a brief, sudden, and self-limited loss of consciousness. The patient may just stare into space or may exhibit rapid blinking, which could last 3 to 5 seconds. Many people are not aware that a seizure is happening. This type of seizure frequently occurs in children, starting at about 3 years of age, and usually disappears by puberty.

Succinimides

The drugs that are most frequently used to treat these seizures are different from the drugs used to treat or prevent tonic–clonic seizures. The succinimides and drugs that modulate the inhibitory neurotransmitter GABA are most frequently used. The succinimides include the following agents:

• Ethosuximide (*Zarontin*) is the drug of choice for treating absence seizures. It has relatively few adverse effects compared with many other antiepileptic drugs. Ethosuximide is available for oral use. The established therapeutic serum level for ethosuximide is 40 to 100 μg/mL.
• Methsuximide (*Celontin*), another oral drug, is used to treat absence seizures that are resistant to other drugs. It has been associated with bone marrow suppression.
• Phensuximide (*Milontin*) is also used in the treatment of absence seizures that are resistant to other agents.

Therapeutic Actions and Indications
Although the exact mechanism of action is not understood, the succinimides suppress the abnormal electrical activity in the brain that is associated with absence seizures. The action may be related to activity in inhibitory neural pathways in the brain (see Figure 23–1).

Ethosuximide, phensuximide, and methsuximide are all indicated for the control of absence seizures. Ethosuximide should be tried first; phensuximide and methsuximide should be reserved for the treatment of seizures that are refractory to other agents, because they are associated with more severe adverse effects.

Pharmacokinetics
The succinimides are readily absorbed from the GI tract, reaching peak levels in 1 to 7 hours, depending on the drug. They are metabolized in the liver and excreted in the urine. The half-life of ethosuximide is 30 hours in children and 60 hours in adults; the half-life of phensuximide is 4 hours, and that of methsuximide is 2.6 to 4 hours. These drugs cross the placenta and enter breast milk. Use during pregnancy should be discussed with the woman because of the potential for adverse effects on the fetus. Another method of feeding the baby should be used if one of these drugs is needed during lactation.

Contraindications and Cautions
The succinimides are contraindicated in the presence of allergy to any of these drugs. Caution should be used with suc-

NURSING CARE GUIDE

Antiepileptic Agents (Hydantoins)

Assessment	Nursing Diagnoses	Implementation	Evaluation
HISTORY Allergies to any of these drugs; hypotension; arrhythmias; bone marrow suppression; coma; psychoses; pregnancy and lactation; hepatic or renal dysfunction.	Acute Pain related to GI, CNS, GU effects Risk for Injury related to CNS effects Disturbed Thought Processes related to CNS effects Deficient Knowledge regarding drug therapy Impaired Skin Integrity related to dermatological effects	Discontinue drug at first sign of liver dysfunction, skin rash. Provide comfort and safety measures: positioning; give with meals; barrier contraceptives; skin care. Provide support and reassurance to cope with diagnosis and drug effects. Provide patient teaching regarding drug, dosage, drug effects, symptoms to report, need to wear medical alert information.	Evaluate drug effects: decrease in incidence and frequency of seizures; serum drug levels within therapeutic range. Monitor for adverse effects: CNS effects (multiple); bone marrow suppression; rash, skin changes; GI effects—nausea, anorexia; arrhythmias. Monitor for drug–drug interactions: increased depression with CNS depressants, alcohol; varies with individual drug. Evaluate effectiveness of patient teaching program. Evaluate effectiveness of comfort and safety measures.
PHYSICAL EXAMINATION CV: BP, P, peripheral perfusion CNS: orientation, affect, reflexes, strength, EEG Skin: color, lesions, texture, temperature GI: abdominal examination, bowel sounds Resp: respiration, adventitious sounds Laboratory tests: renal and liver function tests			

cinimides in the following conditions: renal or hepatic disease, which could interfere with the metabolism and excretion of these drugs and lead to toxic levels; pregnancy and lactation, because of the potential of adverse effects on the fetus and neonate; and intermittent porphyria, which could be exacerbated by the adverse effects of these drugs.

Adverse Effects
Many of the adverse effects associated with the succinimides are related to their depressing effects in the CNS, including depression, drowsiness, fatigue, ataxia, insomnia, headache, and blurred vision. GI depression with nausea, vomiting, anorexia, weight loss, GI pain, and constipation or diarrhea may also occur. Bone marrow suppression, including potentially fatal pancytopenia, and dermatological reactions such as pruritus, urticaria, alopecia, and Stevens–Johnson syndrome may occur as a result of direct chemical irritation of the skin and bone marrow.

Clinically Important Drug–Drug Interactions
Use of succinimides with primidone may cause a decrease in serum levels of primidone. Patients should be monitored and appropriate dosage adjustments made if these two agents are used together.

Nursing Considerations for Patients Receiving Succinimides

Assessment: History and Examination

Screen for the following conditions, which could be cautions or contraindications to use of the drug: any known allergies to these drugs; pregnancy or lactation; renal or hepatic dysfunction; and intermittent porphyria.

CASE STUDY

Antiepileptic Therapy

THE SITUATION

J. M., an athletic, 18-year-old high school senior, suffered his first seizure during math class. He seemed attentive and alert, and then he suddenly slumped to the floor and suffered a full tonic–clonic (grand mal) seizure. The other students, who were very frightened, did not know what to do. Fortunately, the teacher was familiar with seizures and quickly reacted to protect J. M. from hurting himself and to explain what was happening to the other students.

J. M. received a diagnosis of idiopathic generalized epilepsy with tonic–clonic (grand mal) seizures. The combination of phenytoin and phenobarbital that he began taking made him quite drowsy during the day. These drugs were unable to control the seizures, and he suffered three more seizures in the next month—one at school and two at home. J. M. is now undergoing reevaluation for possible drug adjustment and nursing counseling.

CRITICAL THINKING

What teaching implications should be considered when meeting with J. M.? *Consider his age and the setting of his first seizure.*

What problems might J. M. encounter in school and in athletics related to the diagnosis and the prescribed medication? *Consider measures that may help him avoid some of the unpleasant side effects related to this particular drug therapy. Driving a car may be a central social focus in the life of a high school senior.*

What problems can be anticipated and confronted before they occur concerning laws that forbid new epileptics from driving?

Develop a teaching protocol for J. M. How will you involve the entire family in the teaching plan?

DISCUSSION

On their first meeting, it is important for the nurse to establish a trusting relationship with J. M. and his family. J. M., who is at a sensitive stage of development, requires a great deal of support and encouragement to cope with the diagnosis of epilepsy and the need for drug therapy. He may need to ventilate his feelings and concerns and discuss how he can re-enter school without worrying about having a seizure in class.

The nurse should implement a thorough drug teaching program, including a description of warning signs to watch for that should be reported to a health care professional. J. M. should be encouraged to take the following preventive measures:

- Have frequent oral hygiene to protect the gums.
- Avoid operating dangerous machinery or performing tasks that require alertness while drowsy and confused.
- Pace activities as much as possible to help deal with any fatigue and malaise.
- Take the drugs with meals if gastrointestinal upset is a problem.

This information should be given to both J. M. and his family in written form for future reference, along with the name of a health care professional and a telephone number to call with questions or comments. The importance of continuous medication to suppress the seizures should be stressed. The adverse effects of many of these drugs make it difficult for some patients to remain compliant with their drug regimen.

After the discussion with J. M., the nurse should meet with his family members, who also need support and encouragement to deal with his diagnosis and its implications. They need to know what seizures are, how the prescribed antiepileptic drugs affect the seizures, what they can do when seizures occur, and complete information about the drugs he must take and their anticipated drug effects. In addition, it is important to work with family members to determine whether any particular thing precipitated the seizures. In other words, was there any warning or aura? This may help with adjustment of drug dosages or avoidance of certain situations or stimuli that precipitate seizures. Family members should be encouraged to report and record any seizure activity that occurs.

Most states do not permit newly diagnosed epileptics to drive when first diagnosed, and states have varying regulations about the return of the driver's license after a seizure-free interval. If driving makes up a major part of J. M.'s social activities, this news may be even more unacceptable than his diagnosis. J. M. and his family should be counseled and helped to devise other ways of getting places and coping with this restriction. J. M. may be interested in referral to a support group for teens with similar problems, where he can share ideas, support, and frustrations.

J. M.'s condition is a chronic one that will require continual drug therapy and evaluation. He will need periodic reteaching and should have the opportunity to ask further questions and to ventilate his feelings. J. M. should be encouraged to wear or carry a Medic-Alert tag so that emergency medical personnel are aware of his diagnosis and the medications he is taking.

Include screening for baseline status before beginning therapy and any potential adverse effects. Assess the following: temperature; skin color and lesions; CNS orientation, affect, reflexes, and bilateral grip strength; EEG if appropriate; bowel sounds and reported output; pulse, auscultation, and blood pressure; and urinary output. Check liver and renal function tests.

Nursing Diagnoses

The patient receiving succinimides may have the following nursing diagnoses related to drug therapy:

- Acute Pain related to GI, CNS, dermatological effects
- Disturbed Thought Processes related to CNS effects
- Risk for Infection related to bone marrow suppression

DRUGS IN FOCUS

Drugs for Treating Absence (Petit Mal) Seizures—Succinimides

Drug Name	Dosage/Route	Usual Indications
Ⓟ ethosuximide (*Zarontin*)	Adult and pediatric >6 y: 500 mg/d PO Pediatric (3–6 y): 250 mg/d PO, increase cautiously as needed	Drug of choice for absence (petit mal) seizures
methsuximide (*Celontin*)	Adult: 300 mg/d PO, up to 1.2 g/d Pediatric: determine dosage by age and weight considerations	Treatment of absence (petit mal) seizures refractory to other agents
phensuximide (*Milontin*)	500–1000 mg PO b.i.d.–t.i.d. regardless of age	Treatment of absence (petit mal) seizures refractory to other agents

- Impaired Skin Integrity related to dermatological effects
- Deficient Knowledge regarding drug therapy

Implementation

- Administer the drug with food *to alleviate GI irritation if GI upset is a problem.*
- Monitor complete blood count (CBC) before and periodically during therapy *to detect bone marrow suppression early and provide appropriate interventions.*
- Discontinue the drug if skin rash, bone marrow suppression, or unusual depression or personality changes occur, *to prevent the development of more serious adverse effects.*
- Discontinue the drug slowly, and never withdraw the drug quickly, *because rapid withdrawal may precipitate absence seizures.*
- Arrange for counseling for women of child-bearing age who are taking these drugs. *Because these drugs have the potential to cause serious damage to the fetus, women should understand the risk of birth defects and use barrier contraceptives to avoid pregnancy.*
- Evaluate for therapeutic blood levels (40 to 100 µg/mL) for ethosuximide *to ensure the most appropriate dosage of the drug.*
- Provide thorough patient teaching, including the drug name and prescribed dosage, as well as measures for avoidance of adverse effects, warning signs that may indicate possible problems, and the need for monitoring and evaluation, *to enhance patient knowledge about drug therapy and to promote compliance.*
- Suggest the wearing or carrying of a Medic-Alert bracelet *to alert emergency workers and health care providers about the use of an antiepileptic drug.*
- Offer support and encouragement *to help the patient cope with the drug regimen.*

Evaluation

- Monitor patient response to the drug (decrease in incidence or absence of seizures; serum drug level within therapeutic range).
- Monitor for adverse effects (CNS changes, GI depression, arrhythmias, blood pressure changes, bone marrow suppression, severe dermatological reactions).
- Evaluate the effectiveness of the teaching plan (patient can give the drug name and dosage and name possible adverse effects to watch for and specific measures to prevent adverse effects; patient is aware of the risk of birth defects and the need to carry information about the diagnosis and use of this drug).
- Monitor the effectiveness of comfort measures and compliance with the regimen.

Other Drugs for Treating Absence (Petit Mal) Seizures

Three other drugs that are used in the treatment of absence seizures do not fit into a specific drug class.

One such drug is valproic acid (*Depakene*), which reduces abnormal electrical activity in the brain and may also increase GABA activity at inhibitory receptors. This agent is the drug of choice for the treatment of myoclonic seizures. Because it is sometimes associated with hepatic toxicity and because other agents may have fewer adverse effects, valproic acid is a second-choice drug for the treatment of absence seizures. It is also effective in mania, migraine headaches, and partial seizures. It is readily absorbed from the GI tract, reaching peak levels in 1 to 4 hours. It is metabolized in the liver and excreted in the urine with a half-life of 6 to 16 hours. Valproic acid crosses the placenta and enters breast milk; it should not be used during pregnancy or lactation unless the benefit clearly outweighs the risk to the neonate.

NURSING CHALLENGE

Helping Patients Deal With a Diagnosis of Epilepsy

Epilepsy, with its stigma, is frightening to people who know little about the disease. This condition has long been associated with some sort of brain dysfunction or possession by the devil or evil spirits. In some eras, exorcism was the first choice of treatment for a person with a seizure disorder. A person who receives a diagnosis of epilepsy must deal with this stigma as well as the significance of the diagnosis. What does having epilepsy mean? Individuals who are newly diagnosed with epilepsy must consider restrictions on their independence as well as the prospect of chronic therapy for control of this problem.

In our society, the ability to be readily mobile—to drive to appointments, work, or religious obligations—is very important to many people. Most states require physicians to report new diagnoses of epilepsy. In most cases, the driving privileges of affected individuals are revoked, at least temporarily. The conditions for recovering the license vary with the diagnosis and the laws of each state.

The person who is newly diagnosed with epilepsy has to cope not only with the stigma of epilepsy but also with the loss of a driver's license. The nurse may be in the best position to help the patient adjust to both of these problems through patient education and referrals to community resources. Thorough patient teaching should include the following:

- Explanations of old stigmas
- Ways in which people may react to the diagnosis
- Ways in which patients can educate family, friends, and employers about the realities of the condition and its treatment
- Actions to take if a seizure happens so that no injuries occur and no panic develops
- Information about the availability of public transportation
- Contact information regarding other community support services

Many communities have epilepsy support groups that can supply information on valuable resources as well as updated facts about the laws in each area. While patients are first adjusting to epilepsy and its implications, it may help to put them in contact with such organizations. The local chapter of the Epilepsy Foundation of America may be able to offer support groups, lists of resources, and support. Individuals with epilepsy should have several options for getting around without feeling that they are being a burden or an imposition.

Acetazolamide (*Diamox*) is a sulfonamide drug that is especially effective for treatment of absence seizures in children. It is also used to treat open-angle and secondary glaucoma, as prophylaxis and treatment of acute mountain sickness, and to decrease edema associated with congestive heart failure and drug use. It is readily absorbed from the GI tract and is excreted unchanged in the urine with a half-life of 2.5 to 6 hours. It is known to cross the placenta and enter breast milk and should not be used during pregnancy or lac-

tation unless the benefit clearly outweighs the risk to the neonate.

Another sulfonamide, zonisamide (*Zonegran*), is a newer agent that inhibits voltage-sensitive sodium and calcium channels, thus stabilizing nerve cell membranes and modulating calcium-dependent presynaptic release of excitatory neurotransmitters. It is used as an adjunct to other drugs for the treatment of absence seizures. Zonisamide is well absorbed from the GI tract, reaching peak levels in 2 to 6 hours. It is primarily excreted unchanged in the urine, with a half-life of 63 hours. It crosses the placenta and has been shown to be teratogenic in animal studies. Women of child-bearing age should be advised to use contraception while taking this drug. It is not known whether zonisamide enters breast milk, but because of the potential for serious adverse effects on the baby, it should not be used during lactation. When it is discontinued, zonisamide should be tapered over 2 weeks because of a risk of precipitating seizures. Patients who take this drug should be very well hydrated; there is a risk of renal calculi development.

DRUGS FOR TREATING PARTIAL (FOCAL) SEIZURES

Focal seizures, or partial seizures, are so called because they involve only part of the brain and usually originate from one site or focus. The presenting symptoms depend on exactly where in the brain the excessive electrical discharge is occurring. Partial seizures can be simple, involving only a single muscle or reaction, or complex, involving a series of reactions or emotional changes.

Drugs used in the treatment of partial seizures include the following.

- Carbamazepine (*Tegretol, Atretol,* and others) is often the drug of choice for treatment of partial seizures. Chemically related to the tricyclic antidepressants, it has also been used in the treatment of tonic–clonic seizures and trigeminal neuralgia. It has the ability to inhibit polysynaptic responses and to block sodium channels to prevent the formation of repetitive action potentials in the abnormal focus. Carbamazepine is absorbed from the GI tract and metabolized in the liver by the cytochrome P450 system. It is excreted in the urine. Carbamazepine can cause fetal harm and should not be used during pregnancy. Women of child-bearing age should be advised to use contraception. It also enters breast milk and can cause serious adverse effects in the baby. If the drug is needed during lactation, another method of feeding the baby should be used.
- Clorazepate (*Tranxene, Gen-Xene,* and others), a benzodiazepine that is indicated for anxiety and alcohol withdrawal, is also used as adjunctive therapy for partial seizures. It is rapidly absorbed from the GI tract, reaching peak levels in 1 to 2 hours. After metabolism in the liver, it is excreted in the urine with a half-life of 30 to 100 hours.

DRUGS IN FOCUS
Other Drugs for Treating Absence (Petit Mal) Seizures

Drug Name	Dosage/Route	Usual Indications
acetazolamide (*Diamox*)	8–30 mg/kg per day PO regardless of age; 250 mg PO q.d. if used with other antiepileptics	Absence (petit mal) seizures; also glaucoma, mountain sickness, edema
valproic acid (*Depakene*)	Adult: 10–15 mg/kg per day PO up to a maximum 60 mg/kg per day Pediatric: use extreme caution, determine dosage by age and weight	Absence (petit mal) seizures, mania, migraine headaches, partial (focal) seizures
zonisamide (*Zonegran*)	Adults >16 y: 100 mg PO q.d., up to 600 mg/d	Adjunct for treating absence (petit mal) seizures

As with the other benzodiazepines, it should not be used during pregnancy or lactation because of the potential for adverse effects on the neonate when the drug crosses the placenta and enters breast milk.

• Felbamate (*Felbatol*) has been associated with severe liver failure and aplastic anemia. Its use should be reserved for those cases that are unresponsive to other therapies. It is used for the treatment of partial seizures and for the seizures associated with Lennox–Gastaut syndrome in children. Felbamate is absorbed well from the GI tract and is primarily excreted unchanged in the urine with a half-life of 20 to 23 hours. There are no clear studies about the effects of the drug during pregnancy and lactation. Therefore, it should not be used during pregnancy or lactation unless the benefits to the mother clearly outweigh potential adverse effects in the neonate.

• Gabapentin (*Neurontin*), is used as adjunctive therapy in the treatment of partial seizures in adults and children age 3 to 12 years. It is also being studied for the treatment of tremors associated with multiple sclerosis, for neuropathic pain, for bipolar disorder, and for migraine prophylaxis. Gabapentin is well absorbed from the GI tract and widely distributed in the body. It is excreted unchanged in the urine with a half-life of 5 to 7 hours. Patients with renal dysfunction are at higher risk for toxic effects of the drug and need a lower dosage. Gabapentin crosses the placenta and enters breast milk. It was found to be toxic to the fetus in animal studies. Use during pregnancy and lactation should be reserved for those situations in which the benefit to the mother clearly outweighs the potential risk to the neonate.

• Lamotrigine (*Lamictal*) is also used as adjunctive therapy in the treatment of focal seizures and in the treatment of the seizures associated with Lennox–Gastaut syndrome in adults and children. It is being studied for use in tonic–clonic seizures, absence seizures, myoclonic seizures, and drug-resistant seizures of multiple types. It may inhibit voltage-sensitive sodium and calcium channels, stabilize nerve cell membranes, and modulate calcium-dependent presynaptic release of excitatory neurotransmitters. Lamotrigine is rapidly absorbed from the GI tract, metabolized in the liver, and primarily excreted in the urine. The half-life of lamotrigine is approximately 25 hours. It has been associated with very serious to life-threatening rashes and the drug should be discontinued at the first sign of any rash. There are no clear studies about the effects of the drug during pregnancy or lactation, although it was shown to be toxic to the fetus in animal studies. It should not be used during pregnancy or lactation unless the benefits to the mother clearly outweigh the potential adverse effects in the neonate.

• Levetiracetam (*Keppra*) is a newer drug that is approved as an adjunctive therapy in the treatment of partial seizures in adults. Its mechanism of action is not understood; its antiepileptic action does not seem to be associated with any known mechanisms of inhibitory or excitatory neurotransmission. It is rapidly absorbed from the GI tract, reaching peak levels in 1 hour. It goes through very little metabo-

CULTURAL CONSIDERATIONS
Altered Metabolism of Antiepileptic Drugs

Because of differences in liver enzyme functioning among Arab Americans and Asian Americans, patients in these ethnic groups may not metabolize antiepileptic drugs in the same way as patients in other ethnic groups. They may require not only lower doses to achieve the same therapeutic effects but also frequent dose adjustment. Nurses need to be aware that the therapeutic range for patients in these ethnic groups may differ from standard norms and that these patients may be more apt to show adverse or toxic reactions to antiepileptic drugs at lower doses. As with all medications, the lowest possible dose should be used. Serum drug levels should be closely monitored and titrated carefully and slowly to achieve the maximum benefits with the fewest adverse effects.

lism, with most of the drug being excreted unchanged in the urine with a half-life of 6 to 8 hours. Patients with renal dysfunction are more likely to experience toxic effects of the drug, and the dosage for these patients needs to be decreased accordingly. There are no clear studies about the effects of the drug during pregnancy or lactation, although it was shown to be toxic to the fetus in animal studies. It should not be used during pregnancy or lactation unless the benefits to the mother clearly outweigh the potential adverse effects in the neonate.

- Oxcarbazepine (*Trileptal*) was approved in 2000 for the treatment of partial seizures in adults and children 4 to 16 years of age. The exact mechanism of antiseizure activity is not known. It does inhibit voltage-sensitive sodium channels, stabilizing hyperexcited nerve cell membranes. It also increases potassium conductance and modulates calcium-dependent presynaptic release of excitatory neurotransmitters. Any or all of these effects may be responsible for the antiseizure effects of the drug. Oxcarbazepine is completely absorbed from the GI tract and extensively metabolized in the liver. It is excreted in the urine with a half-life of 2 and then 9 hours. Oxcarbazepine is teratogenic in animal studies and should not be used during pregnancy. It is found in breast milk; if the drug is needed during lactation, another method of feeding the baby should be used.

- Tiagabine (*Gabitril*) is used as adjunctive therapy in the treatment of partial seizures in adults and in children 12 to 18 years of age. It has also been associated with serious skin rash. It binds to GABA reuptake receptors, causing an increase in GABA levels in the brain. Because GABA is an inhibitory neurotransmitter, the result is a stabilizing of nerve membranes and a decrease in excessive activity. Tiagabine is rapidly absorbed from the GI tract, reaching peak levels in 45 minutes. It is metabolized in the liver by the cytochrome P450 system. It is excreted in the urine with a half-life of 4 to 7 hours. There are no clear studies about the effects of the drug during pregnancy or lactation, although it was shown to be toxic to the fetus in animal studies. It should not be used during pregnancy or lactation unless the benefits to the mother clearly outweigh the potential adverse effects in the neonate.

- Topiramate (*Topamax*) is a newer drug that is used as adjunctive therapy for partial seizures in adults. It is also approved for treatment of clonic–tonic seizures and is being studied for use in cluster headaches, infantile spasms, and Lennox–Gastaut syndrome. Topiramate is rapidly absorbed from the GI tract, reaching peak levels in 2 hours. It is widely distributed and excreted unchanged in the urine. Patients with renal impairment should receive a reduced dosage of the drug. It has been associated with marked CNS depression. It may interfere with sodium channels, causing a stabilizing of nerve membranes, and it also may increase GABA activity. There are no clear studies about the effects of the drug during pregnancy or lactation, although it was shown to be toxic to the fetus in animal studies. It should not be used during pregnancy or lactation un-

less the benefits to the mother clearly outweigh the potential adverse effects in the neonate.

Therapeutic Actions and Indications

The drugs used to control partial seizures stabilize nerve membranes in two ways—either directly, by altering sodium and calcium channels, or indirectly, by increasing the activity of GABA, an inhibitory neurotransmitter, and thereby decreasing excessive activity (see Figure 21–1). Each of these drugs has a slightly different mechanism of action, as noted earlier.

These drugs are indicated for the treatment of partial seizures. Carbamazepine, oxcarbazepine, and felbamate are used as monotherapy, and the other drugs are used as adjunctive therapy.

Contraindications and Cautions

Contraindications to the drugs used to control partial seizures include the following conditions: presence of any known allergy to the drug; bone marrow suppression, which could be exacerbated by the drug effects; and severe hepatic dysfunction, which could be exacerbated and could interfere with the metabolism of the drugs.

Caution should be used in the following situations: in pregnancy or lactation, because of the potential adverse effects on the fetus or neonate; with renal or hepatic dysfunction, which could alter the metabolism and excretion of the drugs; and with renal stones, which could be exacerbated by the effects of some of these agents.

Adverse Effects

The most frequently occurring adverse effects associated with the drugs used for partial seizures relate to the CNS depression that results. The following conditions may occur: drowsiness, fatigue, weakness, confusion, headache, and insomnia; GI depression, with nausea, vomiting, and anorexia; and upper respiratory infections. These antiepileptics can also be directly toxic to the liver and the bone marrow, causing dysfunction. The exact effects of each drug vary.

Clinically Important Drug–Drug Interactions

If any of these drugs are taken with other CNS depressants or alcohol, a potential for increased CNS depression exists. Patients should be cautioned to avoid alcohol while taking drugs for partial seizures, or to take extreme precautions if such combinations cannot be avoided.

In addition, numerous drug–drug interactions are associated with carbamazepine. A drug reference should be consulted whenever a drug is added or withdrawn from a carbamazepine-containing regimen. Dosage adjustments may be necessary.

Nursing Considerations for Patients Receiving Drugs to Treat Partial (Focal) Seizures

Assessment: History and Examination

Screen for the following conditions, which could be cautions or contraindications for the use of the drug: any known allergies to these drugs; pregnancy or lactation; bone marrow

DRUGS IN FOCUS
Drugs for Treating Partial (Focal) Seizures

Drug Name	Dosage/Route	Usual Indications
Ⓟ carbamazepine (*Tegretol, Atretol*)	Adult: 800–1200 mg/d PO in divided doses q6–8h Pediatric (>12 y): adult doses, do not exceed 1000 mg/d Pediatric (6–12 y): 20–30 mg/kg per day PO in divided doses t.i.d.–q.i.d. Pediatric (<6 y): safety not established	Drug of choice for partial (focal) seizures; tonic–clonic (grand mal) seizures, trigeminal neuralgia
clorazepate (*Tranxene, Gen-Xene*)	Adult: 7.5 mg PO t.i.d., up to 90 mg/d Pediatric (9–12 y): 7.5 mg PO b.i.d., up to 60 mg/d	Adjunct for partial seizures, anxiety, alcohol withdrawal
felbamate (*Felbatol*)	Adult and children >14 y: 2600 mg/d PO Pediatric (2–14 y): 15 mg/kg per day PO in divided doses three to four times per day	Monotherapy or adjunctive therapy for partial seizures; adjunctive therapy for Lennox–Gastaut syndrome in children
gabapentin (*Neurontin*)	Adult: 900–1800 mg/d PO in divided doses t.i.d. Pediatric: 10–15 mg/kg per day PO in divided doses	Adjunct in treating partial seizures
lamotrigine (*Lamictal*)	Adult: 300–500 mg/d PO in divided doses b.i.d. Pediatric (2–12 y): 1–5 mg/kg per day PO in divided doses b.i.d. Pediatric (>12 y): 100–400 mg/d PO in divided doses b.i.d.	Adjunct in treating partial seizures; adjunct for Lennox–Gastaut syndrome in children
levetiracetam (*Keppra*)	500 mg PO b.i.d. up to 3000 mg/d	Adjunctive treatment of partial seizures in adults
oxcarbazepine (*Trileptal*)	Adult: 600 mg PO b.i.d. Pediatric (4–16 yr): 8–10 mg/kg/d PO, do not exceed 600 mg/d	Monotherapy or adjunctive therapy of partial seizures in adults; adjunct in treating partial seizures in children 4 to 16 years of age
tiagabine (*Gabitril*)	Adult: 4 mg PO qd, up to 56 mg/d in 2–4 divided doses Pediatric (12–18 yr): 4 mg PO qd up to a maximum 32 mg/d in two to four divided doses	Adjunct in treating partial seizures
topiramate (*Topamax*)	Adult: 400 mg PO qd in 2 divided doses; reduce dosage in renal impairment Pediatric (2–16 yr): 5–9 mg/kg per day PO in 2 divided doses	Adjunct in treating partial seizures in adults

suppression; hepatic dysfunction; renal dysfunction; and renal stones.

Include screening for baseline status before beginning therapy and any potential adverse effects. Assess the following: temperature; skin color and lesions; CNS orientation, affect, reflexes, and bilateral grip strength; EEG; pulse and blood pressure; respiration and adventitious sounds; and bowel sounds and reported output. Check liver and renal function tests, urinalysis, and CBC with differential.

Nursing Diagnoses

The patient taking a drug to treat partial seizures may have the following nursing diagnoses related to drug therapy:

- Acute Pain related to GI, CNS effects
- Disturbed Thought Processes related to CNS effects
- Risk for Injury related to CNS, bone marrow effects
- Deficient Knowledge regarding drug therapy

Implementation

- Administer the drug with food *to alleviate GI irritation if GI upset is a problem.*
- Monitor CBC before and periodically during therapy, *to detect and prevent serious bone marrow suppression.*
- Discontinue the drug if skin rash, bone marrow suppression, unusual depression, or personality changes occur, *to prevent further serious adverse effects.*
- Discontinue the drug slowly, and never withdraw the drug quickly, *because rapid withdrawal may precipitate seizures.*
- Arrange for counseling for women of child-bearing age who are taking these drugs. *Because these drugs have the potential to cause serious damage to the fetus, women should understand the risk of birth defects and use barrier contraceptives to avoid pregnancy.*
- Evaluate for therapeutic blood levels of carbamazepine (4 to 12 μg/mL) *to ensure that the most effective dosage is being used.*

- Provide thorough patient teaching, including drug name and prescribed dosage, as well as measures for avoidance of adverse effects, warning signs that may indicate possible problems, and the need for monitoring and evaluation, *to enhance patient knowledge about drug therapy and to promote compliance.*
- Suggest that the patient wear or carry a Medic-Alert bracelet *to alert emergency workers and health care providers about the use of an antiepileptic drug.*
- Offer support and encouragement *to help the patient cope with the drug regimen.*

Evaluation

- Monitor patient response to the drug (decrease in incidence or absence of seizures).
- Monitor for adverse effects (CNS changes, GI depression, bone marrow suppression, severe dermatological reactions, liver toxicity, renal stones).
- Evaluate effectiveness of teaching plan (patient can give the drug name and dosage and name possible adverse effects to watch for, and specific measures to prevent adverse effects; patient is aware of the risk of birth defects and the need to carry information about the diagnosis and use of this drug).

◻◼◉◼ WEB LINKS

Health care providers and patients may want to consult the following Internet sources:

Information on epilepsy, including support groups, research, treatment:
  http://www.aesnet.org
Information on education programs, research, and other information related to seizure disorders:
  http://www.ninds.nih.gov
Information about epilepsy research, treatment, and laws:
  http://webmd.lycos.com/content/article/1680.51194

CHAPTER SUMMARY

- Epilepsy is a collection of different syndromes, all of which have the same characteristic: a sudden discharge of excessive electrical energy from nerve cells located within the brain. This event is called a seizure.
- Seizures can be divided into two groups: generalized and partial (focal).
- Generalized seizures can be further classified as tonic–clonic (grand mal); absence (petit mal); myoclonic; febrile; and rapidly recurrent (status epilepticus).
- Partial (focal) seizures can be further classified as simple or complex.
- Drug treatment depends on the type of seizure that the patient has experienced and the toxicity associated with the available agents.

- Drug treatment is directed at stabilizing the overexcited nerve membranes and/or increasing the effectiveness of GABA, an inhibitory neurotransmitter.
- Adverse effects associated with antiepileptics (eg, insomnia, fatigue, confusion, GI depression, bradycardia) reflect the CNS depression caused by the drugs.
- Patients being treated with an antiepileptic should be advised to wear or carry a Medic-Alert notification to alert emergency medical professionals to their epilepsy and their use of antiepileptic drugs.

Review Questions

1. Epilepsy is
   a. always characterized by grand mal seizures.
   b. only a genetic problem.
   c. the most prevalent neurological disorder.
   d. the name given to one brain disorder.
2. Generalized seizures could include all of the following except
   a. petit mal seizures.
   b. febrile seizures.
   c. grand mal seizures.
   d. complex seizures.
3. Patients who are maintained on an antiepileptic drug should be encouraged to
   a. give up their driver's license.
   b. wear or carry a Medic-Alert notice.
   c. take antihistamines to help dry up secretions.
   d. keep the diagnosis a secret to avoid prejudice.
4. Drugs that are commonly used to treat grand mal seizures include
   a. barbiturates, benzodiazepines, and hydantoins.
   b. barbiturates, antihistamines, and local anesthetics.
   c. hydantoins, phenobarbital, and phensuximide.
   d. benzodiazepines, phensuximide, and valproic acid.
5. The drug of choice for the treatment of petit mal seizures is
   a. valproic acid.
   b. methsuximide.
   c. phensuximide.
   d. ethosuximide.
6. Focal or partial seizures
   a. start at one point and spread quickly throughout the brain.
   b. are best treated with benzodiazepines.
   c. involve only part of the brain.
   d. are easily diagnosed and recognized.
7. One drug that is used alone in the treatment of partial seizures is
   a. carbamazepine.
   b. topiramate.
   c. lamotrigine.
   d. topiramate.
8. Treatment of epilepsy is directed at
   a. blocking the transmission of nerve impulses into the brain.

b. stabilizing overexcited nerve membranes and/or increasing the inhibitory neurotransmitter GABA.

c. blocking peripheral nerve terminals.

d. thickening the meninges to damper brain electrical activity.

9. A patient has been stabilized on phenytoin (*Dilantin*) for several years and has not experienced a grand mal seizure in more than 3 years. The patient decides to stop the drug because it no longer seems to be needed. The patient should be counseled that

a. he will always need this drug.

b. this drug needs to be slowly tapered to avoid potentially serious adverse effects and seizures.

c. he is probably correct and the drug is not needed.

d. the drug should not be stopped until appropriate tests are done.

10. The most common adverse effects associated with antiepileptic therapy reflect the depression of the CNS and would not include

a. hypertension.

b. insomnia.

c. confusion.

d. GI depression.

BIBLIOGRAPHY

Bailey, K. (1998). *Psychotropic drug facts*. Philadelphia: Lippincott-Raven.

Bullock, B. L. (2000). *Focus on pathophysiology*. Philadelphia: Lippincott Williams & Wilkins.

Drug facts and comparisons. (2002). St. Louis: Facts and Comparisons.

Gilman, A., Hardman, J. G., & Limbird, L. E. (Eds.) (2002). *Goodman and Gilman's the pharmacological basis of therapeutics* (10th ed.). New York: McGraw-Hill.

Karch, A. M. (2002). *2003 Lippincott nursing drug guide*. Philadelphia: Lippincott Williams & Wilkins.

Professional's guide to patient drug facts. (2002). St. Louis: Facts and Comparisons.

24

Antiparkinsonism Agents

319

In the 1990s, several prominent figures—former heavyweight boxing champion Mohammed Ali, former United States Attorney General Janet Reno, and actor Michael J. Fox—revealed that they had **Parkinson's disease,** a progressive, chronic neurological disorder. In general, Parkinson's disease may develop in people of any age, but it usually affects those who are past middle age and entering their 60s or even older. Therefore, the occurrence of Parkinson's disease in these leading individuals who at the time of diagnosis were relatively young people is that much more interesting. The cause of the condition is not known.

At this time, there is no cure for Parkinson's disease. Therapy is aimed at management of signs and symptoms to provide optimal functioning for as long as possible.

PARKINSON'S DISEASE AND PARKINSONISM

Lack of coordination is characteristic of Parkinson's disease or parkinsonism. Rhythmic tremors develop, insidiously at first. In some muscle groups, these tremors lead to rigidity, and in others, weakness. Affected patients may have trouble maintaining position or posture, and they may develop the condition known as **bradykinesia,** marked by difficulties in performing intentional movements and extreme slowness or sluggishness.

As Parkinson's disease progresses, walking becomes a problem; a shuffling gait is a hallmark of the condition. In addition, patients may drool, and their speech may be slow and slurred. As the cranial nerves are affected, they may develop a mask-like expression. Parkinson's disease does not affect the higher levels of the cerebral cortex, so a very alert and intelligent person may be trapped in a progressively degenerating body.

Causal Theories

Although the cause of Parkinson's disease is not known, it is known that the signs and symptoms of the disease relate to damage to neurons in the basal ganglia of the brain (Figure 24–1). Theories about the cause of the degeneration range from viral infection, blows to the head, brain infection, atherosclerosis, and exposure to certain drugs and environmental factors.

Even though the actual cause is not known, the mechanism that causes the signs and symptoms of Parkinson's disease is understood. In a part of the brain called the **substantia nigra,** a dopamine-rich area, nerve cell bodies begin to degenerate. This process results in a reduction of the number of impulses sent to the **corpus striatum** in the basal ganglia. This area of the brain, in conjunction with the substantia nigra, helps maintain muscle tone not related to any particular movement. The corpus striatum is connected to the substantia nigra by a series of neurons that use the inhibitory neurotransmitter γ-aminobutyric acid (GABA). The substantia nigra sends nerve impulses back into the corpus stratum using the inhibitory neurotransmitter dopamine. The two areas then mutually inhibit activity in a balanced manner.

Higher neurons from the cerebral cortex secrete acetylcholine in the area of the corpus stratum as an excitatory neurotransmitter to coordinate intentional movements of the body. When there is a decrease in dopamine in the area, it causes a chemical imbalance in this area of the brain that allows the cholinergic or excitatory cells to dominate. This affects the functioning of the basal ganglia and of the cortical and cerebellar components of the extrapyramidal motor system. The extrapyramidal system is one that provides coordination for unconscious muscle movements, including those that control position, posture, and movement. The result of this imbalance in the motor system is apparent as the manifestations of Parkinson's disease (see Figure 24–1).

Drug Therapy

At this time, there is no treatment that arrests the neuron degeneration of Parkinson's disease and the eventual decline in patient function. Surgical procedures involving the basal ganglia have been tried with varying success at prolonging the degeneration caused by this disease. Drug therapy remains the primary treatment (Figure 24–2).

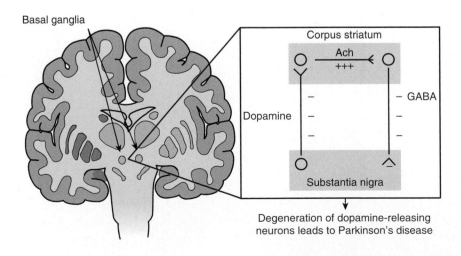

FIGURE 24–1. Schematic representation of the degeneration of neurons that leads to Parkinson's disease. Cells in the corpus striatum send impulses to the substantia nigra using γ-aminobutyric acid (GABA) to inhibit activity. In turn, the substantia nigra sends impulses to the corpus striatum, using dopamine, to inhibit activity. Cortical areas use acetylcholine (Ach) to stimulate intentional movements.

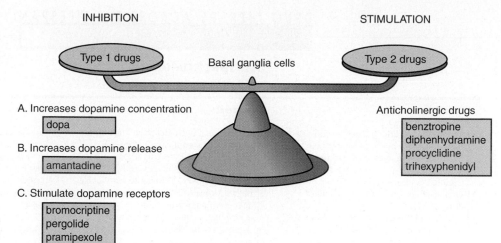

INHIBITION   STIMULATION

Type 1 drugs   Basal ganglia cells   Type 2 drugs

A. Increases dopamine concentration

dopa

B. Increases dopamine release

amantadine

C. Stimulate dopamine receptors

bromocriptine
pergolide
pramipexole
ropinirole

Anticholinergic drugs

benztropine
diphenhydramine
procyclidine
trihexyphenidyl

FIGURE 24-2. Goals of therapy in treating Parkinson's disease. Drug therapy is aimed at achieving a balance between the stimulating cholinergic effects and the inhibitory effects of dopamine in the basal ganglia. Type 1 drugs affect dopamine and are inhibitory. Type 2 drugs block cholinergic effects, preventing stimulation.

Today, therapy is aimed at restoring the balance between the declining levels of dopamine, which has an inhibitory effect on the neurons in the basal ganglia, and the now-dominant cholinergic neurons, which are excitatory. This may help reduce the signs and symptoms of parkinsonism and restore normal function.

Total management of patient care in individuals with Parkinson's disease presents a challenge. Patients should be encouraged to be as active as possible, to perform exercises to prevent the development of skeletal deformities, and to attend to their own care as long as they can. Both patients and family need instruction about following drug protocols and monitoring adverse effects as well as encouragement and support for coping with the progressive nature of the disease. Because of the degenerative effects of this disease, patients may be depressed and emotional. They may require a great deal of psychological as well as physical support.

ANTICHOLINERGICS

Anticholinergics are drugs that oppose the effects of acetylcholine at receptor sites in the substantia nigra and the corpus striatum, thus helping restore chemical balance in the area. At this time, the anticholinergics used to treat parkinsonism are synthetic drugs that have been developed to have a greater affinity for cholinergic receptor sites in the central nervous system (CNS) than for those in the peripheral nervous system. However, they still block, to some extent, the cholinergic receptors that are responsible for stimulation of the parasympathetic nervous system's postganglionic effec-

tors and are associated with the adverse effects resulting from this blockage (see Chapter 33), including slowed gastrointestinal (GI) motility and secretions with dry mouth and constipation, urinary retention, blurred vision, and dilated pupils.

Anticholinergics used to treat Parkinson's disease include the following.

- Benztropine (*Cogentin*) is available in oral and intramuscular/intravenous forms. This agent is used to treat parkinsonism and parkinson-like symptoms that occur as a result of drug effects of phenothiazines.
- Biperiden (*Akineton*) is available in oral and intramuscular forms. This medication is used for the adjunctive treatment of parkinsonism and to treat the drug-induced parkinsonism associated with phenothiazine use.
- Diphenhydramine (*Benadryl*), also used for many other purposes, is often used in combination with other agents to treat Parkinson's disease. This agent is indicated for the treatment of parkinsonism, including drug-induced disease, especially in elderly patients who cannot tolerate more potent drugs and in patients at the early stages of disease.
- Procyclidine (*Kemadrin*) is available only in the oral form. This agent is used for the treatment of any type of parkinsonism. In severe cases, it is combined with other drugs, and it is often the drug of choice to control of the excessive salivation that occurs with the use of neuroleptic medication.
- Trihexyphenidyl (*Artane*) is used as adjunct therapy with levodopa. It can be used alone for the control of drug-induced extrapyramidal disorders.

DRUG THERAPY ACROSS THE LIFESPAN

Antiparkinsonism Agents

Children	Adults	Older Adults
The safety and effectiveness of most of these drugs has not been established in children. The incidence of Parkinson's disease in children is very small. Children do, however, experience parkinsonian symptoms as a result of drug effects. If a child needs an antiparkinsonian drug, diphenhydramine would be the drug of choice. If further relief is needed and another drug is tried, careful dosage calculations should be done based on age and weight and the child should be monitored very closely for adverse effects.	The eventual dependence and lack of control that accompany Parkinson's disease are devastating to all patients and their families but may be particularly overwhelming to individuals in their prime of life who value high degrees of autonomy, self-determination, and independence. Although these characteristics are not associated with any particular ethnic group, they are valued more highly among certain cultures than others. For example, Latinos—who traditionally have strong extended family ties—may not have the same problems adjusting to a chronic, debilitating illness in a relative as members of other ethnic groups. It is important for the nurse to assess all families with sensitivity to determine what convictions they hold and plan nursing care accordingly. Adults diagnosed with Parkinson's disease require extensive teaching and support and help coping with the disease as well as with the effects of the drugs. With the increasing interest in herbal and alternative therapies, it is important to stress the need to inform the health care provider about any other treatment being used. Vitamin B_6 can pose a serious problem for patients who are taking some of these drugs. Women of child-bearing age should be advised to use contraception when they are on these drugs. If a pregnancy does occur, or is desired, they need counseling about the potential for adverse effects. Women who are nursing should be encouraged to find another method of feeding the baby because of the potential for adverse drug effects on the baby.	Although Parkinson's disease may affect individuals of any age, gender, or nationality, the frequency of the disease increases with age. This debilitating condition, which affects more men than women may be one of many chronic problems associated with aging. The drugs that are used to manage Parkinson's disease are associated with more adverse effects in older people with long-term problems. Both anticholinergic and dopaminergic drugs aggravate glaucoma, benign prostatic hypertrophy, constipation, cardiac problems, and chronic obstructive pulmonary diseases. Special precautions and frequent follow-up visits are necessary for older patients with Parkinson's disease, and their drug dosages may need to be adjusted frequently to avoid serious problems. In many cases, other agents are given to counteract the effects of these drugs, and patients then have complicated drug regimens with many associated adverse effects and problems. Consequently, it is essential for these patients to have extensive written drug-teaching protocols.

THERAPEUTIC ACTIONS AND INDICATIONS

The anticholinergics block the action of acetylcholine in the CNS to help normalize the acetylcholine–dopamine imbalance. As a result, these drugs reduce the degree of rigidity and, to a lesser extent, the tremors associated with Parkinson's disease. The peripheral anticholinergic effects that sometimes occur with the use of these drugs help alleviate some of the other adverse effects associated with Parkinson's disease, including drooling.

Anticholinergic drugs are indicated for the treatment of parkinsonism, whether idiopathic, atherosclerotic, or postencephalitic, and for the relief of symptoms of extrapyramidal disorders associated with the use of some drugs, including phenothiazines. Although these drugs are not as effective as levodopa in the treatment of advancing cases of the disease, they may be useful as adjunctive therapy and for patients who no longer respond to levodopa.

Pharmacokinetics

The anticholinergic drugs are variably absorbed from the GI tract, reaching peak levels in 1 to 4 hours. They are metabolized in the liver and excreted by cellular pathways. All of them cross the placenta and enter breast milk. They should be used during pregnancy and lactation only if the benefit to the mother clearly outweighs the potential risk to the neonate. The safety and efficacy for use in children have not been established.

Contraindications and Cautions

Anticholinergics are contraindicated in the presence of allergy to any of these agents. In addition, they are contraindicated in narrow-angle glaucoma, GI obstruction, genitourinary (GU) obstruction, and prostatic hypertrophy, all of which could be exacerbated by the peripheral anticholinergic effects of these drugs, and in myasthenia gravis, which could be exacerbated by the blocking of acetylcholine receptor sites at neuromuscular synapses.

Caution should be used in the presence of the following conditions: tachycardia and other arrhythmias; hypertension or hypotension, because the blocking of the parasympathetic system may cause a dominance of sympathetic stimulatory activity; hepatic dysfunction, which could interfere with the metabolism of the drugs and lead to toxic levels; lactation, because the drugs cross into breast milk and may cause adverse effects in infants; and pregnancy, because these drugs do cross the placenta.

In addition, these agents should be used with caution in individuals who work in hot environments, because reflex sweating may be blocked. These people are at risk for heat prostration.

Adverse Effects

The use of anticholinergics for parkinsonism is associated with CNS effects that relate to the blocking of central acetylcholine receptors, such as disorientation, confusion, and memory loss. Agitation, nervousness, delirium, dizziness, lightheadedness, and weakness may also occur.

Anticipated peripheral anticholinergic effects include dry mouth, nausea, vomiting, paralytic ileus, and constipation related to decreased GI secretions and motility. In addition, other adverse effects may occur, including the following: tachycardia, palpitations, and hypotension related to the blocking of the suppressive cardiac effects of the parasympathetic nervous system; urinary retention and hesitancy related to a blocking of bladder muscle activity and sphincter relaxation; blurred vision and photophobia related to pupil dilation and blocking of lens accommodation; and flushing and reduced sweating related to a blocking of the cholinergic sites that stimulate sweating and blood vessel dilation in the skin.

Clinically Important Drug–Drug Interactions

When these anticholinergic drugs are used with other drugs that have anticholinergic properties, including the tricyclic antidepressants and the phenothiazines, there is a risk of potentially fatal paralytic ileus and an increased risk of toxic psychoses. If such combinations must be given, patients should be monitored closely. Dosage adjustments should be made, and supportive measures should be taken.

In addition, when antipsychotic drugs are combined with anticholinergics, there is a risk for decreased therapeutic effect of the antipsychotics, possibly because of a central antagonism of the two agents.

Nursing Considerations for Patients Receiving Anticholinergic Antiparkinsonism Drugs
Assessment: History and Examination

Screen for the following conditions, which could be contraindications or cautions to the use of the drug: any known allergies to these drugs; GI depression or obstruction; urinary hesitancy or obstruction; benign prostatic hypertrophy; cardiac arrhythmias or hypotension; glaucoma; myasthenia gravis; pregnancy or lactation; hepatic dysfunction; and exposure to a hot environment.

DRUGS IN FOCUS
Anticholinergic Antiparkinsonism Drugs

Drug Name	Dosage/Route	Usual Indications
benztropine (*Cogentin*)	0.5–6 mg/d PO may be needed; 1–2 mg IM or IV; reduce dosage in older patients	Parkinsonism, drug-induced parkinsonism
Ⓟ biperiden (*Akineton*)	2 mg PO t.i.d.–q.i.d. to a maximum of 16 mg/d; 2 mg IM or IV, repeated in ½ hour as needed, do not give more than four doses per day	Parkinsonism, drug-induced parkinsonism
diphenhydramine (*Benadryl*)	Adult: 25–50 mg PO t.i.d.–q.i.d.; 10–50 mg IM or IV, maximum dose 400 mg/d Pediatric: 12.5–25 mg PO t.i.d.–q.i.d; do not exceed 300 mg/d; 5 mg/kg per day IM or IV divided into four equal doses; maximum daily dose, 300 mg	Parkinsonism, particularly in the elderly and in those with mild forms
procyclidine (*Kemadrin*)	2.5–5 mg PO t.i.d.	Parkinsonism; control of excessive salivation
trihexyphenidyl (*Artane*)	1–2 mg PO q.d. initially, titrate up to 6–10 mg/d; up to 15 mg/d may be needed	Adjunct to levodopa in treatment of parkinsonism

Include screening for baseline status before beginning therapy and to monitor for any potential adverse effects. Assess the following: temperature; skin color and lesions; CNS orientation, affect, reflexes, bilateral grip strength, and spasticity evaluation; respiration and adventitious sounds; pulse, blood pressure, and cardiac output; bowel sounds and reported output; urinary output, bladder palpation; and liver and renal function tests.

Nursing Diagnoses

The patient taking an anticholinergic antiparkinsonism drug may have the following nursing diagnoses related to drug therapy:

- Acute Pain related to GI, CNS, GU effects
- Disturbed Thought Processes related to CNS effects
- Risk for Injury related to CNS effects
- Deficient Knowledge regarding drug therapy

Implementation

- Arrange to decrease dosage or discontinue the drug *if dry mouth becomes so severe that swallowing becomes difficult. Provide sugarless lozenges to suck and frequent mouth care to help with this problem.*
- Give the drug with caution and arrange for a decrease in dosage in hot weather or with exposure to hot environments, *because patients are at increased risk for heat prostration.*
- Give the drug with meals if GI upset is a problem, before meals if dry mouth is a problem, and after meals if drooling occurs and the drug causes nausea, *to facilitate compliance with drug therapy.*
- Monitor bowel function and institute a bowel program *if constipation is severe.*
- Ensure that the patient voids before taking the drug *if urinary retention is a problem.*
- Establish safety precautions if CNS or vision changes occur, *to prevent patient injury.*
- Provide thorough patient teaching about topics such as the drug name and prescribed dosage, measures to help avoid adverse effects, warning signs that may indicate problems, and the need for periodic monitoring and evaluation, *to enhance patient knowledge about drug therapy and to promote compliance.*
- Offer support and encouragement *to help the patient cope with the disease and drug regimen.*

Evaluation

- Monitor patient response to the drug (improvement in signs and symptoms of parkinsonism).
- Monitor for adverse effects (CNS changes, urinary retention, GI depression, tachycardia, decreased sweating, flushing).
- Evaluate the effectiveness of the teaching plan (patient can give the drug name and dosage, name possible adverse ef-

fects to watch for and specific measures to prevent adverse effects, and discuss the importance of continued follow-up).
- Monitor the effectiveness of comfort measures and compliance with the regimen.

▄▐●▌ WEB LINKS

Health care providers and patients may want to consult the following Internet sources:

Information on parkinsonism, ataxia, and related disorders including support groups, research, treatment:
http://www.ataxia.org
Information on education programs, research, other information related to parkinsonism:
http://www.ninds.nih.gov
Information on neurosciences, including current research and theories:
http://www.neuroguide.com
Information on support services and aids for activities of daily living:
http://www.accessunlimited.com/links.html

DOPAMINERGICS

Dopaminergics, drugs that increase the effects of dopamine at receptor sites, have been proven to be even more effective than anticholinergics in the treatment of parkinsonism. Dopamine itself does not cross the blood–brain barrier; other drugs that act like dopamine or increase dopamine concentrations indirectly must be used to increase dopamine levels in the brain. These drugs are effective as long as enough intact neurons remain in the substantia nigra to respond to increased levels of dopamine. After the neural degeneration has progressed beyond a certain point, patients no longer respond to these drugs.

Levodopa (*Dopar*) is the mainstay of treatment for parkinsonism. This precursor of dopamine crosses the blood–brain barrier, where it is converted to dopamine. In this way, it acts like a replacement therapy. Levodopa is almost always given in combination form with carbidopa as a fixed-combination drug (*Sinemet*). In this combination form, carbidopa inhibits the enzyme dopa decarboxylase in the periphery, diminishing the metabolism of levodopa in the GI tract and in peripheral tissues and leading to higher levels crossing the blood–brain barrier. Because it decreases the amount of levodopa needed to reach a therapeutic level in the brain, the dosage of levodopa can be decreased, which reduces the incidence of adverse side effects.

Therefore, in combination with carbidopa, smaller doses of levodopa are needed to achieve the same therapeutic effect. Carbidopa is not the only agent that is used primarily to improve the effectiveness of levodopa therapy (Box 24–1).

Other dopaminergics that are used in the treatment of parkinsonism include the following.

- Amantadine (*Symmetrel*), which is an antiviral drug that also seems to increase the release of dopamine. This drug

BOX 24-1
Adjuncts to Levodopa Therapy

Entacapone (*Comtan*) is used with carbidopa–levodopa to increase the plasma concentration and duration of action of levodopa. It does this by inhibiting catecholamine O-methyl transferase (COMT), a naturally occurring enzyme that eliminates catecholamines, including dopamine. It is given with the carbidopa–levodopa at a dose of 200 mg PO, with a maximum of eight doses a day. It is readily absorbed from the gastrointestinal (GI) tract, metabolized in the liver, and excreted in urine and feces. Women of child-bearing age should be encouraged to use barrier contraceptives while taking this drug, which crosses the placenta and could have adverse effects on the fetus.

Tolcapone (*Tasmar*) works in a similar way with carbidopa–levodopa to further increase plasma levels of levodopa. Tolcapone also blocks the enzyme COMT, which is responsible for the breakdown of dopamine. Because this drug has been associated with fulminant and potentially fatal liver damage, it is contraindicated in the presence of liver disease. Tolcapone is reserved for use in later stages of Parkinson's disease, when carbidopa-levodopa is losing its effectiveness. It undergoes hepatic metabolism after GI absorption and is excreted in the urine and feces. It is given in doses of 100 or 200 mg PO t.i.d., up to a maximum of 600 mg/d. Women of child-bearing age should be encouraged to use barrier contraceptives while taking this drug, which crosses the placenta and could have adverse effects on the fetus.

Selegiline (*Carbex, Eldepryl*) is used with carbidopa–levodopa after patients have shown signs of deteriorating response to this treatment. Its mechanism of action is not understood. It does irreversibly inhibit monoamine oxidase (MAO), which has an important role in the breakdown of catecholamines, including dopamine. The maximum daily dose of the drug is 10 mg, and the dose of levodopa needs to be reduced when this drug is started. It is well absorbed from the GI tract, extensively metabolized in the liver, and excreted in urine. It is not known whether this drug crosses the placenta, but it should be used in pregnancy only if the benefits to the mother clearly outweigh any potential risks to the fetus. Because of the risk of MAO inhibitor–induced hypertensive effects, patients should be urged to immediately report severe headache and any other unusual symptoms that they have not experienced before.

can be effective as long as there is a possibility of more dopamine release.

- Bromocriptine (*Parlodel*), which acts as a direct dopamine agonist on dopamine receptor sites in the substantia nigra. Because this drug does not depend on cells in the area to biotransform it or to increase release of already produced dopamine, it may be effective longer than levodopa or amantadine.
- Pergolide (*Permax*), which is used as an adjunct to carbidopa–levodopa therapy. It directly stimulates postsynaptic dopamine receptors in the substantia nigra, an effect that also may lead to inhibition of prolactin secretion and a rise in growth hormone levels.

- Pramipexole (*Mirapex*), which directly stimulates dopamine receptors in the substantia nigra. It may be effective after levodopa effects have weakened.
- Ropinirole (*Requip*), a newer drug that directly stimulates dopamine receptors. It has proved useful in both early and later stages of Parkinson's disease in conjunction with levodopa, when the effects of levodopa are no longer sufficient to provide symptomatic relief.

Therapeutic Actions and Indications

The dopaminergics work by increasing the levels of dopamine in the substantia nigra or directly stimulating the dopamine receptors in that area. This action helps restore the balance between the inhibitory and stimulating neurons. The dopaminergics are indicated for the relief of the signs and symptoms of idiopathic Parkinson's disease. Amantadine, which is also used as an antiviral agent, may be effective in treating drug-induced Parkinson's disease as well.

After neurodegeneration has progressed to the extent that the nerves are damaged or gone, these drugs are no longer effective. These drugs control Parkinson's disease only so long as functioning dopamine receptors remain in the substantia nigra.

Pharmacokinetics

The dopaminergics are generally well absorbed from the GI tract and widely distributed in the body. They are metabolized in the liver and peripheral cells and excreted in the urine. They cross the placenta, but there are no adequate studies of use of these drugs in pregnancy. They should be used during pregnancy only if the benefits to the mother clearly outweigh the potential risks to the fetus. Dopaminergics enter breast milk and should not be used during lactation because of the potential for adverse effects in the baby.

Contraindications and Cautions

The dopaminergics are contraindicated in the presence of any known allergy to the drug or drug components. They are also contraindicated in the following conditions: angle-closure glaucoma, which could be exacerbated by these drugs; history or presence of suspicious skin lesions with levodopa, because this drug has been associated with the development of melanoma; and lactation, because of potential adverse effects on the baby.

Caution should be used with any condition that could be exacerbated by dopamine receptor stimulation, such as cardiovascular disease, including myocardial infarction, arrhythmias, and hypertension; bronchial asthma; history of peptic ulcers; urinary tract obstruction; and psychiatric disorders. Care should also be taken in pregnancy, because these drugs cross the placenta and could adversely affect the fetus, and in renal and hepatic disease, which could interfere with the metabolism and excretion of the drug.

Adverse Effects

The adverse effects associated with the dopaminergics usually result from stimulation of dopamine receptors. CNS effects may include anxiety, nervousness, headache, malaise, fatigue, confusion, mental changes, blurred vision, muscle twitching, and ataxia. Peripheral effects may include anorexia, nausea, vomiting, dysphagia, and constipation or diarrhea; cardiac arrhythmias, hypotension, palpitations; bizarre breathing patterns; urinary retention; and flushing, increased sweating, and hot flashes. Bone marrow depression and hepatic dysfunction have also been reported.

Clinically Important Drug–Drug Interactions

If dopaminergics are combined with monoamine oxidase (MAO) inhibitors, therapeutic effects increase and a risk of hypertensive crisis exists. The MAO inhibitor should be stopped 14 days before beginning therapy with a dopaminergic.

The combination of levodopa with vitamin B_6 or with phenytoin may lead to decreased efficacy. Reduced effectiveness may also result if dopaminergics are combined with dopamine antagonists. In addition, patients who take dopaminergics should be cautioned to avoid over-the-counter vitamins; if such medications are used, the patient should be monitored closely, because a decrease in effectiveness can result.

Nursing Considerations for Patients Receiving Dopaminergic Antiparkinsonism Drugs

Assessment: History and Examination

Screen for the following conditions, which could be contraindications or cautions for the use of the drug: any known allergies to these drugs or drug components; GI depression or obstruction; urinary hesitancy or obstruction; cardiac arrhythmias or hypertension; glaucoma; respiratory disease; pregnancy or lactation; and renal or hepatic dysfunction. With levodopa, check for skin lesions or history of melanoma.

Include screening for baseline status before beginning therapy and to monitor for any potential adverse effects. Assess

the following: temperature; skin color and lesions; CNS orientation, affect, reflexes, bilateral grip strength, and spasticity evaluation; vision; respiration and adventitious sounds; pulse, blood pressure, and cardiac output; bowel sounds and reported output; and urinary output and bladder palpation. Check liver and renal function tests and complete blood count (CBC) with differential.

Nursing Diagnoses

The patient taking a dopaminergic antiparkinsonism drug may have the following nursing diagnoses related to drug therapy:

- Acute Pain related to GI, CNS, GU effects
- Disturbed Thought Processes related to CNS effects
- Risk for Injury related to CNS effects and incidence of orthostatic hypertension
- Deficient Knowledge regarding drug therapy

IMPLEMENTATION

- Arrange to decrease dosage of the drug if therapy has been interrupted for any reason, *to prevent acute peripheral dopaminergic effects.*
- Evaluate disease progress and signs and symptoms periodically and record *for reference of disease progress and drug response.*
- Give the drug with meals *to alleviate GI irritation if GI upset is a problem.*
- Monitor bowel function and institute a bowel program *if constipation is severe.*

DRUGS IN FOCUS
Dopaminergic Antiparkinsonism Drugs

Drug Name	Dosage/Route	Usual Indications
amantadine (Symmetrel)	100 mg PO b.i.d.; up to 400 mg/d has been used	Antiviral; idiopathic and drug-induced parkinsonism in adults
bromocriptine (Parlodel)	1.25 mg PO b.i.d; titrate up to 10–40 mg/d	Idiopathic Parkinson's disease; may be beneficial in later stages when response to levodopa decreases
Ⓟ levodopa (Dopar)	0.5–1 g/d PO in two divided doses; titrate up to 8 g/d; most often given in combination with carbidopa as Sinemet: 25 mg carbidopa/100 mg levodopa PO t.i.d.	Idiopathic Parkinson's disease
pergolide (Permax)	0.05 mg/d PO for 2 days, then slowly titrate to 3 mg/d in three equally divided doses	Adjunct with carbidopa–levodopa for idiopathic Parkinson's disease
pramipexole (Mirapex)	0.125 mg PO t.i.d. up to 1.5 mg PO t.i.d.	Idiopathic Parkinson's disease
ropinirole (Requip)	0.25 mg PO t.i.d.; titrate up to maximum dose of 24 mg/d	Idiopathic Parkinson's disease in early stages and in later stages combined with levodopa

- Ensure that the patient voids before taking the drug *if urinary retention is a problem.*
- Establish safety precautions if CNS or vision changes occur, *to prevent patient injury.*
- Monitor hepatic, renal, and hematological tests periodically during therapy *to detect early signs of dysfunction and consider re-evaluation of drug therapy.*
- Provide support services and comfort measures as needed, *to improve patient compliance.*
- Provide thorough patient teaching about topics such as the drug name and prescribed dosage, measures to help avoid adverse effects, warning signs that may indicate problems, and the need for periodic monitoring and evaluation, *to enhance patient knowledge about drug therapy and to promote compliance.* (See Patient Teaching Checklist: Levodopa.)
- Offer encouragement *to help the patient cope with the disease and drug regimen.*

Evaluation

- Monitor patient response to the drug (improvement in signs and symptoms of parkinsonism).
- Monitor for adverse effects (CNS changes, urinary retention, GI depression, tachycardia, increased sweating, flushing).
- Evaluate the effectiveness of the teaching plan (patient can give the drug name and dosage, name possible adverse effects to watch for and specific measures to prevent adverse effects, and discuss the importance of continued follow-up).
- Monitor the effectiveness of comfort measures and compliance with the regimen (see Nursing Care Guide: Levodopa).

CHAPTER SUMMARY

- Parkinson's disease is a progressive, chronic neurological disorder for which there is no cure.
- Signs and symptoms of Parkinson's disease include tremor, changes in posture and gait, slow and deliberate movements (bradykinesia), and eventually drooling and changes in speech.
- Loss of dopamine-secreting neurons in the substantia nigra is characteristic of Parkinson's disease. Destruction of dopamine-secreting cells leads to an imbalance between excitatory cholinergic cells and inhibitory dopaminergic cells.
- Drug therapy for Parkinson's disease is aimed at restoring the dopamine–acetylcholine balance. The signs and symptoms of the disease can be managed until the degeneration of neurons is so extensive that a therapeutic response no longer occurs.
- Anticholinergic drugs are used to block the excitatory cholinergic receptors, and dopaminergic drugs are used to increase dopamine levels or to directly stimulate dopamine receptors.
- Many adverse effects are associated with the drugs used for treating Parkinson's disease, including CNS changes, anticholinergic (atropine-like) effects, and dopamine stimulation in the peripheral nervous system.

PATIENT TEACHING CHECKLIST

Levodopa

Create customized patient teaching materials for levodopa from the CD-ROM. Patient teaching should stress the following points:

- Levodopa increases the levels of dopamine in central areas of the brain, helping to reduce the signs and symptoms of Parkinson's disease. Often this drug is combined with carbidopa, which allows the correct levels of levodopa to reach the brain.
- People who take this drug must have their individual dosage needs adjusted over time.

Common effects of this drug include

- *Fatigue, weakness, and drowsiness*—Try to space activities evenly throughout the day and allow rest periods to avoid these sometimes very discouraging side effects. Take safety precautions and avoid driving or operating dangerous machinery if these conditions occur.
- *Dizziness, fainting*—Changing position slowly to avoid dizzy spells.
- *Increased sweating, darkening of urine*—This is a normal reaction. Avoid very hot environments.
- *Headaches, difficulty sleeping*—These usually pass as the body adjusts to the drug. If they become too uncomfortable and persist, consult with your health care provider.

Report any of the following conditions to your health care provider: uncontrolled movements of any part of the body; chest pain, palpitations; depression or mood changes; difficulty in voiding; or severe or persistent nausea and vomiting.

Be aware that vitamin B_6 interferes with the effects of levodopa. If you feel that you need a vitamin product, consult with your health care provider about using an agent that does not contain vitamin B_6. In addition, avoid eating large quantities of health foods that contain vitamin B_6, such as grains and brans. If you are taking a carbidopa–levodopa combination, these precautions are not as important.

Tell any doctor, nurse, or other health care provider that you are taking this drug.

Keep this drug and all medications out of the reach of children.

Do not overexert yourself when you begin to feel better. Pace yourself.

Take this drug exactly as prescribed. Be sure to obtain regular medical follow-up, which is necessary to evaluate the effects of this drug.

This Teaching Checklist reflects general patient teaching guidelines. It is not meant to be a substitute for drug-specific teaching information, which is available in nursing drug guides.

Review Questions

1. Parkinson's disease is a progressive, chronic neurological disorder that is usually
   a. associated with severe head injury.
   b. associated with chronic diseases.
   c. associated with old age.
   d. known to affect people of all ages with no known cause.

NURSING CARE GUIDE

Levodopa

Assessment	Nursing Diagnoses	Implementation	Evaluation
HISTORY Allergies to any of these drugs; COPD; arrhythmias; hypotension; hepatic or renal dysfunction; pregnancy and lactation; psychoses; peptic ulcer; glaucoma.	Acute Pain related to GI, GU, CNS effects Risk for Injury related to CNS effects Disturbed Thought Processes related to CNS effects Deficient Knowledge regarding drug therapy	Ensure safe and appropriate administration of drug. Provide comfort and safety measures: positioning, slow changes; orientation; safety measures; pain medication as needed; give drug with food; administer with carbidopa; void before each dose. Provide support and reassurance to deal with disease and drug effects. Provide patient teaching regarding drug, dosage, drug effects, symptoms to report.	Evaluate drug effects: relief of signs and symptoms of Parkinson's disease. Monitor for adverse effects: CNS effects; renal changes; GI effects (constipation); urinary retention; increased sweating, flushing. Monitor for drug–drug interactions: hypertensive crisis with MAO inhibitors; decreased effects with vitamin B_6, or phenytoin. Evaluate effectiveness of patient teaching program. Evaluate effectiveness of comfort and safety measures.
PHYSICAL EXAMINATION CV: blood pressure, pulse, peripheral perfusion, ECG CNS: orientation, affect, reflexes, grip strength Renal: output, bladder palpation GI: abdominal examination, bowel sounds Resp: respiration, adventitious sounds Laboratory tests: renal and liver function tests, CBC			

2. Parkinson's disease reflects an imbalance between inhibitory and stimulating activity of nerves in the
   a. reticular activating system.
   b. cerebellum.
   c. basal ganglia.
   d. limbic system.
3. The main, underlying problem with Parkinson's disease seems to be a decrease in the neurotransmitter
   a. acetylcholine.
   b. norepinephrine.
   c. dopamine.
   d. serotonin.
4. No therapy is available that will stop the loss of neurons and the eventual decline of function in Parkinsonism patients. As a result, nursing care should involve all of the following except

   a. regular exercises to slow loss of function.
   b. support and education as drugs fail and new therapy is needed.
   c. community and family support networking.
   d. discontinuation of drug therapy to test for a cure.
5. Anticholinergic drugs are effective in early Parkinson's disease. They act
   a. to block the stimulating effects of acetylcholine in the brain to bring activity back into balance.
   b. to block the signs and symptoms of the disease, making it more acceptable.
   c. to inhibit dopamine effects in the brain.
   d. to increase the effectiveness of GABA.
6. A patient receiving an anticholinergic drug for Parkinson's disease is planning a winter trip to Tahiti. The temperature in Tahiti is 70 degrees warmer than at

CASE STUDY

Effects of Vitamin B₆ Intake on Levodopa Levels

THE SITUATION

S. S., a 58-year-old man with well-controlled Parkinson's disease, presents with severe nausea, anorexia, fainting spells, and heart palpitations. He has been maintained on levodopa for the Parkinson's disease, and he claims to have followed his drug regimen religiously.

According to S. S., the only change in his lifestyle has been the addition of several health foods and vitamins. His daughter, who recently returned from her freshman year in college, has begun a new "health" regimen, including natural foods and plenty of supplemental vitamins. She was so enthusiastic about her new approach that everyone in the family agreed to give this diet a try.

CRITICAL THINKING

• Based on S. S.'s signs and symptoms, what has probably occurred?
• In Parkinson's disease, is it possible to differentiate a deterioration of illness from a toxic drug reaction?
• What nursing implications should be considered when teaching S. S. and his family about the effects of vitamin B₆ on levodopa levels?
• In what ways can the daughter cope with her role in this crisis?
• *Develop a new care plan for S. S. that involves all family members, including drug teaching.*

DISCUSSION

The presenting symptoms reflect an increase in parkinsonism symptoms as well as an increase in peripheral dopamine reactions (eg, palpitations, fainting, anorexia, nausea). It is necessary to determine whether the problem involves a further degeneration in the neurons in the substantia nigra or the particular medication that S. S. has been taking. Many patients lose their responsiveness to levodopa as the neural degeneration continues.

The explanation of the new lifestyle—full of grains, natural foods, and vitamins—alerted a nurse to the possibility of excessive vitamin B₆ intake. In reviewing the vitamin bottles and some of the food packages supplied by S. S., it seemed that too much vitamin B₆, which speeds the conversion of levodopa to dopamine before it can cross the blood–brain barrier, might be the reason the signs and symptoms of parkinsonism recurred.

S. S. should be evaluated regarding the status of his Parkinson's disease and then be restarted on levodopa. The smallest dose possible should be used to begin drug therapy, with slow increases to achieve the maximum benefit with the least side effects. It would be wise to consider combining the drug with carbidopa to prevent some of the patient's recent problems.

In addition, S. S. should receive thorough drug teaching in a written form for future reference, including the need to avoid vitamin B₆. His entire family should be involved in an explanation of what happened and how this situation can be avoided in the future. Because the daughter may feel especially guilty about her role, she should have the opportunity to discuss her feelings and explore the positive impact of healthy food on nutrition and quality of life. This situation can serve as a good teaching example for staff, as well as presenting them with an opportunity to review drug therapy in Parkinson's disease and the risks and benefits of more extreme diets.

---

home. What precautions should the patient be urged to take?

a. Take the drug with plenty of water to stay hydrated.
b. Reduce dosage and take extreme precautions because you are at increased risk for heat stroke due to the anticholinergic effects of the drug.
c. Wear sunglasses and use sunscreen because of photophobia that will develop.
d. Avoid drinking the water.

7. Replacing dopamine in the brain would seem to be the best treatment for Parkinson's disease. This is difficult because dopamine
a. is broken down in gastric acid.
b. is not available in drug form.
c. cannot cross the blood–brain barrier.
d. is used up in the periphery before it can reach the brain.

8. A patient taking levodopa and over-the-counter megavitamins might experience
a. cure from Parkinson's disease.
b. return of Parkinsonism symptoms and increased blood pressure, pulse, respirations, sweating, and feeling of tension.
c. improved health and well-being.
d. a resistance to viral infections.

9. A patient who has been diagnosed with Parkinson's disease for many years and was controlled using *Sinemet* has started to exhibit increasing signs of Parkinson's disease. Possible treatment might include
a. increased exercise program.
b. addition of pergolide to the drug regimen.
c. combination therapy with an anticholinergic or other dopaminergic drug.
d. changes in diet to eliminate vitamin B₆.

10. Possible causes of parkinsonism could include all of the following except
a. adverse effect of drug therapy.
b. head injury.
c. viral infection.
d. dementia.

BIBLIOGRAPHY

Bailey, K. (1998). *Psychotropic drug facts*. Philadelphia: Lippincott-Raven.

Bullock, B. L. (2000). *Focus on pathophysiology*. Philadelphia: Lippincott Williams & Wilkins.

Drug facts and comparisons. (2002). St. Louis: Facts and Comparisons.

Gilman, A., Hardman, J. G., & Limbird, L. E. (Eds.) (2002). *Goodman and Gilman's the pharmacological basis of therapeutics* (10th ed.). New York: McGraw-Hill.

Karch, A. M. (2002). *2003 Lippincott's nursing drug guide*. Philadelphia: Lippincott Williams & Wilkins.

Professional's guide to patient drug facts. (2002). St. Louis: Facts and Comparisons.

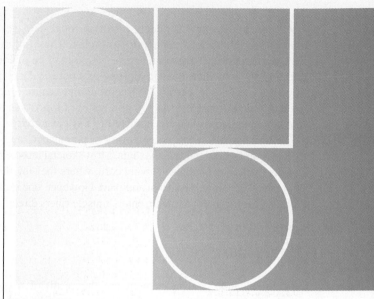

CHAPTER

25

Muscle Relaxants

Key Terms
basal ganglia
cerebellum
extrapyramidal tract
hypertonia
interneuron
pyramidal tract
spasticity

331

Centrally Acting Skeletal Muscle Relaxants

 baclofen
carisoprodol
chlorphenesin
chlorzoxazone
cyclobenzaprine
metaxalone
methocarbamol
orphenadrine
tizanidine

Direct-Acting Skeletal Muscle Relaxants

botulinum toxin type B
 dantrolene

Many injuries and accidents result in local damage to muscles or the skeletal anchors of muscles. These injuries may lead to muscle spasm and pain, which may be of long duration and may interfere with normal functioning. Damage to central nervous system (CNS) neurons may cause a permanent state of muscle spasticity as a result of loss of nerves that help maintain balance in controlling muscle activity.

Neuron damage, whether temporary or permanent, may be treated with skeletal muscle relaxants. Most skeletal muscle relaxants work in the brain and spinal cord, where they interfere with the cycle of muscle spasm and pain. However, one skeletal muscle relaxant, dantrolene, enters muscle fibers directly.

NERVES AND MOVEMENT

Posture, balance, and movement are the result of a constantly fluctuating sequence of muscle contraction and relaxation. The nerves that regulate these actions are the spinal motor neurons. These neurons are influenced by higher-level brain activity in the cerebellum and basal ganglia, which provide coordination of contractions, and in the cerebral cortex, which allows conscious thought to regulate movement.

Spinal Reflexes

The spinal reflexes are the simplest nerve pathways that monitor movement and posture (Figure 25–1). Spinal reflexes can be simple, involving an incoming sensory neuron and an outgoing motor neuron, or more complex, involving interneurons that communicate with the related centers in the brain. Simple reflex arcs involve sensory receptors in the periphery and

spinal motor nerves. Such reflex arcs make up what is known as the spindle gamma loop system; they respond to stretch receptors on muscle fibers to cause a muscle fiber contraction that relieves the stretch. In this system, nerves from stretch receptors form a synapse with gamma nerves in the spinal cord, which send an impulse to the stretched muscle fibers to stimulate their contraction. These reflexes are responsible for maintaining muscle tone and keeping an upright position against the pull of gravity. Other spinal reflexes may involve synapses with **interneurons** within the spinal cord, which adjust movement and response based on information from higher brain centers and coordinate movement and position.

Brain Control

Many areas within the brain influence the spinal motor nerves. Areas of the brainstem, the **basal ganglia,** and the **cerebellum** modulate spinal motor nerve activity and help coordinate activity among various muscle groups, thereby allowing coordinated movement and control of body muscle motions. Nerve areas within the cerebral cortex allow conscious, or intentional, movement. Nerves within the cortex send signals down the spinal cord, where they cross to the opposite side of the spinal cord before sending out nerve impulses to cause muscle contraction. In this way, each side of the cortex controls muscle movement on the opposite side of the body.

Different fibers control different types of movements. These fibers that control precise, intentional movement make up the **pyramidal tract** within the CNS. The **extrapyramidal tract** is composed of cells from the cerebral cortex as well as from several subcortical areas, including the basal ganglia and the cerebellum. This tract modulates or coordinates unconsciously controlled muscle activity, and it allows the body to make automatic adjustments in posture or

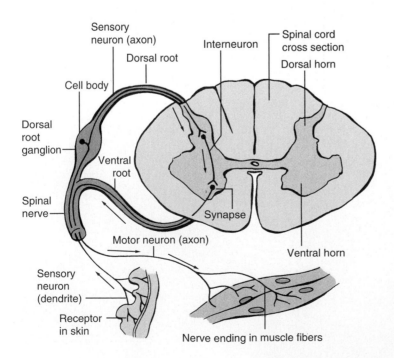

FIGURE 25–1. Reflex arc showing the pathway of impulses.

position and balance. The extrapyramidal tract controls lower-level, or crude, movements.

NEUROMUSCULAR ABNORMALITIES

All of the areas mentioned work together to allow for a free flow of impulses into and out of the CNS to coordinate posture, balance, and movement. When injuries, diseases, and toxins affect the normal flow of information into and out of the CNS motor pathways, many clinical signs and symptoms may develop, ranging from simple muscle spasms to **spasticity,** or sustained muscle spasm, and paralysis.

Muscle Spasm

Muscle spasms often result from injury to the musculoskeletal system—for example, overstretching a muscle, wrenching a joint, or tearing a tendon or ligament. These injuries can cause violent and painful involuntary muscle contractions. It is thought that these spasms are caused by the flood of sensory impulses coming to the spinal cord from the injured area. These impulses can be passed through interneurons to spinal motor nerves, which stimulate an intense muscle contraction. The contraction cuts off blood flow to the muscle fibers in the injured area, causing lactic acid to accumulate, resulting in pain. The new flood of sensory impulse caused by the pain may lead to further muscle contraction, and a vicious cycle may develop.

Muscle Spasticity

Muscle spasticity is the result of damage to neurons within the CNS rather than injury to peripheral structures. Because the spasticity is caused by nerve damage in the CNS, it is a permanent condition. Spasticity may result from an increase in excitatory influences or a decrease in inhibitory influences within the CNS. The interruption in the balance among all of these higher influences within the CNS may lead to excessive stimulation of muscles, or **hypertonia,** in opposing muscle groups at the same time, a condition that may cause contractures and permanent structural changes. This control imbalance also results in a loss of coordinated muscle activity.

For example, the signs and symptoms of cerebral palsy and paraplegia are related to the disruption in the nervous control of the muscles. The exact presentation of any chronic neurologi-

DRUG THERAPY ACROSS THE LIFESPAN

Skeletal Muscle Relaxants

Children	Adults	Older Adults
The safety and effectiveness of most of these drugs have not been established in children. If a child older than 12 years of age requires a skeletal muscle relaxant after an injury, metaxalone has an established pediatric dosage. Other agents have been used, with adjustments to the adult dosage based on the child's age and weight. Baclofen is often used to relieve the muscle spasticity associated with cerebral palsy. A caregiver needs intensive education in the use of the intrathecal infusion pump and how to monitor the child for therapeutic as well as adverse effects. Methocarbamol is the drug of choice if a child needs to be treated for tetanus. Dantrolene is used to treat upper motor neuron spasticity in children. The dosage is based on body weight and increases over time. The child should be screened regularly for central nervous system (CNS) and gastrointestinal (including hepatic) toxicity.	Adults being treated for acute musculoskeletal pain should be cautioned to avoid driving and to take safety precautions against injury because of the related CNS effects, including dizziness and drowsiness. Adults complaining of muscle spasm pain that may be related to anxiety often respond very effectively to diazepam, which is a muscle relaxant and anxiolytic. Women of child-bearing age should be advised to use contraception when they are taking these drugs. If a pregnancy does occur, or is desired, they need counseling about the potential for adverse effects. Women who are nursing should be encouraged to find another method of feeding the baby because of the potential for adverse drug effects on the baby. Premenopausal women are also at increased risk for the hepatotoxicity associated with dantrolene and should be monitored very closely for any change in hepatic function and should be given written information about the prodrome syndrome that often occurs with the hepatic toxicity.	Older patients are more likely to experience the adverse effects associated with these drugs—CNS, gastrointestinal, and cardiovascular. Because older patients often also have renal or hepatic impairment, they are also more likely to have toxic levels of the drug related to changes in metabolism and excretion. Carisoprodol is the centrally acting skeletal muscle relaxant of choice for older patients and for those with hepatic or renal impairment. If dantrolene is required for an older patient, lower doses and more frequent monitoring are needed to assess for potential cardiac, respiratory, and liver toxicity. Older women who are receiving hormone replacement therapy are at the same risk for development of hepatotoxicity as premenopausal women and should be monitored accordingly.

cal disorder depends on the specific nerve centers and tracts that are damaged and how the control imbalance is manifested.

CENTRALLY ACTING SKELETAL MUSCLE RELAXANTS

The centrally acting skeletal muscle relaxants work in the CNS to interfere with the reflexes that are causing the muscle spasm. Because these drugs lyse or destroy spasm, they are often referred to as spasmolytics. They work in the upper levels of the CNS, so possible depression must be anticipated with their use. These drugs include

- Baclofen (*Lioresal*), which is used for the treatment of muscle spasticity associated with neuromuscular diseases such as multiple sclerosis, muscle rigidity, and spinal cord injuries. This agent, which is available in oral and intrathecal forms, can be administered via a delivery pump for the treatment of central spasticity.
- Carisoprodol (*Soma*), which is indicated for the relief of discomfort associated with musculoskeletal pain. It may be safer in older patients and in those with renal or hepatic dysfunction.
- Chlorphenesin (*Malate*), which has the same indication as carisoprodol.
- Chlorzoxazone (*Paraflex*), which is also indicated for the relief of discomfort associated with musculoskeletal pain.
- Cyclobenzaprine (*Flexeril*), which is recommended for the relief of discomfort associated with painful, acute musculoskeletal conditions. This agent, available only in an oral form, is associated with few adverse effects.
- Metaxalone (*Skelaxin*), which is recommended as an adjunct for the relief of discomfort associate with acute, painful musculoskeletal conditions. Caution must be used

with this drug in patients with any hepatic impairment. This is one of the few skeletal muscle relaxants with an established pediatric dose for children older than 12 years of age.
- Methocarbamol (*Robaxin*), which is used to relieve the same conditions as cyclobenzaprine and also to alleviate signs and symptoms of tetanus. It is available only in the parenteral form.
- Orphenadrine (*Banflex, Flexoject*), another parenteral drug, which is available for the relief of acute, painful musculoskeletal conditions. This agent is also being tried for the relief of quinidine-induced leg cramps.
- Tizanidine (*Zanaflex*), which is approved for the acute and intermittent management of increased muscle tone associated with spasticity. It has been associated with liver toxicity and should be used with caution if a patient has hepatic dysfunction. It is also associated with hypotension in some patients.

Diazepam (*Valium*), a drug widely used as an anxiety agent (see Chapter 20), also has been shown to be an effective centrally acting skeletal muscle relaxant. It may be advantageous in situations in which anxiety may precipitate the muscle spasm.

Other measures in addition to these drugs should be used to alleviate muscle spasm and pain. Such modalities as rest of the affected muscle, heat applications to increase blood flow to the area to remove the pain-causing chemicals, physical therapy to return the muscle to normal tone and activity, and anti-inflammatory agents (including nonsteroidal anti-inflammatory drugs [NSAIDs]) if the underlying problem is related to injury or inflammation may help (Box 25–1).

Therapeutic Actions and Indications

Although the exact mechanism of action of these skeletal muscle relaxants is not known, it is thought to involve action in the upper or spinal interneurons. Tizanidine is an α-adrenergic ag-

---

BOX 25-1

Fixed-Combination Skeletal Muscle Relaxants

There are some products available that combine a centrally acting muscle relaxant with an anti-inflammatory or analgesic agent. These products tend to facilitate relief of the discomfort associated with acute painful musculoskeletal conditions. They should be used as adjuncts to rest, physical therapy, and other measures.

Drug Name	Composition	Dosage
Robixisal	400 mg methocarbamol/325 mg aspirin	2 tablets PO q.i.d.
Soma Compound	200 mg carisoprodol/325 mg aspirin	1–2 tablets PO q.i.d.
Soma Compound with codeine	200 mg carisoprodol/325 mg aspirin/16 mg codeine	1–2 tablets PO q.i.d
Flexaphen[a]	250 mg chlorzoxazone/300 mg acetaminophen	2 capsules PO q.i.d.
Lobac[a]	200 mg salicylamide/20 mg phenyltoloxamine/300 mg acetaminophen	2 capsules PO q.i.d.
Norgesic[a]	25 mg orphenadrine/385 mg aspirin/30 mg caffeine	1–2 tablets PO t.i.d.–q.i.d.
Norgesic Forte[a]	50 mg orphenadrine/770 mg aspirin/60 mg caffeine	1 tablet PO t.i.d.–q.i.d.

[a]Rated by the U.S. Food and Drug Administration as "possibly effective" for this indication.

onist and is thought to increase inhibition of presynaptic motor neurons in the CNS. The primary indication for the use of centrally acting skeletal muscle agents is the relief of discomfort associated with acute, painful musculoskeletal conditions as an adjunct to rest, physical therapy, and other measures.

Pharmacokinetics

Most of these agents are rapidly absorbed and metabolized in the liver. Baclofen is not metabolized, but, like the other skeletal muscle relaxants, it is excreted in the urine. No good studies exist regarding the effects of these agents during pregnancy and lactation; therefore, use should be limited to those situations in which the benefit to the mother clearly outweighs any potential risk to the neonate.

Contraindications and Cautions

Centrally acting skeletal muscle relaxants are contraindicated in the presence of any known allergy to any of these drugs and with skeletal muscle spasms resulting from rheumatic disorders. In addition, baclofen should not be used to treat any spasticity that contributes to locomotion, upright position, or increased function. Blocking this spasticity results in loss of these functions.

All centrally acting skeletal muscle relaxants should be used cautiously in the following circumstances: with a history of epilepsy, because the CNS depression and imbalance caused by these drugs may exacerbate the seizure disorder; with cardiac dysfunction, because muscle function may be depressed; with any condition marked by muscle weakness that the drugs could make much worse; and with hepatic or renal dysfunction, which could interfere with the metabolism and excretion of the drugs, leading to toxic levels. These agents should be used with caution in pregnancy or lactation, because the fetus or neonate may suffer adverse effects.

Adverse Effects

The most frequently seen adverse effects associated with these drugs relate to the associated CNS depression: drowsiness, fatigue, weakness, confusion, headache, and insomnia. Gastrointestinal (GI) disturbances, which may be linked to CNS depression of the parasympathetic reflexes, include nausea, dry mouth, anorexia, and constipation. In addition, hypotension and arrhythmias may occur, again as a result of depression of normal reflex arcs. Urinary frequency, enuresis, and feelings of urinary urgency reportedly may occur. Chlorzoxazone may discolor the urine, becoming orange to purple-red when metabolized and excreted. Patients should be warned about this effect to prevent any fears of blood in the urine.

Clinically Important Drug–Drug Interactions

If any of the centrally acting skeletal muscle relaxants are taken with other CNS depressants or alcohol, CNS depression

---

DRUGS IN FOCUS
Centrally Acting Skeletal Muscle Relaxants

Drug Name	Dosage/Route	Usual Indications
℗ baclofen (*Lioresal*)	Adult: 40—80 mg PO q.d. 300–800 μg/d per intrathecal infusion pump Pediatric: intrathecal infusion pump, 24–1199 μg/d — base dosage on patient response	Muscle spasticity, spinal cord injuries
carisoprodol (*Soma*)	350 mg PO t.i.d.–q.i.d.	Relief of discomfort of acute musculoskeletal conditions in adults
chlorphenesin (*Malate*)	800 PO t.i.d. until desired effect is seen; then 400 mg PO q.i.d. may be sufficient	Relief of discomfort of acute musculoskeletal conditions
chlorzoxazone (*Paraflex*)	250 mg PO t.i.d.–q.i.d.	Relief of discomfort of acute musculoskeletal conditions in adults
cyclobenzaprine (*Flexeril*)	10 mg PO t.i.d., do not exceed 60 mg/d	Relief of discomfort of acute musculoskeletal conditions in adults
metaxalone (*Skelaxin*)	Adults and children >12 y: 800 mg PO t.i.d.–q.i.d.; reduce dosage with hepatic impairment	Relief of discomfort of acute musculoskeletal conditions
methocarbamol (*Robaxin*)	Adult: 1.5 g PO q.i.d. 1–2 g IV or IM for tetanus Pediatric: 15 mg/kg IV for tetanus	Relief of discomfort of acute musculoskeletal conditions in adults; tetanus
orphenadrine (*Banflex, Flexoject*)	100 mg PO, AM and h.s. or 60 mg IV or IM q12h	Relief of discomfort of acute musculoskeletal conditions in adults; quinidine-induced leg cramps (100 mg PO h.s.)
tizanidine (*Zanaflex*)	8 mg PO as a single dose may be repeated q6–8h as needed	Relief of discomfort of acute musculoskeletal conditions in adults

may increase. Patients should be cautioned to avoid alcohol while taking these muscle relaxants; if this combination cannot be avoided, they should take extreme precautions.

Nursing Considerations for Patients Receiving Centrally Acting Skeletal Muscle Relaxants

Assessment: History and Examination

Screen for the following conditions, which could be cautions or contraindications for the use of the drug: any known allergies to these drugs; cardiac depression, epilepsy, muscle weakness, rheumatic disorder; pregnancy or lactation; and renal or hepatic dysfunction.

Include screening for baseline status before beginning therapy and for any potential adverse effects. Assess the following: temperature; skin color and lesions; CNS orientation, affect, reflexes, bilateral grip strength, and spasticity evaluation; bowel sounds and reported output; and liver and renal function tests.

Nursing Diagnoses

The patient who is receiving a centrally acting skeletal muscle relaxant may have the following nursing diagnoses related to drug therapy:

- Acute Pain related to GI, CNS effects
- Disturbed Thought Processes related to CNS effects
- Risk for Injury related to CNS effects
- Deficient Knowledge regarding drug therapy

Implementation

- Provide additional measures to relieve discomfort—heat, rest for the muscle, NSAIDs, positioning—*to augment the effects of the drug at relieving the musculoskeletal discomfort.*
- Discontinue the drug at any sign of hypersensitivity reaction or liver dysfunction, *to prevent severe toxicity.*
- If using baclofen, taper drug slowly over 1 to 2 weeks *to prevent the development of psychoses and hallucinations.* Use baclofen cautiously in patients whose spasticity contributes to mobility, posture, or balance, *to prevent loss of this function.*
- If the patient is receiving baclofen through a delivery pump, the patient should understand the pump, the reason for frequent monitoring, and how to adjust the dose and program the unit, *to enhance patient knowledge and promote compliance.*
- Monitor respiratory status *to evaluate adverse effects and arrange for appropriate dosage adjustment or discontinuation of the drug.*
- Provide thorough patient teaching, including drug name, prescribed dosage, measures for avoidance of adverse effects, warning signs that may indicate possible problems, and the need for monitoring and evaluation, *to enhance patient knowledge about drug therapy and to promote compliance.*
- Offer support and encouragement *to help the patient cope with the drug regimen.*

Evaluation

- Monitor patient response to the drug (improvement in muscle spasm and relief of pain; improvement in muscle spasticity).
- Monitor for adverse effects (CNS changes, GI depression, urinary urgency).
- Evaluate the effectiveness of the teaching plan (patient can give the drug name and dosage, name possible adverse effects to watch for and specific measures to prevent adverse effects, and describe, if necessary, proper intrathecal administration).
- Monitor the effectiveness of comfort measures and compliance with the regimen.

▢▰●▰ WEB LINKS

Health care providers and patients may want to consult the following Internet sources:

Information on muscle physiology and muscle disorders and diseases:
http://www1.umn.edu/cmmd/cmmd.html
Information on malignant hyperthermia:
http://www.mhaus.org
Information for patients and health care professionals about cerebral palsy research, treatment:
http://www.ucppgmc.com/index.html
Patient information regarding cerebral palsy:
http://www.spinalcord.org

DIRECT-ACTING SKELETAL MUSCLE RELAXANTS

One drug is currently available for use in treating (general) spasticity that directly affects peripheral muscle contraction. This drug, dantrolene (*Dantrium*), has become important in the management of spasticity associated with neuromuscular diseases such as cerebral palsy, multiple sclerosis, muscular dystrophy, polio, tetanus, quadriplegia, and amyotrophic lateral sclerosis (ALS). This agent is not used for the treatment of muscle spasms associated with musculoskeletal injury or rheumatic disorders.

Therapeutic Actions and Indications

Dantrolene acts within skeletal muscle fibers, interfering with the release of calcium from the muscle tubules (Figure 25–2; see Box 25–1). This action prevents the fibers from contracting. Dantrolene does not interfere with neuromuscular transmissions, and it does not affect the surface membrane of skeletal muscle.

Dantrolene is indicated for the control of spasticity resulting from upper motor neuron disorders, including spinal cord injury, myasthenia gravis, muscular dystrophy, and cerebral palsy (oral form). Continued long-term use is justified as long as the drug reduces painful and disabling spasticity. Long-term use results in a decrease of the amount and intensity of required nursing care.

Dantrolene is also indicated for the prevention of malignant hyperthermia, a state of intense muscle contraction and resulting hyperpyrexia. Malignant hyperthermia may occur

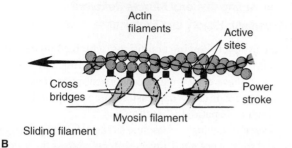

FIGURE 25–2. Sliding filament mechanism of muscle contraction. *A:* The relationship between the myosin filament and the actin filament projections. *B:* The bridges formed by the myosin filament move along successive sites on the actin filaments, as outlined in Box 25–1. (From Bullock, B. L. [2000]. *Focus on pathophysiology.* Philadelphia: Lippincott Williams & Wilkins.)

BOX 25-2

Summary of Muscle Contraction and Relaxation

Stimulus from nerve axon to myoneural junction
↓
Acetylcholine release in synaptic gutter
↓
Increased permeability of muscle cell membrane to sodium
↓
Rise in membrane potential (action potential generation)
↓
Transmission of action potential through T tubules
↓
Release of calcium from sarcoplasmic reticulum
↓
Binding of calcium with troponin–tropomyosin
↓
Sliding of actin on myosin with shortening of sarcomere unit
↓
Contraction of the muscle fiber
↓
Calcium pump moves calcium back to sarcoplasmic reticulum
↓
Unbinding of troponin–tropomyosin
↓
Inhibition of actin and myosin
↓
Lengthening of sarcomere unit
↓
Relaxation of muscle fiber

(From Bullock, B. L. (2000). *Focus on pathophysiology.* Philadelphia: Lippincott Williams & Wilkins.)

---

as an adverse reaction to certain neuromuscular junction blockers that are used to induce paralysis during surgery. (This occurs more often with succinylcholine than with other neuromuscular junction blockers [see Chapter 28].) Dantrolene is used orally as preoperative prophylaxis in susceptible patients who must undergo anesthesia and after acute episodes to prevent recurrence. The agent is also used parenterally to treat malignant hyperthermia crisis.

Botulinum toxin type B (*Myobloc*) is a newer direct acting skeletal muscle relaxant that is approved for the reduction of the severity of abnormal head position and neck pain associated with cervical dystonia. An injection of 5,000–10,000 units is given IM into the affected muscles, causing muscle relaxation and relieving the tight spasm that can distort head position and cause pain. In April, 2002, the FDA approved botulinum toxin type A (*Botox Cosmetic*), a similar drug, to improve the appearance of glabellar lines—or frown lines—between the eyebrows. Four units of the drug is injected between the eyebrows, relaxing the muscles and relieving the appearance of lines. The injection needs to be repeated every 3 months. Adverse effects associated with this use include headache, respiratory infections, flu-like syndrome and droopy eyelids, in severe cases. Pain, redness and muscle weakness were also reported. The reactions tended to be temporary, but there have been reports of reactions that lasted several months. The FDA strongly reminds providers that this is a prescription drug and should be used only under close medical supervision not just injected at the trendy *Botox* parties.

Pharmacokinetics

Dantrolene is slowly absorbed from the GI tract. It is metabolized in the liver with a half-life of 4 to 8 hours. Excretion is through the urine. Dantrolene crosses the placenta and was found to be embryotoxic in animal studies. Use should be reserved for those situations in which the benefit to the mother clearly outweighs the risk to the fetus. Dantrolene enters breast milk and is contraindicated for use during lactation. Safety for use in children younger than 5 years of age has not been established; because the long-term effects are not known, careful consideration should be given to use of the drug in children.

Contraindications and Cautions

Dantrolene is contraindicated in the presence of any known allergy to the drug. It is also contraindicated in the following conditions: spasticity that contributes to locomotion, upright position, or increased function, which would be lost if that spasticity were blocked; active hepatic disease, which might interfere with metabolism of the drug and because of known liver toxicity; and lactation, because the drug may cross into breast milk and cause adverse effects in the infant.

Caution should be used in the following circumstances: in women and in all patients older than 35 years of age, because of increased risk of potentially fatal hepatocellular disease; in patients with a history of liver disease or previous dysfunction, which could make the liver more susceptible to cellular toxicity; in those with respiratory depression, which could be exacerbated by muscular weakness; in those with

GENDER CONSIDERATIONS
Understanding the Risks of Liver Damage With Dantrolene

Dantrolene (*Dantrium*) is associated with potentially fatal hepatocellular injury. When liver damage begins to occur, patients often experience a prodrome, or warning syndrome, which includes anorexia, nausea, and fatigue. The incidence of such hepatic injury is greater in women and in patients older than 35 years of age.

In women, a combination of dantrolene and estrogen seems to affect the liver, thus posing a greater risk. Women of all ages may be at increased risk, because those entering menopause may be taking hormone replacement therapy to protect them from heart disease and osteoporosis. Patients older than 35 years of age are at increasing risk of liver injury because of the changing integrity of the liver cells that comes with age and exposure to toxins over time.

If a particular woman needs dantrolene for relief of spasticity, she should not be taking any estrogens (eg, birth control pills, hormone replacement therapy), and she should be monitored closely for any sign of liver dysfunction. For safer relief of spasticity in these patients, baclofen may be helpful.

cardiac disease, because cardiac muscle depression may be a risk; and during pregnancy, because of the potential for adverse effects on the fetus.

Adverse Effects

The most frequently seen adverse effects associated with this drug relate to drug-caused CNS depression: drowsiness, fatigue, weakness, confusion, headache and insomnia, and visual disturbances. GI disturbances may be linked to direct irritation or to alterations in smooth muscle function caused by the drug-induced calcium effects. Such adverse GI effects may include GI irritation, diarrhea, constipation, and abdominal cramps. Dantrolene may also cause direct hepatocellular damage and hepatitis that can be fatal. Urinary frequency, enuresis, and feelings of urinary urgency reportedly occur,

and crystalline urine with pain or burning on urination may result. In addition, several unusual adverse effects may occur, including acne, abnormal hair growth, rashes, photosensitivity, abnormal sweating, chills, and myalgia.

Clinically Important Drug–Drug Interactions

If dantrolene is combined with estrogens, the incidence of hepatocellular toxicity is apparently increased. If possible, this combination should be avoided.

Nursing Considerations for Patients Receiving a Direct-Acting Skeletal Muscle Relaxant
Assessment: History and Examination

Screen for the following conditions, which could be cautions or contraindications for the use of the drug: any known allergies to these drugs; cardiac depression; epilepsy; muscle weakness; respiratory depression; pregnancy and lactation; and renal or hepatic dysfunction.

Include screening for baseline status before beginning therapy and for any potential adverse effects. Assess the following: temperature; skin color and lesions; CNS orientation, affect, reflexes, bilateral grip strength, and spasticity; respiration and adventitious sounds; pulse, ECG, and cardiac output; bowel sounds and reported output; and liver and renal function tests.

Nursing Diagnoses

The patient taking a direct-acting skeletal muscle relaxant may have the following nursing diagnoses related to drug therapy:

• Acute Pain related to GI, CNS effects
• Disturbed Thought Processes related to CNS effects
• Risk for Injury related to CNS effects
• Deficient Knowledge regarding drug therapy

Implementation

• Discontinue the drug at any sign of liver dysfunction. *Early diagnosis of liver damage may prevent permanent dysfunction. Arrange for the drug to be discontinued if signs of liver damage appear.* A prodrome, with nausea, anorexia, and fa-

DRUGS IN FOCUS
Direct-Acting Skeletal Muscle Relaxant

Drug Name	Dosage/Route	Usual Indications
dantrolene (*Dantrium*)	Adult: initially 25 mg PO; increase based on spinal cord injuries; prevention and management of response to a maximum 400 mg/d for spasticity Prevention of malignant hyperthermia: 4–8 mg/kg per day PO for 1–2 d before surgery, or 2.5 mg/kg IV, over 1 h, given 1 hour before surgery; postcrisis, 4–8 mg/kg per day PO for 1–3 d Pediatric: initially 0.5 mg/kg PO b.i.d., titrate to a maximum 100 mg PO q.i.d. for spasticity; for malignant hyperthermia, follow adult dosage	Upper motor neuron–associated muscle spasticity; malignant hyperthermia

tigue, is present in 60% of patients with evidence of hepatic injury.

- Monitor intravenous access sites for potential extravasation, *because the drug is alkaline and very irritating to tissues.*
- Institute other supportive measures (eg, ventilation, anticonvulsants as needed, cooling blankets) for the treatment of malignant hyperthermia, *to support patient through the reaction.*
- Periodically discontinue the drug for 2 to 4 days *to monitor therapeutic effectiveness.* A clinical impression of exacerbation of spasticity indicates a positive therapeutic effect and justifies continued use of the drug.
- Establish a therapeutic goal before beginning oral therapy (eg, to gain or enhance the ability to engage in a therapeutic exercise program; to use braces; to accomplish transfer maneuvers) *to promote patient compliance and a sense of success with therapy.*
- Discontinue the drug if diarrhea becomes severe, *to prevent dehydration and electrolyte imbalance.* The drug may be restarted at a lower dose.
- Provide thorough patient teaching, including drug name, prescribed dosage, measures for avoidance of adverse effects, warning signs that may indicate possible problems, and the need for monitoring and evaluation *to enhance patient knowledge about drug therapy and to promote compliance.* (See Patient Teaching Checklist: Direct-Acting Skeletal Muscle Relaxant.)
- Offer support and encouragement *to help the patient cope with the drug regimen.*

Evaluation

- Monitor patient response to the drug (improvement in spasticity, improvement in movement and activities).
- Monitor for adverse effects (CNS changes, diarrhea, liver toxicity, urinary urgency).
- Evaluate the effectiveness of the teaching plan (patient can give the drug name and dosage, possible adverse effects to watch for and specific measures to prevent adverse effects, and therapeutic goals).
- Monitor the effectiveness of comfort measures and compliance with the regimen (see Nursing Care Guide: Direct-Acting Skeletal Muscle Relaxant).

CHAPTER SUMMARY

- Movement and control of muscles is regulated by spinal reflexes and influences from upper-level central nervous system areas, including the basal ganglia, cerebellum, and cerebral cortex.
- Spinal reflexes can be simple, involving an incoming sensory neuron and an outgoing motor neuron; or more complex, involving interneurons that communicate with the related centers in the brain.
- Upper-level controls of muscle activity include the pyramidal tract in the cerebellum, which regulates coordination of intentional muscle movement, and the extrapyramidal tract in the cerebellum and basal ganglia, which coordinates crude movements related to unconscious muscle activity.
- Damage to a muscle or anchoring skeletal structure may result in the arrival of a flood of impulses to the spinal cord. Such overstimulation may lead to a muscle spasm or a state of increased contraction.
- Damage to motor neurons can cause muscle spasticity, with a lack of coordination between muscle groups and loss of coordinated activity, including the ability to perform intentional tasks and maintain posture, position, and locomotion.
- Centrally acting skeletal muscle relaxants are used to relieve the effects of muscle spasm, and dantrolene, a direct-acting skeletal muscle relaxant, is used to control spasticity and prevent malignant hyperthermia.

PATIENT TEACHING CHECKLIST
Direct-Acting Skeletal Muscle Relaxant

Create customized patient teaching materials for a specific direct-acting skeletal muscle relaxant from the CD-ROM. Patient teaching should stress the following points for drugs within this class:

- Direct-acting skeletal muscle relaxants cause muscles that are clinically spastic to relax.
- Because these drugs could have serious effects on the liver, it is important that you receive regular medical evaluation.

Common effects of these drugs include

- *Fatigue, weakness, and drowsiness*—Try to space activities evenly throughout the day and allow rest periods to avoid these sometimes very discouraging side effects. If they become too severe, consult your health care provider.
- *Dizziness and fainting*—Change position slowly to avoid dizzy spells. If these effects should occur, avoid driving, operating dangerous machinery, or performing delicate tasks.
- *Diarrhea*—Be sure to be near bathroom facilities if this occurs. This effect usually subsides after a few weeks.

Report any of the following to your health care provider: fever, chills, rash, itching, changes in the color of urine or stool, or yellowish tint to the eyes or skin.

Avoid the use of alcohol or other depressants while you are taking this drug. Serious weakness and muscle depression could occur.

Tell any doctor, nurse, or other health care provider that you are taking these drugs.

Keep this drug and all other medications out of the reach of children.

Take this drug exactly as prescribed. Regular medical follow-up is necessary to evaluate the effects of this drug on your body.

This Teaching Checklist reflects general patient teaching guidelines. It is not meant to be a substitute for drug-specific teaching information, which is available in nursing drug guides.

Review Questions

1. A muscle spasm often results from
   a. damage to the basal ganglia.

NURSING CARE GUIDE

Direct-Acting Skeletal Muscle Relaxant

Assessment	Nursing Diagnoses	Implementation	Evaluation
HISTORY Allergies to any of these drugs, respiratory depression, muscle weakness, hepatic or renal dysfunction, pregnancy and lactation	Acute Pain related to GI, CNS, effects Risk for Injury related to CNS effects Disturbed Thought Processes related to CNS effects Deficient Knowledge regarding drug therapy	Discontinue drug at first sign of liver dysfunction. Provide comfort and safety measures: positioning, orientation, safety measures, pain medication as needed, monitor for extravasation, institute other measures for treatment of malignant hyperthermia. Provide support and reassurance to deal with spasticity and drug effects. Provide patient teaching concerning drug, dosage, drug effects, symptoms to report.	Evaluate drug effects: relief of spasticity, improvement in function. Monitor for adverse effects: CNS effects (multiple), respiratory depression, rash, skin changes, GI effects (diarrhea, liver toxicity), urinary urgency, weakness. Monitor for drug–drug interactions: increased depression with CNS depressant, alcohol; increased liver toxicity with estrogens. Evaluate effectiveness of patient teaching program. Evaluate effectiveness of comfort and safety measures. Periodically discontinue drug for 2–4 d to evaluate therapeutic effectiveness.
PHYSICAL EXAMINATION CV: blood pressure, pulse, peripheral perfusion, ECG CNS: orientation, affect, reflexes, grip strength Skin: color, lesions, texture, temperature GI: abdominal exam, bowel sounds Respiratory: respiration, adventitious sounds Laboratory tests: renal and liver function tests			

b. central nervous system damage.
c. injury to the musculoskeletal system.
d. chemical imbalance within the CNS.
2. Muscle spasticity is the result of
a. direct damage to a muscle cell.
b. overstretching of a muscle.
c. tearing of a ligament.
d. damage to neurons within the CNS.
3. Spasmolytics or centrally acting muscle relaxants block the reflexes in the central nervous system that lead to spasm. While a patient taking one of these drugs, other measures should also be taken, which would not include
a. rest of the affected muscle.
b. heat to the affected area.
c. ice packs to the affected area.

d. use of anti-inflammatory agents.
4. Signs and symptoms of tetanus, which includes severe muscle spasm, are best treated with
a. baclofen.
b. diazepam.
c. carisoprodol.
d. methocarbamol.
5. The drug of choice for a patient experiencing severe muscle spasms and pain precipitated by anxiety would be
a. methocarbamol.
b. baclofen.
c. diazepam.
d. carisoprodol.
6. Dantrolene (*Dantrium*) differs from the other skeletal muscle relaxants because

CASE STUDY

Dantrolene Therapy for a Patient With Cerebral Palsy

THE SITUATION

L. G., a 26-year-old man, was diagnosed with cerebral palsy shortly after birth. He is currently living in a community maintenance home with six other affected individuals under the supervision of two adult caregivers. During the past few months, his spasticity has become progressively more severe, making it impossible for him to carry on his activities of daily living without extensive assistance.

After clinical evaluation, his health care team decided to try a course of dantrolene therapy. After a discussion of the risks of hepatic dysfunction, L. G. decided that the potential benefit was much more important to him at this stage in his life than the risks of hepatotoxicity. He received a baseline complete physical examination, including analysis of liver enzymes. He started taking the drug, and a clinic staff member scheduled L. G. for a visit by a public health nurse 4 days later.

CRITICAL THINKING

• What basic principles must be included in the nursing care plan for L. G. for the visiting nurses? *Think about the importance of including the adult caregivers in any teaching or evaluation programs. Consider specific problems that could develop that L. G. would not be able to handle on his own.*
• What therapeutic goals might the nurse set with L. G. and his caregivers? How might these be evaluated?
• What additional drug-related information should be posted in the community home and reviewed with L. G. and his caregivers?

DISCUSSION

On the first visit to his home, it is important for the nurse to establish a relationship with L. G. and with his caregivers.

They should all realize that drug therapy, together with other measures, is needed to help him attain his full potential and make use of his existing assets. Step-by-step therapeutic goals should be established and written down for future reference. Small, reachable goals, such as partially dressing himself, walking to the table for meals, and managing parts of his daily hygiene routine are best at the beginning. Written goals provide a good basis for future evaluation when the drug is stopped for a few days to determine its therapeutic effectiveness. It also helps L. G. to see progress and improvement.

In addition, the nurse should perform a complete examination to obtain baseline data. The patient should be asked about any noticeable changes or problems since starting the drug. If improvement appears to have occurred, the dosage may be slowly increased until the optimal level of functioning has been achieved. The nurse is in a position to evaluate this and report it to his primary care giver.

While in the home, the nurse should evaluate resources and limitations in the patient's environment and suggest improvements (eg, use of leg braces, environmental controls). L. G. and his caregivers should receive a drug teaching card that includes a telephone number for expression of questions or concerns, highlights warning signs of liver disease, and lists findings to report. The nurse should discuss anticipated return dates for liver function testing to ensure that L. G. is able to keep the appointments. The health care team should work closely with the patient to maximize his involvement in his care and to minimize unnecessary problems and confusion. Because the treatment involves a long-term commitment, a good working relationship among all members of the health care team is important to ensure continuity of care and optimal results.

a. it acts in the highest levels of the CNS.
b. it is used to treat muscle spasms as well as muscle spasticity.
c. it cannot be used to treat neuromuscular disorders.
d. it acts directly within the skeletal muscle fiber and not within the CNS.

7. Muscle relaxants should not be used to treat spasticity
   a. that is associated with spinal cord injury.
   b. that contributes to locomotion, upright position, or increase in function.
   c. that is related to toxins, such as tetanus.
   d. that is a result of neuromuscular degeneration.

8. The use of neuromuscular junction blockers may sometimes cause a condition known as malignant hyperthermia. The drug of choice for prevention or treatment of this condition is
   a. baclofen.
   b. diazepam.
   c. dantrolene.
   d. methocarbamol.

9. Dantrolene is associated with potentially fatal cellular damage. Any patient who is taking dantrolene should
   a. have repeated CBCs during therapy.
   b. have renal function tests done monthly.
   c. be monitored for signs of liver damage and have liver function tests done regularly.
   d. have a thorough eye examination before and periodically during therapy.

BIBLIOGRAPHY

Bullock, B. L. (2000). *Focus on pathophysiology.* Philadelphia: Lippincott Williams & Wilkins.
Drug facts and comparisons. (2002.) St. Louis: Facts and Comparisons.
Gilman, A., Hardman, J. G., & Limbird, L. E. (Eds.) (2002). *Goodman and Gilman's the pharmacological basis of therapeutics* (10th ed.). New York: McGraw-Hill.
Karch, A. M. (2002). *2003 Lippincott's nursing drug guide.* Philadelphia: Lippincott Williams & Wilkins.
Professional's guide to patient drug facts. (2002). St. Louis: Facts and Comparisons.

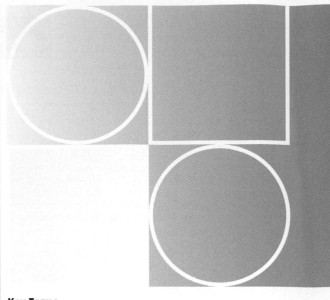

CHAPTER 26

Narcotics and Antimigraine Agents

342

Key Terms

A fibers
A-delta and C fibers
ergot derivatives
gate control theory
migraine headache
narcotics
narcotic agonists
narcotic agonists-antagonists
narcotic antagonists
opioid receptors
spinothalamic tracts
triptan

Narcotics

Narcotic Agonists
codeine
fentanyl
hydrocodone
hydromorphone
levomethadyl
levorphanol
meperidine
methadone
Ⓟ morphine
opium
oxycodone

oxymorphone
propoxyphene
remifentanil
sufentanil
Narcotic Agonists-Antagonists
buprenorphine
butorphanol
nalbuphine
Ⓟ pentazocine
Narcotic Antagonists
nalmefene
Ⓟ naloxone
naltrexone

Antimigraine Drugs

Ergot Derivatives
dihydroergotamine
Ⓟ ergotamine
methysergide
Triptans
almotriptan
frovatriptan
naratriptan
rizatriptan
Ⓟ sumatriptan
zolmitriptan

Pain, by definition, is a sensory and emotional experience associated with actual or potential tissue damage. The perception of pain is part of the clinical presentation in many disorders and is one of the hardest sensations for patients to cope with during the course of a disease or dysfunction. The drugs involved in the management of severe pain, whether acute or chronic, are discussed in this chapter. These agents all work in the central nervous system (CNS)—the brain and the spinal cord—to alter the way that pain impulses arriving from peripheral nerves are processed. These agents can change the perception and tolerance of pain. Two major types of drugs are considered here: the **narcotics,** the opium derivatives that are used to treat many types of pain, and the antimigraine drugs, which are reserved for the treatment of **migraine headaches,** a type of severe headache.

PAIN PERCEPTION

Pain occurs whenever tissues are damaged. The injury to cells releases many chemicals, including kinins and prostaglandins, which stimulate specific sensory nerves (Figure 26–1). Two small-diameter sensory nerves, called the **A-delta and C fibers,** respond to stimulation by generating nerve impulses that produce pain sensations. Pain impulses from the skin, subcutaneous tissues, muscles, and deep visceral structures are conducted to the dorsal, or posterior, horn of the spinal cord on these fibers. In the spinal cord, these nerves form synapses with spinal cord nerves that then send impulses to the brain.

In addition, large-diameter sensory nerves enter the dorsal horn of the spinal cord. These so-called **A fibers** do not transmit pain impulses; instead, they transmit sensations associated with touch and temperature. The A fibers, which are larger and conduct impulses more rapidly than the smaller fibers, can actually block the ability of the smaller fibers to transmit their signals to the secondary neurons in the spinal cord. The dorsal horn, therefore, can be both excitatory and inhibitory with pain impulses that are transmitted from the periphery.

The impulses reaching the dorsal horn are transmitted upward toward the brain by a number of specific ascending nerve pathways. These pathways run from the spinal cord into the thalamus, where they form synapses with various nerve cells that transmit the information to the cerebral cortex, along the **spinothalamic tracts.** According to the **gate control theory,** the transmission of these impulses can be modulated all along these tracts (Figure 26–2). All along the spinal cord, the interneurons can act as "gates" by blocking the ascending transmission of pain impulses. It is thought that the gates can be closed by stimulation of the larger A fibers and by descending impulses coming down the spinal cord from higher levels in such areas as the cerebral cortex, the limbic system, and the reticular activating system.

The inhibitory influence of the higher brain centers on the transmission of pain impulses helps explain much of the mystery associated with pain. Several factors, including learned experiences, cultural expectations, individual toler-

FIGURE 26–1. Neural pathways of pain. (Bullock, B. L. [2000]. *Focus on pathophysiology.* Philadelphia: Lippincott Williams & Wilkins.)

ance, and the placebo effect, can activate the descending inhibitory nerves from the upper central nervous system. Pain management usually involves the use of drugs, but it may also incorporate these other factors. The placebo effect, stress reduction, acupuncture, and back rubs (which stimulate the A fibers) all can play an important role in the effective management of pain.

Narcotics

The narcotics, or opioids, were first derived from the opium plant. Although most narcotics are now synthetically prepared, their chemical structure resembles that of the original plant alkaloids. All drugs in this class are similar in that they occupy specific **opioid receptors** in the CNS.

Opioid Receptors

These receptors respond to naturally occurring peptins, the endorphins and the enkephalins. These receptors are found

FIGURE 26–2. Gate control theory of pain. Narcotics occupy opioid receptors to block pain response. Ergot derivatives constrict cranial blood vessels, and triptans bind serotonin receptors to cause cranial vasoconstriction.

in the CNS, on nerves in the periphery, and on cells in the gastrointestinal (GI) tract. In the brainstem, opioid receptors help control blood pressure, pupil diameter, GI secretions, and the chemoreceptor trigger zone (CTZ) that regulates nausea and vomiting, cough, and respiration. In the spinal cord and thalamus, these receptors help integrate and relate incoming information about pain. In the hypothalamus, they may interrelate the endocrine and neural response to pain. In the limbic system, the receptors incorporate emotional aspects of pain and response to pain. At peripheral nerve sites, the opioids may block the release of neurotransmitters that are related to pain and inflammation.

The narcotic drugs that are used vary with the type of opioid receptors with which they react. This accounts for a change in pain relief as well as a variation in the side effects that can be anticipated. Four types of opioid receptors have been identified: mu (μ), kappa (κ), beta (β), and sigma (σ). The μ-receptors are primarily pain-blocking receptors. Besides analgesia, μ-receptors also account for respiratory depression, a feeling of euphoria, decreased GI activity, pupil constriction, and the development of physical dependence. The κ-receptors have been associated with some analgesia and with pupil constriction, sedation, and dysphoria. Enkephalins react with β-receptors in the periph-

ery to modulate pain transmission. The σ-receptors cause pupil dilation and may be responsible for the hallucinations, dysphoria, and psychoses that can occur with narcotic use.

NARCOTIC AGONISTS

The **narcotic agonists** are drugs that react with the opioid receptors throughout the body to cause analgesia, sedation, or euphoria. Anticipated effects other than analgesia are mediated by the types of opioid receptors affected by each drug. Because of the potential for the development of physical dependence while taking these drugs, the narcotic agonists are classified as controlled substances. The degree of control is determined by the relative ability of each drug to cause physical dependence. The narcotic agonists that are available are listed in Table 26–1.

Therapeutic Actions and Indications

The narcotic agonists act at specific opioid receptor sites in the CNS to produce analgesia, sedation, and a sense of well being. They are used as antitussives and as adjuncts to general anesthesia to produce rapid analgesia, sedation, and respiratory depression. Indications for narcotic agonists include relief of severe acute or chronic pain; preoperative medication; analgesia during anesthesia; and specific individual indications depending on their receptor affinity. Table 26–1 indicates the available routes for each drug, the onset and duration of action, and the degree to which the various opioid effects are stimulated by each drug. If known, the equianalgesic dosage is also given. This is the dose of each drug that would be required to achieve the same level of analgesia as the corresponding dose of the other narcotic agents.

In deciding which narcotic to use in any particular situation, it is important to consider all of these aspects and to select the drug that will be most effective in each situation with the least adverse effects for the patient. For instance, if an analgesic that is long-acting but not too sedating is desired for an outpatient, hydrocodone might fit those objectives (see Table 26–1).

Pharmacokinetics

Intravenous (IV) administration is the most reliable way to achieve therapeutic levels of narcotics. Intramuscular (IM) and subcutaneous (SC) administration offer varying rates of absorption, and absorption is slower in female than in male patients. These drugs undergo hepatic metabolism and are generally excreted in the urine and bile. Half-life periods vary widely depending on the drug being used. These agents cross the placenta and should be used during pregnancy only if the benefit to the mother clearly outweighs the potential risk to the fetus. Oxycodone is classified as Pregnancy Category B, whereas all of the other narcotic agonists are in category C, so it might be the drug of choice if one is needed during pregnancy. Extended release oxycodone (Oxycontin) has been associated with abuse because when the tablet is cut, crushed, or chewed, the entire dose of the drug is released at once. Pregnant women must be cautioned not to

DRUG THERAPY ACROSS THE LIFESPAN

Narcotics and Antimigraine Agents

Children	Adults	Older Adults
The safety and effectiveness of many of these drugs has not been established in children. If a narcotic is used, the dosage should be calculated very carefully and the child should be monitored closely for the adverse effects associated with narcotic use. Narcotics that have an established pediatric dose include codeine, fentanyl (but not transdermal fentanyl), hydrocodone, meperidine, and morphine. Narcotics that are not recommended for children are levomethadyl, levorphanol, oxymorphone, oxycodone, and propoxyphene. Methadone is not recommended as an analgesic. If a child older than 13 years of age requires a narcotic antagonist-agonist, buprenorphine is the drug of choice. Naloxone is the drug of choice for reversal of narcotic effects and narcotic overdose in children. None of the drugs used to treat migraines are recommended for use in children. The ergot derivatives can have many adverse effects in children, and the triptans do not have the clinical experience to recommend them for use in children.	Adults being treated for acute pain should be reassured that the risk of addiction to a narcotic during treatment is remote. They should be encouraged to ask for pain medication before the pain is acute, to get better coverage for their pain. Many institutions allow patients to self-regulate intravenous drips to control their own pain postoperatively. Adults requesting treatment for migraine headaches should be carefully evaluated before one of the antimigraine drugs is used to ensure that the headache being treated is of the type that can benefit from these drugs. The narcotics are contraindicated or should only be used with caution during pregnancy because of the potential for adverse effects on the fetus. These drugs enter breast milk and can cause opioid effects in the baby, so caution should be used during lactation. Morphine, meperidine, and oxymorphone are often used for analgesia during labor. The mother should be monitored closely for adverse reactions and, if the drug is used over a prolonged labor, the newborn infant should be monitored for opioid effects. The ergots and the statins are contraindicated during pregnancy because of the potential for adverse effects in the mother and fetus. Women of child-bearing age should be advised to use contraception while they are taking these drugs. Women who are nursing should be encouraged to find another method of feeding the baby because of the potential for adverse drug effects on the baby.	Elderly patients should be specifically asked whether they require pain medication. Because many older patients can recall a time when nurses were able to spend more time with patients, they may tend to believe that the nurse will meet their needs. Older patients are more likely to experience the adverse effects associated with these drugs, including central nervous system, gastrointestinal, and cardiovascular effects. Because older patients often have renal or hepatic impairment, they are also more likely to have toxic levels of the drug related to changes in metabolism and excretion. The older patient should have safety measures in effect—siderails, call light, assistance to ambulate—when receiving one of these drugs in the hospital setting.

cut, crush, or chew these tablets. The narcotics are known to enter breast milk, but there are no documented adverse effects on the baby. Many sources recommend waiting 4 to 6 hours after receiving a narcotic to feed the baby.

Contraindications and Cautions

The narcotic agonists are contraindicated in the following conditions: presence of any known allergy to any narcotic agonist; pregnancy, labor, or lactation because of potential adverse effects on the fetus or neonate, including respiratory depression; diarrhea caused by poisons, because depression of GI activity could lead to increased absorption and toxicity; and after biliary surgery or surgical anastomoses, because of the adverse effects associated with GI depression and narcotics.

Caution should be used in patients with respiratory dysfunction, which could be exacerbated by the respiratory depression caused by these drugs; recent GI or genitourinary

(GU) surgery; acute abdomen or ulcerative colitis, which could become worse with the depressive effects of the narcotics; head injuries, alcoholism, delirium tremens, or cerebral vascular disease, which could be exacerbated by the CNS effects of the drugs; and liver or renal dysfunction, which could alter the metabolism and excretion of the drugs.

Adverse Effects

The most frequently seen adverse effects associated with narcotic agonists relate to their effects on various opioid receptors. Respiratory depression with apnea, cardiac arrest, and shock may result from narcotic-caused CNS respiratory depression. Orthostatic hypotension is commonly seen with some narcotics. Such GI effects as nausea, vomiting, constipation, and biliary spasm may occur as a result of CTZ stimulation and negative effects on GI motility. Neurological effects such as lightheadedness, dizziness, psychoses, anxiety, fear, hallucina-

TABLE 26-1 Comparison of Narcotic Agonist Analgesics

Drug	Brand Name(s)	Routes	Onset	Duration	Analgesia	Sedation	Depressed Respiration	Constipation	Antitussive	Dependence	Equianalgesic Dose
codeine	—	oral, IM, IV	10–30 min	4–6 h	x	x	x	x	xx	x	PO 200 mg / IM 120 mg
fentanyl	Duragesic	oral, IM, IV, transdermal	7–8 min	1–2 h	xx	x	—	—	—	?	IM 0.1 mg / Transdermal 25 µg/h
hydrocodone	Hycodan	oral	10–20 min	4–6 h	x	—	x	—	xx	x	PO 30 mg
hydromorphone	Dilaudid	oral, SC, IM	15–30 min	4–5 h	xx	x	xx	x	xx	xx	PO 7.5 mg / IM 1.3–1.5 mg
levomethadyl	ORLAAM	oral	slow	72 h	x	x	x	x	x	x	NA
levorphanol	Levo-Dromoran	oral, SC	30–90 min	6–8 h	xx	xx	xx	xx	xx	xx	PO 4 mg / IM 2 mg
meperidine	Demerol	oral, SC, IM, IV	10–15 min	2–4 h	xx	x	xx	x	x	xx	PO 300 mg / IM 75 mg
methadone	Dolophine	oral, SC, IM	10–60 min	4–12 h	xx	x	xx	xx	xx	x	PO 10–20 mg / IM 10 mg
Ⓟ morphine	Roxanol, Astramorph	oral, PR, SC, IM, IV	20–60 min	3–7 h	xx	xx	xx	xx	xx	xx	PO 30–60 mg / IM 10 mg
opium	Paregoric	oral	varies	3–7 h	x	x	x	xx	—	x	NA
oxycodone	OxyContin	oral	15–30 min	4–6 h	xx	xx	xx	xx	xx	xx	PO 30 mg / IM 10–15 mg
oxymorphone	Numorphan	PR, SC, IM, IV	5–30 min	3–6 h	xx	—	xx	xx	x	xx	PR 5–10 mg / IM 1 mg
propoxyphene	Darvon	oral	varies	4–6 h	x	x	x	—	x	x	PO 130 mg
remifentanil	Ultiva	IV	immediate	5 min	xx	xx	xx	x	xx	—	NA
sufentanil	Sufenta	IV	immediate	5 min	xx	xx	xx	x	x	—	IM 0.01–0.04 mg

NA, not applicable.

x, effect seen.

xx, stronger effect seen.

tions, pupil constriction, and impaired mental processes may occur as a result of the stimulation of CNS opioid receptors in the cerebrum, limbic system, and hypothalamus. GU effects, including ureteral spasm, urinary retention, hesitancy, and loss of libido, may be related to direct receptor stimulation or to CNS activation of sympathetic pathways. In addition, sweating and dependence (both physical and psychological) are possible, more so with some agents than with others.

Clinically Important Drug–Drug Interactions

When narcotic agonists are given with the barbiturate general anesthetics, or with some phenothiazines and monoamine oxidase (MAO) inhibitors, the likelihood of respiratory depression, hypotension, and sedation or coma is increased. If these drug combinations cannot be avoided, patients should be monitored closely and appropriate supportive measures taken.

Nursing Considerations for Patients Receiving Narcotic Agonists

Assessment: History and Examination

Screen for the following conditions, which could be cautions or contraindications for the use of the drug: any known allergies to these drugs; pregnancy; respiratory dysfunction; GI or biliary surgery; psychoses; convulsive disorders; diarrhea caused by toxins; alcoholism or delirium tremens; and renal or hepatic dysfunction.

Include screening for baseline status before beginning therapy and for any potential adverse effects. Assess the following: CNS orientation, affect, reflexes, pupil size; respiration and adventitious sounds; pulse, blood pressure, and cardiac output; bowel sounds and reported output; bladder palpation, voiding pattern. Check liver and renal function tests, as well as electroencephalogram (EEG) and electrocardiogram (ECG) as appropriate.

Nursing Diagnoses

The patient receiving a narcotic agonist may have the following nursing diagnoses related to drug therapy:

- Acute Pain related to GI, CNS, GU effects
- Disturbed Sensory Perception (Visual, Auditory, and Kinesthetic) related to CNS effects
- Impaired Gas Exchange related to respiratory depression
- Constipation related to GI effects
- Deficient Knowledge regarding drug therapy

Implementation

- Provide a narcotic antagonist and equipment for assisted ventilation on standby during IV administration, *to support the patient in case severe reaction occurs.*
- Monitor injection sites for irritation and extravasation *in order to provide appropriate supportive care if needed.*
- Monitor timing of analgesic doses. *Prompt administration may provide a more acceptable level of analgesia and lead to quicker resolution of the pain.*
- Use extreme caution when injecting a narcotic into any

body area that is chilled or has poor perfusion or shock, *because absorption may be delayed. After repeated doses, an excessive amount is absorbed all at once.*
- Use additional measures for relief of pain, such as back rubs, stress reduction, hot packs, and ice packs, *to increase the effectiveness of the narcotic and reduce pain.*
- Reassure patients that the risk of addiction is minimal. *Most patients who receive narcotics for medical reasons do not develop dependency syndromes.*
- Provide thorough patient teaching, including drug name and prescribed dosage, measures for avoidance of adverse effects, warning signs that may indicate possible problems, and the need for monitoring and evaluation, *to enhance patient knowledge about drug therapy and to promote compliance.* (See Patient Teaching Checklist: Narcotics.)

PATIENT TEACHING CHECKLIST
Narcotics

Create customized patient teaching materials for a specific narcotic from the CD-ROM. Patient teaching should stress the following points for drugs within this class:

- A narcotic is used to relieve pain. Do not hesitate to take this drug if you feel uncomfortable. It is important to use the drug before the pain becomes severe and thus more difficult to treat.

  Common effects of these drugs include

- *Constipation*—Your health care provider will suggest an appropriate bowel program to alleviate this common problem.
- *Dizziness, drowsiness, and visual changes*—If any of these occur, avoid driving, operating dangerous machinery, or performing delicate tasks. If these effects occur in the hospital, the siderails on the bed may be put up for your own protection
- *Nausea and loss of appetite*—Taking the drug with food may help. Lying quietly until these sensations pass may also help alleviate this problem.

  Report any of the following to your health care provider: severe nausea or vomiting, skin rash, or shortness of breath or difficulty breathing.
  Avoid the use of alcohol, antihistamines, and other over-the-counter drugs while taking this drug. Many of these drugs could interact with this narcotic.
  Tell any doctor, nurse, or other health care provider that you are taking this drug.
  Keep this drug and all medications out of the reach of children.
  Do not take any leftover medication for other disorders, and do not let anyone else take your medication.
  Take this drug exactly as prescribed. Regular medical follow-up is necessary to evaluate the effects of this drug on your body.

This Teaching Checklist reflects general patient teaching guidelines. It is not meant to be a substitute for drug-specific teaching information, which is available in nursing drug guides.

DRUGS IN FOCUS
Narcotic Agonists

Drug Name	Dosage/Route	Usual Indications
codeine	Adult: 15–60 mg PO, IM, IV, or SC q4–6h; 10–20 mg PO q4–6h for cough Pediatric: 0.5 mg/kg PO, IM, or SC q4–6h; 2.5–10 mg PO q4–6h for cough	Relief of mild to moderate pain; coughing induced by mechanical or chemical irritation of the respiratory tract
fentanyl (*Duragesic*)	Adult: 0.05–0.1 mg IM, 30–60 min before surgery; 0.002 mg/kg IV or IM during surgery; 0.05–0.1 mg postoperatively; 5 µg/kg transmucosal; for transdermal patch, calculate the previous day's narcotics need and use table to convert to patch strength Pediatric (>2 y): 2–3 µg/kg IM or IV; base transmucosal dose on weight and do not exceed 400 µg	For analgesia before, during, and after surgery; transdermal patch for management of chronic pain
hydrocodone (*Hycodan*)	Adult: 5–10 mg PO q4h in combination products for pain: 5–10 mg PO q4–6h for cough Pediatric (2–12 y): 1.25–5 mg PO q4–6h	Relief of cough; relief of moderate pain in combination products
hydromorphone (*Dilaudid*)	2–4 mg PO q4–6h *or* 3 mg PR q6–8h *or* 1–4 mg SC or IM q4–6h	Relief of moderate to severe pain in adults
levomethadyl (*ORLAAM*)	20–40 mg PO initially, then 60–90 mg PO three times a week for maintenance	Management of opiate dependence in adults
levorphanol (*Levo-Dromoran*)	1 mg IV by slow injection *or* 1–2 mg IM or SC q6–8h *or* 2 mg PO q6–8h	Management of moderate to severe pain in adults; postoperative pain in adults
meperidine (*Demerol*)	Adult: 50–150 mg PO IM, or SC q3–4h; during labor, 100 mg IM or SC q1–3h Pediatric: 1–1.8 mg/kg IM, SC, or PO q3–4h	Relief of moderate to severe pain, preoperative analgesia and support of anesthesia, and obstetrical analgesia
methadone (*Dolophine*)	2.5–10 mg IM, SC, or PO q3–4h for pain; 15–20 mg PO for withdrawal, then 20 mg PO q4–8h for maintenance treatment	Relief of severe pain; detoxification and temporary maintenance treatment of narcotic addiction in adults
morphine (*Roxanol, Astramorph*)	Adult: 10–20 mg solution PO or 15–30 mg tablets PO q4h *or* 10 mg SC or IM q4h *or* 2.5–15 mg/70kg IV over 4–5 min *or* 10–20 mg PR q4h Pediatric: 0.05–0.2 mg/kg IM or SC q4h	Relief of moderate to severe chronic and acute pain; preoperatively and postoperatively and during labor
opium (*Paregoric*)	Adult: 0.6 mL liquid PO q.i.d. *or* 5–10 mL camphorated tincture one to four times per day PO Pediatric: 0.005–0.02 mg/kg PO q3–4h *or* 0.25–0.5 mL/kg PO q.d.–q.i.d. of camphorated tincture	Treatment of diarrhea, relief of moderate pain
oxycodone (*OxyContin*)	10–30 mg PO q4h as needed	Relief of moderate to severe pain in adults
oxymorphone (*Numorphan*)	0.5 mg IV initially; 1–1.5 mg IM or SC q4–6h as needed; 0.5–1 mg IM for labor; 5 mg PR q4–6h	Relief of moderate to severe pain in adults; preoperative medication; obstetrical analgesia
propoxyphene (*Darvon, Darvon-N*)	65 mg PO q4h as needed; *Darvon N*—100 mg PO q4h as needed	Relief of mild to moderate pain in adults **Special considerations:** limit use in suicidal or addiction-prone patients
remifentanil (*Ultiva*)	Adult and children >2 y: dosage determined by general anesthetic being used	Analgesic for use during general anesthesia **Special considerations:** must be under the direct supervision of anesthesia practitioner
sufentanil (*Sufental*)	Adult: 1–2 µg/kg IV with general anesthesia Pediatric: 10–25 µg/kg IV	Analgesic for use during general anesthesia; used as an epidural agent in labor and delivery **Special considerations:** must be under the direct supervision of anesthesia practitioner

- Offer support and encouragement *to help the patient cope with the drug regimen.*

Evaluation

- Monitor patient response to the drug (relief of pain, cough suppression, sedation).
- Monitor for adverse effects (CNS changes, GI depression, respiratory depression, constipation).
- Evaluate the effectiveness of the teaching plan (patient can give the drug name and dosage and describe possible adverse effects to watch for, specific measures to prevent adverse effects, and warning signs to report).
- Monitor the effectiveness of comfort measures and compliance with the regimen (see Nursing Care Guide: Narcotic Agonists).

NARCOTIC AGONISTS-ANTAGONISTS

The **narcotic agonists-antagonists** stimulate certain opioid receptors but block other such receptors. These drugs, which have less abuse potential than the pure narcotic agonists, all have about the same analgesic effect as morphine. Like morphine, they may cause sedation, respiratory depression, and constipation. They have also been associated with more psychotic-like reactions, and they may even induce a withdrawal syndrome in patients who have been taking narcotics for a long period.

Available narcotic agonists-antagonists include the following:

- Buprenorphine (*Buprenex*), which is recommended for treatment of mild to moderate pain; it is available for use in IM and IV forms.

NURSING CARE GUIDE

Narcotic Agonists

Assessment	Nursing Diagnoses	Implementation	Evaluation
HISTORY Allergies to any of these drugs, respiratory depression, GI or biliary surgery, hepatic or renal dysfunction, pregnancy and lactation, alcoholism, convulsive disorders	Acute Pain related to GI, CNS, GU effects Disturbed Sensory Perceptions (Visual, Auditory, Kinesthetic) related to CNS effects Impaired Gas Exchange related to respiratory depression Deficient Knowledge regarding drug therapy Constipation	Provide a narcotic antagonist, facilities for assisted ventilation during IV administration. Provide comfort and safety measures: orientation, safety measures, accurate timing of doses, monitor for extravasation, use additional measures for pain relief to increase effects. Provide support and reassurance to deal with drug effects, addiction potential. Provide patient teaching about drug, dosage, drug effects, symptoms to report.	Evaluate drug effects: relief of pain, sedation, cough suppression. Monitor for adverse effects: CNS effects (multiple), respiratory depression, rash, skin changes, GI depression, constipation. Monitor drug–drug interactions: increased respiratory depression, sedation, coma with barbiturate anesthetics, monoamine oxidase inhibitors, phenothiazines. Evaluate effectiveness of patient teaching program. Evaluate effectiveness of comfort and safety measures.
PHYSICAL EXAMINATION CV: blood pressure, pulse, peripheral perfusion, ECG CNS: orientation, affect, reflexes, grip strength Skin: color, lesions, texture, temperature GI: abdominal examination, bowel sounds Respiratory: respiration, adventitious sounds Laboratory tests: renal and liver function tests			

- Butorphanol (*Stadol, Stadol NS*), which is used as a preoperative medication to relieve moderate to severe pain. This drug is formulated in IM and IV preparations and as a nasal spray. It is effective in the treatment of migraine headaches, with fewer peripheral adverse effects than many of the traditional antimigraine drugs.
- Nalbuphine (*Nubain*), which is used to treat moderate to severe pain, as an adjunct for general anesthesia, and to relieve pain during labor and delivery. This drug, which is formulated in SC, IM, and IV preparations, should not be given to patients who are allergic to sulfites.
- Pentazocine (*Talwin*), which is also available in an oral form, making it the preferred drug for patients who will be switched from parenteral to oral forms after surgery or labor. This drug has been abused in combination with tripelennamine ("Ts and Blues") because of an hallucino-

genic, euphoric effect of the two drugs, with potentially fatal complications.

Therapeutic Actions and Indications

The narcotic agonists-antagonists act at specific opioid receptor sites in the CNS to produce analgesia, sedation, euphoria, and hallucinations. In addition, they block opioid receptors that may be stimulated by other narcotics. These drugs have three functions: (1) relief of moderate to severe pain, (2) adjuncts to general anesthesia, and (3) relief of pain during labor and delivery.

Pharmacokinetics

These drugs are readily absorbed after IM administration and reach rapid peak levels when given intravenously. They are metabolized in the liver and are excreted in urine or feces. They are known to cross the placenta, but no adequate studies are available regarding their effects during preg-

CASE STUDY

Using Morphine to Relieve Pain

THE SITUATION

L. M., a 25-year-old businessman, was in a serious automobile accident and suffered a fractured pelvis, a fractured left tibia, a fractured right humerus, and multiple contusions and abrasions. For the first 2 days after surgery to reduce the fractures, L. M. was heavily sedated. As healing progressed, he was given intramuscular injections of morphine every 4 hours as needed for pain. L. M. requested medication every 2 to 3 hours and became very agitated by the end of the prescribed 4 hours. L. M.'s physician decided to switch him to meperidine given intramuscularly every 3 hours for 2 days and then to oral dosage in an attempt to wean him from the narcotics.

CRITICAL THINKING

What basic principles must be included in the nursing care plan for this patient? *Think about the difficult position the floor nurse is in when L. M. begins demanding pain relief before the prescribed time limit.*

What implications will his agitation have on the way that the staff responds to him and on other patients in the area?

What other nursing measures could be used to help relieve pain and make the narcotic more effective?

What plans could the health team make with L. M. to give him more control over his situation and increase the chances that the pain relief will be effective?

DISCUSSION

In assessing L. M.'s response to drug therapy, it is apparent that the morphine was not providing the desired therapeutic effect. Numerous research studies have shown that, in general, the dosage of narcotics prescribed for acute pain relief provides inadequate analgesic coverage. It could be that the dose of morphine ordered for L. M. is just not sufficient to relieve his pain. This patient

has many causes of acute pain and will heal more quickly if the pain is managed better. He has requested more drugs because the dosage is too small or the intervals between doses are too long to effectively relieve his pain. Intravenous morphine could be added to complement his pain management. Other measures may be successful in helping the morphine relieve the pain; back rubs, environmental controls to decrease excessive stimuli (eg, noise, lighting, temperature, interruptions), and stress reduction may all be useful.

L. M. may be very anxious about his injuries, and the opportunity to ventilate his feelings and concerns may alleviate some of the tension associated with pain. He may fear that if he does not request the medication early, he will not get it by the prescribed time. The nursing staff can work on this concern and figure out a way to reassure him that the medication will be delivered on time. Changing from morphine to meperidine may improve the analgesic effects, partly because of a placebo reaction that may occur when he is told that this drug will be more effective and partly because people respond differently to different narcotics.

The health care team should try to discuss the concerns with L. M., including the concern about the physical dependence. L. M. is a businessman and may respond positively to having some input into his care; he may even offer suggestions as to how he could cope better and adjust to his situation. Cortical impulses can close gates as effectively as descending inhibitory pathways, and stimulation of the cortical pathways through patient education and active involvement should be considered an important aspect of pain relief. Because L. M.'s injuries are extensive, a long-term approach should be taken to his care. The sooner that L. M. can be involved, the better the situation will be for everyone involved.

nancy. They should be used during pregnancy only if the benefit to the mother clearly outweighs the risk to the fetus. They are used to relieve pain during labor, which provides a short-term exposure to the fetus. They are known to enter breast milk and should be used with caution during lactation because of the potential for adverse effects on the baby.

Contraindications and Cautions

Narcotic agonists-antagonists are contraindicated in the presence of any known allergy to any narcotic agonist-antagonist and during pregnancy and lactation because of potential adverse effects on the neonate, including respiratory depression. (However, these drugs may be used to relieve pain during labor and delivery.)

Caution should be used in cases of physical dependence on a narcotic, because a withdrawal syndrome may be precipitated; the narcotic antagonistic properties can block the analgesic effect and intensify the pain. Narcotic agonists-antagonists may be desirable for relieving chronic pain in patients who are susceptible to narcotic dependence, but extreme care must be used if patients are switched directly from a narcotic agonist to one of these drugs.

Caution should also be exercised in the following conditions: chronic obstructive pulmonary disease or other respiratory dysfunction, which could be exacerbated by respiratory depression; acute myocardial infarction (MI), documented coronary artery disease (CAD), or hypertension that could be exacerbated by cardiac stimulatory effects of these drugs; and renal or hepatic dysfunction that could interfere with the metabolism and excretion of the drug.

Pentazocine also may cause cardiac stimulation including arrhythmias, hypertension, and increased myocardial oxygen consumption, which could lead to angina, MI, or congestive heart failure. Care must be taken in patients with known heart disease.

Adverse Effects

The most frequently seen adverse effects associated with narcotic agonists-antagonists relate to their effects on various opioid receptors. Respiratory depression with apnea and suppression of the cough reflex is associated with the respiratory depression caused by the narcotics. Nausea, vomiting, constipation, and biliary spasm may occur as a result of CTZ stimulation and the negative effects on GI motility. Lightheadedness, dizziness, psychoses, anxiety, fear, hallucinations, and impaired mental processes may occur as a result of the stimulation of CNS opioid receptors in the cerebrum, limbic system, and hypothalamus. GU effects, including ureteral spasm, urinary retention, hesitancy, and loss of libido, may be related to direct receptor stimulation or to CNS activation of sympathetic pathways. Although sweating and dependence, both physical and psychological, are possible, their occurrence is considered less likely than with narcotic agonists.

Clinically Important Drug–Drug Interactions

When narcotic agonists-antagonists, like narcotic agonists, are given with barbiturate general anesthetics, the likelihood of respiratory depression, hypotension, and sedation or coma increases. If this combination cannot be avoided, patients should be monitored closely and appropriate supportive measures taken.

Use of narcotic agonists-antagonists in patients who have previously received narcotics puts these patients at risk. When such a sequence of drugs is used, patients require support and monitoring.

DRUGS IN FOCUS
Narcotic Agonists-Antagonists

Drug Name	Dosage/Route	Usual Indications
buprenorphine (*Buprenex*)	Adults and children >13 y: 0.3 mg IM or slow IV q6h as needed	Mild to moderate pain
butorphanol (*Stadol*)	Adult: 0.5–2 mg IV q3–4h *or* 1–4 mg IM q3–4h; 1 mg nasal spray, repeated in 60–90 minutes, then in 3–4h as needed. Geriatric: use one half of the adult dose at twice the usual interval. Pediatric: not recommended for children <18 y	Preoperative medication, moderate to severe pain, migraine headache
nalbuphine (*Nubain*)	10 mg/70 kg IM, SC, or IV q3–6h as needed, do not exceed 160 mg/d	Labor and delivery, adjunct to general anesthesia, moderate to severe pain in adults
℗ pentazocine (*Talwin*)	Adults and children >12 y: 30 mg IM, SC, or IV q3–4h as needed or 50mg PO q3–4h as needed do not exceed 360 mg/d; 30 mg IM most common for labor	Moderate to severe pain, labor and delivery, postpartum pain, adjunct to general anesthesia

Nursing Considerations for Patients Receiving Narcotic Agonists-Antagonists

Assessment: History and Examination

Screen for the following conditions, which could be cautions or contraindications for the use of the drug: any known allergies to these drugs or to sulfites if using nalbuphine; pregnancy or lactation; respiratory dysfunction; MI or CAD; and renal or hepatic dysfunction.

Include screening for baseline status before beginning therapy and for any potential adverse effects. Assess the following: CNS orientation, affect, reflexes, and pupil size; respiration and adventitious sounds; pulse, blood pressure, and cardiac output; bowel sounds and reported output; and liver and renal function tests as well as ECG.

Nursing Diagnoses

The patient receiving a narcotic agonist-antagonist may have the following nursing diagnoses related to drug therapy:

- Acute Pain related to GI, CNS effects
- Disturbed Sensory Perception (Visual, Auditory, Kinesthetic) related to CNS effects
- Impaired Gas Exchange related to respiratory depression
- Deficient Knowledge regarding drug therapy

Implementation

- Provide a narcotic antagonist and equipment for assisted ventilation on standby during IV administration, *to provide patient support in case of severe reaction.*
- Monitor injection sites for irritation and extravasation, in order *to provide appropriate supportive care if needed.*
- Monitor timing of analgesic doses. *Prompt administration may provide a more acceptable level of analgesia and lead to quicker resolution of the pain.*
- Use extreme caution when injecting these drugs into any body area that is chilled or has poor perfusion or shock, *because absorption may be delayed, and after repeated doses an excessive amount is absorbed all at once.*
- Use additional measures to relieve pain (eg, back rubs, stress reduction, hot packs, ice packs) *to increase the effectiveness of the narcotic being given and reduce pain.*
- Institute comfort and safety measures, such as siderails and assistance with ambulation, *to ensure patient safety;* bowel program as needed *to treat constipation;* environmental controls *to decrease stimulation;* and small, frequent meals *to relieve GI distress if GI upset is severe.*
- Reassure patients that the risk of addiction is minimal. *Most patients who receive these drugs for medical reasons do not develop dependency syndromes.*
- Provide thorough patient teaching, including drug name and prescribed dosage, as well as measures for avoidance of adverse effects, warning signs that may indicate possible problems, and the need for monitoring and evaluation, *to enhance patient knowledge about drug therapy and to promote compliance.* (See Patient Teaching Checklist: Narcotics.)

- Offer support and encouragement *to help the patient cope with the drug regimen.*

Evaluation

- Monitor patient response to the drug (relief of pain, sedation).
- Monitor for adverse effects (CNS changes, GI depression, respiratory depression, arrhythmias, hypertension).
- Evaluate the effectiveness of the teaching plan (patient can give the drug name and dosage and describe possible adverse effects to watch for, specific measures to prevent adverse effects, and warning signs to report).
- Monitor the effectiveness of comfort measures and compliance with the regimen.

NARCOTIC ANTAGONISTS

The **narcotic antagonists** are drugs that bind strongly to opioid receptors, but they do not activate the receptors. These agents are useful in blocking unwanted adverse effects associated with narcotics, such as respiratory depression, and they play a role in the treatment of narcotic overdose. These drugs do not have an appreciable effect in most people, but individuals who are addicted to narcotics experience the signs and symptoms of withdrawal when rapidly receiving these drugs.

The narcotic antagonists in use today include the following:

- Nalmefene (*Revex*), which can be given by the IV, IM, or SC route to reverse the effects of narcotics and to manage known or suspected narcotic overdose.

CULTURAL CONSIDERATIONS
Differences in Responses to Narcotic Therapy

Because of physical and cultural differences among various ethnic groups, patients from certain groups respond differently to particular medications. Nurses should keep in mind that patients in some ethnic groups are genetically predisposed to metabolize medications differently. For example, Arab Americans may not achieve the same pain relief from narcotics as patients in other ethnic groups; their inborn differences in metabolism may require larger doses to achieve therapeutic effects.

Some African American patients seem to have a decreased sensitivity to the pain-relieving qualities of some narcotics, although the reason for this is unknown. Moreover, increasing the dosage of these medications may not increase the level of pain relief and actually may be toxic. In such cases, another class of medication might be used to "boost" the pain-relieving qualities of the narcotic.

Among some immigrant and first-generation Asian Americans, it may not be socially acceptable to show strong emotion, such as that associated with pain. The sensitive nurse will frequently ask such patients if they are comfortable or require additional medication.

• Naloxone (*Narcan*) which is used IV, IM, or SC to reverse adverse effects of narcotics and to diagnose suspected acute narcotic overdose.

• Naltrexone (*ReVia*), which is used orally in the management of alcohol or narcotic dependence as part of a comprehensive treatment program.

Therapeutic Actions and Indications

The narcotic antagonists block opioid receptors and reverse the effects of opioids, including respiratory depression, sedation, psychomimetic effects, and hypotension. Their effects are seen in people who have been using narcotics or are dependent on narcotics.

These agents are indicated for reversal of the adverse effects of narcotic use, including respiratory depression and sedation, and for treatment of narcotic overdose. Naloxone is used to diagnose narcotic overdose (the naloxone challenge), and naltrexone is used as part of a comprehensive program to treat narcotic and/or alcoholic dependence.

Pharmacokinetics

These agents are well absorbed after injection and are widely distributed in the body. They undergo hepatic metabolism and are excreted primarily in the urine. There are no well controlled studies during pregnancy, so they should be used during pregnancy only if the benefit to the mother clearly outweighs any potential risk to the fetus. They enter breast milk and should be used with caution during lactation because of the potential adverse effects on the baby.

Contraindications and Cautions

Narcotic antagonists are contraindicated in the presence of any known allergy to any narcotic antagonist. Caution should be used in the following circumstances: during pregnancy and lactation, because of potential adverse effects on the fetus and neonate; with narcotic addiction, because of the

precipitation of a withdrawal syndrome; and with cardiovascular (CV) disease, which could be exacerbated by the reversal of the depressive effects of narcotics.

Adverse Effects

The most frequently seen adverse effects associated with these drugs relate to the blocking effects of the opioid receptors. The most common effect is an acute narcotic abstinence syndrome that is characterized by nausea, vomiting, sweating, tachycardia, hypertension, tremulousness, and feelings of anxiety. CNS excitement and reversal of analgesia is especially common postoperatively. CV effects related to the reversal of the opioid depression can include tachycardia, blood pressure changes, arrhythmias, and pulmonary edema.

Nursing Considerations for Patients Receiving Narcotic Antagonists

Assessment: History and Examination

Screen for the following conditions, which could be cautions or contraindications to the use of the drug: any known allergies to these drugs; pregnancy and lactation; MI or CAD; and narcotic addiction.

Include screening for baseline status before beginning therapy and for any potential adverse effects. Assess the following: CNS orientation, affect, reflexes, and pupil size; respiration and adventitious sounds; pulse, blood pressure, and cardiac output; and ECG.

Nursing Diagnoses

The patient receiving a narcotic antagonist may have the following nursing diagnoses related to drug therapy:

• Acute Pain related to withdrawal, CV effects
• Decreased Cardiac Output related to CV effects
• Deficient Knowledge regarding drug therapy

DRUGS IN FOCUS
Narcotic Antagonists

Drug Name	Dosage/Route	Usual Indications
nalmefene (*Revex*)	Adult: for reversal of postoperative opioid depression, 0.25 μg/kg IV q2–5 min until desired reversal is obtained; for management of overdose, 0.5 mg/70 kg IV, then 1 mg IV 2–5 min later, reduce dosage in renal and hepatic disease	Reversal of opioid effects, management of narcotic overdose
Ⓟ naloxone (*Narcan*)	Adult: for overdose, 0.4–2 mg IV, may repeat at 2–3 min intervals; for reversal of opioid effects, 0.1–0.2 mg IV, may repeat at 2–3 min intervals Pediatric: for overdose, 0.01 mg/kg IV, repeat as needed; for reversal of opioid effects, 0.005–0.01 mg IV at 2–3 min intervals	Diagnosis of narcotic overdose, reversal of opioid effects
naltrexone (*ReVia, Depade*)	Adult: 50 mg/d PO	Adjunct treatment of alcohol or narcotic dependence in adults

Implementation

- Maintain open airway and provide artificial ventilation and cardiac massage *as needed to support the patient. Administer vasopressors as needed to manage narcotic overdose.*
- Administer naloxone challenge before giving naltrexone, *because of the serious risk of acute withdrawal.*
- Monitor the patient continually, *adjusting the dosage as needed, during treatment of acute overdose.*
- Provide comfort and safety measures *to help the patient cope with the withdrawal syndrome.*
- Ensure that patients receiving naltrexone have been narcotic free for 7 to 10 days, *to prevent severe withdrawal syndrome. Check urine opioid levels if there is any question.*
- If the patient is receiving naltrexone as part of a comprehensive narcotic or alcohol withdrawal program, the patient should be advised to wear or carry a Medic-Alert warning *so that medical personnel know how to treat the patient in an emergency.*
- Institute comfort and safety measures, such as siderails and assistance with ambulation, *to ensure patient safety;* institute bowel program as needed *for treatment of constipation;* use environmental controls *to decrease stimulation;* and provide, small frequent meals *to relieve GI irritation if GI upset is severe.*
- Provide thorough patient teaching, including drug name and prescribed dosage, as well as measures for avoidance of adverse effects, warning signs that may indicate possible problems, and the need for monitoring and evaluation *to enhance patient knowledge about drug therapy and to promote compliance.* (See Patient Teaching Checklist: Narcotics.)
- Offer support and encouragement *to help the patient cope with the drug regimen.*

Evaluation

- Monitor patient response to the drug (reversal of opioid effects, treatment of alcohol dependence).
- Monitor for adverse effects (CV changes, arrhythmias, hypertension).
- Evaluate the effectiveness of the teaching plan (patient can give the drug name and dosage and describe possible adverse effects to watch for, specific measures to prevent adverse effects, and warning signs to report).
- Monitor the effectiveness of comfort measures and compliance with the regimen.

MIGRAINE HEADACHES AND THEIR TREATMENT

The term *migraine headache* is used to describe several different syndromes, all of which include severe, throbbing headaches on one side of the head. This pain can be so severe that it can cause widespread disturbance, affecting GI and CNS function, including mood and personality changes.

Migraine headaches should be distinguished from cluster headaches and tension headaches. Cluster headaches usually begin during sleep and involve sharp, steady eye pain that lasts 15 to 90 minutes with sweating, flushing, tearing, and nasal congestion. Tension headaches, which usually occur at times of stress, feel like a dull band of pain around the entire head and last from 30 minutes to 1 week. They are accompanied by anorexia, fatigue, and a mild intolerance to light or sound.

There are at least two types of migraine headaches. Common migraines, which occur without an aura, cause severe, unilateral, pulsating pain that is frequently accompanied by nausea, vomiting, and sensitivity to light and sound. Such migraine headaches are often aggravated by physical activity. Classic migraines are usually preceded by an aura, or a sensation involving sensory or motor disturbances, that usually occurs about one-half hour before the pain begins. The pain and adverse effects are the same as those of the common migraine.

It is believed that the underlying cause of migraine headaches is arterial dilation. Headaches accompanied by an aura are associated with a hypoperfusion of the brain during the aura stage, followed by reflex arterial dilation and a hyperperfusion. The underlying cause and continued state of arterial dilation are not clearly understood, but they may be related to the release of bradykinins, serotonin, or a response to other hormones and chemicals.

For many years, the one standard treatment for migraine headaches was acute analgesia, often involving a narcotic, together with control of lighting and sound and the use of **ergot derivatives.** In the late 1990s, a new class of drugs, the triptans, was found to be extremely effective in treating migraine headaches without the adverse effects associated with ergot derivative use.

ERGOT DERIVATIVES

The ergot derivatives cause constriction of cranial blood vessels and decrease the pulsation of cranial arteries. As a result, they reduce the hyperperfusion of the basilar artery vascular bed. Because these agents are associated with many systemic adverse effects, their usefulness is limited in some patients.

Available ergot derivatives include the following:

- Dihydroergotamine (*Migranal*), which can be used in the IM or IV form or as a nasal spray to provide rapid relief from migraine headache. This agent is the drug of choice if the oral route of administration is not possible.
- Ergotamine (generic), the prototype drug in this class, was the mainstay of migraine headache treatment before the triptans became available. This agent is administered sublingually for rapid absorption. *Cafergot,* the very popular oral form, combines ergotamine with caffeine to increase its absorption from the GI tract.
- Methysergide (*Sansert*), which is not used for acute attacks but to prevent attacks or to decrease the intensity and frequency of attacks. It is an oral drug with a very slow onset and long duration of action.

GENDER CONSIDERATIONS
Headache Distribution

Headaches are distributed in the general population in a definite gender-related pattern. For example:

- Migraine headaches are three times more likely to occur in women than men.
- Cluster headaches are more likely to occur in men than in women.
- Tension headaches are more likely to occur in women than in men.

There is some speculation that the female predisposition to migraine headaches may be related to the vascular sensitivity to hormones. Some women can directly plot migraine occurrence to periods of fluctuations in their menstrual cycle. The introduction of the triptan class of antimigraine drugs has been beneficial for many of these women.

Therapeutic Actions and Indications

The ergot derivatives block α-adrenergic and serotonin receptor sites in the brain to cause a constriction of cranial vessels, a decrease in cranial artery pulsation, and a decrease in the hyperperfusion of the basil artery bed. These drugs are indicated for the prevention or abortion of migraine or vascular headaches. Methysergide is indicated only for the prevention of vascular headaches.

Pharmacokinetics

The ergot derivatives are rapidly absorbed from many routes, with an onset of action ranging from 15 to 30 minutes. They are metabolized in the liver and primarily excreted in the bile. These drugs cannot be used during pregnancy because they cause serious adverse effects on the fetus and can have oxytocic effects on the mother. They are excreted in breast milk and can cause vomiting and diarrhea in the baby, so they should be used with extreme caution in nursing mothers.

Contraindications and Cautions

Ergot derivatives are contraindicated in the following circumstances: presence of allergy to ergot preparations; CAD, hypertension, or peripheral vascular disease, which could be exacerbated by the CV effects of these drugs; impaired liver function, which could alter the metabolism and excretion of these drugs; and pregnancy or lactation, because of the potential for adverse effects on the fetus and neonate—ergotism (vomiting, diarrhea, seizures) has been reported in affected infants.

Caution should be used in two instances: with pruritus, which could become worse with drug-induced vascular constriction; and with malnutrition, because ergot derivatives stimulate the CTZ and can cause severe GI reactions, possibly worsening malnutrition.

Adverse Effects

The adverse effects of ergot derivatives can be related to the drug-induced vascular constriction. CNS effects include numbness, tingling of extremities, and muscle pain; CV effects such as pulselessness, weakness, chest pain, arrhythmias, localized edema and itching, and MI may also occur. In addition, the direct stimulation of the CTZ can cause GI upset, nausea, vomiting, and diarrhea. Ergotism, a syndrome associated with the use of these drugs, causes nausea, vomiting, severe thirst, hypoperfusion, chest pain, blood pressure changes, confusion, drug dependency (with prolonged use), and a drug withdrawal syndrome.

Clinically Important Drug–Drug Interactions

If these drugs are combined with β-blockers, the risk of peripheral ischemia and gangrene is increased. Such combinations should be avoided.

DRUGS IN FOCUS
Antimigraine Ergots

Drug Name	Dosage/Route	Usual Indications
dihydroergotamine (*Migranal, D.H.E. 45*)	1 spray (0.5 mg) in each nostril, may repeat in 15 min for a total of four sprays *or* 1 mg IM at first sign of headache, repeat in 1 h for a total of 3 mg *or* 2 mg IV, do not exceed 6 mg/wk	Rapid treatment of acute attacks of migraines in adults
Ⓟ ergotamine (generic)	1 tablet SL at the first sign of headache, repeat at 30-min intervals for a total of three tablets *or* 1 inhalation at first sign of headache, repeat in 5 min to a total of 6 inhalations per day	Prevention and abortion of migraine attacks in adults
methysergide (*Sansert*)	4–8 mg PO q.d. with meals	Prophylaxis of migraines for adults

Nursing Considerations for Patients Receiving Ergot Derivatives

Assessment: History and Examination

Screen for the following conditions, which could be cautions or contraindications to the use of the drug: any known allergies to ergot derivatives; pregnancy or lactation; MI, CAD, or hypertension; impaired renal or hepatic function; pruritus; and malnutrition.

Include screening for baseline status before beginning therapy and for any potential adverse effects. Assess the following: temperature; skin color, and lesions; CNS orientation, affect, and reflexes; respiration and adventitious sounds; pulse, blood pressure, and cardiac output; ECG and liver and renal function tests.

Nursing Diagnoses

The patient receiving an ergot derivative may have the following nursing diagnoses related to drug therapy:

- Acute Pain related to GI, vasoconstrictive effects
- Decreased Cardiac Output related to CV effects
- High Risk for Injury related to loss of peripheral sensation
- Deficient Knowledge regarding drug therapy

Implementation

- Avoid prolonged use or excessive dosage, *to prevent severe adverse effects.*
- Arrange for the use of atropine or phenothiazines if nausea and vomiting are severe, *because these are the appropriate drugs to relieve nausea and vomiting.*
- Provide comfort and safety measures, such as environmental controls and stress reduction, *for the prevention of headache and to provide additional pain relief as needed.*
- Assess extremities carefully to ensure that no decubitus ulcer or gangrene is present *when using drugs that cause peripheral vasoconstriction, which could further aggravate these conditions.*
- Provide supportive measures *to ensure patient safety if acute overdose should occur.*
- Provide thorough patient teaching, including drug name and prescribed dosage, as well as measures for avoidance of adverse effects, warning signs that may indicate possible problems, and the need for monitoring and evaluation, *to enhance patient knowledge about drug therapy and to promote compliance.*
- Offer support and encouragement *to help the patient cope with the drug regimen.*

Evaluation

- Monitor patient response to the drug (prevention or abortion of migraine headaches).
- Monitor for adverse effects (CV changes, arrhythmias, hypertension, peripheral vasoconstriction).

- Evaluate the effectiveness of the teaching plan (patient can give the drug name and dosage and describe possible adverse effects to watch for, specific measures to prevent adverse effects, and warning signs to report).
- Monitor the effectiveness of comfort measures and compliance with the regimen.

◼◼◉◼ WEB LINKS

Health care providers and patients may want to consult the following Internet sources:

Information on pain, physiology, and management:
  http://www.ampainsoc.org
Information on education programs, research, other information related to pain management:
  http://www.aapainmanage.org
Information on chronic pain and the use of narcotics:
  http://www.mayohealth.org
Information on migraines—support groups, treatment, and research:
  www.nih.gov/health
Information for patients and families on migraine headaches—understanding them, treatments, support groups:
  http://www.geocities.com/HotSprings/Spa/7379/migraine.html

TRIPTANS

The triptans are a new class of drugs that cause cranial vascular constriction and relief of migraine headache pain in many patients. These drugs are not associated with all of the vascular and GI effects of the ergot derivatives. The triptan of choice for a particular patient depends on personal experience and other pre-existing medical conditions. A patient may have a poor response to one triptan and respond well to another.

Available triptans include the following:

- Sumatriptan (*Imitrex*), the first drug of this class, which is used for the treatment of acute migraine attacks. It can be given orally, subcutaneously, or by nasal spray; when given by the SC route, it has proved very effective against cluster headaches. It is not recommended for use in elderly patients. It has been found that older patients are more susceptible to the adverse effects of the drug, including decreased hepatic function, increased risk of hypertension, and increased risk of coronary artery disease.
- Naratriptan (*Amerge*), which is used orally only for the treatment of acute migraines. It has been associated with severe birth defects and is not recommended for patients with severe renal or hepatic dysfunction.
- Rizatriptan (*Maxalt*), which is used orally for the treatment of acute migraine attacks with or without aura. This drug is also available as a fast-dissolving tablet that is placed in the mouth. Because this agent seems to have more angina-

related effects, it is not recommended for patients with a history of CAD. It has also been shown to cause fetal abnormalities in animal studies and should not be used during pregnancy.

- Zolmitriptan (*Zomig*), which is used orally only for the treatment of acute migraine.
- Almotriptan (*Axert*), which is a newly approved agent for the treatment of acute migraine with or without aura in adults. This drug, released in 2001, is reported to have fewer side effects than the other triptans, but long-term use studies are not available.
- Frovatriptan (*Frova*) was approved in late 2001 and has the advantage of a long half-life. It is used orally as a treatment of acute migraines with or without aura. Although long-term studies are not available, it is thought that the longer half-life of this drug will prevent the rebound headaches that may be seen with other triptans.

Therapeutic Actions and Indications

The triptans bind to selective serotonin receptor sites to cause vasoconstriction of cranial vessels, relieving the signs and symptoms of migraine headache. They are indicated for the treatment of acute migraine and are not used for prevention of migraines. Sumatriptan injection is also indicated for the treatment of cluster headaches.

Pharmacokinetics

The triptans are rapidly absorbed from many sites; they are metabolized in the liver, sumatriptan by monoamine oxidase (MAO), and are primarily excreted in the urine. They cross the placenta and have been shown to be toxic to the fetus in animal studies. They should be used in pregnancy only if the benefit to the mother clearly outweighs any potential risks to the fetus. They have also been shown to enter breast milk

and should be used with caution during lactation. The safety and efficacy of use in children have not been established.

Contraindications and Cautions

Triptans are contraindicated with any of the following conditions: allergy to any triptan; pregnancy, because of the possibility of severe adverse effects on the fetus; and active CAD, which could be exacerbated by the vessel-constricting effects of these drugs. These drugs should be used with caution in elderly patients because of the possibility of underlying vascular disease; in patients with risk factors for CAD; in lactating women, because of the possibility of adverse effects on the infant; and in patients with renal or hepatic dysfunction, which could alter the metabolism and excretion of the drug.

Adverse Effects

The adverse effects associated with the triptans are related to the vasoconstrictive effects of the drugs. CNS effects may include numbness, tingling, burning sensation, feelings of coldness or strangeness, dizziness, weakness, myalgia, and vertigo. GI effects such as dysphagia and abdominal discomfort may occur. CV effects can be severe and include blood pressure alterations and tightness or pressure in the chest.

Clinically Important Drug–Drug Interactions

Combining triptans with ergot-containing drugs results in a risk of prolonged vasoactive reactions.

There is a risk of severe adverse effects if these drugs are used within 2 weeks after discontinuation of an MAO inhibitor because of the increased vasoconstrictive effects that occur. If triptans are to be given, it should be clear that the patient has not received an MAO inhibitor in more than 2 weeks.

DRUGS IN FOCUS
Antimigraine Triptans

Drug Name	Dosage/Route	Usual Indications
Almotriptan (*Axert*)	6.25–12.5 mg PO at onset of aura or symptoms, may repeat in 2h	Acute migraines in adults
frovatriptan (*Frova*)	2.5 mg PO at first sign of migraine; may repeat in 2 h	Acute migraines in adults
naratriptan (*Amerge*)	1–2.5 mg PO with fluid, may repeat in 4 h if needed	Acute migraines in adults
rizatriptan (*Maxalt*)	5–10 mg PO, may repeat in 2 h, do not exceed 30 mg/d	Acute migraines in adults
Ⓟ sumatriptan (*Imitrex*)	25–100 mg PO at first sign of headache, may repeat in 2 h, do not exceed 200 mg/d; *or* 6 mg SC; *or* 5, 10, or 20 mg by nasal spray in one nostril, may repeat in 2 h, do not exceed 40 mg/d	Acute migraines, cluster headaches in adults
zolmitriptan (*Zomig*)	2.5 mg PO, may repeat in 2 h, do not exceed 10 mg/d	Acute migraines in adults

Nursing Considerations for Patients Receiving Triptans

Assessment: History and Examination

Screen for the following conditions, which could be cautions or contraindications for the use of the drug: any known allergies to triptans; pregnancy; MI, CAD, or hypertension; and hepatic or renal dysfunction.

Include screening for baseline status before beginning therapy and for any potential adverse effects. Assess the following: temperature; skin color and lesions; CNS orientation, affect, and reflexes; respiration and adventitious sounds; pulse, blood pressure, and cardiac output; ECG and liver and renal function tests.

Nursing Diagnoses

The patient receiving a triptan may have the following nursing diagnoses related to drug therapy:

- Acute Pain related to CV, vasoconstrictive effects
- Decreased Cardiac Output related to CV effects
- Disturbed Sensory Perception (Visual, Auditory, Kinesthetic, and Tactile) related to CNS effects
- Deficient Knowledge regarding drug therapy

Implementation

- Administer the drug to relieve acute migraines; *these drugs are not used for prevention.*
- Arrange for safety precautions if CNS or visual changes occur, *to prevent patient injury.*
- Provide comfort and safety measures, such as environmental controls and stress reduction, *for the relief of headache.* Provide additional pain relief as needed.
- Monitor the blood pressure of any patient with a history of CAD, and discontinue the drug if any sign of angina or prolonged hypertension occurs, *to prevent severe vascular effects.*
- Provide thorough patient teaching, including drug name and prescribed dosage, as well as measures for avoidance of adverse effects, warning signs that may indicate possible problems, and the need for monitoring and evaluation, *to enhance patient knowledge about drug therapy and to promote compliance.*
- Offer support and encouragement *to help the patient cope with the drug regimen.*

Evaluation

- Monitor patient response to the drug (relief of acute migraine headaches).
- Monitor for adverse effects (CV changes, arrhythmias, hypertension, CNS changes).
- Evaluate the effectiveness of the teaching plan (patient can give the drug name and dosage and describe possible adverse effects to watch for, specific measures to prevent adverse effects, and warning signs to report).
- Monitor the effectiveness of comfort measures and compliance with the regimen.

CHAPTER SUMMARY

- Pain occurs any time that tissue is injured and various chemicals are released. The pain impulses are carried to the spinal cord by small-diameter A-delta and C fibers, which form synapses with interneurons in the dorsal horn of the spinal cord.
- Pain impulses travel from the spine to the cortex via spinothalamic tracts that can be modulated along the way at specific gates. These gates can be closed to block transmission of pain impulses by descending nerves from the upper CNS, which relate to emotion, culture, placebo effect, and stress, and by large-diameter sensory A fibers, which are associated with touch.
- Opioid receptors, which are found throughout various tissues in the body, react with endogenous endorphins and enkephalins to modulate the transmission of pain impulses.
- Narcotics, derived from the opium plant, react with opioid receptors to relieve pain. In addition, they lead to constipation, respiratory depression, sedation, and suppression of the cough reflex, and they stimulate feelings of well-being or euphoria.
- Because narcotics are associated with the development of physical dependence, they are controlled substances.
- The effectiveness and adverse effects associated with specific narcotics are associated with their particular affinity for various types of opioid receptors.
- Narcotic agonists react with opioid receptor sites to stimulate their activity.
- Narcotic agonists-antagonists react with some opioid receptor sites to stimulate activity and block other opioid receptor sites. These drugs are not as addictive as pure narcotic agonists.
- Narcotic antagonists, which work to reverse the effects of narcotics, are used to treat narcotic overdose or to reverse unacceptable adverse effects.
- Migraine headaches are severe, throbbing headaches on one side of the head that may be associated with an aura or warning syndrome. These headaches are thought to be caused by arterial dilation and hyperperfusion of the brain vessels.
- Treatment of migraines may involve either ergot derivatives or triptans. Ergot derivatives cause vasoconstriction and are associated with sometimes severe systemic vasoconstrictive effects, whereas triptans, a new class of selective serotonin receptor blockers, cause CNS vasoconstriction but are not associated with as many adverse systemic effects.

Review Questions
1. According to the gate control theory, pain
    a. is caused by gates in the CNS.

b. can be blocked or intensified by the opening or closing of gates in the CNS.

c. is caused by gates in peripheral nerve sensors.

d. cannot be affected by learned experiences.

2. Opioid receptors are found throughout the body

   a. only in people who have become addicted to opiates.

   b. in increasing numbers with chronic pain conditions.

   c. and incorporate pain perception and blocking.

   d. and cause endorphin release.

3. Narcotics are drugs that react with opioid receptors throughout the body and are not associated with

   a. hypnosis.

   b. sedation.

   c. analgesia.

   d. euphoria.

4. A narcotic would not be the analgesic of choice in a patient

   a. with severe postoperative pain.

   b. with severe chronic obstructive pulmonary disease and difficulty breathing.

   c. with severe, chronic pain.

   d. with a productive and irritating cough.

5. Most narcotics are controlled substances because

   a. they are very expensive.

   b. they can cause respiratory depression.

   c. they can be addictive.

   d. they can be used only in a hospital setting.

6. Injecting a narcotic into an area of the body that is chilled can be dangerous because

   a. an abscess will form.

   b. the injection will be very painful.

   c. absorption may be delayed and an excessive amount absorbed all at once.

   d. narcotics are inactivated in cold temperatures.

7. Proper administration of an ordered narcotic

   a. can lead to addiction.

b. should be done promptly to prevent increased pain and the need for larger doses.

c. would include holding the drug as long as possible until the patient really needs it.

d. should rely on the patient's request for medication.

8. Migraine headaches

   a. occur during sleep and involve sweating and eye pain.

   b. occur with stress and feel like a dull band around the entire head.

   c. often occur when drinking coffee.

   d. are throbbing headaches on one side of the head.

9. The triptans are a class of drugs that bind to selective serotonin receptor sites and cause

   a. cranial vascular dilation.

   b. cranial vascular constriction.

   c. depression.

   d. nausea and vomiting.

10. The only triptan that has been approved for use in treating cluster headaches as well as migraines is

   a. naratriptan.

   b. rizatriptan.

   c. sumatriptan.

   d. zolmitriptan.

BIBLIOGRAPHY

Bullock, B. L. (2000). *Focus on pathophysiology.* Philadelphia: Lippincott Williams & Wilkins.

Drug facts and comparisons. (2002). St. Louis: Facts and Comparisons.

Gilman, A., Hardman, J. G., & Limbird, L. E. (Eds.) (2002). *Goodman and Gilman's the pharmacological basis of therapeutics* (10th ed.). New York: McGraw-Hill.

Karch, A. M. (2002). *2003 Lippincott's nursing drug guide.* Philadelphia: Lippincott Williams & Wilkins.

Professional's guide to patient drug facts. (2002). St. Louis: Facts and Comparisons.

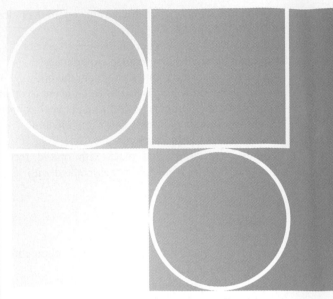

General and Local Anesthetic Agents

360

Anesthetics are drugs that are used to cause complete or partial loss of sensation. The anesthetics can be subdivided into general and local anesthetics depending on their site of action.

General anesthetics are central nervous system (CNS) depressants used to produce loss of pain sensation and consciousness. **Local anesthetics** are drugs used to cause loss of pain sensation and feeling in a designated area of the body without the systemic effects associated with severe CNS depression. This chapter discusses various general and local anesthetics.

GENERAL ANESTHETICS

When administering general anesthetics, several different drugs are combined to achieve the following goals: **analge-**

DRUG THERAPY ACROSS THE LIFESPAN

Anesthetic Agents

Children	Adults	Older Adults
Children are at greater risk for complications after anesthesia—laryngospasm, bronchospasm, aspiration, and even death. They require very careful monitoring and support, and the anesthetist needs to be very skilled at calculating dosage and balance during the procedure. Propofol is widely used for diagnostic tests and short procedures in children older than 3 years of age because of its rapid onset and metabolism and generally smooth recovery. Halothane is widely used for children, especially those with respiratory dysfunction, because it tends to dilate bronchi. It cannot be used with any increase in intracranial pressure, which it increases. Sevoflurane has a minimal impact on intracranial pressure and allows a very rapid induction and recovery with minimal sympathetic reaction. It is still quite expensive, however, which may limit its use. The dosage of anesthetics may need to be higher in children, and that factor will be considered by the anesthetist. Nursing care after general anesthesia should include support and reassurance; assessment of the child for any skin breakdown related to immobility, and safety precautions until full recovery has occurred. Local anesthetics are used in children in much the same way that they are used in adults. Bupivacaine, dyclonine, levobupivacaine, and tetracaine do not have established doses for children younger than 12 years of age. Benzocaine should not be used in children younger than 1 year of age. When topically applying a local anesthetic, it is important to remember that there is greater risk of systemic absorption and toxicity with infants. Tight diapers can act like occlusive dressings and increase systemic absorption. Children need to be cautioned not to bite themselves when receiving dental anesthesia.	Adults require a considerable amount of teaching and support when receiving anesthetics, including what will happen, what they will feel, how it will feel when they recover, and the approximate time to recovery. Adults should be monitored closely until fully recovered from general anesthetics and should be cautioned to prevent injury when receiving local anesthetics. It is important to remember to reassure and talk to adults who may be aware of their surroundings yet unable to speak. Most of the general anesthetics are not recommended for use during pregnancy because of the potential risk to the fetus. Short-onset and local anesthetics are frequently used at delivery. Use of a regional or other local anesthetic is usually preferred if surgery is needed during pregnancy. During lactation, it is recommended that the mother wait 4 to 6 hours to feed the baby after the anesthetic is used.	Older patients are more likely to experience the adverse effects associated with these drugs, including central nervous system, cardiovascular, and dermatological effects. Thinner skin and the possibility of decreased perfusion to the skin makes them especially susceptible to skin breakdown during immobility. Because older patients often also have renal or hepatic impairment, they are also more likely to have toxic levels of the drug related to changes in metabolism and excretion. The older patient should have safety measures in effect, such as siderails, a call light, and assistance to ambulate; special efforts to provide skin care to prevent skin breakdown are especially important with older skin. The older patient may require longer monitoring and regular orienting and reassuring. After general anesthesia, it is very important to promote vigorous pulmonary toilet to decrease the risk of pneumonia.

sia, or loss of pain perception; **unconsciousness**, or loss of awareness of one's surroundings; and **amnesia**, or inability to recall what took place. General anesthetics also block the body's reflexes. Blockage of autonomic reflexes prevents the response of involuntary reflexes to injury to the body that might compromise a patient's cardiac, respiratory, gastrointestinal (GI), and immune status. Blockage of muscle reflexes prevents jerking movements that might interfere with the success of the surgical procedure.

Risk Factors Associated With General Anesthetics

Use of general anesthetics involves a widespread CNS depression, which is not without risks. Several factors must be taken into consideration before the use of general anesthesia, which usually involves a series of drugs aimed at achieving the best effect with the fewest side effects. Because of the wide systemic effects of general anesthetics, patients should be evaluated for potential risks. When anesthetic drugs are selected, these factors are kept in mind so that the potential risk to each particular patient is minimized.

CNS factors: presence of any underlying neurological disease (eg, epilepsy, stroke, myasthenia gravis) that presents a risk for abnormal reaction to the CNS-depressing and muscle-relaxing effects of these drugs.

Cardiovascular factors: presence of underlying vascular disease, coronary artery disease, or hypotension, which put patients at risk for severe reactions to anesthesia, including hypotension and shock, arrhythmias, and ischemia.

Respiratory factors: presence of obstructive pulmonary disease (eg, asthma, chronic obstructive pulmonary disease, bronchitis), which can complicate the delivery of gas anesthesia as well as the intubation and mechanical ventilation that must be used in most cases of general anesthesia.

Renal and hepatic function: conditions that interfere with the metabolism and excretion of anesthetics (eg, acute renal failure, hepatitis) and could result in prolonged anesthesia and the need for continued support during recovery. Toxic reactions to the accumulation of abnormally high levels of anesthetic agents may even occur.

Balanced Anesthesia

With the wide variety of drugs available, the anesthesiologist has the opportunity to try to balance the therapeutic effects needed with the potential for adverse effects by ordering a variety of anesthetic drugs. **Balanced anesthesia** is the use of a combination of drugs, each with a specific effect, to achieve analgesia, muscle relaxation, unconsciousness, and amnesia, rather than the use of a single drug.

Balanced anesthesia commonly involves the following agents:

Preoperative medications, which may include the use of anticholinergics that decrease secretions to facilitate

intubation and prevent bradycardia associated with neural depression.

Sedative/hypnotics to relax the patient, facilitate amnesia, and decrease sympathetic stimulation.

Antiemetics to decrease the nausea and vomiting associated with GI depression.

Antihistamines to decrease the chance of allergic reaction and to help dry up secretions.

Narcotics to aid analgesia and sedation.

Many of these drugs are given before the anesthetic to facilitate the process, and some are maintained during surgery to aid the anesthetic, allowing therapeutic effects at lower doses. For example, patients may receive a neuromuscular junction (NMJ) blocker and a rapid-acting intravenous anesthetic to induce anesthesia, and then a gas anesthetic to balance it during the procedure and allow easier recovery. Careful selection of appropriate anesthetic agents, along with monitoring and support of the patient, helps to alleviate many problems.

Administration of General Anesthetics

Anesthesia is delivered by a physician or nurse anesthetist trained in the delivery of these potent drugs with equipment for intubation, mechanical ventilation, and full life support. During the delivery of anesthesia, the patient can go through predictable stages, referred to as the depth of anesthesia. These stages are as follows:

Stage 1, the analgesia stage, refers to the loss of pain sensation, with the patient still conscious and able to communicate.

Stage 2, the excitement stage, is a period of excitement and often combative behavior, with many signs of sympathetic stimulation (eg, tachycardia, increased respirations, blood pressure changes).

Stage 3, surgical anesthesia, involves relaxation of skeletal muscles, return of regular respirations, and progressive loss of eye reflexes and pupil dilation. Surgery can be safely performed in stage 3.

Stage 4, medullary paralysis, is very deep CNS depression with loss of respiratory and vasomotor center stimuli, in which death can occur rapidly.

Induction

Induction is the period from the beginning of anesthesia until stage 3, or surgical anesthesia is reached. The danger period for many patients during induction is stage 2 because of the systemic stimulation that occurs. Many times a rapid-acting anesthetic is used to move quickly through this phase and into stage 3. NMJ blockers may be used during induction to facilitate intubation, which is necessary to support the patient with mechanical ventilation during anesthesia.

Maintenance

Maintenance is the period from stage 3 until the surgical procedure is complete. A slower, more predictable anesesters or amides. The esters are broken down immediately in the plasma by enzymes known as **plasma esterases.** The amides are metabolized more slowly in the liver, and serum levels of these drugs can increase and lead to toxicity.

Modes of Administration

The way in which a local anesthetic is administered helps increase its effectiveness by delivering it directly to the area that is causing or will cause the pain, thereby decreasing systemic absorption and related toxic effects (Figure 27–2). There are five types of local anesthetic administration: topical, infiltration, field block, nerve block, and intravenous regional anesthesia.

Topical Administration

Topical anesthesia involves applying a cream, lotion, ointment, or drop of a local anesthetic to traumatized skin to relieve pain. It can also involve applying the lotion, cream, ointment, or drops to the mucous membranes in the eye, nose, throat, mouth, urethra, anus, or rectum to relieve pain or to anesthetize the area to facilitate a medical procedure. Although systemic absorption is rare with topical application, it can occur if there is damage or breakdown of the tissues in the area.

Infiltration

Infiltration anesthesia involves injecting the anesthetic directly into the tissues to be treated (eg, sutured, drilled, cut). This injection brings the anesthetic into contact with the nerve endings in the area and prevents them from transmitting nerve impulses to the brain.

Field Block

Field block anesthesia involves injecting the anesthetic all around the area that will be affected by the operation. This is more intense than infiltration anesthesia because the anesthetic agent comes in contact with all of the nerve endings surrounding the area. This type of block is often used for tooth extractions.

Nerve Block

Nerve block anesthesia involves injecting the anesthetic at some point along the nerve or nerves that run to and from the region in which the loss of pain sensation or muscle paralysis is desired. These blocks are performed not in the surgical field but at some distance from the field; they involve a greater area with potential for more adverse effects. Several types of nerve blocks are possible. A peripheral nerve block blocks the sensory and motor aspects of a particular nerve for relief of pain or for diagnostic purposes. With a central nerve block, the anesthetic is injected into the roots of the nerves in the spinal cord. In epidural anesthesia, the drug is injected into the space where the nerves emerge from the spinal cord. A caudal block involves injection into the sacral canal, below the epidural area.

Intravenous Regional Anesthesia

Intravenous regional anesthesia involves carefully draining all of the blood from the patient's arm or leg, securing a

FIGURE 27–2. Mechanism of action of local anesthetics. *Top:* An injury produces pain impulses (action potentials) that are conducted and transmitted in an area of the brain in which pain is perceived. *A:* Conduction of the pain impulse has been blocked by infiltration anesthesia at the site of the injury. *B:* A nerve block at some distance from the injury. Local anesthetics block the movement of sodium into the nerve and prevent nerve depolarization, stopping the transmission of the pain impulse.

tourniquet to prevent the anesthetic from entering the general circulation, and then injecting the anesthetic into the vein of the arm or leg. This technique is used for very specific surgical procedures.

Characteristics of Local Anesthetics

Several agents may be used as local anesthetics. The agent of choice depends on the method of administration, the length of time for which the area is to be anesthetized, and consideration of potential adverse effects.

Therapeutic Actions and Indications

Local anesthetics work by causing a temporary interruption in the production and conduction of nerve impulses. They affect the permeability of nerve membranes to sodium ions, which normally infuse into the cell in response to stimulation. By preventing the sodium ions from entering the nerve, they stop the nerve from depolarizing. A particular section of the nerve cannot be stimulated, and nerve impulses directed toward that section are lost when they reach that area. Local anesthetics are indicated for infiltration anesthesia, peripheral nerve block, spinal anesthesia, and the relief of local pain.

Pharmacokinetics

The ester local anesthetics are broken down immediately in the plasma by enzymes known as plasma esterases. The amide local anesthetics are metabolized more slowly in the liver, and serum levels of these drugs can increase and lead to toxicity. They should be used during pregnancy and lactation only if the benefit outweighs any potential risk to the neonate, which could occur if the drug is inadvertently absorbed systemically.

Contraindications and Cautions

The local anesthetics are contraindicated with any of the following conditions: history of allergy to any one of these agents or to parabens; heart block, which could be greatly exacerbated with systemic absorption; shock, which could alter the local delivery and absorption of these drugs; and decreased plasma esterases, which could result in toxic levels of the ester-type local anesthetics.

Adverse Effects

The adverse effects of these drugs may be related to their local blocking of sensation (eg, skin breakdown, self-injury, biting oneself). Other problematic effects are associated with the route of administration and the amount of drug that is absorbed systemically. These effects are related to the blockade of nerve depolarization throughout the system. Effects that may occur include CNS effects such as headache, restlessness, anxiety, dizziness, tremors, blurred vision, and backache; GI effects such as nausea and vomiting; cardiovascular effects such as peripheral vasodilation, myocardial depression, arrhythmias, and blood pressure changes, all of which may lead to fatal cardiac arrest; and respiratory arrest.

Clinically Important Drug–Drug Interactions

When local anesthetics and succinylcholine are given concurrently, increased and prolonged neuromuscular blockade occurs.

There is also less risk of systemic absorption and increased local effects if these drugs are combined with epinephrine.

Nursing Considerations for Patients Receiving Local Anesthetics

Assessment: History and Examination

Screen for the following conditions, which could be cautions or contraindications to the use of the drug: any known allergies to these drugs or to parabens; impaired liver function; low plasma esterases; heart block; shock; and pregnancy or lactation.

Include screening for baseline status before beginning therapy and for any potential adverse effects. Assess the following: body temperature and weight; skin color and lesions; affect, orientation, reflexes, pupil size and reaction, and muscle tone and response; pulse, blood pressure, and ECG; respiration and adventitious sounds; and liver function tests and plasma esterases (if appropriate).

Nursing Diagnoses

The patient receiving a local anesthetic may have the following nursing diagnoses related to drug therapy:

- Disturbed Sensory Perception (Kinesthetic, Tactile) related to anesthetic effect
- Impaired Skin Integrity related to immobility
- Risk for Injury related to loss of sensation and mobility
- Deficient Knowledge regarding drug therapy

Implementation

- Have equipment on standby *to maintain airway and provide mechanical ventilation if needed.*
- Ensure that drugs for managing hypotension, cardiac arrest, and CNS alterations are on standby *in case of severe reaction and toxicity.*
- Ensure that patients receiving spinal anesthesia are well hydrated and remain lying down for up to 12 hours after the anesthesia, *to minimize headache.*
- Establish safety precautions *to prevent skin breakdown and injury during the time that the patient has a loss of sensation and/or mobility.*
- Provide comfort measures *to help the patient tolerate drug effects.* Provide pain relief as appropriate; reassurance and support *to deal with the effects of anesthesia and loss of control;* skin care and turning *to prevent skin breakdown;* and supportive care for hypotension *to prevent shock or serious hypoxia.*
- Provide thorough patient teaching *to explain what to expect, safety precautions that will be needed, and when to expect return of function.* (See Patient Teaching Checklist: Local Anesthetics.)

DRUGS IN FOCUS
Local Anesthetics

Drug Name	Administration	Notes
Esters		
benzocaine (*Dermoplast, Lanacane, Unguentine*)	Skin, mucous membranes	**Onset:** 1 min **Duration:** 30–60 min **Special considerations:** Avoid tight bandages with skin preparation
butamben (*Butesin Picrate*)	Skin, mucous membranes	**Onset:** slow **Duration:** 30–60 min **Special considerations:** Swallowing may be difficult if used in throat
chloroprocaine (*Nesacaine*)	Nerve block, caudal, epidural	**Onset:** 6–15 min **Duration:** 15–75 min **Special considerations:** Do not use with subarachnoid administration
procaine (*Novocain*)	Infiltration, peripheral, spinal, dental	**Onset:** 2–25 min **Duration:** 15–75 min **Special considerations:** Monitor skin condition if immobile; keep supine to avoid headache after spinal
tetracaine (*Pontocaine*)	Spinal, prolonged spinal, skin	**Onset:** 15–30 min **Duration:** 2–2.5 h **Special considerations:** Monitor skin condition if immobile, provide reassurance if prolonged; keep supine to avoid headache after spinal
Amides		
bupivacaine (*Marcaine, Sensorcaine*)	Local, epidural, dental, caudal, subarachnoid, sympathetic, retrobulbar	**Onset:** 5–20 min **Duration:** 2–7 h **Special considerations:** Do not use Bier Block—deaths have occurred
dibucaine (*Nupercainal*)	Skin, mucous membranes	**Onset:** <15 min **Duration:** 3–4 h **Special considerations:** Monitor for local reactions
levobupivacaine (*Chirocaine*)	Regional block, obstetric, postoperative pain	**Onset:** 5–20 min **Duration:** 2–7 h **Special considerations:** Less cardiac and central nervous system toxicity than bupivacaine, suggesting safer use in some patients
Lidocaine (*Dilocaine, Solarcaine, Xylocaine, Lidoderm, Octocaine*)	Caudal, epidural, spinal, cervical, dental, skin, mucous membrane, topical patch	**Onset:** <2 min **Duration:** 30–90 min **Special considerations:** Short-acting; preferred for short procedures; danger is absorbed systemically
mepivacaine (*Carbocaine, Isocaine, Polocaine*)	Nerve block, obstetrical, cervical, epidural, dental, local infiltration	**Onset:** 3–15 min **Duration:** 45–90 min **Special considerations:** Caution with renal impairment
prilocaine (*Citanest*)	Nerve block, dental	**Onset:** 1–15 min **Duration:** 0.5–3 h **Special considerations:** Advise patients not to bite themselves
ropivacaine (*Naropin*)	Nerve block, epidural, caudal	**Onset:** 1–20 min **Duration:** 2–6 h **Special considerations:** Avoid rapid infusion; offers good management postoperative and obstetrical pain
Other		
dyclonine (*Dyclone*)	Mucous membranes	**Onset:** <10 min **Duration:** < 60 min **Special considerations:** Used for diagnostic and preparation for medical procedures
pramoxine (*Tronothane, PrameGel, Itch-X, Prax*)	Skin, mucous membranes	**Onset:** 3–5 min **Duration:** <60 min **Special considerations:** Do not cover with tight bandages; protect patient from injury

PATIENT TEACHING CHECKLIST
Local Anesthetics

Create customized patient teaching materials for a specific anesthetic from the CD-ROM. Patient teaching should stress the following points for drugs within this class:
 Discussion of the procedure:

• What it will feel like (any numbness, tingling, inability to move, pressure, pain, choking?)
• Any anticipated discomfort
• How long it will last
• Concerns during the procedure: report any discomfort and ask any questions as they arise

 Discussion of the recovery:

• How long it will take
• Feelings to anticipate: tingling, numbness, pressure, itching
• Pain that will be felt as the anesthesia wears off
• Measures to reduce pain in the area
• Signs and symptoms to report (eg, pain along a nerve route, palpitations, feeling faint, disorientation)

This Teaching Checklist reflects general patient teaching guidelines. It is not meant to be a substitute for drug-specific teaching information, which is available in nursing drug guides.

• Offer support and encouragement *to help the patient cope with the procedure and drugs being used.*

Evaluation

• Monitor patient response to the drug (loss of feeling in designated area).
• Monitor for adverse effects (respiratory depression, blood pressure changes, arrhythmias, GI upset, skin breakdown, injury, CNS alterations).
• Evaluate the effectiveness of the teaching plan (patient can relate the anticipated effects of the drug and the recovery process) (see Nursing Care Guide: Local Anesthetics).

CHAPTER SUMMARY

• General anesthetics are drugs used to produce pain relief, analgesia, amnesia, and unconsciousness and to block muscle reflexes that could interfere with a surgical procedure or put the patient at risk for harm.
• The use of general anesthetics involves a widespread CNS depression that could be harmful, especially in patients with underlying CNS, cardiovascular, or respiratory diseases.

CASE STUDY

Spinal Anesthesia

THE SITUATION
A. M., a 32-year-old male athlete with a prior history of asthma (which could indicate pulmonary dysfunction), was admitted to the hospital for an inguinal hernia repair. At the patient's request, the surgeon elected to use a local anesthetic employing spinal anesthesia. Because the extent of the repair was unknown (A. M. had undergone two previous repairs), levobupivacaine, a long-acting anesthetic, was selected. He remained alert (BP 120/64, P 62, R 10) and stable throughout the procedure.

Two hours after the conclusion of the procedure, A. M. appeared agitated (BP 154/68, P 88, R 12). Although he did not complain of discomfort, he did state that he still had no feeling and had only limited movement of his legs.

CRITICAL THINKING
• What safety precautions need to be taken?
• What nursing interventions should be done at this point?
• How could the patient be reassured? *Think about the anxiety level of the patient—an athlete who elected to have local anesthesia may have a problem with control and feel somewhat invincible. Consider the anxiety that loss of mobility and sensation in the legs may cause in a person who makes his living as an athlete.*
• In addition, consider the expected duration of action of levobupivacaine and the rate of return of function.

DISCUSSION
Levobupivacaine is a long-acting anesthetic with effects that may persist for several hours. The timing of the drug's effects should be explained to A. M., and he should be monitored for a period of time to determine whether his agitated state and slightly elevated vital signs are a result of anxiety or an unanticipated reaction to the surgery or the drug. Life-support equipment should be on standby in case his condition is a toxic drug reaction or some unanticipated problem occurring after surgery.

The nurse is in the best position to perform the following interventions: explaining the effects of the drug and the anticipated recovery schedule; keeping the patient as flat as possible to decrease the headache usually associated with spinal anesthesia; encouraging the patient to turn from side to side periodically to allow skin care to be performed and to alleviate the risk of pressure sore development; and staying with the patient as much as possible to reassure him, to answer questions, and to encourage him to talk about his feelings and reaction.

If the agitated state is caused by a stress reaction, the patient should return to normal; comfort measures, teaching, and reassurance should be provided. An elevated systolic pressure with a normal diastolic pressure is often an indication of a sympathetic stress response. An athlete is more likely than most people to suffer great anxiety and fear if his legs become numb and he is unable to move them. The teaching and comfort measures may be all that is needed to relieve the anxiety and ensure a good recovery.

NURSING CARE GUIDE

Local Anesthetics

Assessment	Nursing Diagnoses	Implementation	Evaluation
HISTORY Allergies to any of these drugs or to parabens, cardiac disorders, vascular problems, hepatic dysfunction	Disturbed Sensory Perception (Kinesthetic, Tactile) related to anesthesia Impaired Skin Integrity related to immobility Risk for Injury related to loss of sensation, mobility Deficient knowledge regarding drug therapy	Administer drug under strict supervision. Provide comfort and safety measures: positioning, skin care, side rails, pain medication as needed, maintain airway, ventilate patient, antidotes on standby. Provide support and reassurance to deal with loss of sensation and mobility. Provide patient teaching about procedure being performed, what to expect. Provide life support as needed.	Evaluate drug effects: loss of sensation, loss of movement. Monitor for adverse effects: cardiovascular effects (BP changes, arrhythmias), respiratory depression, GI upset, CNS alterations, skin breakdown, anxiety, fear. Monitor for drug–drug interactions as indicated for each drug. Evaluate effectiveness of patient teaching program. Evaluate effectiveness of comfort and safety measures. Constantly monitor vital signs and return to normal muscular function and sensation.
PHYSICAL EXAMINATION CV: blood pressure, pulse, peripheral perfusion, ECG CNS: orientation, affect, reflexes, vision Skin: color, lesions, texture, sweating Respiratory: respiration, adventitious sounds Laboratory tests: liver function tests, plasma esterases			

- Anesthesia proceeds through predictable stages from loss of sensation to total CNS depression and death.
- Induction of anesthesia is the period of time from the beginning of anesthesia administration until the patient reaches surgical anesthesia.
- Balanced anesthesia involves giving a variety of drugs, including anticholinergics, rapid intravenous anesthetics, inhaled anesthetics, NMJ blockers, and narcotics.
- Patients receiving general anesthetics should be monitored for any adverse effects and to provide reassurance and safety precautions until the recovery of sensation, mobility, and ability to communicate.
- Local anesthetics block the depolarization of nerve membrane, preventing the transmission of pain sensations and motor stimuli.
- Local anesthetics are administered to deliver the drug directly to the desired area and to prevent systemic absorption, which could lead to serious interruption of nerve impulses and response.
- Ester-type local anesthetics are immediately destroyed by plasma esterases. Amide local anesthetics are destroyed in the liver and have a greater risk of accumulation and systemic toxicity.
- Nursing care of patients receiving anesthetics should include safety precautions, to prevent injury and skin breakdown; support and reassurance, to deal with the loss of sensation and mobility; and patient teaching regarding what to expect, to decrease stress and anxiety.

Review Questions

1. General anesthetics are used for all of the following except
   a. to produce analgesia.

b. to produce amnesia.

c. to activate the reticular activating system.

d. to block muscle reflexes.

2. The most dangerous period for many patients undergoing general anesthesia is during

a. stage 1, when communication becomes difficult.

b. stage 2, when systemic stimulation occurs.

c. stage 3, when skeletal muscles relax.

d. there is no real danger during general anesthesia.

3. Recovery after a general anesthetic refers to the period of time

a. from the beginning of the anesthesia until the patient is ready for surgery.

b. during the surgery when anesthesia is maintained at a certain level.

c. from the discontinuation of the anesthetic until the patient has regained consciousness, movement, and the ability to communicate.

d. when the patient is in the most danger of CNS depression.

4. Balanced anesthesia combines different classes of drugs to achieve the best effects with the least adverse effects. Balanced anesthesia does not usually involve the use of

a. anticholinergics.

b. narcotics.

c. sedative/hypnotics.

d. adrenergic β-blockers.

5. While a patient is receiving a general anesthetic, he or she must be continually monitored because

a. the patient has no pain sensation.

b. generalized CNS depression affects all body functions and could cause problems for patients with CNS, CV, or respiratory disorders.

c. the patient cannot move.

d. the patient cannot communicate.

6. Because of the risks to the patient, general anesthetics are administered

a. under the watchful eye of a nursing supervisor.

b. only by graduate nurses.

c. only by trained personnel (usually an anesthesiologist).

d. by surgeons.

7. Local anesthetics are used to block feeling in specific body areas. If given in increasing concentrations, local anesthetics can cause loss, in order, of the following:

a. temperature sensation, touch sensation, proprioception, and skeletal muscle tone.

b. touch sensation, skeletal muscle tone, temperature sensation, and proprioception.

c. proprioception, skeletal muscle tone, touch sensation, and temperature sensation.

d. skeletal muscle tone, touch sensation, temperature sensation, and proprioception.

8. Comfort measures that are important for a patient receiving a local anesthetic would not include

a. skin care and turning.

b. reassurance over loss of control and sensation.

c. use of antihypertensive agents.

d. use of analgesics as needed.

BIBLIOGRAPHY

Bullock, B. L. (2000). *Focus on pathophysiology*. Philadelphia: Lippincott Williams & Wilkins.

Drug facts and comparisons. (2002). St. Louis: Facts and Comparisons.

Gilman, A., Hardman, J. G., & Limbird, L. E. (Eds.) (2002). *Goodman and Gilman's the pharmacological basis of therapeutics* (10th ed.). New York: McGraw-Hill.

Karch, A. M. (2002). *2003 Lippincott's nursing drug guide*. Philadelphia: Lippincott Williams & Wilkins.

Professional's guide to patient drug facts. (2002). St. Louis: Facts and Comparisons.

Neuromuscular Junction Blocking Agents

Key Terms
acetylcholine receptor site
depolarizing
malignant hyperthermia
nondepolarizing
paralysis
sarcomere
sliding filament theory

373

Nondepolarizing Neuromuscular Blockers

atracurium
cisatracurium
doxacurium
mivacurium
pancuronium
pipercuronium
rocuronium
Ⓟ tubocurarine
vecuronium

Depolarizing Neuromuscular Blocker
Ⓟ succinylcholine

Drugs that affect the neuromuscular junction (NMJ), the NMJ blockers, can be divided into two groups. One group, the **nondepolarizing** NMJs, includes those agents that act as antagonists to acetylcholine (ACh) at the NMJ and prevent depolarization of muscle cells. The other group, the **depolarizing** NMJs (of which there is one drug), act as an ACh agonist at the junction, causing stimulation of the muscle cell and then preventing it from repolarizing. Both of these types of drugs are used to cause **paralysis,** or loss of muscular function, for performance of surgical procedures or facilitation of mechanical ventilation.

THE NEUROMUSCULAR JUNCTION

The NMJ blockers affect the normal functioning of muscles by interfering with the normal processes that occur at the junction of nerve and muscle cell. The functional unit of a muscle, called a **sarcomere,** is made up of light and dark filaments formed by actin and myosin molecules arranged in orderly stacks that give the sarcomere a striated or striped appearance (Figure 28–1). Normal muscle function involves the arrival of a nerve impulse at the motor nerve terminal, followed by the release of ACh into the synaptic cleft. At the **acetylcholine receptor site** on the effector side of the synapse, the ACh interacts with the nicotinic cholinergic receptors, causing depolarization of the muscle membrane. This depolarization allows the release of calcium ions, stored in tubules, into the cell. The calcium binds to troponin, a chemical found throughout the sarcomere, and the binding of troponin causes the release of actin and myosin binding sites, allowing them to react with each other.

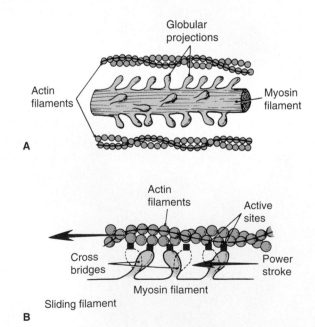

FIGURE 28–1. Sliding filament theory of muscle contraction. (From Bullock, B. L. [2000]. *Focus on pathophysiology.* Philadelphia: Lippincott Williams & Wilkins, with permission.)

The actin and myosin molecules react with each other again and again, sliding along the filament and making it shorter. This is a contraction of the muscle fiber according to the **sliding filament theory.** As the calcium is removed from the cell during repolarization of the muscle membrane, the troponin is freed and prevents the actin and myosin from reacting with each other. The muscle filament then relaxes or slides back to the resting position. Muscle tone results from a dynamic balance between excitatory and inhibitory impulses to the muscle. Muscle paralysis may occur when ACh cannot react with the cholinergic muscle receptor or when the muscle cells cannot repolarize to allow new stimulation and muscle contraction.

NONDEPOLARIZING NEUROMUSCULAR JUNCTION BLOCKERS

The first nondepolarizing NMJ blocker to be discovered was curare, a poison used on the tips of arrows or spears by primitive hunters to paralyze their game. Animals died when their respiratory muscles became paralyzed. Because the poison was destroyed by the cooking process, or by gastric acid if the meat were eaten raw, it was safe for humans. Curare was first purified for clinical use as the NMJ blocker tubocurarine.

All nondepolarizing NMJ blockers are similar in structure to ACh and occupy the muscular cholinergic receptor site, preventing ACh from reacting with the receptor. These agents do not cause activation of muscle cells, and consequently muscle contraction does not occur. Because they are not broken down by acetylcholinesterase, their effect is more long-lasting than that of ACh. NMJ blockers are used when clinical situations require muscle paralysis.

DEPOLARIZING NEUROMUSCULAR JUNCTION BLOCKER: SUCCINYLCHOLINE

Succinylcholine, a depolarizing NMJ blocker, attaches to the ACh receptor site on the muscle cell, depolarizing the muscle. This depolarization causes stimulation of the muscle and muscle contraction. Unlike ACh, succinylcholine is not broken down instantly, and the result is a prolonged contraction of the muscle, which cannot be restimulated. Eventually a gradual repolarization occurs as continually stimulated channels in the cell membrane close.

Therapeutic Actions and Indications
All of the NMJ blockers are structurally similar to ACh and compete with ACh for muscle ACh receptor sites. They are hydrophilic, instead of lipophilic, so they do not readily cross the blood–brain barrier. The nondepolarizing NMJ blockers act by blocking the ACh receptor so that it cannot be stimulated. Depolarizing NMJ blockers prevent muscle movement by prohibiting the depolarization of the muscle membrane. The depolarizing NMJ blocker succinylcholine

DRUG THERAPY ACROSS THE LIFESPAN

Neuromuscular Junction Blocking (NMJ) Agents

Children	Adults	Older Adults
Children require very careful monitoring and support after the use of NMJ blockers. These agents are used by anesthetists who are skilled in their use and with full support services available. The nondepolarizing NMJs are preferable because of the lack of muscle contraction with its resultant discomfort on recovery. Succinylcholine is usually preferred when a very short-acting, rapid-onset blocker is needed (eg, for intubation).	Adults need to be monitored closely for full return of muscle function. If succinylcholine is used, they need to be told that they will experience muscle pain and discomfort when the procedure is over. The NMJs are used during pregnancy and lactation only if the benefit to the mother outweighs the potential risk to the fetus.	Because older patients often also have renal or hepatic impairment, they are more likely to have toxic levels of the drug related to changes in metabolism and excretion. The older patient should receive special efforts to provide skin care to prevent skin breakdown, which is more likely with older skin. The older patient may require longer monitoring and regular orienting and reassuring.

(*Anectine, Quelicin*) works by reacting with the ACh receptor and causing a prolonged depolarization, which causes first muscle contraction and then flaccid paralysis. Both effects cause muscles to stop responding to stimuli, and paralysis occurs. Clinically, muscle twitching occurs when the drug is first given and is followed by flaccid paralysis. Succinylcholine has a rapid onset and a short duration of action because it is broken down by cholinesterase in the plasma (Figure 28–2).

These drugs are indicated for any situation in which muscle paralysis is desired. The therapeutic uses of NMJ blocking are as follows:

- To serve as an adjunct to general anesthetics during surgery, when reflex muscle movement could interfere with the surgical procedure or the delivery of gas anesthesia.
- To facilitate mechanical intubation by preventing resistance to passing of the endotracheal tube and in situations in which patients "fight" or resist the respirator.
- To facilitate electroconvulsive therapy when intense skeletal muscle contractions as a result of electric shock could cause the patient broken bones or other injury.

Several NMJ blockers are available, with different times of onset and durations of activity. The drug of choice in any given situation is determined by the procedure being performed, including the estimated time involved (Figure 28–3).

Pharmacokinetics

In general, the NMJs are metabolized in the serum, although metabolism is dependent on the liver to produce the needed plasma cholinesterases. Patients with hepatic impairment may experience prolonged effects of the drugs. Most of the metabolites are excreted in the urine. Patients with renal impairment may be at risk for increased toxicity from the drugs. There are no well-controlled studies regarding the effects of these drugs during pregnancy, and they should be used during pregnancy only if they are clearly needed and

the benefits outweigh the potential risks to the fetus. Succinylcholine is often used during cesarean sections, where it does cross the placenta but accurate timing prevents serious effects on the fetus. Effects during lactation are not known.

Contraindications and Cautions

The NMJ blockers are contraindicated in the following conditions: known allergy to any of these drugs; myasthenia gravis, because blocking of the ACh cholinergic receptors aggravates the neuromuscular disease (which results from a destruction of the ACh receptor sites) and increases the muscular effects (see Chapter 32); renal or hepatic disease, which could interfere with the metabolism or excretion of these drugs, leading to toxic effects; and pregnancy (some of these drugs are used in cesarean sections, but the dose needs to be decreased to protect the fetus).

Caution should be used in patients with any family or personal history of **malignant hyperthermia,** a serious adverse effect associated with these drugs that is characterized by extreme muscle rigidity, severe hyperpyrexia, acidosis, and death in some cases. Caution should also be used in the following circumstances: pulmonary or cardiovascular dysfunction, which could be made worse by the paralysis of the respiratory muscles and resulting changes in perfusion and respiratory function; altered fluid and electrolyte imbalance, which could affect membrane stability and muscular function; some respiratory conditions that could be made worse by the histamine release associated with some of these agents; and lactation, because of the potential for adverse effects on the baby.

In addition, succinylcholine should be used with caution in patients with fractures, because the muscle contractions it causes might lead to additional trauma; in those with narrow-angle glaucoma or penetrating eye injuries, because intraocular pressure increases; and in those with paraplegia or spinal cord injuries, which could cause loss of potassium from the overstimulated cells and hyperkalemia. Extr

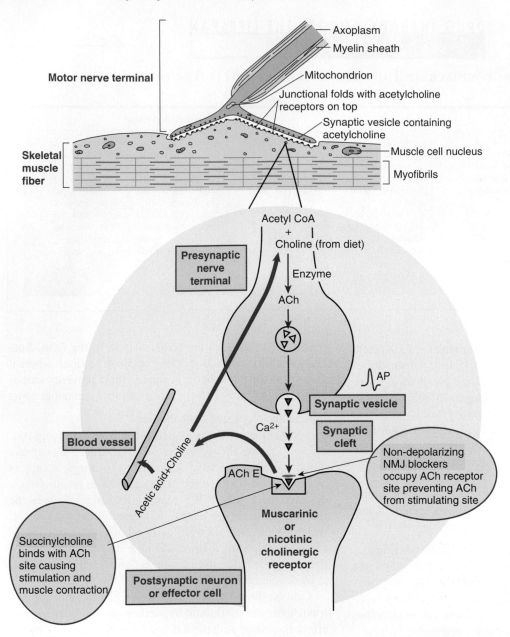

FIGURE 28-2. Sites of action of the neuromuscular junction (NMJ) blockers. ACh, acetylcholine.

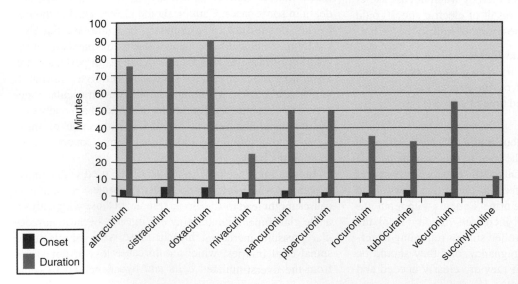

FIGURE 28-3. Onset and duration of neuromuscular junction blockers.

caution should be taken in the presence of genetic or disease-related conditions causing low plasma cholinesterase levels, such as cirrhosis, metabolic disorders, carcinoma, burns, dehydration, malnutrition, hyperpyrexia, thyroid toxicosis, collagen diseases, and exposure to neurotoxic insecticides. Low plasma cholinesterase levels may result in a very prolonged paralysis because succinylcholine is not broken down in the plasma and continues to stimulate the receptor site, leading to a need for prolonged support after the drug is discontinued.

◻◼◉ WEB LINKS

Health care providers and patients may want to consult the following Internet sources:

Information on cholinesterase deficiencies—research, diagnosis, and so on:
http://www.anesthesia.wisc.edu

Information on the physiology of the NMJ, effects of blocking the junction:
http://www.ohsu.edu/cliniweb/A11/A11.195.443.780.550.html

Information on paralysis of ventilator patients, particularly the use of pancuronium:
http://www.sccm.org

Patient guides to general anesthetics, what to expect, how they work:
http://www.asr.net

Adverse Effects

The adverse effects related to the use of NMJ blockers are associated with the paralysis of muscles. Profound and prolonged muscle paralysis is always possible, and patients must be supported until they are able to resume voluntary and involuntary muscle movement. When the respiratory muscles are paralyzed, depressed respiration, bronchospasm, and apnea are anticipated adverse effects. NMJ blockers are never used without an anesthesiologist or nurse anesthetist present who can provide artificial respiration and deliver oxygen under positive pressure. Intubation is an anticipated procedure with these drugs.

The histamine release associated with many of the NMJ blockers can cause respiratory obstruction with wheezing and bronchospasm. The NMJ rapacuronium (*Raplon*) was withdrawn in 2001 after a very short time on the market because of deaths associated with severe bronchospasm. It was decided that the risks associated with use of the drug were too great. Hypotension and cardiac arrhythmias may occur in patients who do not adapt to the drugs effectively, use the drugs for prolonged periods, have certain underlying conditions, or take certain drugs (eg, vecuronium) that are known to affect cardiovascular receptors. Prolonged drug use may also result in gastrointestinal (GI) dysfunction related to paralysis of the muscles in the GI tract; constipation, vomiting, regurgitation, and aspiration may occur. Decubitus ulcers may develop because the patient loses reflex muscle movement that protects the body from pressure sores. Hyperkalemia may occur as a result of muscle membrane alterations.

CULTURAL CONSIDERATIONS
Succinylcholine and Paralysis

Succinylcholine is broken down in the body by cholinesterase, an enzyme found in the plasma. Several conditions may cause the body to produce less of this enzyme, including cirrhosis, metabolic disorders, carcinoma, burns, dehydration, malnutrition, hyperpyrexia, thyrotoxicosis, collagen diseases, and exposure to neurotoxic insecticides. If plasma cholinesterase levels are low, the serum levels of succinylcholine remain elevated, and the paralysis can last much longer than anticipated. These patients need support and ventilation for long periods after surgery.

There is also a genetic predisposition to low plasma cholinesterase levels. Patients should be asked whether they or any family member has a history of either low plasma cholinesterase levels or prolonged recovery from anesthetics. Alaskan Eskimos belong to such a genetic group, and they are especially likely to suffer prolonged paralysis and inability to breathe for several hours after succinylcholine has been used for surgery. If there is no other drug of choice for these patients, special care must be taken to monitor their response and ensure their breathing for an extended postoperative period.

In addition, succinylcholine is associated with muscle pain, related to the contraction of the muscles as a first reaction. A nondepolarizing NMJ blocker may be given first to prevent some of these contractions and the associated discomfort. Aspirin also alleviates much of this pain after the procedure. Malignant hyperthermia, which may occur in susceptible patients, is a very serious condition characterized by massive muscle contraction, sharply elevated body temperature, severe acidosis, and, if uncontrolled, death. This reaction is most likely with succinylcholine, and treatment involves dantrolene (see Chapter 25) to inhibit the muscle effects of the NMJ blocker (Table 28–1).

Clinically Important Drug–Drug Interactions

Many drugs are known to react with the NMJ blockers. Some drug combinations result in an increased neuromuscular effect. Halogenated hydrocarbon anesthetics such as halothane cause a membrane stabilizing effect, which greatly enhances the paralysis induced by the NMJ blockers. If these drugs are used together for a procedure, dosage adjustments are necessary, and patients should be monitored closely until they recover fully. A combination of NMJ blockers and aminoglycoside antibiotics (eg, gentamicin) also leads to increased neuromuscular blockage. Patients who receive this drug combination require a lower dose of NMJ blocker and prolonged support and monitoring after the procedure.

Calcium channel blockers may also increase the paralysis caused by NMJ blockers greatly because of their effects on the calcium channels in the muscle. If the combination of NMJ blockers and calcium channel blockers cannot be avoided, the dose of the NMJ agent should be lowered and

TABLE 28-1 Neuromuscular Junction Blockers

Drug Name	Preferred Uses	Potential Problems
atracurium (*Tracrium*)	Mechanical ventilation; long duration of action; surgical procedures	Has no effect on pain perception or consciousness; do not use before induction of anesthesia; bradycardia is more common with this drug; reduce dose in renal failure
cisatracurium (*Nimbex*)	Intermediate action; used for surgical procedures and to facilitate intubation	No known effect on pain perception or consciousness; contains benzyl alcohol, avoid use in neonates
doxacurium (*Nuromax*)	Surgical procedures; facilitates intubation; mechanical ventilation	No known effect on pain perception or consciousness; contains benzyl alcohol, avoid use with neonates
mivacurium (*Mivacron*)	Short surgical procedures; rapid recovery; facilitates endotracheal intubation	No known effect on pain perception or consciousness; dosage may be affected by renal or hepatic impairment
pancuronium (*Pavulon*)	Surgical procedures; mechanical ventilation	Vagalytic effect, associated with increased heart rate; long-term use for mechanical ventilation, monitor for prolonged adverse effects
pipercuronium (*Arduan*)	Surgical procedures of ≤90 min; facilitates endotracheal intubation	Not as likely as tubocurarine to cause bradycardia; not recommended for long-term use; no known effect on pain perception or consciousness
rocuronium (*Zemuron*)	Rapid onset; preferred for rapid intubation; short outpatient surgical procedures	No known effect on pain perception or consciousness; may be associated with pulmonary hypertension; use caution with hepatic impairment
tubocurarine (generic)	Surgical procedures; electroshock therapy; diagnosis of myasthenia gravis when neostigmine or edrophonium is not conclusive	May cause histamine release and increase secretions; may cause neuroganglia blockade and cause hypotension
vecuronium (*Norcuron*)	Short surgical procedures; intubation; mechanical ventilation	May contain benzyl alcohol; avoid use in neonates, can cause fatalities in premature infants; monitor with long-term use during ventilation; if response does not occur with first twitch test, discontinue, may be associated with permanent muscle damage
succinylcholine (*Anectine, Quelicin*)	Surgical procedures; intubation; mechanical ventilation	May cause myalgia secondary to muscle contraction; associated with increased intraocular pressure; increased intragastric pressure which may cause vomiting; more likely to cause malignant hyperthermia

the patient should be monitored closely until complete recovery occurs.

If NMJ blockers are combined with cholinesterase inhibitors, the effectiveness of the NMJ blockers is decreased because of a buildup of ACh in the synaptic cleft. Combination with xanthines (eg, theophylline, aminophylline) could result in reversal of the neuromuscular blockage. Patients receiving this combination of drugs should be monitored very closely during the procedure for the potential of early arousal and return of muscle function.

Nursing Considerations for Patients Receiving Neuromuscular Junction Blockers

Assessment: History and Examination

Screen for the following conditions, which could be cautions or contraindications to use of the drug: any known allergies to these drugs; impaired liver or kidney function; myasthenia gravis; pregnancy or lactation; impaired cardiac or respiratory function; personal or family history of malignant hyperthermia; and fractures, narrow-angle glaucoma, or paraplegia.

Include screening for baseline status before beginning therapy and for any potential adverse effects. Assess the following: body temperature; skin color and lesions; affect, orientation, reflexes, pupil size and reactivity, and muscle tone and response; pulse, blood pressure, and electrocardiogram

(ECG); respiration and adventitious sounds; bowel sounds and abdominal examination; renal and liver function tests and serum electrolytes.

Nursing Diagnoses

The patient receiving an NMJ blocker may have the following nursing diagnoses related to drug therapy:

- Impaired Gas Exchange related to depressed respirations
- Impaired Skin Integrity related to immobility
- Impaired Verbal Communication, Fear related to paralysis
- Deficient Knowledge regarding drug therapy

Implementation

- Administration of the drug should be performed by trained personnel (usually an anesthesiologist) *because of the potential for serious adverse effects and the need for immediate ventilatory support.*
- Have supplies and equipment on standby *to maintain airway and provide mechanical ventilation.*
- Do not mix the drug with any alkaline solutions such as barbiturates, *because a precipitate may form, making it inappropriate for use.*

- Test patient response and recovery periodically if the drug is being given over a long period, *to maintain mechanical ventilation. Discontinue the drug if response does not occur or is greatly delayed.*
- Monitor patient temperature *for prompt detection and treatment of malignant hyperthermia.*
- Maintain dantrolene on standby *for treatment of malignant hyperthermia if it should occur.*
- Arrange for a small dose of a nondepolarizing NMJ blocker before the use of succinylcholine, *to reduce adverse effects associated with muscle contraction.*
- Maintain a cholinesterase inhibitor on standby *to overcome excessive neuromuscular blockade caused by nondepolarizing NMJ blockers.*
- Provide a peripheral nerve stimulator on standby *to assess the degree of neuromuscular blockade, if appropriate.*
- Provide comfort measures *to help the patient tolerate drug effects,* such as pain relief as appropriate; reassurance, support, and orientation *for conscious patients unable to move or communicate;* skin care and turning *to prevent skin breakdown;* and supportive care for *emergencies such as hypotension and bronchospasm.*
- Monitor patient response closely (blood pressure, temperature, pulse, respiration, reflexes) *and adjust dosage accordingly to ensure the greatest therapeutic effect with minimal risk of toxicity.*
- Incorporate information on this drug into a thorough preoperative patient teaching plan, *because most patients who receive the drug will be receiving teaching about a particular procedure and will be unconscious when the drug is given.* (See Patient Teaching Checklist: Neuromuscular Junction Blockers.)
- Offer support and encouragement *to help the patient cope with drug effects.*

Evaluation

- Monitor patient response to the drug (adequate muscle paralysis).
- Monitor for adverse effects (respiratory depression, hypotension, bronchospasm, GI slowdown, skin breakdown, fear related to helplessness and inability to communicate).
- Evaluate the effectiveness of the teaching plan (patient can relate anticipated effects of the drug and the recovery process).
- Monitor the effectiveness of comfort measures and compliance with the regimen (see Nursing Care Guide: Neuromuscular Junction Blockers).

PATIENT TEACHING CHECKLIST

Neuromuscular Junction Blockers

Create customized patient teaching materials for a specific neuromuscular junction blocker from the CD-ROM. Patient teaching should stress the following points for drugs within the class:

Before the _____ (surgery, ventilation, intubation), you will be given a drug to paralyze your muscles called a neuromuscular blocking agent. It is important that your muscles do not move at this time because it could interfere with the procedure.

Common effects of these drugs include complete paralysis:

- You will not be able to move or to speak while you are receiving this drug.
- You will not be able to breathe on your own, and you will receive assistance in breathing.
- This drug may not affect your level of consciousness, and it can be very frightening to be unable to communicate with anyone around you. Someone will be with you, will try to anticipate your needs, and will explain what is going on at all times.
- This drug may have no effect on your pain perception. Every effort will be made to make sure that you do not experience pain.
- If you receive the drug succinylcholine, you may experience back and throat pain related to muscle contractions that occur. You will be able to take aspirin to relieve this discomfort.
- Recovery of your muscle function may take _____, and someone will be nearby at all times until you have recovered from the paralysis.

This Teaching Checklist reflects general patient teaching guidelines. It is not meant to be a substitute for drug-specific teaching information, which is available in nursing drug guides.

CHAPTER SUMMARY

- The nerves communicate with muscles at a point called the neuromuscular junction (NMJ), using acetylcholine (ACh) as the neurotransmitter.
- NMJ blockers prevent skeletal muscle function.
- Nondepolarizing NMJ blockers prevent ACh from exciting the muscle, and paralysis ensues because the muscle is unable to respond.
- Depolarizing NMJ blockers cause muscle paralysis by acting like ACh and exciting the muscle (depolarization), preventing repolarization and further stimulation of that muscle cell.
- NMJ blockers are primarily used as adjuncts to general anesthesia, to facilitate endotracheal intubation, to facilitate mechanical ventilation, and to prevent injury during electroconvulsive therapy.
- Adverse effects of NMJ blockers, such as prolonged paralysis, inability to breathe, weakness, muscle pain and soreness, and effects of immobility, are related to muscle function blocking.
- Care of patients receiving NMJ blockers must include support and reassurance, because communication is decreased with paralysis; vigilant maintenance of airways and respiration; prevention of skin breakdown; and monitoring for return of function.

C A S E   S T U D Y

Using Succinylcholine in an Elderly Patient

THE SITUATION

S. N., an 82-year-old white woman in very good health, has been admitted to the hospital for an exploratory laparotomy to evaluate a probable abdominal mass. On admission, health care practitioners learned that she had a history of mild hypertension that was well regulated by diuretic therapy. She received a baseline physical examination and preoperative instruction. On the morning of the surgery, it was noted that the anesthesiologist planned to give her a general anesthetic and succinylcholine to ensure muscle paralysis.

CRITICAL THINKING

- What nursing care plans should be made for S. N.? *Consider the patient's age and associated chronic problems that often occur with aging. Also consider the support that she has available and potential physical and emotional support that she might need before and after this procedure. Use of a neuromuscular junction (NMJ) blocker in the elderly presents some nursing challenges that may not be seen with younger patients. What particular nursing care activities should be considered with S. N.?*
- *Because S. N. has been maintained on long-term diuretic therapy, she is at special risk for electrolyte imbalance.*
- What, if any, complications could arise if S. N. has electrolyte disturbances before surgery?

DISCUSSION

Before surgery, the preoperative teaching protocol should be reviewed with the patient. S. N. should be advised that she may experience back, neck, and throat pain after the procedure. Reassure her that this is normal and that aspirin will be made available to alleviate the discomfort. Review deep breathing and coughing; she may need encouragement to clear secretions from her lungs and ensure full inflation. This is usually easier to do if it is a familiar activity. S. N.'s serum electrolytes should be evaluated before surgery, because potassium imbalance can cause unexpected effects with succinylcholine. Renal and hepatic function tests should also be performed to ensure that the dosage of the NMJ blocker is not excessive.

During the procedure, S. N.'s cardiac and respiratory status should be monitored carefully for any potential problems; such effects are more common in people with underlying physical problems. Because of S. N.'s age and potential circulatory problems, she should receive meticulous skin care and turning as soon as the procedure allows this kind of movement. She should be turned frequently during the recovery period, and her skin should be checked for any breakdown. Nursing personnel must be near the patient until she has regained muscle control and the ability to communicate. She should be evaluated for the need for pain medication and position adjustments.

S. N. will require further teaching about her diagnosis and potential treatment. This should wait until she has regained full ability to communicate and is able to respond and participate in any discussion that may be held. At that time, she may require emotional support and encouragement. It may be necessary to contact available family or social service agencies regarding her physical and medical needs.

Review Questions

1. Nondepolarizing NMJ blockers
   a. antagonize acetylcholine to prevent depolarization of muscle cells.
   b. act as agonists of acetylcholine and cause depolarization of muscle cells.
   c. prevent the repolarization of muscle cells.
   d. are associated with painful muscle contractions on administration.

2. Curare is used as a poison on arrow tips in some cultures. Curare
   a. is a depolarizing NMJ blocker.
   b. causes muscle paralysis in the brain, leading to respiratory arrest and death.
   c. is not affected by cooking.
   d. has no clinical use today.

3. Succinylcholine has a rapid onset of action and a short duration of activity because it
   a. does not bind well to receptor sites.
   b. rapidly crosses the blood–brain barrier and is lost.

   c. is broken down by acetylcholinesterase that is found in the plasma.
   d. is very unstable.

4. Whenever NMJ blockers are used, the patient
   a. must be in an intensive care unit.
   b. must be intubated to ensure continuation of respirations.
   c. will have no memory of any events.
   d. will have no adverse effects after the drug is stopped.

5. Malignant hyperthermia can occur with any NMJ blocker, but it most often occurs with succinylcholine. This disorder is treated with
   a. barbiturates.
   b. ice packs.
   c. dantrolene.
   d. diazepam.

6. Patient recovery from an NMJ blocker
   a. is predictable, based on the drug given.
   b. can be affected by genetic enzyme deficiency.
   c. can always be ensured because of the drug half-life.
   d. can be shortened by administration of oxygen.

NURSING CARE GUIDE

Neuromuscular Junction Blockers

Assessment	Nursing Diagnoses	Implementation	Evaluation
HISTORY Allergies to any of these drugs, COPD, cardiac disorders, myasthenia gravis, pregnancy and lactation, hepatic or renal dysfunction, fractures, glaucoma	Impaired Gas Exchange related to depressed respirations Impaired Skin Integrity related to immobility Deficient Knowledge regarding drug therapy Impaired Verbal Communication, fear related to paralysis and inability to communicate	Administer drug under strict supervision. Provide comfort and safety measures: positioning, skin care, temperature control, pain medication as needed, maintain airway, ventilate patient, antidotes on standby. Provide support and reassurance to deal with paralysis and inability to communicate. Provide patient teaching about procedure being performed, what to expect. Provide life support as needed.	Evaluate drug effects: muscle paralysis. Monitor for adverse effects: CV effects (tachycardia, hypotension, respiratory distress, increased respiratory secretions), GI effects (constipation, nausea), skin breakdown, anxiety, fear. Monitor for drug–drug interactions as indicated for each drug. Evaluate effectiveness of patient teaching program. Evaluate effectiveness of comfort and safety measures. Constantly monitor vital signs and return of normal muscular function.
PHYSICAL EXAMINATION CV: BP, P, peripheral perfusion, ECG CNS: orientation, affect, reflexes, vision Skin: color, lesions, texture, sweating GU: urinary output, bladder tone GI: abdominal exam Resp: R, adventitious sounds			

7. When preparing NMJ blockers for administration, it is important that they
   a. are not mixed in with any alkaline solutions, because a precipitate may form.
   b. are not exposed to light.
   c. are not mixed with any other drug.
   d. are not mixed with heparin.
8. An NMJ blocker would not be used to
   a. facilitate endotracheal intubation.
   b. facilitate mechanical ventilation.
   c. prevent injury during electroconvulsive therapy.
   d. relieve pain during labor and delivery.

BIBLIOGRAPHY

Bullock, B. L. (2000). *Focus on pathophysiology.* Philadelphia: Lippincott Williams & Wilkins.

Drug facts and comparisons. (2002). St. Louis: Facts and Comparisons.

Gilman, A., Hardman, J. G., & Limbird, L. E. (Eds.) (2002). *man and Gilman's the pharmacological basis of* Phila. (10th ed.). New York: McGraw-Hill.

Karch, A. M. (2002). *2003 Lippincott's nu* delphia: Lippincott Williams & Wilki

Professional's guide to patient dru and Comparisons.

V

Drugs Acting on the Autonomic Nervous System

CHAPTER

29

Introduction to the Autonomic Nervous System

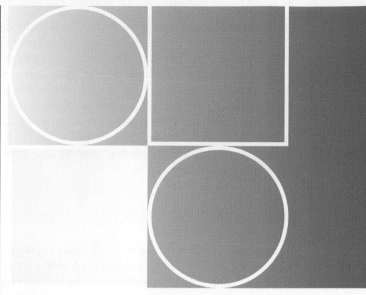

385

The **autonomic nervous system** (ANS) is sometimes called the involuntary or visceral nervous system because it mostly functions with little conscious awareness of its activity. Working closely with the endocrine system, the ANS helps to regulate and integrate the body's internal functions within a relatively narrow range of normal, on a minute-to-minute basis. The ANS integrates parts of the central nervous system (CNS) and peripheral nervous system to automatically react to changes in the internal and external environment (Figure 29–1).

GENERAL FUNCTIONS

The main nerve centers for the ANS are located in the hypothalamus, the medulla, and the spinal cord. Nerve impulses that arise in peripheral structures are carried to these centers by afferent nerve fibers. These integrating centers in the CNS respond by sending out efferent impulses along the autonomic nerve pathways. These impulses adjust the functioning of various internal organs in ways that keep the body's internal environment constant, or homeostatic.

The ANS works to regulate blood pressure, heart rate, respiration, body temperature, water balance, urinary excretion, and digestive functions, among other things. The minute-to-minute control exerted by this system results from an interrelationship between opposing divisions of the autonomic system: the sympathetic and the parasympathetic divisions (Figure 29–2).

◼◼●◼ WEB LINKS
To explore the virtual ANS, consult the following Internet sources:

http://www.InnerBody.com

DIVISIONS OF THE AUTONOMIC NERVOUS SYSTEM

Throughout the ANS, nerve impulses are carried from the CNS to the outlying organs by way of a two-neuron system. In most peripheral nervous system activities, the CNS nerve body sends an impulse directly to an effector organ or muscle. The ANS does not send impulses directly to the periphery. Instead, axons from CNS neurons end in **ganglia,** or groups of nerve bodies that are packed together, located outside the CNS. These ganglia receive information from the preganglionic neuron that started in the CNS and relay that information along postganglionic neurons. The postganglionic neurons transmit impulses to the neuroeffector cells—muscles, glands, and organs. The ANS is divided into two branches (sympathetic and parasympathetic) that differ in three basic ways: (1) the location of the originating cells in the CNS, (2)

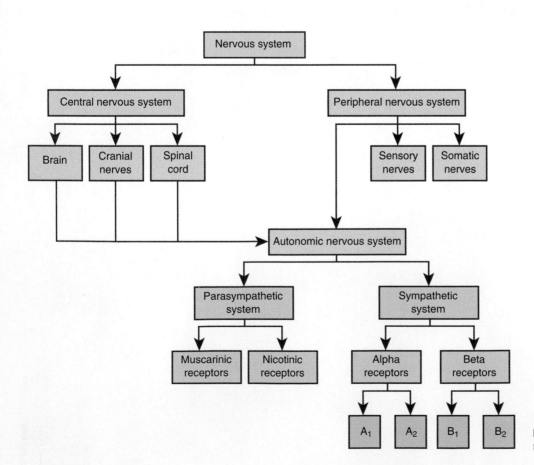

FIGURE 29-1. Organization of the nervous system.

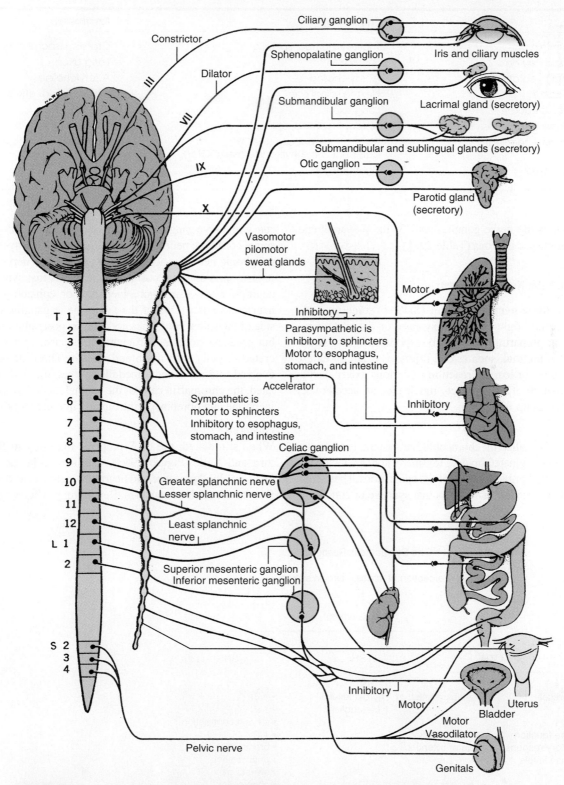

FIGURE 29–2. The autonomic nervous system. The parasympathetic, or craniosacral, division sends long preganglionic fibers that synapse with a second nerve cell in ganglia located close to or within the organs that are then innervated by short postganglionic fibers. The sympathetic, or thoracolumbar, division sends relatively short preganglionic fibers to the chains of paravertebral ganglia and to certain outlying ganglia. The second cell shown sends relatively long postganglionic fibers to the organs it innervates.

TABLE 29-1 Comparison of the Sympathetic and Parasympathetic Nervous Systems

Characteristic	Sympathetic	Parasympathetic
CNS nerve origin	Thoracic, lumbar spinal cord	Cranium, sacral spinal cord
Preganglionic neuron	Short axon	Long axon
Preganglionic neurotransmitter	Acetylcholine	Acetylcholine
Ganglia location	Next to spinal cord	Within or near effector organs
Postganglionic neuron	Long axon	Short axon
Postganglionic neurotransmitter	Norephinephrine, epinephrine	Acetylcholine
Neurotransmitter terminator	Monoamine oxidase (MAO), catechol-O-methyltransferase (COMT)	Acetylcholinesterase
General response	Fight or flight	Rest and digest

the location of the nerve ganglia, and (3) the preganglionic and postganglionic neurons (Table 29–1).

The Sympathetic Nervous System

The **sympathetic nervous system** (SNS) is sometimes referred to as the "fight or flight" system, or the system responsible for preparing the body to respond to stress. Stress can either be internal, such as cell injury or death, or external, a perceived or learned reaction to various external situations or stimuli. The SNS acts much like an accelerator, speeding things up for action.

Anatomy

The SNS is also called the thoracolumbar system, because the CNS cells that originate impulses for this system are located in the thoracic and lumbar sections of the spinal cord. These cells send out short preganglionic fibers that synapse or communi-

cate with nerve ganglia located in chains running alongside the spinal cord. The neurotransmitter that is released by these preganglionic nerves is acetylcholine (ACh). The nerve ganglia, in turn, send out long postganglionic fibers that synapse with neuroeffectors, using norepinephrine or epinephrine as the neurotransmitter. One of the sympathetic ganglia, on either side of the spinal cord, does not develop postganglionic axons but produces norepinephrine and epinephrine, which are secreted directly into the blood stream. These ganglia have evolved into the adrenal medullae. When the SNS is stimulated, the chromaffin cells of the adrenal medullae secrete epinephrine and norepinephrine directly into the bloodstream.

Functions

When stimulated, the SNS prepares the body to flee or to turn and fight (Figure 29–3). Cardiovascular activity increases; blood pressure and heart rate increase, as does blood flow to the skeletal muscles. Respiratory efficiency also in-

FIGURE 29–3. The "fight or flight" response: the sympathetic stress reaction. ACTH, adrenocorticotropic hormone; ADH, antidiuretic hormone; BP, blood pressure; GI, gastrointestinal; P, pulse; R, heart rate; SNS, sympathetic nervous system; TSH, thyroid stimulating hormone.

creases; bronchi are dilated to allow more air to enter with each breath, and the respiratory rate increases. Pupils dilate to permit more light to enter the eye, to improve vision in darkened areas (which helps a person to see in order to fight or flee). Sweating increases, to dissipate heat generated by the increased metabolic activity.

Piloerection (hair standing on end) also occurs. In lower animals, this important protection mechanism makes the fur stand up on end, so that an attacking larger animal is often left with a mouthful of fur while the intended victim scurries away. The actual benefit to humans is not known, except that this activity helps to generate heat when the core body temperature is too low.

SNS stimulation causes blood to be diverted away from the gastrointestinal tract, because there is no real need to digest food during a flight-or-fight situation. Because of this, bowel sounds decrease and digestion slows dramatically; sphincters are constricted, and no bowel evacuation can occur. Blood is also diverted away from other internal organs, including the kidneys, resulting in activation of the renin–angiotensin system (Chapter 42) and a further increase in blood pressure and blood volume as water is retained by the kidneys. Sphincters in the urinary bladder are also constricted, precluding urination.

Several other metabolic activities occur that prepare the body to fight or flee. For example, glucose is formed by glycogenolysis, to increase blood glucose levels and provide energy. The immune and inflammatory reactions are suppressed, to preserve energy that otherwise might be used by these activities. The corticosteroid hormones are released to regulate glucose activity and balance electrolytes. Together, all of these activities prepare the body to flee or to fight more effectively. When overstimulated, however, they can lead to system overload and a variety of diseases.

Adrenergic Transmission

Sympathetic postganglionic nerves that synthesize, store, and release norepinephrine are referred to as adrenergic nerves. Adrenergic nerves are also found within the CNS. The chromaffin cells of the adrenal medulla also are adrenergic, because they synthesize, store, and release norepinephrine as well as epinephrine.

Norepinephrine Synthesis and Storage

Norepinephrine belongs to a group of structurally related chemicals called catecholamines. Dopamine and epinephrine are also catecholamines. Norepinephrine is made by the nerve cells using tyrosine, which is obtained in the diet. Dihydroxyphenylalanine (dopa) is produced by a nerve, using tyrosine from the diet and other chemicals. With the help of the enzyme dopa decarboxylase, it is converted to dopamine, which in turn is converted to norepinephrine in adrenergic cells. The norepinephrine then is stored in granules or storage vesicles within the cell. These vesicles move down the nerve axon to the terminals of the axon, where they line up along the cell membrane. To be an adrenergic nerve, the

nerve must contain all of the enzymes and building blocks necessary to produce norepinephrine (Figure 29–4).

Norepinephrine Release

When the nerve is stimulated, the action potential travels down the nerve axon and arrives at the axon terminal (see Chapter 19). The action potential then depolarizes the axon membrane. This action allows calcium into the nerve, causing the membrane to contract and the storage vesicles to fuse with the cell membrane, then dump their load of norepinephrine into the synaptic gap or cleft. The norepinephrine travels across the very short gap to very specific adrenergic receptor sites on the effector cell on the other side of the synaptic gap.

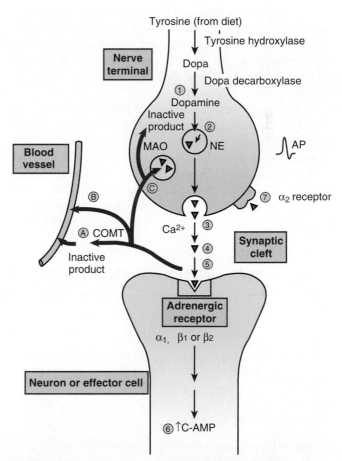

FIGURE 29–4. Sequence of events at an adrenergic synapse. *1*, Dopamine, a precursor of norepinephrine (NE), is synthesized from tyrosine in several steps. Metyrosine inhibits tyrosine hydroxylase; a drug given with dopa to parkinsonian patients inhibits dopa decarboxylase. *2*, Dopamine is taken into the storage vesicle and converted to NE. *3*, Release of neurotransmitter by action potential (AP) in presynaptic nerve. *4*, Diffusion of neurotransmitter across synaptic cleft. *5*, Combination of neurotransmitter with receptor. The events resulting from NE's occupying of receptor sites depend on the nature of the postsynaptic cell. *6*, Interaction of NE with many β-receptors leads to increased synthesis of cyclic adenosine monophosphate (C-AMP). *7*, Feedback control at α₂-receptor leads to decreased NE relapse from presynaptic neuron. An enzyme, catechol O-methyl transferase (COMT), inactives the NE (A), but the most important way in which the action of NE is terminated is by reuptake into the presynaptic neuron (C), where it may be reused or inactivated by another enzyme, monoamine oxidase (MAO). The neurotransmitter may also diffuse away from the synaptic cleft (B).

Adrenergic Receptors

The receptor sites that react with neurotransmitters at adrenergic sites have been classified as **α-receptors** and **β-receptors;** further classifications include α_1-, α_2-, β_1-, and β_2-receptors (Table 29–2). The distinction arises because different drugs that are known to affect the SNS may affect parts of the sympathetic response but not all of it. It is thought that receptors may respond to different concentrations of norepinephrine or different ratios of norepinephrine and epinephrine. **Adrenergic receptors** can be stimulated by the neurotransmitter released from the axon in the immediate vicinity, and they can be further stimulated by circulating norepinephrine and epinephrine secreted directly into the bloodstream by the adrenal medulla.

α-Receptors

α_1-Receptors are found in blood vessels, in the iris, and in the urinary bladder. In blood vessels, they can cause vasoconstriction and increase peripheral resistance, thus raising blood pressure. In the iris, they cause pupil dilation. In the urinary bladder, they cause the increased closure of the internal sphincter.

α_2-Receptors are located on nerve membranes and act as modulators of norepinephrine release. When norepinephrine is released from a nerve ending, it crosses the synaptic cleft to react with its specific receptor site. Some of it also flows back to react with the α-receptor on the nerve membrane. This causes a reflex decrease in norepinephrine release. In this way, the α_2-receptor helps to prevent overstimulation of effector sites. These receptors are also found on the beta cells in the pancreas, where they help to moderate the insulin release stimulated by SNS activation.

β-Receptors

β_1-Receptors are found in cardiac tissue, where they can stimulate increased myocardial activity and increased heart rate. They are also responsible for increased lipolysis in peripheral tissues.

β_2-Receptors are found in the smooth muscle in blood vessels, in the bronchi, in the periphery, and in uterine muscle. In blood vessels, β_2-stimulation leads to vasodilation. β_2-Receptors also cause dilation in the bronchi. In the periphery, they can cause increased muscle and liver breakdown of glycogen and increased release of glucagon from the alpha cells of the pancreas. Stimulation of β_2-receptors in the uterus results in relaxed uterine smooth muscle.

Termination of Transmission

Once norepinephrine has been released into the synaptic cleft, stimulation of the receptor site is terminated only when any extra norepinephrine, as well as the neurotransmitter that has reacted with the receptor site, is disposed of. Most of the free norepinephrine molecules are taken up by the nerve terminal that released them. This neurotransmitter is then repackaged into vesicles to be released later with nerve stimulation. This is an effective recycling effort by the nerve. Enzymes are also in the area, as well as in the liver, to metabolize or biotransform any remaining norepinephrine or any norepinephrine that is absorbed into circulation. These enzymes are **monoamine oxidase (MAO)** and catechol O-methyl transferase (COMT).

TABLE 29-2 | **Physiological Effects of Specific Receptor Sites in the Autonomic Nervous System**

Sympathetic System	Parasympathetic System
α_1-Receptors 　Vasoconstriction 　Increased peripheral resistance with increased blood pressure 　Contracted piloerection muscles 　Pupil dilation 　Thickened salivary secretions 　Closure of urinary bladder sphincter 　Male sexual emmission	Muscarinic receptors 　Pupil constriction 　Accommodation of the lens 　Decreased heart rate 　Increased GI motility 　Increased GI secretions 　Increased urinary bladder contraction 　Male erection 　Sweating
α_2-Receptors 　Negative feedback control of norepinephrine release from presynaptic neuron 　Moderation of insulin release from the pancreas	Nicotinic receptors 　Muscle contractions 　Release of norepinephrine from the adrenal medulla 　Autonomic ganglia stimulation
β_1-Receptors 　Increased heart rate 　Increased conduction through the atrioventricular node 　Increased myocardial contraction 　Lipolysis in peripheral tissues	
β_2-Receptors 　Vasodilation 　Bronchial dilation 　Increased breakdown of muscle and liver glycogen 　Release of glucagon from the pancreas 　Relaxation of uterine smooth muscle 　Decreased gastrointestinal (GI) muscle tone and activity 　Decreased GI secretions 　Relaxation of urinary bladder detrusor muscle	

The Parasympathetic Nervous System

In many areas, the **parasympathetic nervous system** (PSNS) works in opposition to the SNS. This allows the autonomic system to maintain a fine control over internal homeostasis. For instance, the SNS increases heart rate, and the parasympathetic system decreases it. Therefore, the ANS can influence heart rate by increasing or decreasing sympathetic activity, or by increasing or decreasing parasympathetic activity. This is very much like controlling the speed of a car by moving between the accelerator and the brake or combining the two. Whereas the SNS is associated with the stress reaction and expenditure of energy, the PSNS is associated with activities that help the body to store up or conserve energy, a "rest and digest" response (Table 29–3).

Anatomy

The PSNS is sometimes called the craniosacral system, because the CNS neurons that originate parasympathetic impulses are found in the cranium (one of the most important being the vagus or tenth cranial nerve) and in the sacral area of the spinal cord (see Figure 29–1). The PSNS has long preganglionic axons that meet in ganglia located close to or within the organ that will be affected. The postganglionic axon is very short, going directly to the effector cell. The neurotransmitter used by both the preganglionic and postganglionic neurons is ACh.

Functions

PSNS stimulation results in the following actions:

- Increased motility and secretions in the gastrointestinal tract, to promote digestion and absorption of nutrients.
- Decreased heart rate and contractility, to conserve energy and provide rest for the heart.
- Constriction of the bronchi, with increased secretions.
- Relaxation of the gastrointestinal and urinary bladder sphincters, allowing evacuation of waste products.
- Pupillary constriction, which decreases the light entering the eye and decreases stimulation of the retina.

These activities are aimed at increasing digestion, absorption of nutrients, and building of essential proteins as well as a general conservation of energy.

Cholinergic Transmission

Neurons that use ACh as their neurotransmitter are called cholinergic neurons. There are four basic kinds of cholinergic nerves:

1. All preganglionic nerves in the ANS, both sympathetic and parasympathetic
2. Postganglionic nerves of the PSNS and a few SNS nerves, such as those that re-enter the spinal cord and cause general body reactions like sweating

TABLE 29-3 | Effects of Autonomic Stimulation

Effector Site	Sympathetic Reaction	Parasympathetic Reaction
Eye structures		
Iris radial muscle	Contraction (pupil dilates)	—
Iris sphincter muscle	—	Contraction (pupil constricts)
Ciliary muscle	—	Contraction (lens accommodates for near vision)
Lacrimal glands	—	↑ Secretions
Heart	↑ Rate, contractility	↓ Rate
	↑ Atrioventricular conduction	↓ atrioventricular conduction
Blood vessels		
Skin, mucous membranes	Constriction	—
Skeletal muscle	Dilation	
Bronchial muscle	Relaxation (dilation)	Constriction
Gastrointestinal system		
Muscle motility and tone	↓ Activity	↑ Activity
Sphincters	Contraction	Relaxation
Secretions	↓ Secretions	↑ Activity
Salivary glands	Thick secretions	Copious, watery secretions
Gallbladder	Relaxation	Contraction
Liver	Glyconeogenesis	—
Urinary bladder		
Detrusor muscle	Relaxation	Contraction
Trigone muscle and sphincter	Contraction	Relaxation
Sex organs		
Male	Emission	Erection (vascular dilation)
Female	Uterine relaxation	—
Skin structures		
Sweat glands	↑ Sweating	—
Piloerector muscles	Contracted (goosebumps)	—

—, no reaction or response.

3. Motor nerves on skeletal muscles
4. Cholinergic nerves within the CNS

Acetylcholine Synthesis and Storage

ACh is an ester of acetic acid and an organic alcohol called choline. Cholinergic nerves use choline, obtained in the diet, to produce ACh. The last step in the production of the neurotransmitter involves choline acetyltransferase, an enzyme that is also produced within cholinergic nerves. Just like norepinephrine, the ACh is produced in the nerve and travels to the end of the axons, where it is packaged into vesicles. To be a cholinergic nerve, the nerve must contain all of the enzymes and building blocks necessary to produce ACh.

Acetylcholine Release

The vesicles full of ACh move to the nerve membrane; when an action potential reaches the nerve terminal, calcium entering the cell causes the membrane to contract and secrete the neurotransmitter into the synaptic cleft. The ACh travels across the synaptic cleft and reacts with very specific **cholinergic receptor** sites on the effector cell (Figure 29–5).

ACh receptors are found on organs and muscles. They have been classified as **muscarinic receptors** and **nicotinic receptors.** This classification is based on very early research of the ANS that used muscarine (a plant alkaloid from mushrooms) and nicotine (a plant alkaloid found in tobacco plants) to study the actions of the PSNS.

Muscarinic Receptors

As the name implies, muscarinic receptors are receptors that can be stimulated by muscarine. They are found in visceral effector organs, in sweat glands, and in some vascular smooth muscle. Stimulation of muscarinic receptors causes pupil constriction, increased gastrointestinal motility and secretions (including saliva), increased urinary bladder contraction, and a slowing of the heart rate.

Nicotinic Receptors

Nicotinic receptors are located in the CNS, the adrenal medulla, the autonomic ganglia, and the neuromuscular junction. Stimulation of nicotinic receptors causes muscle contractions, autonomic responses, and release of norepinephrine and epinephrine from the adrenal medulla.

Termination of Transmission

Once the effector cell has been stimulated by ACh, it is important to stop the stimulation and get rid of the ACh. The destruction of ACh is carried out by the enzyme **acetylcholinesterase.** This enzyme reacts with the ACh to form a chemically inactive compound. The breakdown of the released ACh is accomplished in a thousandth of a second and the receptor is vacated, allowing the effector membrane to repolarize and be ready for the next stimulation.

CHAPTER SUMMARY

• The autonomic nervous system (ANS) works with the endocrine system to regulate internal functioning and maintain homeostasis.

FIGURE 29–5. Sequence of events at a cholinergic synapse. *1,* Synthesis of acetylcholine (ACh) from choline (a substance in the diet) and a cofactor (the enzyme is choline acetyltransferase, CoA). *2,* Uptake of neurotransmitter into storage (synaptic) vesicle. *3,* Release of neurotransmitter by action potential (AP) in presynaptic nerve. *4,* Diffusion of neurotransmitter across synaptic cleft. *5,* Combination of neurotransmitter with receptor. The events resulting from ACh's occupying of receptor sites depend on the nature of the postsynaptic cell. ACh excites some cells and inhibits others. An enzyme, acetylcholinesterase (AChE), found in the tissues and on the postsynaptic cell, inactivates ACh (A). Some of the products diffuse into the circulation, but most of the choline formed is taken up and reused by the cholinergic neuron.

• The ANS is divided into two branches, the sympathetic nervous system (SNS) and the parasympathetic nervous system (PSNS).
• The two branches of the ANS work in opposition to maintain minute-to-minute regulation of the internal environment and to allow rapid response to stress situations.
• The SNS, when stimulated, is responsible for the "fight or flight" response. It prepares the body for immediate reaction to stressors by increasing metabolism, diverting blood to big muscles, and increasing cardiac and respiratory function.
• The PSNS, when stimulated, acts as a "rest and digest" response. It increases the digestion, absorption, and metabolism of nutrients and slows metabolism and function to save energy.
• The SNS is composed of CNS cells arising in the thoracic or lumbar area of the spinal cord, short preganglionic ax-

ons, ganglia located near the spinal cord, and long postganglionic axons that react with effector cells. The neurotransmitter used by the preganglionic cells is acetylcholine (ACh); the neurotransmitter used by the postganglionic cells is norepinephrine.

- One SNS ganglion on either side of the spinal cord does not develop postganglionic axons but instead secretes norepinephrine directly into the bloodstream to travel throughout the body to react with adrenergic receptor sites. These ganglia evolved into the adrenal medulla.
- The PSNS comprises CNS cells that arise in the cranium and sacral region of the spinal cord, long preganglionic axons that secrete ACh, ganglia located very close to or within the effector tissue, and short postganglionic axons that also secrete ACh.
- Norepinephrine is made by adrenergic nerves using tyrosine from the diet. It is packaged in storage vesicles that align on the axon membrane and is secreted into the synaptic cleft when the nerve is stimulated. It reacts with specific receptor sites and is then broken down by MAO or COMT to relax the receptor site and recycle the building blocks of norepinephrine.
- ACh is made by choline from the diet and packaged into storage vesicles to be released by the cholinergic nerve into the synaptic cleft. ACh is broken down to an inactive form almost immediately by acetylcholinesterase.
- SNS adrenergic receptors are classified as being α_1-, α_2-, β_1-, or β_2-receptors based on the effectors that they stimulate.
- PSNS receptors are classified as muscarinic or nicotinic, depending on what response they have to these plant alkaloids.

Review Questions

1. The autonomic nervous system functions to
   a. maintain balance and posture.
   b. maintain the special senses.
   c. regulate and integrate internal functions of the body.
   d. coordinate peripheral and central nerve pathways.
2. The autonomic nervous system differs from other systems in the CNS in that
   a. it uses only peripheral pathways.
   b. it affects organs and muscles by way of a two-neuron system.
   c. it uses a unique one-neuron system.
   d. it bypasses the CNS in all of its actions.
3. The sympathetic nervous system
   a. is not called the thoracolumbar system.
   b. is not called the "fight or flight" system.
   c. is not called the craniosacral system.
   d. uses acetylcholine as its sole neurotransmitter.
4. If you suspect that a person is very stressed and is experiencing a sympathetic stress reaction, you would expect to find
   a. increased bowel sounds and urinary output.
   b. constricted pupils and warm, flushed skin.
   c. slow heart rate and decreased systolic blood pressure.
   d. dilated pupils and elevated systolic blood pressure.
5. Stimulating only the β_2-receptors in the sympathetic nervous system would result in
   a. increased heart rate.
   b. increased myocardial contraction.
   c. vasodilation and bronchial dilation.
   d. uterine contraction.
6. The sympathetic system uses catecholamines at the postganglionic receptors. Which of the following is not considered to be a catecholamine?
   a. dopamine.
   b. norepinephrine.
   c. acetylcholine.
   d. epinephrine.
7. Once a postganglionic receptor site has been stimulated, the neurotransmitter must be broken down immediately. The sympathetic system breaks down postganglionic neurotransmitters by using
   a. liver enzymes and acetylcholinesterase.
   b. acetylcholinesterase and MAO.
   c. COMT and liver enzymes.
   d. MAO and COMT.
8. The parasympathetic nervous system, in most situations, opposes the actions of the sympathetic nervous system, allowing the autonomic nervous system to
   a. generally have no effect.
   b. maintain a fine control over internal homeostasis.
   c. promote digestion.
   d. respond to stress most effectively.
9. Cholinergic neurons, those using acetylcholine as their neurotransmitter, can be found in all but which of the following?
   a. motor nerves on skeletal muscles.
   b. preganglionic nerves in the sympathetic and parasympathetic systems.
   c. postganglionic nerves in the parasympathetic system.
   d. the adrenal medulla.
10. Stimulation of the parasympathetic nervous system would cause
    a. slower heart rate and increased gastrointestinal secretions.
    b. faster heart rate and urinary retention.
    c. vasoconstriction and bronchial dilation.
    d. pupil dilation and muscle paralysis.

BIBLIOGRAPHY

Bullock, B. L. (2000). *Focus on pathophysiology*. Philadelphia: Lippincott Williams & Wilkins.
Fox, S. (1991). *Perspectives on human biology*. Dubuque, IA: Wm. C. Brown.
Ganong, W. (1999). *Review of medical physiology* (15th ed.). Norwalk, CT: Appleton & Lange.
Guyton, A., & Hall, J. (2000). *Textbook of medical physiology*. Philadelphia: W. B. Saunders.
Gilman, A., Hardman, J. G., & Limbird, L. E. (Eds.) (2002). *Goodman and Gilman's the pharmacological basis of therapeutics* (10th ed.). New York: McGraw-Hill.

CHAPTER

30

Adrenergic Agents

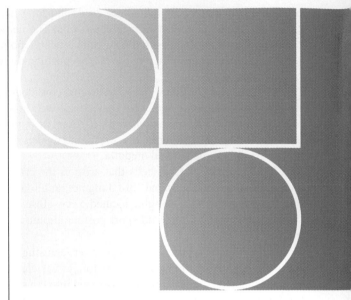

Key Terms
adrenergic agonist
α-agonist
β-agonist
glycogenolysis
sympathomimetic

dreneric agonists are also called **sympathomimetic** drugs because they mimic the effects of the sympathetic nervous system (SNS). The therapeutic and adverse effects associated with these drugs are related to their stimulation of adrenergic receptor sites. The use of adrenergic agonists varies from ophthalmic preparations for dilating pupils to systemic preparations used to support people who are in shock.

ADRENERGIC AGONISTS

The therapeutic and adverse effects associated with these drugs are related to their stimulation of adrenergic receptors sites (Figure 30–1). That stimulation can be either direct, by occupation of the adrenergic receptor, or indirect, by modulation of the release of neurotransmitter from the axon. Some drugs act in both ways.

α- and β-Adrenergic Agonists

Drugs that are generally sympathomimetic (that is, they stimulate all of the adrenergic receptors) are called α- and β-agonists. Some of these drugs are preparations of catecholamines.

Epinephrine (*Adrenalin, Sus-Phrine,* and others) is a naturally occurring catecholamine that interacts with both α- and β-adrenergic receptors. It is used therapeutically in the treatment of shock, when increased blood pressure and heart contractility is essential; as one of the primary treatments for bronchospasm, by direct dilation of the bronchi; as an ophthalmic agent, to reduce intraocular pressure in glaucoma and decrease the production of aqueous humor; and to produce a local vasoconstriction that prolongs the effects of local anesthetics.

Norepinephrine (*Levophed*), another naturally occurring catecholamine, is not used as frequently. It is given intravenously to treat shock or during cardiac arrest to get sympathetic activity, but it has been replaced in recent years by dopamine.

Dopamine (*Intropin*) is the sympathomimetic of choice for the treatment of shock. It stimulates the heart and blood pressure but also causes a renal and splanchnic arteriole dilation that increases blood flow to the kidney, preventing the diminished renal blood supply and possible renal shutdown that can occur with epinephrine or norepinephrine.

Dobutamine (*Dobutrex*) is a synthetic catecholamine that has a slight preference for β_1-receptor sites. It is used in the treatment of congestive heart failure, because it can increase myocardial contractility without much change in rate and does not increase oxygen demand of the cardiac muscle, an advantage over all of the other sympathomimetic drugs.

Ephedrine (Pretz-D) is a synthetically produced plant alkaloid that stimulates the release of norepinephrine from nerve endings and directly acts on adrenergic receptor sites. Although ephedrine was once used for everything from the

DRUG THERAPY ACROSS THE LIFESPAN

Adrenergic Agents

Children	Adults	Other Adults
Children are at greater risk for complications associated with the use of adrenergic agents, including tachycardia, hypertension, tachypnea, and gastrointestinal complications. The dosage for these agents needs to calculated from the child's body weight and age. It is good practice to have a second person check the dosage calculation before administering the drug to avoid potential toxic effects. Children should be carefully monitored and supported during the use of these drugs. Phenylephrine is often found in over-the-counter (OTC) allergy and cold preparations, and parents need to be instructed to be very careful with the use of these drugs—they should check the labels for ingredients, monitor the recommended dosage, and avoid combining drugs that contain similar ingredients.	Adults being treated with adrenergic agents for shock or shock-like states require constant monitoring and dosage adjustments based on their response. Patients who may be at increased risk for cardiac complications should be monitored very closely and started on a lower dose. Adults using these agents for glaucoma or for seasonal rhinitis need to be cautioned about the use of OTC drugs and alternative therapies that might increase the drug effects and cause serious adverse effects. Many of these drugs are used in emergency situations and may be used during pregnancy and lactation. In general, there are no adequate studies about their effects during pregnancy and lactation, and in those situations they should be used only if the benefit to the mother is greater than the risk to the fetus or neonate.	Older patients are more likely to experience the adverse effects associated with these drugs—central nervous system, cardiovascular, gastrointestinal, and respiratory. Because older patients often have renal or hepatic impairment, they are also more likely to have toxic levels of the drug related to changes in metabolism and excretion. Older patients should be started on lower doses of the drugs and should be monitored very closely for potentially serious arrhythmias or blood pressure changes. They too should be cautioned about the use of OTC drugs and complementary therapies that could increase drug effects and cause serious adverse reactions.

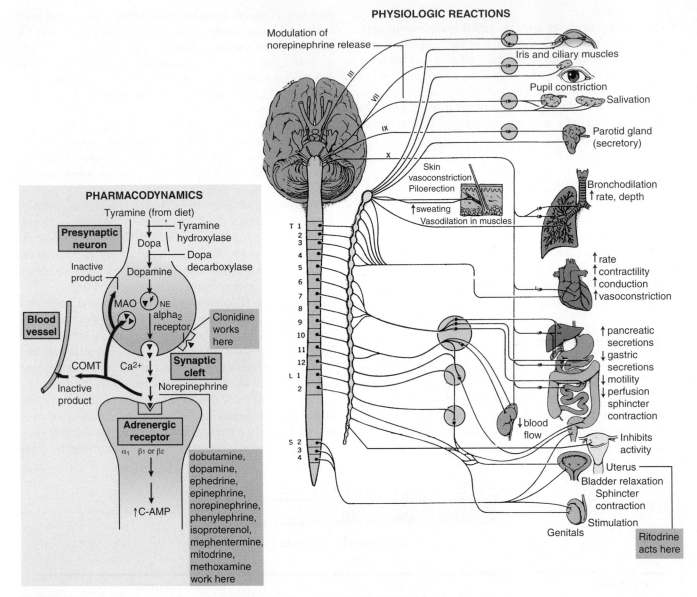

FIGURE 30-1. Pharmacodynamics of adrenergic agonists and associated physiologic reactions.

treatment of shock to chronic management of asthma and allergic rhinitis, its use in many areas is declining because of the availability of less toxic drugs with more predictable onset and action. It is heavily used as a nasal decongestant in a topical, nasal form.

Mephentermine (*Wyamine Sulfate*) is mainly used to treat hypertension that occurs secondary to ganglionic blockade and to spinal anesthesia. It can be used for a short period during emergency treatment of shock due to hemorrhage to maintain blood pressure until blood or blood substitutes are available. Mephentermine has the advantage of not causing tissue irritation, so it can be given intramuscularly and does not cause irritation if extravasation occurs with intravenous use.

Metaraminol (*Aramine*) is a synthetic agent that is very similar to norepinephrine. It is given as a single parenteral injection to prevent hypotension by increasing myocardial contractility and causing peripheral vasoconstriction. Its use

is limited to situations in which dopamine or norepinephrine cannot be used.

◻◼●◼ **WEB LINKS**

Health care providers and patients may want to consult the following Internet sources:

Information on epinephrine and basic sympathomimetic effects:
http://www.healthgate.com

Information on the current treatment of shock:
http://www.healthanswers.com

Information on the acute nursing care of patients in shock as well as research articles:
http://www.aacn.org

Information on cardiovascular research, treatments, and heart transplantation:
http://www.acc.org

Therapeutic Actions and Indications

The effects of the sympathomimetic drugs are mediated by the adrenergic receptors in target organs: heart rate increases with increased myocardial contractility, bronchi dilate and respirations increase in rate and depth, vasoconstriction occurs with increase in blood pressure, intraocular pressure decreases, **glycogenolysis** (breakdown of glucose stores so that the glucose can be used as energy) occurs throughout the body, pupils dilate, and sweating can increase (see Figure 30–1). These drugs are indicated for the treatment of hypotensive states or shock, bronchospasm, and some types of asthma. As noted earlier, dopamine has become the drug of choice for the treatment of shock and hypotensive states, because it causes an increase in renal blood flow and does not cause the renal shutdown that has been associated with other agents. Ephedrine is also widely used as a local nasal drug for the treatment of seasonal rhinitis.

Pharmacokinetics

These drugs are generally absorbed rapidly after injection or passage through mucous membranes. They are metabolized in the liver and excreted in the urine. Because the sympathomimetic drugs stimulate the SNS, they should be used during pregnancy and lactation only if the benefits to the mother clearly outweigh any potential risks to the fetus.

Contraindications and Cautions

The α- and β-agonists are contraindicated in patients with pheochromocytoma, because the systemic overload of catecholamines could be fatal; with tachyarrhythmias or ventricular fibrillation, because the increased heart rate and oxygen consumption usually caused by these drugs could exacerbate these conditions; with hypovolemia, for which fluid replacement would be the treatment for the associated hypotension; and with halogenated hydrocarbon general anesthetics, which sensitize the myocardium to catecholamines and could cause serious cardiac effects. Caution should be used with any kind of peripheral vascular disease (eg, atherosclerosis, Raynaud's disease, diabetic endarteritis), which could be exacerbated by systemic vasoconstriction.

Adverse Effects

The adverse effects associated with the use of α- and β-adrenergic agonists may be associated with the drug's effects on the SNS: arrhythmias, hypertension, palpitations, angina, and dyspnea related to the effects on the heart and cardiovascular (CV) system; nausea and vomiting, related to the depressant effects on the gastrointestinal (GI) tract; and headache, sweating, and piloerection, related to the sympathetic stimulation.

Clinically Important Drug–Drug Interactions

Increased effects of tricyclic antidepressants and monoamine oxidase (MAO) inhibitors can occur because of the increased norepinephrine levels or increased receptor stimulation that occurs with both drugs.

There is an increased risk of hypertension if α- and β-adrenergic agonists are given with any other drugs that cause hypertension.

Nursing Considerations for Patients Receiving α- and β-Adrenergic Agonists

Assessment: History and Examination

Screen for the following conditions, which could be cautions or contraindications to use of the drug: any known allergies to these drugs; pheochromocytoma, tachyarrhythmias or ventricular fibrillation, hypovolemia; general anesthesia with halogenated hydrocarbon anesthetics, which would be contraindications to the use of the drug; and the presence of vascular disease, which would require cautious use of the drug.

Include screening for baseline status before beginning therapy and for any potential adverse effects: skin color, temperature; pulse, blood pressure, ECG; respiration, adventitious sounds; urine output and electrolytes.

Nursing Diagnoses

The patient receiving an α- and β-agonist may have the following nursing diagnoses related to drug therapy:

- Acute Pain related to CV and systemic effects
- Decreased Cardiac Output related to CV effects
- Ineffective Tissue Perfusion related to CV effects
- Deficient Knowledge regarding drug therapy

Implementation

- Use extreme caution in calculating and preparing doses of these drugs, *because even small errors could have serious effects.* Always dilute drug before use, if it is not prediluted, *to prevent tissue irritation on injection.*
- Monitor patient response closely (blood pressure, ECG, urine output, cardiac output) and adjust dosage accordingly, *to ensure most benefit with least amount of toxicity.*
- Maintain phentolamine on standby *in case extravasation occurs; infiltration of the site with 10 mL saline containing 5 to 10 mg phentolamine is usually effective in saving the area.*
- Provide thorough patient teaching, including measures to avoid adverse effects, warning signs of problems, and the need for monitoring and evaluation, *to enhance patient knowledge about drug therapy and to promote compliance.*
- Offer support and encouragement *to deal with the drug regimen.* (See Patient Teaching Checklist: Adrenergic Agonists.)

Evaluation

- Monitor patient response to the drug (improvement in blood pressure, ocular pressure, bronchial airflow).
- Monitor for adverse effects (cardiovascular changes, decreased urine output, headache, GI upset).
- Evaluate the effectiveness of the teaching plan (patient can name the drug, dosage, adverse effects to watch for, specific measures to avoid adverse effects).
- Monitor the effectiveness of comfort measures and com-

DRUGS IN FOCUS
α- and β-Adrenergic Agonists

Drug Name	Dosage/Route	Usual Indications
dobutamine (*Dobutrex*)	2.5–10 µg/kg per minute IV with dosage adjusted based on patient response	Treatment of congestive heart failure
🅿 dopamine (*Intropin*)	Initially 2–10 µg/kg per minute IV with incremental increases up to 20–50 µg/kg per minute based on patient response	Treatment of shock
ephedrine (*Pretz-D*)	Adult: 25–50 mg IM, SC, or IV for acute treatment; 12.5–25 mg PO for asthma maintenance; instill solution in each nostril q4h for seasonal rhinitis Pediatric: 25–100 mg/m² IM or SC in four to six divided doses; 3 mg/kg per day in four to six divided doses PO, SC, or IV for bronchodilation; instill in each nostril q4h for seasonal rhinitis in children >6 y	Treatment of signs and symptoms of seasonal rhinitis; hypotensive episodes
epinephrine (*Adrenalin, Sus-Phrine*)	Adult: 0.5–1.0 mg IV for acute treatment; 0.3–0.5 mg SC or IM for respiratory distress; 1–2 gtts per affected eye q.d.–b.i.d. for glaucoma; may be used in nebulizer or as topical nasal drops Pediatric: 0.01–0.75 mg/kg SC, base dose on age, weight, and response; do not repeat more than q6h; topical nasal drops for children >6 y as needed	Treatment of shock; glaucoma; to prolong effects of regional anesthetic
mephentermine (*Wyamine Sulfate*)	30–45 mg IM or IV may be repeated every 20–30 doses of 30 mg as needed	Treatment of hypotension secondary to ganglionic blockade or spinal anesthesia in adults
metaraminol (*Aramine*)	Adult: 2–10 mg SC or IM to prevent hypotension; 15–100 mg IV in 250–500 mL sodium chloride or dextrose solution to treat hypotension Pediatric: 0.01 mg/kg IV as a single dose	Treatment of shock if norepinephrine or dopamine cannot be used; prevention of hypotension with spinal anesthesia
norepinephrine (*Levophed*)	8–12 µg base/min IV; base rate and dosage on patient response	Treatment of shock; cardiac arrest

pliance to regimen (see Nursing Care Guide: Adrenergic Agonists).

α-Specific Adrenergic Agonists

α-Specific adrenergic agonists, or **α-agonists,** are drugs that bind primarily to α-receptors rather than to β-receptors. Currently, four drugs are in this class: phenylephrine (*Neo-Synephrine, Allerest, AK-Dilate,* and others), methoxamine (*Vasoxyl*), midodrine (*ProAmatine*), and clonidine (*Catapres*).

Phenylephrine, a potent vasoconstrictor with little or no effect on the heart or bronchi, is used in many combination cold and allergy products. Parenterally it is used to treat shock or shock-like states, to overcome paroxysmal supraventricular tachycardia, to prolong local anesthesia, and to maintain blood pressure during spinal anesthesia. Topically it is used to treat allergic rhinitis and to relieve the symptoms of otitis media. Ophthalmically it is used to dilate the pupils for eye examination, before surgery, or to relieve elevated eye pressure associated with glaucoma.

Methoxamine is used primarily to support, restore, and maintain blood pressure during anesthesia. It has also been

used to terminate some episodes of supraventricular tachycardia. It has a prolonged vasopressor effect caused by its α-adrenergic agonist activity leading to increased peripheral resistance. It does not cause an increase in heart rate; in fact, many times it causes a bradycardia, thought to be caused by a carotid sinus reflex.

Midodrine is an oral drug that is used to treat orthostatic hypotension in patients who do not respond to traditional therapy. It activates α-adrenergic receptors, leading to peripheral vasoconstriction and an increase in vascular tone and blood pressure. This effect can cause a serious supine hypertension. Patients need to be monitored in the standing, sitting, and supine positions to determine whether this will be a problem.

Clonidine specifically stimulates CNS α_2-receptors. This leads to decreased sympathetic outflow from the CNS, because the α_2-receptors moderate the release of norepinephrine from the nerve axon. Clonidine is used to treat essential hypertension as a step 2 drug, to treat chronic pain in cancer patients in combination with opiates and other drugs, and to ease withdrawal from opiates. Because of its centrally acting effects, clonidine is associated with many more CNS effects (bad dreams, sedation, drowsiness, fatigue, headache) than

PATIENT TEACHING CHECKLIST
Adrenergic Agonists

Create customized patient teaching materials for a specific adrenergic agonist from the CD-ROM. Patient teaching should stress the following points for drugs within this class:

• An adrenergic agonist, or a sympathomimetic drug, acts by mimicking the effects of the sympathetic nervous system, a particular part of your nervous system that is responsible for your "fight or flight" response. Because this drug causes many effects in the body, you may experience some undesired adverse effects. It is crucial to discuss the effects of the drug with your health care provider and to try to make them as tolerable as possible.
• If your drug is in solution, you should check the solution before each use. If the solution is pink, brown, or black, it should be discarded.
• If you are a man with known prostate problems, it might help to void before each dose of the drug.
• If your drug is to be taken sublingually (under the tongue), you must be careful to avoid swallowing the tablet; do not swallow until the tablet is completely dissolved. If the tablet is swallowed, it will be destroyed in your stomach and you will not receive any of the beneficial effects of the drug.
• If your drug is taken with an inhaler, check the manufacturer's instructions that come with the inhaler, because each one is slightly different.

Some of the following adverse effects may occur:

• *Restlessness, shaking*—If these occur, avoid driving, operating heavy machinery, or performing delicate tasks.
• *Flushing, sweating*—Avoid warm temperatures and heavy clothing; frequent washing with cool water may help.
• *Heart palpitations*—If you feel that your heart is beating too fast or skipping beats, sit down for a while and rest. If the feeling becomes too uncomfortable, notify your health care provider.
• *Sensitivity to light*—Avoid glaring lights or wear sunglasses if in bright light. Be careful when moving between extremes of light, because your vision may not adjust quickly.

Report any of the following to your health care provider: difficulty voiding, chest pain, difficulty breathing, dizziness, headache, changes in vision.

Do not stop taking this drug suddenly; make sure you have enough of your prescription. This drug should be tapered over 2 to 4 days when you are instructed to discontinue it by your health care provider.

Avoid over-the-counter medications, including cold and allergy remedies and diet pills. If you feel that you need one of these, check with your health care provider first.

Tell any doctor, nurse, or other health care provider that you are taking these drugs.

Keep this drug, and all medications, out of the reach of children. Do not share these drugs with other people.

This Teaching Checklist reflects general patient teaching guidelines. It is not meant to be a substitute for drug-specific teaching information, which is available in nursing drug guides.

other sympathomimetics. Because it can also cause extreme hypotension, congestive heart failure, and bradycardia owing to its centrally mediated effects, it should be used carefully with any patient who is susceptible to such conditions. It is available in an oral and transdermal form and in injection form for epidural infusion to control pain.

Therapeutic Actions and Indications

The therapeutic effects of the α-specific adrenergic agonists come from the stimulation of α-receptors within the SNS (see Figure 30–1). The uses are varied, depending on the route of the drug and the drug being used. Clonidine is frequently used to treat essential hypertension. Phenylephrine is found in many cold and allergy products because it is so effective in constricting topical vessels and decreasing the swelling, signs, and symptoms of rhinitis. Midodrine is reserved for use in patients with orthostatic hypotension who do not respond to other therapies because it can cause supine hypertension. Methoxamine is used primarily to support, restore, and maintain blood pressure during anesthesia and to terminate some episodes of supraventricular tachycardia.

Pharmacokinetics

These drugs are generally well absorbed and reach peak levels in a short period—20 to 45 minutes. They are widely distributed in the body, metabolized in the liver, and primarily excreted in the urine. There are no adequate studies about use during pregnancy and lactation, so use should be reserved for situations in which the benefit to the mother outweighs any potential risk to the neonate.

Contraindications and Cautions

The α-specific adrenergic agonists are contraindicated in the presence of allergy to the specific drug; severe hypertension or tachycardia, because of possible additive effects; narrow-angle glaucoma, which could be exacerbated by arterial constriction; or pregnancy, because of potential adverse effects on the fetus.

They should be used with caution in the presence of cardiovascular disease or vasomotor spasm, because these conditions could be aggravated by the vascular effects of the drug; thyrotoxicosis or diabetes, because of the thyroid-stimulating and glucose-elevating effects of sympathetic stimulation; lactation, because the drug may be passed to the infant and cause α-specific adrenergic stimulation; or renal or hepatic impairment, which could interfere with metabolism and excretion of the drug.

Adverse Effects

Patients receiving these drugs often experience adverse effects that are extensions of the therapeutic effects or other sympathetic stimulatory reactions. CNS effects include feelings of anxiety, restlessness, depression, fatigue, strange dreams, blurred vision, and personality changes. Cardiovascular effects can include arrhythmias, ECG changes, blood pressure changes, and peripheral vascular problems. Nausea, vomiting, and anorexia can occur, related to the GI-depressing effects of the sympathetic system. Genitourinary effects can include decreased urinary output, difficulty uri-

NURSING CARE GUIDE

Adrenergic Agonists

Assessment	Nursing Diagnoses	Implementation	Evaluation
HISTORY Allergies to any of these drugs, cardiovascular dysfunction, pheochromocytoma, pregnancy and lactation, narrow angle glaucoma, prostatic hypertrophy, thyroid-disease, diabetes	Decreased Cardiac Output related to CV effects Acute Pain related to CV and systemic effects Impaired Tissue Perfusion related to CV effects Deficient Knowledge regarding drug therapy	Ensure safe and appropriate administration of drug. Provide comfort and safety measures; assistance/siderails, temperature control, lighting control, mouth care, skin care. Monitor BP, P, respiratory status throughout drug therapy. Provide support and reassurance to deal with drug effects and discomfort. Provide patient teaching regarding drug name, dosage, side effects, precautions, and warning signs to report.	Evaluate drug effects: relief of signs and symptoms being treated. Monitor for adverse effects: CV effects, dizziness, confusion; headache, rash; difficulty voiding; sweating, flushing; pupil dilation. Monitor for drug–drug interactions as indicated for each drug. Evaluate effectiveness of patient teaching program. Evaluate effectiveness of comfort and safety measures.
PHYSICAL EXAMINATION CV: BP, P, peripheral perfusion, ECG CNS: orientation, affect, reflexes, vision Skin: color, lesions, texture GU: urinary output GI: abdominal, liver evaluation Resp: R, adventitious sounds			

nating, dysuria, and changes in sexual function related to the sympathetic stimulation of these systems.

Clinically Important Drug–Drug Interactions

Phenylephrine combined with MAO inhibitors can cause severe hypertension, headache, and hyperpyrexia; this combination should be avoided. Increased sympathomimetic effects occur when phenylephrine is combined with tricyclic antidepressants (TCAs); if this combination must be used, the patient should be monitored very closely.

Clonidine has a decreased antihypertensive effect if taken with TCAs, and a paradoxical hypertension occurs if it is combined with propranolol. If these combinations are used, the patient response should be monitored closely and dosage adjustment made as needed.

Midodrine can precipitate increased drug effects of digoxin, β-blockers, and many antipsychotics. Such combinations should be avoided.

Methoxamine in combination with guanethidine, bretylium,

or TCAs has reportedly caused increased vasopressor effects. Patients should be monitored closely and dosage adjustments made as needed.

Nursing Considerations for Patients Receiving α-Specific Adrenergic Agonists

Assessment: History and Examination

Screen for the following conditions, which could be cautions or contraindications to use of the drug: any known allergies to the drug; presence of any cardiovascular diseases, thyrotoxicosis, or diabetes, which would require cautious use; pregnancy or lactation; and chronic renal failure, which could be exacerbated by drug use.

Include screening for baseline status before beginning therapy and for any potential adverse effects: orientation, affect, reflexes, and vision, to monitor for CNS changes related to drug therapy; blood pressure, pulse, ECG, peripheral perfusion, and cardiac output, to establish a baseline and to monitor drug effects and adverse cardiovascular effects; and

CASE STUDY

Adrenergic Agonist Toxicity

THE SITUATION

M. C. is a 26-year-old man who has recently moved to the northeastern United States from New Mexico. He has been suffering from sinusitis, runny nose, and cold-like symptoms for 2 weeks. He appears at an outpatient clinic with complaints of headache, "jitters," inability to sleep, loss of appetite, and a feeling of impending doom. He states that he feels "on edge" and has not been productive in his job as a watch repairman and jewelry maker. According to his history, M. C. has been treated with several different drugs for nocturnal enuresis, a persisting childhood problem. Only ephedrine, which he has been taking for 2 years, has been successful. He has no other significant health problems. He denies any side effects from the use of ephedrine but does admit to self-medicating his nagging cold with over-the-counter (OTC) preparations—a nasal spray used four times a day and a combination decongestant–pain reliever. A physical examination reveals a pulse of 104, BP 154/86, R 16. The patient appears flushed and slightly diaphoretic.

CRITICAL THINKING

• What are the important nursing implications for M. C.? *Think about the problems that confront a patient in a new area seeking health care for the first time.*
• What could be causing the problems that M. C. presents with? *The diagnosis of ephedrine overdose was eventually made based on the patient history of OTC drug use and the presenting signs and symptoms.*
• Keeping in mind that this diagnosis means M. C. has an overstimulated sympathetic stress reaction; what other physical problems can be anticipated? *Overwhelming feelings of anxiety and stress are influencing M. C.'s response to work and health care.*
• Given this fact, how may the nurse best deal with explaining the problem and how it could have happened—without making the patient feel uninformed or that the practice of his former health care provider is being questioned?
• What treatment should be planned and what teaching points should be covered for M. C.?

DISCUSSION

The first step in caring for M. C. is establishing a trusting relationship to help alleviate some of the anxiety he is feeling. Being in a new state and seeking health care in a new setting can be very stressful for patients under normal circumstances. In M. C.'s case, the sympathomimetic effects of the drugs that he has been taking make him feel even more anxious and jittery.

A careful patient history will help determine whether there are any underlying medical problems that could be exacerbated by these drug effects. A review of M. C.'s nocturnal enuresis and the treatments that have been tried will enhance understanding of his former health care and suggest possible implications for further study. This questioning will also give M. C. reassurance that he is an important member of the health team and that the information he has to offer is important and valuable.

A careful review of the OTC drugs that M. C. has been using will be informative for the patient as well as for the health care providers who have not actually checked OTC drugs for those specific ingredients, but combining them to ease signs and symptoms often results in toxic levels and symptoms of overdose. M. C. will need a full teaching program about the effects of his ephedrine and which OTC drugs to avoid. The treatment for his current problems involves withdrawal of the OTC drugs; when these drug levels fall, the signs and symptoms will disappear. M. C. may also wish to avoid nicotine and caffeine, because these stimulants could increase his "jitters."

To build trust and ensure that the underlying cause of the problem was drug toxicity, M. C. should receive written patient instructions that highlight warning signs to report, including chest pain, palpitations, and difficulty voiding. He also should be given the health care provider's telephone number with instructions to call the next day and report on his health status. Finally, the sinusitis should be cultured and antibiotic treatment prescribed, if appropriate.

---

urinary output and renal function tests, to monitor drug effects on the renal system.

Nursing Diagnoses

The patient receiving an α-agonist may have the following nursing diagnoses related to drug therapy:

• Disturbed Sensory Perception (Visual, Kinesthetic, Tactile) related to CNS effects
• Risk for Injury related to CNS, CV effects of drug
• Decreased Cardiac Output related to blood pressure changes, arrhythmias, vasoconstriction
• Deficient Knowledge regarding drug therapy

Implementation

• Do not discontinue drug abruptly, *because sudden withdrawal can result in rebound hypertension, arrhythmias, flushing, and even hypertensive encephalopathy and death; taper drug over 2 to 4 days.*
• Do not discontinue drug before surgery; mark the patient's chart and monitor blood pressure carefully during surgery. *Sympathetic stimulation may alter the normal response to anesthesia as well as recovery from anesthesia.*
• Monitor blood pressure, pulse, rhythm, and cardiac output regularly, even with ophthalmic preparations, *in order to adjust dosage or discontinue the drug if cardiovascular effects are severe.*

DRUGS IN FOCUS
α-Specific Adrenergic Agonists

Drug Name	Dosage/Route	Usual Indications
clonidine (*Catapres*)	0.1 mg PO b.i.d. initially up to a maximum 2.4 mg/d if needed; transdermal system may increase from 0.1 to 0.3 mg/d	Treatment of essential hypertension, chronic pain, to ease opiate withdrawal; used only for adults
methoxamine (*Vasoxyl*)	3–5 mg IV, injected slowly for emergency use; 5–15 mg IM preoperatively, during, and postoperatively depending on response; 10 mg IV, injected slowly to terminate tachycardia	Supporting, restoring, and maintaining blood pressure during anesthesia; treatment of supraventricular tachycardia
midodrine (*ProAmantine*)	10 mg PO t.i.d. during daytime hours when patient is upright	Treatment of orthostatic hypotension
Ⓟ phenylephrine (*Neo-Synephrine*)	1–10 mg SC or IV or 0.1–0.5 mg IV as a starting dose; 0.5 mg IV by rapid injection to convert tachycardias: 1–2 gtt in affected eye or eyes for glaucoma	Cold and allergies; shock and shock-like states; supraventricular tachycardias; glaucoma; allergic rhinitis; otitis media

- When giving phenylephrine intravenously, maintain an α-blocking agent on standby *in case severe reaction occurs;* infiltrate any area of extravasation with phentolamine within 12 hours after extravasation *to preserve tissue.*
- Arrange for supportive care and comfort measures, including rest and environmental control, *to decrease CNS irritation;* headache medication *to relieve discomfort;* safety measures if CNS effects occur *to protect the patient from injury;* and protective measures *if CNS effects are severe.*
- Provide thorough patient teaching, including dosage, potential adverse effects, safety measures, warning signs of problems, and proper administration for each route used, *to enhance patient knowledge about drug therapy and to promote compliance.* (See Patient Teaching Checklist: Adrenergic Agonists.)
- Offer support and encouragement *to help the patient deal with the drug regimen.*

Evaluation

- Monitor patient response to the drug (improvement in condition being treated).
- Monitor for adverse effects (GI upset, CNS and cardiovascular changes).
- Evaluate the effectiveness of the teaching plan (patient can name drug, dosage, adverse effects to watch for, and specific measures to avoid adverse effects).
- Monitor the effectiveness of comfort measures and compliance to the regimen (see Nursing Care Guide: Adrenergic Agonists).

β-Specific Adrenergic Agonists

Most of the drugs that belong to the class of β-specific adrenergic agonists, or **β-agonists,** are β₂-specific agonists, which are used to manage and treat bronchial spasm, asthma, and other obstructive pulmonary conditions. These drugs, including albuterol, bitolterol, isoetharine, metaproterenol, pirbuterol, salmeterol, and terbutaline, are covered in Chapter 55, which deals with drugs used to treat obstructive pulmonary diseases.

Two other β-agonists are available for use. Ritodrine (*Yutopar*) is used to manage preterm labor. Isoproterenol (*Isuprel, Medihaler-Iso*) is used in an inhaled form to treat obstructive pulmonary disease; as an injection to treat shock and cardiac standstill and to prevent bronchospasm during anesthesia; and in a sublingual form to treat bronchospasm, heart block, and some ventricular arrhythmias.

Therapeutic Actions and Indications

The therapeutic effects of these drugs are related to their stimulation of the β-adrenergic receptors. Increased heart rate, conductivity, and contractility; bronchodilation; increased blood flow to skeletal muscles and splanchnic beds; and relaxation of the uterus are the desired effects of these drugs. Ritodrine is indicated for the management of preterm labor because of its relaxing effects on the uterus, stopping uterine contractions. Isoproterenol is indicated for the treatment of shock to increase cardiac activity; with cardiac arrest and certain ventricular arrhythmias to stimulate cardiac activity and conduction; and to prevent bronchospasm, if used in the sublingual or inhaled forms. It is especially effective in treating heart blocks in transplanted hearts.

Pharmacokinetics

These drugs are rapidly distributed after injection; they are metabolized in the liver and excreted in the urine. The half-life of these drugs is relatively short, less than 1 hour. Isoproterenol should be used during pregnancy and lactation only if the benefits to the mother clearly outweigh potential risks to the fetus. Ritodrine is used only to manage preterm labor.

Contraindications and Cautions

The β-specific adrenergic agonists are contraindicated in the presence of allergy to the drug or any components of the drug; with pulmonary hypertension; during anesthesia with halogenated hydrocarbons, which sensitize the myocardium to catecholamines and could cause a severe reaction; with eclampsia, uterine hemorrhage, and intrauterine death, which could be complicated by uterine relaxation or increased blood pressure; and during pregnancy and lactation, because of potential effects on the fetus or neonate, unless used cautiously to manage preterm labor. Caution should be used with diabetes, thyroid disease, vasomotor problems, degenerative heart disease, or history of stroke, all of which could be exacerbated by the sympathomimetic effects of the drugs.

Adverse Effects

Patients receiving these drugs often experience adverse effects related to the stimulation of sympathetic adrenergic receptors. CNS effects include restlessness, anxiety, fear, tremor, fatigue, and headache. Cardiovascular effects can include tachycardia, angina, myocardial infarction, and palpitations. Pulmonary effects can be severe, ranging from difficulty breathing, coughing, and bronchospasm to severe pulmonary edema. GI upset, nausea, vomiting, and anorexia can occur as a result of the slowdown of the GI system by the SNS. Other anticipated effects can include sweating, pupil dilation, rash, and muscle cramps.

Clinically Important Drug–Drug Interactions

Increased sympathomimetic effects can be expected if these drugs are taken with other sympathomimetic drugs. Decreased therapeutic effects can occur if these drugs are combined with β-adrenergic blockers.

Ritodrine has been associated with the increased risk of potentially fatal pulmonary hypertension when it is combined with corticosteroids, so this combination should be avoided.

Nursing Considerations for Patients Receiving β-Specific Adrenergic Agonists
Assessment: History and Examination

Screen for the following conditions, which could be cautions or contraindications to the use of the drug: any known allergies to any drug or any components of the drug; pulmonary hypertension; anesthesia with halogenated hydrocarbons, which sensitize the myocardium to catecholamines and could cause severe reaction; eclampsia, uterine hemorrhage, and intrauterine death, which could be complicated by uterine relaxation or increased blood pressure; pregnancy and lactation, because of potential effects on the fetus or neonate, unless used cautiously to manage preterm labor; diabetes, thyroid disease, vasomotor problems, degenerative heart disease, or history of stroke, all of which could be exacerbated by the sympathomimetic effects of the drugs.

Physical assessment should include screening for baseline status before beginning therapy and for any potential adverse effects: skin color, temperature; pulse, blood pressure, and ECG; respiration, adventitious sounds; and urine output and electrolytes.

Nursing Diagnoses

The patient receiving β-agonists may have the following nursing diagnoses related to drug therapy:

- Acute Pain related to CV and systemic effects
- Decreased Cardiac Output related to CV effects
- Ineffective Tissue Perfusion related to CV effects
- Deficient Knowledge regarding drug therapy

Implementation

- Monitor patient pulse and blood pressure carefully during administration, *in order to arrange to discontinue the drug at any sign of pulmonary edema.*
- Have patients receiving ritodrine lie in the left lateral position during administration, *to decrease risk of hypotension.*

DRUGS IN FOCUS
β-Specific Adrenergic Agonists

Drug Name	Dosage/Route	Usual Indications
ⓟ isoproterenol (*Isuprel*)	Adult: IV injection—0.02–0.06 mg; IV infusion—2–5 μg/min; 0.2 mg IM or SC Pediatric: 0.1–1.0 μg/kg/min has been used	Treatment of shock, cardiac standstill; treatment of heart block in transplanted hearts; prevention of bronchospasm during anesthesia; inhaled to treat bronchospasm
ritodrine (*Yutopar*)	0.05 mg/min IV; up to 0.35 mg/min may be needed	Management of preterm labor

- Maintain a β-adrenergic blocker on standby when giving parenteral isoproterenol, *in case severe reaction occurs.*
- Use minimal doses of isoproterenol needed to achieve desired effects, *because drug tolerance can occur over time.*
- Arrange for supportive care and comfort measures, including rest and environmental control, *to relieve CNS effects;* provide headache medication and safety measures if CNS effects occur, *to provide comfort and prevent injury;* avoid overhydration, *to prevent pulmonary edema.*
- Provide thorough patient teaching, including the name of the drug, dosage, anticipated adverse effects, measures to avoid drug-related problems, warning signs of problems, and proper administration techniques, *to enhance patient knowledge about drug therapy and to promote compliance.* (See Patient Teaching Checklist: Adrenergic Agonists.)
- Offer support and encouragement *to help the patient deal with the drug regimen.*

Evaluation

- Monitor patient response to the drug (improvement in condition being treated, stabilization of blood pressure, prevention of preterm labor, cardiac stimulation).
- Monitor for adverse effects (GI upset, CNS changes, respiratory problems).
- Evaluate the effectiveness of the teaching plan (patient can name drug, dosage, adverse effects to watch for, specific measures to avoid adverse effects).
- Monitor the effectiveness of comfort measures and compliance to the regimen (see Nursing Care Guide: Adrenergic Agonists).

■ CHAPTER SUMMARY

- Adrenergic agonists are drugs used to stimulate the adrenergic receptors within the SNS. They are also called sympathomimetic drugs, because they mimic the effects of the SNS.
- Sympathomimetic drugs are used when sympathetic stimulation is needed. The adverse effects associated with these drugs are usually also a result of sympathetic stimulation.
- α- and β-Adrenergic agonists stimulate all of the adrenergic receptors in the SNS. They are used to induce a "fight or flight" response and are frequently used to treat shock.
- α-Specific adrenergic agonists stimulate only the α-receptors within the SNS. Clonidine stimulates α_2-receptors and is used to treat hypertension because its action blocks release of norepinephrine from nerve axons. Phenylephrine is used in many cold and allergy remedies because it is a powerful local vasoconstrictor. Midodrine is reserved for use in patients with orthostatic hypotension who do not respond to other therapies, and methoxamine is used to manage blood pressure during anesthesia and sometimes to convert tachycardia.
- Many of the β_2-specific adrenergic agonists are used to

manage and treat asthma, bronchospasm, and other obstructive pulmonary diseases.
- Ritodrine, a β_2-specific agonist, is used to manage preterm labor because of its relaxing effect on the uterus.
- Isoproterenol, a β-specific adrenergic agonist, is used to treat shock, cardiac standstill, and certain arrhythmias when used systemically; it is especially effective in the treatment of heart block in transplanted hearts and is also used to treat bronchospasm and asthma when used in an inhaled form.

Review Questions

1. Adrenergic drugs, because of their action in the body, are also called
   a. sympatholytic agents.
   b. cholinergic agents.
   c. sympathomimetic agents.
   d. anticholinergic agents.
2. The adrenergic agent of choice for treating the signs and symptoms of seasonal rhinitis would be
   a. norepinephrine.
   b. ephedrine.
   c. dobutamine.
   d. Intropin.
3. An adrenergic agent that is being used to treat shock is being given intravenously and it infiltrates. The nurse should
   a. watch the area for any signs of necrosis.
   b. notify the physician and decrease the rate of infusion.
   c. pull the IV and have phentolamine ready to infuse into the area.
   d. apply ice and elevate the arm.
4. Phenylephrine, an α-agonist, is found in many cold and allergy preparations. Adverse effects that should be watched for would include
   a. urinary retention and pupil constriction.
   b. hypotension and slow heart rate.
   c. cardiac arrhythmias and increased appetite.
   d. cardiac arrhythmias and difficulty urinating.
5. Isoproterenol, a pure β-agonist, might be used to treat all of the following except
   a. preterm labor.
   b. bronchospasm.
   c. cardiac standstill.
   d. shock.
6. Use of adrenergic agonists is not recommended with the concurrent use of
   a. anticholinergic drugs.
   b. halogenated hydrocarbon anesthetics.
   c. β-blockers.
   d. benzodiazepines.
7. Adverse effects associated with adrenergic agents are related to the generalized stimulation of the sympathetic nervous system and could include
   a. slowed heart rate.
   b. constriction of the pupils.

c. hypertension.

d. increased GI secretions.

8. A patient has elected to take an over-the-counter cold preparation that contains phenylephrine. The patient should be advised not to take that drug if

a. the patient has known thyroid or cardiovascular disease.

b. the patient has a cough and runny nose.

c. the patient has chronic obstructive pulmonary disease.

d. the patient has hypotension.

BIBLIOGRAPHY

Bullock, B. L. (2000). *Focus on pathophysiology*. Philadelphia: Lippincott Williams & Wilkins.

Gilman, A., Hardman, J. G., & Limbird, L. E. (Eds.) (2002). *Goodman and Gilman's the pharmacological basis of therapeutics* (10th ed.). New York: McGraw-Hill.

Karch, A. M. (2002). *2003 Lippincott's nursing drug guide*. Philadelphia: Lippincott Williams & Wilkins.

Drug facts and comparisons. (2002). St. Louis: Facts and Comparisons.

Professional's guide to patient drug facts. (2002). St. Louis: Facts and Comparisons.

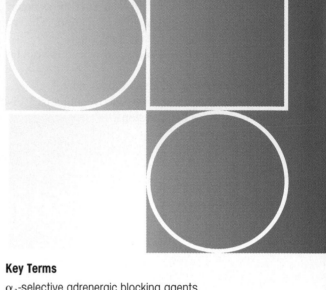

CHAPTER

31

Adrenergic Blocking Agents

Key Terms

α_1-selective adrenergic blocking agents
β-adrenergic blocking agents
β_1-selective adrenergic blocking agents
bronchodilating effect
pheochromocytoma
specific adrenergic receptor sites
sympatholytic

Adrenergic blocking agents are also called **sympatholytic** drugs because they lyse, or block, the effects of the sympathetic nervous system (SNS). The therapeutic and adverse effects associated with these drugs are related to their ability to react with **specific adrenergic receptor sites** without activating them. By occupying the adrenergic receptor site, they prevent norepinephrine released from the nerve terminal or from the adrenal medulla from activating the receptor, thus blocking the SNS effects.

ADRENERGIC BLOCKERS

Both the therapeutic and the adverse effects associated with these drugs are related to their ability to prevent the signs and symptoms associated with SNS activation. The adrenergic blockers have varying degrees of specificity for the adrener-

gic receptor sites. For example, some can interact with all of the adrenergic sites (both α- and β-receptors). Some are specific to α-receptors or even to just α_1-receptors. Some adrenergic blockers are specific to both β_1- and β_2-receptors, whereas others interact with just one type of β-receptor, either β_1- or β_2-receptors only. This specificity allows the clinician to select a drug that will have the desired therapeutic effects without the undesired effects that occur when the entire SNS is blocked. In general, however, the specificity of these drugs depends on the concentration of drug in the body. Most specificity is lost with higher serum levels (Figure 31–1).

α- AND β-ADRENERGIC BLOCKING AGENTS

Drugs that block all adrenergic receptors are primarily used to treat cardiac-related conditions. Amiodarone (*Cordarone*) and bretylium, both α- and β-adrenergic blockers, are only

DRUG THERAPY ACROSS THE LIFESPAN

Adrenergic Blocking Agents

Children	Adults	Older Adults
Children are at greater risk for complications associated with the use of adrenergic blocking agents, including bradycardia, difficulty breathing, and changes in glucose metabolism. The safety and efficacy for use of these drugs has not been established for children younger than 18 years of age. If one of these drugs is used, the dosage for these agents needs to be calculated from the child's body weight and age. It is good practice to have a second person check the dosage calculation before administering the drug to avoid potential toxic effects. Three adrenergic blocking agents have established pediatric dosages, and they might be the drugs to consider when one is needed: guanethidine and prazosin, both used to treat hypertension, and phentolamine, which is used during surgery for pheochromocytoma. Children should be carefully monitored and supported during the use of these drugs.	Adults being treated with adrenergic blocking agents should be cautioned about the many adverse effects associated with the drugs. Patients with diabetes need to be re-educated about ways to monitor themselves for hyperglycemia and hypoglycemia, because the sympathetic reaction usually alerts patients that there is a problem with their glucose levels. Patients with severe thyroid disease are also at high risk when taking these drugs, and if one of them is needed, the patient should be monitored very closely. Propranolol and metoprolol are associated with more central nervous system (CNS) adverse effects than other adrenergic blockers, and patients who have CNS complications already or who develop CNS problems while taking an adrenergic blocker might do better with a different agent. In general, there are no adequate studies about the effects of adrenergic blockers during pregnancy and lactation, and they should be used only in those situations in which the benefit to the mother is greater than the risk to the fetus or neonate. Adrenergic blockers can affect labor, and babies born to mothers taking these drugs may exhibit the adverse cardiovascular, respiratory, and CNS effects. Many of these drugs were teratogenic in animal studies. Because of a similar risk of adverse reactions on the baby, nursing mothers should find another way to feed the baby if an adrenergic blocking drug is needed.	Older patients are more likely to experience the adverse effects associated with these drugs—CNS, cardiovascular, GI, and respiratory. Because older patients often also have renal or hepatic impairment, they are more likely to have toxic levels of the drug related to changes in metabolism and excretion. The older patient should be started on lower doses of the drugs and should be monitored very closely for potentially serious arrhythmias or blood pressure changes. Bisoprolol is often a drug of choice for older patients who require an adrenergic blocker for hypertension, because it is not associated with as many problems in the elderly and regular dosing profiles can be used.

FIGURE 31-1. Site of action of adrenergic blockers and resultant physiologic responses. A bar indicates blocking of the effects indicated by those receptors.

used as antiarrhythmics (see Chapter 45). Carvedilol (*Coreg*) is used as part of combination therapy in the treatment of hypertension and congestive heart failure (CHF). Guanadrel (*Hylorel*), an older drug, is used to treat hypertension that does not respond to thiazide diuretics. Guanethidine (*Ismelin*), another older drug, is used to treat hypertension and renal hypertension (high blood pressure caused by changes in renal blood flow or response). A newer drug, labetalol (*Normodyne, Trandate*), is used intravenously and orally to treat hypertension and can be used in conjunction with diuretics. Labetalol has also been used to treat hypertension associated with pheochromocytoma and clonidine withdrawal hypertension.

Therapeutic Actions and Indications

Adrenergic blocking agents competitively block the effects of norepinephrine at both α- and β-receptors throughout the SNS. This action prevents the signs and symptoms associated with a sympathetic stress reaction and results in lower blood pressure, slower pulse, and increased renal perfusion with decreased renin levels. These drugs are indicated to treat essential hypertension, alone or in combination with diuretics.

Pharmacokinetics

These drugs are well absorbed and distributed throughout the body. They are metabolized in the liver and excreted in feces and urine. The half-life varies with the particular drug and preparation. There are no well-defined studies on the use of these drugs during pregnancy and lactation, so use should be reserved for those situations in which the benefit to the mother outweighs the potential risk to the neonate. The adrenergic blockers are not recommended for use in children younger than 18 years of age.

Contraindications and Cautions

The α- and β-adrenergic blocking agents are contraindicated in the presence of bradycardia or heart blocks, which could be worsened by the slowed heart rate and conduction; asthma, which could be exacerbated by the loss of norepinephrine's **bronchodilating effect;** shock or CHF, which could become worse with the loss of the sympathetic reaction; and pregnancy or lactation, because of the potential adverse effects on the fetus or neonate.

These drugs should be used with caution in patients with diabetes, because the disorder could be aggravated by the blocked sympathetic response and because the usual signs and symptoms of hypoglycemia and hyperglycemia are lost when the SNS cannot respond. Caution also should be used with bronchospasm, which could progress to respiratory distress with the loss of norepinephrine's bronchodilating actions.

Adverse Effects

The adverse effects associated with the use of α- and β-adrenergic blocking agents are usually associated with the drug's effects on the SNS. These effects can include dizziness, paresthesias, insomnia, depression, fatigue, and vertigo, which are related to the blocked effects of norepinephrine in the central nervous system (CNS). Nausea, vomiting, diarrhea, anorexia, and flatulence are associated with the loss of the balancing sympathetic effect on the gastrointestinal (GI) tract and increased parasympathetic dominance. Cardiac arrhythmias, hypotension, CHF, pulmonary edema, and cerebrovascular accident, or stroke, are related to the lack of stimulatory effects and loss of vascular tone in the cardiovascular (CV) system. Bronchospasm, cough, rhinitis, and bronchial obstruction are related to loss of the bronchodilating effects on the respiratory tract and vasodilation of the mucous membrane vessels. Other effects reported include decreased exercise tolerance, hypoglycemia, and rash.

Clinically Important Drug–Drug Interactions

There is increased risk of excessive hypotension if any of these drugs are combined with enflurane, halothane, or isoflurane anesthetics.

There also is an increased effectiveness of diabetic agents, leading to hypoglycemia when such agents are used with these drugs; patients should be monitored closely and dosage adjustments made as needed.

In addition, carvedilol has been associated with potentially dangerous conduction system disturbances when combined with verapamil or diltiazem; if this combination is used, the patient should be continuously monitored.

Nursing Considerations for Patients Receiving α- and β-Adrenergic Blocking Agents
Assessment: History and Examination

Screen for the following conditions, which could be cautions or contraindications to use of the drug: any known allergies to these drugs; presence of bradycardia or heart blocks, which could be worsened by the slowing of heart rate and conduction; asthma, which could be exacerbated by the loss of the bronchodilating effect of norepinephrine; shock or CHF, which could become worse with the loss of the sympathetic reaction; pregnancy or lactation, because of the potential adverse effects on the fetus or neonate; diabetes, which could be aggravated by the blocking of the sympathetic response and because the usual signs and symptoms of hypoglycemia and hyperglycemia are lost when the SNS cannot respond; and bronchospasm, which could progress to respiratory distress with the loss of the bronchodilating actions of norepinephrine.

Include screening for baseline status and any potential adverse effects: skin color, temperature; pulse, blood pressure, cardiac output, electrocardiogram (ECG); respiration, adventitious sounds; and blood glucose levels and electrolytes.

Nursing Diagnoses

The patient receiving an α- and β-adrenergic blocker may have the following nursing diagnoses related to drug therapy:

DRUGS IN FOCUS
α- and β-Adrenergic Blocking Agents

Drug Name	Dosage/Route	Usual Indications
carvedilol (*Coreg*)	6.25–12.5 mg PO b.i.d. for hypertension; 3.125–6.25 mg PO b.i.d. for congestive heart failure	Treatment of hypertension, congestive heart failure in adults
guanadrel (*Hylorel*)	20–75 mg PO in divided doses b.i.d.; reduce dosage with renal impairment	Treatment of hypertension in adults that does not respond to thiazide diuretics
guanethidine (*Ismelin*)	Adult: 25–50 mg PO q.d.; reduce dosage with renal impairment	Treatment of hypertension, renal hypertension
Ⓟ labetalol (*Normodyne, Trandate*)	100 mg PO b.i.d. initially, maintenance 200–400 mg PO b.i.d.; 20 mg IV, slowly with additional doses given at 10-min intervals to a maximum dose of 300 mg for severe hypertension	Treatment of hypertension, pheochromocytoma, clonidine withdrawal, hypertension in adults

- Acute Pain related to CV and systemic effects
- Decreased Cardiac Output related to CV effects
- Ineffective Airway Clearance related to lack of bronchodilating effects
- Deficient Knowledge regarding drug therapy

Implementation

- Do not discontinue abruptly after chronic therapy, *because hypersensitivity to catecholamines may develop and the patient could have a severe reaction; taper drug slowly over 2 weeks, monitoring patient.*
- Consult with the physician about withdrawing the drug before surgery, *because withdrawal is controversial; effects on the sympathetic system after surgery can cause problems.*
- Encourage the patient to adapt lifestyle changes, including diet, exercise, stopping smoking, and decreasing stress, *to aid in lowering blood pressure.*
- Monitor for orthostatic hypotension and provide safety precautions if this occurs, *to prevent injury to the patient.*
- Monitor for any sign of liver failure, *in order to arrange to discontinue the drug if this occurs (this effect is more likely to happen with carvedilol).*
- Provide thorough patient teaching, including measures to avoid adverse effects, warning signs of problems, and the need for monitoring and evaluation, *to enhance patient knowledge about drug therapy and to promote compliance.*
- Offer support and encouragement *to help the patient deal with the drug regimen.*

Evaluation

- Monitor patient response to the drug (improvement in blood pressure and CHF).
- Monitor for adverse effects (CV changes, headache, GI upset, bronchospasm, liver failure).

- Evaluate the effectiveness of the teaching plan (patient can name drug, dosage, adverse effects to watch for, specific measures to avoid adverse effects).
- Monitor the effectiveness of comfort measures and compliance to the regimen.

α-ADRENERGIC BLOCKING AGENTS

Some adrenergic blocking agents have a specific affinity for α-receptor sites. Their use is somewhat limited because of the development of even more specific and safer drugs.

Only one of these drugs is still used. A **pheochromocytoma** is a tumor of the chromaffin cells of the adrenal medulla that periodically releases large amounts of norepinephrine and epinephrine into the system, with resultant severe hypertension and tachycardia. Phentolamine (*Regitine*) is used to diagnose pheochromocytoma and to prevent severe hypertension reactions caused by manipulation of the pheochromocytoma before and during surgery. Phentolamine is most frequently used to prevent cell death and tissue sloughing after extravasation of intravenous norepinephrine or dopamine.

Therapeutic Actions and Indications

These drugs block the postsynaptic α_1-adrenergic receptors, decreasing sympathetic tone in the vasculature and causing vasodilation, which leads to a lowering of blood pressure. They also block presynaptic α_2-receptors, preventing the feedback control of norepinephrine release. The result is an increase in the reflex tachycardia that occurs when blood pressure is lowered. These drugs are used to diagnose and manage episodes of pheochromocytoma. Phentolamine is used to rescue cells injured by norepinephrine or dopamine extravasation; it causes vasodilation and a return of blood flow.

DRUGS IN FOCUS
α-Adrenergic Blocking Agents

Drug Name	Dosage/Route	Usual Indications
P phentolamine (*Regitine*)	Adult: 5 mg IV or IM 1–2 h before surgery; 5–10 mg in 10 mL saline injected into area of extravasation within 12 h after extravasation Pediatric: 1 mg IM or IV 1–2 h before surgery; treat extravasation as in the adult	Diagnosis of pheochromocytoma, management of severe hypertension during pheochromocytoma surgery; to prevent cell death with intravenous infiltration of norepinephrine or dopamine

Pharmacokinetics

Phentolamine is rapidly absorbed after injection and is excreted in the urine. There are few data on its metabolism and distribution. Use of phentolamine during pregnancy or lactation should be reserved for those situations in which the benefit to the mother outweighs any potential risk to the neonate.

Contraindications and Cautions

The α-adrenergic blocking agents are contraindicated in the presence of allergy to these or similar drugs and in the presence of coronary artery disease or myocardial infarction (MI), because of the potential exacerbation of these conditions; they should be used cautiously in pregnancy or lactation because of the potential adverse effects on the fetus or neonate.

Adverse Effects

Patients receiving these drugs often experience extensions of the therapeutic effects, including hypotension, orthostatic hypotension, angina, MI, cerebrovascular accident, flushing, tachycardia, and arrhythmia—all of which are related to vasodilation and decreased blood pressure. Weakness and dizziness often occur as a reaction to the hypotension. Nausea, vomiting, and diarrhea may also occur.

Clinically Important Drug–Drug Interactions

There may be decreased hypertensive and vasoconstrictive effects of ephedrine and epinephrine if they are taken concomitantly with phentolamine, because these agents work in opposing ways in the body.

Increased hypotension may occur if these drugs are combined with alcohol, which is also a vasodilator.

Nursing Considerations for Patients Receiving α-Adrenergic Blocking Agents
Assessment: History and Examination

Screen for the following conditions, which could be cautions or contraindications to the use of the drug: any known allergies to either drug; presence of any cardiovascular diseases, which may be contraindications to the use of these drugs; and pregnancy or lactation, which require caution for drug use.

Include screening for baseline status and for any potential adverse effects: assess orientation, affect, and reflexes to monitor for CNS changes related to drug therapy; blood pressure, pulse, ECG, peripheral perfusion, and cardiac output; and urinary output.

Nursing Diagnoses

The patient receiving an α-adrenergic blocking agent may also have the following nursing diagnoses related to drug therapy:

• Risk for Injury related to CNS, CV effects of drug
• Decreased Cardiac Output related to blood pressure changes, arrhythmias, vasodilation
• Deficient Knowledge regarding drug therapy

Implementation

• Monitor heart rate and blood pressure very carefully *in order to arrange to discontinue the drug if adverse reactions are severe; provide supportive management if needed.*
• Inject phentolamine directly into the area of extravasation of epinephrine or dopamine *to prevent local cell death.*
• Arrange for supportive care and comfort measures such as rest, environmental control, and other measures, *to decrease CNS irritation;* provide headache medication, *to alleviate patient discomfort;* arrange safety measures if CNS effects or orthostatic hypotension occur, *to prevent patient injury.*
• Provide thorough patient teaching, including dosage, potential adverse effects, measures to avoid adverse effects, and warning signs of problems, *to enhance patient knowledge about drug therapy and to promote compliance.*
• Offer support and encouragement *to help the patient deal with the drug regimen.*

Evaluation

• Monitor patient response to the drug (improvement in signs and symptoms of pheochromocytoma, improvement in tissue condition after extravasation).
• Monitor for adverse effects (orthostatic hypotension, arrhythmias, CNS effects).
• Evaluate the effectiveness of the teaching plan (patient can name drug, dosage, adverse effects to watch for, specific measures to avoid adverse effects).
• Monitor the effectiveness of comfort measures and compliance to the regimen.

α₁-SELECTIVE ADRENERGIC BLOCKING AGENTS

α₁-Selective adrenergic blocking agents are drugs that have a specific affinity for α₁-receptors. Doxazosin (*Cardura*) is used to treat hypertension and is also effective in the treatment of benign prostatic hypertrophy (BPH) (see Chapter 52). Prazosin (*Minipress*) is used to treat hypertension, alone or in combination with other drugs. Terazosin (*Hytrin*) is used to treat hypertension as well as BPH (see Chapter 52). Tamsulosin (*Flomax*) and alfuzosin (*Xatral*) are used only in the treatment of BPH and are discussed later (see Chapter 52).

Therapeutic Actions and Indications

The therapeutic effects of the α₁-selective adrenergic blocking agents come from their ability to block the postsynaptic α₁-receptor sites. This causes a decrease in vascular tone and vasodilation, which leads to a fall in blood pressure. Because these drugs do not block the presynaptic α₂-receptor sites, the reflex tachycardia that accompanies a fall in blood pressure does not occur. These drugs can be used to treat BPH or to treat hypertension, alone or as part of a combination therapy.

Pharmacokinetics

The α₁-selective adrenergic blocking agents are well absorbed and undergo extensive hepatic metabolism. They therefore must be used with caution in patients with hepatic impairment. They are excreted in the urine. Use during pregnancy and lactation should be limited to those situations in which the benefits to the mother outweigh the potential risks to the neonate, because these drugs cross the placenta and are known to enter breast milk. Safety for use in children has not been established.

Contraindications and Cautions

The α_1-selective adrenergic blocking agents are contraindicated in the presence of allergy to any of these drugs, and also with lactation, because the drugs cross into breast milk and could have adverse effects on the neonate. They should be used cautiously in the presence of CHF or renal failure, because their blood pressure–lowering effects could exacerbate these conditions, and with hepatic impairment, which could alter the metabolism of these drugs. Caution also should be used during pregnancy, because of the potential for adverse effects on the fetus.

Adverse Effects

The adverse effects associated with the use of these drugs are usually related to their effects of blocking the SNS. CNS effects include dizziness, weakness, fatigue, drowsiness, and depression. Nausea, vomiting, abdominal pain, and diarrhea may occur as a result of direct effects on the GI tract and sympathetic blocking. Anticipated cardiovascular effects include arrhythmias, hypotension, edema, CHF, and angina. The vasodilation caused by these drugs can also cause flushing, rhinitis, reddened eyes, nasal congestion, and priapism.

Clinically Important Drug–Drug Interactions

Increased hypotensive effects may occur if these drugs are combined with any other vasodilating or antihypertensive drugs.

Nursing Considerations for Patients Receiving α_1-Selective Adrenergic Blocking Agents

Assessment: History and Examination

Screen for the following conditions, which could be cautions or contraindications to use of the drug: any known allergies to either drug; pregnancy or lactation, which could be contraindications or cautions for drug use; and CHF or renal failure, which could be exacerbated by drug use.

Include screening for baseline status and for any potential adverse effects: assess orientation, affect, and reflexes to monitor for CNS changes related to drug therapy; blood pressure, pulse, ECG, peripheral perfusion, and cardiac output. Monitor cardiovascular effects as well as urinary output and renal function to monitor effects on the renal system.

Nursing Diagnoses

The patient receiving an α_1-selective adrenergic blocking agent may have the following nursing diagnoses related to drug therapy:

• Acute Pain related to headache, GI upset, flushing, nasal congestion
• Risk for Injury related to CNS, CV effects of drug
• Decreased Cardiac Output related to blood pressure changes, arrhythmias, vasodilation
• Deficient Knowledge regarding drug therapy

Implementation

• Monitor blood pressure, pulse, rhythm, and cardiac output regularly, *in order to arrange to adjust dosage or discontinue the drug if cardiovascular effects are severe.*
• Establish safety precautions if CNS effects or orthostatic hypotension occurs, *to prevent patient injury.*

DRUGS IN FOCUS
α_1-Selective Adrenergic Blocking Agents

Drug Name	Dosage/Route	Usual Indications
alfuzosin (*Xatral OD*)	10 mg/d PO	Treatment of benign prostatic hypertrophy (BPH)
Ⓟ doxazosin (*Cardura*)	1 mg PO q.d. up to 16 mg PO q.d. for hypertension; 1–8 mg PO q.d. for BPH	Treatment of hypertension and BPH
prazosin (*Minipress*)	Adult: 1 mg PO b.i.d.–t.i.d. with maintenance at 6–15 mg/d PO in divided doses Pediatric: 0.5–7 mg PO t.i.d.	Treatment of hypertension
tamsulosin (*Flomax*)	0.4–0.8 mg PO q.d. 30 min after the same meal each day	Treatment of BPH
terazosin (*Hytrin*)	1–5 mg PO q.d., preferably at bedtime for hypertension; 10 mg/d PO for BPH	Treatment of hypertension and BPH

- Arrange for small, frequent meals if GI upset is severe, *to relieve discomfort and maintain nutrition.*
- Arrange for supportive care and comfort measures (rest, environmental control, other measures), *to decrease CNS irritation;* provide headache medication, *to alleviate patient discomfort;* arrange safety measures if CNS effects occur, *to prevent patient injury.*
- Provide thorough patient teaching, including dosage, adverse effects to anticipate, measures to avoid adverse effects, and warning signs of problems, *to enhance patient knowledge about drug therapy and to promote compliance.*
- Offer support and encouragement *to help the patient deal with the drug regimen.*

Evaluation

- Monitor patient response to the drug (lowering of blood pressure).
- Monitor for adverse effects (GI upset, CNS or cardiovascular changes).
- Evaluate the effectiveness of the teaching plan (patient can name drug, dosage, adverse effects to watch for, specific measures to avoid adverse effects).
- Monitor the effectiveness of comfort measures and compliance to the regimen.

β-ADRENERGIC BLOCKING AGENTS

The **β-adrenergic blocking agents** are used to treat cardiovascular problems (hypertension, angina, migraine headaches) and to prevent reinfarction after MI. These drugs are widely used today; in fact, propranolol (*Inderal*) was once the most prescribed drug in the country.

Propranolol has been approved for multiples uses, which include treatment of hypertension, angina, idiopathic hypertrophic subaortic stenosis (IHSS)–induced palpitations, angina and syncope, and certain cardiac arrhythmias induced by catecholamines or digoxin; prevention of reinfarction after MI; treatment of pheochromocytoma; prophylaxis for migraine headache (which may be caused by vasodilation and is relieved by vasoconstriction); prevention of stage fright (which is a sympathetic stress reaction to a particular situation); and treatment of essential tremors. It is very effective in blocking all of the β-receptors in the SNS and was one of the first drugs of the class.

Since the introduction of propranolol, newer and more selective drugs have become available that are not associated with some of the adverse effects seen with total blockade of the SNS β-receptors. Carteolol (*Cartrol*) is used for the treatment of hypertension, alone or in combination with other drugs. Penbutolol (*Levator*) and pindolol (*Visken*) are also used for the treatment of hypertension. The drug of choice would depend mostly on personal experience. Nadolol (*Corgard*) is used to treat hypertension and also for the chronic management of angina. It would be a drug of choice in an angina patient who is also hypertensive. Sotalol (*Betapace*) is reserved for use in the treatment of potentially life-threatening arrhythmias and is not recommended for any other use; *Betapace AF,* a newer preparation of the drug, is used in the treatment of atrial fibrillation. Timolol (*Blocadren, Timoptic*), a newer β-adrenergic blocker, has several recommended uses, including treatment of hypertension, prevention of reinfarction after MI, prophylaxis for migraine, and, in ophthalmic form, reduction of intraocular pressure in patients with open-angle glaucoma.

Therapeutic Actions and Indications

The therapeutic effects of these drugs are related to their competitive blocking of the β adrenergic receptors in the SNS. The blockade of the β-receptors in the heart and in the juxtaglomerular apparatus of the nephron account for most of the therapeutic benefit of these drugs. Decreased heart rate, contractility, and excitability, as well as a membrane-stabilizing effect, lead to a decrease in arrhythmias, a decreased cardiac workload, and decreased oxygen consumption. The juxtaglomerular cells are not stimulated to release renin, which further decreases the blood pressure. These effects are useful in treating hypertension and chronic angina and can help to prevent reinfarction after an MI by decreasing cardiac workload and oxygen consumption.

Blocking of other SNS effects accounts for the use of propranolol to prevent stage fright. The decreased feelings of anxiety, decreased pulse and blood pressure, and decreased sweating and flushing help to alleviate situational anxiety. The mechanism of action in treating migraines is not clearly understood.

Timolol is used topically to reduce intraocular pressure through its relaxing effects on the eye muscles. Because it is applied topically, it is usually not absorbed systemically from this route.

Pharmacokinetics

These drugs are absorbed from the GI tract and undergo hepatic metabolism. Food has been found to increase the bioavailability of propranolol, although this effect was not found with other β-adrenergic blocking agents. Absorption of sotalol is decreased by the presence of food. Propranolol also crosses the blood–brain barrier, but carteolol, nadolol, and sotalol do not, making them a better choice if CNS effects occur with propranolol. These drugs are excreted in the urine, requiring caution in patients with renal impairment. Teratogenic effects have occurred in animal studies with all of these drugs except sotalol. The use of any β-adrenergic blocker during pregnancy should be reserved for situations in which the benefit to the mother outweighs the risk to the fetus. In general, they should not be used during lactation because of the potential for adverse effects on the baby. The safety and efficacy for use of these drugs in children have not been established.

Contraindications and Cautions

β-Adrenergic blocking agents are contraindicated in the presence of allergy to any of these drugs or any components of the drug being used; with bradycardia or heart blocks, shock, or CHF, which could be exacerbated by the cardiac suppressing effects of these drugs; with bronchospasm, chronic obstructive pulmonary disease (COPD), or acute asthma, which could be made worse by the blocking of the sympathetic bronchodilation; with pregnancy, because neonatal apnea, bradycardia, and hypoglycemia could occur; and with lactation, because of the potential effects on the neonate, which could include slowed heart rate, hypotension, and hypoglycemia. These drugs should be used cautiously in patients with diabetes and hypoglycemia, because of the blocking of the normal signs and symptoms of hypoglycemia and hyperglycemia; with thyrotoxicosis, because of the adrenergic blocking effects on the thyroid gland; or with hepatic dysfunction, which could interfere with the metabolism of these drugs.

Adverse Effects

Patients receiving these drugs often experience adverse effects related to the blocking of the SNS's β-receptors. CNS effects include fatigue, dizziness, depression, paresthesias, sleep disturbances, memory loss, and disorientation. Cardiovascular effects can include bradycardia, heart block, CHF, hypotension, and peripheral vascular insufficiency. Pulmonary effects can range from difficulty breathing, coughing, and bronchospasm to severe pulmonary edema and bronchial obstruction. GI upset, nausea, vomiting, diarrhea, gastric pain, and even colitis can occur as a result of

unchecked parasympathetic activity and the blocking of the sympathetic receptors. Genitourinary effects can include decreased libido, impotence, dysuria, and Peyronie's disease. Other effects that can occur include decreased exercise tolerance (patients often report that their "get up and go" is gone), hypoglycemia or hyperglycemia, and liver changes.

Clinically Important Drug–Drug Interactions

A paradoxical hypertension occurs when β-blockers are given with clonidine, and an increased rebound hypertension with clonidine withdrawal may also occur. It is best to avoid this combination.

A decreased antihypertensive effect occurs when β-blockers are given with nonsteroidal anti-inflammatory drugs (NSAIDs); if this combination is used, the patient should be monitored closely and dosage adjustment should be made to achieve the desired control of blood pressure.

An initial hypertensive episode followed by bradycardia may occur if these drugs are given with epinephrine.

There also is a possibility of peripheral ischemia if the β-blockers are taken in combination with ergot alkaloids.

When these drugs are given with insulin or antidiabetic agents, there is a potential for change in blood glucose levels. The patient also will not display the usual signs and symptoms of hypoglycemia or hyperglycemia, which are caused by activation of the SNS. Because these effects are

DRUGS IN FOCUS
β-Adrenergic Blocking Agents

Drug Name	Dosage/Route	Usual Indications
carteolol (*Cartrol*)	Initially 2.5 mg PO, titrate to 5–10 mg PO based on patient response; reduce dosage with renal impairment	Treatment of hypertension in adults
nadolol (*Corgard*)	Angina: 40–80 mg/d PO Hypertension: 40–80 mg/d PO, up to 320 mg/d may be needed; reduce dosage in renal impairment	Treatment of hypertension, management of angina in adults
penbutolol (*Levator*)	Initially 20 mg/d PO, titrate up to 40–80 mg/d PO based on patient response	Treatment of hypertension in adults
pindolol (*Visken*)	Initially 5 mg PO b.i.d., to a maximum of 60 mg/d PO	Treatment of hypertension in adults
Ⓟ propranolol (*Inderal*)	Dosage varies widely based on indication; check your drug guide for specific information	Treatment of hypertension, angina, idiopathic hypertrophic subaortic stenosis, certain cardiac arrhythmias, pheochromocytoma; prophylaxis for migraine headache, prevention of stage fright
sotalol (*Betapace, Betapace AF*)	*Betapace:* 80 mg PO b.i.d. up to 160 mg PO b.i.d. may be needed *Betapace AF:* 80 mg/d PO based on QT interval and patient response Reduce dosage of both with renal impairment	Treatment of potentially life threatening ventricular arrhythmias (*Betapace*); maintenance of normal sinus rhythm in patients with atrial fibrillation/flutter
timolol (*Blocadren, Timoptic*)	10 mg PO b.i.d., increases based on patient response; 1–2 gtt in affected eye(s) for glaucoma	Treatment of hypertension; prevention of reinfarction after myocardial infarction; prophylaxis for migraine; in ophthalmic form, reduction of intraocular pressure in open-angle glaucoma

blocked, the patient will need new indications to alert him or her to potential problems. If this combination is used, the patient should monitor blood glucose levels frequently throughout the day and should be alert to new warnings about glucose imbalance.

Nursing Considerations for Patients Receiving β-Adrenergic Blocking Agents

Assessment: History and Examination

Screen for the following conditions, which could be cautions or contraindications to the use of the drug: known allergy to any drug or to any components of the drug; bradycardia or heart blocks, shock, or CHF, which could be exacerbated by the cardiac suppressing effects of these drugs; bronchospasm, COPD, or acute asthma, which could be made worse by the blocking of the sympathetic bronchodilation; pregnancy and lactation, because of the potential effects on the fetus or neonate; diabetes or hypoglycemia; thyrotoxicosis; and hepatic dysfunction, which could interfere with the metabolism of these drugs.

Include screening for baseline status and for any potential adverse effects: skin color, temperature; pulse, blood pressure, ECG; respiration, adventitious sounds; abdominal examination, liver function tests, urine output, and electrolytes.

Nursing Diagnoses

The patient receiving β-adrenergic blocking agents may have the following nursing diagnoses related to drug therapy:

- Acute Pain related to CNS, GI, and systemic effects
- Decreased Cardiac Output related to CV effects
- Ineffective Tissue Perfusion related to CV effects
- Deficient Knowledge regarding drug therapy

Implementation

- Do not stop these drugs abruptly after chronic therapy but taper gradually over 2 weeks, *because long-term use of these drugs can sensitize the myocardium to catecholamines and severe reactions could occur.*
- Continuously monitor any patient receiving an intravenous form of these drugs, *to avert serious complications caused by rapid sympathetic blockade.*
- Arrange for supportive care and comfort measures (rest, environmental control, other measures), *to relieve CNS effects;* institute safety measures if CNS effects occur, *to prevent patient injury;* provide small, frequent meals and mouth care, *to help relieve the discomfort of GI effects.*
- Provide thorough patient teaching, including name of the drug, dosage, anticipated adverse effects, measures to avoid drug-related problems, warning signs of problems, and proper administration techniques as needed, *to enhance patient knowledge about drug therapy and to promote compliance.* (See Patient Teaching Checklist: β-Adrenergic Blocking Agents.)
- Offer support and encouragement, *to help the patient deal with the drug regimen.*

PATIENT TEACHING CHECKLIST
β-Adrenergic Blocking Agents

Create customized patient teaching materials for a specific beta adrenergic blocking agent from the CD-ROM. Patient teaching should stress the following for drugs within this class:

- A β-adrenergic blocking agent works to prevent certain stimulating activities that normally occur in your body in response to such factors as stress, injury, or excitement.
- You should learn to take your own pulse and monitor it daily, writing the pulse rate on your calendar. Your current pulse rate is _____.
- Never discontinue this medication suddenly. If you find that your prescription is running out, notify your health care provider at once. This drug needs to be taped over time to prevent severe reactions when it is discontinued.

Some of the following adverse effects may occur:

- *Fatigue, weakness*—Try to space your activities throughout the day and allow rest periods.
- *Dizziness, drowsiness*—If these should occur, take care to avoid driving, operating dangerous machinery, or doing delicate tasks. Change position slowly to avoid dizzy spells.
- *Change in sexual function*—Be assured that this is a drug effect and discuss it with your health care provider.
- *Nausea, diarrhea*—These gastrointestinal discomforts often diminish over time. If they become too uncomfortable or do not improve, talk to your health care provider.
- *Dreams, confusion*—These are drug effects. If they become too uncomfortable, discuss them with your health care provider.

Report any of the following to your health care provider: very slow pulse, need to sleep on more pillows at night, difficulty breathing, swelling in the ankles or fingers, sudden weight gain, mental confusion or personality change, fever, or rash.

Avoid over-the-counter medications, including cold and allergy remedies and diet pills. Many of these preparations contain drugs that could interfere with this medication. If you feel that you need one of these, check with your health care provider first.

Tell any doctor, nurse, or other health care provider that you are taking these drugs.

Keep this drug, and all medications, out of the reach of children. Do not share these drugs with other people.

This Teaching Checklist reflects general patient teaching guidelines. It is not meant to be a substitute for drug-specific teaching information, which is available in nursing drug guides.

Evaluation

- Monitor patient response to the drug (lowering of blood pressure, decrease in anginal episodes, improvement in condition being treated).
- Monitor for adverse effects (GI upset, CNS changes, respiratory problems, CV effects, loss of libido, and impotence).

- Evaluate effectiveness of teaching plan (patient can name drug, dosage, adverse effects to watch for, specific measures to avoid adverse effects).
- Monitor the effectiveness of comfort measures and compliance to the regimen (see Nursing Care Guide: β-Adrenergic Blocking Agents).

β₁-SELECTIVE ADRENERGIC BLOCKING AGENTS

β₁-Selective adrenergic blocking agents have an advantage over the nonselective β-blockers in some cases. Because they do not usually block β₂-receptor sites, they do not block the sympathetic bronchodilation that is so important for patients with lung diseases or allergic rhinitis. Conse-quently, these drugs are preferred for patients who smoke or who have asthma, any other obstructive pulmonary disease, or seasonal or allergic rhinitis. These selective β-blockers are also used for treating hypertension, angina, and some cardiac arrhythmias.

Acebutolol (*Sectral*) is used for treating hypertension and premature ventricular contractions. Atenolol (*Tenormin*), which is more widely used, is prescribed to treat MI, chronic angina, and hypertension. Betaxolol (*Kerlone*) is used to treat hypertension; it is also available as an ophthalmic agent (*Betoptic*) to treat ocular hypertension and open-angle glau-coma. Bisoprolol (*Zebeta*) is reserved for use in treating hy-pertension. Esmolol (*Brevibloc*) is available as an intra-venous agent for the treatment of supraventricular tachycardias (eg, atrial flutter, atrial fibrillation) and noncompensatory

N U R S I N G   C A R E   G U I D E

β-Adrenergic Blocking Agents

Assessment	Nursing Diagnoses	Implementation	Evaluation
HISTORY Allergies to any of these drugs, CHF, shock, brady-cardia, heart block, hy-potension, COPD, preg-nancy and lactation, thyroid disease, diabetes	Decreased Cardiac Out-put related to CV effects Acute pain related to CNS, GI, systematic effects Impaired Tissue Perfusion, related to CV effects Deficient Knowledge re-garding drug therapy	Ensure safe and appropri-ate administration of drug. Provide comfort and safety measures: assis-tance/siderails; tempera-ture control; rest periods; mouth care; small, fre-quent meals. Monitor BP, P, respiratory status throughout drug therapy. Provide support and reas-surance to deal with drug effects and discomfort, sexual dysfunction, fa-tigue. Provide patient teaching regarding drug name, dosage, side effects, pre-cautions, and warning signs to report.	Evaluate drug effects: BP within normal limit, de-crease in anginal episodes, stabilized car-diac rhythm. Monitor for adverse ef-fects: CV effects: CHF, block; dizziness, confusion; sexual dysfunction; GI ef-fects; hypoglycemia; respi-ratory problems. Monitor for drug–drug in-teractions as indicated for each drug. Evaluate effectiveness of patient teaching program. Evaluate effectiveness of comfort and safety mea-sures.
PHYSICAL EXAMINATION CV: BP, P, peripheral perfu-sion, ECG CNS: orientation, affect, reflexes, vision Skin: color, lesions, texture GU: urinary output, sexual function GI: abdominal, liver evalu-ation Resp: R, adventitious sounds			

C A S E   S T U D Y

Nonspecific β-Blockers

THE SITUATION
M. R., a 59-year-old man suffered a diaphragmatic myocardial infarction (MI) last August. He recovered well and returned to work as a salesman within 8 weeks. Shortly after he resumed working, he began to suffer vague, pressure-type chest pains. He was maintained on propranolol (*Inderal*) 10 mg q.i.d. with no further problems. The following June, M. R. developed acute respiratory distress while picnicking in a state park with his family. On the way to the emergency room, he suffered an apparent respiratory arrest. He was admitted to the hospital and placed in the respiratory intensive care unit. It was found that M. R. had a history of hay fever and allergic rhinitis during the pollen season but had never experienced such a severe reaction.

CRITICAL THINKING
Why did M. R. have such a severe reaction? What appropriate measures should be taken to ensure that M. R. recovers fully and does not re-experience this event?

What sort of support will M. R. and his family need after going through such a frightening experience? Think about the children who may have witnessed the respiratory arrest and how they should be reassured, depending on their ages. *Think about the support M. R.'s wife may need and the fear that may now be associated with M. R.'s condition. M. R. has been taking propranolol for several months and needs to be weaned from it, because the drug is somewhat responsible for the reaction that M. R. experienced.*

What kind of teaching program will need to be developed to help M. R. deal with his drugs, their effects, and his underlying cardiac problem?

DISCUSSION
Propranolol, a nonspecific β-blocker, was prescribed to decrease the workload and oxygen consumption of

M. R.'s heart and to prevent reinfarction after his MI. He did well on the drug until pollen season arrived. That is because propranolol, a nonspecific β-blocker, prevented the compensatory bronchodilation that occurs when the sympathetic nervous system is stimulated. When the pollen reacted with M. R.'s airways, causing them to swell and become narrower, his body was unable to dilate the bronchi to allow airflow through the swollen bronchial tubes. The result was bronchial constriction and respiratory distress that, in M. R.'s case, progressed to a respiratory arrest. Before he began taking propranolol, M. R. had probably been effectively compensating for the swelling of the bronchi through bronchodilation and had never experienced such a reaction. The propranolol needs to be weaned from M. R.'s system. M. R. should then be started on a specific β-adrenergic blocker, which should give him the decreased cardiac workload that he needs without interfering with his reflex bronchodilation.

M. R. may want to discuss this frightening incident with his health care provider. He also may want to include his family in this discussion. It should be stressed that he did so well up to this point because he had not been exposed to pollen and therefore had not had the problem that brought him into the hospital this time. M. R. probably never reported the occurrence of hay fever to his health care provider when the drug was prescribed because it had never been a problem and probably did not seem significant to him. M. R. and his family should receive support and be encouraged to talk about what happened and how they reacted to it. It is normal to feel frightened and unsure when a loved one is in distress. A full teaching program, including information on M. R.'s heart disease and details about his new specific β-adrenergic blocker, should be undertaken. M. R. should receive written information about the drug, including warning signs to watch for and adverse effects that may occur.

tachycardia when the heart rate must be slowed. Metoprolol (*Lopressor, Toprol XL*) is used to treat hypertension and has an extended-release form that only needs to be taken once a day. It is also used to treat angina, to treat stable and symptomatic CHF, and to prevent reinfarction after MI. The β_1-selective blocker of choice depends on the condition or combination of conditions being treated and personal experience with the drugs.

Therapeutic Actions and Indications
The therapeutic effects of these drugs are related to their ability to selectively block β_1-receptors in the SNS. That selectivity occurs at therapeutic doses, but the selectivity is lost with doses higher than the recommended range. The blockade of the β_1-receptors in the heart and in the juxtaglomerular apparatus account for most of the therapeutic benefit of these drugs. Decreased heart rate, contractility, and excitability, as well as a membrane-stabilizing effect, lead to a decrease in ar-

rhythmias, decreased cardiac workload, and decreased oxygen consumption. The juxtaglomerular cells are not stimulated to release renin, which further decreases blood pressure. These effects are useful in treating hypertension and chronic angina and can help to prevent reinfarction after an MI by decreasing cardiac workload and oxygen consumption. At therapeutic doses, these drugs do not block the β_2-receptors and therefore do not prevent sympathetic bronchodilation. These drugs are used to treat cardiac arrhythmias, hypertension, and angina; to prevent reinfarction after MI; and, in ophthalmic form, to decrease intraocular pressure and to treat open-angle glaucoma. Metoprolol is also approved in the extended-release form for the treatment of stable, symptomatic CHF.

Pharmacokinetics
The β_1-selective adrenergic blockers are absorbed from the GI tract. The bioavailability of metoprolol is increased if it is taken in the presence of food. These drugs are metabolized

in the liver and excreted in the urine. Metoprolol readily crosses the blood–brain barrier and may cause more CNS effects than acebutolol and atenolol, which do not cross. Because of the potential for adverse effects on the fetus and neonate, these drugs should not be used during pregnancy and lactation unless the benefit to the mother outweighs the potential risk to the fetus. The safety and efficacy of the use of these drugs in children have not been established.

Contraindications and Cautions

The β_1-selective adrenergic blockers are contraindicated in the presence of allergy to the drug or any components of the drug; with sinus bradycardia, heart block, cardiogenic shock, CHF, or hypotension, all of which could be exacerbated by the cardiac-depressing and blood pressure–lowering effects of these drugs; and with lactation, because of the potential adverse effects on the neonate. They should be used with caution in patients with diabetes, thyroid disease, or COPD, because of the potential for adverse effects on these diseases with sympathetic blockade; and in pregnancy, because of the potential for adverse effects on the fetus.

Adverse Effects

Patients receiving these drugs often experience adverse effects related to the blocking of β_1-receptors in the SNS. CNS effects include fatigue, dizziness, depression, paresthesias, sleep disturbances, memory loss, and disorientation. CV effects can include bradycardia, heart block, CHF, hypotension, and peripheral vascular insufficiency. Pulmonary effects ranging from rhinitis to bronchospasm and dyspnea can occur; these effects are not as likely to occur with these drugs as with the nonselective β-blockers. GI upset, nausea, vomiting, diarrhea, gastric pain, and even colitis can occur as a result of unchecked parasympathetic activity and the blocking of the sympathetic receptors. Genitourinary effects can include decreased libido, impotence, dysuria, and Peyronie's disease. Other effects that can occur include decreased exercise tolerance (patients often report that their "get up and go" is gone), hypoglycemia or hyperglycemia, and liver changes that are reflected in increased concentrations of liver enzymes.

Clinically Important Drug–Drug Interactions

A decreased hypertensive effect occurs if these drugs are given with clonidine, NSAIDs, rifampin, or barbiturates. If such a combination is used, the patient should be monitored closely and dosage adjustment made.

There is an initial hypertensive episode followed by bradycardia if these drugs are given with epinephrine.

Increased serum levels and increased toxicity of intravenous lidocaine will occur if it is given with these drugs.

An increased risk for postural hypotension occurs if these drugs are taken with prazosin. If this combination is used, the patient must be monitored closely and safety precautions taken.

There are increased effects of the selective β_1 blockers if they are taken with verapamil, cimetidine, methimazole, or propylthiouracil. The patient should be monitored closely and appropriate dosage adjustment made.

Nursing Considerations for Patients Receiving β_1-Selective Adrenergic Blocking Agents
Assessment: History and Examination

Screen for the following conditions, which could be cautions or contraindications to the use of the drug: known allergies to

---

DRUGS IN FOCUS
β_1-Selective Adrenergic Blocking Agents

Drug Name	Dosage/Route	Usual Indications
acebutolol (*Sectral*)	400 mg/d PO, up to 1200 mg/d may be used; decrease dosage in elderly patients and in those with renal and hepatic impairment	Treatment of hypertension and premature ventricular contractions in adults
P atenolol (*Tenormin*)	Initially 50 mg/d PO, may increase to 200 mg/d; reduce dosage with renal impairment	Treatment of myocardial infarction (MI), chronic angina, hypertension in adults
betaxolol (*Kerlone, Betoptic*)	10–20 mg/d PO; reduce to 5 mg/d PO with the elderly; 1–2 gtts in affected eye(s) for glaucoma	Treatment of hypertension in adults; treatment of ocular hypertension, open-angle glaucoma
bisoprolol (*Zebeta*)	Initially 5 mg/d PO, up to 20 mg/d PO may be needed; reduce dosage with renal or hepatic impairment	Treatment of hypertension in adults
esmolol (*Brevibloc*)	50–200 µg/kg per minute IV with dosage based on patient response	Treatment of supraventricular tachycardias in adults
metoprolol (*Lopressor, Toprol XL*)	100–450 mg/d PO, based on patient response; XL preparations: 50–200 mg/d PO based on patient response	Treatment of hypertension, angina; prevention of reinfarction after MI; treatment of stable, symptomatic congestive heart failure (extended-release preparation only)

any drug or any components of the drug; bradycardia or heart blocks, shock, or CHF, which could be exacerbated by the cardiac-suppressing effects of these drugs; bronchospasm or COPD; pregnancy or lactation, because of the potential effects on the fetus or neonate; diabetes or hypoglycemia; and thyrotoxicosis.

Include screening for baseline status and for any potential adverse effects: skin color, temperature; pulse, blood pressure, ECG; respiration, adventitious sounds; abdominal examination, urine output, and electrolytes.

Nursing Diagnoses

The patient receiving β_1-adrenergic blockers may have the following nursing diagnoses related to drug therapy:

- Acute Pain related to CNS, GI, and systemic effects
- Decreased Cardiac Output related to cardiovascular effects
- Ineffective Tissue Perfusion related to cardiovascular effects
- Deficient Knowledge regarding drug therapy

Implementation

- Do not stop these drugs abruptly after chronic therapy but taper gradually over 2 weeks, *to prevent the possibility of severe reactions. Long-term use of these drugs can sensitize the myocardium to catecholamines and severe reactions could occur.*
- Consult with the physician about discontinuing these drugs before surgery, *because withdrawal is controversial.*
- Give oral forms of the drug with food, *to facilitate absorption.*
- Continuously monitor any patient receiving an intravenous form of these drugs, *to detect severe reactions to sympathetic blockade and to ensure rapid response if these reactions occur.*
- Arrange for supportive care and comfort measures, including rest, environmental control, and other measures, *to relieve CNS effects;* safety measures if CNS effects occur, *to protect the patient from injury;* and small, frequent meals and mouth care, *to relieve the discomfort of GI effects.*
- Provide thorough patient teaching, including the name of the drug, dosage, anticipated adverse effects, measures to avoid drug-related problems, and warning signs of problems, as well as proper administration, as needed *to enhance patient knowledge about drug therapy and to promote compliance.*
- Offer support and encouragement *to help the patient deal with the drug regimen.*

Evaluation

- Monitor patient response to the drug (lowering of blood pressure, decrease in anginal episodes, lowered intraocular pressure).
- Monitor for adverse effects (GI upset, CNS changes, cardiovascular effects, loss of libido and impotence, potential respiratory effects).
- Evaluate the effectiveness of the teaching plan (patient can

name drug, dosage, adverse effects to watch for, specific measures to avoid adverse effects).
- Monitor the effectiveness of comfort measures and compliance to the regimen.

WEB LINKS

Health care providers and patients may want to consult the following Internet sources:

Information on research, alternative methods of therapy, and pharmacology from the National Heart, Lung and Blood Institute:
http://www.heartinfo.org/news98/jnvi42398.htm
Patient information, support groups, diet, exercise, research information on hypertension and other cardiovascular diseases:
http://amhrt.org
Information on cardiovascular research, treatments, hypertension, arrhythmias:
http://www.acc.org/login

CHAPTER SUMMARY

- Adrenergic blocking agents, or sympatholytic drugs, lyse or block the effects of the sympathetic nervous system (SNS).
- Both the therapeutic and the adverse effects associated with these drugs are related to their blocking of the normal responses of the SNS.

CULTURAL CONSIDERATIONS
Alternative Therapies and Adrenergic Blocking Effects

Patients who use alternative therapies as part of their daily regimen should be cautioned about potential increased adrenergic blocking effects if the following alternative therapies are combined with adrenergic blocking agents:

- *Ginseng, sage*—increased antihypertensive effects (risk of hypotension and increased central nervous system effects)
- *Xuan seng, nightshade*—slow heart rate (risk of severe bradycardia and reflex arrhythmias)
- *Celery, coriander, Di huang, fenugreek, goldenseal, Java plum, xuan seng*—lower blood glucose (increased risk of severe hypoglycemia)
- *Saw palmetto*—increased urinary tract complications

Patients who are prescribed an adrenergic blocking drug should be cautioned about the use of herbs, teas, and alternative medicines. If a patient feels that one of these agents is needed, the health care provider should be consulted and appropriate precautions should be taken to ensure that the patient is able to achieve the most therapeutic effects with the least adverse effects while taking the drug.

- The α- and β-adrenergic blocking agents block all of the receptor sites within the SNS, which results in lower blood pressure, slower pulse, and increased renal perfusion with decreased renin levels. These drugs are indicated for the treatment of essential hypertension. They are associated with many adverse effects, including lack of bronchodilation, cardiac suppression, and diabetic reactions.
- Selective adrenergic blocking agents have been developed that, at therapeutic levels, have specific affinity for α- or β-receptors or for specific α_1-, β_1-, or β_2-receptor sites. This specificity is lost at levels higher than the therapeutic range.
- α-Adrenergic drugs specifically block the α-receptors of the SNS. At therapeutic levels, they do not block β-receptors.
- Nonspecific α-adrenergic blocking agents are used to treat pheochromocytoma, a tumor of the adrenal medulla.
- α_1-Selective adrenergic blocking agents block the postsynaptic α_1-receptor sites, causing a decrease in vascular tone and a vasodilation that leads to a fall in blood pressure without the reflex tachycardia that occurs when the presynaptic α_2-receptor sites are also blocked.
- β-Blockers are drugs used to block the β-receptors within the SNS. These drugs are used for a wide range of problems, including hypertension, stage fright, migraines, angina, and essential tremors.
- Blockade of all β-receptors results in a loss of the reflex bronchodilation that occurs with sympathetic stimulation. This limits the use of these drugs in patients who smoke or have allergic or seasonal rhinitis, asthma, or COPD.
- β_1-Selective adrenergic blocking agents do not block the β_1-receptors that are responsible for bronchodilation and therefore are preferred in patients with respiratory problems.

Review Questions

1. Adrenergic blocking drugs, because of their clinical effects, are also known as
   a. anticholinergics.
   b. sympathomimetics.
   c. parasympatholytics.
   d. sympatholytics.
2. Drugs that generally block all adrenergic receptor sites are used to treat
   a. signs and symptoms of allergic rhinitis.
   b. COPD.
   c. cardiac-related conditions.
   d. premature labor.
3. Phentolamine (*Regitine*), an α-adrenergic blocker, is most frequently used
   a. to prevent cell death after extravasation of intravenous dopamine or norepinephrine.
   b. to treat COPD.
   c. to treat hypertension.
   d. to block bronchoconstriction during acute asthma attacks.
4. α_1-Selective adrenergic blocking agents are therapeutically useful in the treatment of
   a. COPD.
   b. hypertension and BPH.
   c. erectile dysfunction.
   d. shock states and bronchospasm.
5. The β-adrenergic blocker propranolol is approved for a wide variety of uses, but it is not approved to treat
   a. migraine headaches.
   b. stage fright or situational anxiety.
   c. bronchospasm.
   d. reinfarction after an MI.
6. The β-blocker of choice for a patient who is hypertensive and suffers from angina would be
   a. nadolol.
   b. pindolol.
   c. timolol.
   d. carteolol.
7. The β_1-selective adrenergic blockers would not be recommended for the treatment of
   a. cardiac arrhythmias.
   b. hypertension.
   c. cardiogenic shock.
   d. open-angle glaucoma.
8. A smoker who is being treated for hypertension with a β-blocker should be treated with a
   a. nonspecific β-blocker.
   b. β_2-specific β-blocker.
   c. β- and α-blocker.
   d. β_1-specific blocker.
9. Patients who are taking adrenergic blockers should be cautioned
   a. to avoid exposure to infection.
   b. to stop the drug if they develop flu-like symptoms.
   c. never to stop the drug abruptly, because it needs to be tapered slowly.
   d. to avoid exposure to the sun.
10. Selective adrenergic blockers
   a. may lose their selectively at higher-than-normal doses.
   b. are designed to react very specifically with only one receptor.
   c. are never absorbed systemically if given ophthalmically.
   d. have fewer associated adverse effects than other adrenergic blockers do.

BIBLIOGRAPHY

Andrews, M. & Boyle, J. (1999). *Transcultural concepts in nursing care.* Philadelphia: Lippincott Williams & Wilkins.

Bullock, B. L. (2000). *Focus on pathophysiology.* Philadelphia: Lippincott Williams & Wilkins.

Drug facts and comparisons. (2002). St. Louis: Fact and Comparisons.

Gilman, A., Hardman, J. G., & Limbird, L. E. (Eds.) (2002). *Goodman and Gilman's the pharmacological basis of therapeutics* (10th ed.). New York: McGraw-Hill.

Karch, A. M. (2002). *2003 Lippincott's nursing drug guide.* Philadelphia: Lippincott Williams & Wilkins.

The medical letter on drugs and therapeutics. (2002). New Rochelle, NY: Medical Letter.

Porth, C. M. (2002). *Pathophysiology: Concepts of altered health states* (6th ed.). Philadelphia: Lippincott Williams & Wilkins.

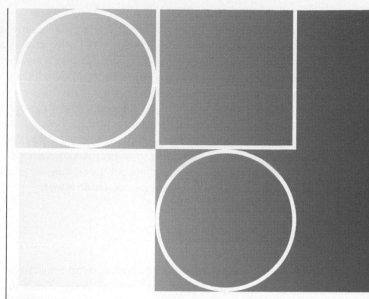

Key Terms
acetylcholinesterase
Alzheimer's disease
cholinergic
miosis
myasthenia gravis
nerve gas
parasympathomimetic

Cholinergic Agents

421

Direct-Acting Cholinergic Agonists
🅟 bethanechol
carbachol
pilocarpine
Indirect-Acting Cholinergic Agonists
ambenonium
🅟 donepezil
edrophonium
galantamine
neostigmine
🅟 pyridostigmine
rivastigmine
tacrine

Reversing Agent
pralidoxime

Cholinergic drugs are chemicals that act at the same site as the neurotransmitter acetylcholine (ACh). Because these sites are found extensively throughout the parasympathetic nervous system (PSNS), the stimulation of these sites produces a response similar to what is seen when the parasympathetic system is activated. As a result, these drugs are often called **parasympathomimetic** drugs, because their action mimics the action of the PSNS. Because the action of these drugs cannot be limited to a specific site, their effects can be widespread throughout the body, and they are usually associated with many undesirable systemic effects.

CHOLINERGIC AGONISTS

Cholinergic agonists are drugs that increase the activity of the ACh receptor sites throughout the body. These drugs work either directly or indirectly. Direct-acting cholinergic agonists occupy receptor sites for ACh on the membranes of the effector cells of the postganglionic cholinergic nerves, causing increased stimulation of the cholinergic receptor. In contrast, indirect-acting cholinergic agonists cause increased stimulation of the ACh receptor sites by reacting with the enzyme **acetylcholinesterase** and preventing it from breaking down the ACh that was released from the nerve. These drugs produce their effects indirectly by producing an increase in the level of ACh in the synaptic cleft, leading to increased stimulation of the cholinergic receptor site (Figure 32–1).

DIRECT-ACTING CHOLINERGIC AGONISTS

The direct-acting cholinergic agonists are similar to ACh and react directly with receptor sites to cause the same reaction as ACh. These drugs tend to cause stimulation of the muscarinic receptors within the parasympathetic system. They are used to increase bladder tone and urinary excretion and as ophthalmic agents, which are not usually absorbed systemically. Their use today is infrequent: because they can cause widespread parasympathetic activity, the more specific and less toxic drugs that are now available are preferred.

The agent bethanechol (*Duvoid, Urecholine*) is available for use orally and subcutaneously to treat nonobstructive postoperative and postpartum urinary retention and to treat neurogenic bladder atony by directly increasing muscle tone and relaxing the sphincters. It has also been used to diagnose and treat reflux esophagitis. Though not indicated for use in children, this drug has been used orally in infants and children for the treatment of esophageal reflux. The drugs carbachol (*Miostat*) and pilocarpine (*Pilocar* and others) are available only as ophthalmic agents; they are used to induce **miosis,** or pupil constriction; to relieve the increased intraocular pressure of glaucoma; and to allow surgeons to perform certain surgical procedures.

DRUG THERAPY ACROSS THE LIFESPAN

Cholinergic Agents

Children	Adults	Older Adults
Children may be more susceptible to the adverse effects associated with the cholinergic agents, including gastrointestinal (GI) upset, diarrhea, increased salivation that could lead to choking, and loss of bowel and bladder control, a problem that could cause stress in the child. Children should be monitored closely if these agents are used and should receive appropriate supportive care.	Adults should be cautioned about the many adverse effects that can be anticipated when using a cholinergic agent. Flushing, increased sweating, increased salivation and GI upset, and urinary urgency often occur. The patient also needs to be aware that dizziness, drowsiness, and blurred vision may occur and that driving and operating dangerous machinery should be avoided.	Older patients are more likely to experience the adverse effects associated with these drugs—central nervous system, cardiovascular, GI, respiratory, and urinary. Because older patients often have renal or hepatic impairment, they are also more likely to have toxic levels of the drug related to changes in metabolism and excretion.
Bethanechol is approved for the treatment of neurogenic bladder in children older than 8 years of age.	In general, there are no adequate studies about the effects of these drugs during pregnancy and lactation. Therefore, the cholinergic agents should be used only in those situations in which the benefit to the mother is greater than the risk to the fetus or neonate. Nursing mothers who require one of these drugs should find another way to feed the baby.	The older patient should be started on lower doses of the drugs and should be monitored very closely for potentially serious arrhythmias or hypotension. Safety precautions should be established if the drug causes dizziness or drowsiness. Special efforts may also be needed to help the patient maintain fluid intake and nutrition if the GI effects become uncomfortable.
Neostigmine and pyridostigmine are used in the control of myasthenia gravis and for reversal of neuromuscular junction blocker effects in children. Care should be taken in determining the appropriate dose based on weight.		Taking the drug with food and offering the patient several small meals throughout the day may alleviate some of these problems.
Edrophonium is used for diagnosis of myasthenia gravis only.		

PHYSIOLOGIC RESPONSES TO CHOLINERGIC DRUGS

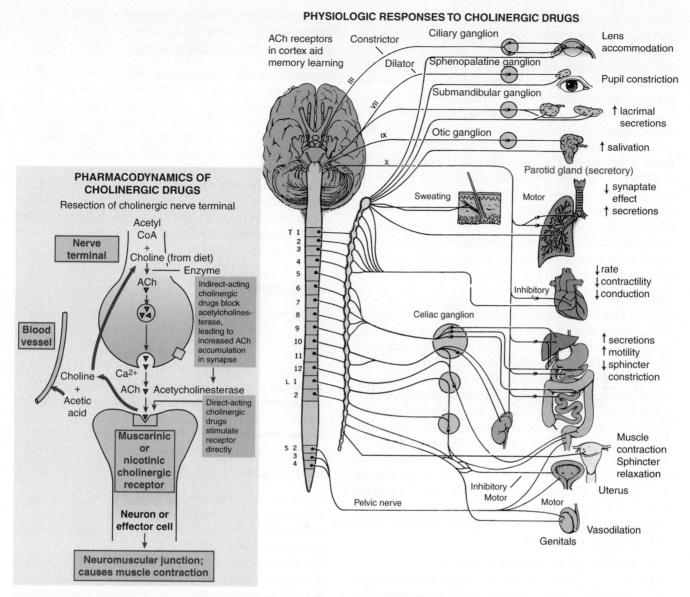

FIGURE 32-1. Pharmacodynamics of cholinergic drugs and associated physiologic responses.

Therapeutic Actions and Indications

The direct-acting cholinergic agonists act at cholinergic receptors in the peripheral nervous system to mimic the effects of ACh and parasympathetic stimulation. These parasympathetic effects include slowed heart rate and decreased myocardial contractility, vasodilation, bronchoconstriction and increased secretions from bronchial mucus, increased gastrointestinal (GI) activity and secretions, increase in bladder tone, relaxation of GI and bladder sphincters, and pupil constriction (see Figure 32–1).

The only drug of this type that is used systemically is bethanechol. Bethanechol has an affinity for the cholinergic receptors in the urinary bladder; it increases the tone of the detrusor muscle of the bladder and relaxes the bladder sphincter to improve bladder emptying. Because this drug is not destroyed by acetylcholinesterase, the effects on the receptor site are longer than with stimulation by ACh. Carba-

chol and pilocarpine are topical drugs that are not generally absorbed systemically, so they are not associated with severe adverse effects.

Pharmacokinetics

The direct-acting cholinergic agonists are generally well absorbed and have relatively short half-lives, ranging from 1 to 6 hours. The metabolism and excretion of these drugs is not known but is believed to occur at the synaptic level. It is not known whether these drugs cross the placenta or enter breast milk, but because of the potential for serious adverse effects on the fetus and neonate, they should not be used during pregnancy or lactation unless the benefit to the mother outweighs the potential risk to the neonate.

Contraindications and Cautions

These drugs are used sparingly because of the potential undesirable systemic effects of parasympathetic stimulation.

They are contraindicated in the presence of any condition that would be exacerbated by parasympathetic effects. For example, bradycardia, hypotension, vasomotor instability, and coronary artery disease could be made worse by the cardiac- and cardiovascular-suppressing effects of the parasympathetic system. Peptic ulcer, intestinal obstruction, or recent GI surgery could be negatively affected by the GI-stimulating effects of the peripheral nervous system. Asthma could be exacerbated by the increased parasympathetic effect, overriding the protective sympathetic bronchodilation. Bladder obstruction or healing sites from recent bladder surgery could be aggravated by the stimulatory effects on the bladder. Epilepsy and parkinsonism could be affected by the stimulation of ACh receptors in the brain. Caution should be used during pregnancy and lactation because of the potential adverse effects on the fetus or neonate.

Adverse Effects

Patients should be cautioned about the potential adverse effects of these drugs. Even if the drug is being given as a topical ophthalmic agent, there is always a possibility that it will be absorbed. The adverse effects associated with these drugs are related to PSNS stimulation. GI effects can include nausea, vomiting, cramps, diarrhea, increased salivation, and involuntary defecation related to the increase in GI secretions and activity. Cardiovascular effects can include bradycardia, heart block, hypotension, and even cardiac arrest related to the cardiac-suppressing effects of the PSNS. Urinary tract effects can include a sense of urgency related to the stimulation of the bladder muscles and sphincter relaxation. Other effects may include flushing and increased sweating secondary to stimulation of the cholinergic receptors in the sympathetic nervous system.

Clinically Important Drug–Drug Interactions

There is an increased risk of cholinergic effects if these drugs are combined or given with acetylcholinesterase inhibitors. The patient should be monitored and appropriate dosage adjustments made.

Nursing Considerations for Patients Receiving Direct-Acting Cholinergic Agonists
Assessment: History and Examination

Screen for the following conditions, which could be cautions or contraindications to use of the drug: known allergies to these drugs; bradycardia, vasomotor instability, peptic ulcer, obstructive urinary or GI diseases; recent GI or genitourinary surgery; asthma; parkinsonism or epilepsy; and pregnancy or lactation, all of which could be exacerbated or complicated by parasympathetic stimulation.

Include screening for baseline status before beginning therapy and for any potential adverse effects: skin color, lesions, temperature; pulse, blood pressure, electrocardiogram (ECG); respiration, adventitious sounds; and urine output and bladder tone.

Nursing Diagnoses

The patient receiving a direct-acting cholinergic agonist may have the following nursing diagnoses related to drug therapy:

- Acute Pain related to GI effects
- Decreased Cardiac Output related to cardiovascular effects
- Impaired Urinary Elimination related to effects on the bladder
- Deficient Knowledge regarding drug therapy

Implementation

- Ensure proper administration of ophthalmic preparations, *to increase effectiveness of drug therapy.*
- Administer oral drug on an empty stomach, *to decrease nausea and vomiting.*
- Monitor patient response closely, including blood pressure, ECG, urine output, and cardiac output, *and arrange to adjust dosage accordingly to ensure the most benefit with the least amount of toxicity.* Maintain atropine on standby *to reverse overdose or counteract severe reactions.*

DRUGS IN FOCUS
Direct-Acting Cholinergic Agonists

Drug Name	Dosage/Route	Usual Indications
P bethanechol (*Duvoid, Urecholine*)	10–50 mg PO b.i.d.–q.i.d. or 2.5–5 mg SC t.i.d.–q.i.d.	Nonobstructive urinary retention, neurogenic bladder in adults and children >8 y
carbachol (*Miostat*)	1–2 gtt in affected eye(s) up to three times a day as needed	Glaucoma, miosis
pilocarpine (*Pilocar*)	1–2 gtt in affected eye(s) as needed, up to six times per day	Glaucoma, miosis

PATIENT TEACHING CHECKLIST
Cholinergic Agents

Create customized patient teaching materials for a specific cholinergic agent from the CD-ROM. Patient teaching should stress the following points for drugs within this class:

Cholinergic drugs get this name because they act at certain nerve–nerve and nerve–muscle junctions in the body that are called cholinergic sites.

• If your drug is given as eye drops, it is important to make sure that you are storing them properly. Eye drops should be clear and kept sterile; if you have any doubts about the drug, discard it.

• Proper administration of eye drops helps to decrease the adverse effects that you might experience. To administer the drops, follow these instructions: Tilt the head backward slightly. Pull down the lower eyelid, maintaining pressure over the opening of the tear duct in the corner of the eye. Administer the correct number of drops. Do not touch the eyedropper to your eye. Maintain pressure over the tear duct opening for a full minute after putting in the drops.

Some of the following adverse effects may occur.

• *Nausea, excessive gas, diarrhea*—It is wise to be near bathroom facilities after taking your drug. If these symptoms become too severe, consult with your health care provider.

• *Flushing, sweating*—Staying in a cool environment and wearing lightweight clothing may help.

• *Urgency to void*—Maintaining access to a bathroom may relieve some of this discomfort.

• *Headache*—Aspirin or another headache medication (if not contraindicated in your particular case) will help to alleviate this pain.

Report any of the following to your health care provider: very slow pulse, light-headedness, fainting, excessive salivation, abdominal cramping or pain, weakness or confusion, blurring of vision.

Tell any doctor, nurse, or other health care provider that you are taking these drugs.

Keep this drug, and all medications, out of the reach of children. Do not share these drugs with other people.

This Teaching Checklist reflects general patient teaching guidelines. It is not meant to be a substitute for drug-specific teaching information, which is available in nursing drug guides.

• Provide safety precautions if the patient reports poor visual acuity in dim light, *to prevent injury*.

• Provide thorough patient teaching, including measures to avoid adverse effects and warning signs of problems, as well as the need for monitoring and evaluation, *to enhance patient knowledge about drug therapy and to promote compliance*. (See Patient Teaching Checklist: Cholinergic Agents.)

• Offer support and encouragement *to help the patient deal with the drug regimen*.

Evaluation

• Monitor patient response to the drug (improvement in bladder function, miosis).

• Monitor for adverse effects (cardiovascular changes, GI stimulation, urinary urgency, respiratory distress).

• Evaluate the effectiveness of the teaching plan (patient can name drug, dosage, adverse effects to watch for, specific measures to avoid adverse effects, proper administration of ophthalmic drugs).

• Monitor the effectiveness of comfort and safety measures and compliance to the regimen (see Nursing Care Guide: Cholinergic Agents).

INDIRECT-ACTING CHOLINERGIC AGONISTS

The indirect-acting cholinergic agonists do not react directly with ACh receptor sites; instead, they react chemically with acetylcholinesterase (the enzyme responsible for the breakdown of ACh) in the synaptic cleft to prevent it from breaking down ACh. As a result, the ACh that is released from the presynaptic nerve remains in the area and accumulates, stimulating the ACh receptors. These drugs work at all ACh receptors, in the PSNS, in the central nervous system (CNS), and at the neuromuscular junction. All of these drugs bind reversibly to acetylcholinesterase, so their effects will pass with time. (Certain drugs, however, are irreversible acetylcholinesterase-inhibiting agents, requiring special considerations—Boxes 32–1 and 32–2.)

The indirect-acting cholinergic agents fall into two main categories: (1) agents used to treat myasthenia gravis and (2) newer agents used to treat Alzheimer's disease.

Myasthenia Gravis Agents

Myasthenia gravis is a chronic muscular disease that is caused by a defect in neuromuscular transmission. It is thought to be an autoimmune disease in which patients make antibodies to their ACh receptors. These antibodies cause gradual destruction of the ACh receptors, causing the patient to have fewer and fewer receptor sites available for stimulation. The disease is marked by progressive weakness and lack of muscle control with periodic acute episodes. The disease can progress to paralysis of the diaphragm, which prevents the patient from breathing and would prove fatal without intervention.

Drugs used to help patients with this progressive disease are acetylcholinesterase inhibitors. These drugs cause an accumulation of ACh in the synaptic cleft, providing a longer period of time for ACh to stimulate whatever receptors are still available.

Neostigmine (*Prostigmine*) is a synthetic drug that does not cross the blood–brain barrier but has a strong influence at the neuromuscular junction. It has a duration of action of 2 to 4 hours and therefore must be given every few hours, based on patient response, to maintain a therapeutic level.

Pyridostigmine (*Regonol, Mestinon*), which has a longer duration of action than neostigmine (3 to 6 hours), is pre-

NURSING CARE GUIDE

Cholinergic Agents

Assessment	Nursing Diagnoses	Implementation	Evaluation
HISTORY Allergies to any of these drugs, coronary artery disease, hypotension, bradycardia, heart block, bowel or urinary obstruction, pregnancy and lactation, epilepsy, parkinsonism, recent GI or urinary surgery	Decreased Cardiac Output related to CV effects Acute Pain related to GI, systemic effects Impaired Urinary Elimination related to GI effects Deficient Knowledge regarding drug therapy	Ensure safe and appropriate administration of drug. Provide comfort and safety measures: assistance/siderails; temperature control; pain relief; small, frequent meals. Monitor cardiac status and urine output throughout drug therapy. Provide support and reassurance to deal with drug effects, discomfort, and GI effects. Provide patient teaching regarding drug name, dosage, side effects, precautions, and warning signs to report.	Evaluate drug effects: miosis; decrease in signs and symptoms of myasthenia gravis, Alzheimer's disease. Monitor for adverse effects: CV effects—bradycardia, heart block, hypotension; urinary problems; GI effects; respiratory problems. Monitor for drug–drug interactions as indicated for each drug. Evaluate effectiveness of patient teaching program. Evaluate effectiveness of comfort and safety measures.
PHYSICAL EXAMINATION CV: BP, P, peripheral perfusion, ECG CNS: orientation, affect, reflexes, vision Skin: color, lesions, texture GU: urinary output, bladder tone GI: abdominal exam Resp: R, adventitious sounds			

BOX 32-1

Pralidoxime Chloride: Antidote for Irreversible Acetylcholinesterase-Inhibiting Drugs

Pralidoxime (*Protopam Chloride*), the antidote for irreversible acetylcholinesterase-inhibiting drugs, is given intramuscularly or intravenously to reactivate the acetylcholinesterase that has been blocked by these drugs. Freeing up the acetylcholinesterase allows it to break down accumulated acetylcholine that has overstimulated acetylcholine receptor sites, causing paralysis.

Pralidoxime does not readily cross the blood–brain barrier, and it is most useful for treating peripheral drug effects. It reacts within minutes after injection and should be available for any patient receiving indirect-acting cholinergic agonists to treat myasthenia gravis. The patient and a significant other should understand when to use the drug and how to administer it.

Pralidoxime is also used with atropine (which does cross the blood–brain barrier and will block the effects of accumulated acetylcholine at central nervous system sites) to treat organophosphate pesticide poisonings and nerve gas exposure (see Box 32-2), both of which cause inactivation of acetylcholinesterase.

Adverse effects associated with the use of pralidoxime include dizziness, blurred vision, diplopia, headache, drowsiness, hyperventilation, and nausea. These effects are also seen with exposure to nerve gas and organophosphate pesticides, so it can be difficult to differentiate drug effects from the effects of the poisoning.

BOX 32-2

Nerve Gas: An Irreversible Acetylcholinesterase Inhibitor

Recent worldwide events and conflicts have made the potential use of **nerve gas** a major news story. Developed as a weapon, nerve gas is an irreversible acetylcholinesterase inhibitor. The drug is inhaled and quickly spreads throughout the body, where it permanently binds with acetylcholinesterase. This causes an accumulation of acetylcholine at nerve endings and a massive cholinergic response. The heart rate slows and becomes ineffective, pupils and bronchi constrict, the gastrointestinal tract increases activity and secretions, and muscles contract and remain that way. The muscle contraction soon freezes the diaphragm, causing breathing to stop. The bodies of people who are killed by nerve gas have a characteristic rigor of muscle contraction.

If the presence of nerve gas is expected, individuals who may be exposed are given intramuscular injections of atropine (to temporarily block cholinergic activity and to activate acetylcholine sites in the central nervous system) and pralidoxime (to free up the acetylcholinesterase to start breaking down acetylcholine). An autoinjection is provided to military personnel who may be at risk. The injector is used to give atropine and then pralidoxime. The injections are repeated in 15 minutes. If symptoms of nerve gas exposure exist after an additional 15 minutes, the injections are repeated. If symptoms still persist after a third set of injections, medical help should be sought.

ferred in some cases for the management of myasthenia gravis because it does not need to be taken as frequently. It is available in oral and parenteral forms; the latter can be used if the patient is having trouble swallowing.

Ambenonium (*Mytelase*) is a newer drug that is similar to pyridostigmine in that it is taken only four times a day. Its main disadvantage is that it is available only in an oral preparation and cannot be used if the patient is unable to swallow tablets.

Edrophonium (*Tensilon, Enlon*) has a very short duration of action (10 to 20 minutes). Its primary use is as a diagnostic agent for myasthenia gravis. If a patient has a temporary reversal of symptoms after injection with edrophonium, it indicates a problem with the ACh neuromuscular receptors.

Alzheimer's Disease Drugs

Alzheimer's disease is a progressive disorder involving neural degeneration in the cortex that leads to a marked loss of memory and of the ability to carry on activities of daily living. The cause of the disease is not yet known, but there is a progressive loss of ACh-producing neurons and their target neurons. Four drugs are currently available to slow the progression of this disease: tacrine (*Cognex*), the first drug developed for the treatment of mild to moderate Alzheimer's dementia; galantamine (*Reminyl*) which is recommended for use with mild to moderate Alzheimer's dementia to delay progression of the disease; rivastigmine (*Exelon*), which is

available in capsule and solution forms to help with patients who have swallowing difficulties, and donepezil (*Aricept*), which has once-a-day dosing. The once-a-day dosing offers a great advantage in a disease that affects memory and the patient's ability to remember to take pills throughout the day.

Therapeutic Actions and Indications

All of the indirect-acting cholinergic agonists work by blocking acetylcholinesterase at the synaptic cleft. This blocking allows the accumulation of ACh released from the nerve endings and leads to increased and prolonged stimulation of ACh receptor sites at all of the postsynaptic cholinergic sites. These drugs can work to relieve the signs and symptoms of myasthenia gravis and increase muscle strength by accumulating ACh in the synaptic cleft at neuromuscular junctions.

The drugs preferred for use with myasthenia gravis are those that do not cross the blood–brain barrier. Drugs that do cross the blood–brain barrier and seem to affect mostly the cells in the cortex to increase ACh concentration are used in the treatment of mild to moderate Alzheimer's disease. Neostigmine and edrophonium, because of their rapid onset of action, are also used to reverse toxicity from nondepolarizing neuromuscular junction blocking drugs, which are used to paralyze muscles during surgery (see Chapter 28).

Pharmacokinetics

These drugs are well absorbed and distributed throughout the body. The drugs used to treat myasthenia gravis do not cross the blood–brain barrier, and their sites of metabolism and excretion are not known. The drugs used for Alzheimer's disease are metabolized in the liver by the cytochrome P450 system, so caution must be used with hepatic impairment and with many interacting drugs. They are excreted in the urine. Because there are no definitive studies on the effects of these drugs during pregnancy and lactation, they should be used during those times only if the benefit to the mother clearly outweighs the potential risks to the fetus.

Contraindications and Cautions

These drugs are contraindicated in the presence of allergy to any of these drugs; with bradycardia or intestinal or urinary tract obstruction, which could be exacerbated by the stimulation of cholinergic receptors; and in pregnancy (the uterus could be stimulated and labor induced) and lactation, because of the potential effects on the baby.

Caution should be used with any condition that could be exacerbated by cholinergic stimulation. Although the effects of these drugs are generally more localized to the cortex and the neuromuscular junction, the possibility of parasympathetic effects should be considered carefully in patients with asthma, coronary disease, peptic ulcer, arrhythmias, epilepsy, or parkinsonism.

Adverse Effects

The adverse effects associated with these drugs are related to the stimulation of the PSNS. GI effects can include nausea, vomiting, cramps, diarrhea, increased salivation, and involuntary defecation related to the increase in GI secretions and

DRUGS IN FOCUS
Indirect-Acting Cholinergic Agonists

Drug Name	Dosage/Route	Usual Indications
ambenonium (*Mytelase*)	5–25 mg PO t.i.d.–q.i.d.	Myasthenia gravis in adults
(P) donepezil (*Aricept*)	5–10 mg PO q.d. at bed time	Alzheimer's disease
edrophonium (*Tensilon, Enlon*)	Diagnosis: 2 mg IV over 15–30 sec, then 8 mg IV if response was seen or 10 mg IM, repeat with 2 mg IM in ½ hour to rule out false-negative results Antidote: 10 mg IV over 30–45 sec, repeat as needed, maximum dose—40 mg Pediatric (diagnosis only): 0.5–2 mg IV based on weight, or 2–5 mg IM	Myasthenia gravis diagnosis, antidote to neuromuscular junction blockers
galantamine (*Reminyl*)	4–12 mg PO b.i.d.; reduce dosage to 16 mg/d maximum with renal or hepatic impairment	Alzheimer's disease
neostigmine (*Prostigmine*)	Adult: 0.5 mg SC or IM for control; 0.022 mg/kg IM for diagnosis; 0.5–2 mg IV as antidote, maximum dose 5 mg Pediatric: 0.01–0.04 mg/kg per dose IM, IV, or SC for control q2–3h; 0.04 mg/kg IM for diagnosis; 0.07–0.08 mg/kg IV, slowly, for antidote	Myasthenia gravis diagnosis and control, antidote to neuromuscular junction blockers
(P) pyridostigmine (*Regonol, Mestinon*)	Adult: average, 60–1,500 mg q.d. PO for myasthenia gravis; 0.1–0.25 mg/kg IV for antidote Pediatric: 7 mg/kg per day PO in five or six divided doses for myasthenia gravis	Myasthenia gravis, antidote to neuromuscular junction blockers
rivastigmine (*Exelon*)	1.5–6 mg PO b.i.d., based on patient response and tolerance	Alzheimer's disease
tacrine (*Cognex*)	10–40 mg PO q.i.d., based on patient response and tolerance	Alzheimer's disease

activity caused by PSNS stimulation. Cardiovascular effects can include bradycardia, heart block, hypotension, and even cardiac arrest, related to the cardiac-suppressing effects of the PSNS. Urinary tract effects can include a sense of urgency related to stimulation of the bladder muscles and sphincter relaxation. Miosis and blurred vision, headaches, dizziness, and drowsiness can occur related to CNS cholinergic effects. Other effects may include flushing and increased sweating secondary to stimulation of the cholinergic receptors in the sympathetic nervous system.

Clinically Important Drug–Drug Interactions
There may be an increased risk of GI bleeding if these drugs are used with nonsteroidal anti-inflammatory drugs (NSAIDs) because of the combination of increased GI secretions and the GI mucosal erosion associated with use of NSAIDs. If this combination is used, the patient should be monitored closely for any sign of GI bleeding.

The effect of anticholinesterase drugs is decreased if they are taken in combination with any cholinergic drugs, because these work in opposition to each other.

Theophylline levels can be increased up to twofold if combined with the tacrine; if that combination is used, the

dosage of theophylline should be reduced accordingly and the patient monitored closely.

Nursing Considerations for Patients Receiving Indirect-Acting Cholinergic Agonists
Assessment: History and Examination

Screen for the following conditions, which could contraindications or cautions to use of the drug: known allergies to any of these drugs; arrhythmias, coronary artery disease, hypotension, urogenital or GI obstruction, peptic ulcer, pregnancy, lactation, or recent GI or genitourinary surgery, which could limit use of the drugs; and regular use of NSAIDs, cholinergic drugs, or theophylline, which could cause a drug–drug interaction.

Include screening for baseline status before beginning therapy and for any potential adverse effects: assess orientation, affect, reflexes, ability to carry on activities of daily living (Alzheimer's drugs), and vision, to monitor for CNS changes related to drug therapy; blood pressure, pulse, ECG, peripheral perfusion, and cardiac output; urinary output, and renal and liver function tests, to monitor drug effects on the renal system and liver, which could change the metabolism and excretion of the drugs.

NURSING CHALLENGE
Myasthenic Crisis Versus Cholinergic Crisis

Myasthenia gravis is an autoimmune disease that runs an unpredictable course throughout the patient's life. Some patients have a very mild presentation (eg, drooping eyelid) and go into remission with no further signs or symptoms for several years. Others have a more severe course, with progressive muscle weakness, confinement to a wheelchair, and so on. Many times, the disease goes through an intense phase called a myasthenic crisis, marked by extreme muscle weakness and respiratory difficulty.

Because of the variability of the disease and the tendency to have crises and periods of remission, management of the drug dosage for a patient with myasthenia gravis is a genuine nursing challenge. If a patient goes into remission, a smaller dosage will be needed. If a patient has a crisis, an increased dosage will be needed. To further complicate the clinical picture, the presentation of a cholinergic overdose or cholinergic crisis is similar to the presentation of a myasthenic crisis. The patient with a cholinergic crisis presents with progressive muscle weakness and respiratory difficulty as the accumulation of acetylcholine at the cholinergic receptor site leads to reduced impulse transmission and muscle weakness. This is a crisis when the respiratory muscles are involved.

For a myasthenic crisis, the correct treatment is increased cholinergic drug. However, treatment of a cholinergic crisis requires withdrawal of the drug. The patient's respiratory difficulty usually necessitates acute medical attention. At this point, the drug edrophonium can be used as a diagnostic agent to distinguish the two conditions. If the patient improves immediately after the edrophonium injection, the problem is a myasthenic crisis, which is improved by administration of the cholinergic drug. If the patient gets worse, the problem is probably a cholinergic crisis, and withdrawal of the patient's cholinergic drug along with intense medical support is indicated. Atropine helps to alleviate some of the parasympathetic reactions to the cholinergic drug. However, because atropine is not effective at the neuromuscular junction, only time will reverse the drug toxicity.

The patient and a significant other will need support, teaching, and encouragement to deal with the tricky regulation of the cholinergic medication throughout the course of the disease. Nurses in the acute care setting need to be mindful of the difficulty in distinguishing drug toxicity from the need for more drug—and be prepared to respond appropriately.

Nursing Diagnoses

The patient receiving an indirect-acting cholinergic agonist may also have the following nursing diagnoses related to drug therapy:

- Disturbed Thought Processes related to CNS effects
- Acute Pain related to GI effects
- Decreased Cardiac Output related to blood pressure changes, arrhythmias, vasodilation
- Deficient Knowledge regarding drug therapy

Implementation

- If the drug is given intravenously, administer it slowly, *to avoid severe cholinergic effects.*
- Maintain atropine sulfate on standby *as an antidote in case of overdose or severe cholinergic reaction.*
- Discontinue the drug if excessive salivation, diarrhea, emesis, or frequent urination becomes a problem, *to decrease the risk of severe adverse reactions.*
- Administer the oral drug with meals, *to decrease GI upset if it is a problem.*
- Mark the patient's chart and notify the surgeon if the patient is to undergo surgery, *because prolonged muscle relaxation may occur if succinylcholine-type anesthetics are*

CULTURAL CONSIDERATIONS
Alzheimer's Disease

Alzheimer's disease was diagnosed increasingly in the 1990s. In the past, many people with Alzheimer's disease would have been diagnosed with senile dementia or dementia. This disease can affect individuals at any age, but it is seen mainly in elderly people and more often men than in women. Currently, the only accurate way to diagnose Alzheimer's disease is at autopsy. However, many companies are working to develop a diagnostic test to permit preautopsy diagnosis.

Alzheimer's is a chronic, progressive disease on the brain's cortex. Eventually it results in memory loss so severe the patients may not remember how to perform basic activities of daily living and may not recognize close family members. Although Alzheimer's disease primarily strikes the elderly, it has a tremendous impact on family members of all ages. For example, adult children of Alzheimer's patients, many of whom are busy raising children of their own, may find themselves in the role of caregivers—in essence, becoming parents of their parent. This new role can put tremendous stress on individuals who are trying to struggle with work, family, and issues related to their parent's care.

When caring for an Alzheimer's patient and family, the nurse must remember that the patient's cultural background can affect how the family copes with the progressive, debilitating nature of the disease. For instance, those who tend to have solid extended families or who are part of communities that offer strong social support and interdependence may be better equipped to deal with the tremendous burden of caring for the patient as the disease progresses. In contrast, families that are more goal and achievement oriented and who value autonomy and independence may find themselves overwhelmed by the patient's needs and may require more support and referrals to community resources.

The nurse is in the best position to evaluate the family situation. By approaching each situation as unique and striving to incorporate cultural and social norms into the considerations for care, the nurse can help ease the family's burden while also maintaining the dignity of the patient and the family through this difficult experience.

used. The patient will require prolonged support and monitoring.

- Monitor the patient being treated for Alzheimer's disease for any progress. *The drug is not a cure and only slows progression; refer families to supportive services.*
- The patient who is being treated for myasthenia gravis and a significant other should receive instruction in drug administration, warning signs of drug overdose, and signs and symptoms to report immediately, *to enhance patient knowledge about drug therapy and to promote compliance.*
- Arrange for supportive care and comfort measures, including rest, environmental control, and other measures, *to decrease CNS irritation;* headache medication, *to relieve pain;* safety measures if CNS effects occur, *to prevent injury;* protective measures if CNS effects are severe, *to prevent patient injury;* and small, frequent meals if GI upset is severe, *to decrease discomfort and maintain nutrition.*
- Provide thorough patient teaching, including dosage and adverse effects to anticipate, measures to avoid adverse ef-

fects, and warning signs of problems as well as proper administration for each route used, *to enhance patient knowledge about drug therapy and to promote compliance.* (See Patient Teaching Checklist: Cholinergic Agents.)
- Offer support and encouragement *to help the patient deal with the drug regimen.*

Evaluation

- Monitor patient response to the drug (improvement in condition being treated).
- Monitor for adverse effects (GI upset, CNS changes, cardiovascular changes, genitourinary changes).
- Evaluate the effectiveness of the teaching plan (patient can name drug, dosage, adverse effects to watch for, specific measures to avoid adverse effects, proper administration).
- Monitor the effectiveness of comfort measures and compliance to the regimen (see Nursing Care Guide: Cholinergic Agents).

C A S E   S T U D Y

Cholinergic Drugs as Causes of Postoperative Abdominal Distention

THE SITUATION

A. J. has been returned to your unit after a lengthy abdominal surgery. She has not eaten since the previous evening but has no desire for the ice chips that have been offered. Her abdomen appears distended, and no bowel sounds are heard on auscultation. The harried house officer who is called decides that A. J. is probably suffering from either paralytic ileus or atonic bladder and orders an intramuscular injection of neostigmine (to reverse the effects of a neuromuscular junction blocker used during surgery) and several oral doses of bethanechol.

CRITICAL THINKING

What could be responsible for A. J.'s symptoms? After abdominal surgery, it is not unusual to have some reflex intestinal atony because of the intestinal manipulation during surgery.

Do the ordered medications seem to be reasonable? What are the potential adverse effects to consider when giving two cholinergic drugs?

What are the potential complications from these drugs after gastrointestinal surgery? *Outline a care plan for A. J. considering her postoperative status, the potential problem she is encountering, the potential effects of the prescribed drug therapy, and the stress and anxiety she may be experiencing as a result of these complications.*

Do you think you would give the ordered medications? If not, what else should be done?

DISCUSSION

The cholinergic drugs that have been ordered would produce some anticipated adverse effects related to their stimulation of the parasympathetic nervous system. These

effects include increased bronchial secretions and bronchoconstriction, which could cause a problem in recovery from general anesthesia, requiring vigorous pulmonary toilet; increased gastric secretions and activity, which could cause major problems after abdominal surgery, including rupture or obstruction; hypotension and bradycardia, which could further complicate recovery from anesthesia and result in poor perfusion to the operative site; and increased tone and contractions of the bladder, which could cause some problems in the postoperative patient, depending on the site of the surgery and use of a catheter.

The most appropriate action in this case would be to question the drugs ordered and to refuse to give the medications until further tests are done to evaluate the actual cause of the abdominal distention. An abdominal radiograph or ultrasound study would be helpful in determining the cause of the problem, which could just as easily be internal bleeding.

In the meantime, A. J. should receive support and comfort measures (eg, positioning, medication). Baseline assessment should be done on all of those parameters most affected by anticholinergic drugs. If the cholinergic drugs are the most appropriate treatment in this case, baseline information will be in place to evaluate for any adverse effects of the drugs. If these drugs are used, very careful patient assessment will be necessary to ensure the safety of the patient in the postoperative phase and full recovery later on.

Teaching plans should include the reason for the concerns, the reasons for additional tests, and the actions and anticipated side effects of the drugs, as well as supportive measures that will be taken to help A. J. cope with the therapy and recover fully.

◼◼◼◼ **WEB LINKS**

Health care providers and patients may want to consult the following Internet sources:

Information on Alzheimer's disease research, conferences:
   http://www.alzheimers.org
Information on resources, medical treatments, outreach
   programs, and local support groups involved with
   Alzheimer's disease:
   http://www.alz.org
Information on current research on myasthenia gravis,
   treatments:
   http://www.myasthenia.org
Information on myasthenia gravis educational programs,
   local support groups, and resources:
   http://www.lowvision.org/myasthenia_gravis.htm
Information on nerve gas treatment protocols:
   http://www.defenselink.mil

CHAPTER SUMMARY

- Cholinergic drugs are chemicals that act at the same site as the neurotransmitter acetylcholine (ACh), stimulating the parasympathetic nerves, some nerves in the brain, and the neuromuscular junction.
- Direct-acting cholinergic drugs react with the ACh receptor sites to cause cholinergic stimulation.
- Use of direct-acting cholinergic drugs is limited by the systemic effects of the drug. They are used to cause miosis and to treat glaucoma, and one agent is available to treat neurogenic bladder and bladder atony postoperatively or postpartum.
- Indirect-acting cholinergic drugs are acetylcholinesterase inhibitors. They block acetylcholinesterase to prevent it from breaking down ACh in the synaptic cleft.
- Cholinergic stimulation by acetylcholinesterase inhibitors is caused by an accumulation of the ACh released from the nerve ending.
- Myasthenia gravis is an autoimmune disease characterized by antibodies to the ACh receptors. This results in a loss of ACh receptors and eventual loss of response at the neuromuscular junction.
- Acetylcholinesterase inhibitors are used to treat myasthenia gravis because they are able to cause the accumulation of ACh in the synaptic cleft, prolonging stimulation of any ACh sites that remain.
- Alzheimer's disease is a progressive dementia characterized by a loss of ACh-producing neurons and ACh receptor sites in the neurocortex.
- Acetylcholinesterase inhibitors that cross the blood–brain barrier are used to manage Alzheimer's disease by increasing ACh levels in the brain and slowing the progression of the disease.
- Side effects associated with the use of these drugs are related to stimulation of the parasympathetic nervous system (bradycardia, hypotension, increased GI secretions and activity, increased bladder tone, relaxation of GI and genitourinary sphincters, bronchoconstriction, pupil constriction) and may limit the usefulness of some of these drugs.
- Nerve gas is an irreversible acetylcholinesterase inhibitor that leads to toxic accumulations of ACh at cholinergic receptor sites and can cause parasympathetic crisis and muscle paralysis.
- Pralidoxime is an antidote for the irreversible acetylcholinesterase inhibitors; it frees the acetylcholinesterase that was inhibited.

Review Questions

1. Indirect acting cholinergic agents
   a. react with acetylcholine receptor sties on the membranes of effector cells.
   b. react chemically with acetylcholinesterase to increase acetylcholine concentrations around effector cell receptor sites.
   c. are used to increase bladder tone and urinary excretion.
   d. should be given with food to decrease nausea.
2. Pilocarpine (*Pilocar*) is a frequently used drug in the clinical setting and would be indicated for the treatment of
   a. myasthenia gravis.
   b. neurogenic bladder.
   c. glaucoma.
   d. Alzheimer's disease.
3. Myasthenia gravis is not
   a. thought to be an autoimmune disease.
   b. associated with destruction of acetylcholine receptor sites.
   c. best treated with potent antibiotics.
   d. a chronic and progressive muscular disease.
4. Myasthenia gravis is treated with indirect-acting cholinergic agents that
   a. lead to accumulation of acetylcholine in the synaptic cleft and eventual stimulation of the muscle.
   b. block the GI effects of the disease.
   c. directly stimulate the remaining acetylcholine receptors.
   d. can be given only by injection.
5. The cholinergic drug of choice for a patient with myasthenia gravis who is no longer able to swallow would be
   a. tacrine.
   b. ambenonium.
   c. pyridostigmine.
   d. edrophonium.
6. Alzheimer's disease is marked by a progressive loss of memory and is associated with
   a. degeneration of dopamine-producing cells in the basal ganglia.
   b. loss of acetylcholine-producing neurons and their target neurons in the CNS.
   c. loss of acetylcholine receptor sites in the parasympathetic nervous system.
   d. increased levels of acetylcholinesterase in the CNS.
7. Donepezil (*Aricept*) would be the Alzheimer's disease drug of choice for a patient who
   a. cannot remember family members' names.

b. is mildly inhibited and can still follow medical dosing regimens.

c. is able to carry on normal activities of daily living.

d. has memory problems and would benefit from once-a-day dosing.

8. Adverse effects associated with the use of cholinergic drugs would include

a. constipation and insomnia.

b. diarrhea and urinary urgency.

c. tachycardia and hypertension.

d. dry mouth and tachycardia.

9. Nerve gas is an irreversible acetylcholinesterase inhibitor that can cause muscle paralysis and death. An antidote to such an agent is

a. atropine.

b. propranolol.

c. pralidoxime.

d. neostigmine.

BIBLIOGRAPHY

Andrews, M. & Boyle, J. (1999). *Transcultural concepts in nursing care*. Philadelphia: Lippincott Williams & Wilkins.

Bullock, B. L. (2000). *Focus on pathophysiology*. Philadelphia: Lippincott Williams & Wilkins.

Drug facts and comparisons. (2002). St. Louis: Facts and Comparisons.

Gilman, A., Hardman, J. G., & Limbird, L. E. (Eds.) (2002). *Goodman and Gilman's the pharmacological basis of therapeutics* (10th ed.). New York: McGraw-Hill.

Karch, A. M. (2002). *2003 Lippincott's nursing drug guide*. Philadelphia: Lippincott Williams & Wilkins.

The medical letter on drugs and therapeutics. (2002). New Rochelle, NY: Medical Letter.

Porth, C. M. (2002). *Pathophysiology: Concepts of altered health states* (6th ed.). Philadelphia: Lippincott Williams & Wilkins.

33

Anticholinergic Agents

Key Terms

anticholinergic

belladonna

cycloplegia

mydriasis

parasympatholytic

Anticholinergic Agents/Parasympatholytics

P atropine

dicyclomine

glycopyrrolate

propantheline

scopolamine

Drugs that are used to block the effects of acetylcholine are called **anticholinergic** drugs. Because this action lyses, or blocks, the effects of the parasympathetic nervous system, they are also called **parasympatholytic** agents. This class of drugs was once very widely used to decrease gastrointestinal (GI) activity and secretions in the treatment of ulcers and to decrease other parasympathetic activities to allow the sympathetic system to become more dominant. Today, more specific and less systemically toxic drugs are available for many of the conditions that would benefit from these effects, so this class of drugs is less commonly used. Atropine remains the only widely used anticholinergic drug.

ANTICHOLINERGICS/PARASYMPATHOLYTICS

Atropine (generic) has been used for many years and is derived from the plant **belladonna.** (Belladonna was once used by fashionable ladies of the European court to dilate the pupils in an effort to make them more innocent-looking and alluring.)

Both atropine and scopolamine (*Transderm-Scop* and generic) work by blocking only the muscarinic effectors in the parasympathetic nervous system and those few cholinergic receptors in the sympathetic nervous system (SNS), such as those that control sweating. They act by competing with acetylcholine for the muscarinic acetylcholine receptor sites. They do not block the nicotinic receptors and therefore have little or no effect at the neuromuscular junction.

Atropine is available for parenteral, oral, and topical use to block parasympathetic effects in a variety of situations. Scopolamine is available in a transdermal form as well as oral and parenteral forms (Table 33–1). Dicyclomine (*Antispas, Dibent,* and others) is an oral drug used to relax the GI tract in the treatment of hyperactive or irritable bowel. Glycopyrrolate (*Robinul*), available in oral and parenteral forms, can be used orally as an adjunct in the treatment of ulcers, although it is not a drug of choice. It is widely used systemically to decrease secretions before anesthesia or intubation and to protect the patient from the peripheral effects of cholinergic drugs used to reverse neuromuscular blockade. Propantheline (*Pro-Banthine*), an oral drug, was once widely used as an adjunct in the treatment of ulcers but now has been replaced, for the most part by the histamine-2 blockers.

Flavoxate (see Chapter 52), ipratropium (see Chapter 55), and methscopolamine (see Chapter 58) are anticholinergic drugs with very specific indications that are discussed in relation to the systems they affect.

DRUG THERAPY ACROSS THE LIFESPAN

Anticholinergic Agents

Children	Adults	Older Adults
The anticholinergic agents are often used in children. Children are often more sensitive to the adverse effects of the drugs, including constipation, urinary retention, heat intolerance, and confusion. If a child is given one of these drugs, the child should be closely watched and monitored for adverse effects, and appropriate supportive measures should be instituted. Dicyclomine is not recommended for use in children.	Adults need to be made aware of the potential for adverse effects associated with the use of these drugs. They should be encouraged to void before taking the medication if urinary retention or hesitancy is a problem. They should be encouraged to drink plenty of fluids and to avoid hot temperatures, because heat intolerance can occur and it will be important to maintain hydration should this happen. Safety precautions may be needed if blurred vision and dizziness occur. The patient should be urged not to drive or perform tasks that require concentration and coordination. These drugs should not be used during pregnancy, because they cross the placenta and could cause adverse effects on the fetus. If the benefit to the mother clearly outweighs the potential risk to the fetus, they should be used with caution. Nursing mothers should find another method of feeding the baby if an anticholinergic drug is needed because of the potential for serious adverse effects on the baby.	Older adults are more likely to experience the adverse effects associated with these drugs; dosage should be reduced, and the patient should be monitored very closely. Because older patients are more susceptible to heat intolerance owing to decreased body fluid and decreased sweating, extreme caution should be used when an anticholinergic drug is given. The patient should be urged to drink plenty of fluids and to avoid extremes of temperature on exertion in warm temperatures. Safety precautions may be needed if central nervous system effects are severe. The older adult is more likely to experience confusion, hallucinations, and psychotic syndromes when taking an anticholinergic drug. Older adults may also have renal impairment, making them more likely to have problems excreting these drugs. Further reduction in dosage may be needed in the older patient who also has renal dysfunction.

TABLE 33-1   Available Forms of Anticholinergic Drugs

Drug	Available Forms					
	Oral	IM	IV	SC	Transdermal Patch	Ophthalmic
atropine	×	×	×	×	—	×
dicyclomine	×	×	—	—	—	—
glycopyrrolate	×	×	×	×	—	—
propantheline	×	—	—	—	—	—
scopolamine	—	×	×	×	×	×

Therapeutic Actions and Indications

The anticholinergic drugs competitively block the acetylcholine receptors at the muscarinic cholinergic receptor sites that are responsible for mediating the effects of the parasympathetic postganglionic impulses (Figure 33–1). This means that atropine is used to depress salivation and bronchial secretions and to dilate the bronchi, but it can thicken respiratory secretions (causing obstruction of airways). Atropine also is used to inhibit vagal responses in the heart, to relax the GI and genitourinary tracts, to inhibit GI secretions, to

FIGURE 33–1. Pharmacodynamics of anticholinergic drugs and associated physiologic responses. A bar indicates blockade of that activity.

cause **mydriasis** or relaxation of the pupil of the eye (also called a mydriatic effect), and to cause **cycloplegia** or inhibition of the ability of the lens in the eye to accommodate to near vision (also called a cycloplegic effect). Anticholinergic drugs also are thought to block the effects of acetylcholine in the central nervous system (CNS).

Anticholinergic drugs can be used to decrease secretions before anesthesia; to treat parkinsonism; to restore cardiac rate and blood pressure after vagal stimulation during surgery; to relieve bradycardia caused by a hyperactive carotid sinus reflex; to relieve pylorospasm and hyperactive bowel; to relax biliary and ureteral colic; to relax bladder detrusor muscles and tighten sphincters; to help to control crying or laughing episodes in patients with brain injuries; to relax uterine hypertonicity; to help in the management of peptic ulcer; to control rhinorrhea associated with hay fever; as an antidote for cholinergic drugs and for poisoning by certain mushrooms; and as an ophthalmic agent to cause mydriasis or cycloplegia in acute inflammatory conditions.

Scopolamine is also used to decrease the nausea and vomiting associated with motion sickness and has been used to induce obstetric amnesia and relax the mother. Other agents are used for specific indications, as noted earlier and summarized in Table 33–2.

Pharmacokinetics

The anticholinergics are well absorbed after administration. They are widely distributed throughout the body and cross the blood–brain barrier. Their half-lives vary with route and drug. They are excreted in the urine. These drugs should be used in pregnancy and lactation only if the benefit clearly outweighs the potential risk to the fetus or baby. Nursing mothers should find another way of feeding the baby if an anticholinergic drug is needed.

Contraindications and Cautions

Anticholinergics are contraindicated in the presence of known allergy to any of these drugs. They are also contraindicated with any condition that could be exacerbated by a blocking of the parasympathetic nervous system. These conditions include glaucoma, because of the possibility of increased pressure with pupil dilation; stenosing peptic ulcer, intestinal atony, paralytic ileus, GI obstruction, severe ulcerative colitis, and toxic megacolon, all of which could be intensified with a further slowing of GI activity; prostatic hy-

TABLE 33-2 | Effects of Parasympathetic Blockade and Associated Therapeutic Uses

Physiological Effect	Therapeutic Uses
GASTROINTESTINAL Smooth muscle: blocks spasm, blocks peristalsis Secretory glands: decreases acid and digestive enzyme production	Decreases motility and secretory activity in peptic ulcer, gastritis, cardiospasm, pylorospasm, enteritis, diarrhea, hypertonic constipation
URINARY TRACT Decreases tone and motility in the ureters and fundus of the bladder; increases tone in the bladder sphincter	Increases bladder capacity in children with enuresis, spastic paraplegics; decreases urinary urgency and frequency in cystitis; antispasmodic in renal colic and to counteract bladder spasm caused by morphine
BILIARY TRACT Relaxes smooth muscle, antispasmodic	Relief of biliary colic; counteracts spasms caused by narcotics
BRONCHIAL MUSCLE Weakly relaxes smooth muscle	Aerosol form may be used in asthma; may counteract bronchoconstriction caused by drugs
CARDIOVASCULAR SYSTEM Increases heart rate (may decrease heart rate at very low doses); causes local vasodilation and flushing	Counteracts bradycardia caused by vagal stimulation, carotid sinus syndrome, surgical procedures; used to overcome heart blocks following MI; used to counteract hypotension caused by cholinergic drugs.
OCULAR EFFECTS Pupil dilation, cycloplegia	Allows ophthalmological examination of the retina, optic disk; relaxes ocular muscles and decreases irritation in iridocyclitis, choroiditis
SECRETIONS Reduces sweating, salivation, respiratory tract secretions	Preoperatively before inhalation anesthesia; reduces nasal secretions in rhinitis, hay fever; may be used to reduce excessive sweating in hyperhidrosis
CENTRAL NERVOUS SYSTEM Decreases extrapyramidal motor activity Atropine may cause excessive stimulation, psychosis, delirium, disorientation Scopolamine causes depression, drowsiness	Decreases tremor in parkinsonism; helps to prevent motion sickness; scopolamine may be in OTC sleep aids

pertrophy and bladder obstruction, which could be further compounded by a blocking of bladder muscle activity and a blocking of sphincter relaxation in the bladder; cardiac arrhythmias, tachycardia, and myocardial ischemia, which could be exacerbated by the increased sympathetic influence, including tachycardia and increased contractility that occurs when the parasympathetic nervous system is blocked; impaired liver or kidney function, which could alter the metabolism and excretion of the drug; and myasthenia gravis, which could worsen with further blocking of the cholinergic receptors (low doses of atropine are sometimes used in myasthenia gravis to block unwanted GI and cardiovascular effects of the cholinergic drugs used to treat that condition).

Caution should be used in the presence of lactation, because of possible suppression of lactation; hypertension, because of the possibility of additive hypertensive effects from the sympathetic system's dominance with parasympathetic nervous system blocking; and spasticity and brain damage, which could be exacerbated by cholinergic blockade within the CNS.

Adverse Effects

The adverse effects associated with the use of anticholinergic drugs are caused by the systemic blockade of cholinergic receptors. What are adverse effects in some cases may be the desired therapeutic effects in others. The intensity of adverse effects is related to drug dosage: the more of the drug in the system, the greater the systemic effects. These adverse effects could include the CNS effects of blurred vision, pupil dilation and resultant photophobia, cycloplegia, and increased intraocular pressure, all of which are related to the blocking of the parasympathetic effects in the eye. Weakness, dizziness, insomnia, mental confusion, and excitement are effects related to the blocking of the cholinergic receptors within the CNS. Dry mouth results from the blocking of GI secretions. Altered taste perception, nausea, heartburn, constipation, bloated feelings, and paralytic ileus are related to a slowing of GI activity. Tachycardia and palpitations are possible effects related to blocking of the parasympathetic effects on the heart. Urinary hesitancy and retention are related to the blocking of bladder muscle activity and relaxation of the sphincter. Decreased sweating and an increased

CULTURAL CONSIDERATIONS
Mydriatric Effects

Nurses working in eye clinics or administering preoperative medications for eye surgery should be aware that mydriatics (including atropine) are much less effective in African Americans than in the general population. Increased dosage may be needed, and there may be a prolonged time to peak effect. This effect, although somewhat less pronounced, is seen in any individual with dark-pigmented eyes.

NURSING CHALLENGE
Atropine Toxicity

Atropine is used in a large variety of clinical settings to

- Decrease secretions, as a preoperative agent
- Treat parkinsonism (relieves tremor and rigidity)
- Restore cardiac rate and arterial pressure during general anesthesia when increased vagal stimulation causes a rapid parasympathetic response
- Relieve bradycardia and syncope with hyperreactive carotid sinus
- Relieve pylorospasm and hypertonic intestine
- Relax the spasm of biliary and ureteral colic and bronchospasm
- Relax the urinary bladder
- Control crying and laughing episodes in patients with brain lesions
- Treat closed head injuries that cause acetylcholine release
- Relax uterine hypertonicity
- Manage peptic ulcer
- Control rhinorrhea or acute rhinitis from hay fever
- Induce mydriasis for ophthalmic procedures

It also is used as an antidote to overdose with cholinergic drugs or cholinesterase inhibitors and as an antidote to poisoning with certain mushrooms.

Atropine can be a poison, causing severe toxicity. Because it is found in many natural products, including the belladonna plant, and may be present in herbal or alternative therapy products, atropine toxicity can occur inadvertently. Atropine toxicity should be considered whenever a patient receiving an anticholinergic drug presents with a sudden onset of bizarre mental and neurological symptoms. Toxicity is dose related and usually progresses as follows:

0.5 mg atropine—slight cardiac slowing, dryness of mouth, inhibition of sweating

1.0 mg atropine—definite mouth and throat dryness, thirst, rapid heart rate, pupil dilation

2.0 mg atropine—rapid heart rate, palpitations; marked mouth dryness; dilated pupils; some blurring of vision

5.0 mg atropine—all of the above and marked speech disturbances; difficulty swallowing; restlessness, fatigue, headache; dry and hot skin; difficulty voiding; reduced intestinal peristalsis

10.0 mg atropine—all of the above symptoms, more marked; pulse rapid and weak; iris nearly gone; vision blurred; skin flushed, hot, dry, and scarlet; ataxia; restlessness and excitement; hallucinations; delirium and coma

Treatment is as follows. If the poison was taken orally, immediate gastric lavage should be done to limit absorption. Physostigmine can be used as an antidote. A slow intravenous injection of 0.5 to 4 mg (depending on the size of the patient and the severity of the symptoms) usually reverses the delirium and coma of atropine toxicity. Physostigmine is metabolized rapidly, so the injection may need to be repeated every 1 to 2 hours until the atropine has been cleared from the system. Diazepam is the drug of choice if an anticonvulsant is needed. Cool baths and alcohol sponging may relieve the fever and hot skin. In extreme cases, respiratory support may be needed. It is important to remember that the half-life of atropine is 2.5 hours; at extremely high doses, several hours may be needed to clear the atropine from the body.

predisposition to heat prostration are related to the inability to cool the body by sweating, a result of blocking of the sympathetic cholinergic receptors responsible for sweating. Suppression of lactation is related to anticholinergic effects in the breasts and in the CNS (see Table 33–2).

Clinically Important Drug–Drug Interactions

There is an increased incidence of anticholinergic effects if these drugs are combined with any other drugs with anticholinergic activity, including antihistamines, antiparkinsonism drugs, monoamine oxidase (MAO) inhibitors, and tricyclic antidepressants (TCAs). If such combinations must be used, the patient should be monitored closely and dosage adjustments made. Patients should be advised to avoid over-the-counter products that might contain these drugs.

There is a decreased effectiveness of phenothiazines if they are combined with anticholinergic drugs, and there is an increased risk of paralytic ileus. This combination should be avoided.

Nursing Considerations for Patients Receiving Anticholinergic Agents

Assessment: History and Examination

Screen for the following conditions, which could be cautions or contraindications to use of the drug: any known allergies to these drugs; glaucoma; stenosing peptic ulcer, intestinal atony, paralytic ileus, GI obstruction, severe ulcerative colitis, and toxic megacolon; prostatic hypertrophy and bladder obstruction; cardiac arrhythmias, tachycardia, and myocardial ischemia, all of which could be exacerbated by parasympathetic blockade; impaired liver or kidney function, which could alter the metabolism and excretion of the drug; myasthenia gravis, which could become much worse with further blocking of the cholinergic receptors; lactation, because of possible suppression of lactation; hypertension; and spasticity and brain damage, which require cautious use of these drugs.

Include screening for baseline status before beginning therapy and for any potential adverse effects: skin color, le-

CASE STUDY

Anticholinergic Drugs and Heart Disease

THE SITUATION

E. K., a 64-year-old woman with a long history of heart disease, has suffered from repeated bouts of cystitis. With this infection, her course was marked by severe pain, frequency, urgency, and even nocturnal enuresis. She was treated with an antibiotic deemed appropriate after a culture and sensitivity tests were done on her urine, and she was given atropine to relax the bladder spasm and alleviate some of the unpleasant side effects that she was experiencing. Within the next few days, she plans to travel south for the winter and wants any information that she should have before she goes

CRITICAL THINKING

E. K. presents many nursing care problems. What are the implications of giving an anticholinergic drug to a person with a long history of heart disease?

Repeated bouts of cystitis are not normal; what potential problems should be addressed in this area?

E. K. is about to leave for her winter home in the south; what teaching plans will be essential for her if she is taking atropine when she leaves?

What are the medical problems that can arise with people who live in different areas at different times of the year?

Considering her age, what written information should E. K. take with her as she travels?

DISCUSSION

E. K. is doing well with her cardiac problems at the moment, but she could develop problems as a result of the anticholinergic drug that has been prescribed. The anticipated adverse effect of tachycardia could tip the balance in a compensated heart, leading to congestive heart failure or oxygen delivery problems. She will need to

be carefully evaluated for the status of her heart disease and potential problems.

E. K. should be further evaluated for the cause of her repeated bouts with cystitis. Does she have a structural problem, a dietary problem, or a simple hygiene problem? She should receive instruction on ways to avoid bladder infections, such as wiping only from front to back, voiding after sexual intercourse, avoiding baths, avoiding citrus juices and other alkaline ash foods that decrease the acidity of the urine and promote bacterial growth, and pushing fluids as much as possible.

E. K. also should be evaluated to establish a baseline for vision, reflexes, the possibility of glaucoma, gastrointestinal problems, and so on. She should receive thorough teaching about her atropine, especially adverse effects to anticipate, safety measures to take if vision changes occur, and a bowel program that she can follow to avoid constipation.

Because E. K. is leaving a cold climate and traveling to a warm climate, she will need to be warned that atropine decreases sweating. This means that she may be susceptible to heat stroke in the warmer climate. She should be encouraged to take precautions to avoid these problems.

It will be difficult to monitor E. K. while she is away. It should be anticipated that patients such as E. K. might have two sets of health care providers who may not communicate with each other. It is important to give E. K. written information about her current diagnosis, including test results; details about her drugs, including dosages; information about the adverse effects she may experience and ways to deal with them; and ways to avoid cystitis in the future. It may be useful to include a telephone number that E. K. can use or can give to her southern health care provider to use if further tests or follow-up is indicated.

DRUGS IN FOCUS
Anticholinergic Agents

Drug Name	Dosage/Route	Usual Indications
ⓟ atropine (generic)	0.4–0.6 mg IM, SC, or IV; use caution with older patients Pediatric: 0.1–0.4 mg IV, IM, or SC based on weight	Decrease secretions, bradycardia, pylorospasm, ureteral colic, relaxing of bladder, emotional lability with head injuries, antidote for cholinergic drugs, pupil dilation
dicyclomine (*Antispas, Dibent*)	160 mg/d PO in four divided doses; 80 mg/d IM in four divided doses—do not give IV	Irritable or hyperactive bowel in adults
glycopyrrolate (*Robinul*)	Adult: 1–2 mg PO b.i.d.–t.i.d. for ulcers; 0.004 mg/kg IM 30–60 min before surgery, then 0.1 mg IV during surgery Pediatric: 0.002–0.004 mg/kg IM 30–60 min before surgery, then 0.004 mg/kg IV during surgery	Decrease secretions, antidote for neuromuscular blockers
propantheline (*Pro-Banthine*)	Adult: 15 mg PO 30 min before meals and at bedtime Pediatric: as antisecretory agent, 1.5 mg/kg per day PO in divided doses t.i.d.–q.i.d. as antispasmodic, 2–3 mg/kg per day PO in divided doses q4–6h and at bedtime	Adjunctive therapy for ulcers; antisecretory, antispasmodic
scopolamine (*Transderm Scop*)	Adult: 0.32–0.65 mg SC or IM; 1–2 gtts in eye(s) for refraction; 1.5 mg transdermal every 3 d for motion sickness; use caution with older patients. Pediatric: Do not use PO or transdermal system with children; 0.006 mg/kg SC, IM, or IV	Motion sickness, decrease secretions, obstetric amnesia, relief of urinary problems, adjunctive for ulcers, pupil dilation

sions, temperature; affect, orientation, reflexes, pupil response; pulse, blood pressure, electrocardiogram; respiration, adventitious sounds; urine output, bladder tone; and bowel sounds and abdominal examination.

Nursing Diagnoses

The patient receiving anticholinergic drugs may have the following nursing diagnoses related to drug therapy:

- Acute Pain related to GI, CNS, genitourinary, cardiovascular effects
- Decreased Cardiac Output related to cardiovascular effects
- Constipation, related to GI effects
- Noncompliance related to adverse drug effects
- Deficient Knowledge regarding drug therapy

Implementation

- Ensure proper administration of the drug, *to ensure effective use and decrease the risk of adverse effects.*
- Ensure adequate hydration and temperature control, *to prevent hyperpyrexia.*
- Provide comfort measures, *to help the patient tolerate drug effects:* sugarless lozenges to suck and frequent mouth

care, *to alleviate problems associated with dry mouth;* lighting control, *to alleviate photophobia;* small and frequent meals, *to alleviate GI discomfort;* bowel program, *to alleviate constipation;* safety precautions, *to prevent injury* if CNS effects are severe; analgesics, *to relieve pain* if headaches occur; and voiding before taking medication, *if urinary retention is a problem* (commonly occurs with benign prostatic hypertrophy).
- Monitor patient response closely (blood pressure, electrocardiogram, urine output, cardiac output) in order *to arrange to adjust dosage accordingly to ensure benefit with the least amount of toxicity.*
- Provide thorough patient teaching, including measures to avoid adverse effects, warning signs of problems, and the need for monitoring and evaluation, *to enhance patient knowledge about drug therapy and to promote compliance.* (See Patient Teaching Checklist: Anticholinergic Agents.)
- Offer support and encouragement, *to help the patient deal with the drug regimen.*

Evaluation

- Monitor patient response to the drug (improvement in disorder being treated).

PATIENT TEACHING CHECKLIST
Anticholinergic Agents

Create customized patient teaching materials for a specific anticholinergic agent from the CD-ROM. Patient teaching should stress the following points for drugs within this class:

Parasympathetic blockers, parasympatholytics, or anticholinergics block or stop the actions of a group of nerves that are part of the parasympathetic nervous system. These drugs may decrease the activity of your GI tract, dilate your pupils, or speed up your heart.

Some of the following adverse effects may occur:

• *Dry mouth, difficulty swallowing*—Frequent mouth care will help to remove dried secretions and keep the mouth fresh. Sucking on sugarless candies will help to keep the mouth moist. Taking lots of fluids with meals (unless you are on fluid restriction) will help swallowing.
• *Blurring vision, sensitivity to light*—If your vision is blurred, avoid driving, operating hazardous machinery, or doing close work that requires attention to details until your vision returns to normal. Dark glasses will help protect your eyes from the light.
• *Retention of urine*—Take the drug just after you have emptied your bladder. Moderate your fluid intake while the drug's effects are the highest; if possible, take the drug before bedtime, when this effect will not be a problem.
• *Constipation*—Include fluid and roughage in your diet, and follow any bowel regimen that you may have. Monitor your bowel movements so that appropriate laxatives can be taken if necessary.
• *Flushing, intolerance to heat, decreased sweating*—This drug blocks sweating, which is your body's way of cooling off. This places you at increased risk for heat stroke. Avoid extremes of temperature, dress coolly on very warm days, and avoid exercise as much as possible.

Report any of the following to your health care provider: eye pain, skin rash, fever, rapid heartbeat, chest pain, difficulty breathing, agitation or mood changes, impotence (a dosage adjustment may help alleviate this problem).

Avoid the use of over-the-counter medications, especially for sleep and nasal congestion; avoid antihistamines, diet pills, and cold capsules. These products may contain drugs that cause similar anticholinergic effects, which could cause a severe reaction. Consult with your health care provider if you feel that you need medication for symptomatic relief.

Tell any doctor, nurse, or other health care provider that you are taking these drugs.

Keep this drug, and all medications, out of the reach of children. Do not share these drugs with other people.

This Teaching Checklist reflects general patient teaching guidelines. It is not meant to be a substitute for drug-specific teaching information, which is available in nursing drug guides.

• Monitor for adverse effects (cardiovascular changes, GI problems, CNS effects, urinary hesitancy and retention, pupil dilation and photophobia, decrease in sweating and heat intolerance).

• Evaluate the effectiveness of the teaching plan (patient can name drug, dosage, adverse effects to watch for, specific measures to avoid adverse effects, proper administration of ophthalmic drugs).
• Monitor the effectiveness of comfort measures and compliance with the regimen (see Nursing Care Guide: Anticholinergic Agents).

▢▇●▇ WEB LINKS

Health care providers and patients may want to consult the following Internet sources:

Information on atropine and related anticholinergics: http://www.infoplease.com/ce5/CE003568.html

CHAPTER SUMMARY

• Anticholinergic drugs are drugs that block the effects of acetylcholine at cholinergic receptor sites.
• Anticholinergic drugs are also called parasympatholytic drugs because they block the effects of the parasympathetic nervous system.
• Blocking of the parasympathetic system causes an increase in heart rate, decrease in GI activity, decrease in urinary bladder tone and function, and pupil dilation and cycloplegia.
• These drugs also block cholinergic receptors in the CNS and sympathetic postganglionic cholinergic receptors, including those that cause sweating.
• There are many systemic adverse effects associated with the use of anticholinergic drugs; they are caused by the systemic cholinergic blocking effects that can also produce the desired therapeutic effect.
• Atropine is the most commonly used anticholinergic drug. It is indicated for a wide variety of conditions and is available in oral, parenteral, and topical forms.
• Patients receiving anticholinergic drugs must be monitored for dry mouth, difficulty swallowing, constipation, urinary retention, tachycardia, pupil dilation and photophobia, cycloplegia and blurring of vision, and heat intolerance caused by a decrease in sweating.

Review Questions

1. Anticholinergic drugs are used
   a. to block the parasympathetic system to allow the sympathetic system to dominate.
   b. to block the parasympathetic system which is commonly hyperactive.
   c. as the drugs of choice for treating ulcers.
   d. to stimulate GI activity.
2. Atropine and scopolamine work by blocking
   a. nicotinic receptors only.
   b. muscarinic and nicotinic receptors.
   c. muscarinic receptors only.
   d. adrenergic receptors to allow cholinergic receptors to dominate.

NURSING CARE GUIDE

Anticholinergic Agents

Assessment	Nursing Diagnoses	Implementation	Evaluation
HISTORY Allergies to any of these drugs, COPD, narrow-angle glaucoma, myasthenia gravis, bowel or urinary obstruction, pregnancy and lactation, tachycardia, prostatic hypertrophy, recent GI or urinary surgery	Decreased Cardiac Output related to CV effects Acute Pain related to GI, GU, CNS, CV effects Constipation related to GI effects Deficient Knowledge regarding drug therapy Noncompliance related to adverse effects	Ensure safe and appropriate administration of drug. Provide comfort, safety measures: assistance/siderails; temperature control; dark glasses; small, frequent meals; artificial saliva, fluids; sugarless lozenges, mouth care; bowel program. Provide support and reassurance to deal with drug effects, discomfort, and GI effects. Provide patient teaching regarding drug name, dosage, adverse effects, precautions, and warnings to report. Monitor blood pressure and pulse and adjust dosage as needed.	Evaluate drug effects: pupil dilation, decrease in signs and symptoms being treated. Monitor for adverse effects: CV effects—tachycardia, CHF; CNS—confusion, dreams; urinary retention; GI effects—constipation; visual blurring, photophobia. Monitor for drug–drug interactions as indicated for each drug. Evaluate effectiveness of patient teaching program. Evaluate effectiveness of comfort and safety measures.
PHYSICAL EXAMINATION CV: BP, P, peripheral perfusion, ECG CNS: orientation, affect, reflexes, vision Skin: color, lesions, texture, sweating GU: urinary output, bladder tone GI: abdominal exam Resp: R, adventitious sounds			

3. Atropine is not used to
   a. depress salivation.
   b. dry up bronchial secretions.
   c. block parasympathetic effects on the heart.
   d. promote uterine contractions.
4. Because of their blocking effects of the parasympathetic nervous system, anticholinergics should not be used with
   a. ulcerative colitis, glaucoma, or prostatic hypertrophy.
   b. antihistamines.
   c. bradycardia.
   d. inner ear imbalance.
5. Sweating is blocked by anticholinergic agents, so nursing interventions should include
   a. covering the head at extremes of temperature.
   b. assuring hydration and temperature control.
   c. changing position slowly and protection from the sun.
   d. monitoring for difficulty swallowing.
6. Teaching patients who are taking anticholinergic drugs would not include
   a. encouraging the patient to void before dosing.
   b. bowel program to deal with constipation.
   c. encouragement to suck sugarless lozenges to avoid the discomfort of dry mouth.
   d. exercise measures to increase the heart rate.

BIBLIOGRAPHY
Andrews, M. & Boyle, J. (1999). *Transcultural concepts in nursing care*. Philadelphia: Lippincott Williams & Wilkins.

Bullock, B. L. (2000). *Focus on pathophysiology.* Philadelphia: Lippincott Williams & Wilkins.

Drug facts and comparisons. (2002). St. Louis: Facts and Comparisons.

Gilman, A., Hardman, J. G., & Limbird, L. E. (Eds.) (2002). *Goodman and Gilman's the pharmacological basis of therapeutics* (10th ed.). New York: McGraw-Hill.

Karch, A. M. (2002). *2003 Lippincott's nursing drug guide.* Philadelphia: Lippincott Williams & Wilkins.

The medical letter on drugs and therapeutics. (2002). New Rochelle, NY: Medical Letter.

Porth, C. M. (2002). *Pathophysiology: Concepts of altered health states* (6th ed.). Philadelphia: Lippincott Williams & Wilkins.

VI

Drugs Acting on the Endocrine System

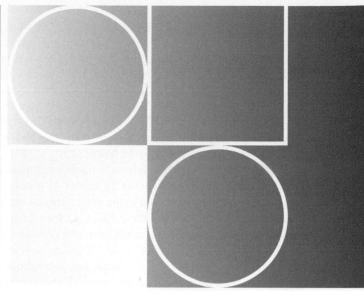

CHAPTER 34

Introduction to the Endocrine System

Key Terms

anterior pituitary
diurnal rhythm
hormones
hypothalamic–pituitary axis
hypothalamus
negative feedback system
neuroendocrine system
pituitary gland
posterior pituitary
releasing hormones or factors

445

The nervous system and the endocrine system work together to maintain internal homeostasis and to integrate the body's response to the external environment. Their activities and functions are so closely related that it is probably more correct to refer to them as the **neuroendocrine system.** However, this section deals with drugs affecting the traditional endocrine system, which includes glands that secrete **hormones,** or chemical messengers, directly into the bloodstream to communicate within the body.

It is important to note that certain hormones that influence body functioning are not secreted by endocrine glands. For example, tissue hormones such as the prostaglandins are produced in various tissues and have effects at their local site. Neurotransmitters such as norepinephrine and dopamine also can be classified as hormones because they are secreted directly into the bloodstream for dispersion throughout the body. There also are many gastrointestinal (GI) hormones that are produced in GI cells and act locally. All of these hormones are addressed in the sections most related to their effects.*

HORMONES

Hormones are chemicals that are produced in the body and that meet specific criteria. The following are characteristic of all hormones:

- They are produced in very small amounts.
- They are secreted directly into the bloodstream.
- They travel through the blood to specific receptor sites throughout the body.
- They act to increase or decrease the normal metabolic processes of cells when they react with their specific receptor sites.
- They are immediately broken down.

Hormones may react with specific receptor sites on a cell membrane to stimulate the nucleotide cyclic adenosine monophosphate (cAMP) within the cell to cause an effect. For example, when insulin reacts with an insulin receptor site, it activates intracellular enzymes that cause many effects, including changing the cell membrane's permeability to glucose. Hormones such as insulin that do not enter the cell act very quickly, often within seconds, to produce an effect.

---

*Gastrointestinal hormones are discussed in Part XI: Drugs Acting on the Gastrointestinal System. Neurotransmitters acting like hormones are discussed in Chapter 29: Introduction to the Autonomic Nervous System. The reproductive hormones are discussed in Chapter 39: Introduction to the Reproductive System. Hormones active in the inflammatory and immune responses are discussed in Part III: Drugs Acting on the Immune System. Specific traditional endocrine glands and hormones are discussed in Chapter 35 (hypothalamic and pituitary hormones), Chapter 36 (adrenocortical hormones), Chapter 37 (thyroid and parathyroid hormones), and Chapter 38 (pancreatic hormones).

Other hormones, such as estrogen, actually enter the cell and react with a receptor site inside the cell to change messenger RNA and affect the cell's function. These hormones take quite a while to produce an effect. The full effects of estrogen may not be seen for months to years, as evidenced by the changes that occur at puberty. Because the neuroendocrine system tightly regulates the body's processes within a narrow range of normal limits, overproduction or underproduction of any hormone can affect the body's activities and other hormones within the system.

THE HYPOTHALAMUS

The **hypothalamus** is the coordinating center for the nervous and endocrine responses to internal and external stimuli. The hypothalamus constantly monitors the body's homeostasis by analyzing input from the periphery and the central nervous system (CNS) and coordinating responses through the autonomic, endocrine, and nervous systems. In effect, it is the "master gland" of the neuroendocrine system. This title was once given to the pituitary gland because of its many functions (see later discussion).

Situated at the base of the forebrain, the hypothalamus receives input from virtually all other areas of the brain, including the limbic system and the cerebral cortex. Because of its positioning, the hypothalamus is able to influence, and be influenced by, emotions and thoughts. The hypothalamus is located in an area of the brain that is poorly protected by the blood–brain barrier, so it is able to act as a sensor to various electrolytes, chemicals, and hormones that are in circulation and do not affect other areas of the brain. The hypothalamus has various neurocenters, areas specifically sensitive to certain stimuli, that regulate a number of body functions, including body temperature, thirst, hunger, water retention, sleep and waking, blood pressure, respiration, reproduction, and emotional reactions.

The hypothalamus maintains internal homeostasis by sensing blood chemistries and by stimulating or suppressing endocrine, autonomic, and CNS activity. In essence, it can turn the autonomic nervous system and its effects on or off. The hypothalamus also produces and secretes a number of **releasing hormones or factors** that stimulate the pituitary gland to stimulate or inhibit various endocrine glands throughout the body (Figure 34–1). These releasing hormones include growth hormone–releasing hormone (GHRH), thyrotropin-releasing hormone (TRH), gonadotropin-releasing hormone (GnRH), corticotropin-releasing hormone (CRH), and prolactin-releasing hormone (PRH). The hypothalamus also produces two inhibiting factors that act as regulators to shut off the production of hormones when levels become too high: growth hormone release–inhibiting factor (somatostatin) and prolactin-inhibiting factor (PIF) (Table 34–1).

Recent research has indicated that PIF may actually be dopamine, a neurotransmitter. Patients who are taking dopamine-blocking drugs often develop galactorrhea (inap-

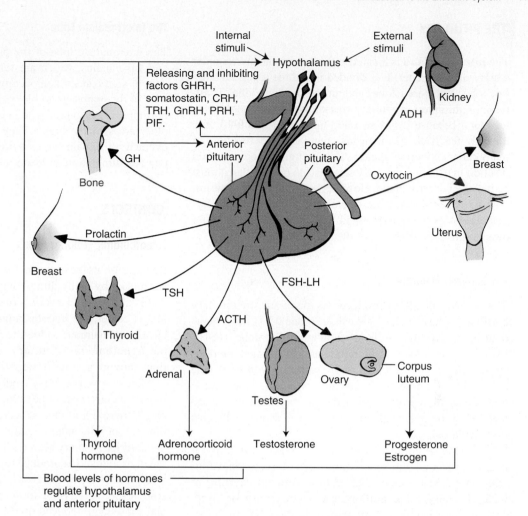

FIGURE 34-1. The traditional endocrine system.

propriate milk production) and breast engorgement, theoretically because PIF also is blocked. Research is ongoing about the actual chemical structure of several of the releasing factors.

The hypothalamus produces two other hormones, antidiuretic hormone (ADH) and oxytocin, which are stored in the posterior pituitary to be released when stimulated by the hypothalamus. The hypothalamus is connected to the pituitary gland by two networks: a vascular network carries the hypothalamic releasing factors directly into the anterior pituitary, and a neurological network delivers ADH and oxytocin to the posterior pituitary to be stored.

TABLE 34-1 | **Hypothalamic Releasing and Inhibiting Hormones and Associated Anterior Pituitary and Endocrine Gland Response**

Hypothalamus Hormones	Anterior Pituitary Hormones	Target Organ Response
STIMULATING HORMONES		
CRH (corticotropin-releasing hormone)	ACTH (adrenocorticotropic hormone)	Adrenal corticosteriod hormones
TRH (thyroid-releasing hormone)	TSH (thyroid-stimulating hormone)	Thyroid hormone
GHRH (growth hormone–releasing hormone)	GH (growth hormone)	Cell growth
GnRH (gonadotropin-releasing hormone)	LH and FSH (leutinizing hormone, follicle-stimulating hormone)	Estrogen and progesterone (females), Testosterone (males)
PRH (prolactin-releasing hormone)	Prolactin	Milk production
INHIBITING HORMONES		
Somatostatin (growth hormone–inhibiting factor)		Stops release of GH
PIF (prolactin inhibiting factors)		Stops release of prolactin

THE PITUITARY

The **pituitary gland** is located in the bony sella turcica under a layer of dura mater. It is divided into three lobes: an anterior lobe, a posterior lobe, and an intermediate lobe. Traditionally, the anterior pituitary was known as the body's master gland because it has so many important functions and, through feedback mechanisms, regulates the function of many other endocrine glands. Also, its unique and protected position in the brain led early scientists to believe that it must be the chief control gland. However, as knowledge of the endocrine system has grown, scientists now designate the hypothalamus as the master gland because it has even greater direct regulatory effects over the neuroendocrine system.

The Anterior Pituitary

The **anterior pituitary** produces six major anterior pituitary hormones. These include growth hormone (GH), adrenocorticotropin (ACTH), follicle-stimulating hormone (FSH), luteinizing hormone (LH), prolactin (PRL), and thyroid-stimulating hormone (TSH, also called thyrotropin) (see Figure 34–1). These hormones are essential for the regulation of growth, reproduction, and some metabolic processes. Deficiency or overproduction of these hormones disrupts this regulation.

The anterior pituitary hormones are released in a rhythmic manner into the bloodstream. Their secretion varies with time of day (often referred to as **diurnal rhythm**) or with physiological conditions such as exercise or sleep. Their release is affected by activity in the CNS; by hypothalamic hormones; by hormones of the peripheral endocrine glands; by certain diseases that can alter endocrine functioning; and by a variety of drugs, which can directly or indirectly upset the homeostasis in the body and cause an endocrine response.

The anterior pituitary also produces melanocyte-stimulating hormone (MSH) and lipotropins. MSH plays an important role in animals that use skin color changes as an adaptive mechanism. It also might be important for nerve growth and development in humans. Lipotropins stimulate fat mobilization but have not been clearly isolated in humans.

The Posterior Pituitary

The **posterior pituitary** stores two hormones that are produced by the hypothalamus and deposited in the posterior lobe via the nerve axons where they are produced. These two hormones are ADH, also referred to as vasopressin, and oxytocin. ADH is directly released in response to increased plasma osmolarity or decreased blood volume (which often results in increased osmolarity). The osmoreceptors in the hypothalamus stimulate the release of ADH. Oxytocin stimulates uterine smooth muscle contraction in late phases of pregnancy and also causes milk release or "let down" in lactating women.

The Intermediate Lobe

The intermediate lobe of the pituitary produces endorphins and enkephalins, which are released in response to severe pain or stress and which occupy specific endorphin-receptor sites in the brainstem to block the perception of pain. These hormones are also produced in tissues in the periphery and in other areas of the brain. They are released in response to overactivity of pain nerves, sympathetic stimulation, transcutaneous stimulation, guided imagery, and vigorous exercise.

CONTROLS

Hypothalamic–Pituitary Axis

Because of its position in the brain, the hypothalamus is stimulated by many things, such as light, emotion, cerebral cortex activity, and a variety of chemical and hormonal stimuli. Together, the hypothalamus and the pituitary function closely to maintain endocrine activity along what is called the **hypothalamic–pituitary axis** (HPA). This axis functions through a series of **negative feedback systems.**

Here is how a negative feedback system works. When the hypothalamus senses a need for a particular hormone, for example thyroid hormone, it secretes a releasing factor (TRH) directly into the anterior pituitary. In response to the TRH, the anterior pituitary secretes TSH, which in turn stimulates the thyroid gland to produce thyroid hormone. When the hypothalamus senses the rising levels of thyroid hormone, it stops secreting TRH, resulting in decreased TSH production and subsequent reduced thyroid hormone levels. The hypothalamus, sensing the falling thyroid hormone levels, secretes TRH again. The negative feedback system continues in this fashion, maintaining the levels of thyroid hormone within a relatively narrow range of normal (Figure 34–2).

It is thought that this feedback system is more complex than once believed. The hypothalamus probably also senses TRH and TSH levels and regulates TRH secretion within a narrow range, even if thyroid hormone is not produced. The anterior pituitary may also be sensitive to TSH levels and thyroid hormone, regulating its own production of TSH.

FIGURE 34–2. Negative feedback system. Regulation of thyroid hormone levels is done by a series of negative feedback systems influencing thyrotropin-releasing hormone (TRH), thyrotropin (TSH), and thyroid hormone levels.

This complex system provides backup controls and regulation if any part of the HPA fails. This system also can create complications, especially when there is a need to override or interact with the total system, as is the case with replacement therapy or treatment of endocrine disorders.

Two of the traditional anterior pituitary hormones, growth hormone and prolactin, do not have a target organ and so cannot be regulated by the same type of feedback mechanism. Growth hormone release and prolactin release are directly inhibited by the hypothalamic inhibiting factors somatostatin and PIF, respectively. The hypothalamus may be stimulated to release inhibiting factors by increased circulating levels of hormones or by some mediating factor that is stimulated by these hormones. The HPA functions constantly to keep these particular hormones regulated.

Other Controls

Other hormones are released in response to stimuli other than stimulating hormones. For example, the endocrine pancreas produces and releases insulin, glucagon, and somatostatin from different cells in response to varying blood glucose levels. The parathyroid glands release parathormone in response to local calcium levels. The juxtaglomerular cells in the kidney release erythropoietin and renin in response to decreased pressure or decreased oxygenation of the blood flowing into the glomerulus. GI hormones are released in response to local stimuli in the area, such as acid, proteins, or calcium. The thyroid gland produces and secretes another hormone, called calcitonin, in direct response to serum calcium levels. Many different prostaglandins are released throughout the body in response to local stimuli in the tissues that produce them. Activation of the sympathetic nervous system directly causes release of ACTH, and the adrenocorticoid hormones to prepare the body for fight or flight. Aldosterone, an adrenocorticoid hormone, is released in response to ACTH but also is released directly in response to high potassium levels.

As more is learned about the interactions of the nervous and endocrine systems, new ideas are being formed about how the body controls its intricate homeostasis. When administering any drug that affects the endocrine or nervous systems, it is important for the nurse to remember how closely related all of these activities are. Expected or unexpected adverse effects involving areas of the endocrine and nervous systems often occur.

◻◼◧◼ WEB LINKS
Students may want to explore up-to-date information from the following source:

Travel through the virtual endocrine system:
http://www.innerbody.com/image/endoov.html

CHAPTER SUMMARY

- The endocrine system is a regulatory system that communicates through the use of hormones.

- Because the endocrine and nervous systems are tightly intertwined in the regulation of body homeostasis, they are often referred to as the neuroendocrine system.
- A hormone is a chemical that is produced within the body, is needed in only small amounts, travels to specific receptor sites to cause an increase or decrease in cellular activity, and is broken down immediately.
- The hypothalamus is the "master gland" of the neuroendocrine system. It helps regulate the central and autonomic nervous systems and the endocrine system to maintain homeostasis.
- The pituitary is made up of three lobes: anterior, posterior, and intermediate. The anterior lobe produces stimulating hormones in response to hypothalamic stimulation. The posterior lobe stores two hormones produced by the hypothalamus, ADH and oxytocin. The intermediate lobe produces endorphins and enkephalins to modulate pain perception.
- The hypothalamus and pituitary operate by a series of negative feedback mechanisms called the hypothalamic–pituitary axis (HPA). The hypothalamus secretes releasing factors to cause the anterior pituitary to release stimulating hormones, which act with specific endocrine glands to cause the release of hormones or, in the case of growth hormone and prolactin, to stimulate cells directly. This stimulation shuts down the production of releasing factors, which leads to decreased stimulating factors and, subsequently, decreased hormone release.
- Growth hormone and prolactin are released by the anterior pituitary and directly influence cell activity. These hormones are regulated by the release of hypothalamic inhibiting factors in response to hormone levels or a cellular mediator.
- Some hormones are not influenced by the HPA and are released in response to direct, local stimulation.
- When any drug that affects either the endocrine or the nervous system is given, adverse effects may occur throughout both systems because they are closely interrelated.

Review Questions

1. Hormones do not exert their influence on human cells by influencing
   a. enzyme controlled reactions.
   b. messenger RNA.
   c. lysosome activity.
   d. cellular DNA.
2. Aldosterone
   a. causes the loss of sodium and water from the renal tubules.
   b. is under direct hormonal control from the hypothalamus.
   c. is released into the bloodstream in response to angiotensin I.
   d. is released into the bloodstream in response to high potassium levels.
3. Antidiuretic hormone (ADH)
   a. is produced by the anterior pituitary.
   b. causes the retention of water by the kidneys.

c. is released by the hypothalamus.

d. causes the retention of sodium by the kidneys.

4. The endocrine glands
   a. form part of the communication system of the body.
   b. cannot be stimulated by hormones circulating in the blood.
   c. cannot be viewed as integrating centers of reflex arcs.
   d. are all controlled by the hypothalamus.

5. The specific criteria that define a hormone would not include which of the following?
   a. It is produced in very small amounts.
   b. It is secreted directly into the bloodstream.
   c. It is slowly metabolized in the liver and lungs.
   d. It reacts with a very specific receptor set on a target cell.

6. The hypothalamus maintains internal homeostasis and could be considered the master endocrine gland because
   a. it releases stimulating hormones that cause endocrine glands to produce their hormones.
   b. no hormone-releasing gland responds unless stimulated by the hypothalamus.
   c. it secretes releasing hormones that are an important part of the hypothalamic–pituitary axis that finely regulates the traditional endocrine system.
   d. it regulates temperature control and arousal as well as hormone release.

7. The posterior lobe of the pituitary gland
   a. secretes a number of stimulating hormones.
   b. produces endorphins to modulate pain perception.
   c. has no function that has yet been identified.
   d. stores ADH and oxytocin, which are produced in the hypothalamus.

8. Some endocrine glands do not respond to the hypothalamic–pituitary axis. These glands would not include the
   a. thyroid gland.
   b. ovaries.
   c. parathyroid glands.
   d. adrenal cortex.

9. An example of a negative feedback system would be
   a. growth hormone control.
   b. prolactin control.
   c. melanocyte-stimulating hormone control.
   d. thyroid hormone control.

10. Internal body homeostasis and communication are regulated by
    a. the cardiovascular and respiratory systems.
    b. the nervous and cardiovascular systems.
    c. the endocrine and nervous systems.
    d. the endocrine and cardiovascular systems.

BIBLIOGRAPHY

Bullock, B. L. (2000). *Focus on pathophysiology*. Philadelphia: Lippincott Williams & Wilkins.

Girard, J. (1991). *Endocrinology of puberty*. Farmington, CT: Karger Publishers.

Guyton, A. & Hall, J. (2000). *Textbook of medical physiology*. Philadelphia: W. B. Saunders.

Joseph, R. (1996). *Neuropsychiatry, neuropsychology and clinical neurosciences* (2nd ed.). Baltimore: Williams & Wilkins.

Karch, A. M. (2002). *2003 Lippincott's nursing drug guide*. Philadelphia: Lippincott Williams & Wilkins.

North, W. G., Moses, A. M., & Shafe, L. (eds) (1993). The neurohypophysis: A window on brain function. *Annals of the New York Academy of Sciences, 689*.

Porth, C. (2001). *Pathophysiology: Concepts of altered health states* (6th ed.). Philadelphia: Lippincott Williams & Wilkins.

35

Hypothalamic and Pituitary Agents

451

As described in Chapter 34, the endocrine system's main function is to maintain homeostasis. This is achieved through a complex balance of glandular activities that either stimulate or suppress hormone release. Too much or too little glandular activity disrupts the body's homeostasis, leading to various disorders and interfering with the normal functioning of other endocrine glands. The drugs presented in this chapter are those used to either replace or interact with the hormones or factors produced by the hypothalamus and pituitary.

HYPOTHALAMIC RELEASING FACTORS

The hypothalamus uses a number of releasing hormones or factors to stimulate or inhibit the release of hormones from the anterior pituitary. These releasing hormones are growth hormone–releasing hormone (GHRH), thyrotropin-releasing hormone (TRH), gonadotropin-releasing hormone (GnRH), corticotropin-releasing hormone (CRH), and prolactin-releasing hormone (PRH). The hypothalamus also releases two inhibiting factors, somatostatin (growth hormone—inhibiting factor) and prolactin-inhibiting factor (PIF). These hormones are found in such minute quantities that their actual chemical structures have not been clearly identified. Not all of the hypothalamic hormones are used as pharmacological agents. A number of the hypothalamic releasing factors described here are used for diagnostic purposes only, and others are used primarily as antineoplastic agents.

CRH stimulates the release of adrenocorticotropin (ACTH) from the anterior pituitary and is used to diagnose Cushing's disease (a condition characterized by hypersecretion of adrenocortical hormones in response to excessive ACTH release). It is being studied for the treatment of peritumoral brain edema.

Goserelin (*Zoladex*) is an analog of GnRH. After an initial burst of follicle-stimulating hormone (FSH) and luteinizing hormone (LH) release, goserelin inhibits pituitary gonadotropin secretion with a resultant drop in the production of the sex hormones. This drug currently is used as an antineoplastic agent to treat prostatic cancers.

Histrelin (*Supprelin*) is a GnRH agonist. With chronic use, it inhibits gonadotropin secretion and decreases the levels of steroid sex hormones. It is used to treat precocious puberty in children.

Leuprolide (*Lupron*) occupies pituitary GnRH receptor sites so that they no longer respond to GnRH. As a result, there is no stimulation for release of LH and FSH. This drug is used primarily as an antineoplastic agent to treat specific cancers. It is also used to treat endometriosis and precocious puberty that results from hypothalamic activity.

Nafarelin (*Synarel*), a potent agonist of GnRH, is used to decrease the production of gonadal hormones through repeated stimulation of their receptor sites. After about 4

DRUG THERAPY ACROSS THE LIFESPAN

Hypothalmic and Pituitary Agents

Children	Adults	Older Adults
Children who receive any of the hypothalamic or pituitary agents need to be monitored closely for adverse effects associated with changes in overall endocrine function, particularly growth and development and metabolism. Periodic radiograph of the long bones as well as monitoring of blood sugar levels and electrolytes should be a standard part of the treatment plan. Children receiving growth hormone pose many challenges (see the Nursing Challenge) Children who are using desmopressin for diabetes insipidus need to have the administration technique monitored and should have an adult responsible for the overall treatment protocol.	Adults also need frequent monitoring of electrolytes and blood sugar levels when receiving any of these agents. Adults using nasal forms of drugs to control diabetes insipidus should review the proper administration of the drug with the primary care provider periodically; inappropriate administration can lead to complications and lack of therapeutic effect. Adults receiving regular injections of these drugs should learn the proper storage, preparation, and administration of the drug, including rotation of injection sites. These drugs should not be used during pregnancy or lactation unless the benefit to the mother clearly outweighs any risk to the fetus or neonate, because of the potential for severe adverse effects associated with the use of these drugs.	Older adults may be more susceptible to the imbalances associated with alterations in the endocrine system. They should be evaluated periodically during treatment for hydration and nutrition as well as for electrolyte balance. Proper administration technique should be reviewed, and nasal mucus membranes should be evaluated regularly, because older patients are more apt to develop dehydrated membranes and possibly ulcerations, leading to improper dosing of drugs delivered nasally.

weeks of therapy, gonadal hormone levels fall and the cells they normally stimulate are quiet. This drug is used to treat endometriosis and precocious puberty.

TRH (protirelin) is used only for diagnostic purposes. It stimulates the pituitary to produce thyrotropin (thyroid-stimulating hormone, TSH), which in turn stimulates the thyroid to produce thyroid hormones (see Chapter 37). A TRH infusion test is the most sensitive method for diagnosing mild hypothyroidism and hyperthyroidism. TRH has orphan drug status when it is used to prevent infant respiratory distress syndrome associated with prematurity. TRH is also under investigation for improving the outcome of spinal cord injuries when it is given within a very specific time frame.

GHRH (sermorelin) stimulates the production of growth hormone (GH) by the anterior pituitary. It is used for diagnostic purposes in short children to determine the presence of hypothalamic or pituitary dysfunction. It is also used to evaluate the therapeutic response in patients undergoing surgery or irradiation. It has orphan drug status with gonadotropin to induce ovulation and to treat cachexia associated with the acquired immunodeficiency syndrome (AIDS).

Figure 35–1 displays the sites of action of hypothalamic releasing factors and other hypothalamic and pituitary agents.

Nursing Considerations for Patients Receiving Hypothalamic Releasing Factors

The specific nursing care of the patient who is receiving a hypothalamic releasing factor is related to the hormone (or hormones) that the drug is affecting (see Chapter 36 for adrenocorticoid hormones, Chapter 37 for thyroid hormones, and Chapters 40 and 41 for sex hormones). Drugs used for diagnostic purposes are short-lived; information about these agents should be included in any patient teaching about the diagnostic procedure. Nursing process guidelines for other agents can be found with the therapeutic drug class to which they belong (eg, antineoplastic agents, Chapter 14).

ANTERIOR PITUITARY HORMONES

Agents that affect pituitary function are used mainly to mimic or antagonize the effects of specific pituitary hormones. They may be used either as replacement therapy for conditions resulting from a hypoactive pituitary or for diagnostic purposes. The anterior pituitary hormones that are in use today include seven different drugs (see Figure 35–1).

• Chorionic gonadotropin (*Chorex*) acts like LH and stimulates the production of testosterone and progesterone. It is

DRUGS IN FOCUS
Hypothalamic Releasing Factors

Drug Name	Dosage/Route	Usual Indications
corticotropin-releasing hormone (CRH) (generic)	10–25 units in 500mL, DSW infused over 8 h	Diagnosis of Cushing's disease
goserelin (*Zoladex*)	3.6 mg SC every 28 d or 10.8 mg SC every 3 mo	Treatment of prostatic cancers
histrelin (*Supprelin*)	10 µg/kg per day SC	Treatment of precocious puberty in children
Ⓟ leuprolide (*Lupron*)	Prostate cancer: 1 mg/d SC or various depot preparations: 3.75 mg IM once a month—endometriosis Precocious puberty—5–10 µg/kg per day SC	Treatment of specific cancers, endometriosis, precocious puberty
nafarelin (*Synarel*)	400 µg/d divided as one spray in left nostril AM or PM; one spray in right nostril AM or PM; Precocious puberty—1,600–1,800 µ/d per nasal spray	Treatment of endometriosis and precocious puberty
thyrotropin-releasing hormone (TRH) (*Protirelin, Thypinone*)	500 µg IV Pediatric: 7 µg/kg IV, up to 500 µg	Diagnosis of thyroid dysfunction; prevention of respiratory distress of prematurity (orphan drug use)
growth hormone–releasing hormone (GHRH) (*sermorelin, Geref*)	1 µg/kg IV	Diagnosis of hypothalamic or pituitary dysfunction in short children; evaluation of response to surgery or irradiation; ovulation induction, AIDS-associated cachexia (orphan drug uses)

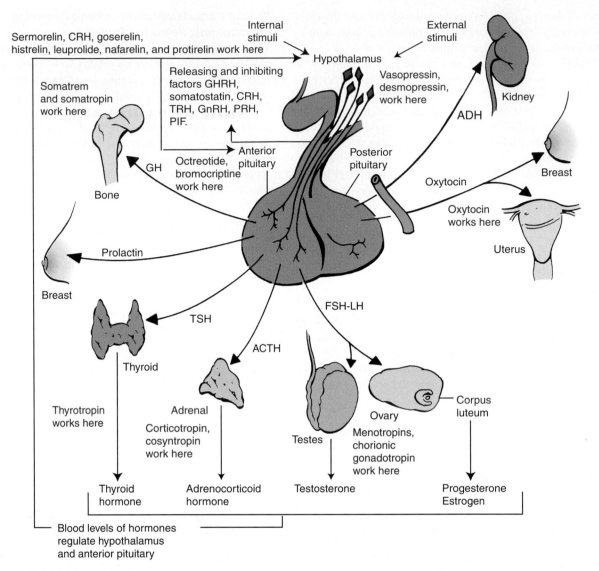

FIGURE 35-1. Sites of action of hypothalamic/pituitary agents.

used to treat hypogonadism in males, to induce ovulation in females with functioning ovaries, and to treat prepubertal cryptorchidism when there is no anatomical obstruction to testicular movement. (See Chapters 40 and 41 for nursing implications.)

- Corticotropin (*Acthar*), or ACTH, is used for diagnostic purposes to test adrenal function and responsiveness. Because it stimulates steroid release and anti-inflammatory effects, it also is used to treat various inflammatory disorders.
- Cosyntropin (*Cortrosyn*) is used to diagnose adrenal dysfunction. Because it has a rapid onset and a short duration of activity, it is not used for therapeutic purposes.
- Menotropins (*Pergonal*) is a purified preparation of gonadotropins. It is used as a fertility drug to stimulate ovulation in women and spermatogenesis in men. (See Chapters 40 and 41 for nursing implications.)
- Somatropin (*Nutropin, Saizen, Genotropin, Serostim,* and

others) is a GH that is produced with the use of recombinant DNA technology. It is used in the treatment of children with growth failure.
- Somatrem (*Protropin*) is a genetically engineered GH with an added amino acid, making it longer acting and purer than animal-derived GH. This drug is also used to treat children with growth failure.
- Thyrotropin (*Thytropar*) is equivalent to TSH and is used as a diagnostic agent to evaluate thyroid function.

In clinical practice, the agents that are used purely as replacements for anterior pituitary hormones are those acting as GH—somatropin and somatrem. These are discussed further.

Growth Hormone

GH is responsible for linear skeletal growth, the growth of internal organs, protein synthesis, and the stimulation of many other processes that are required for normal growth. **Hypopituitarism** is often seen as GH deficiency before any other signs and symptoms occur. Hypopituitarism may occur as a result of developmental abnormalities or congenital defects of the pituitary, circulatory disturbances (eg, hemorrhage, infarction), acute or chronic inflammation of the pituitary, and pituitary tumors. GH deficiency in children results in short stature (**dwarfism**). Adults with somatropin deficiency syndrome (SDS) may have hypopituitarism as a result of pituitary tumors or trauma, or they may have been treated for GH deficiency as children, resulting in a shutdown of the pituitary production of somatotropin.

GH deficiency was once treated with GH injections extracted from the pituitary glands of cadavers. The supply of GH was therefore rather limited and costly. Synthetic human GH is now available from recombinant DNA sources using genetic engineering. Synthetic GH is expensive, but it is thought to be safer than cadaver GH and is being used increasingly to treat GH deficiencies. Somatropin and somatrem are the two GH replacement drugs in use today (see Figure 35–1).

Therapeutic Actions and Indications

As noted previously, somatropin and somatrem are hormones of recombinant DNA origin that are equivalent to human GH.

Somatrem is indicated only for the treatment of children with growth failure due to lack of endogenous GH. It has orphan drug status for the treatment of short stature associated with Turner's syndrome in girls.

Somatropin is indicated for the treatment of growth failure due to lack of GH or to chronic renal failure, for long-term treatment of growth failure in children born small for gestational age who do not achieve catch-up growth by 2 years of age, and for the treatment of short stature associated with Turner's syndrome. It has orphan drug status for use to increase protein production and growth in various AIDS-related states. Box 35–1 discusses a new delivery system for somatropin.

Pharmacokinetics

These drugs are injected and reach peak levels within 7 hours. They are widely distributed in the body and localize in highly perfused tissues, particularly the liver and kidney. Excretion occurs through the urine and feces. Patients with liver or renal dysfunction may experience reduced clearance and increased concentrations of the drug. These drugs should be avoided in pregnancy and lactation because of the potential for adverse effects on the fetus or neonate.

Contraindications and Cautions

These drugs are contraindicated with any known allergy to the drug or ingredients in the drug. They also are contraindicated in the presence of closed epiphyses or with underlying cranial lesions.

Adverse Effects

The adverse effects that most often occur when using GH include the development of antibodies to GH and subsequent signs of inflammation and autoimmune-type reactions (much more common with somatrem); swelling and joint pain; and the endocrine reactions of hypothyroidism and insulin resistance.

Nursing Considerations for Patients Receiving Growth Hormone

Assessment: History and Examination

Screen for the following conditions, which could be contraindications to use of the drug: history of allergy to any GH or binder, and closed epiphyses or underlying cranial lesions, which are contraindications to the use of the drug.

Include screening for baseline status before beginning therapy and for any potential adverse effects: height, weight, thyroid function tests, glucose tolerance tests, and GH levels.

Nursing Diagnoses

The patient receiving any GH may have the following nursing diagnoses related to drug therapy:

- Imbalanced Nutrition: Less than Body Requirements, related to metabolic changes
- Acute Pain related to need for injections
- Deficient Knowledge regarding drug therapy

Implementation

- Reconstitute the drug following manufacturer's directions, *because individual products vary;* administer intramuscularly or subcutaneously *for appropriate delivery of drug.*
- Monitor response carefully when beginning therapy, *to allow appropriate dosage adjustments as needed.*
- Monitor thyroid function, glucose tolerance, and GH levels periodically, *to monitor endocrine changes and to institute treatment as needed.*

BOX 35-1
New Delivery System for Growth Hormone

Saizen (somatropin) is a preparation of recombinant DNA–produced human growth hormone that is used to treat children with growth failure due to lack of growth hormone. The drug must be given by injection six or seven times a week. A new delivery form is now available to ease the discomfort and trauma of the frequent injections. The *cool.click* delivery system is a neon-colored, needle-free system that delivers the drug through the skin using a fine mist. Tests have shown a bioequivalency of this method with standard injection techniques, and the young patients who must use this drug are much less resistant to the dosing. Other drug companies are working on similar delivery systems which will provide therapeutic dose of drugs without the associated discomfort of intramuscular or subcutaneous injection.

DRUGS IN FOCUS
Anterior Pituitary Hormones

Drug Name	Dosage/Route	Usual Indications
chorionic gonadotropin (*Chorex, others*)	Dosage varies with indication; 4,000–10,000 IU IM once to three times per week is not unusual	Treatment of male hypogonadism, induction of ovulation, treatment of prepubertal cryptorchidism
Ⓟ corticotropin (*Acthar*)	Diagnosis: 10–25 U IV over 8 h Treatment: 20 IU IM or SC q.i.d.	Diagnosis of adrenal function, treatment of various inflammatory disorders
cosyntropin (*Cortrasyn*)	0.25–0.75 mg IV or IM	Diagnosis of adrenal function
menotropins (*Pergonal*)	75 IU FSH/75 IU LH per day IM for 9–12 d	Stimulation of ovulation and spermatogenesis
somatropin (*Nutropin, Saizen, Humatrope*)	Dosage varies with each product, check manufacturer's instructions; must be given SC or IM	Treatment of children with growth failure
somatrem (*Protropin*)	Up to 0.1 mg/kg IM or SC given three times per week	Treatment of children with growth failure
thyrotropin (*Thytropar*)	0.9 mg IM q24h for 2 doses	Diagnosis of thyroid function

• Provide thorough patient teaching, including measures to avoid adverse effects, warning signs of problems, and the need for regular evaluation (including blood tests), *to enhance patient knowledge about drug therapy and promote compliance*. Instruct a family member or caregiver in proper preparation and administration techniques, *to ensure proper administration of the drug*.

Evaluation

• Monitor patient response to the drug (return of GH levels to normal; growth and development).
• Monitor for adverse effects (hypothyroidism, glucose intolerance, nutritional imbalance).
• Evaluate the effectiveness of the teaching plan (patient can name drug, dosage, adverse effects to watch for, specific measures to avoid adverse effects; family member can demonstrate proper technique for preparation and administration of drug).
• Monitor the effectiveness of comfort measures and compliance to the regimen.

▢▮●▮ WEB LINKS
Patients and health care providers may want to consult the following Internet sources:

Information on GH therapy, pediatric challenges, and research—the Pediatric Endocrinology Nursing Society: http://www.pens.org

Information on disease research and development, latest drug therapy, and links to other resources—National Institutes of Health: http://www.nih.gov

GROWTH HORMONE ANTAGONISTS

GH hypersecretion can occur at any time of life. This is often referred to as hyperpituitarism. If it occurs before the epiphyseal plates of the long bones fuse, it causes an acceleration in linear skeletal growth, producing **gigantism** of 7 to 8 feet in height with fairly normal body proportions. In adults after epiphyseal closure, linear growth is impossible. Instead, hypersecretion of GH causes enlargement in the peripheral parts of the body, such as the hands and feet, and the internal organs, especially the heart. **Acromegaly** is the term used to describe the onset of excessive GH secretion that occurs after puberty and epiphyseal plate closure.

Most conditions of GH hypersecretion are caused by pituitary tumors and are treated by radiation therapy or surgery. Drug therapy for GH excess can be used for those patients who are not candidates for surgery or radiation therapy. The drugs used to treat GH excess include a somatostatin analog (octreotide acetate *[Sandostatin]*) and a dopamine agonist (bromocriptine *[Parlodel]*) (see Figure 35–1).

Therapeutic Actions and Indications
Somatostatin is an inhibitory factor released from the hypothalamus. It is not used to decrease GH levels, although

NURSING CHALLENGE
Growth Hormone Therapy

In the past, growth hormone therapy was very expensive and rather unsafe. The use of cadaver pituitaries resulted in unreliable hormone levels and, in many cases, hypersensitivity reactions to the proteins found in the drug. With the advent of genetic engineering and the development of safer, more reliable forms of growth hormone, there has been a surge in use of the drug to treat children with short stature. Even so, the drug is still costly and not without adverse effects.

Growth hormone can be used to treat growth failure caused either by lack of growth hormone or by renal failure. It also can help children with normal growth hormone levels who are just genetically small. Before the drug is prescribed, the child must undergo screening procedures and specific testing (including radiographs and blood tests) and must display a willingness to have regular injections. The child taking this drug will need to have pretherapy and periodic tests of thyroid function, blood sugar levels, glucose tolerance, and tests for growth hormone antibodies (a risk that increases with the length of time the drug is given). In addition, radiographs of the long bones will be taken to monitor for closure of the epiphyses, a sign that the drug must be stopped. Because the child who is taking growth hormone may experience sudden growth, he or she will need to be monitored for nutritional needs as well as psychological trauma that may occur with the sudden change in body image. Insulin therapy and replacement thyroid therapy may be needed, depending on the child's response to the drug.

The child's family or caregivers will need instructions on the following points:

• Storage of the drug (refrigeration is required)
• Preparation of the drug (the reconstitution procedure varies depending on the brand name product used)
• Administration of the drug (sterile technique, need to rotate injection sites, and need to monitor injection sites for atrophy or extravasation)

They also must be advised to report any lack of growth as well as signs of glucose intolerance (thirst, hunger, voiding pattern changes) or thyroid dysfunction (fatigue, thinning hair, slow pulse, puffy skin, intolerance to the cold).

The use of growth hormone involves an interrelationship among many subspecialists and expensive and regular medical evaluation and care. The key to the success of this therapy may be the attitude and cooperation of the young patient.

Bromocriptine, a semisynthetic ergot alkaloid, is a dopamine agonist frequently used to treat acromegaly. It may be used alone or as an adjunct to irradiation. Dopamine agonists inhibit GH secretion in some patients with acromegaly; the opposite effect occurs in normal individuals. Bromocriptine's GH-inhibiting effect may be explained by the fact that dopamine increases somatostatin release from the hypothalamus. Both of these drugs are indicated for the treatment of acromegaly in patients who are not candidates for or cannot tolerate other therapy.

Pharmacokinetics
Octreotide is rapidly absorbed and widely distributed throughout the body. It is metabolized in the tissues, and about 30% is excreted unchanged in the urine. Patients with renal dysfunction may accumulate higher levels of the drug. There are no adequate studies of effects in pregnancy and during lactation, and use should be reserved for situations in which the benefits to the mother clearly outweigh any potential risks to the fetus or neonate.

Bromocriptine is effectively absorbed from the gastrointestinal (GI) tract and undergoes extensive first-pass metabolism in the liver. It is primarily excreted in the bile. The drug should not be used during pregnancy or lactation because of effects on the fetus and because it blocks lactation.

Contraindications and Cautions
These drugs are contraindicated in the presence of any known allergy to the drug. They should be used cautiously in the presence of any other endocrine disorder (eg, diabetes, thyroid dysfunction) and in pregnancy or lactation.

Adverse Effects
Octreotide is associated with many GI complaints because of its effects on the GI tract. Constipation or diarrhea, flatulence, and nausea are not uncommon. Octreotide has also been associated with the development of acute cholecystitis, cholestatic jaundice, biliary tract obstruction, and pancreatitis. Patients must be assessed for the possible development of any of these problems. Other, less common adverse effects include headache, sinus bradycardia or other cardiac arrhythmias, and decreased glucose tolerance. Octreotide must be administered subcutaneously, and it can be associated with discomfort and/or inflammation at injection sites.

Bromocriptine is given orally and is also associated with GI disturbances. Because of its dopamine-blocking effects, it may cause drowsiness and postural hypotension. It blocks lactation and should not be used by nursing mothers.

Clinically Important Drug–Drug Interactions
Increased serum bromocriptine levels and increased toxicity occur if this drug is combined with erythromycin. This combination should be avoided.

There also may be a decreased effectiveness of bromocriptine if it is combined with phenothiazines. If this combination is used, the patient should be monitored carefully.

it does do that very effectively. Because it has multiple effects on many secretory systems (for example, it inhibits release of gastrin, glucagon, and insulin) and a short duration of action, it is not desirable as a therapeutic agent. An analog of somatostatin, octreotide acetate, is considerably more potent in inhibiting GH release with less of an inhibitory effect on insulin release. Consequently, it is used instead of somatostatin.

*Nursing Considerations for Patients Receiving
Growth Hormone Antagonists*

Assessment: History and Examination

Screen for the following conditions, which could be cautions or contraindication to use of the drug: history of allergy to any GH antagonist or binder; other endocrine disturbances; and pregnancy and lactation, which are contraindications to the use of the drug.

Include screening for baseline status before beginning therapy and for any potential adverse effects: orientation, affect, reflexes; blood pressure, pulse, orthostatic blood pressure; abdominal examination; glucose tolerance tests, GH levels.

Nursing Diagnoses

The patient receiving any GH antagonist may have the following nursing diagnoses related to drug therapy:

- Imbalanced Nutrition: More than Body Requirements, related to metabolic changes
- Acute Pain related to need for injections (octreotide)
- Deficient Knowledge regarding drug therapy

Implementation

- Reconstitute octreotide following manufacturer's directions; administer the drug subcutaneously and rotate injection sites regularly, *to prevent skin breakdown and to ensure proper delivery of the drug.*
- Monitor thyroid function, glucose tolerance, and GH levels periodically, *to detect problems and to institute treatment as needed.*
- Arrange for baseline and periodic ultrasound evaluation of the gallbladder if using octreotide, *to detect any gallstone development and to arrange for appropriate treatment.*
- Provide thorough patient teaching, including measures to avoid adverse effects, warning signs of problems, and need for regular evaluation (including blood tests), *to enhance*

patient knowledge about drug therapy and promote compliance. Instruct a family member in proper preparation and administration techniques to ensure that there is another responsible person to administer the drug if needed.

Evaluation

- Monitor patient response to the drug (return of GH levels to normal, growth and development).
- Monitor for adverse effects (hypothyroidism, glucose intolerance, nutritional imbalance, GI disturbances, cholecystitis).
- Evaluate the effectiveness of the teaching plan (patient can name drug, dosage, adverse effects to watch for, specific measures to avoid adverse effects; family member can demonstrate proper technique for preparation and administration of drug).
- Monitor the effectiveness of comfort measures and compliance with the regimen.

POSTERIOR PITUITARY HORMONES

The posterior pituitary stores two hormones produced in the hypothalamus: antidiuretic hormone (ADH, also known as vasopressin) and oxytocin. Oxytocin stimulates milk ejection or "let down" in lactating women. In pharmacological doses, it can be used to initiate or improve uterine contractions in labor. This drug is discussed in Chapter 40.

ADH possesses antidiuretic, hemostatic, and vasopressor properties. Posterior pituitary disorders can occur secondary to metastatic cancer, lymphoma, disseminated intravascular coagulation (discussed in Chapter 48), or septicemia. Posterior pituitary disorders that are seen clinically involve ADH release and include **diabetes insipidus,** which results from insufficient secretion, and syndrome of inappropriate antidiuretic hormone (SIADH), which occurs with excessive secretion of ADH. Diabetes insipidus can be treated pharmacologically.

Diabetes insipidus is characterized by the production of a

DRUGS IN FOCUS
Growth Hormone Antagonists

Drug Name	Dosage/Route	Usual Indications
Ⓟ bromocriptine (*Parlodel*)	1.25–2.5 mg/d PO; 20–30 mg per day may be needed	Treatment of acromegaly in patients who are not candidates for or cannot tolerate other therapy; not recommended for children <15 y
octreotide (*Sandostatin*)	100–600 mcg SC t.i.d.; adjust dose in elderly patients	Treatment of acromegaly in adults who are not candidates for or cannot tolerate other therapy

large amount of dilute urine containing no glucose. Blood glucose levels are higher than normal, and the body responds with polyuria (lots of urine), polydipsia (lots of thirst), and dehydration. With this rare metabolic disorder, patients produce large quantities of dilute urine and are constantly thirsty. Diabetes insipidus is caused by a deficiency in the amount of posterior pituitary ADH and may result from pituitary disease or injury (eg, head trauma, surgery, tumor). The condition can be acute and short in duration, or it can be a chronic, lifelong problem.

ADH itself is never used as therapy for diabetes insipidus. Instead, synthetic preparations of ADH, which are purer and have fewer adverse effects, are used. The ADH preparations that are available include vasopressin (*Pitressin Synthetic*), which is available in parenteral and nasal spray forms, and desmopressin (*DDAVP*) (see Figure 35–1). The drug of choice depends on the individual response to the drug and the patient's ability or willingness to use a particular dosage form.

Therapeutic Actions and Indications

ADH is released in response to increases in plasma osmolarity or decreases in blood volume. It produces its antidiuretic activity in the kidney, causing the cortical and medullary parts of the collecting duct to become permeable to water, thereby increasing water reabsorption and decreasing urine formation. These activities reduce plasma osmolarity and increase blood volume.

The ADH preparations that are available are indicated for the treatment of neurogenic diabetes insipidus. Desmopressin is also indicated for the treatment of hemophilia A and von Willebrand's disease, and it is used as a nasal spray for the treatment of nocturnal enuresis (bed wetting). Because of vasopressin's actions to increase GI motility, it is also indicated for the prevention and treatment of postoperative abdominal distention and to dispel gas formation before abdominal tests.

C A S E   S T U D Y

Teaching Plan for Diabetes Insipidus

THE SITUATION
B. T. is a 56-year-old teacher who developed diabetes insipidus. Her condition was eventually regulated on vasopressin nasal spray, one or two sprays per nostril four times a day. B. T. seemed highly interested in her disease and therapy and learned to control her own dosage by symptom control. For several years, B. T. maintained good control of her symptoms. At her last clinical visit, it was noted that she had developed postnasal ulcerations and nasal rhinitis. She also complained of several gastrointestinal symptoms including upset stomach, abdominal cramps, and diarrhea.

CRITICAL THINKING
• *Think about the pathophysiology of diabetes insipidus.* What are the effects of vasopressin on the body, and what adverse effects might occur if the drug were being absorbed inappropriately?
• *Because B. T. has used the drug for so many years, she may have forgotten some of the teaching points about her disease and drug administration. Outline a care plan for B. T. that includes necessary teaching points and takes into consideration her long experience with her disease and her drug therapy. Think about specific warning signs that should be highlighted for B. T. and ways to involve her in the teaching program that might make it more pertinent to her and her needs.*

DISCUSSION
An essential aspect of the ongoing nursing process is continual evaluation of the effectiveness of the drug therapy. An evaluation of this situation shows that B. T.'s postnasal mucosa was ulcerated, possibly as a result of overexposure to the vasoconstrictive properties of the

drug. B. T.'s gastrointestinal tract also seemed to show evidence of increased antidiuretic hormone effects. These factors seem to indicate that perhaps the drug was being administered incorrectly, resulting in excessive exposure of the nasal mucosa to the drug, increased absorption, and increased levels of the drug reaching the systemic circulation.

The nurse should ask B. T. to administer a dose of the drug to herself, then discuss the signs and symptoms of problems that B. T. should watch for. In this case, B. T. remembered most of the details of her drug teaching. But when administering the drug, she tiled her head back, tipped the bottle upside down, and then squirted the drug into each nostril. When the nurse questioned B. T. about her technique, she explained that she had seen an advertisement on TV about nasal sprays and realized that she had been doing it wrong all these years. The nurse explained the difference in the types of nasal sprays and reviewed the entire teaching plan with B. T. The drug was discontinued and B. T. was placed on subcutaneous antidiuretic hormone until the nasal ulcerations healed.

As a patient becomes more familiar with drug therapy, the details about the drug may be forgotten. It is important to remember that patient teaching needs regular updating and evaluation. This point is often forgotten when dealing with patients who have been taking a drug for years. However, remembering to assess the patient's knowledge about the drug can prevent problems such as B. T.'s from developing. Because B. T. is a teacher, she might be interested in developing a teaching protocol that will meet her needs and serve as an appropriate reminder about the disease and drug therapy. If B. T. is actively involved in preparing such a plan, it will be more effective and might be remembered much longer.

Pharmacokinetics

These drugs are rapidly absorbed and metabolized; they are excreted in the liver and kidneys. They should not be used during pregnancy because of the risk of uterine contractions that would harm the fetus. The effects of these drugs during lactation are not clear, so caution should be used with nursing mothers.

Contraindications and Cautions

ADH preparations are contraindicated with any known allergy to the drug or its components or with severe renal dysfunction. Caution should be used with any known vascular disease (because of its effects on vascular smooth muscle); epilepsy; asthma; and pregnancy or lactation.

Adverse Effects

The adverse effects associated with the use of ADH preparations include water intoxication (drowsiness, lightheadedness, headache, coma, convulsions), related to the shift to water retention; tremor, sweating, vertigo, and headache, related to water retention (a "hangover" effect); abdominal cramps, flatulence, nausea, and vomiting, related to stimulation of GI motility; and local nasal irritation, related to nasal administration. Hypersensitivity reactions have also been reported, ranging from rash to bronchial constriction.

Nursing Considerations for Patients Receiving Posterior Pituitary Hormones

Assessment: History and Examination

Screen for the following conditions, which could be cautions or contraindications to use of the drug: history of allergy to any ADH preparation or components; vascular diseases; epilepsy; renal dysfunction; pregnancy; and lactation.

Include screening for baseline status before beginning therapy and for any potential adverse effects: skin, lesions; orientation, affect, reflexes; blood pressure, pulse; respiration, adventitious sounds; abdominal examination; renal function tests; and serum electrolytes.

Nursing Diagnoses

The patient receiving any posterior pituitary hormone may have the following nursing diagnoses related to drug therapy:

- Impaired Urinary Elimination
- Excess Fluid Volume related to water retention
- Deficient Knowledge regarding drug therapy

Implementation

- Monitor patient fluid volume, *to watch for signs of water intoxication and fluid excess;* arrange to decrease dosage as needed.
- Monitor patients with vascular disease for any sign of exacerbation, *to provide for immediate treatment.*
- Monitor condition of nasal passages if given intranasally, *to observe for nasal ulceration, which can occur and could affect absorption of the drug.*
- Provide thorough patient teaching, including measures to avoid adverse effects, warning signs of problems, and the need for regular evaluation, including blood tests, *to enhance patient knowledge about drug therapy and promote compliance.* (See Patient Teaching Checklist: Antidiuretic Hormone.)

Evaluation

- Monitor patient response to the drug (maintenance of fluid balance).

DRUGS IN FOCUS
Posterior Pituitary Hormones

Drug Name	Dosage/Route	Usual Indications
desmopressin (DDAVP)	Adult: 0.1–0.4 mL/d PO, IV, SC, intranasal for diabetes insipidus; 0.3 μg/kg IV over 15–30 min for von Willebrand's disease; 20 μg intranasal h.s. for nocturnal enuresis Pediatric: 0.05–0.3 mL/d intransal for diabetes insipidus; 0.3 μg/kg IV over 15–30 min for von Willebrand's disease; 20 μg intranasal h.s. for nocturnal enuresis	Diabetes insipidus, von Willebrand's disease, hemophilia A, treatment of nocturnal enuresis
Ⓟ vasopressin (Pitressin Synthetic)	5–10 IU IM or SC b.i.d.–t.i.d. or administer on cotton pledgets by nasal spray or dropper	Diabetes insipidus, prevention of postoperative abdominal distention, to dispel gas for abdominal examination

PATIENT TEACHING CHECKLIST
Antidiuretic Hormone

Create customized patient teaching materials for a specific antidiuretic hormone from the CD-ROM. Patient teaching should stress the following points for drugs within this class:

• Antidiuretic hormone, or ADH, works in the kidneys to limit the loss of water in the urine.
• If the drug is to be injected, you and a significant other will need to learn how to prepare and inject the drug and how to rotate injection sites
• If the drug is to be used intranasally, it should be administered with the head held upright and the bottle also held upright.

When taking the drug, you might experience the following adverse effects:

• *Nasal irritation and congestion*—Your nasal passages may adjust to the drug over time. If the irritation becomes severe, check with your health care provider.
• *Heartburn and gastrointestinal upset*—These symptoms often occur when the nasal preparation drips down the pharynx and may be eliminated with careful administration.
• *Abdominal cramps*—These symptoms occur because the drug acts to increase gastrointestinal activity and will have to be tolerated. If the cramping becomes severe, talk to your health care provider.

Report any of the following to your health care provider: drowsiness, listlessness, headache; chest pain, shortness of breath; severe abdominal cramps; prolonged nasal congestion; return of the signs of diabetes insipidus, (eg, large volumes of urine, excessive thirst).
Tell any doctor, nurse or other health care provider that you are taking this drug.
Keep this drug, and all medications, out of the reach of children.

This Teaching Checklist reflects general patient teaching guidelines. It is not meant to be a substitute for drug-specific teaching information, which is available in nursing drug guides.

• Monitor for adverse effects (GI problems, water intoxication, headache, skin rash).
• Evaluate the effectiveness of the teaching plan (patient can name drug, dosage, adverse effects to watch for, specific measures to avoid adverse effects; patient can demonstrate proper administration of nasal preparations).
• Monitor the effectiveness of comfort measures and compliance with the regimen (see Nursing Care Guide: Antidiuretic Hormone).

CHAPTER SUMMARY

• Hypothalamic releasing factors stimulate the anterior pituitary to release hormones.

• The hypothalamic releasing factors are used mostly for diagnostic testing and for treating some forms of cancer.
• Anterior pituitary hormones stimulate endocrine glands or cell metabolisms.
• Growth hormone (GH) deficiency can cause dwarfism in children and somatropin deficiency syndrome in adults.
• GH replacement is done with drugs produced by recombinant DNA processes; these agents are more reliable and cause fewer problems than drugs used in the past.
• GH excess causes gigantism in patients whose epiphyseal plates have not closed and acromegaly in patients with closed epiphyseal plates.
• GH antagonists include octreotide and bromocriptine. Blockage of other endocrine activity may occur when these drugs are used.
• Posterior pituitary hormones are produced in the hypothalamus and stored in the posterior pituitary. They include oxytocin and antidiuretic hormone (ADH).
• Lack of antidiuretic hormone produces diabetes insipidus, which is characterized by large amounts of dilute urine and excessive thirst.
• ADH replacement uses analogs of ADH and can be administered parenterally or intranasally.
• Fluid balance needs to be monitored when patients are taking ADH replacement drugs, because water intoxication and dilution of essential electrolytes can occur.

Review Questions

1. Hypothalamic hormones are normally present in very small amounts. When used therapeutically, their main indication is
   a. diagnosis of endocrine disorders and treatment of specific cancers.
   b. treatment of multiple endocrine disorders.
   c. treatment of CNS-related abnormalities.
   d. treatment of autoimmune-related problems.
2. Somatropin (*Nutropin* and others) is a genetically engineered growth hormone that is used
   a. to diagnose hypothalamic failure.
   b. to treat precocious puberty.
   c. in the treatment of children with growth failure.
   d. to stimulate pituitary response.
3. Growth hormone deficiencies
   a. occur only in children.
   b. always result in dwarfism.
   c. are treated only in children because GH is usually produced only until puberty.
   d. can occur in adults as well as children.
4. A father brought his 15-year-old son to the endocrine clinic because the boy was only 5 feet tall. He wanted his son to receive growth hormone therapy because short stature would be a real detriment to his success as an adult. The boy would not be a candidate for this therapy if
   a. he was adverse to the use of cadaver parts.
   b. his epiphyses were closed.

NURSING CARE GUIDE

Antidiuretic Hormone (ADH)

Assessment	Nursing Diagnosis	Implementation	Evaluation
HISTORY Allergies to any ADH preparation, pregnancy, lactation, vascular disease, chronic renal disease	Impaired Urinary Elimination related to antidiuretic effect Excess Fluid Volume related to antidiuretic effect Deficient Knowledge regarding drug therapy	Prepare and safely administer drug as ordered. Monitor and limit fluid intake as needed. Provide patient teaching regarding drug name, dosage, adverse effects, precautions, proper administration, warning signs to report.	Evaluate drug effects: regulation of fluid volume. Monitor for adverse effects: water intoxication, nasal congestion, GI problems. Monitor for drug–drug interactions as indicated for each drug. Evaluate effectiveness of patient teaching program. Evaluate effectiveness of comfort and safety measures.
PHYSICAL EXAMINATION Neurological: orientation Skin: color, lesions CV: P, cardiac auscultation, BP Respiratory: R, adventitious sounds GI: bowel sounds Renal: output, urinalysis Lab tests: serum electrolytes			

c. his GH levels were very low.

d. he was also diabetic.

5. Patients who are receiving growth hormone replacement therapy must be monitored very closely. Routine follow-up examinations would include
a. bowel program to deal with constipation.
b. tests of thyroid function and glucose tolerance.
c. calorie check to control weight gain.
d. tests of adrenal hormone levels.

6. Acromegaly and gigantism are both conditions related to excessive secretion of
a. thyroid hormone.
b. melanin-stimulating hormone.
c. growth hormone.
d. oxytocin

7. Octreotide (Sandostatin) would not be the drug of choice in the treatment of acromegaly in a patient with known
a. diabetes.
b. gall bladder disease.
c. adrenal insufficiency.
d. hypothalamic lesions.

8. Diabetes insipidus is a relatively rare disease characterized by
a. excessive secretion of ADH.
b. renal damage.
c. the production of large amounts of dilute urine containing no glucose.
d. insufficient pancreatic activity.

9. Treatment with ADH preparations is associated with adverse effects including
a. constipation and paralytic ileus.
b. cholecystitis and bile obstruction.
c. nocturia and bed wetting.
d. "hangover" symptoms including headache, sweating, and tremors.

10. A patient who is receiving an ADH preparation for diabetes insipidus may need instruction in administering the drug
a. orally or intramuscularly.
b. orally or intranasally.
c. rectally or orally.
d. intranasally or by dermal patch.

BIBLIOGRAPHY

Andrews, M. & Boyle, J. (1999). *Transcultural concepts in nursing care*. Philadelphia: Lippincott Williams & Wilkins.

Bullock, B. L. (2000). *Focus on pathophysiology*. Philadelphia: Lippincott Williams & Wilkins.

Drug facts and comparisons. (2002). St. Louis: Facts and Comparisons.

Girard, J. (1991). *Endocrinology of puberty*. Farmington, CT: Karger Publishers.

Guyton, A. & Hall, J. (2000). *Textbook of medical physiology*. Philadelphia: W. B. Saunders.

Gilman, A., Hardman, J. G., & Limbird, L. E. (Eds.) (2002). *Goodman and Gilman's the pharmacological basis of therapeutics* (10th ed.). New York: McGraw-Hill.

Karch, A. M. (2002). *2003 Lippincott's nursing drug guide*. Philadelphia: Lippincott Williams & Wilkins.

The medical letter on drugs and therapeutics. (2002). New Rochelle, NY: Medical Letter.

North, W. G., Moses, A. M., & Share, L. (eds.) (1993). The neurohypophysis: A window on brain function. *Annals of the New York Academy of Sciences*, 689.

Porth, C. (2002). *Pathophysiology: Concepts of altered health states* (6th ed.). Philadelphia: Lippincott Williams & Wilkins.

36

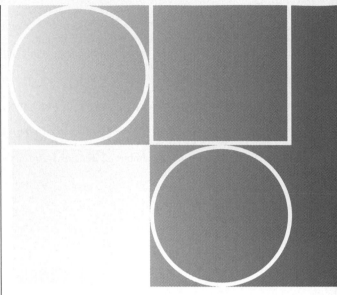

Key Terms

adrenal cortex
adrenal medulla
corticosteroids
diurnal rhythm
glucocorticoids
mineralocorticoids

Adrenocortical Agents

464

Glucocorticoids	Mineralocorticoids
beclomethasone	cortisone
betamethasone	fludrocortisone
budesonide	hydrocortisone
cortisone	
dexamethasone	
flunisolide	
hydrocortisone	
methylprednisolone	
℗ prednisolone	
prednisone	
triamcinolone	

Adrenocortical agents are widely used to suppress the immune system and actually help people to feel better. These drugs do not, however, cure any inflammatory disorders. Once widely used to treat a number of chronic problems, adrenocortical agents are now reserved for short-term use to relieve inflammation during acute stages of illness.

THE ADRENAL GLANDS

The two adrenal glands are flattened bodies that sit on top of each kidney. Each gland is made up of an inner core or **adrenal medulla** and an outer shell called the **adrenal cortex.**

The adrenal medulla is actually part of the sympathetic nervous system (SNS). It is a ganglion of neurons that releases the neurotransmitters norepinephrine and epinephrine into circulation when the SNS is stimulated. The secretion of these neurotransmitters directly into the bloodstream allows them to act as hormones, traveling from the adrenal medulla to react with specific receptor sites throughout the body. This is thought to be a backup system for the sympathetic system, adding an extra stimulus to the "fight or flight" response.

The adrenal cortex surrounds the medulla and consists of three layers of cells, each of which synthesizes chemically different types of steroid hormones that exert physiological effects throughout the body. The adrenal cortex produces hormones called **corticosteroids.** There are three types of corticosteroids: androgens, glucocorticoids, and mineralocorticoids.

Androgens (male and female sex hormones) actually have little effect compared with the sex hormones produced by the testes and ovaries. They are able to maintain a certain level of cellular stimulation and can contribute to cell-sensitive growth in some forms of cancers, particularly prostate, breast, and ovarian cancers. These drugs are addressed in Part VII: Drugs Acting on the Reproductive System.

Glucocorticoids are so named because they stimulate the increase of glucose levels for energy. They also increase the rate of protein breakdown and decrease the rate of protein formation from amino acids, another way of preserving energy. Glucocorticoids also cause lipogenesis, or the formation and storage of fat in the body. This stored fat will then be available to be broken down for energy when needed.

Mineralocorticoids affect electrolyte levels and homeostasis. These steroid hormones, such as aldosterone, directly affect the levels of electrolytes in the system. Potassium is lost and sodium and water are retained in response to aldosterone. Hydrocortisone and cortisone also have the same effects when present in high levels.

Figure 36–1 displays the sites of action of the glucocorticoids and the mineralocorticoids.

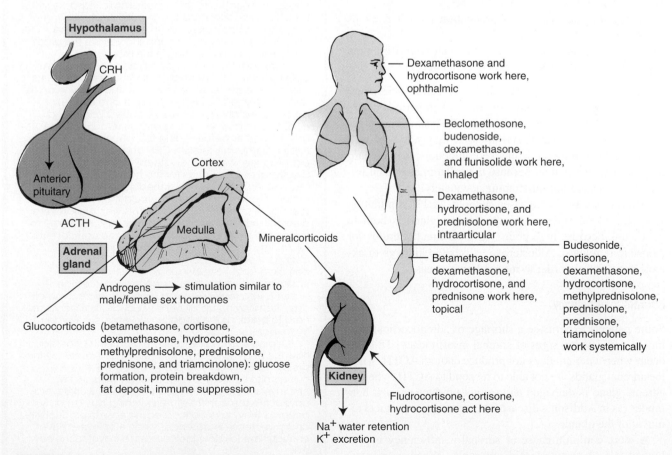

FIGURE 36–1. Sites of action of the adrenocortical agents.

Controls

The adrenal cortex responds to adrenocorticotropic hormone (ACTH) released from the anterior pituitary. ACTH, in turn, responds to corticotropin-releasing hormone (CRH) released from the hypothalamus. This happens during a normal day in what is called **diurnal rhythm.** A person who has a regular cycle of sleep and wakefulness will produce high levels of CRH during sleep, usually around midnight. A resulting peak response of increased ACTH and adrenocortical hormones occurs sometime early in the morning, around 6 to 9 AM. This high level of hormones then suppresses any further CRH or ACTH release. The corticosteroids are metabolized and excreted slowly throughout the day and fall to low levels by evening. At this point, the hypothalamus and pituitary sense low levels of the hormones and begin the production and release of CRH and ACTH again. This peaks around midnight, and the cycle starts again.

Activation of the stress reaction through the SNS bypasses the usual diurnal rhythm and cause release of ACTH and secretion of the adrenocortical hormones—an important aspect of the stress ("fight or flight") response. The stress response is activated with cellular injury or when a person perceives fear or feels anxious. These hormones have many actions, including the following:

- Increasing the blood volume (aldosterone effect)
- Causing the release of glucose for energy
- Slowing the rate of protein production (which reserves energy)
- Blocking the activities of the inflammatory and immune systems (which reserves a great deal of energy)

These actions are important during an acute stress situation, but they can cause adverse reactions in periods of extreme or prolonged stress. For instance, a postoperative patient who is very fearful and stressed may not heal well because protein building is blocked; infections may be hard to treat in such a patient because the inflammatory and immune systems are not functioning adequately.

Aldosterone is also released without ACTH stimulation when the blood surrounding the adrenal gland is high in potassium, because high potassium is a direct stimulus for aldosterone release. Aldosterone causes the kidneys to excrete potassium in order to restore homeostasis.

Adrenal Insufficiency

Some patients experience a shortage of adrenocortical hormones and develop signs of adrenal insufficiency. This can occur when a patient does not produce enough ACTH, when the adrenal glands are not able to respond to ACTH, when an adrenal gland is damaged and cannot produce enough hormones (as in Addison's disease), or secondary to surgical removal of the glands.

A more common cause of adrenal insufficiency is prolonged use of corticosteroid hormones. When exogenous corticosteroids are used, they act to negate the regular feedback systems (Figure 36–2). The adrenal glands begin to atrophy because ACTH release is suppressed by the exogenous hormones, so the glands are no longer stimulated to produce or secrete hormones. It takes several weeks to recover from the atrophy caused by this lack of stimulation. To prevent this from happening, patients should receive only short-term steroid therapy and should be weaned slowly from the hormones so that the adrenals have time to recover and start producing hormones again.

NURSING CHALLENGE
Diurnal Rhythm

The adrenocortical hormones are released in a pattern called the diurnal rhythm. The secretion of corticotropin-releasing hormone (CRH), adrenocorticotropin (ACTH), and cortisol are high in the morning in day-oriented people (those who have a regular cycle of wakefulness during the day and sleep during the night). In such individuals, the peak levels of cortisol usually come between 6 and 8 AM. The levels then fall off slowly (with periodic spurts) and reach a low in the late evening, with lowest levels around midnight. It is thought that this cycle is related to the effects of sleeping on the hypothalamus, and that the hypothalamus regulating its stimulation of the anterior pituitary in relation to sleep and activity. The cycle may also be connected to the hypothalamic response to light. This is important to keep in mind when treating patients with corticosteroids. In order to mimic the normal diurnal pattern, patients should take the drugs immediately on awakening in the morning.

Complications to this pattern arise, however, when patients work shifts or change their sleeping patterns (eg, college students). In response, the hypothalamus shifts its release of CRH to correspond to the new cycle. For instance, if a person works all night and goes to bed at 8 AM, arising at 3 PM to carry on the day's activities before going to work at 11 PM, the hypothalamus will release CRH at about 3 PM in accordance with the new sleep–wake cycle. It usually takes 2 or 3 days for the hypothalamus to readjust. A patient on this schedule who is taking replacement corticosteroids would then need to take them at 3 PM, or on arising. Patients who work several different shifts in a single week may not have time to reregulate their hypothalamus, and the corticosteroid cycle may be thrown off. Patients who have to change their sleep patterns repeatedly often complain about feeling weak, getting sick more easily, or having trouble concentrating. College students frequently develop a pattern of sleeping all day, then staying up all night—a cycle that becomes hard to break as their bodies and endocrine systems try to readjust.

It is a nursing challenge to help patients understand how the body works and to offer ways to decrease the stress of changing sleep patterns—especially if the nurse is also working several different shifts. Many employers are willing to have employees work several days of the same shift before switching back, mainly because they have noticed an increase in productivity and a decrease in absences when employees have enough time to allow their bodies to adjust to the new shift.

FIGURE 36–2. *A.* Normal controls of adrenal gland. The hypothalamus releases corticotropin-releasing hormone (CRH), which causes release of corticotropin (ACTH) from the anterior pituitary. ACTH stimulates the adrenal cortex to produce and release corticosteroids. Increasing levels of corticosteroids inhibit the release of CRH and ACTH. *B.* Exogenous corticosteroids act to inhibit CRH and ACTH release; the adrenal cortex is no longer stimulated and atrophies. Sudden stopping of steroids results in a crisis of adrenal hypofunction until hypothalamic–pituitary axis (HPA) controls stimulate the adrenal gland again.

Adrenal Crisis

Patients who have an adrenal insufficiency may do quite well until they experience a period of extreme stress, such as a motor vehicle accident, a surgical procedure, or a massive infection. Because they are not able to supplement the energy-consuming effects of the sympathetic reaction, they enter an adrenal crisis, which can include physiological exhaustion, hypotension, fluid shift, shock, and even death. Patients in adrenal crisis are treated with massive infusion of replacement steroids, constant monitoring, and life support procedures.

GLUCOCORTICOIDS

Several glucocorticoids are available for pharmacological use. They differ mainly by route of administration and duration of action.

Beclomethasone (*Beclovent*) is available as a respiratory inhalant and nasal spray to block inflammation locally in the respiratory tract.

Betamethasone (*Celestone* and others) is a long-acting steroid. It is available for systemic, parenteral use in acute

DRUG THERAPY ACROSS THE LIFESPAN

Corticosteroids

Children	Adults	Older Adults
Corticosteroids are used in children for the same indications as in adults. The dosage for children is determined by the severity of the condition being treated and the response to the drug, not on a weight or age formula. Children need to be monitored closely for any effects on growth and development, and dosage adjustments should be made or drug discontinued if growth is severely retarded. Topical use of corticosteroids should be limited in children; because their body surface area is comparatively large, the amount of the drug absorbed in relation to weight is greater than in an adult. Apply sparingly and do not use in the presence of open lesions. Do not occlude treated areas with dressings or diapers, which may increase the risk of systemic absorption. Children need to be supervised when using nasal sprays or respiratory inhalants to ensure that proper technique is being used. Children receiving long-term therapy should be protected from exposure to infection, and special precautions should be instituted to avoid injury. If injuries or infections do occur, the child should be seen by a primary care provider as soon as possible.	Adults should be reminded of the importance of taking these drugs in the morning, to approximate diurnal rhythm. They should also be cautioned about the importance of tapering the drug, rather than stopping abruptly. Several over-the-counter topical preparations contain corticosteroids, and adults should be cautioned to avoid combining these preparations with prescription topical corticosteroids. They also should be cautioned to apply any of these sparingly and to avoid applying them to open lesions or excoriated areas. With long-term therapy, the importance of avoiding exposure to infection—crowded areas, people with colds or the flu, activities associated with injury—should be stressed. If an injury or infection should occur, the patient should be encouraged to seek medical care. These drugs should not be used during pregnancy because they cross the placenta and could cause adverse effects on the fetus. If the benefit to the mother clearly outweighs the potential risk to the fetus, they should be used with caution. Nursing mothers should find another method of feeding the baby if corticosteroids are needed, because of the potential for serious adverse effects on the baby.	Older adults are more likely to experience the adverse effects associated with these drugs, and the dosage should be reduced and the patient monitored very closely. Older adults are more likely to have hepatic and/or renal impairment which could lead to accumulation of drug and resultant toxic effects. They are also more likely to have medical conditions that could be imbalanced by changes in fluid and electrolytes, metabolism changes, and other drug effects. Such conditions include diabetes, congestive heart failure, osteoporosis, coronary artery disease, and immune suppression. Careful monitoring of drug dosage and response to the drug should be done on a regular basis.

situations. It also is available orally for short-term relief of inflammation and as a topical application for local inflammatory conditions.

Budesonide (*Rhinocort, Entocort EC*) is a relatively new steroid for intranasal use. It relieves the signs and symptoms of allergic or seasonal rhinitis with few side effects. It was approved in 2001 as an oral agent for the treatment of mild-to-moderate active Crohn's disease.

Cortisone (*Cortone Acetate*) was one of the first corticosteroids made available. It is used orally and parenterally for replacement therapy in adrenal insufficiency as well as acute inflammatory situations.

Dexamethasone (*Decadron* and others) is widely used and available in multiple forms for dermatological, ophthalmological, intra-articular, parenteral, and inhalational uses. It peaks quickly, and effects can last for 2 to 3 days.

Flunisolide (*Aero-Bid, Nasalide*) is another drug that has proved to be very successful as a respiratory inhalant or intranasal drug.

Hydrocortisone (*Cortef* and others) is a powerful corticosteroid that has both glucocorticoid and mineralocorticoid activity. For that reason, it is used as replacement therapy in patients with adrenal insufficiency. It has largely been replaced for other uses (eg, intra-articular, intravenous) by other steroid hormones with less mineralocorticoid effect. It may be preferred for use as a topical or ophthalmic agent.

Methylprednisolone (*Medrol*) has little mineralocorticoid activity at therapeutic doses. Because it has significant anti-inflammatory and immunosuppressive effects, it is a drug of choice for inflammatory and immune disorders and is available in multiple forms, including oral, parenteral, intra-articular, and retention enema preparations.

Prednisolone (*Delta-Cortef* and others) is an intermediate-acting corticosteroid with effects lasting only a day or so. It is used for intralesional and intra-articular injection, and is also available in oral and topical forms.

Prednisone (*Deltasone* and others) is available only as an oral agent and can be used as replacement therapy in cases of adrenal insufficiency. It is also used for short-term and acute therapy to decrease inflammation.

Triamcinolone (*Aristocort, Kenaject,* and others) is available in many forms for use in acute inflammatory conditions. It has been used to treat adrenal insufficiency when combined with a mineralocorticoid.

Therapeutic Actions and Indications

Glucocorticoids enter target cells and bind to cytoplasmic receptors, initiating many complex reactions that are responsible for anti-inflammatory and immunosuppressive effects. Hydrocortisone, cortisone, and prednisone also have some mineralocorticoid activity and affect potassium, sodium, and water levels in the body (Table 36–1).

Glucocorticoids are indicated for the short-term treatment of many inflammatory disorders, to relieve discomfort and to give the body a chance to heal from the effects of inflammation. They block the actions of arachidonic acid, which leads to a decrease in the formation of prostaglandins and leukotrienes. Without these chemicals, the normal inflammatory reaction is blocked. They also impair the ability of phagocytes to leave the bloodstream and move to injured tissues, and they inhibit the ability of lymphocytes to act within the immune system, including a blocking of the production of antibodies. They can be used to treat local inflammation as topical agents, intranasal or inhaled agents, intra-articular injections, and ophthalmic agents. Systemic use is indicated for the treatment of some cancers, hypercalcemia associated with cancer, hematological disorders, and some neurological infections. When combined with mineralocorticoids, some of these drugs can be used in replacement therapy for adrenal insufficiency.

Pharmacokinetics

These drugs are absorbed well from many sites. They are metabolized by natural systems, mostly within the liver, and are excreted in the urine. The glucocorticoids are known to cross the placenta and to enter breast milk; they should be used during pregnancy and lactation only if the benefits to the mother clearly outweigh the potential risks to the fetus or neonate.

TABLE 36-1 | Selected Corticosteroids: Equivalent Strength, Glucocorticoid and Mineralocorticoid Effects, and Duration of Effects by Drug

Drug	Equivalent Dose (mg)	Glucocorticoid Effects	Mineralocorticoid Effects	Duration of Effects
SHORT-ACTING CORTICOSTEROIDS				
cortisone	25	+	++++	8–12 h
hydrocortisone	20	+	++++	8–12 h
INTERMEDIATE-ACTING CORTICOSTEROIDS				
prednisone	5	++++	++	18–36 h
prednisolone	5	++++	++	18–36 h
triamcinolone	4	+++++	—	18–36 h
methylprednisolone	4	+++++	—	18–36 h
LONG-ACTING CORTICOSTEROIDS				
dexamethasone	0.75	+++++++++	—	36–54 h
betamethasone	0.75	+++++++++	—	35–54 h

CULTURAL CONSIDERATIONS
Steroid Toxicity in the African Americans

African Americans develop increased toxicity to the corticosteroid methylprednisolone—particularly when it is used for immunosuppression after renal transplantation. This toxicity can include severe steroid-induced diabetes mellitus. African Americans are almost four times as likely as whites to develop end-stage renal disease, so this complication is not an unusual problem. If an African American patient is being treated with methylprednisolone, extreme care should be taken to adjust dosages appropriately and to treat adverse effects as they arise.

Contraindications and Cautions

These drugs are contraindicated in the presence of any known allergy to any steroid preparation; in the presence of an acute infection, which could become serious or even fatal if the immune and inflammatory responses are blocked; and with lactation, because the anti-inflammatory and immuno-suppressive actions could be passed to the baby.

Caution should be used in patients with diabetes (the glucose-elevating effects disrupt glucose control), acute peptic ulcers (steroid use is associated with the development of ulcers); other endocrine disorders (which could be sent into imbalance), or pregnancy.

Adverse Effects

The adverse effects associated with the glucocorticoids are related to the route of administration that is used. Systemic use is associated with endocrine disorders; fluid retention and potential congestive heart failure (CHF); increased appetite and weight gain; fragile skin and loss of hair; weakness and muscle atrophy as protein breakdown occurs and protein is not built; and increased susceptibility to infections and the development of cancers (with long-term use). Children are at risk for growth retardation associated with suppression of the hypothalamic–pituitary system. Local use is associated with local inflammations and infections, as well as burning and stinging sensations (Box 36–1).

Clinically Important Drug–Drug Interactions

There are increased therapeutic effects and toxic effects if corticosteroids are given with erythromycin, ketoconazole, or troleandomycin.

There is a risk of decreased serum levels and decreased effectiveness if corticosteroids are combined with salicylates, barbiturates, phenytoin, or rifampin.

Nursing Considerations for Patients Receiving Glucocorticoids

Assessment: History and Examination

Screen for the following conditions, which could be cautions or contraindications to use of the drug: history of allergy to any steroid preparations; acute infections; peptic ulcer dis-

BOX 36-1
Adverse Effects of Corticosteroid Use Associated With Varying Routes of Administration

Systemic: Systemic effects are most likely to occur when the corticosteroid is given by the oral, intravenous, intramuscular, or subcutaneous route. Systemic absorption is possible, however, if other routes of administration are not used correctly or if tissue breakdown or injury allows direct absorption.

Central nervous system: vertigo, headache, parethesias, insomnia, convulsions, psychosis

Gastrointestinal: peptic or esophageal ulcers, pancreatitis, abdominal distention, nausea, vomiting, increased appetite, weight gain

Cardiovascular: hypotension, shock, congestive heart failure secondary to fluid retention, thromboembolism, thrombophlebitis, fat embolism, arrhythmias secondary to electrolyte disturbances

Hematological: sodium and fluid retention, hypokalemia, hypocalcemia, increased blood sugar, increased serum cholesterol, decreased thyroid hormone levels

Musculoskeletal: muscle weakness, steroid myopathy, loss of muscle mass, osteoporosis, spontaneous fractures

Eyes, ears, nose, and throat: cataracts, glaucoma

Dermatological: frail skin, petechiae, ecchymoses, purpura, striae, subcutaneous fat atrophy

Endocrine: Amenorrhea, irregular menses, growth retardation, decreased carbohydrate tolerance, diabetes

Other: immunosuppression, aggravation or masking of infections, impaired wound healing, suppression of hypothalamic–pituitary axis

Intramuscular repository injections: atrophy at the injection site

Retention enema: local pain, burning; rectal bleeding

Intra-articular injection: osteonecrosis, tendon rupture, infection

Intraspinal: meningitis, adhesive arachnoiditis, conus medullaris syndrome

Intrathecal administration: arachnoiditis

Topical: local burning, irritation, acneform lesions, striae, skin atrophy

Respiratory inhalant: oral, laryngeal, and pharyngeal irritation; fungal infections

Intranasal: headache, nausea, nasal irritation, fungal infections, epistaxis, rebound congestion, perforation of the nasal septum, anosmia, urticaria

Ophthalmic: infections, glaucoma, cataracts

Intralesional: blindness when used on the face and head (rare)

ease; pregnancy; lactation; endocrine disturbances; and renal dysfunction.

Include screening for baseline status before beginning therapy and for any potential adverse effects: weight; temperature; orientation, affect, grip strength, eye examination;

DRUGS IN FOCUS
Glucocorticoids

Drug Name	Dosage/Route	Usual Indications
beclomethasone (*Beclovent*)	Nasal spray, respiratory inhalant Adult: two inhalations (84–168 µg) t.i.d.–q.i.d. for respiratory inhalant; one inhalation (42–84 µg) in each nostril b.i.d.–q.i.d. for nasal spray Pediatric (6–12 y): one or two inhalations t.i.d.–q.i.d. for respiratory inhalant Pediatric (>12 y): one inhalation in each nostril b.i.d.–q.i.d. for nasal spray	Blocking inflammation in the respiratory tract
betamethasone (*Celestone*)	Oral, IM, IV intra-articular, topical Adult: 0.6–7.2 mg/d PO, up to 9 mg/d IV; 0.5–9.0 mg/d IM; apply topical preparation sparingly Pediatric: individualize dose based on severity and response, and monitor closely	Management of allergic intra-articular, topical, and inflammatory disorders
budesonide (*Rhinocort, Entocort EC*)	Intranasal—Adult and children >6 y: 256 µg/d given as two sprays in each nostril AM and PM Oral—Adult: 9 mg/d for up to 8 wk	Relief of symptoms of seasonal and allergic rhinitis (intranasal); treatment of mild to moderate active Crohn's disease (oral)
cortisone (*Cortisone Acetate*)	Oral, IM Adult: 25–300 mg/d PO; 20–330 mg IM Pediatric: base dosage on response, monitor patient closely	Replacement therapy in adrenal insufficiency; treatment of allergic and inflammatory disorders
dexamethasone (*Decadron*)	Oral, IV, IM, inhalation, intranasal, ophthalmic, topical Adult and pediatric: individualize dosage based on response and severity—0.75–9 mg/d PO; 8–16 mg/d IM; 0.5–9 mg/d IV; two to three inhalations per day for inhalation; one to two sprays in each nostril b.i.d. for nasal spray; 1 gtt t.i.d.–q.i.d. for ophthalmic solutions; apply topical preparation sparingly	Management of allergic and topical inflammatory disorders, adrenal hypofunction
flunisolide (*Nasalide, Aero–Bid*)	Inhalant, intranasal Adult: 200 µg intranasal Pediatric: 300–400 µg b.i.d. via diskhaler	Control of bronchial asthma; relief of symptoms of seasonal and allergic rhinitis
hydrocortisone (*Cortef*)	Oral, IV, IM, topical, ophthalmic, rectal, intra-articular Adult: 100–500 mg IM or IV q2–6h; 100 mg h.s. by retention enema for 21 d; one applicatorful q.d.–b.i.d. intrarectal; apply topical sparingly; 5–20 mg/d PO based on response Pediatric: 20–240 mg/d PO, IM or SC; 100 mg h.s. by retention enema for 21 d; one applicatorful q.d.–b.i.d. intrarectal; apply topical sparingly; 5–20 mg/d PO based on response	Replacement therapy, treatment of allergic and inflammatory disorders
methylprednisolone (*Medrol*)	Oral, IV, IM, intra-articular Adult: 40–120 mg/d PO or IM; 40 mg IV slowly Pediatric: base dosage on severity and response	Treatment of allergic and inflammatory disorders
ⓟ prednisolone (*Delta-Cortef*)	Oral, IV, IM, ophthalmic, intra-articular Adult: 5–60 mg/d PO; 4–60 mg IM or IV; 1–2 gtt in affected eye t.i.d.–q.i.d. Pediatric: base dosage on severity and response	Treatment of allergic and inflammatory disorders
prednisone (*Deltasone*)	Oral Adult: 0.1–0.15 mg/kg per day PO Pediatric: base dosage on severity and response	Replacement therapy for adrenal insufficiency; treatment of allergic and inflammatory disorders
triamcinolone (*Aristocort*)	Oral, IM, inhalant, intra-articular, topical Adult: 4–60 mg/d PO; 2.5–60 mg/d IM; two inhalations t.i.d.–q.i.d. Pediatric: individualize dosage based on severity and response; 6–12 y, one to two inhalations t.i.d.–q.i.d.	Treatment of allergic and inflammatory disorders, management of asthma

blood pressure, pulse, peripheral perfusion, vessel evaluation; respiration, adventitious breath sounds; glucose tolerance, renal function, serum electrolytes, and endocrine function tests as appropriate.

Nursing Diagnoses

The patient receiving any glucocorticoid may have the following nursing diagnoses related to drug therapy:

• Decreased Cardiac Output related to fluid retention
• Excess Fluid Volume related to water retention
• Disturbed Sensory Perception (Visual, Kinesthetic)
• Risk for Infection related to immunosuppression
• Ineffective Coping related to body changes caused by the drug
• Deficient Knowledge regarding drug therapy

Implementation

• Administer drug daily at 8 to 9 AM, *to mimic normal peak diurnal concentration levels and thereby minimize suppression of the hypothalamic–pituitary axis.*
• Space multiple doses evenly throughout the day, *to try to achieve homeostasis.*
• Use minimal dose for minimal amount of time, *to minimize adverse effects.*
• Taper doses when discontinuing from high doses or from long-term therapy, *to give the adrenal glands a chance to recover and produce adrenocorticoids.*
• Arrange for increased dosage when the patient is under stress, *to supply increased demand for corticosteroids associated with the stress reaction.*
• Use alternate-day maintenance therapy with short-acting drugs whenever possible, *to decrease the risk of adrenal suppression.*
• Do not give live virus vaccines when the patient is immunosuppressed, *because there is an increased risk of infection.*
• Protect the patient from unnecessary exposure to infection and invasive procedures, *because the steroids suppress the immune system and the patient is at increased risk for infection.*
• Assess the patient carefully for any potential drug–drug interactions, *to avoid adverse effects.*
• Provide thorough patient teaching, including measures to avoid adverse effects; warning signs of problems; and the need for regular evaluation, including blood tests, *to enhance patient knowledge of drug therapy and promote compliance.* Explain the need to protect the patient from exposure to infections. (See Patient Teaching Checklist: Corticosteroids.)

Evaluation

• Monitor patient response to the drug (relief of signs and symptoms of inflammation, return of adrenal function to within normal limits).

PATIENT TEACHING CHECKLIST
Corticosteroids

Create customized patient teaching materials for a specific corticosteroid from the CD-ROM. Patient teaching should stress the following points for drugs within this class:

• Corticosteroids are similar to steroids produced naturally in your body, and they affect a number of bodily functions.
• You should never stop taking your drug suddenly. If your prescription is low or you are unable to take the medication for any reason, notify your health care provider.

Some of the following adverse effects may occur:

• *Increased appetite*—This may be a welcome change, but if you notice a continual weight gain, you may want to watch your calories.
• *Restlessness, trouble sleeping*—Some people experience elation and a feeling of new energy; frequent rest periods should be taken.
• *Increased susceptibility to infection*—Because your body's normal defenses will be decreased, you should avoid crowded places and people with known infections. If you notice any signs of illness or infection, notify your health care provider at once.

If you are taking this drug for a prolonged period, limit your intake of salt and salted products and add proteins to your diet.

Avoid the use of any over-the-counter medication without first checking with your health care provider. Several of these medications can interfere with the effectiveness of this drug.

Tell any doctor, nurse, or other health care provider that you are taking this drug.

Because this drug affects your body's natural defenses, you will need special care during any stressful situations. You may want to wear or carry a Medic-Alert tag showing that you are taking this medication. This tag alerts any medical personnel taking care of you in an emergency to the fact that you are taking this drug.

Report any of the following to your health care provider: sudden weight gain; fever or sore throat; black, tarry stools; swelling of the hands or feet; any signs of infection; easy bruising.

It is important to have regular medical follow-up. If you are being tapered from this drug, notify your health care provider if any of the following occur: fatigue; nausea, vomiting; diarrhea; weight loss; weakness; dizziness.

Keep this drug out of the reach of children. Do not give this medication to anyone else or take any similar medication that has not been prescribed for you.

This Teaching Checklist reflects general patient teaching guidelines. It is not meant to be a substitute for drug-specific teaching information, which is available in nursing drug guides.

• Monitor for adverse effects (increased susceptibility to infections, skin changes, endocrine dysfunctions, fatigue, fluid retention, peptic ulcer, psychological changes).
• Evaluate the effectiveness of the teaching plan (patient can

name drug, dosage, adverse effects to watch for, specific measures to avoid adverse effects).

- Monitor the effectiveness of comfort measures and compliance with the regimen (see Nursing Care Guide: Corticosteroids).

MINERALOCORTICOIDS

The classic mineralocorticoid is aldosterone. Aldosterone holds sodium—and with it, water—in the body and causes the excretion of potassium. Aldosterone is no longer available for pharmacological use. When used in high doses, the glucocorticoids cortisone and hydrocortisone have a mineralocorticoid effect. However, this effect usually is not enough to maintain electrolyte balance in adrenal insufficiency. Fludrocortisone (*Florinef*) is a more powerful mineralocorticoid and is preferred for replacement therapy, in combination with a glucocorticoid.

Therapeutic Actions and Indications

The mineralocorticoids increase sodium reabsorption in renal tubules and increase potassium and hydrogen excretion, leading to water and sodium retention (see Figure 36–1). These drugs are indicated, in combination with a glucocorticoid, for replacement therapy in primary and secondary adrenal insufficiency. They are also indicated for the treatment of salt-wasting adrenogenital syndrome when taken with appropriate glucocorticoids. Fludrocortisone is being tried for

N U R S I N G   C A R E   G U I D E

Corticosteroids

Assessment	Nursing Diagnoses	Implementation	Evaluation
HISTORY Allergies to any steroids, CHF, pregnancy, lactation, hypertension, acute infection, peptic ulcer, vaccination with a live virus, endocrine disorders	Decreased Cardiac Output related to fluid retention Disturbed Sensory Perception related to CNS effects Risk for Infection related to immunosuppression Ineffective Coping related to body changes caused by drug Excess Fluid Volume related to water retention Deficient Knowledge regarding drug therapy	Administer around 9 A.M. to mimic normal diurnal rhythm. Use minimal dose for minimal period of time dosage is needed. Arrange for increased doses during times of stress. Taper gradually to allow adrenal glands to recover and produce own steroids. Protect patient from unnecessary exposure to infection. Provide support and reassurance to deal with drug therapy. Provide patient teaching regarding drug name, dosage, adverse effects, precautions, and warning signs to report.	Evaluate drug effects: relief of signs and symptoms of inflammation; adrenal replacement as appropriate. Monitor for adverse effects: infection, peptic ulcer, fluid retention, hypertension, electrolyte imbalance, endocrine changes. Monitor for drug–drug interactions as indicated for each drug. Evaluate effectiveness of patient teaching program. Evaluate effectiveness of comfort and safety measures.
PHYSICAL EXAMINATION Neurological: orientation, reflexes, affect General: T, weight CV: P, cardiac auscultation, BP, edema Respiratory: R, adventitious sounds Lab tests: urinalysis, blood glucose, stool guaiac test, renal function tests			

the treatment of severe orthostatic hypotension because its sodium and water retention effects can lead to increased blood pressure.

Pharmacokinetics

These drugs are absorbed slowly and distributed throughout the body. They undergo hepatic metabolism to inactive forms. They are known to cross the placenta and to enter breast milk. They should be avoided during pregnancy and lactation because of the potential for adverse effects in the fetus or baby.

Contraindications and Cautions

These drugs are contraindicated in the presence of any known allergy to the drug; with severe hypertension, CHF, or cardiac disease, because of the resultant increased blood pressure; and lactation. Caution should be used in pregnancy, in the presence of any infection, and with high sodium intake (severe hypernatremia could occur).

Adverse Effects

Adverse effects commonly associated with the use of mineralocorticoids are related to the increased fluid volume seen with sodium and water retention (eg, headache, edema, hypertension, CHF, arrhythmias, weakness, hypokalemia). Allergic reactions, ranging from skin rash to anaphylaxis, have also been reported.

Clinically Important Drug–Drug Interactions

Decreased effectiveness of salicylates, barbiturates, hydantoins, rifampin, and anticholinesterases has been reported when these drugs are combined with mineralocorticoids. Such combinations should be avoided if possible, but if they

are necessary, the patient should be monitored closely and the dosage increased as needed.

■●■ WEB LINKS

Patients and health care providers may want to consult the following Internet sources:

Information on where to go to learn about diseases, drugs, other therapies:
http://www.healthfinder.gov

Information on disease research and development, latest drug therapy, and links to other resources—National Institutes of Health:
http://www.nih.gov

Information on where to go to find support groups, information on specific diseases, and treatments:
http://www.medicinenet.com

Information on rheumatoid and inflammatory diseases:
http://www.arthritis.org
http://www.arthritis.about.com

Nursing Considerations for Patients Receiving Mineralocorticoids

Assessment: History and Examination

Screen for the following conditions, which could be cautions or contraindications to use of the drug: allergy to these drugs; history of CHF, hypertension, infections; high sodium intake; lactation, and pregnancy.

Include screening for baseline status before beginning therapy and for any potential adverse effects: blood pressure, pulse, adventitious breath sounds; weight, temperature; tissue turgor; reflexes and bilateral grip strength; and serum electrolyte levels.

DRUGS IN FOCUS
Mineralocorticoids

Drug Name	Dosage/Route	Unusual Indications
cortisone (*Cortisone Acetate*)	Oral, IM Adult: 25–300 mg/d PO or 20–330 mg/d IM Pediatric: base dosage on severity and response	Replacement therapy in adrenal insufficiency, treatment of allergic and inflammatory disorders
Ⓟ fludrocortisone (*Florinef*)	Adult: 0.1–0.2 mg/d PO	Replacement therapy and treatment of salt-losing adrenogenital syndrome with a glucocorticoid; not recommended for children
hydrocortisone (*Cortef*)	Oral, IV, IM, topical, ophthalmic, rectal, intra-articular Adult: 20–240 mg/d PO; 100–500 mg IM or IV q2–6h; 100 mg h.s. by retention enema; one applicatorful rectal foam q.i.d.–b.i.d.; apply topical preparation sparingly Pediatric: base dosage on response and severity; 20–240 mg/d PO; 20–240 mg/d IM or SC; 100 mg h.s. by retention enema; one applicatorful rectal foam q.i.d.–b.i.d.; apply topical preparation sparingly	Replacement therapy, treatment of allergic and inflammatory disorders

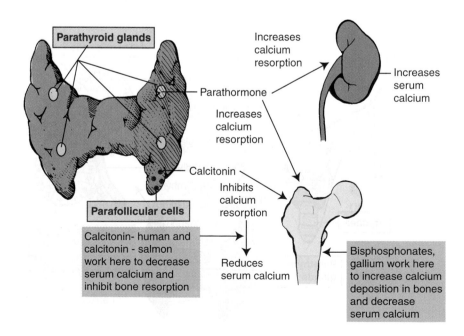

FIGURE 37-2. In response to low blood serum levels of thyroid hormone, the hypothalamus sends the thyrotropin-releasing hormone (TRH) to the anterior pituitary, which responds by releasing the thyroid-stimulating hormone (TSH) to the thyroid gland; it, in turn, responds by releasing the thyroid hormone (T$_3$ and T$_4$) into the bloodstream. The anterior pituitary is also sensitive to the increase in blood serum levels of the thyroid hormone and responds by decreasing production and release of TSH. As thyroid hormone production and release subside, the hypothalamus senses the lower serum levels and the process is repeated by the release of TRH again. This intricate series of negative feedback mechanisms keep the level of thyroid hormone within normal limits.

of carbohydrates, fats, and proteins. Thyroid hormone is also an important regulator of growth and development, especially within the reproductive and nervous systems. Because the thyroid has such widespread effects throughout the body, any dysfunction of the thyroid gland will have numerous systemic effects.

Cells found around the follicle of the thyroid gland, called parafollicular cells, produce another hormone, called **calcitonin.** This hormone affects calcium levels and acts to balance the effects of the parathyroid hormone parathormone. The release of calcitonin is not controlled by the hypothalamic–pituitary axis but is regulated locally at the cellular level. The cells release calcitonin when the concentration of calcium around them rises. The calcitonin released into the

bloodstream works to reduce calcium levels by blocking bone resorption and enhancing bone formation, pulling calcium out of the serum for deposit into bone (Figure 37–3). When the calcium level surrounding the cells falls, they will no longer produce calcitonin.

THYROID DYSFUNCTION

Thyroid dysfunction involves either underactivity, called **hypothyroidism,** or overactivity, called **hyperthyroidism.**

Hypothyroidism

Hypothyroidism is a lack of sufficient levels of thyroid hormones to maintain a normal metabolism. This condition occurs in a number of pathophysiological states:

- Absence of the thyroid gland
- Lack of sufficient iodine in the diet to produce the needed level of thyroid hormone
- Lack of sufficient functioning thyroid tissue due to tumor or autoimmune disorders
- Lack of TSH due to pituitary disease
- Lack of TRH related to a tumor or disorder of the hypothalamus

Hypothyroidism is the most common type of thyroid dysfunction. It is estimated that approximately 5% to 10% of women older than 50 years of age are hypothyroid. Hypothyroidism is also a common finding in the elderly. The symptoms of hypothyroidism can be varied and vague and are frequently overlooked. The signs and symptoms of hypothyroidism are often mistaken for signs of normal aging. Goiter, or enlargement of the thyroid gland, occurs when the thyroid is overactive. This effect frequently occurs when the

FIGURE 37-3. Calcium control. Parathormone and calcitonin work to maintain calcium homostasis in the body.

thyroid is overstimulated by TSH, which can happen if the thyroid gland does make sufficient thyroid hormones to turn off the hypothalamus and anterior pituitary. In the body's attempt to produce the needed amount of thyroid hormone, the thyroid is continually stimulated by increasing levels of TSH.

Children who are born without a thyroid gland or who have a nonfunctioning gland develop a condition called **cretinism.** If untreated, these children will have poor growth and development and mental retardation because of the lack of thyroid hormone stimulation. Severe adult hypothyroidism is called **myxedema.** Myxedema usually develops gradually as the thyroid slowly stops functioning. It can develop as a result of autoimmune thyroid disease (Hashimoto's disease), viral infection, or overtreatment with antithyroid drugs or because of surgical removal or irradiation of the thyroid gland. Patients with myxedema exhibit many signs and symptoms of decreased metabolism, including lethargy, hypoactive reflexes, hypotension, bradycardia, pale and coarse skin, loss of hair, intolerance to the cold, decreased appetite, decreased body temperature, thickening of the tongue and vocal chords, decreased sexual function, and even sterility. Patients with hypothyroidism are treated with replacement thyroid hormone therapy.

Hyperthyroidism

Hyperthyroidism occurs when excessive amounts of thyroid hormones are produced and released into the circulation. Graves' disease, a poorly understood condition that is thought to be an autoimmune problem, is the most common cause of hyperthyroidism. Patients with hyperthyroidism may exhibit many signs and symptoms of overactive cellular metabolism, including increased body temperature, tachycardia, palpitations, hypertension, flushing, thin skin, an intolerance to heat, amenorrhea, weight loss, and goiter.

Treatment of hyperthyroidism may involve surgical removal of the gland or portions of the gland; treatment with radiation to destroy parts or all of the gland; or drug treatment to block the production of **thyroxine** in the thyroid gland or to destroy parts or all of the gland. These patients then must be regulated with replacement thyroid hormone therapy.

Table 37–1 outlines the signs and symptoms of thyroid dysfunction.

THYROID HORMONE

Several replacement hormone products are available for treating hypothyroidism. These products contain both natural and synthetic thyroid hormone. Replacement hormones act to replace low or absent levels of the thyroid hormones and to suppress overproduction of TSH by the pituitary (see Figure 37–1).

Levothyroxine (*Synthroid, Levoxyl, Levo-T, Levothroid*), a synthetic salt of T_4, is the most frequently used replacement hormone because of its predictable bioavailability and reliability.

Thyroid desiccated (*Armour Thyroid* and others) is prepared from dried animal thyroid glands and contains both T_3 and T_4. Although the ratio of the hormones is unpredictable and the required dosage and effects vary widely, this drug is inexpensive, making it attractive to some.

Liothyronine (*Cytomel*) is a synthetic salt of T_3. Because it contains only T_3, liothyronine has a rapid onset and a long duration of action. It also has a greater incidence of cardiac side effects and is not recommended for use in patients with potential cardiac problems.

Liotrix (*Thyrolar*) is a synthetic preparation of T_4 and T_3 in a standard 4:1 ratio. Because it is associated with several

TABLE 37-1 | Signs and Symptoms of Thyroid Dysfunction

System	Hypothyroidism	Hyperthyroidism
Central nervous system	Depressed—hypoactive reflexes, lethargy, sleepiness, slow speech, emotional dullness	Stimulated—hyperactive reflexes, anxiety, nervousness, insomnia, tremors, restlessness
Cardiovascular	Depressed—bradycardia, hypotension, anemia, oliguria, decreased sensitivity to catecholamine	Stimulated—tachycardia, palpitations, increased pulse pressure, systolic hypertension, increased sensitivity to catecholamines
Skin, hair, nails	Pale, coarse, dry, thickened; puffy eyes and eyelids; hair coarse and thin; nails thick and hard	Flushed, warm, thin, moist, sweating; hair fine and soft; nails soft and thin
Metabolic rate	Decreased—lower body temperature; intolerance to cold; decreased appetite, higher levels of fat and cholesterol, weight gain, and hypercholesterolemia	Increased—low-grade fever; intolerance to heat; increased appetite with weight loss; muscle wasting and weakness, thyroid myopathy
Generalized myxedema	Accumulation of mucopolysaccharides in the heart, tongue, vocal chords; periorbital edema, cardiomyopathy, hoarseness, and thickened speech	Localized with accumulation of mucopolysaccharides in eyeballs, ocular muscles; periobital edema, lid lag, exophthalmos; pretibial edema
Ovaries	Decreased function—menorrhagia, habitual abortion, sterility	Altered; tendency toward oligomenorrhea, amenorrhea
Goiter	Rare; simple nontoxic type may occur	Diffuse, highly vascular; very frequent

DRUG THERAPY ACROSS THE LIFESPAN

Thyroid and Parathyroid Agents

Children

Thyroid replacement therapy is required when a child is hypothyroid. Levothyroxine is the drug of choice in children. Dosage is determined based on serum thyroid hormone levels and the response of the child, including growth and development. Dosage in children tends to be higher than in adults because of the higher metabolic rate of the growing child. Usually, the starting dose to consider is 10 to 15 μg/kg per day.

Regular monitoring, including growth records, is necessary to determine the accurate dosage as the child grows. Maintenance levels at the adult dosage usually occurs after puberty and when active growing stops.

If an antithyroid agent is needed, propylthiouracil (*PTU*) is the drug of choice because it is less toxic. Radioactive agents are not used in children, unless other agents are ineffective, because of the effects of radiation on chromosomes and developing cells.

Hypercalcemia is relatively rare in children, although may be seen with certain malignancies. If a child develops a malignancy-related hypercalcemia, the bisphosphonates may be used, with dosage adjustments based on age and weight. Serum calcium levels should be monitored very closely in the child and dosage adjustments made as necessary.

Adults

Adults who require thyroid replacement therapy need to understand that this will be a lifelong replacement need. An established routine of taking the tablet first thing in the morning may help the patient comply with the drug regimen. Levothyroxine is the drug of choice for replacement, but in some cases other agents may be needed. Periodic monitoring of thyroid hormone levels is necessary to ensure that dosage needs have not changed.

If antithyroid drugs are needed, the patient's underlying problems should be considered. Methimazole is associated with bone marrow suppression and more gastrointestinal and central nervous system effects than *PTU* is. Radioactive iodine should not be used in adults in their reproductive years unless they are aware of the possibility of adverse effects on fertility.

Alendronate and risendronate are commonly used drugs for osteoporosis and calcium lowering. Serum calcium levels need to be monitored carefully with any of the drugs that affect calcium levels. Patients should be encouraged to take calcium and vitamin D in their diet or as supplements in cases of hypocalcemia, and also for prevention and treatment of osteoporosis.

Thyroid replacement therapy is necessary during pregnancy for women who have been maintained on this regimen. It is not uncommon for hypothyroidism to develop during pregnancy. Levothyroxine is again the drug of choice.

If an antithyroid drug is essential during pregnancy, *PTU* is the drug of choice because it is less likely to cross the placenta and cause problems for the fetus. Radioactive agents should not be used. Bisphosphonates should be used during pregnancy only if the benefit to the mother clearly outweighs the potential risk to the fetus. Nursing mothers who need thyroid replacement therapy should continue with their prescribed regimen and report any adverse reactions in the baby. Bisphosphonates and antithyroid drugs should not be used during lactation because of the potential for adverse reactions in the baby—another method of feeding the baby should be used.

Older Adults

Because the signs and symptoms of thyroid disease mimic many other problems that are common to older adults—hair loss, slurred speech, fluid retention, congestive heart failure, and so on—it is important to screen older adults for thyroid disease carefully before beginning any therapy. The dosage should be started at a very low level and increased based on the patient response. Levothyroxine is the drug of choice for hypothyroidism. Periodic monitoring of thyroid hormone levels as well as cardiac and other responses is essential with this age group.

If antithyroid agents are needed, radioactive iodine may be the drug of choice because it has fewer adverse effects than the other agents and surgery. The patient should be monitored closely for the development of hypothyroidism, which usually occurs within a year after initiation of antithyroid therapy.

Older adults may have dietary deficiencies related to calcium and vitamin D. They should be encouraged to eat dairy products and foods high in calcium and to supplement their diet if necessary. Postmenopausal women, who are prone to develop osteoporosis, may want to consider hormone replacement therapy and calcium supplements to prevent osteoporosis. Many postmenopausal women, and some older men, respond well to the effect of bisphosphonates in moving calcium back into the bone. They need specific instructions on the proper way to take these drugs and may not be able to comply with the restrictions about staying upright and swallowing the tablet with a full glass of water.

Older adults have a greater incidence of renal impairment and kidney function should be evaluated before starting any of these drugs. Bisphosphonates should be used in lower doses in patients with moderate renal impairment and are not recommended for those who have severe renal impairment. With any of these drugs, regular monitoring of calcium levels is important to ensure that therapeutic effects are achieved with a minimum of adverse effects.

cardiac and central nervous system (CNS) effects, it may not be the drug of choice for patients who have cardiac problems or are prone to anxiety reactions.

Therapeutic Actions and Indications

The thyroid replacement hormones increase the metabolic rate of body tissues, increasing oxygen consumption, respiration, heart rate, growth and maturation, and the metabolism of fats, carbohydrates, and proteins. They are indicated for replacement therapy in hypothyroid states, treatment of myxedema coma, suppression of TSH in the treatment and prevention of goiters, and management of thyroid cancer. In conjunction with antithyroid drugs, they also are indicated to treat thyroid toxicity, prevent goiter formation during thyroid overstimulation, and treat thyroid overstimulation during pregnancy.

Pharmacokinetics

These drugs are well absorbed from the GI tract and bound to serum proteins. Deiodination of the drugs occurs at several sites, including the liver, kidney, and other body tissues. Elimination is primarily in the bile. Thyroid hormone does not cross the placenta and seems to have no effect on the fetus. Thyroid replacement therapy should not be discontinued during pregnancy, and the need for thyroid replacement often becomes apparent during pregnancy. Thyroid hormone does enter breast milk in small amounts. Caution should be used during lactation.

Contraindications and Cautions

These drugs should not be used with any known allergy to the drugs or their binders, during acute thyrotoxicosis (unless used in conjunction with antithyroid drugs), or during acute myocardial infarction (unless complicated by hypothyroidism), because the thyroid hormones could exacerbate these conditions. Caution should be used during lactation, because the drug enters breast milk and could suppress the infant's own thyroid production, and with hypoadrenal conditions such as Addison's disease.

Adverse Effects

When the correct dosage of the replacement therapy is being used, there are few if any adverse effects associated with these drugs. Skin reactions and loss of hair are sometimes seen, especially during the first few months of treatment in children. Symptoms of hyperthyroidism may occur as the drug dose is regulated. Some of the less predictable effects are associated with cardiac stimulation (arrhythmias, hypertension) and CNS effects (anxiety, sleeplessness, headache).

Clinically Important Drug–Drug Interactions

Decreased absorption of the thyroid hormones occurs if they are taken concurrently with cholestyramine. If this combination is needed, the drugs should be taken 2 hours apart.

The effectiveness of oral anticoagulants is increased if they are combined with thyroid hormone. Because this may lead to increased bleeding, the dosage of the oral anticoagulant should be reduced and the bleeding time checked periodically.

NURSING CHALLENGE
Thyroid Hormones for Obesity

Treatment trends for obesity have changed over the years. Not long ago, one of the suggested treatments was the use of thyroid hormone. The thinking was that obese people had slower metabolisms and therefore would benefit from a boost in metabolism from extra thyroid hormone.

If an obese patient is truly hypothyroid, this might be a good idea. Unfortunately, many of the patients who received thyroid hormone for weight loss were not tested for thyroid activity and ended up with excessive thyroid hormone in their systems. This situation triggered a cascade of events. The exogenous thyroid hormone disrupted the hypothalamic–pituitary–thyroid control system, resulting in decreased production of thyrotropin-releasing hormone (TRH) and thyroid-stimulating hormone (TSH) as the hypothalamus and pituitary sensed the rising levels of thyroid hormone. Because the thyroid was no longer stimulated to produce and secrete thyroid hormone, thyroid levels would actually fall. Lacking stimulation by TSH, the thyroid gland would start to atrophy. If exogenous thyroid hormone were stopped, the atrophied thyroid would not be able to immediately respond to the TSH stimulation and produce thyroid hormone. Ultimately, these patients experienced an endocrine imbalance. What's more, they also did not lose weight—and in the long run may actually have gained weight as the body's compensatory mechanisms tried to deal with the imbalances.

Today, thyroid hormone is no longer considered a good choice for treating obesity. Other drugs have come and gone, and new drugs are released each year to attack other aspects of the problem. Many patients, especially middle-aged people who may recall that thyroid was once used for weight loss, ask for thyroid hormone as an answer to their weight problem. Patients have even been know to "borrow" thyroid replacement hormones from others for a quick weight loss solution.

Obese patients need reassurance, understanding, and education about the risks of borrowed thyroid hormone. Insistent patients should undergo thyroid function tests. If the results are normal, patients should receive teaching about the controls and actions of thyroid hormone in the body and an explanation of why taking these hormones can cause problems. Obesity is a chronic and frustrating problem that poses continual challenges for health care providers.

Decreased effectiveness of digitalis glycosides can occur when these drugs are combined. Consequently, digitalis levels should be monitored and increased dosage may be required.

Theophylline clearance is decreased in hypothyroid states. As the patient approaches normal thyroid function, theophylline dosage may need to be adjusted frequently.

Nursing Considerations for Patients Receiving Thyroid Hormones

Assessment: History and Examination

Screen for the following conditions, which could be contraindications or cautions to use of the drug: history of al-

DRUGS IN FOCUS
Thyroid Hormones

Drug Name	Dosage/Route	Usual Indications
Ⓟ levothyroxine (*Synthroid, Levoxyl, Levo-T,* others)	Adult: 0.05–0.2 mg/d PO Pediatric: 0.025–0.4 mg/d PO	Replacement therapy in hypothyroidism; suppression of thyroid-stimulating hormone (TSH) release; treatment of myxedema coma and thyrotoxicosis
liothyronine (*Cytomel*)	Adult: 25–75 µg/d PO Pediatric: 20–50 µg/d PO	Replacement therapy in hypothyroidism; suppression of TSH release; treatment of thyrotoxicosis; synthetic hormone used in patients allergic to dessicated thyroid **Special considerations:** not for use with cardiac or anxiety problems
liotrix (*Thyrolar*)	Adult: 60–120 mg/d PO Pediatric: 25–150 µg/d PO based on age and weight	Replacement therapy in hypothyroidism; suppression of TSH release; treatment of thyrotoxicosis **Special considerations:** not for use with cardiac dysfunction
thyroid desiccated (*Armour Thyroid*)	Adult: 60–120 mg/d PO Pediatric: 15–90 mg/d PO	Replacement therapy in hypothyroidism; suppression of TSH release; treatment of thyrotoxicosis

C A S E   S T U D Y

Hypothyroidism

THE SITUATION
H. R., a 38-year-old white woman, is seen in the clinic with complaints of "exhaustion, lethargy, and sleepiness." Her past history is sketchy, her speech seems slurred, and her attention span is limited. Mr. R., her husband, reports feeling frustrated with H. R., stating that she has become increasingly lethargic, disorganized, and uninvolved at home. He also notes that she has gained weight and lost interest in her appearance. Physical examination reveals the following remarkable findings: pulse, 52; blood pressure, 90/62; temperature 96.8°F (oral); skin, pale, dry, thick; periorbital edema; tongue thick and asymmetric; height, 5 ft 5 in; weight, 165 lb. The immediate impression is that of hypothyroidism. Laboratory tests confirm this, revealing elevated thyroid-stimulating hormone (TSH) and very low levels of triiodothyronine (T_3) and thyroxine (T_4). *Synthroid,* 0.2 mg qd PO, is prescribed.

CRITICAL THINKING
- What teaching plans should be developed for this patient?
- What interventions would be appropriate in helping Mr. and Mrs. R. accept her diagnosis and the pathophysiological basis for her complaints and the problems they are having?
- What body image changes will H. R. experience as her body adjusts to the thyroid therapy?
- How can H. R. be helped to adjust to these changes and re-establish her body image and self-concept?

DISCUSSION
Hypothyroidism develops slowly. With it comes fatigue, lethargy, and lack of emotional affect—conditions that result in the patient's losing interest in appearance, activities, and responsibilities. In this case, the patient's husband, not knowing that there was a physical reason for the problem, became increasingly frustrated and even angry. Mr. R. should be involved in the teaching program so that his feelings can be taken into consideration. Any teaching content should be written down for later reference. (When H. R. starts to return to normal, her attention span and interest should return; anything that was missed or forgotten can be referred to in the written teaching program.)

H. R. should be encouraged to bring a picture of herself from a year or so ago to help her to understand and appreciate the changes that have occurred. Many patients are totally unaware of changes in their appearance and activity level because the disease progresses so slowly and brings on lethargy and lack of emotional affect.

The teaching plan should include information about the function of the thyroid gland and the anticipated changes that will be occurring to H. R. over the next week and beyond. The importance of taking the medication daily should be emphasized. The need to return for follow-up to evaluate the effectiveness of the medication and the effects on her body should also be stressed. Both H. R. and her husband will need support and encouragement to deal with past frustrations and the return to normal. Lifelong therapy will probably be needed, so further teaching will be important once things have stabilized.

lergy to any thyroid hormone or binder; lactation; Addison's disease; acute myocardial infarction not complicated by hypothyroidism; and thyrotoxicosis.

Include screening for baseline status before beginning therapy and for any potential adverse effects: presence of any skin lesions; orientation and affect: baseline pulse and blood pressure, baseline electrocardiogram (ECG); respiration, adventitious sounds; and thyroid function tests.

Nursing Diagnoses

The patient receiving any thyroid hormone may have the following nursing diagnoses related to drug therapy:

• Decreased Cardiac Output related to cardiac effects
• Imbalanced Nutrition: Less than Body Requirements, related to changes in metabolism
• Ineffective Tissue Perfusion related to thyroid activity
• Deficient Knowledge regarding drug therapy

Implementation

Administer a single daily dose before breakfast each day, *to ensure consistent therapeutic levels.*

Monitor response carefully when beginning therapy, *to adjust dosage according to patient response.*

Monitor cardiac response, *to detect cardiac adverse effects.*

Assess the patient carefully, *to detect any potential drug–drug interactions if giving thyroid hormone in combination with other drugs.*

Arrange for periodic blood tests of thyroid function, *to monitor the effectiveness of the therapy.*

Provide thorough patient teaching, including measures to avoid adverse effects, warning signs of problems, and the need for regular evaluation if used for longer than recommended, *to enhance patient knowledge of drug therapy and promote compliance.* (See Patient Teaching Checklist: Thyroid Hormone.)

Evaluation

• Monitor patient response to the drug (return of metabolism to normal, prevention of goiter).
• Monitor for adverse effects (tachycardia, hypertension, anxiety, skin rash).
• Evaluate the effectiveness of the teaching plan (patient can name drug, dosage, adverse effects to watch for, specific measures to avoid adverse effects).
• Monitor the effectiveness of comfort measures and compliance to the regimen (see Nursing Care Guide: Thyroid Hormone).

ANTITHYROID AGENTS

Drugs used to block production of thyroid hormone and to treat hyperthyroidism include the **thioamides** and iodide so-

PATIENT TEACHING CHECKLIST
Thyroid Hormone

Create customized patient teaching materials for a specific thyroid hormone from the CD-ROM. Patient teaching should stress the following points for drugs within this class:

• This hormone is designed to replace the thyroid hormone that your body is not able to produce. The thyroid hormone is responsible for regulating your body's metabolism, or the speed with which your body's cells burn energy. Because of this action of the thyroid hormone, it affects many body systems. It is very important that you take this medication only as prescribed.
• Never stop taking this drug without consulting with your health care provider. The drug is used to replace a very important hormone and will probably have to be taken for life. Stopping the medication can lead to serious problems.

The drug usually causes no adverse effects. You may notice a slight skin rash or hair loss in the first few months of therapy. You should notice the signs and symptoms of your thyroid deficiency disappearing, and you will feel "back to normal."

Report any of the following to your health care provider: chest pain, difficulty breathing, sore throat, fever, chills, weight gain, sleeplessness, nervousness, unusual sweating or intolerance to heat.

Avoid the use of any over-the-counter medication without first checking with your health care provider. Several of these medications can interfere with the effectiveness of this drug.

Tell any doctor, nurse, or other health care provider that you are taking this drug. You may want to wear or carry a Medic-Alert tag showing that you are taking this medication. This would alert any medical personnel taking care of you in an emergency to the fact that you are taking this drug.

While you are taking this drug, it is important to have regular medical follow-up, including blood tests to check the activity of your thyroid gland, to evaluate your response to the drug and any possible underlying problems.

Keep this drug, and all medications, out of the reach of children. Do not give this medication to anyone else or take any similar medication that has not been prescribed for you.

This Teaching Checklist reflects general patient teaching guidelines. It is not meant to be a substitute for drug-specific teaching information, which is available in nursing drug guides.

lutions. Although not chemically related, both groups of drugs block the formation of thyroid hormones within the thyroid gland (see Figure 37–1).

The Thioamides

Propylthiouracil (*PTU*) is the most frequently used thioamide. The other available thioamide is methimazole (*Tapazole*). Hematological adverse effects are more common with methi-

NURSING CARE GUIDE

Thyroid Hormone

Assessment	Nursing Diagnoses	Implementation	Evaluation
HISTORY Allergies to any of these drugs, Addison's disease; acute myocardial infarction not complicated by hypothyroidism; lactation; thyrotoxicosis	Decreased Cardiac Output related to cardiac effects Imbalanced Nutrition: Less than Body Requirements, related to effects on metabolism Ineffective Tissue Perfusion related to thyroid effects. Deficient Knowledge regarding drug therapy	Administer once a day at breakfast. Provide comfort, safety measures (eg, temperature control, rest as needed, safety precautions). Provide support and reassurance to deal with drug effects and lifetime need. Provide patient teaching regarding drug name, dosage, adverse effects, precautions, and warning signs to report.	Evaluate drug effects: return of metabolism to normal; prevention of goiter. Monitor for adverse effects: anxiety, tachycardia, hypertension, skin reaction. Monitor for drug–drug interactions as indicated for each drug. Evaluate effectiveness of patient teaching program. Evaluate effectiveness of comfort and safety measures.
PHYSICAL EXAMINATION Neurological: orientation, affect Skin: color, lesions CV: P, cardiac auscultation, BP, ECG Respiratory: R, adventitious sounds Hematological: thyroid function tests			

mazole, so the patient needs to have a complete blood count and differential monitored regularly. Gastrointestinal (GI) effects are somewhat less pronounced with methimazole, so it may be the drug of choice in patients who are unable to tolerate *PTU*.

Therapeutic Actions and Indications

The thioamides prevent the formation of thyroid hormone within the thyroid cells, lowering the serum levels of thyroid hormone. They also partially inhibit the conversion of T_4 to T_3 at the cellular level. Thioamides are indicated for the treatment of hyperthyroidism.

Pharmacokinetics

These drugs are well absorbed from the GI tract and are then concentrated in the thyroid gland. Some excretion can be detected in the urine. Methimazole crosses the placenta and is found in a high ratio in breast milk. *PTU* has a low potential for crossing the placenta and for entering breast milk. If an antithyroid drug is needed during pregnancy, *PTU* is the drug of choice but caution should still be used. Another method of feeding the baby should be chosen if an antithy-

roid drug is needed during lactation because of the potential for adverse effects on the baby, including the development of neonatal goiter.

Contraindications and Cautions

Thioamides are contraindicated in the presence of any known allergy to antithyroid drugs and during pregnancy. (If an antithyroid drug is absolutely essential and the mother has been informed about the risk of cretinism in the infant, propylthiouracil is the drug of choice.) These drugs should be used cautiously during lactation because of the risk of antithyroid activity in the infant. (Again, if an antithyroid drug is needed, propylthiouracil is the drug of choice.)

Adverse Effects

The adverse effects most commonly seen with these drugs are the effects of thyroid suppression: drowsiness, lethargy, bradycardia, nausea, skin rash, and so on. Propylthiouracil is associated with nausea, vomiting, and GI complaints. Methimazole is also associated with bone marrow suppression, so the patient using this drug must have frequent blood tests to monitor for this effect.

CHAPTER 37 Thyroid and Parathyroid Agents 485

Iodine Solutions

Low doses of iodine are needed in the body for the formation of thyroid hormone. High doses, however, act to block thyroid function. Therefore, iodine preparations are sometimes used to treat hyperthyroidism. Radioactive iodine (I^{131}) is sometimes used as a diagnostic agent or to destroy thyroid tissue in cases of severe Graves' disease. It is usually reserved for use in patients who are older than 30 years of age because of the adverse effects associated with the radioactivity. Strong iodine solution, potassium iodide and sodium iodide (Thyro Block) are taken orally and have a rapid onset of action, with effects seen within 24 hours and peak effects seen in 10 to 15 days. The effects are short-lived and may even precipitate further thyroid enlargement and dysfunction. For this reason, and because of the availability of the more predictable thioamides, iodides are not used as often as they once were in the clinical setting.

Therapeutic Actions and Indications

These drugs cause the thyroid cells to become oversaturated with iodine and stop producing thyroid hormone. In some cases, the thyroid cells are actually destroyed. The iodine solutions are reserved for presurgical suppression of the thyroid gland, for treatment of acute thyrotoxicosis until thioamide levels can take effect, or for thyroid blocking during radiation therapy.

The iodine solutions are also used to block thyroid function in radiation emergencies. Radioactive iodine is taken up into the thyroid cells, which are then destroyed by the β-radiation given off by the radioactive iodine. Except during radiation emergencies. The use of radioactive iodine is reserved for those patients who are not candidates for surgery, women who cannot become pregnant, and elderly patients with such severe, complicating conditions that immediate thyroid destruction is needed.

Pharmacokinetics

These drugs are rapidly absorbed from the GI tract and widely distributed throughout the body fluids. Excretion occurs through the urine. Radioactive iodine can cause serious fetal harm and is rated Pregnancy Category X. It enters breast milk, and another method of feeding the baby should be used if radioactive iodine is needed. The iodide solutions cross the placenta and can cause hypothyroidism and goiter in the fetus or newborn. They should not be used during pregnancy unless the benefit to the mother clearly outweighs the potential risk to the fetus. They are known to enter breast milk, but the effects on the neonate are not known. Caution should be used.

Contraindications and Cautions

The use of iodine solutions is contraindicated in the presence of pregnancy, because of the effect on the thyroid glands of the mother and the fetus, and with pulmonary edema or pulmonary tuberculosis.

Adverse Effects

The most common adverse effect of these drugs is hypothyroidism; the patient will need to be started on replacement thyroid hormone to maintain homeostasis. Other adverse effects

---

DRUGS IN FOCUS
Antithyroid Agents

Drug Name	Dosage/Route	Usual Indications
Thioamides		
methimazole (Tapazole)	Adult: 15 mg/d PO initially, up to 30–60 mg/d may be needed; maintainence, 5–15 mg/d PO Pediatric: 0.4 mg/kg per day PO initially; maintenance, 15–20 mg/m² per day PO in three divided doses	Treatment of hyperthyroidism
℗ propylthiouracil (PTU)	Adult: 300–900 mg/d PO initially; maintenance, 100–150 mg/d PO Pediatric: 50–300 mg/d PO based on age and response	Treatment of hyperthyroidism
Iodines		
sodium iodide I¹³¹ (generic)	Adult (>30 y): 4–10 millicuries PO as needed	Treatment of hyperthyroidism, destruction of thyroid tissue in patients who are not candidates for surgery and thyroid destruction is needed
strong iodine solution, potassium iodide (Thyro-Block)	Adult: 1 tablet, or 2–6 gtt PO q.d. to t.i.d. Pediatric (>1 y): adult dose Pediatric (<1 y): 1/2 tablet or 3 gtt PO q.d. to t.i.d.	Treatment of hyperthyroidism, thyroid blocking in radiation emergencies

include iodism (metallic taste and burning in the mouth, sore teeth and gums, diarrhea, cold symptoms, and stomach upset), staining of teeth, skin rash, and the development of goiter.

Clinically Important Drug–Drug Interactions

Because the use of drugs to destroy thyroid function reverts the patient from hyperthyroidism to hypothyroidism, patients who are taking drugs that are metabolized differently in hypothyroid and hyperthyroid states, or drugs that have a small margin of safety which could be altered by the change in thyroid function, should be monitored closely. These drugs include anticoagulants, theophylline, digoxin, metoprolol, and propranolol.

Nursing Considerations for Patients Receiving Antithyroid Agents

Assessment: History and Examination

Screen for the following conditions, which could be cautions or contraindications to use of the drug: history of allergy to any antithyroid drug, pregnancy, and lactation.

Include screening for baseline status before beginning therapy and for any potential adverse effects: the presence of any skin lesions; orientation and affect; baseline pulse and blood pressure, baseline ECG; respiration, adventitious sounds; and thyroid function tests.

Nursing Diagnoses

The patient receiving any antithyroid drug may have the following nursing diagnoses related to drug therapy:

- Decreased Cardiac Output related to cardiac effects
- Imbalanced Nutrition: More than Body Requirements, related to changes in metabolism
- Risk for Injury related to bone marrow suppression
- Deficient Knowledge regarding drug therapy

Implementation

- Administer propylthiouracil three times a day, around the clock, *to ensure consistent therapeutic levels.*
- Give iodine solution through a straw, *to decrease staining of teeth;* tablets can be crushed.
- Monitor response carefully, and arrange for periodic blood tests, *to assess patient response and to monitor for adverse effects.*
- Monitor patients receiving iodine solution for any sign of iodism, *so drug can be stopped immediately if such signs appear.*
- Provide thorough patient teaching, including measures to avoid adverse effects, warning signs of problems, and the need for regular evaluation if used for longer than recommended, *to enhance patient knowledge of drug therapy and promote compliance.*

Evaluation

- Monitor patient response to the drug (lowering of thyroid hormone levels).

- Monitor for adverse effects (bradycardia, anxiety, blood dyscrasias, skin rash).
- Evaluate the effectiveness of the teaching plan (patient can name drug, dosage, adverse effects to watch for, specific measures to avoid adverse effects).
- Monitor the effectiveness of comfort measures and compliance to the regimen.

THE PARATHYROID GLANDS

Structure and Function

The parathyroid glands are actually four very small groups of glandular tissue located on the back of the thyroid gland. These cells produce parathyroid hormone (PTH) or **parathormone.** PTH is the most important regulator of serum calcium levels in the body. PTH has many actions, including the following:

- Stimulation of osteoclasts or bone cells to release calcium from the bone
- Increased intestinal absorption of calcium
- Increased calcium resorption from the kidneys
- Stimulation of cells in the kidney to produce calcitriol, the active form of vitamin D, which stimulates intestinal transport of calcium into the blood

Control

Calcium is an electrolyte that is used in many of the body's metabolic processes. These processes include membrane transport systems, conduction of nerve impulses, muscle contraction, and blood clotting. To achieve all of these effects, serum levels of calcium must be maintained between 9 and 11 mg/dL. This is achieved through regulation of serum calcium by two hormones, PTH and calcitonin (Figure 37–4).

Calcitonin is released when serum calcium levels rise. Calcitonin, produced in the thyroid gland, works to reduce calcium levels by blocking bone resorption and enhancing bone formation. This action pulls calcium out of the serum for deposit into the bone. PTH secretion is also directly regulated by serum calcium levels. When serum calcium levels

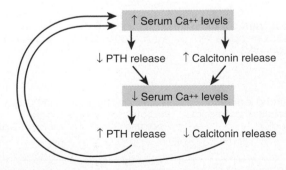

FIGURE 37–4. Control of serum Ca^{++} levels by parathormone (PTH) and calcitonin, showing the negative feedback cycle in effect.

are low, PTH release is stimulated. When serum calcium levels are high, PTH release is blocked.

Another electrolyte, magnesium, also affects PTH secretion by mobilizing calcium and inhibiting the release of PTH when concentrations rise above or fall below normal. An increased serum phosphate level indirectly stimulates parathyroid activity. Renal tubular phosphate reabsorption is balanced by calcium secretion into the urine, which causes a drop in serum calcium, stimulating PTH secretion. The hormones PTH and calcitonin work together to maintain the delicate balance of serum calcium levels in the body and to keep serum calcium levels within the normal range.

PARATHYROID DYSFUNCTION AND RELATED DISORDERS

The absence of parathormone, a condition called **hypoparathyroidism,** is relatively rare. It is most likely to occur with the accidental removal of the parathyroid glands during thyroid surgery. The treatment of hypoparathyroidism consists of calcium and vitamin D therapy to increase serum calcium levels. There is currently no replacement PTH available.

The excessive production of parathormone, called **hyperparathyroidism,** can occur as a result of parathyroid tumor or certain genetic disorders. Patients with hyperparathyroidism may present with decalcification of bone and deposits of calcium in body tissues including the kidney, resulting in kidney stones. Primary hyperparathyroidism occurs more often in women in their 60s and 70s. Secondary hyperparathyroidism occurs most frequently in patients with chronic renal failure. When plasma concentrations of calcium are elevated secondary to high PTH levels, inorganic phosphate levels are usually decreased. Pseudorickets (renal fibrocystic osteosis or renal rickets) may occur as a result of this phosphorus retention (hyperphosphatemia), which results from increased stimulation of the parathyroid glands and increased PTH secretion.

The genetically linked disorder **Paget's disease** is a condition of overactive osteoclasts that are eventually replaced by enlarged and softened bony structures. Patients with this disease complain of deep bone pain, headaches, and hearing loss and usually have cardiac failure and bone malformation.

Postmenopausal osteoporosis can occur when dropping levels of estrogen allow calcium to be pulled out of the bone, resulting in weakened and honeycombed bone structure. Estrogen normally causes calcium deposits in the bone; osteoporosis is one of the many complications that accompany the loss of estrogen at menopause.

ANTIHYPOCALCEMIC AGENTS

Deficient levels of parathyroid hormone result in **hypocalcemia,** or calcium deficiency. Vitamin D stimulates calcium absorption from the intestine and restores the serum

calcium to a normal level. Hypoparathyroidism is treated primarily with vitamin D and, if necessary, dietary supplements of calcium. Calcitriol (*Rocaltrol*) is the most commonly used form of vitamin D. Dihydrotachysterol (*Hytakerol*) is also used.

Therapeutic Actions and Indications
Vitamin D compounds regulate the absorption of calcium and phosphate from the small intestine, mineral resorption in bone, and reabsorption of phosphate from the renal tubules. Working along with PTH and calcitonin to regulate calcium homeostasis, vitamin D actually functions as a hormone. Use of these agents is indicated for the management of hypocalcemia in patients undergoing chronic renal dialysis and for the treatment of hypoparathyroidism.

Pharmacokinetics
These drugs are well absorbed from the GI tract and widely distributed throughout the body. They are stored in the liver, fat, muscle, skin, and bones. After being metabolized in the liver, they are primarily excreted in the urine. Patients with liver and/or renal dysfunction may experience increased levels of the drugs and experience toxic effects. At therapeutic levels, these drugs should be used during pregnancy only if the benefit to the mother clearly outweighs the potential for adverse effects on the fetus. Calcitriol has been associated with hypercalcemia in the baby when used by nursing mothers. Another method of feeding the baby should be used if these drugs are needed during lactation.

Contraindications and Cautions
These drugs should not be used in the presence of any known allergy to vitamin D, hypercalcemia, vitamin D toxicity, or pregnancy. Caution should be used with a history of renal stones or during lactation, when high calcium levels could cause problems.

Adverse Effects
The adverse effects most commonly seen with these drugs are related to GI effects: metallic taste, nausea, vomiting, dry mouth, constipation, and anorexia. CNS effects such as weakness, headache, somnolence, and irritability may also occur. These are possibly related to the changes in electrolytes that occur with these drugs.

Clinically Important Drug–Drug Interactions
There is increased risk of hypermagnesemia if these drugs are taken with magnesium-containing antacids. This combination should be avoided.

Reduced absorption of these compounds may occur if they are taken with cholestyramine or mineral oil, because they are fat-soluble vitamins. If this combination is used, the drugs should be separated by at least 2 hours.

Nursing Considerations for Patients Receiving Antihypocalcemic Agents
Assessment: History and Examination

Screen for the following conditions, which could be cautions or contraindications to use of the drug: history of allergy to

DRUGS IN FOCUS
Antihypocalcemic Agents

Drug Name	Usual Dosage	Usual Indications
(P) calcitriol (Rocaltrol)	0.5–2 µg/d PO in the morning	Management of hypocalcemia and reduction of parathormone levels
dihydrotachysterol (Hytakerol)	0.8–2.4 mg/d PO initially, maintenance 0.2–1 mg/d PO based on serum calcium levels	Management of hypocalcemia

vitamin D; hypercalcemia; vitamin toxicity; renal stone; and pregnancy or lactation.

Include screening for baseline status before beginning therapy and for any potential adverse effects: the presence of any skin lesions; orientation and affect; liver evaluation; serum calcium, magnesium, and alkaline phosphate levels; and radiographs of bones as appropriate.

Nursing Diagnoses

The patient receiving any antihypocalcemic drug may have the following nursing diagnoses related to drug therapy:

- Acute Pain related to GI, CNS effects
- Imbalanced Nutrition: Less than Body Requirements related to GI effects
- Deficient Knowledge regarding drug therapy

Implementation

- Monitor serum calcium concentration before and periodically during treatment, *to allow for adjustment of dosage to maintain calcium levels within normal limits.*
- Provide supportive measures *to help the patient deal with GI and CNS effects of the drug* (analgesics, small and frequent meals, help with activities of daily living).
- Arrange for a nutritional consultation if GI effects are severe, *to ensure nutritional balance.*
- Provide thorough patient teaching, including measures to avoid adverse effects, warning signs of problems, and the need for regular evaluation, *to enhance the patient's knowledge about drug therapy and promote compliance.*

Evaluation

- Monitor patient response to the drug (return of serum calcium levels to normal).
- Monitor for adverse effects (weakness, headache, GI effects).
- Evaluate the effectiveness of the teaching plan (patient can name drug, dosage, adverse effects to watch for, specific measures to avoid adverse effects).

- Monitor the effectiveness of comfort measures and compliance to the regimen.

ANTIHYPERCALCEMIC AGENTS

Drugs used to treat parathyroid hormone excess or high levels of serum calcium (hypercalcemia) include the **bisphosphonates,** calcitonin (human and salmon), and gallium. These drugs act on the serum levels of calcium and not directly on the parathyroid gland or parathyroid hormone.

Bisphosphonates

The bisphosphonates include etidronate (*Didronel*), pamidronate (*Aredia*), risedronate (*Actonel*), tiludronate (*Skelid*), alendronate (*Fosamax*), and zoledronic acid (*Zometa*). These drugs act to slow or block bone resorption; by doing this, they help to lower serum calcium levels.

Therapeutic Actions and Indications
The bisphosphonates slow normal and abnormal bone resorption but do not inhibit normal bone formation and mineralization. These drugs are used in the treatment of Paget's disease and of postmenopausal osteoporosis in women, and alendronate is also used to treat osteoporosis in men. Pamidronate, etidronate, and zoledronic acid are also used for the treatment of hypercalcemia of malignancy and osteolytic bone lesions in certain cancer patients. Tiludronate is reserved for use in the treatment of Paget's disease if there is no response to other therapy. Risedronate is used daily for 2 months to treat Paget's disease in symptomatic people who are at risk for complications.

Pharmacokinetics
These drugs are well absorbed from the small intestine and do not undergo metabolism. They are excreted relatively unchanged in the urine. Patients with renal dysfunction may experience toxic levels of the drug and should be evaluated for a dosage reduction. Fetal abnormalities have been associated with these drugs in animal trials, and they should not be used during pregnancy unless the benefit to the mother

clearly outweighs the potential risk to the fetus. Extreme caution should be used when nursing because of the potential for adverse effects on the baby. Alendronate should not be used by nursing mothers.

Contraindications and Cautions

These drugs should not be used in the presence of hypocalcemia, which could be made worse by lowering calcium levels; during pregnancy or lactation, because of the potential for adverse effects on the fetus or neonate; or with a history of any allergy to bisphosphonates. Caution should be used in patients with renal dysfunction, which could interfere with excretion of the drug, or with upper GI disease, which could be aggravated by the drug. Alendronate and risedronate should not be given to anyone who is unable to remain upright for 30 minutes after taking the drug. Serious esophageal erosion can occur, and taking the drug with a full glass of water and remaining upright for at least 30 minutes facilitates delivery of the drug to the stomach. These drugs need to be taken on arising in the morning, with a full glass of water, fully 30 minutes before any other food or beverage. The patient must then remain upright for at least 30 minutes. Zoledronic acid should be used cautiously in aspirin-sensitive asthmatic patients. Alendronate and risedronate are now available in a once-a-week formulation to decrease the number of times the patient must take the drug, which should increase compliance with the drug regimen.

Adverse Effects

The most common adverse effects seen with bisphosphonates are headache, nausea, and diarrhea. There is also an increase in bone pain in patients with Paget's disease, but this effect usually passes after a few days to a few weeks.

Esophageal erosion has been associated with alendronate and risedronate if the patient has not remained upright for at least 30 minutes after taking the tablets.

Clinically Important Drug–Drug Interactions

Oral absorption of bisphosphonates is decreased if they are taken concurrently with antacids, calcium products, iron, or multiple vitamins. If these drugs need to be taken, they should be separated by at least 30 minutes.

There may also be increased GI distress if bisphosphonates are combined with aspirin; this combination should be avoided if possible.

Calcitonins

The calcitonins are hormones secreted by the thyroid gland to balance the effects of parathyroid hormone. They are available as synthetic human calcitonin (*Cibacalcin*) or salmon calcitonin (*Calcimar* and others).

Therapeutic Actions and Indications

These hormones inhibit bone resorption; lower serum calcium levels in children and in patients with Paget's disease; and increase the excretion of phosphate, calcium, and sodium from the kidney. Human calcitonin is now approved only for orphan drug use in treating Paget's disease. Salmon calcitonin, which has a longer duration of action, has more approved uses. For example, it is also recommended for the treatment of Paget's disease, for the treatment of postmenopausal osteoporosis in conjunction with vitamin D and calcium supplements, and for the emergency treatment of hypercalcemia. Both of these drugs must be given by injection.

DRUGS IN FOCUS
Bisphosphonates

Drug Name	Dosage/Route	Usual Indications
(P) alendronate (*Fosamax*)	10 mg PO q.d.; for postmenopausal osteoporosis, 70 mg PO every week or 10 mg/d PO for treatment, 35 mg PO every week or 5 mg/d PO for prevention	Treatment of Paget's disease, postmenopausal osteoporosis treatment and prevention, treatment of glucocorticoid-induced osteoporosis, osteoporosis in men
etidronate (*Didronel*)	5–10 mg/kg/d PO; 7.5 mg/kg per day IV for 3 d for hypercalcemia of malignancy	Treatment of Paget's disease, postmenopausal osteoporosis, hypercalcemia of malignancy, osteolytic bone lesions in cancer patients
pamidronate (*Aredia*)	60–90 mg IV	Treatment of hypercalcemia of malignancy, osteolytic bone lesions in cancer patients
risedronate (*Actonel*)	30 mg PO q.d. for 2 mo; reduce dosage in renal dysfunction; 5 mg/d PO for osteoporosis	Treatment of symptomatic Paget's disease; osteoporosis
tiludronate (*Skelid*)	400 mg PO q.d. for 3 mo; reduce dosage with renal impairment	Treatment of Paget's disease that is not responsive to other treatment
zoledronic acid (*Zometa*)	4 mg IV as a single infusion over not less than 15 min	Treatment of hypercalcemia of malignancy

GENDER CONSIDERATIONS
Osteoporosis

Osteoporosis is the most common bone disease found in adults. It results from a lack of bone-building cell (osteoclast) activity and a decrease in bone matrix and mass, with less calcium and phosphorous being deposited in the bone. This can occur with advancing age, when the endocrine system is slowing down and the stimulation to build bone is absent; with menopause, when the calcium-depositing effects of estrogen are lost; with malnutrition states, when vitamin C and proteins essential for bone production are absent from the diet; and with a lack of physical stress on the bones from lack of activity, which promotes calcium removal and does not stimulate osteoclast activity. The inactive, elderly, postmenopausal woman with a poor diet is a prime candidate for osteoporosis. Fractured hips and wrists, shrinking size, and curvature of the spine are all evidence of osteoporosis in this age group. Besides the use of bisphosphonates to encourage calcium deposition in the bone, several other interventions can help prevent severe osteoporosis in this group or in any other people with similar risk factors.

• *Aerobic exercise*—Walking, even 10 minutes a day, has been shown to help increase osteoclast activity. Encourage people to walk around the block or to park their car far from the door and walk. Exercise does not have to involve vigorous gym activity to be beneficial.
• *Proper diet*—Calcium and proteins are essential for bone growth. The person who eats only pasta and avoids milk products could benefit from calcium supplements and encouragement to eat protein at least 2 to 3 times a week. Weight loss can also help to improve activity and decrease pressure on bones at rest.
• *Hormone replacement therapy (HRT)*—For women, HRT has been very successful in decreasing the progression of osteoporosis. Women who are at high risk for breast cancer and do not elect to take HRT may be good candidates for bisphosphonates.

The risk of osteoporosis should be taken into consideration as part of the health care regimen for all people as they age. Prevention can save a great deal of pain and debilitation in the long run.

Pharmacokinetics

These drugs are metabolized in the body tissues to inactive fragments, which are excreted by the kidney. They cross the placenta and have been associated with adverse effects on the fetus in animal studies. They should be used in pregnancy only if the benefit to the mother clearly outweighs the potential risk to the fetus. These drugs inhibit lactation in animals; it is not known whether they are excreted in breast milk.

Contraindications and Cautions

These drugs should not be used during lactation, because the calcium-lowering effects could cause problems for the baby. Salmon calcitonin should not be used with a known allergy to salmon or fish products. Caution should be used in patients with renal dysfunction or pernicious anemia, which could be exacerbated by these drugs.

Adverse Effects

The most common adverse effects seen with these drugs are flushing of the face and hands; skin rash; nausea and vomiting; urinary frequency; and local inflammation at the site of injection. Many of these side effects lessen with time, the time varying with each individual patient.

▢▮◖◼ WEB LINKS

Patients and health care providers may want to consult the following Internet sources:

Information on thyroid diseases, support groups, treatments, research:
  http://the-thyroid-society.org
Information on endocrine diseases, screening, treatment:
  http://www.endo-society.org
Information on osteoporosis—support groups, screening, treatment, research:
  http://www.nof.org
Information on national and international research on osteoporosis and related bone diseases:
  http://www.osteorec.com

DRUGS IN FOCUS
Calcitonins

Drug Name	Dosage/Route	Usual Indications
calcitonin, human (*Cibacalcin*)	0.5 mg/d SC	Treatment of Paget's disease
℗ calcitonin, salmon (*Calcimar* and others)	Paget's disease: 50–100 IU/d SC or IM Postmenopausal osteoporosis: 100 IU/d SC or IM with calcium and vitamin D Hypercalcemia: 4–8 IU/kg SC or IM q12h	Treatment of Paget's disease, postmenopausal osteoarthritis, emergency treatment of hypercalcemia

Other Antihypercalcemic Agents

Gallium (*Ganite*) is another drug that is used as an antihypercalcemic agent. It does not fit into either of the previous categories.

Therapeutic Actions and Indications

Gallium inhibits calcium resorption from bone and reduces bone turnover, producing a lowered serum calcium concentration. Gallium is administered intravenously for a period of 5 days to treat cancer-related hypercalcemia that is symptomatic and does not respond to conventional treatment.

Pharmacokinetics

Gallium is slow to reach its peak level, usually taking 2 days. It is not thought to be metabolized, and it is excreted in the urine. It may cross the placenta and enter breast milk and should not be used during pregnancy or lactation unless the benefit to the mother clearly outweighs the potential risk to the fetus or neonate.

Contraindications and Cautions

Gallium is contraindicated in the presence of severe renal dysfunction or lactation. Caution should be used in patients with mild hypocalcemia and in pregnant patients.

Adverse Effects

Because there is a risk of acute renal failure with this drug, renal function tests must be monitored closely for any sign of renal failure. It is crucial to maintain adequate hydration in patients receiving gallium and to closely monitor serum electrolytes. Other adverse effects that occur often are hypocalcemia and decreased serum bicarbonate, which could lead to acidosis.

Clinically Important Drug–Drug Interactions

Because of the risk of renal failure, extreme caution should be used if other nephrotoxic drugs are used concurrently, including the aminoglycosides and amphotericin B.

Nursing Considerations for Patients Receiving Antihypercalcemic Agents

Assessment: History and Examination

Screen for the following conditions, which could be cautions or contraindications to use of the drug: history of al-lergy to any of these products, or to fish products with salmon calcitonin; pregnancy or lactation; hypocalcemia; and renal dysfunction.

Include screening for baseline status before beginning therapy and for any potential adverse effects: presence of any skin lesions; orientation and affect; abdominal examination; serum electrolytes; and renal function tests.

Nursing Diagnoses

The patient receiving any antihypercalcemic agent may have the following nursing diagnoses related to drug therapy:

- Acute Pain related to GI, skin effects
- Imbalanced Nutrition: Less than Body Requirements, related to GI effects
- Anxiety related to need for parenteral injections (specific drugs)
- Deficient Knowledge regarding drug therapy

Implementation

Ensure adequate hydration with any of these agents, *to reduce risk of renal complications.*

Arrange for concomitant vitamin D, calcium supplements, and hormone replacement therapy *if used to treat postmenopausal osteoporosis.*

Rotate injection sites and monitor for inflammation if using calcitonins, *to prevent tissue breakdown and irritation.*

Monitor serum calcium regularly, *to allow for dosage adjustment as needed.*

Assess the patient carefully for any potential drug–drug interactions if giving in combination with other drugs, *to prevent serious effects.*

Arrange for periodic blood tests of renal function if using gallium, *to monitor for renal dysfunction.*

Provide comfort measures and analgesics, *to relieve bone pain if it returns as treatment begins.*

Provide thorough patient teaching, including measures to avoid adverse effects, warning signs of problems, and the need for regular evaluation if used for longer than recommended, *to enhance patient knowledge about drug therapy and promote compliance.*

DRUGS IN FOCUS
Other Antihypercalcemic Agents

Drug Name	Usual Dosage	Usual Indications
gallium (*Ganite*)	100–200 mg/m^2/d IV for 5 consecutive days	Treatment of cancer-related hypercalcemia unresponsive to other treatments in adults

Evaluation

- Monitor patient response to the drug (return of calcium levels to normal; prevention of complications of osteoporosis; control of Paget's disease).
- Monitor for adverse effects (skin rash; nausea and vomiting; hypocalcemia; renal dysfunction).
- Evaluate the effectiveness of the teaching plan (patient can name drug, dosage, adverse effects to watch for, specific measures to avoid adverse effects).
- Monitor the effectiveness of comfort measures and compliance to the regimen.

CHAPTER SUMMARY

- The thyroid gland uses iodine to produce thyroid hormones. Thyroid hormones control the rate at which most body cells use energy (metabolism).
- Control of the thyroid gland is an intricate balance between TRH, released by the hypothalamus; TSH, released by the anterior pituitary; and circulating levels of thyroid hormone.
- Hypothyroidism, or lower-than-normal levels of thyroid hormone, is treated with replacement thyroid hormone.
- Hyperthyroidism, or higher-than-normal levels of thyroid hormone, is treated with thioamides, which block the thyroid from producing thyroid hormone, or with iodines, which prevent thyroid hormone production or destroy parts of the gland.
- The parathyroid glands are located behind the thyroid gland and produce parathormone, which works with calcitonin, produced by thyroid cells, to maintain the calcium balance in the body.
- Hypocalcemia, or low levels of calcium, is treated with vitamin D products and calcium replacement therapy.
- Hypercalcemia and hypercalcemic states include postmenopausal osteoporosis and Paget's disease, as well as hypercalcemia related to malignancy.
- Hypercalcemia is treated with bisphosphonates, calcitonin, or gallium. Bisphosphonates slow or block bone resorption, which lowers serum calcium levels. Calcitonin inhibits bone resorption; lowers serum calcium levels in children and patients with Paget's disease; and increases the excretion of phosphate, calcium, and sodium from the kidney. Gallium inhibits calcium resorption from bone and reduces bone turnover, producing a lowered serum calcium concentration.

Review Questions

1. The thyroid gland produces the thyroid hormones T_3 and T_4, which are dependent on the availability of:
   a. iodine produced in the liver.
   b. iodine found in the diet.
   c. iron absorbed from the GI tract.
   d. parathyroid hormone to promote iodine binding.
2. The thyroid gland is dependent on the hypothalamic–pituitary axis for regulation. Increasing the levels of thyroid hormone (by taking thyroid replacement) would
   a. increase hypothalamic release of TRH.
   b. increase pituitary release of TSH.
   c. suppress hypothalamic release of TRH.
   d. stimulate the thyroid gland to produce more T_3 and T_4.
3. Hypothyroidism is a very common and often missed disorder. Signs and symptoms of hypothyroidism would not include
   a. increased body temperature.
   b. thickening of the tongue.
   c. bradycardia.
   d. loss of hair.
4. Goiter, or enlargement of the thyroid gland, is usually associated with
   a. hypothyroidism.
   b. iodine deficiency.
   c. hyperthyroidism.
   d. underactive thyroid tissue.
5. Thyroid replacement therapy is indicated for the treatment of
   a. obesity.
   b. myxedema.
   c. Graves' disease.
   d. acute thyrotoxicosis.
6. Assessing a patient's knowledge of his or her thyroid replacement therapy would show good understanding if the patient stated:
   a. "My wife may use some of my drug, since she wants to lose weight."
   b. "I should only need this drug for about 3 months."
   c. "I can stop taking this drug as soon as I feel like my old self."
   d. "I should call if I experience unusual sweating, weight gain, or chills and fever."
7. Administration of propylthiouracil would include giving the drug
   a. once a day in the morning.
   b. around the clock to assure therapeutic levels.
   c. once a day at bedtime to decrease adverse effects.
   d. if the patient is experiencing slow heart rate, skin rash, or excessive bleeding.
8. The parathyroid glands produce parathyroid hormone, important in the body as
   a. a modulator of thyroid hormone.
   b. a regulator of potassium.
   c. a regulator of calcium.
   d. an activator of vitamin D.
9. A drug of choice for the treatment of postmenopausal osteoporosis would be
   a. risendronate.
   b. alendronate.
   c. tiludronate.
   d. calcitriol.
10. A patient who is receiving a bisphosphonate for the treatment of postmenopausal osteoporosis should be taught
    a. to also take vitamin D, calcium, and hormone replacement.
    b. to restrict fluids as much as possible.
    c. that severe bone pain can occur.
    d. to avoid exercise which could aggravate the condition.

BIBLIOGRAPHY

AMA drug evaluations. (2001). Chicago: American Medical Association.

Bullock, B. L. (2000). *Focus on pathophysiology.* Philadelphia: Lippincott Williams & Wilkins.

Drug facts and comparisons. (2002). St. Louis: Fact and Comparisons.

Gilman, A., Hardman, J. G., & Limbird, L. E. (Eds.) (2002). *Goodman and Gilman's the pharmacological basis of therapeutics* (10th ed.). New York: McGraw-Hill.

Karch, A. M. (2002). *2003 Lippincott's nursing drug guide.* Philadelphia: Lippincott Williams & Wilkins.

The medical letter on drugs and therapeutics. (2002). New Rochelle, NY: Medical Letter.

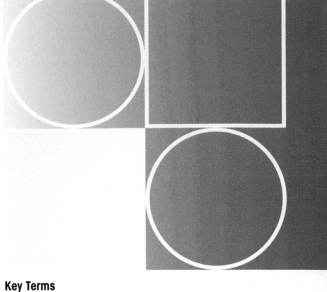

C H A P T E R

38

Antidiabetic Agents

494

Key Terms

diabetes mellitus
glycogen
glycosuria
hyperglycemia
hypoglycemia
insulin
ketosis
polydipsia
polyphagia
sulfonylureas

Parenteral Antidiabetic Agent
insulin

Oral Antidiabetic Agents

Sulfonylureas: First Generation
acetohexamide
🅿 chlorpropamide
tolazamide
tolbutamide

Sulfonylureas: Second Generation
glimepiride
glipizide
🅿 glyburide

Nonsulfonylureas
🅿 acarbose
metformin
miglitol
nateglinide
pioglitazone
repaglinide
rosiglitazone

Glucose-Elevating Agents
diazoxide
glucagon

Diabetes mellitus is the most common of all metabolic disorders. It is estimated that 8 million people in the United States have been diagnosed with diabetes mellitus, and there are many others not yet diagnosed. Diabetes is a complicated disorder that affects many end organs and causes numerous clinical complications. Currently, treatment of diabetes is aimed at tightly regulating the blood sugar level through the use of insulin or insulin-stimulating drugs.

GLUCOSE REGULATION

Glucose is the leading energy source for the human body. Glucose is stored in the body for rapid release in times of stress and so that the serum concentration of glucose can be maintained at a level that provides a constant supply of glucose to the neurons. The minute-to-minute control of glucose levels is the function of the endocrine pancreas gland.

The Pancreas Gland

The pancreas is both an endocrine gland, producing hormones, and an exocrine gland, releasing sodium bicarbonate and pancreatic enzymes directly into the common bile duct to be released into the small intestine, where they neutralize the acid chyme from the stomach and aid digestion. The endocrine part of the pancreas produces hormones in collections of tissue called the islets of Langerhans. These islets contain endocrine cells that produce specific hormones. The alpha cells release glucagon in response to low glucose levels. The beta cells release **insulin** in response to high glucose levels. Delta cells produce somatostatin, which blocks the secretion of insulin and glucagon. These hormones work together to maintain the serum glucose level within normal limits.

Insulin

Insulin is the hormone produced by the beta cells of the islets of Langerhans. The hormone is released into circulation when the levels of glucose around these cells rise. Insulin circulates through the body and reacts with specific insulin receptor sites to stimulate the transport of glucose into the cells to be used for energy, a process called facilitated diffusion. Insulin also stimulates the synthesis of **glycogen** (glucose stored for immediate release during times of stress or low glucose), the conversion of lipids into fat stored in the form of adipose tissue, and the synthesis of needed proteins from amino acids.

Insulin is released after a meal, when the blood glucose levels rise. It circulates and affects metabolism, allowing the body to either store or use the nutrients from the meal effectively. As a result of the insulin release, blood glucose levels fall and insulin release drops off. Sometimes, an insufficient amount of insulin is released. This may occur because the

pancreas cannot produce enough insulin, the insulin receptor sites have lost their sensitivity to insulin, or the person does not have enough receptor sites to support his or her body size, as in obesity.

When an insufficient amount of insulin is released, several metabolic changes occur, beginning with hyperglycemia or increased blood sugar. Hyperglycemia results in glycosuria: sugar is spilled into the urine because the concentration of glucose in the blood is too high for complete reabsorption. Because this sugar-rich urine is an ideal environment for bacteria, cystitis is a common finding. The patient experiences fatigue because the body's cells cannot use the glucose that is there; they need insulin to facilitate transport of the glucose into the cells. **Polyphagia** (increased hunger) occurs because the hypothalamic centers cannot take in glucose and sense that they are starving. **Polydipsia** (increased thirst) occurs because the tonicity of the blood is increased owing to the increased glucose and waste products in the blood and the loss of fluid with glucose in the urine. (The hypothalamic cells that are sensitive to fluid levels sense a need to increase fluid in the system, and the patient feels thirsty.) Lipolysis, or fat breakdown, occurs as the body breaks down stored fat for energy because glucose is not usable. The patient experiences **ketosis** as metabolism shifts to the use of fat and the ketone wastes cannot be removed effectively. Acidosis also occurs because the liver cannot remove all of the waste products (acid being a primary waste product) that result from the breakdown of glucose, fat, and proteins. Muscles break down because proteins are no longer being built and because the body breaks down proteins for their essential amino acids. The breakdown of proteins results in an increase in nitrogen wastes, which is seen in an elevated blood urea nitrogen (BUN) concentration and sometimes in protein in the urine. Patients with hyperglycemia do not heal quickly because of this breakdown of proteins and the lack of a stimulus to build proteins. All of these actions eventually contribute to development of the complications associated with chronic hyperglycemia or diabetes.

DIABETES MELLITUS

Diabetes mellitus (literally, "honey urine") is characterized by complex disturbances in metabolism. Diabetes affects carbohydrate, protein, and fat metabolism. The most frequently recognized clinical signs of diabetes are **hyperglycemia** (fasting blood sugar level greater than 126 mg/dL) and **glycosuria** (the presence of sugar in the urine). The alterations in the body's ability to effectively deal with carbohydrate, fat, and protein metabolism over a long term result in a thickening of the basement membrane (a thin layer of collagen filament that lies just below the endothelial lining of blood vessels) in large and small blood vessels. This thickening leads to changes in oxygenation of the lining of the vessel; damage to the vessel lining, which leads to narrowing and decreased blood flow through the vessel; and an inability of oxygen to rapidly diffuse across the membrane to the tissues. These changes result in increased incidence of a number of disorders, including the following:

Atherosclerosis—heart attacks and strokes related to the development of atherosclerotic plaques in the vessel lining

Retinopathy—with resultant loss of vision as tiny vessels in the eye are narrowed and closed

Neuropathies—with motor and sensory changes in the feet and legs and progressive changes in other nerves as the oxygen supply to these nerves is slowly cut off

Nephropathy—with renal dysfunction related to changes in the basement membrane of the glomerulus

The overall metabolic disturbances associated with diabetes are thought to be caused by a lack of the hormone insulin. There is debate over whether lack of insulin leads to the basement membrane changes and complications of diabetes, or whether the basement membrane thickening is the initial problem that leads to lack of insulin. Whichever comes first, replacement or stimulation of insulin release is the mainstay for treating diabetes mellitus. The diagnosis of diabetes mellitus has involved monitoring of fasting blood glucose levels and sometimes challenging the system with glucose for a glucose tolerance test. Recent research indicates that the body's response to food may be a more important indicator of impending diabetes, and it is now believed that a fasting blood glucose level may not be as important as a postprandial blood glucose level, which reveals the body's ability to response to a glucose challenge. Researchers believe that very early intervention—diet, exercise, and lifestyle changes—may delay the onset of diabetes and the complications, including coronary artery disease, that come with it.

Diabetes mellitus is classified as either type 1, insulin-dependent diabetes mellitus (IDDM) or type 2, non–insulin-dependent diabetes mellitus (NIDDM). Type 1 diabetes is usually associated with rapid onset, mostly in younger people, and is connected in many cases to viral destruction of the beta cells of the pancreas. Type 1 diabetes always requires insulin replacement.

Type 2 diabetes usually occurs in mature adults and has a slow and progressive onset. However, studies released in 2001 reported that the incidence of type 2 diabetes in teenagers and young adults is increasing markedly. The treatment of type 2 diabetes usually begins with changes in diet and exercise. Dieting controls the amount and timing of glucose introduction into the body, and weight loss decreases the number of insulin receptor sites that need to be stimulated. Exercise increases the movement of glucose into the cells by activation of the sympathetic nervous system and by the increase of potassium in the blood that occurs directly after exercising. Potassium acts as part of a polarizing system during exercise that pushes glucose into the cells.

When diet and exercise no longer work, oral agents (discussed later) are tried, to stimulate the production of insulin in the pancreas, increase the sensitivity of the insulin receptor sites, or control the entry of glucose into the system. In-

CULTURAL CONSIDERATIONS
Diabetes and Blood Glucose Variations

Certain cultures tend to have a genetically predetermined variation in routine blood glucose levels, possibly caused by a variation in metabolism. For example, American Indians, Hispanic Americans, and Japanese Americans have higher blood glucose levels than white Americans do. The clinical importance of this fact relates to proper screening of patients for hypoglycemia and diabetes mellitus. Patients in these cultural groups who have fasting glucose tolerance tests and need to have the standard readjusted before a diagnosis is made. Such patients also require an understanding of potential differences in normal levels on home glucose monitoring units when they are regulating insulin at home.

Cultural groups that are more likely to develop diabetes mellitus include African Americans and Hispanic Americans. People in these groups should be screened regularly for diabetes. They also can benefit from teaching about warning signs of diabetes.

jection of insulin may eventually be needed to replace the missing insulin. This concept is often confusing to patients who are learning about diabetes. NIDDM (type 2) often evolves until insulin is needed. Timing of the injections is correlated with food intake and anticipated increases in blood glucose levels.

Hyperglycemia

Hyperglycemia, or high blood sugar, results when there is insufficient insulin to deal with the glucose in the system. Clinical signs and symptoms of hyperglycemia include fatigue, lethargy, irritation, glycosuria, polyphagia, polydipsia, and itchy skin (from accumulation of wastes that the liver cannot clear). If the hyperglycemia goes unchecked, the patient will experience ketoacidosis and central nervous system (CNS) changes that can progress to coma. Signs of impending dangerous complications of hyperglycemia include the following:

- Fruity breath as the ketones build up in the system and are excreted through the lungs
- Dehydration as fluid and important electrolytes are lost through the kidneys
- Slow, deep respirations (Kussmaul's respirations) as the body tries to rid itself of high acid levels
- Loss of orientation and coma

This level of hyperglycemia needs to be treated immediately with insulin.

Hypoglycemia

Hypoglycemia, or a blood sugar concentration lower than 40 mg/dL, occurs in a number of clinical situations, includ-

TABLE 38-1 | Signs and Symptoms of Hypoglycemia and Hyperglycemia

System	Hypoglycemia	Hyperglycemia
Central nervous system	Headache, blurred vision, diplopia; drowsiness progressing to coma; ataxia; hyperactive reflexes	Decreased level of consciousness, sluggishness progressing to coma; hypoactive reflexes
Neuromuscular	Paresthesias; weakness; muscle spasms; twitching progressing to seizures	Weakness, lethargy
Cardiovascular	Tachycardia; palpitations; normal to high blood pressure	Tachycardia; hypotension
Respiratory	Rapid, shallow respirations	Rapid, deep respirations (Kussmaul's); acetone-like or fruity breath
Gastrointestinal	Hunger, nausea	Nausea; vomiting; thirst
Other	Diaphoresis; cool and clammy skin; normal eyeballs	Dry, warm, flushed skin; soft eyeballs
Laboratory tests	Urine glucose—negative; blood glucose low	Urine glucose—strongly positive; urine ketone levels—positive; blood glucose levels—high
Onset	Sudden; patient appears anxious, drunk; associated with overdose of insulin, missing a meal, increased stress	Gradual; patient is slow and sluggish; associated with lack of insulin, increased stress

ing starvation, and if treatment of hyperglycemia with insulin or oral agents lowers the blood sugar too far. The body immediately reacts to lowered blood sugar because the cells require glucose to survive, the neurons being among the cells most sensitive to the lack of glucose. The initial reaction to falling blood sugar is parasympathetic stimulation—increased gastrointestinal (GI) activity to increase digestion and absorption. Rather rapidly, the sympathetic nervous system (SNS) responds with a "fight or flight" reaction that increases blood glucose levels by initiating the breakdown of fat and glycogen to release glucose for rapid energy. The pancreas releases glucagon, a hormone that counters the effects of insulin and works to increase glucose levels. In many cases, the response to the hypoglycemic state causes a hyperglycemic state. Balancing the body's responses to glucose is sometimes difficult when one is trying to treat and control diabetes. Table 38–1 offers a comparison of the signs and symptoms of hyperglycemia and hypoglycemia.

REPLACEMENT INSULIN

Replacement insulin is used to treat diabetes mellitus in adults who have no response to diet, exercise, and oral agents, and for type I diabetics who require replacement insulin. Originally, insulin was prepared from pork and beef pancreas. Today, virtually all insulin is prepared by recombinant DNA technology and is human insulin produced by genetically altered bacteria. This more pure form of insulin is not associated with the sensitivity problems that many patients developed with the animal products. Animal insulins may still be obtained for patients who are most responsive to them, but they are not generally used.

Box 38–1 describes the various forms of insulin delivery that are currently available or under study for future use.

Therapeutic Actions and Indications

Insulin is a hormone that promotes the storage of the body's fuels; facilitates the transport of various metabolites and ions across cell membranes; and stimulates the synthesis of glycogen from glucose, of fats from lipids, and of proteins from amino acids. Insulin does these things by reacting with specific receptor sites on the cell. Figure 38–1 shows the sites of action of replacement insulin and other drugs used to treat diabetic conditions.

Replacement insulin is used to treat diabetes mellitus; type 2 diabetes mellitus in patients whose diabetes cannot be controlled by diet or other agents; severe ketoacidosis or diabetic coma; and hyperkalemia with infusion of glucose to produce a shift of potassium into the cells (polarizing solution). It also is used for short courses of therapy during periods of stress (eg, surgery, disease) in type 2 diabetics, for newly diagnosed patients getting stabilized, for patients with poor control of glucose levels, and for patients with gestational diabetes. Various preparations of insulin are available to provide short- and long-term coverage (Table 38–2). Frequently, patients use more than one preparation to provide insulin coverage at different times during the day.

Pharmacokinetics

The various insulins available are processed within the body like endogenous insulin. The peak, onset, and duration of the different preparations vary with each type of insulin because of the placement or addition of glycine and/or arginine chains. Insulin does not cross the placenta, and it is the drug of choice for managing diabetes during pregnancy. Insulin does enter breast milk, but it is destroyed in the GI tract and does not affect the nursing baby. Insulin-dependent mothers may have inhibited milk production, however, and the effectiveness of nursing should be evaluated periodically.

DRUG THERAPY ACROSS THE LIFESPAN

Antidiabetic Agents

Children	Adults	Older Adults
Oral antidiabetic agents have not been proven to be safe or effective for use in children. With the increasing number of children being diagnosed with type 2 diabetes, the use of these agents in children may be tested.

Treatment of diabetes in children is a difficult challenge of balancing diet, activity, growth and stress needs, and insulin requirements. Children need to be carefully monitored for any sign of hypoglycemia or hyperglycemia and treated quickly, because their fast metabolism and lack of body reserves can push them into a severe state quickly.

Insulin dosage, especially in infants, may be so small that the dose is difficult to calibrate. Insulin often needs to be diluted to a volume that can be detected on the syringe. A second person should always check the calculations and dosage of insulin being given to small children.

Teenage children often present a real challenge for diabetes management. The desire to be "normal" often leads to a resistance to dietary restrictions and insulin injections. The metabolism of the teenager is also in flux, leading to complications in regulating insulin dosage. A team approach, including the child, family members, teachers, coaches, and even friends, may be the best way to help the child deal with the disease and the required therapy. New delivery methods for insulin may help this age group cope with the drug therapy in the future. | Adults need extensive education about the disease as well as the drug therapy. Warning signs and symptoms should be stressed repeatedly as the adult learns to juggle insulin needs with exercise, stressors, other drug effects, and diet. Adults maintained on oral agents need to be monitored for changes in response to the drugs. Often additional drugs are added or dosages are changed as the disease progresses over time.

Exercise and diet should always be emphasized as the mainstay of dealing with diabetes. Adults need to be cautioned about the use of over-the-counter and herbal or alternative therapies. Many of these products contain agents that alter blood glucose levels and will change insulin or oral agent requirements. Adults should always be asked specifically whether they use any of these agents and adjustments made accordingly.

Insulin therapy is the best choice for diabetics during pregnancy and lactation, times of high stress and metabolic demands. Needs may change on a daily basis, and the mother should have ready support and extensive teaching about what to do if hypoglycemia or hyperglycemia occurs. Labor and delivery is often a critical time in diabetes management because of the stress and sudden changes in body fluid volume and hormone levels. The obstetrician and the endocrinologist or primary care provider should consult frequently about the best way to support the patient through this period. | Older adults can have many underlying problems that complicate diabetic therapy. Poor vision and/or coordination may make it difficult to prepare a syringe. A week's supply of syringes can be prepared and refrigerated for the usual dose of insulin.

Dietary deficiencies related to changes in taste, absorption, or attitude may lead to wide fluctuations in blood sugar levels, making it difficult to control diabetes. Many areas offer nutritional assistance programs for older adults (eg, Meals on Wheels) or can refer patients to appropriate agencies that might be able to offer assistance.

Older adults have a greater incidence of renal or hepatic impairment, and kidney and liver function should be evaluated before starting any of these drugs. Combinations of oral agents may not be feasible with severe dysfunction, and the patient may need to use insulin to control blood glucose levels.

Older adults should still receive periodic educational reminders about diet, the need for exercise, skin and foot care, and warning signs to report to the health care provider.

The older patient is also more likely to experience end organ damage related to the diabetes—loss of vision, kidney problems, coronary artery disease, infections—and the drug regimen of these patients can become quite complex. Careful screening for drug interactions is an important aspect of the assessment of these patients. |

BOX 38-1

Insulin Delivery—Past, Present, and Future

PAST

Subcutaneous injection—The delivery of insulin by subcutaneous injection was first introduced in the 1920s and changed the way that diabetic patients were managed clinically, giving them a chance for a normal lifestyle. Research is ongoing to find more efficient and acceptable ways to deliver insulin to diabetic patients.

PRESENT

Subcutaneous insulin injection—This remains the primary delivery system.

Insulin jet injector—This cylindrical device shoots a fine spray of insulin through the skin under very high pressure. Although it is appealing for people who don't like needles or have problems disposing of needles properly, it can be very expensive.

BOX 38-1 (CONTINUED)

Insulin Delivery—Past, Present, and Future

Insulin pen—This syringe-like device actually looks like a pen. It has a small needle at the tip and a barrel that holds insulin. The patient "dials" the amount of insulin to be given and injects the insulin subcutaneously by pressing on the top of the pen. This is advantageous for people who need insulin two or three times during the day but cannot easily transport syringes and needles. It is a subtle way to give insulin, and is popular with students and business people on the go. It is important to rotate the syringe 15 to 20 times before injecting the insulin, to disperse it. Patients often forget this point after using the pens for awhile, and as a result, may inject far too much or too little insulin when it is needed. Periodic reinforcement of the administration instructions is important.

External insulin pump—This pump device can be worn on a belt or hidden in a pocket and is attached to a small tube inserted into the subcutaneous tissue of the abdomen. The device slowly leaks a base rate of insulin into the abdomen all day; the patient can pump or inject booster doses throughout the day to correspond with meals and activity. The device does have several disadvantages. For example, it is awkward, the tubing poses an increased risk of infection and requires frequent changing, and the patient has to frequently check blood glucose levels throughout the day to monitor response.

Long-acting insulin—The year 2001 brought the release of a subcutaneous insulin that lasts two to three times longer than NPH insulin. This should decrease the need for multiple injections and may increase glucose control, especially for patients with erratic glucose levels during the night. Long-term effects of this type of insulin therapy are not yet known.

FUTURE

Implantable insulin pump—This pump is surgically implanted into the abdomen and delivers base insulin as well as insulin boluses as needed directly into the abdomen to be absorbed by the liver, just as pancreatic insulin is. The disadvantages are risk of infection, mechanical problems with the pump, and lack of long-term data on its effectiveness. This method is not yet available for general use.

Insulin patch—The patch is placed on the skin and delivers a constant low dose of insulin. When the patient eats a meal, tabs are pulled on the patch to release more insulin. The problem with this delivery method is that insulin does not readily pass through the skin, so there is tremendous variability in its effects. This route is not yet commercially available.

Inhaled insulin—The lung tissue is one of the best sites for insulin absorption. An aerosol delivery system has been developed that delivers a powdered insulin formulation directly into the lung tissue. Research has been very promising, suggesting that this may be a more reliable method of delivering insulin in the future. Earlier reports anticipated availability of this type of delivery system within the next few years. However, Phase III studies showed an increase in insulin antibody formation in patients using inhaled insulin in clinical trials, sending the drug back for further refinement and research.

For the most up-to-date information on insulin delivery research, visit the following website: http://www.niddk.nih.gov.

FIGURE 38-1. Sites of action of drugs used to treat diabetic conditions.

TABLE 38-2 Comparison of Insulin Types

Type	Onset	Peak	Duration
Insulin analog (*Humalog*)	<15 min	1 h	3.5–4.5 h
Insulin asparT (*NovoLog*)	5–10 min	30–60 min	2–3 h
Insulin glargine (*Lantus*)	30–60 min	None	8 h
Regular (*Humulin R, Iletin Regular, Novolin R, Velosulin BR*)	30–60 min	2–4 h	6–8 h
NPH (*Humulin N, Iletin NPH, Novolin N*)	1–2 h	6–12 h	18–24 h
Lente (*Humulin L, Iletin L, Novolin L*)	1–2.5 h	6–12 h	18–24 h
PZI (*Humulin U*)	4–8 h	8–20 h	24–48 h
COMBINATION INSULINS			
NPH and Regular (*Humulin 70/30, Novolin 70/30, Humulin 50/50, Humalog 75/25*)	30–60 min, then 1–2 h	2–4 h, then 6–12 h	6–8 h, then 18–24 h

Insulin is available in various preparations with a wide range of peaks and durations of action. A patient may receive a combination of regular and NPH insulin in the morning to cover the glucose peak from breakfast (regular onset, 30–60 min) and the lunch and dinner glucose peaks. The patient may then require another injection before bed. The types of insulin used are determined by the anticipated eating and exercise activities of any particular patient. It is very important to make sure one is using the correct insulin preparation when administering the drug. Insulin glargine (*Lantus*) cannot be mixed in solution with any other drug, including other insulins.

Contraindications and Cautions

Because insulin is used as a replacement hormone, there are no contraindications. Care should be taken during pregnancy and lactation to monitor glucose levels closely and adjust the insulin dosage accordingly. Patients with allergies to beef or pork products should use only human insulins.

Adverse Effects

The most common adverse effects to insulin use are hypoglycemia and ketoacidosis, which can be controlled with proper dosage adjustments, and local reactions at injection sites.

Clinically Important Drug–Drug Interactions

Caution should be used when giving a patient stabilized on insulin any drug that decreases glucose levels (eg, monoamine oxidase inhibitors, β-blockers, salicylates, alcohol). Dosage adjustments are needed when any of these drugs is added or removed.

Care should also be taken when combining insulin with any β-blocker. The blocking of the SNS also blocks many of the signs and symptoms of hypoglycemia, hindering the patient's ability to recognize problems. Patients taking β-blockers need to learn other ways to recognize hypoglycemia.

DRUGS IN FOCUS
Parenteral Antihyperglycemic Agent

Drug Name	Dosage/Route	Usual Indications
Insulin (various types)	Varies based on patient response, diet, and activity level	Treatment of diabetes; treatment of diabetes type 2 that cannot be controlled by other means; treatment of severe ketoacidosis; treatment of newly diagnosed diabetes; treatment of hyperkalemia as part of a polarizing solution; treatment of gestational diabetes

NURSING CHALLENGE
Managing Glucose Levels During Stress

The body has many compensatory mechanisms for ensuring that blood glucose levels stay within a safe range. The sympathetic stress reaction elevates the blood glucose levels to provide ready energy for fight or flight (see Chapter 29). The stress reaction causes the breakdown of glycogen to release glucose, and the breakdown of fat and proteins to release other energy. The stress reaction elevates the blood glucose concentration above the normal range. In severe stress situations—such as an acute myocardial infarction or an automobile accident—the blood glucose level can be very high (300–400 mg/dL). The body uses that energy to either fight the insult or flee from the stressor.

Nurses in acute care situations need to be aware of this reflex elevation in glucose when caring for patients in acute stress, especially patients in emergency situations whose medical history is unknown. The usual medical response to a blood glucose concentration of 400 mg/dL would be the administration of insulin. In many situations, that is exactly what is done, especially if the patient's history is not known and the effects of such a high glucose level could cause severe systemic reactions. Insulin administration causes a drop in the blood glucose level as glucose enters cells to be either used for energy or converted to glycogen for storage.

However, a problem may arise in the acute care setting, particularly in a patient who is not diabetic. Relieving the stress reaction can also drop glucose levels as the stimulus to increase these levels is lost and the glucose that was there is used for energy. A patient in this situation, who has been treated with insulin, is at risk for development of potentially severe hypoglycemia. The body's response to low glucose levels is a sympathetic stress reaction, which again elevates the blood glucose concentration. If treated, the patient potentially can enter a cycle of high and low glucose levels. Nurses are often the ones in closest contact with the highly stressed patient—in the emergency room, the intensive care unit, the postanesthesia room—and should be constantly aware of the normal and reflex changes in blood glucose that accompany stress. Careful monitoring, with awareness of stress and the relief of stress, can prevent a prolonged treatment program to maintain blood glucose levels within the range of normal, a situation that is not "normal" during a stress reaction.

Diabetic patients who are in severe stress situations require changes in their insulin dosages. They should be allowed some elevation of blood glucose, even though their inability to produce sufficient insulin will make it difficult for their cells to make effective use of the increased glucose levels. It is a clinical challenge to balance glucose levels with the needs of the patient because so many factors can affect the glucose level.

Nursing Considerations for Patients Taking Insulin
Assessment: History and Examination

Screen for history of allergy to any insulin and for pregnancy or lactation so that appropriate monitoring and dosage adjustments can be done.

Include screening for baseline status before beginning therapy and for any potential adverse effects: presence of any skin lesions; orientation and reflexes; baseline pulse and blood pressure; respiration, adventitious breath sounds; urinalysis and blood glucose level.

Nursing Diagnoses

The patient receiving insulin may have the following nursing diagnoses related to drug therapy:

- Imbalanced Nutrition: Less than Body Requirements, related to metabolic effects
- Disturbed Sensory Perception (kinesthetic, visual, auditory, tactile) related to glucose levels
- Risk for Infection related to injections and disease process
- Ineffective Coping related to diagnosis and injection therapy
- Deficient Knowledge regarding drug therapy

Implementation

- *Ensure uniform suspension of insulin* by gently rotating vial; avoid vigorous shaking.
- Give maintenance doses by the subcutaneous route only, and rotate injection sites regularly, *to avoid damage to muscles and to prevent subcutaneous atrophy;* give regular insulin intramuscularly or intravenously in emergency situations.
- Monitor response carefully, *to avoid adverse effects;* blood glucose monitoring is the most effective way to evaluate insulin dosage.
- Use caution when mixing types of insulin; administer mixtures of regular and NPH or regular and lente insulins within 15 minutes after combining them, *to prevent precipitation and ineffective dosing.*
- Store insulin in a cool place away from direct sunlight. Predrawn syringes are stable for 1 week if refrigerated; they offer a good way *to ensure the proper dosage for patients* who have limited vision.
- Monitor patients during times of trauma or severe stress *for potential dosage adjustment needs.*
- Instruct patients who are also receiving β-blockers about ways to monitor glucose levels and signs and symptoms of glucose abnormalities, *to prevent hypoglycemic and hyperglycemic episodes when SNS and warning signs are blocked.*
- Provide thorough patient teaching, including measures to avoid adverse effects, warning signs of problems, proper administration techniques, and the need to monitor disease status, *to enhance patient knowledge about drug therapy and promote compliance.* (See Patient Teaching Checklist: Insulin.)

Evaluation

- Monitor patient response to the drug (stabilization of blood glucose levels).
- Monitor for adverse effects (hypoglycemia, ketoacidosis, injection site irritation).
- Evaluate the effectiveness of the teaching plan (patient can name drug, dosage, adverse effects to watch for, specific

CASE STUDY

Type I Diabetes Mellitus

THE SITUATION

M. J. is a 22-year-old woman who has newly diagnosed type I diabetes mellitus. She was stabilized on insulin while hospitalized for diagnosis and management. One week after discharge, M. J. experienced nausea and anorexia. She was unable to eat, but she took her insulin as usual in the morning. That afternoon, she experienced profuse sweating and was tremulous and apprehensive, so she went to the hospital emergency room. The initial diagnosis was insulin reaction from taking insulin and not eating, combined with the stress of her gastrointestinal distress. M. J. was treated at the emergency room with intravenous glucose. After she had rested and her glucose levels returned to normal, she was discharged to home.

CRITICAL THINKING

• What instructions should M. J. receive before she leaves? *Think about the ways that stress can alter the blood glucose levels. Then consider the stress that a newly diagnosed type I diabetic patient undergoes while trying to cope with the diagnosis, learn self-injection, and think about complications of the disease that may arise in the future.*
• What teaching approaches could help M. J. to decrease her stress and to effectively plan her medical regimen?
• What sort of support would be useful for M. J. as she adjusts to her new life?

DISCUSSION

The diagnosis of type 1 diabetes is a life-changing event. M. J. had to learn about the disease and how to test her own blood and give herself injections; manage a new diet and exercise program; and perhaps, cope with the knowledge that the long-term complications of diabetes can be devastating. Many patients who are regulated on

insulin in the hospital experience a change in insulin demand after discharge. The sympathetic nervous system (SNS) is active in the hospital, and one of the effects of SNS activity is increased glucose levels—preparing the body for fight or flight. For some patients, returning home eases the stress that activated the SNS, and glucose levels fall. If the patient continues to use the same insulin dose, hypoglycemia can occur. Other patients may feel protected in the hospital and experience stress when they are sent home. They may feel anxious about taking care of themselves while coping with everyday problems and tensions. These patients need an increased insulin dose because their stress reaction intensifies when they get home, driving their blood glucose level up.

Patients are taught how to measure their own blood glucose levels before they leave the hospital. When they get used to doing this and regulating their own insulin based on glucose concentrations, they usually manage well. The first few days to weeks are often the hardest. The nurse should review with M. J. how to test her glucose, draw up her insulin, and regulate the dose. The nurse also should give M. J. written information that she can refer to later.

In addition, the nurse should give M. J. a chance to talk and to vent her feelings about her diagnosis and her future. To help decrease M. J.'s stress and to avoid problems during this adjustment period, the nurse can give M. J. a telephone number to call if she has problems or questions. M. J. should return in a few days to review her progress and have any questions answered. In the meantime, the nurse should encourage M. J. to write down any questions or problems that arise so that they can be addressed during the follow-up visit. Support and encouragement will be crucial to helping M. J. adjust to her disease and her drug therapy. She can also be referred to the American Diabetic Association, which in many communities offers support services to help diabetics.

---

measures to avoid adverse effects, proper administration technique).
• Monitor the effectiveness of comfort measures and compliance to the regimen (see Nursing Care Guide: Insulin).

ORAL ANTIDIABETIC AGENTS

Oral drugs are successful in controlling type 2 diabetes in patients who still have a functioning pancreas. The **sulfonylureas** were the first oral agents introduced. They stimulate the pancreas to release insulin. Other oral agents, called nonsulfonylureas, have been introduced more recently. The nonsulfonylureas act to decrease insulin resistance or alter

glucose absorption and uptake. They often are combined with a sulfonylurea for effectiveness.

Sulfonylureas

The sulfonylureas bind to potassium channels on pancreatic beta cells to increase insulin secretion. They may improve insulin binding to insulin receptors and increase the number of insulin receptors. They are also known to increase the effect of antidiuretic hormone on renal cells. They are effective only in patients who have functioning beta cells. They are not effective for all diabetics and may lose their effectiveness over time with others. All of the sulfonylureas can cause hypoglycemia.

PATIENT TEACHING CHECKLIST
Insulin

Create customized patient teaching materials for a specific insulin from the CD-ROM. Patient teaching should stress the following points for drugs within this class:

• Insulin is a hormone that is normally produced by your pancreas. It helps to regulate your energy balance by affecting the way the body uses sugar and fats. The lack of insulin produces a disease called diabetes mellitus. By injecting insulin each day, you can help your body use the sugars and fats in your food effectively.
• Check the expiration date on your insulin. Store the insulin at room temperature and avoid extremes of heat and light. Gently rotate the vial between your palms before use to dispense any crystals that may have formed. Do not shake the vial, because vigorous shaking can inactivate the drug.
• A prescription is required to get the syringes that you will need to administer your insulin. Keep the syringes sealed until ready to use, and dispose of them appropriately. Rotate your injection sites regularly to prevent tissue damage and to ensure that the proper amount of insulin is absorbed.
• You should be aware of the signs and symptoms of hypoglycemia (too much insulin). If any of these occur, eat or drink something high in sugar, such as candy, orange juice, honey, or sugar. The signs and symptoms to watch for include the following: nervousness, anxiety, sweating, pale and cool skin, headache, nausea, hunger, shakiness. These may happen if you skip a meal, exercise too much, or experience extreme stress. If these symptoms happen very often, notify your health care provider.
• Avoid the use of any over-the-counter medication without first checking with your health care provider. Several of these medications can interfere with the effectiveness of insulin. Avoid the use of alcohol because it increases the chances of having hypoglycemic attacks.

Tell any doctor, nurse, or other health care provider that you are taking this drug. You may want to wear or carry a Medic-Alert tag showing that you are on this medication. This would alert any medical personnel taking care of you in an emergency to the fact that you are taking this drug.

Report any of the following to your health care provider: loss of appetite, blurred vision, fruity odor to your breath, increased urination, increased thirst, nausea, vomiting.

While you are taking this drug, it is important to have regular medical follow-up, including blood tests to monitor your blood glucose levels, to evaluate you for any adverse effects of your diabetes.

Keep this drug and your syringes out of the reach of children. Do not give this medication to anyone else or take any similar medication that has not been prescribed for you.

This Teaching Checklist reflects general patient teaching guidelines. It is not meant to be a substitute for drug-specific teaching information, which is available in nursing drug guides.

First-Generation Sulfonylureas

The first-generation sulfonylureas include chlorpropamide (*Diabinese*), tolbutamide (*Orinase*), acetohexamide (*Dymelor*), and tolazamide (*Tolinase*). Chlorpropamide is the most frequently used of the group because it has the most predictable effects and has proven to be very reliable. Tolbutamide is preferred for patients with renal dysfunction, who may not be able to excrete chlorpropamide, because it is more easily cleared from the body. Acetohexamide and tolazamide, which are used less frequently, are usually tried after the first two drugs have been shown to be ineffective. They are not as predictably effective in many patients, but they may be very effective in some patients who do not respond to chlorpropamide. Tolbutamide, acetohexamide, and tolazamide are sometimes used in combination with insulin to reduce the insulin dosage and decrease the risk of hypoglycemia in certain type 2 diabetics who have begun to use insulin to control their blood glucose level.

The first-generation sulfonylureas were associated with an increased risk of cardiovascular disease and death in a somewhat controversial study. They are now thought to possibly cause an increase in cardiovascular deaths.

Second-Generation Sulfonylureas

These drugs have several advantages over the first-generation drugs, including the following:

• Second-generation sulfonylureas are excreted in urine and bile, making them safer for patients with renal dysfunction.
• They do not interact with as many protein-bound drugs as the first-generation drugs do.
• They have a longer duration of action, making it possible to take them only once or twice a day, thus increasing compliance.

The second-generation drugs include glimepiride (*Amaryl*), glipizide (*Glucotrol*), and glyburide (*DiaBeta* and others). Glimepiride is a much less expensive drug than most of the other sulfonylureas, which has advantages for some people. Prescribers may try different agents (first- or second-generation drugs) before finding the one that is most effective for a given patient.

Therapeutic Actions and Indications

The sulfonylureas stimulate insulin release from the beta cells in the pancreas (see Figure 38–1). They improve insulin binding to insulin receptors and may actually increase the number of insulin receptors. They are indicated as an adjunct to diet and exercise to lower blood glucose in type 2 diabetes mellitus. They have the unlabeled use of being an adjunct to insulin to improve glucose control in type 2 diabetics.

NURSING CARE GUIDE

Insulin

Assessment	Nursing Diagnoses	Implementation	Evaluation
HISTORY Allergies to any insulins, pregnancy, lactation	Imbalanced Nutrition: Less than Body Requirements, related to metabolic effects Disturbed Sensory Perception (kinesthetic, visual, auditory, tactile) related to effects on glucose levels Risk for Infection related to injections and disease process Ineffective Coping related to diagnosis and injections Deficient Knowledge regarding drug therapy	Administer SC and rotate sites. Store in cool place away from light. Use caution when mixing types. Monitor blood glucose to adjust dosage as needed. Monitor during times of stress and trauma and adjust dosage. Provide support and reassurance to deal with drug injections and lifetime need. Provide patient teaching regarding drug name, dosage, adverse effects, precautions, warning signs to report, and proper administration technique.	Evaluate drug effects: return of glucose levels to normal. Monitor for adverse effects: hypoglycemia, injection site reaction. Monitor for drug–drug interactions as indicated for insulin. Evaluate effectiveness of patient teaching program. Evaluate effectiveness of comfort and safety measures.
PHYSICAL EXAMINATION Neurological: orientation, reflexes Skin: color, lesions CV: P, cardiac auscultation, BP Respiratory: R, adventitious sounds Lab tests: urinalysis, blood glucose			

Pharmacokinetics

These drugs are rapidly absorbed from the GI tract and undergo hepatic metabolism. They are excreted in the urine. The peak effects and duration of effects differ because of the activity of various metabolites of the different drugs. These drugs are not for use during pregnancy. Insulin should be used if an antidiabetic agent is needed during pregnancy. Some of these drugs cross into breast milk, and adequate studies are not available on others. Because of the risk of hypoglycemic effects in the baby, these drugs should not be used during lactation. Another method of feeding the baby should be used.

Contraindications and Cautions

Sulfonylureas are contraindicated in the presence of known allergy to any sulfonylureas and in diabetes complicated by fever, severe infection, severe trauma, major surgery, ketoacidosis, severe renal or hepatic disease, pregnancy, or lactation. These drugs are also contraindicated for use in type I diabetics.

Adverse Effects

The most common adverse effects related to the sulfonylureas are hypoglycemia (caused by an imbalance in levels of glucose and insulin) and GI distress, including nausea, vomiting, epigastric discomfort, heartburn, and anorexia. (Anorexia should be monitored, because affected patients may not eat after taking the sulfonylurea, which could lead to hypoglycemia.) Allergic skin reactions have been reported with some of these drugs and, as mentioned earlier, there may be an increased risk of cardiovascular mortality, particularly with the first-generation agents.

Clinically Important Drug–Drug Interactions

Care should be taken with any drug that acidifies the urine, because excretion of the sulfonylurea may be decreased.

Caution should also be used with β-blockers, which may mask the signs of hypoglycemia, and with alcohol, which can lead to altered glucose levels when combined with sulfonylureas.

The safety and efficacy of these drugs for use in children have not been established.

Nonsulfonylureas

The nonsulfonylureas are oral agents that are structurally unrelated to the sulfonylureas. They frequently are effective when used in combination with sulfonylureas or insulin. These drugs include the α-glucosidase inhibitors acarbose (*Precose*) and miglitol (*Glyset*); the biguanide, metformin (*Glucophage*); the meglitinides, repaglinide (*Prandin*) and

nateglinide (*Starlix*); and the thiazolidinediones, pioglitazone (*Actos*) and rosiglitazone (*Avandia*).

Acarbose and miglitol are inhibitors of α-glucosidase (an enzyme that breaks down glucose for absorption); they delay the absorption of glucose. They have only a mild effect on glucose levels and have been associated with severe hepatic toxicity. They do not enhance insulin secretion, so their effects are additive to those of the sulfonylureas in controlling blood glucose. These drugs are used in combination with other oral agents for patients whose glucose levels cannot be controlled with a single agent.

Metformin decreases the production and increases the uptake of glucose. It is effective in lowering blood glucose levels and does not cause hypoglycemia as the sulfonylureas do. It has been associated with the development of lactic acidosis. Both acarbose and metformin can cause GI distress. Box 38–2 describes a new fixed-combination product containing metformin and glyburide.

DRUGS IN FOCUS
Sulfonylureas

Drug Name	Dosage/Route	Usual Indications
First Generation		
acetohexamide (*Dymelor*)	250 mg to 1.5 g/d PO; start geriatric patients on lower doses because they may be more sensitive to drug effects. Pediatric: safety and efficacy not established	Adjunct to diet for the management of type 2 diabetes; adjunct to insulin for management in certain type 2 diabetics, reducing the insulin dose and decreasing the risks of hypoglycemia
Ⓟ chlorpropamide (*Diabinese*)	100–250 mg/d PO; use lower doses with geriatric patients	Adjunct to diet for the management of type 2 diabetes
tolazamide (*Tolinase*)	100–250 mg/d PO; use lower doses with geriatric patients	Adjunct to diet for the management of type 2 diabetes; adjunct to insulin for management in certain type 2 diabetics, reducing the insulin dose and decreasing the risks of hypoglycemia
tolbutamide (*Orinase*)	0.25–3 g/d PO; use lower doses with geriatric patients	Adjunct to diet for the management of type 2 diabetes; adjunct to insulin for management in certain type 2 diabetics, reducing the insulin dose and decreasing the risks of hypoglycemia
Second Generation		
glimepiride (*Amaryl*)	1–4 mg PO q.d.; use lower doses with geriatric patients	Adjunct to diet for the management of type 2 diabetes; adjunct to insulin for management in certain type 2 diabetics, reducing the insulin dose and decreasing the risks of hypoglycemia
glipizide (*Glucotrol*)	5 mg PO q.d., titrate based on response; do not exceed 15 mg/d; use lower doses with geriatric and hepatic-impaired patients	Adjunct to diet for the management of type 2 diabetes; adjunct to insulin for management in certain type 2 diabetics, reducing the insulin dose and decreasing the risks of hypoglycemia
Ⓟ glyburide (*DiaBeta, Micronase, Glynase PresTab*)	1.25–20 mg/d PO (*DiaBeta, Micronase*), 0.75–12 mg/d PO (*Glynase*); use lower doses with geriatric patients	Adjunct to diet for the management of type 2 diabetes; adjunct to insulin for management in certain type 2 diabetics, reducing the insulin dose and decreasing the risks of hypoglycemia

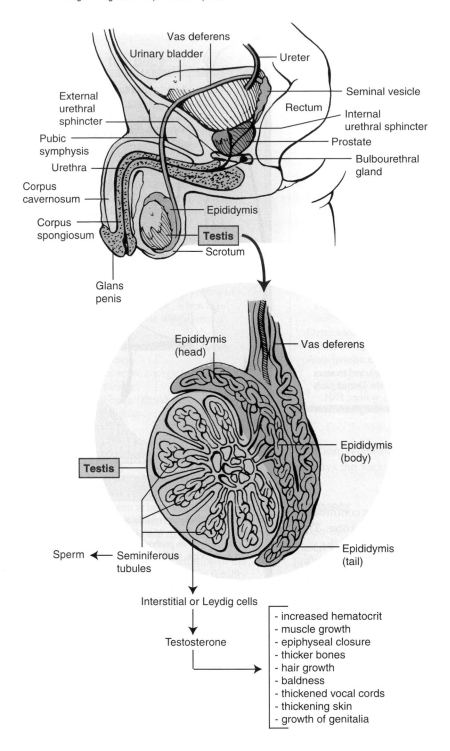

FIGURE 39-4. The male reproductive system.

The LH or ICSH stimulates the interstitial (Leydig) cells to produce testosterone. The concentration of testosterone acts in a similar negative feedback system with the hypothalamus. When the concentration is high enough, the hypothalamus decrease GnRH release, leading to a subsequent decrease in FSH and LH release. The levels of testosterone are thought to remain within a fairly well-defined range of normal. It has been documented, however, that light affects the male sexual hormones in a similar fashion to its effect on female hormones. "Spring fever," with increased exposure time to sunlight, does increase testosterone levels in men. Other factors that may also have an influence on male hormone levels are likely to be identified in the future.

With age, the seminiferous tubules and interstitial cells atrophy and the male climacteric, a period of lessened sexual activity, occurs. This is similar to female menopause, when the hypothalamus and anterior pituitary put out larger amounts of GnRH, FSH, and LH in an attempt to stimulate the gland. When no increase in testosterone or inhibin occurs, the levels of GnRH, FSH, and LH eventually return to normal levels.

FIGURE 39–5. Interaction of the hypothalamic, pituitary, and testicular hormones that underlies the male sexual hormone system. CNS, central nervous system; FSH, follicle-stimulating hormone; GnRH, gonadotropin-releasing hormone; LH, luteinizing hormone.

Hormones

Testosterone is responsible for many sexual and metabolic effects in the male. Like estrogen, testosterone enters the cell and reacts with a cytoplasmic receptor site to influence messenger RNA (mRNA) activity, resulting in the production of proteins for cell structure or function. The effects of testosterone on the body are summarized in Box 39–3.

Castration, or removal of the testes, before puberty results in lack of development of the normal male characteristics as well as sterility. However, once puberty and the physical changes brought about by testosterone have occurred, the androgens released by the adrenal glands are sufficient to sustain the male characteristics. This is important informa-

tion for adult patients undergoing testicular surgery or chemical castration.

THE HUMAN SEXUAL RESPONSE

Humans are the only animals known to be sexually stimulated and responsive at will. Many animals require particular endocrine stimuli, called an estrous cycle, for sexual response to occur. Humans can be sexually stimulated by thoughts, sights, touch, or a variety of combined stimuli. The human sexual response consists of four phases:

- A period of stimulation with mild increases in sensitivity and beginning stimulation of the sympathetic nervous system
- A plateau stage when stimulation levels off
- A climax, which results from massive sympathetic stimulation of the body
- A period of recovery or resolution, when the effects of the sympathetic stimulation are resolved (Figure 39–6)

It was once believed that male and female responses were very different, but it is now thought that the physiology of the responses is very similar. Sexual stimulation and activity are a normal response and, in healthy individuals, are probably necessary for complete health of the body's systems. The sympathetic stimulation causes increased heart rate, increased blood pressure, sweating, pupil dilation, glycogenolysis (breakdown of stored glycogen to glucose for energy), and other sympathetic responses. This stimulation could be dangerous in some cardiovascular conditions that could be exacerbated by the sympathetic effects. In the male, the increased blood flow to the penis causes erection, which is necessary for penetration of the female and depositing of the sperm. Any drug therapy or disease process that interferes with the sympathetic response or the innervation of the sexual organs will change the person's ability to experience the human sexual response. This is important to keep in mind

<table>
<tr><td>

BOX 39-3

Effects of Testosterone on the Body

Growth of male and sexual accessory organs (penis, prostate gland, seminal vesicles, vas deferens)
Growth of testes and scrotal sac
Thickening of vocal chords, producing the deep, male voice
Hair growth on the face, body, arms, legs, and trunk
Male-pattern baldness
Increased protein anabolism and decreased protein catabolism (this causes larger and more powerful muscle development)
Increased bone growth in length and width, which ends when the testosterone stimulates closure of the epiphyses
Thickening of the cartilage and skin, leading to the male gait
Vascular thickening
Increased hematocrit

</td></tr>
</table>

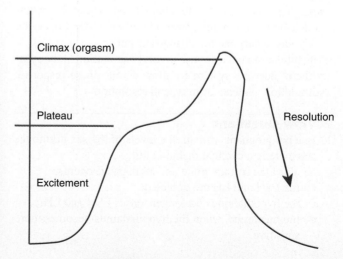

FIGURE 39-6. Human sexual response.

when doing patient teaching and when evaluating the effects of a drug.

WEB LINK
Students may want to explore the following Internet source:

Explore the virtual reproductive system:
 http://www.InnerBody.com

CHAPTER SUMMARY

- Male and female reproductive systems arise from the same fetal cells.
- The female ovary stores ova and produces the sex hormones estrogen and progesterone.
- The male testes produce sperm and the sex hormone testosterone.
- The hypothalamus releases GnRH at puberty to stimulate the anterior pituitary release of FSH and LH, thus stimulating the production and release of the sex hormones. Levels are controlled by a series of negative feedback systems.
- Female sex hormones are released in a cyclical fashion. Male sex hormones are released in a steadier fashion.
- Female sex hormones prepare the body for pregnancy and the maintenance of the pregnancy. Ovulation is the release of an egg for possible fertilization.
- If pregnancy does not occur, the prepared inner lining of the uterus is sloughed off as menstruation in the menstrual cycle, so that the lining can be prepared again when ovulation reoccurs.
- Menopause in women and the male climacteric in men occur when the body can no longer produce sex hormones, and the hypothalamus and anterior pituitary respond by releasing increasing levels of GnRH, FSH, and LH in an attempt to achieve higher levels of sex hormones.
- The testes produce sperm in the seminiferous tubules, in response to FSH stimulation, and testosterone in the interstitial cells, in response to LH stimulation.
- Testosterone is responsible for the development of male sex characteristics. These characteristics can be maintained by the androgens from the adrenal gland once the body has undergone the changes of puberty.
- The human sexual response involves activation of the sympathetic nervous system to allow a four-phase response: stimulation, plateau, climax, and resolution.

Review Questions

1. In a nonpregnant woman, the levels of the sex hormones fluctuate in a cyclical fashion until
   a. all of the ova are gone and menopause occurs.
   b. the FSH and LH are depleted.
   c. the hypothalamus no longer senses FSH and LH.
   d. the menarche, when the hypothalamus becomes more sensitive.

2. A woman develops ova, or eggs
   a. continually until menopause.
   b. during fetal life.
   c. until menopause.
   d. starting with puberty.

3. Control of the female sex hormones starts with the release of GnRH from the hypothalamus. Because of this, the cycling of these hormones may be influenced by
   a. body temperature.
   b. stress, emotional problems.
   c. age.
   d. androgen release.

4. Estrogen has many effects on the body. Estrogenic effects would not include
   a. increased levels of high-density lipoproteins.
   b. calcium resorption from the bone.
   c. closing of the epiphyses.
   d. development of facial hair.

5. The rhythm method of birth control depends on the effects of progesterone
   a. to increase uterine motility.
   b. to decrease and thicken cervical secretions.
   c. to elevate body temperature.
   d. to depress appetite.

6. The menstrual cycle
   a. always repeats itself every 28 days.
   b. is associated with the cyclical effects of the changing hormone levels.
   c. is necessary for a human sexual response.
   d. cannot occur if ovulation does not occur.

7. In the male reproductive system
   a. the seminiferous tubules produce sperm and testosterone.
   b. the interstitial cells produce sperm.
   c. the seminiferous tubules produce sperm and the interstitial cells produce testosterone.
   d. the interstitial cells produce sperm and testosterone.

8. Spring fever occurs as a result of increased light. In males, this increase light causes an increased production of
   a. inhibin.
   b. adrenal androgens.
   c. estrogen.
   d. testosterone.

9. Testosterone has many effects on the body. Testosterone effects would not include
   a. thickening of skin and vocal chords.
   b. development of a wide and flat pelvis.
   c. development of facial hair.
   d. closure of the epiphyses.

10. The human sexual response depends on stimulation of
    a. the sympathetic nervous system.
    b. the parasympathetic nervous system.
    c. the hypothalamic sex drive center.
    d. adrenal androgens.

BIBLIOGRAPHY

Bullock, B. L. (2000). *Focus on pathophysiology.* Philadelphia: Lippincott Williams & Wilkins.

Girard, J. (1991). *Endocrinology of puberty.* Farmington, CT: Karger Publishers.

Guyton, A., & Hall, J. (2000). *Textbook of medical physiology.* Philadelphia: W.B. Saunders.

Karch, A. M. (2002). *2003 Lippincott's nursing drug guide.* Philadelphia: Lippincott Williams & Wilkins.

Muske, L. E. (1993). *The neurobiology of reproductive behavior.* Farmington, CT: Karger Publishers.

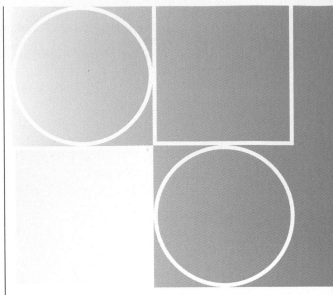

Drugs Affecting the Female Reproductive System

Key Terms

abortifacients

fertility drugs

oxytocics

progestins

tocolytics

Estrogens

dienestrol

🅟 estradiol

estrogens, conjugated

estrogens, esterified

estrone

estropipate

Estrogen Receptor Modulators

🅟 raloxifene

toremifene

Progestins

hydroxyprogesterone

🅟 levonorgestrel

medroxyprogesterone

norethindrone

norgestrel

progesterone

Fertility Drugs

cetrorelix

chorionic gonadotropin

chorionic gonadotropin alpha

🅟 clomiphene

follitropin alfa

follitropin beta

ganirelix

menotropins

urofollitropin

Oxytocics

ergonovine

methylergonovine

🅟 oxytocin

Abortifacients

carboprost

🅟 dinoprostone

mifepristone

Tocolytics

🅟 ritodrine

The female reproductive system uses a cycling balance to maintain homeostasis. Changing any factor in the system can have a wide variety of effects on the entire body. Drugs that are used to affect the female reproductive system include the female steroid hormones estrogen and the **progestins,** which include the endogenous female hormone progesterone and its various derivatives; estrogen receptor modulators, which are not hormones but affect specific estrogen receptor sites; **fertility drugs,** which stimulate the female reproductive system; **oxytocics,** which stimulate uterine contractions and assist labor; **abortifacients,** which are used to induce abortion; and **tocolytics,** which are used to relax the gravid uterus to prolong pregnancy (Figure 40–1).

ESTROGENS

Estrogens are used in many clinical situations. For example, in small doses, they are used for hormone replacement therapy (HRT) when ovarian activity is blocked or absent. They also are useful in palliative and preventive therapy during menopause, when many of the beneficial effects of estrogen

are lost. (Box 40–1 lists combination products used as HRT.) Estrogens produce a wide variety of systemic effects, including protecting the heart from atherosclerosis, retaining calcium in the bones, and maintaining the secondary female sex characteristics. (See Box 39–1 in Chapter 39 for a complete list of estrogen effects.)

Estrogens that are available for use include dienestrol (*Ortho Dienestrol*), which is available only as a topical agent; estradiol (*Estrace, Climara,* and others), which is widely used and is found in combination form as an oral contraceptive; conjugated estrogens (*Premarin*), one of the most popular drugs for postmenopausal treatment; esterified estrogen (*Estratab*); estrone (*Kestrone* and others), which is slow-acting and is available only for intramuscular administration; and estropipate (*Ortho-Est, Ogen*), a slow-acting oral agent that has been associated with severe hepatic effects. Figure 40–2 summarizes the various forms in which estrogens are available.

Therapeutic Actions and Indications
As explained previously, estrogens are important for the development of the female reproductive system and secondary sex characteristics. They affect the release of pituitary follicle-

FIGURE 40–1. Sites of action of drugs affecting the female reproductive system.

DRUG THERAPY ACROSS THE LIFESPAN

Drugs Affecting the Female Reproductive System

Children	Adults	Older Adults
The estrogens and progestins have undergone little testing in children. Because of their effects on closure of the epiphyses, they should be used only with great caution in growing children. If oral contraceptives are prescribed for teenage girls, the smallest dose possible should be used and the child should be monitored carefully for metabolic and other effects.	If any of these drugs are used in males for the treatment of specific cancers, the patient should be advised about the possibility of estrogenic effects and appropriate support should be offered. Women who are receiving any of these drugs should receive an annual medical examination, including breast examination and Pap smear, to monitor for adverse effects and underlying medical conditions. The potential for adverse effects should be discussed and comfort measures provided. Women taking estrogen should be advised not to smoke because of the increased risk of thrombotic events. When combinations of these hormones are used as part of fertility programs, women need a great deal of psychological support and comfort measures to cope with the many adverse effects associated with these drugs. The risk of multiple births should be explained, as should the need for frequent monitoring. When abortifacients are used, patients need a great deal of psychological support. Written lists of signs and symptoms to report and what to expect are more effective than just verbal lists in this time of potential stress. These agents are not for use during pregnancy or lactation because of the potential for adverse effects on the fetus or neonate.	Hormone replacement therapy (HRT) is commonly used by postmenopausal women. Reports of benefits and risks are frequent and conflicting, and patients need support and reliable information to make informed decisions about the use of these drugs. If patients are also using alternative therapies, their effects on the HRT and other possible prescription drugs need to be carefully evaluated.

BOX 40-1

Combination Drugs Used for Menopause

Many fixed-combination drugs containing estrogen and a progestin are available specifically for relieving the signs and symptoms associated with menopause in women with an intact uterus. The benefits include reduction in the risk of osteoporosis and coronary artery disease. These drugs are taken as one tablet, once a day. Patients should receive regular medical follow-up and monitoring while taking these drugs.

Estradiol/norethindrone (*Activella*)
Estradiol/norgestimate (*Ortho-Prefest*)
Ethinyl estradiol/norethindrone acetate (*Femhrt 1/5*)
Estrogen/medoxyprogesterone (*Premphase*)
Estrogen/medoxyprogesterone/conjugated estrogens (*Prempro*)

BOX 40-1 (CONTINUED)

Combination Drugs Used for Menopause

A combination patch is also available. The patch should be changed two times each week.

Estrogen/norethindrone (*Combipatch*)

---

stimulating hormone (FSH) and luteinizing hormone (LH); cause capillary dilatation, fluid retention, and protein anabolism and thin the cervical mucous; conserve calcium and phosphorus and encourage bone formation; inhibit ovulation; and prevent postpartum breast discomfort. Estrogens also are responsible for the proliferation of the endometrial lining. An absence or decrease in estrogen produces the

	Oral	Injection	Vaginal cream or gel	Transdermal patch	Vaginal ring	Implant	Implanted uterine device
Estrogens							
chlorotrianisene	x	–	–	–	–	–	–
dienestrol	–	–	x	–	–	–	–
diethylstilbestrol	x	x	–	–	–	–	–
estradiol	x	x	x	x	x	–	–
estrogens, conjugated	x	x	x	–	–	–	–
estrogens, esterified	x	–	–	–	–	–	–
estrone	–	x	–	–	–	–	–
estropipate	x	–	x	–	–	–	–
Progestins							
etonogestrel	–	–	–	–	x	–	–
hydroxyprogesterone	–	x	–	–	–	–	–
levonorgestrel	–	–	–	–	–	x	x
medroxyprogesterone	x	x	–	–	–	–	–
norelgestromin	–	–	–	x	–	–	–
norethindrone	x	–	–	–	–	–	–
norgestrel	x	–	–	–	–	–	–
progesterone	–	x	x	–	–	–	–

FIGURE 40–2. Available forms of estrogen and progestin products.

signs and symptoms of menopause in the uterus, vagina, breasts, and cervix. Estrogens are known to compete with androgens for receptor sites; this trait makes them beneficial in certain androgen-dependent prostate cancers.

Estrogens are indicated for the palliation of moderate to severe vasomotor symptoms, atrophic vaginitis, and kraurosis vulvae (atrophy of the female genitalia) associated with menopause; in the treatment of female hypogonadism, female castration, and primary ovarian failure; for prevention of postpartum breast engorgement; in combination with progestins as oral contraceptives; as a postcoital contraceptive when taken in a particular sequence; to retard osteoporosis in postmenopausal women; to decrease the risk of coronary artery disease (CAD) in postmenopausal women; and as palliation in certain types of prostatic and mammary cancers (Figure 40–3).

Pharmacokinetics

Oral estrogens are well absorbed through the gastrointestinal (GI) tract and undergo extensive hepatic metabolism. They are excreted in the urine. Estrogens cross the placenta and enter breast milk. They should not be used during pregnancy or lactation because of associated adverse effects on the fetus and neonate.

Contraindications and Cautions

Estrogens are contraindicated in the presence of any known allergies to estrogens and in patients with pregnancy (serious fetal defects have occurred); idiopathic vaginal bleeding; breast cancer; any estrogen-dependent cancer; history of

thromboembolic disorders (because of the increased risk of thrombus and embolus development); or hepatic dysfunction (because of the effects of estrogen on liver function).

Estrogens should be used with caution during lactation, because of possible effects on the neonate; with metabolic bone disease, because of the bone-conserving effect of estrogen; with renal insufficiency, because of the affect on fluid and electrolytes and because estrogens are excreted in the urine; and with hepatic impairment, because of the many effects on the liver and GI tract and because estrogens are metabolized in the liver.

Adverse Effects

Many of the most common adverse effects associated with estrogens involve the genitourinary (GU) tract; they include breakthrough bleeding, menstrual irregularities, dysmenorrhea, amenorrhea, and changes in libido. Other effects can result from the systemic effects of estrogens, including fluid retention, electrolyte disturbances, headache, dizziness, mental changes, weight changes, and edema. GI effects also are fairly common and include nausea, vomiting, abdominal cramps and bloating, and colitis. Potentially serious GI effects of acute pancreatitis, cholestatic jaundice, and hepatic adenoma have been reported with the use of estrogens.

Clinically Important Drug–Drug Interactions

If estrogens are given in combination with drugs that enhance hepatic metabolism of the estrogens (eg, barbiturates, rifampin, tetracyclines, phenytoin), decreased serum levels of estrogens may occur.

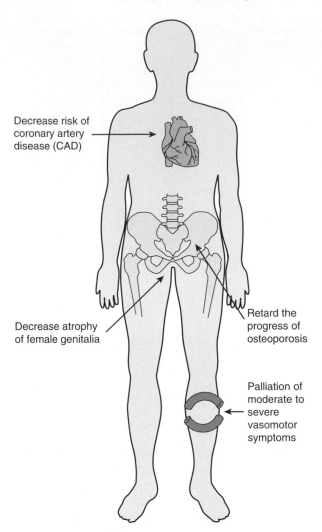

Decrease risk of
coronary artery
disease (CAD)

Decrease atrophy
of female genitalia

Retard the
progress of
osteoporosis

Palliation of
moderate to
severe
vasomotor
symptoms

FIGURE 40-3. Sites of action of the estrogens.

Whenever a drug is added to or removed from a drug regimen that contains estrogens, the nurse should evaluate that drug for possible interactions and consult with the prescriber for appropriate dosage adjustments.

Estrogens have been associated with increased therapeutic and toxic effects of corticosteroids, so patients taking both drugs should be monitored very closely.

Smoking while taking estrogens should be strongly discouraged, because the combination with nicotine increases the risk for development of thrombi and emboli.

Grapefruit juice can inhibit the metabolism of estradiols, leading to increased serum levels. If grapefruit juice is used, it should taken 2 hours before or after estradiol.

ESTROGEN RECEPTOR MODULATORS

Estrogen receptor modulators were developed to produce some of the positive effects of estrogen replacement, yet limit the adverse effects. The two estrogen receptor modulators that are currently available are raloxifene (*Evista*), which is used to prevent and treat osteoporosis, and toremifene (*Fareston*), which is used as an antineoplastic agent because of its effects on estrogen receptor sites (see Chapter 14 for information on this drug). The long-term effects of these two drugs are not yet known.

Therapeutic Actions and Indications
Raloxifene has modulating effects on estrogen receptor sites, stimulating some and blocking others. It is used therapeutically to stimulate specific estrogen receptor sites so as to increase bone mineral density without stimulating the endometrium in women. It is indicated for the treatment of postmenopausal osteoporosis.

Pharmacokinetics
Raloxifene is well absorbed from the GI tract and is metabolized in the liver. Excretion occurs through the feces. It is known to cross the placenta and enter into breast milk. It should not be used during pregnancy or lactation.

Contraindications and Cautions
Raloxifene is contraindicated in the presence of any known allergy to raloxifene, and in pregnancy and lactation (because of potential effects on the fetus or neonate). Caution should be used in patients with a history of venous thrombosis or smoking, because of an increased risk of blood clot formation when smoking and estrogen are combined.

Adverse Effects
Raloxifene has been associated with GI upset, nausea, and vomiting. Changes in fluid balance may also cause headache, dizziness, visual changes, and mental changes. Hot flashes, skin rash, edema, and vaginal bleeding may occur, secondary to specific estrogen receptor stimulation. Venous thromboembolism is a potentially dangerous side effect that has been reported.

Nursing Considerations for Patients Receiving Estrogens or Estrogen Receptor Modulators
Assessment: History and Examination

Screen for the following conditions, which could be cautions or contraindications to use of the drug: history of allergy to any estrogen or estrogen product, pregnancy, lactation, hepatic dysfunction, cardiovascular disease, breast or genital cancer, renal disease, metabolic bone disease, history of thromboembolism, smoking, and idiopathic vaginal bleeding.

Include screening for baseline status before beginning therapy and for any potential adverse effects: skin color, lesions, texture; affect, orientation, mental status, reflexes; blood pressure, pulse, cardiac auscultation, edema, perfusion; abdominal examination, liver examination, pelvic examination, Pap smear, urinalysis, breast examination, and ophthalmic examination (particularly if the patient wears contact lenses).

Nursing Diagnoses

The patient receiving estrogens or estrogen receptor modulators may have the following nursing diagnoses related to drug therapy:

DRUGS IN FOCUS
Estrogens

Drug Name	Dosage/Route	Usual Indications
dienestrol (*Ortho Dienestrol*)	1–2 applicatorsful intravaginally daily for 1–2 wk, then half the initial dose every other day for 1–2 wk, then 1 applicatorful one to three times per week	Palliation of signs and symptoms of menopause
Ⓟ estradiol (*Estrace*)	1–2 mg/d PO; 1–5 mg IM every 3–4 wk; 10–20 mg valerate in oil IM every 4 wk; or 1–5 mg cypionate in oil IM every 3–4 wk; 2–4 g intravaginal cream daily; apply vaginal ring once every 90 d	Palliation of signs and symptoms of menopause, prostate cancer, inoperable breast cancer; treatment of female hypogonadism; postpartum breast engorgement
estrogens, conjugated (*C.E.S.*)	0.3–1.25 mg/d PO	Palliation of signs and symptoms of menopause, prostate cancer, inoperable breast cancer; treatment of female hypogonadism, postpartum breast engorgement; to retard the progress of osteoporosis
estrogens, esterified (*Estratab*)	0.3–1.25 mg/d PO	Palliation of signs and symptoms of menopause, prostate cancer, inoperable breast cancer; treatment of female hypogonadism
estrone (*Kestrone*)	0.1–0.5 mg IM two to three times per week	Palliation of signs and symptoms of menopause, prostate cancer; treatment of female hypogonadism, treatment of abnormal uterine bleeding
estropipate (*Ortho-Est*)	0.625–5 mg/d PO	Palliation of signs and symptoms of menopause; treatment of female hypogonadism

- Excess Fluid Volume related to fluid retention
- Acute Pain related to systemic side effects
- Ineffective Tissue Perfusion (Cerebral, Cardiopulmonary, Peripheral)
- Deficient Knowledge regarding drug therapy

Implementation

- Administer drug as prescribed, *to prevent adverse effects;* administer with food if GI upset is severe, *to relieve GI distress.*
- Provide analgesics *for relief of headache as appropriate.*
- Arrange for at least an annual physical examination, including pelvic examination, Pap smear, and breast examination, *to avert adverse effects and monitor drug effects.*
- Monitor liver function periodically for the patient on long-term therapy, *to ensure that the drug is discontinued at any sign of hepatic dysfunction.*
- Provide support and reassurance *to deal with the drug and drug effects.*
- Provide thorough patient education, including measures to avoid adverse effects, warning signs of problems, and the need for regular evaluation, *to enhance patient knowledge about drug therapy and to promote compliance.*

Evaluation

- Monitor patient response to the drug (palliation of signs and symptoms of menopause, prevention of pregnancy, decreased risk of CAD, palliation of certain cancers).

- Monitor for adverse effects (liver changes, GI upset, edema, changes in secondary sex characteristics, headaches, thromboembolic episodes, breakthrough bleeding).
- Monitor for potential drug–drug interactions as indicated.
- Evaluate the effectiveness of the teaching plan: patient can name drug, dosage, adverse effects to watch for, specific measures to avoid adverse effects. (See Patient Teaching Checklist: Oral Contraceptives.)
- Monitor the effectiveness of comfort measures and compliance to the regimen (see Nursing Care Guide: Estrogens, Progestins).

PROGESTINS

Progestins are used as contraceptives, most effectively in combination with estrogens (Box 40–3 lists the currently available contraceptives); to treat amenorrhea and functional uterine bleeding; and as part of fertility programs. Like the estrogens, some progestins are useful in the treatment of specific cancers with specific receptor site sensitivity (see Chapter 14). A number of progestins are available for use. Hydroxyprogesterone (*Hylutin*) is available in for intramuscular injection to treat amenorrhea and to produce a secretory endometrium. Levonorgestrel (*Norplant System*) is used in an implant system to prevent pregnancy. It also is found in many combination oral contraceptives. Medroxyprogesterone (*Amen, Curretab*, and others) is available

CASE STUDY

Menopause

THE SITUATION
J. M. is a 52-year-old female who is being seen in her gynecologist's office for a routine annual physical and Pap smear. J. M. reports that her periods are closer together and much heavier than they used to be. Her mother went through menopause in her early 50s, so J. M. is anxious to know whether she is about to enter menopause and what to expect.

CRITICAL THINKING
What teaching and counseling issues will be important for J. M. at this time? *Think about myths and stories surrounding menopause and ways that these ideas can affect the experience people have.*

What important issues should be discussed when suggesting the advisability of hormone replacement therapy (HRT) to this patient?

What other measures can be taken to help a patient cope with the signs and symptoms of menopause that do not involve drug therapy?

DISCUSSION
The exact age at which a woman experiences menopause or "the change" varies. The age at which a patient's mother underwent menopause is a good measure for estimating when the patient can expect menopause. The nurse should review with J. M. the cause of menopause (running out of ova, so further production of estrogen and progesterone is drastically reduced). The

nurse also should discuss the physical signs and symptoms that J. M. might experience. These include hot flashes (a sign of vasomotor instability with feelings of heat and sweating unrelated to activity or environment); decreased muscle strength; personality changes; irregular and erratic periods; thin, dry skin; dryness of vaginal area; sleep disturbances; and changes in libido. The nurse also should advise J. M. about changes that she might not be aware of, such as the increased risk of coronary artery disease and heart attack, uterine atrophy, osteoporosis, and possible decrease in cognitive ability.

Nonpharmacological measures to help J. M. through menopause can be explored. Regular exercise can help to protect the heart and to relieve insomnia; environmental control can help to alleviate some of the discomfort of hot flashes; avoiding stimulants like caffeine can be beneficial in alleviating insomnia and in easing some of the mood swings that may occur. J. M. may want to discuss other "remedies" that she has heard about, and these can be explored with the health care provider.

The leading cause of death in postmenopausal women is heart disease, but research has shown that treating women with HRT can greatly decrease that risk. The health care provider should give J. M. information about replacement hormones for women in menopause. J. M. may be aware of the possible increased risk of breast or cervical cancer while taking these drugs, and the data available concerning that risk should be discussed (see Nursing Challenge).

---

orally for treating amenorrhea and by injection for cancer palliation therapy. Norethindrone (*Aygestin*) is used in combination oral contraceptives and alone for the treatment of amenorrhea. Norgestrel (*Ovrette*) is an oral contraceptive that is most effective when used in combination form. Progesterone (*Progestasert* and others) is available in several forms for the treatment of amenorrhea, contraception, and fertility programs. (See Figure 40–2 for a summary of the various forms in which progestins are available.)

Therapeutic Actions and Indications
The progestins transform the proliferative endometrium into a secretory endometrium, inhibit the secretion of FSH and LH, prevent follicle maturation and ovulation, inhibit uterine contractions, and may have some anabolic and estrogenic effects. When they are used as contraceptives, the exact mechanism of action is not known, but it is thought that circulating progestins and estrogens "trick" the hypothalamus and pituitary and prevent the release of gonadotropic releasing hormone (GnRH), FSH, and LH, thus preventing follicle development and ovulation. The low levels of these

hormones do not produce a lush endometrium that is receptive to implantation, and if ovulation and fertilization were to occur, the chances of implantation would be remote.

Progestins are indicated for contraception; as treatment of primary and secondary amenorrhea; as treatment for functional uterine bleeding; and in some fertility protocols. Some progestins are also effective as palliative treatment in specific cancers (see Chapter 14).

Pharmacokinetics
The progestins are well absorbed, undergo hepatic metabolism, and are excreted in the urine. They are known to cross the placenta and to enter breast milk. They are not for use during pregnancy or lactation because of the potential for adverse effects on the fetus or neonate.

Contraindications and Cautions
Progestins are contraindicated in the presence of any known allergies to progestins; pregnancy (serious fetal defects have occurred); idiopathic vaginal bleeding; breast cancer or genital cancer; history of thromboembolic disorders, including

NURSING CHALLENGE

Menopause and Hormone Replacement Therapy

Women experience the menarche, or onset of the menstrual cycle, in their adolescent years and menopause, or cessation of the menstrual cycle, in their middle years. The exact age at which a woman experiences menopause or "the change" varies. The family history of onset of menopause is a good guide for when the effects can be expected. Just as the physical changes associated with puberty can take a few years to be accomplished, the changes associated with menopause may also take a few years. The signs and symptoms of menopause are related to the loss of estrogen and progesterone effects on the body (see Case Study).

For centuries, women have proceeded through this time in their lives without pharmacological intervention. Many herbal and alternative therapies are available to help the transition through menopause (see Box 40–2). Women who rely on these therapies need to be cautioned about potential drug–drug interactions and advised to always report the use of these agents to their health care provider. Today, with more research and safer drugs available to counteract some of the effects of menopause, many women are being advised to use hormone replacement therapy (HRT). The use of HRT can decrease the discomforts associated with menopause and can dramatically decrease the risk of coronary artery disease, the leading cause of death among women older than 50 years of age in the Western world.

Various forms of HRT have been associated over the years with increased risks of breast cancer and cervical cancer, and many women are reluctant to consider HRT because of these effects. The newer drugs used in HRT have been shown to be associated with only a possible increase in risk of breast and cervical cancer. Patients with many risk factors for developing these cancers are at greater risk than patients with no risk factors. Other drugs, the estrogen receptor modulators, have antiestrogen effects on the breast and may remove the cancer risk. But these drugs may be less reliable in their management of the signs and symptoms of menopause and have not been correlated with a reduction in the risk of coronary artery disease.

The woman who is entering menopause should have all of the information available before deciding about the use of HRT. A complete family and personal history of cancer and coronary artery disease risk factors should be completed to help the patient balance the benefits versus the risks of this therapy. This is a very difficult decision for many women to make. The nurse is often in the best position to provide information, listen to concerns, and help the patient decide what is best for her. If the decision is made to use HRT, the patient may need support in dealing with the effects of the drugs and may have to try several different preparations before the one best suited to her is found. This can be a very frustrating time, so the patient will need a consistent, reliable person to turn to with questions and for support. As more research is done in women's health issues, better therapies may be developed to help women through this transition in life.

BOX 40-2

Herbal and Alternative Therapies Used in Menopause

black cohosh—40 mg/d active ingredient, should not be used for longer than 60 d; monitor for dizziness, nausea, vomiting, visual disturbances; contains alcohol, do not combine with disulfiram, metronidazole

borage—90–500 mg PO in softgel capsules, not for long-term use; use caution with seizure disorders or liver impairment

chaste tree—150–325 mg PO q.d.–b.i.d.; may cause increased blood pressure, avoid use with antihypertensives or β-blockers, may cause rash and itching

clary—8 gtt in 1 oz of water q.d. as an atomizer or dissolved in bath water; may cause sedation, avoid use with alcohol; not for internal use

devil's claw—1.5–6 g/d PO depending on preparation; increases stomach acid and may interfere with many prescription drugs, use with caution

dong quai—500 mg PO; causes photosensitivity, avoid exposure to the sun; do not use with warfarin, increased bleeding can occur

false unicorn root—1–2 mL PO t.i.d.; do not use with estrogen or progestins, may alter uterine effects

red clover—4 g PO t.i.d. as tea; 30–60 gtt PO t.i.d. of liquid extract; do not use with heparin or warfarin because of increased bleeding effects; do not combine with hormone replacement therapy because of risk of increased estrogenic effects

soy—25 g/d PO; do not use with calcium, iron, or zinc products; may decrease effects of estrogen, raloxifene, tamoxifen, alert health care provider if combining these drugs

wild yam—1–6 g/d PO; contains progesterone, do not use with hormone replacement therapy; may cause increased blood glucose and other toxic effects; do not combine with disulfiram or metronidazole, severe reaction may occur

cerebrovascular accident (because of the increased risk of thrombus and embolus development); hepatic dysfunction (because of the effects of progestins on the liver function); pelvic inflammatory disease (PID), sexually transmitted diseases, endometriosis, or pelvic surgery (because of the effects of progestins on the uterus); and lactation (because of potential effects on the neonate).

Progestins should be used with caution in patients with epilepsy, migraine headaches, asthma, or cardiac or renal dysfunction, because of the potential exacerbation of these conditions.

Adverse Effects

Adverse effects associated with progestins vary with the administration route used. Oral contraceptives are associated

DRUGS IN FOCUS
Estrogen Receptor Modulators

Drug Name	Dosage/Route	Usual Indications
Ⓟ raloxifene *Evista*	60 mg PO q.d.	Treatment of postmenopausal osteoporosis

with thromboembolic disorders (particularly when combined with nicotine), increased blood pressure, weight gain, and headache. Dermal patch contraceptives are associated with the same systemic effects as well as local skin irritation. Vaginal gel use is associated with headache, nervousness, constipation, breast enlargement, and perineal pain. Intrauterine systems are associated with abdominal pain, endometriosis, abortion, PID, and expulsion of the intrauterine device. Vaginal use is associated with local irritation and swelling. Parenteral routes are associated with breakthrough bleeding, spotting, changes in the menstrual cycle, breast tenderness, thrombophlebitis, vision changes, weight gain, and fluid retention.

Nursing Considerations for Patients Receiving Progestins
Assessment: History and Examination

Screen for the following conditions, which could be cautions or contraindications to use of the drug: history of allergy to any progestin product, pregnancy, lactation, hepatic dysfunction, cardiovascular disease, breast or genital cancer, renal disease, history of thromboembolism, smoking, idiopathic vaginal bleeding, pelvic disease, asthma, and epilepsy.

Include screening for baseline status before beginning therapy and for any potential adverse effects: skin color, le-

PATIENT TEACHING CHECKLIST
Oral Contraceptives

Create customized patient teaching materials for a specific oral contraceptive from the CD-ROM. Patient teaching should stress the following points for drugs within this class:

• An oral contraceptive (OC) or birth control pill contains specific amounts of female sex hormones that work to make the body unreceptive to pregnancy and to prevent ovulation, the release of the egg from the ovary. Because these hormones affect many systems in your body, it is important to have regular physical checkups while you are taking this drug.
• Many drugs affect the way that OCs work. To be safe, avoid the use of over-the counter drugs and other drugs, unless you first check with your health care provider.

Some of the following adverse effects may occur:

• *Headache, nervousness*—Check with your health care provider about the use of an analgesic; this effect usually passes after a few months on the drug.
• *Nausea, loss of appetite*—This usually passes with time; consult your health care provider if it is a problem.
• *Swelling, weight gain*—Water retention is a normal effect of these hormones. Limiting salt intake may help. You may have trouble with contact lenses if you wear them, because the body often retains fluid, which may change the shape of your eye. This usually adjusts over time.

Cigarette smoking can aggravate serious side effects of OCs, such as the formation of blood clots. When taking OCs, it is advisable to cut down, or preferably to stop, cigarette smoking.
Tell any doctor, nurse, or other health care provider that you are taking this drug.
Report any of the following to your health care provider: pain in the calves or groin; chest pain or difficulty breathing; lump in the breast; severe headache, dizziness, visual changes; severe abdominal pain; yellowing of the skin; pregnancy.
Bleeding (a false menstrual period) should occur during the time that the drug is withdrawn.
Report bleeding at *any* other time to your health care provider.
It is important to have regular medical checkups, including Pap smears, while you are taking this drug. If you decide to stop the drug to become pregnant, consult with your health care provider.
Keep this drug and all medications out of the reach of children.
A patient package insert is included with the drug. Read this information and feel free to ask any questions that you might have.

This Teaching Checklist reflects general patient teaching guidelines. It is not meant to be a substitute for drug-specific teaching information, which is available in nursing drug guides.

NURSING CARE GUIDE

Estrogens, Progestins

Assessment	Nursing Diagnoses	Implementation	Evaluation
HISTORY Allergies to any estrogens; pregnancy, lactation; breast or genital cancer; hepatic dysfunction; CAD; thromboembolic disease; renal disease; idiopathic vaginal bleeding; metabolic bone disease; diabetes	Excess Fluid Volume related to fluid retention Acute Pain related to systemic side effects Ineffective Tissue Perfusion Deficient Knowledge regarding drug therapy	Administer as prescribed. Administer with meals. Provide analgesics for headache if appropriate. Provide at least annual physical examination, including Pap smear and breast exam. Provide support and reassurance to deal with drug therapy. Provide patient teaching regarding drug name, dosage, adverse effects, precautions, warnings to report, safe administration.	Evaluate drug effects: prevention of pregnancy; relief of signs and symptoms of menopause; decreased risk of CAD. Monitor for adverse effects: liver changes; GI upset; edema; changes in secondary sex characteristics; headaches; thromboembolic episodes; breakthrough bleeding. Monitor for drug–drug interactions as indicated for each drug. Evaluate effectiveness of patient teaching program. Evaluate effectiveness of comfort and safety measures.
PHYSICAL EXAMINATION Neurological: orientation, reflexes, affect, mental status Skin: color, lesions CV: P, cardiac auscultation, BP, edema, perfusion GI: abdominal exam, liver exam GU: pelvic exam, Pap smear, urinalysis Eye: ophthalmic exam			

BOX 40-3

Contraceptives

Oral contraceptives are available as monophasic, biphasic, and triphasic preparations. One tablet is taken orally for 21 days, beginning on the fifth day of the cycle (day 1 of the cycle is the first day of menstrual bleeding). Inert tablets or no tablets are taken for the next 7 days, and then a new course of 21 days is started.

Missed doses—If one tablet is missed, take it as soon as possible or take 2 tablets the next day. If two consecutive tablets are missed, take 2 tablets daily for the next 2 days, then resume the regular schedule. If three consecutive tablets are missed, begin a new cycle of tablets 7 days after the last tablet was taken, and use an additional method of birth control until the start of the next menstrual period.

Postcoital or emergency contraception ("morning after" regimen)—The dosing regimen must start within 72 hours after unprotected intercourse, and a follow-up dose of the same number of pills must be taken 12 h after the first dose. The dosages are as follows:

Ovral	2 white tablets
Nordette	4 light orange tablets

Box 40–3 continues on page 532

BOX 40-3 (CONTINUED)

Contraceptives

Lo/Ovral	4 white tablets
Triphasil	4 yellow tablets
Levlen	4 light orange tablets
Tri-Levlen	4 yellow tablets
Preven	Postcoital contraception kit includes a pregnancy test, used first to ensure that there is no pregnancy; 4 tablets containing levonorgestrel and ethinyl estradiol are then taken—two within 72 h after intercourse and two 12 h later.
Plan B (levonorgestrel)	Take 1 tablet 72 h after intercourse and a second tablet 12 h later.

MONOPHASIC ORAL CONTRACEPTIVES

Alesse, Avian 28	20 μg estradiol, 0.10 mg levonorgestrel
Brevicon, Modicon	35 μg estradiol, 0.5 mg norethindrone
Demulen 1/50, Zovia 1/50E	50 μg estradiol, 1 mg ethynodiol diacetate
Demulen 1/35, Zovia 1/35E	35 μg ethinyl estradiol, 1 mg ethynodiol diacetate
Desogen, Ortho-Cept	30 μg ethinyl estradiol, 0.15 mg desogestrel
Levlen, Levora 0.15/30, Nordette	30 μg ethinyl estradiol, 0.15 mg levonorgestrel
Levlite	0.10 mg levonorgestrel, 0.2 mg ethinyl estradiol
Loestrin 21 1.5/30	30 μg ethinyl estradiol, 1.5 mg norethindrone
Loestrin 21 1/20	20 μg estradiol, 1 mg norethindrone
Lo/Ovral	30 μg ethinyl estradiol, 0.3 mg norgestrel
Necon 1/50, Norinyl 1+50, Nelova 1/50 M	50 μg mestranol, 1 mg norethindrone
Necon 1/35, Norinyl 1+35, Ortho-Novum 1/35	35 μg ethinyl estradiol, 1 mg norethindrone
Ortho-Cyclen	35 μg ethinyl estradiol, 0.25 mg norgestimate
Ortho-Novum 1/50, Ovcon 50	50 μg ethinyl estradiol, 1 mg norethindrone
Ovcon-35	35 μg ethinyl estradiol, 0.4 mg norethindrone
Ovral-28	50 μg ethinyl estradiol, 0.5 mg norgestrel
Yasmin	30 μg ethinyl estradiol, 3 mg drospirenone

BIPHASIC ORAL CONTRACEPTIVES

Jenest-28	phase 1, 10 tablets: 0.5 mg norethindrone, 35 μg ethinyl estradiol
	phase 2, 11 tablets: 1 mg norethindrone, 35 μg ethinyl estradiol
Necon 10/11, Ortho-Novum 10/11	phase 1, 10 tablets: 0.5 mg norethindrone, 35 μg ethinyl estradiol
	phase 2, 11 tablets: 1 mg norethindrone, 35 μg ethinyl estradiol
Mircette	phase 1, 21 tablets: 0.15 mg desogesinel, 20 μg ethinyl estradiol
	phase 2, 5 tablets: 0.01 mg ethinyl estradiol

TRIPHASIC ORAL CONTRACEPTIVES

Estrostep 21, Estrostep Fe	phase 1, 5 tablets: 1 mg norethindrone, 20 μg ethinyl estradiol
	phase 2, 7 tablets: 1 mg norethindrone, 30 μg ethinyl estradiol
	phase 3, 9 tablets: 1 mg norethindrone, 35 μg ethinyl estradiol
Ortho-Novum 7/7/7	phase 1, 7 tablets: 0.5 mg norethindrone, 35 μg ethinyl estradiol
	phase 2, 7 tablets: 0.75 mg norethindrone, 35 μg ethinyl estradiol
	phase 3, 7 tablets: 1 mg norethindrone, 35 μg ethinyl estradiol
Ortho Tri-Cyclen	phase 1, 7 tablets: 0.18 mg norgestimate, 35 μg ethinyl estradiol
	phase 2, 7 tablets: 0.215 mg norgestimate, 35 μg ethinyl estradiol
	phase 3, 7 tablets: 0.25 mg norgestimate, 35 μg ethinyl estradiol

IMPLANTED SYSTEM
Norplant　　Six Silastic capsules implanted for a period of 3 y or 5 y; releases low-dose levonorgestrel

INTRAUTERINE SYSTEM
Mirena　　Inserted into the uterus, releases low-dose levonorgestrel over a 5-y period

PATCH CONTRACEPTIVE
Ortho Evra　　Three patches per cycle, each worn for 1 wk; releases estrogen and progestin to prevent ovulation; found to be as safe and effective as oral contraceptives and easier to remember to use for some patients

VAGINAL RING
NuvaRing　　Ethinyl estrodial/etonogestrol; ring inserted vaginally once a month and kept in place for 3 wk; after a week's rest, a new ring is inserted

DRUGS IN FOCUS
Progestins

Drug Name	Dosage/Route	Usual Indications
hydroxyprogesterone (*Hylutin*)	375 mg IM, cycle with estradiol	Treatment of amenorrhea; production of a secretory endometrium for fertility treatment
Ⓟ levonorgestrel (*Norplant System*)	Six Silastic capsules, each with 36 mg, inserted during first 7 d after onset of menses, replace every 5 y	Contraception
medroxyprogesterone (*Amen, Curretab*)	5–10 mg/d PO for 5–10 d; 400–1000 mg/wk IM for cancer therapy	Treatment of amenorrhea; palliation of certain cancers
norethindrone (*Aygestin*)	2.5–10 mg/d PO	Contraception, treatment of amenorrhea
norgestrel (*Ovrette*)	0.075–0.35 mg/d PO	Contraception
progesterone (*Progestasert*)	5–10 mg/d IM for 6–8 d; 90 mg/d intravaginally	Contraception, treatment of amenorrhea, fertility programs

sions, texture; affect, orientation, mental status, reflexes; blood pressure, pulse, cardiac auscultation, edema, perfusion; abdominal examination, liver examination, pelvic examination, Pap smear, urinalysis, breast examination, and ophthalmic examination (particularly if the patient wears contact lenses).

Nursing Diagnoses

Follow the same guidelines as for estrogens.

Implementation

Follow the same guidelines as for estrogens.

Evaluation

Follow the same guidelines as for estrogens (see Nursing Care Guide: Estrogens, Progestins).

FERTILITY DRUGS

Women without primary ovarian failure who cannot get pregnant after a year of trying may be candidates for the use of fertility drugs. These drugs act to stimulate follicle development and ovulation in functioning ovaries and are combined with human chorionic gonadotropin (HCG) to maintain the follicles once ovulation has occurred. The following fertility drugs are in use today.

Cetrorelix (*Cetrotide*) an injected drug that inhibits premature LH surges in women undergoing controlled ovarian

stimulation by acting as a GnRH antagonist. Chorionic gonadotropin (*Chorex, Profasi, Pregnyl*) is an injected drug that is used to stimulate ovulation by acting like GnRH and affecting FSH and LH release. Chorionic gonadotropin alpha (*Ovidrel*) is an injected drug that stimulates final follicular development and ovulation in infertile women. Clomiphene (*Clomid* and others) is a commonly used oral agent that is also used for the treatment of male infertility. Follitropin alfa (*Gonal-F*) and follitropin beta (*Follistim*) are FSH molecules produced by recombinant DNA technology; they are injected to stimulate follicular development in infertility and for harvesting ova for in vitro fertilization. Ganirelix (*Antagon*) is an injected drug which inhibits premature LH surges in women undergoing controlled ovarian hyperstimulation as part of a fertility program. Menotropins (*Pergonal, Humegon*) is a purified gonadotropin (similar to FSH and LH) that is also used to stimulate spermatogenesis. Urofollitropin (*Fertinex*) is an injected preparation derived from the urine of postmenopausal women; it has been associated with immune-type reactions. With the development of newer, purer drugs, urofollitropin is used less often.

Therapeutic Actions and Indications

Fertility drugs work either directly or by stimulating the hypothalamus to increase FSH and LH levels and stimulate ovarian follicular development and maturation of ova. Given in sequence with HCG to maintain the follicle and hormone production, these drugs are used to treat infertility in women with functioning ovaries whose partners are fertile. Fertility drugs also may be used to stimulate multiple follicle development for the harvesting of ova for in vitro fertilization. Menotropins also stimulates spermatogenesis in men with low sperm counts and otherwise normally functioning testes.

Pharmacokinetics

These drugs are well absorbed and are treated like endogenous hormones within the body, undergoing hepatic metabolism and renal excretion. They should not be used during pregnancy or lactation because of the potential for adverse hormonal effects on the fetus or neonate.

Contraindications and Cautions

These drugs are contraindicated in the presence of primary ovarian failure (they only work to stimulate functioning ovaries); thyroid or adrenal dysfunction (because of the effects on the hypothalamic–pituitary axis); ovarian cysts; pregnancy (serious fetal defects have occurred); idiopathic uterine bleeding; and known allergy to any fertility drug. Caution should be used with lactation, thromboembolic diseases (because of the risk of increased thrombus formation), and respiratory diseases (because of alterations in fluid volume and blood flow).

Adverse Effects

Adverse effects associated with fertility drugs include a greatly increased risk of multiple births and birth defects; ovarian overstimulation (abdominal pain, distention, ascites, pleural effusion); and headache, fluid retention, nausea, bloating, uterine bleeding, ovarian enlargement, gynecomas-

tia, and febrile reactions (possibly due to stimulation of progesterone release).

Nursing Considerations for Patients Receiving Fertility Drugs

Assessment: History and Examination

Screen for the following conditions, which could be cautions or contraindications to use of the drug: history of allergy to any fertility drug, pregnancy, lactation, ovarian failure, thyroid or adrenal dysfunction, ovarian cysts, idiopathic uterine bleeding, thromboembolic diseases, and respiratory diseases.

Include screening for baseline status before beginning therapy and for any potential adverse effects: skin, lesions; orientation, affect, reflexes; blood pressure, pulse; respiration, adventitious sounds; hormone levels, Pap smear, breast examination.

Nursing Diagnoses

The patient receiving fertility drugs may have the following nursing diagnoses related to drug therapy:

- Disturbed Body Image related to drug treatment and diagnosis
- Acute Pain related to headache, fluid retention, GI upset

DRUGS IN FOCUS
Fertility Drugs

Drug Name	Dosage/Route	Usual Indications
cetrorelix (Cetrotide)	3 mg SC during early follicular phase or 0.25 mg SC on day 5 of 6 of stimulation and then every day until HCG is administered	Inhibition of premature luteinizing hormone (LH) surge in women undergoing controlled ovarian stimulation
chorionic gonadotropin (Chorex, Profasi)	2,000–10,000 IU SC depending on timing and indication	Ovulation induction, hypogonadism, prepubertal cryptorchidism
chorionic gonadotropin alpha (Ovidrel)	250 μg SC, timing depends on indication	Induction of final follicular maturation and ovulation induction
Ⓟ clomiphene (Clomid and others)	50–100 mg/d PO with length of therapy and timing dependent on the particular situation	Treatment of infertility
follitropin alfa (Gonal-F)	75–150 IU/d SC, dosage increases based on response; do not exceed 300 IU/d	Stimulation of follicular development for harvesting of ova
follitropin beta (Follistim)	75–225 IU/d SC, dosage increases based on response; do not exceed 300 IU/d	Stimulation of follicular development for harvesting of ova
ganirelix (Antagon)	250 μg/d SC during early follicular phase	Inhibition of premature LH surges in women undergoing controlled ovarian hyperstimulation
menotropins (Pergonal)	Treatment scheduled with HCG; 150 IU FSH/150 IU LH IM for 9–12 d is often used	Stimulation of ovulation in women and spermatogenesis in men
urofollitropin (Fertinex)	75–150 IU/d IM for 7–12 d cycled with HCG, dosage dependent on response	Stimulation of ovulation for the treatment of infertility and to stimulate follicular development for harvesting of ova

- Sexual Dysfunction
- Deficient Knowledge regarding drug therapy

Implementation

- Assess the cause of dysfunction before beginning therapy, *to ensure appropriate use of the drug.*
- Complete a pelvic examination before each cycle of drug therapy, *to rule out ovarian enlargement, pregnancy, or uterine problems.*
- Check urine estrogen and estradiol levels before beginning therapy, *to verify ovarian function.*
- Administer with an appropriate dosage of HCG as indicated, *to ensure beneficial effects.*
- Discontinue the drug at any sign of ovarian overstimulation, *and arrange for hospitalization if this occurs.*
- Provide women with a calendar of treatment days, explanations of adverse effects to anticipate, and instructions on when intercourse should occur, *to increase the therapeutic effectiveness of the drug.*
- Provide warnings about the risk and hazards of multiple births, *so the patient can make informed decisions about drug therapy.*
- Provide thorough patient education, including measures to avoid adverse effects, warning signs of problems, and the need for regular evaluation *to enhance patient knowledge about drug therapy and to promote compliance.*

Evaluation

- Monitor patient response to the drug (ovulation).
- Monitor for adverse effects (abdominal bloating, weight gain, ovarian overstimulation, multiple births).
- Evaluate the effectiveness of the teaching plan (patient can name drug, dosage, adverse effects to watch for, specific measures to avoid adverse effects).
- Monitor the effectiveness of comfort measures and compliance with the regimen.

OXYTOCICS

Oxytocic drugs are used to stimulate contraction of the uterus, much like the action of the hypothalamic hormone oxytocin, which is stored in the posterior pituitary. These drugs include ergonovine (*Ergotrate*), which is given intramuscularly or intravenously and is used to prevent and treat postpartum and postabortion uterine atony; methylergonovine (*Methergine*), which can be given intramuscularly or intravenously directly after delivery, then continued in the oral form to promote uterine involution; and oxytocin (*Pitocin, Syntocinon*), which is used to induce labor and to promote uterine contractions after labor. Oxytocin is also available in a nasal form to stimulate milk "let down" in lactating women.

Therapeutic Actions and Indications

The oxytocics directly affect neuroreceptor sites to stimulate contraction of the uterus. They are especially effective in the gravid uterus. Oxytocin, a synthetic form of the hypothalamic hormone, also stimulates the lacteal glands in the breast to contract, promoting milk ejection in lactating women.

Oxytocics are indicated for the prevention and treatment of uterine atony after delivery. This is important to prevent postpartum hemorrhage. Ergonovine is being investigated for use in diagnostic tests for angina during arteriography studies because it has been shown to induce coronary artery contraction. Methylergonovine has been successfully used to stimulate the last stage of labor. Oxytocin is used in a nasal form to stimulate milk "let down" in lactating women. It is also being evaluated as a diagnostic agent to test abnormal fetal heart rates (oxytocin challenge) and to treat breast engorgement.

Pharmaockinetics

The oxytocics are rapidly absorbed, metabolized in the liver, and excreted in urine and feces. They cross the placenta and enter breast milk. Because of their effects on the uterus, they are not used during pregnancy. Oxytocin is used during lactation because of its effects on milk ejection, but the baby

DRUGS IN FOCUS
Oxytocics

Drug Name	Dosage/Route	Usual Indications
ergonovine (*Ergotrate*)	0.2 mg IM, may repeat doses q2–4h as needed for no more than 5 doses	Prevention and treatment of postpartum and postabortion uterine atony
methylergonovine (*Methergine*)	0.2 mg IM or IV, may repeat q2–4h; 0.2 mg PO t.i.d. or q.i.d. during the puerperium for up to 1 wk	Promotion of postpartum uterine involution
oxytocin (*Pitocin, Syntocinon*)	1–2 mU/min IV through an infusion pump, increase as needed, do not exceed 20 mU/min; 10 U IM after delivery of the placenta	Induction of labor; promotion of uterine contractions postpartum; nasally to stimulate milk "let down" in lactating women

should be evaluated for any adverse effects associated with the hormone.

Contraindications and Cautions

Oxytocics are contraindicated in the presence of any known allergy to oxytocics and with cephalopelvic disproportion, unfavorable fetal position, complete uterine atony, or early pregnancy. Caution should be used in patients with coronary disease, hypertension, lactation, or previous cesarean section.

Adverse Effects

The adverse effects most often associated with the oxytocics are related to excessive effects (eg, uterine hypertonicity and spasm, uterine rupture, postpartum hemorrhage, decreased fetal heart rate). GI upset, nausea, headache, and dizziness are not uncommon. Ergonovine and methylergonovine can produce ergotism (eg, nausea, blood pressure changes, weak pulse, dyspnea, chest pain, numbness and coldness in extremities, confusion, excitement, delirium, convulsions, and even coma). Oxytocin has caused severe water intoxication with coma and even maternal death when used for a prolonged period. This is thought to occur because of related effects of antidiuretic hormone (ADH), which is also stored in the posterior pituitary and may be released in response to oxytocin activity, causing water retention in the kidney.

Nursing Considerations for Patients Receiving Oxytocics

Assessment: History and Examination

Screen for the following conditions, which could be cautions or contraindications to use of the drug: history of allergy to oxytocics, early pregnancy, lactation, uterine atony, hypertension, history of cesarean section, undesirable fetal position, and cephalopelvic disproportion.

Include screening for baseline status before beginning therapy and for any potential adverse effects: skin, lesions; orientation, affect, reflexes; blood pressure, pulse; respiration, adventitious sounds; fetal position, fetal heartbeat, uterine tone, and timing of contractions; and bleeding studies and complete blood count.

Nursing Diagnoses

The patient receiving oxytocics may have the following nursing diagnoses related to drug therapy:

- Acute Pain related to uterine contractions, headache, fluid retention, GI upset
- Excess Fluid Volume related to ergotism or water intoxication
- Deficient Knowledge regarding drug therapy

Implementation

- Ensure fetal position (if appropriate) and cephalopelvic proportions, *to prevent serious complications of delivery.*
- Regulate oxytocin delivery between contractions if being given *to stimulate labor.*

- Monitor blood pressure periodically during and after administration, *to monitor for adverse effects. Discontinue the drug if blood pressure rises dramatically.*
- Monitor uterine tone and involution and amount of bleeding, *to ensure safe and therapeutic use of the drug.*
- Discontinue the drug at any sign of uterine hypertonicity, *to avoid potentially life-threatening effects; provide life support as needed.*
- Monitor fetal heartbeat if given during labor, *to ensure safety of the fetus.*
- Provide nasal oxytocin at bedside with the bottle sitting upright. The patient should be instructed to invert the squeeze bottle and exert gentle pressure *to deliver the drug just before nursing.*
- Provide thorough patient education, including measures to avoid adverse effects and warning signs of problems to report, *to enhance patient knowledge about drug therapy and to promote compliance.*

Evaluation

- Monitor patient response to the drug (uterine contraction, prevention of hemorrhage, milk "let down").
- Monitor for adverse effects (blood pressure changes, uterine hypertonicity, water intoxication, ergotism).
- Evaluate the effectiveness of the teaching plan (patient can name drug, dosage, adverse effects to watch for, specific measures to avoid adverse effects).
- Monitor the effectiveness of comfort measures and compliance with the regimen.

ABORTIFACIENTS

Abortifacients are drugs used to evacuate the uterus by stimulating intense uterine contractions. These drugs include carboprost (*Hemabate*), dinoprostone (*Cervidil, Prepidil Gel, Prostin E2*), and mifepristone (RU-486, *Mifeprex*). Carboprost is an intramuscular drug used to terminate early pregnancy, evacuate a missed abortion, or control postpartum hemorrhage. Dinoprostone is a prostaglandin that stimulates uterine contractions; it is given by intravaginal suppository. Besides evacuating the uterus, it is also used to stimulate cervical ripening before labor. Mifepristone is a newer, controversial drug that acts as an antagonist of progesterone sites in the endometrium, allowing local prostaglandins to stimulate uterine contractions and dislodge or prevent the implantation of any fertilized egg. This drug is given orally and takes 5 to 7 days to produce the desired effect.

Therapeutic Actions and Indications

The abortifacients stimulate uterine activity, dislodging any implanted trophoblast and preventing implantation of any fertilized egg. These drugs are approved for use to terminate pregnancy 12 to 20 weeks from the date of the last menstrual period. Mifepristone is approved for use during the first 49 days of the pregnancy. Carboprost and dinoprostone are also approved for use to evacuate the uterus after a missed abortion or fetal death. Carboprost also is used to treat postpartum hemorrhage that is not responsive to the usual therapy. Because of its local prostaglandin effects, dinoprostone can also be used to stimulate cervical ripening before induction of labor.

Pharmacokinetics

These drugs are well absorbed, metabolized in the liver, and excreted in the urine. Because of their effects on the uterus, they are used during pregnancy only to end the pregnancy. They are not recommended for use during lactation because of the potential for serious effects on the neonate. If these drugs are to be used by a lactating mother, another method of feeding the baby should be used.

Contraindications and Cautions

Abortifacients should not be used with any known allergy to abortifacients or prostaglandins; after 20 weeks from the last menstrual period; or with active PID or acute cardiovascular, hepatic, renal, or pulmonary disease. Caution should be used with any history of asthma, hypertension, or adrenal disease and with acute vaginitis (inflammation of the vagina) or scarred uterus.

Adverse Effects

Adverse effects associated with abortifacients include abdominal cramping, heavy uterine bleeding, perforated uterus, and uterine rupture, all of which are related to exaggeration of the desired effects of the drug. Other side effects include headache, nausea and vomiting, diarrhea, diaphoresis (sweating), backache, and rash.

Nursing Considerations for Patients Receiving Abortifacients

Assessment: History and Examination

Screen for the following conditions, which could be cautions or contraindications to use of the drug: history of allergy to any abortifacient or prostaglandin preparation; active PID; cardiac, hepatic, pulmonary, or renal disease; history of asthma; and hypotension, hypertension, epilepsy, scarred uterus, or acute vaginitis.

Include screening for baseline status before beginning therapy and for any potential adverse effects: skin, lesions; orientation, affect; blood pressure, pulse; respiration, adventitious sounds; vaginal discharge, pelvic examination, uterine tone; and liver and renal function tests, leukocyte count, and urinalysis.

Nursing Diagnoses

The patient receiving abortifacients may have the following nursing diagnoses related to drug therapy:

- Acute Pain related to uterine contractions, headache, fluid retention, GI upset
- Ineffective Coping related to abortion or fetal death
- Deficient Knowledge regarding drug therapy

Implementation

- Administer via route indicated, following the manufacturer's directions for storage and preparation, *to ensure safe and therapeutic use of the drug.*
- Confirm the age of the pregnancy before administering the drug, *to ensure appropriate use of the drug.*
- Confirm that abortion or uterine evacuation is complete, *to avoid potential bleeding problems; prepare for dilation and curettage if necessary.*
- Monitor blood pressure periodically during and after administration, *to assess for adverse effects; discontinue the drug if blood pressure rises dramatically.*
- Monitor uterine tone and involution and the amount of bleeding during and for several days after use of the drug, *to ensure appropriate response and recovery from the drug.*

DRUGS IN FOCUS
Abortifacients

Drug Name	Dosage/Route	Usual Indications
carboprost (*Hemabate*)	250 μg IM at intervals of 1.5–3.5 h, do not exceed 12 mg total dose; 250 μg IM to control postpartum bleeding, do not exceed 2 mg total dose	Termination of early pregnancy, evacuation of missed abortion, control of postpartum hemorrhage
Ⓟ dinoprostone (*Cerilvid*)	20 mg vaginal suppository, may repeat q3–5h as needed for termination of pregnancy; 0.5 mg gel via cervical catheter, repeated in 6 h if needed for cervical ripening, then wait 6–12h before using oxytocin	Evacuation of the uterus, cervical ripening before labor
mifepristone (*Mifeprex*)	600 mg PO as a single dose; if pregnancy not terminated by day 3, 400 μg misoprostol PO; if not terminated by day 14, surgical intervention in suggested	Termination of early pregnancy

- Provide support and appropriate referrals *to help the patient deal with abortion or fetal death.*
- Provide thorough patient teaching, including measures to avoid adverse effects and warning signs of problems to report, *to enhance patient knowledge about drug therapy and to promote compliance.*

Evaluation

- Monitor patient response to the drug (evacuation of uterus).
- Monitor for adverse effects (GI upset, nausea, blood pressure changes, hemorrhage, uterine rupture).
- Evaluate the effectiveness of the teaching plan (patient can name drug, dosage, adverse effects to watch for, specific measures to avoid adverse effects).
- Monitor the effectiveness of comfort measures and compliance to the regimen.

TOCOLYTICS

Uterine contractions that become strong before term can lead to premature labor and delivery, which can have detrimental effects on the neonate, including death. Drugs used to relax the uterine smooth muscle and prevent contractions leading to premature labor and delivery are called tocolytics. They are usually reserved for use after 20 weeks of gestation, when the neonate has a chance of survival outside the uterus. Only one tocolytic agent is in use today—ritodrine (*Yutopar*).

Therapeutic Actions and Indications

The tocolytics are β_2-specific adrenergic agonists that mimic the effects of the sympathetic nervous system at β_2 sites. These effects include relaxation of the uterine smooth muscle. They are indicated for the management of preterm labor in selected patients at more than 20 weeks' gestation.

Pharmacokinetics

Ritodrine is rapidly absorbed, metabolized in the liver, and excreted in the urine. It has a half-life of 1.7 to 2.6 hours. It crosses the placenta and enters breast milk and can have adverse effects on the fetus and neonate. If the drug is used during lactation, another method of feeding the baby should be

used. Babies born to mothers who have been treated with ritodrine should be closely monitored for cardiovascular and other effects of the drug.

Contraindications and Cautions

Tocolytics are contraindicated in the presence of known allergy to these drugs or components used in their preparation; with pregnancies of less than 20 weeks, because of the low chance of neonatal survival; with antepartum hemorrhage, which could be exacerbated by uterine relaxation; with eclampsia or preeclampsia, which could be exacerbated by sympathetic stimulation; with intrauterine death when uterine evacuation is desirable; and with maternal cardiac disease, uncontrolled diabetes, pulmonary hypertension, or other disorders that could be exacerbated by sympathetic stimulation.

Adverse Effects

Maternal adverse effects associated with these drugs are related to the sympathetic stimulation that they can cause and include headache, tremor, nervousness, nausea, vomiting, tachycardia, hypertension, rash, and potentially fatal postpartum pulmonary edema, a condition that is more likely in patients taking corticosteroids. Fetal effects can include tachycardia, hypotension, hypoglycemia, and paralytic ileus.

Clinically Important Drug–Drug Interactions

There is an increase in sympathetic effects if tocolytics are combined with other sympathomimetic drugs.

Decreased effects occur if tocolytics are combined with β-adrenergic blockers.

The risk of potentially fatal postpartum pulmonary edema is increased if tocolytics are combined with corticosteroids.

Nursing Considerations for Patients Receiving Tocolytics

Assessment: History and Examination

Screen for the following conditions, which could be cautions or contraindications to use of the drug: history of allergy to any tocolytic or components used in the preparation; cardiac or pulmonary disease; history of asthma; gestational age; intrauterine death of fetus <20 weeks; uterine hemorrhage; and eclampsia or preeclampsia.

Include screening for baseline status before beginning therapy and for any potential adverse effects: skin, lesions;

DRUGS IN FOCUS

Tocolytics

Drug Name	Dosage/Route	Usual Indications
ⓟ ritodrine (*Yutopar*)	0.05 mg/min IV, increase as needed, usual effective dose is 0.15–0.35 mg/min IV	Management of preterm labor in selected patients > 20 wk gestation

orientation, affect; blood pressure, pulse; respiration, adventitious sounds; pelvic examination, uterine tone, maternal and fetal heart rates; and blood glucose.

Nursing Diagnoses

The patient receiving tocolytics may have the following nursing diagnoses related to drug therapy:

- Anxiety related to potential premature labor and delivery
- Impaired Gas Exchange related to pulmonary edema
- Deficient Knowledge regarding drug therapy

Implementation

- Monitor maternal pulse and respirations closely; *persistent maternal pulse greater than 140 beats per minute or respirations higher than 20 per minute may be signs of impending pulmonary edema and require immediate action.*
- Avoid fluid overload; *serial hemograms may indicate the state of hydration.*
- Maintain the patient in the left lateral position during infusion, *to minimize hypotension.*
- Provide support and appropriate referrals *to help the patient deal with possible premature labor.*
- Provide thorough patient teaching, including measures to avoid adverse effects and warning signs of problems to report, *to enhance patient knowledge about drug therapy and to promote compliance.*

Evaluation

- Monitor patient response to the drug (stopping of premature labor).
- Monitor for adverse effects (tachycardia, hypertension, headache, pulmonary edema, GI upset, rash).
- Evaluate the effectiveness of the teaching plan (patient can name drug, dosage, adverse effects to watch for, specific measures to avoid adverse effects).
- Monitor the effectiveness of comfort measures and compliance to the regimen.

▭▬●◼ WEB LINKS

Health care providers and patients may want to explore the following Internet sources:

Information on fertility drugs—research, explanations, related information:
http://www.babycenter.com/refcap/4091.html

Information on menopause specifically for patients, and teaching aids with explanations, drugs, choices, support groups:
http://fbhc.org/Patients/BetterHealth/Menopause/home.html

Information on HRT, updated regularly with studies, controversies, and treatment choices, cross-referenced to research studies:
http://www.menopause-online.com
http://www.menopause.org

Information on contraceptives—good teaching guidelines, explanations, choices:
http://www.reproline.jhu.edu/english/1contech/1methods/1methods.htm

Information on estrogens—research, uses, and controversies, for professionals:
http://www.asrm.com

CHAPTER SUMMARY

- Estrogens are female sex hormones that are important in the development of the female reproductive system and secondary sex characteristics.
- Estrogens are used pharmacologically mainly to replace hormones lost at menopause so as to prevent many of the signs and symptoms associated with menopause, including the development of CAD; to stimulate ovulation in woman with hypogonadism; and in combination with progestins for oral contraceptives.
- Progestins are female sex hormones that are responsible for maintenance of a pregnancy and for the development of some secondary sex characteristics.
- Progestins are used in combination with estrogens for contraception, to treat uterine bleeding, and for palliation in certain cancers with sensitive receptor sites.
- Fertility drugs stimulate FSH and LH in women with functioning ovaries to increase follicle development and improve the chances for pregnancy.
- A major adverse effect of fertility drugs is multiple births and birth defects.
- Oxytocic drugs act like the hypothalamic hormone oxytocin to stimulate uterine contractions and induce or speed up labor. They are most frequently used to control bleeding and promote postpartum involution of the uterus.
- Abortifacients are drugs that stimulate uterine activity to cause uterine evacuation. These drugs can be used to induce abortion in early pregnancy or to promote uterine evacuation after intrauterine fetal death.
- Tocolytics are drugs that relax the uterine smooth muscle; they are used to stop premature labor in patients after 20 weeks' gestation.

Review Questions

1. Estrogens produce a wide variety of systemic effects. An effect not attributed to estrogen is
   a. protecting the heart from atherosclerosis.
   b. retaining calcium in the bones.
   c. maintaining the secondary female sex characteristics.
   d. relaxing the gravid uterus to prolong pregnancy.
2. A postmenopausal woman is started on estrogens to control her unpleasant menopausal symptoms. She should be instructed that, as a result of the drug therapy, she may experience
   a. constipation.
   b. breakthrough bleeding.

c. weight loss.

d. persistently elevated body temperature.

3. An estrogen receptor modulator might be the drug of choice in the treatment of postmenopausal osteoporosis in a patient with a family history of breast or uterine cancer. The postmenopausal patient might experience

a. constipation and dry, itchy skin.

b. flushing and dry vaginal mucosa.

c. hot flashes and vaginal bleeding.

d. no associated adverse effects.

4. Combination estrogens and progestins are commonly used as oral contraceptives. It is thought that this combination has its effect by

a. acting like circulating estrogen and progesterone to block the hypothalamic release of FSH and LH, preventing follicle development and ovulation.

b. directly suppressing the ovaries and preventing ovulation.

c. keeping the endometrium constantly lush and blood filled.

d. preventing menstruation, which prevents pregnancy.

5. Any patient who is taking estrogens, progestins, or combination products should be cautioned to avoid smoking because

a. nicotine increases the metabolism of the hormones and they may not be effective.

b. the combination leads to an increased risk of potentially dangerous thromboembolic episodes.

c. nicotine amplifies the adverse effects of the hormones.

d. nicotine blocks hormone receptor sites and they may no longer be effective.

6. A patient is taking *Clomid* (clomiphene) after 6 years of inability to conceive a child. The patient will need to be informed about all of the following except

a. the need for a complete physical and pelvic examination before each course of drug therapy.

b. the risks and hazards of multiple births.

c. the importance of scheduling treatments and intercourse to increase the chance of conception.

d. the need to avoid intercourse during drug therapy.

7. Oxytocin, a synthetic form of the hypothalamic hormone, is used to

a. induce abortion.

b. stimulate milk "let down" in the lactating woman.

c. increase fertility and the chance of conception.

d. relax the gravid uterus and prevent preterm labor.

8. A patient is receiving an oxytocic drug to stimulate labor. The nursing care of this patient would not include

a. monitoring of fetal heartbeat during labor.

b. regulation of drug delivery between contractions.

c. administration of blood pressure–lowering drugs to balance hypertensive effects.

d. monitoring of maternal blood pressure periodically during and after administration.

9. The use of an abortifacient drug would be contraindicated in a woman

a. who is 15 weeks pregnant.

b. who is older than 50 years of age.

c. who has had four cesarean sections in the past.

d. who is 10 weeks pregnant.

10. Because of the risk of potentially fatal pulmonary edema, tocolytic drugs should not be combined with

a. corticosteroids.

b. β-blockers.

c. antibiotics.

d. inhalation anesthetics.

BIBLIOGRAPHY

Abernathy, K. (1997). Hormone replacement therapy. *Professional Nurse, 21*(10), 717–719.

Bullock, B. L. (2000). *Focus on pathophysiology.* Philadelphia: Lippincott Williams & Wilkins.

Crandall, S. G. (1997). Menopause made easier. *RN, 60*(7), 46–50.

Drug facts and comparisons. (2002). St. Louis: Fact and Comparisons.

Greendale, G. A., & Sowers, M. (1997). The menopause transition. *Endocrinology and Metabolism Clinics of North America, 26*(2), 262–277.

Gilman, A., Hardman, J. G., & Limbird, L. E. (Eds.) (2002). *Goodman and Gilman's the pharmacological basis of therapeutics* (10th ed.). New York: McGraw-Hill.

Karch, A. M. (2002). *2003 Lippincott's nursing drug guide.* Philadelphia: Lippincott Williams & Wilkins.

CHAPTER

41

Drugs Affecting the Male Reproductive System

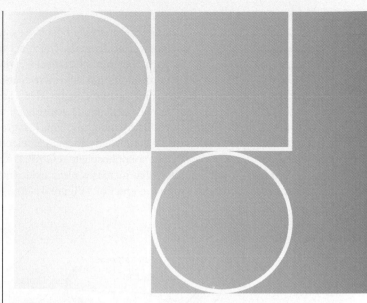

Key Terms
anabolic steroids
androgenic effects
androgens
hirsutism
hypogonadism
penile erectile dysfunction

541

Drugs that are used to affect the male reproductive system include male steroid hormones or **androgens,** which act like testosterone, the male sex hormone; **anabolic steroids,** which are synthetic testosterone preparations that have more anabolic (tissue-building) effects than **androgenic effects** (effects associated with development of male sexual characteristics); and drugs that act to improve penile dysfunction. This last group includes alprostadil, a prostaglandin, and sildenafil, a selective inhibitor of cyclic guanosine monophosphate (cGMP, a reactive tissue enzyme inhibitor) that increases nitric oxide in the corpus cavernosum to improve erection (Figure 41–1).

ANDROGENS

The primary natural androgen, testosterone (*Duratest, Testoderm,* and others) is the classic androgen in use today. It is used for replacement therapy in cases of **hypogonadism** (underdeveloped testes) and to treat certain breast cancers. These drugs are all class III controlled substances. Other androgens include danazol (*Danocrine*), a synthetic androgen that is used primarily to block the release of follicle-stimulating hormone and luteinizing hormone in women; fluoxymesterone (*Halotestin*), an analog of testosterone and a controlled substance used for replacement therapy in hypogonadism

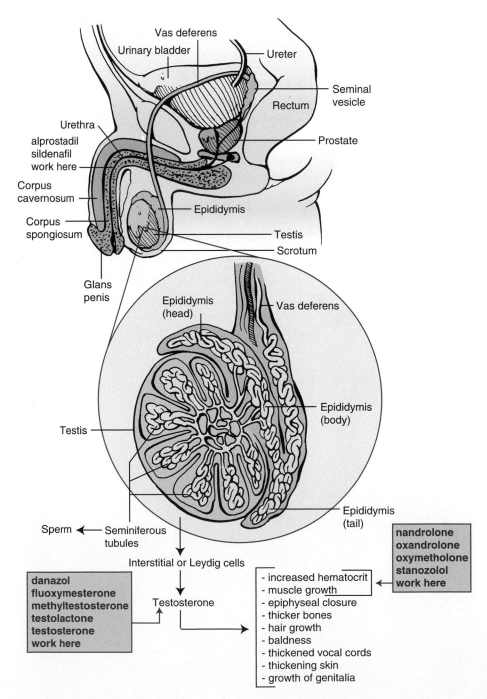

FIGURE 41-1. Sites of action of drugs affecting the male reproductive system.

DRUG THERAPY ACROSS THE LIFESPAN

Drugs Affecting the Male Reproductive System

Children	Adults	Older Adults
These drugs are used in children as replacement therapy and to increase red blood cell production in renal failure. Because of the effects of these hormones on epiphyseal closure, children should be closely monitored with hand and wrist radiographs pretreatment and every 6 months. If precocious puberty occurs, the drug should be stopped. Adolescents who are prescribed androgens should be alerted to the potential for increased acne and other effects. Adolescent athletes need constant education about the risks associated with the use of anabolic steroids to improve athletic prowess and the lack of scientific evidence of beneficial effects.	Adults also need reinforcement of the information about anabolic steroid use and athletics. Women who are prescribed these drugs may experience masculinizing effects and may need support in coping with these body changes. Men who are receiving these drugs for replacement therapy may need to learn self-injection techniques and may benefit from information on depot forms or dermal systems. Periodic liver function tests are important in monitoring the effects of these drugs on the liver. These drugs are not indicated for use in pregnancy or lactation because of the potential for serious effects on the fetus or neonate.	Older adults may have problems with androgen therapy because of underlying conditions that are aggravated by the drug effects. Hypertension, congestive heart failure, and coronary artery disease may be aggravated by the fluid retention associated with these drugs. Benign prostatic hypertrophy, a common problem in older men, may be aggravated by androgenic effects that may enlarge the prostate further, leading to urinary difficulties and increased risk of prostate cancer. Many older adults have hepatic dysfunction, and these drugs can be hepatotoxic. Older patients should be monitored very carefully and dosage should be reduced. If signs of liver failure or hepatitis occur, the drug should be stopped immediately.

and to treat certain breast cancers; and testolactone (*Teslac*), a synthetic androgen used for the treatment of specific breast cancers.

Therapeutic Actions and Indications

The androgens are forms of testosterone. They are responsible for the growth and development of male sex organs and the maintenance of secondary sex characteristics (see Figure 41–1). They act to increase the retention of nitrogen, sodium, potassium, and phosphorus and to decrease the urinary excretion of calcium. Testosterones increase protein anabolism and decrease protein catabolism (breakdown). They also increase the production of red blood cells.

Androgens (testosterone, methyltestosterone, and fluoxymesterone) can be indicated for the treatment of hypogonadism and delayed puberty in male patients. They are also indicated for the treatment of certain breast cancers in postmenopausal women; for the prevention of ovulation to treat endometriosis (danazol); for the prevention of postpartum breast engorgement (testosterone); and for the treatment of hereditary angioedema (danazol). Testosterone is long acting and is available in several forms, including depot (deep, slow-release) injections and a dermal patch. Fluoxymesterone, methyltestosterone, and testolactone are short acting and are available only in oral form. Danazol is long acting and also is available only in oral form.

Pharmacokinetics

The androgens are well absorbed and widely distributed throughout the body. They are metabolized in the liver and excreted in the urine. Androgens are contraindicated for use in pregnancy because of adverse effects on the fetus. It is not known whether androgens enter breast milk, but because of the potential for adverse effects, another method of feeding the baby should be used if these drugs are needed during lactation.

Contraindications and Cautions

These drugs are contraindicated with any known allergy to the drug or ingredients in the drug; during pregnancy and lactation (because of potential effects on the neonate); and in the presence of prostate or breast cancer in men. They should be used cautiously in the presence of any liver dysfunction or cardiovascular disease, because these disorders could be exacerbated by the effects of the hormones.

Adverse Effects

Androgenic effects include acne, edema, **hirsutism** (increased hair distribution), deepening of the voice, oily skin and hair, weight gain, decrease in breast size, and testicular atrophy. Antiestrogen effects—flushing, sweating, vaginitis, nervousness, and emotional lability—can be anticipated when these drugs are used with women. Other common effects include headache (possibly related to fluid and electrolyte changes), dizziness, sleep disorders and fatigue, rash, and altered serum electrolytes. A potentially life-threatening effect that has been documented is hepatocellular cancer. This may occur because of the effect of testosterone on hepatic cells. Patients on long-term therapy should have hepatic function tests monitored regularly—before beginning therapy and every 6 months during therapy.

DRUGS IN FOCUS
Androgens

Drug Name	Usual Dosage	Usual Indications
danazol (*Danocrine*)	100–800 mg/d PO, depending on use and response	Blockade of follicle-stimulating hormone and luteinizing hormone release in women, treatment of endometriosis, prevention of angioedema
fluoxymesterone (*Halotestin*)	5–20 mg/d PO for replacement therapy; 10–40 mg/d PO for certain breast cancers; 2.5 mg PO shortly after delivery and 5–10 mg/d PO for 4–5 d for breast engorgement	Replacement therapy in hypogonadism, certain breast cancers; postpartum breast engorgement
methyltestosterone (*Android, Testred*)	10–40 mg/d PO	Treatment of hypogonadism, postpubertal cryptorchidism, some breast cancers
testolactone (*Teslac*)	250 mg PO q.i.d.	Treatment of specific breast cancers
℗ testosterone (*Duratest, Testoderm*)	50–400 mg IM every 2–4 wk, dose varies with preparation; some long-acting depository forms are available; dermatological patch 4–6 mg/d, replace patch daily	Replacement therapy in hypogonadism, certain breast cancers

Clinically Significant Drug–Laboratory Test Interferences

While a patient is taking androgens, there may be a decrease in thyroid function as well as increased creatinine and creatinine clearance results that are not associated with disease states. These effects can last up to 2 weeks after the discontinuation of therapy.

Nursing Considerations for Patients Receiving Androgens
Assessment: History and Examination

Screen for the following conditions, which could be cautions or contraindications to use of the drug: history of allergy to any testosterone or androgen, pregnancy, lactation, hepatic dysfunction, cardiovascular disease, and breast or prostate cancer in men.

Include screening for baseline status before beginning therapy and for any potential adverse effects: skin color, lesions, texture, hair distribution; affect, orientation, peripheral sensation; abdominal examination; serum electrolytes, serum cholesterol, and liver function tests; and radiographs of the long bones in children.

Nursing Diagnoses

The patient receiving any androgen may also have the following nursing diagnoses related to drug therapy:

- Disturbed Body Image related to androgenic effects
- Acute Pain related to need for injections
- Sexual Dysfunction related to androgenic effects
- Deficient Knowledge regarding drug therapy

Implementation

- Reconstitute the drug according to the manufacturer's directions, *to ensure proper reconstitution and to administer as prescribed.*
- Monitor response carefully when beginning therapy, *so that the dosage can be adjusted accordingly.*
- Monitor liver function periodically with long-term therapy; *arrange to discontinue the drug at any sign of hepatic dysfunction.*
- Provide thorough patient teaching, including measures to avoid adverse effects, warning signs of problems, and the need for regular evaluation, including blood tests. Instruct a family member or caregiver in proper preparation and administration techniques as appropriate, *to enhance patient knowledge about drug therapy and to promote compliance with the drug regimen.*

Evaluation

- Monitor patient response to the drug (onset of puberty; maintenance of male sexual characteristics; palliation of breast cancer; blockage of ovulation; prevention of postpartum breast engorgement; relief of angioedema).
- Monitor for adverse effects (androgenic effects, hypoestrogen effects, serum electrolyte imbalance, headache, sleep disturbances, rash, hepatocellular carcinoma).
- Evaluate the effectiveness of the teaching plan (patient can name drug, dosage, adverse effects to watch for, specific measures to avoid adverse effects; family member or caregiver can demonstrate proper technique for preparation and administration of drug as appropriate).

• Monitor the effectiveness of comfort measures and compliance to the regimen.

ANABOLIC STEROIDS

The anabolic steroids are analogs of testosterone that have been developed to produce the tissue-building effects of testosterone with less androgenic effect. These are controlled substances that are known to be used illegally for the enhancement of athletic performance through increased muscle mass, increased hematocrit, and, theoretically, an increase in strength and endurance. The adverse effects of these drugs can be deadly when used in the amounts needed for enhanced athletic performance. Cardiomyopathy, hepatic carcinoma, personality changes, and sexual dysfunction are all associated with the excessive and nonindicated use of anabolic steroids. There is an increased effort to encourage the use of herbal products to improve athletic performance. These products are advertised as "safe" alternatives (see Box 41–1).

Oxandrolone (*Oxandrin*) is an anabolic steroid that has several uses: to promote weight gain in debilitated patients, to increase protein anabolism in patients receiving prolonged corticosteroid therapy, and to treat certain cancers. Oxymetholone (*Anadrol-50*) is used to treat various anemias. Stanozolol (*Winstrol*) is indicated only for the treatment of hereditary angioedema, because of its toxic effects on the liver.

Therapeutic Actions and Indications
Anabolic steroids promote body tissue-building processes; reverse catabolic or tissue-destroying processes; and increase hemoglobin and red blood cell mass.

Indications for particular anabolic steroids vary with the drug. They can be used to treat anemias, certain cancers, and angioedema, and to promote weight gain and tissue repair in debilitated patients and protein anabolism in patients who are receiving long-term corticosteroid therapy.

Pharmacokinetics
Like the androgens, the anabolic steroids are well absorbed and widely distributed throughout the body. They are metabolized in the liver and excreted in the urine. Anabolic steroids are contraindicated for use in pregnancy because of adverse effects to the fetus. It is not known whether anabolic steroids enter breast milk, but because of the potential for adverse effects, another method of feeding the baby should be used if these drugs are needed during lactation.

Contraindications and Cautions
These drugs are contraindicated in the presence of any known allergy to anabolic steroids; during pregnancy and lactation (because of potential masculinization in the neonate); and in the presence of liver dysfunction (because these drugs are metabolized in the liver and are known to cause liver toxicity), coronary disease (because of cholesterol-raising effects through effects on the liver), or prostate or breast cancer in males.

BOX 41-1
Alternative Therapies Used to Enhance Athletic Performance

With an increasing awareness of the risks associated with anabolic steroid use and increasing pressures to make it difficult to get these drugs, even illegally, there is an increased push in advertising of alternative or "natural" products that are reported to enhance athletic performance.

Bee pollen—Reported to contain amino acids and other minerals and enzymes. There are no scientific studies regarding its effectiveness. Serious allergic reactions have been reported with the use of this product. Random studies have found a wide variety of ingredients in each product, depending on the season, growing conditions, and geographical area.

Creatine—Contains a substance that is found in muscle and naturally occurs in red meats and other dietary sources. No scientific data are available on its actual effects on energy or athletic performance. It interacts with many other drugs, including nonsteroidal anti-inflammatory drugs, cimetidine, probenecid, and trimethoprim, and can cause serious effects on kidney functioning. Users should be advised to drink plenty of fluids while taking this drug and to monitor for swelling, muscle cramps, and dizziness. Suggested only for short-term use.

Damiana—Used to increase muscle strength, as an aphrodisiac, and to boost mental health. It can cause liver toxicity. It interferes with antidiabetic agents and causes elevated blood sugar concentrations. Users should report muscle spasms or hallucinations.

Spirulina—Used to increase energy and boost metabolism. It may contain toxic metals and can cause serious reactions in children and pets. It interferes with vitamin B_{12} absorption. No scientific studies validate the claims of its effectiveness.

Wild yam—Found to have many estrogen-like effects, this herb is used to increase athletic performance because it may contain a constituent of dihydroepiandrosterone (DHEA) used to slow the aging process and to improve energy and stamina. Preparations interact with disulfiram and metronidazole because they contain alcohol. It is known to be toxic to the liver. Users may experience estrogen-like effects including breast pain. Users should be monitored closely and urged to report any adverse effects.

Adverse Effects
In prepubertal males, adverse effects include virilization (eg, phallic enlargement, hirsutism, increased skin pigmentation). Postpubertal males may experience inhibition of testicular function, gynecomastia, testicular atrophy, priapism (a painful and continual erection of the penis), baldness, and change in libido (increased or decreased). Women may experience hirsutism, hoarseness, deepening of the voice, clitoral enlargement, baldness, and menstrual irregularities. As with the androgens, serum electrolyte changes, liver dysfunction (including life-threatening hepatitis), insomnia, and weight gain may occur. There is an increased risk of prostate problems, especially in geriatric patients.

CASE STUDY

Adverse Effects of Anabolic Steroids

THE SITUATION

K. S. is a senior nursing student who recently became engaged to a college senior. He is training as a javelin thrower and hopes to make it to the Olympics. K. S. noticed that her fiancé had been suffering from gastrointestinal upset for the last 3 weeks and more recently had developed tremors and muscle cramps. K. S. first suspected that he was suffering from a viral infection, but when the symptoms did not resolve, she became concerned. K. S. tried to get her fiancé to see a doctor, but he refused. Eventually, he admitted that he had begun using anabolic steroids to develop his muscles and improve his athletic prowess. He said that his friend who gave him the drugs told him that stomach upset was normal. He refuses to see a physician because he knows that the use of these drugs is illegal. He believes that using the anabolic steroids for a while will put him closer to his goal. K. S. accepts his explanation but is upset about the use of anabolic steroids. She consults with her clinical instructor about the effects of these drugs.

CRITICAL THINKING

• What does K. S. need to know? *Think about the systemic effects of anabolic steroids and the possible long-term effects from their abuse.*

• What implications do these effects have for the athlete? *Consider the concern that K. S. must be experiencing. Suggest ways for K. S. to share the information about the actual effects of anabolic steroids with her fiancé, and still cope with her own feelings and concerns.*

• What are the ethical and legal issues involved with a heath care provider knowing about illegal drug use and abuse? *Outline a plan for helping K. S. and her fiancé cope with this issue and its implications for their futures.*

DISCUSSION

Use of anabolic steriods is illegal in almost all organized athletic contests. Random drug testing is done to rule out use of these and other drugs. Not surprisingly, K. S. feels insecure about her fiancé's decision. She needs to know that her discussion will be confidential and that she will receive support for her concerns and her fears. K. S. needs to review the effects of anabolic steroids. Although they do promote muscle development, there has never been any evidence that they actually improve athletic performance. The potential adverse effects of these drugs can be deadly, especially if K. S.'s fiancé is receiving the drugs from a friend and has no medical evaluation or dosage guidance to reduce the risk. Personality changes, cardiomyopathy, liver cancer, and impotence are just a few of the possible adverse effects.

K. S. is in a precarious position, not wanting to interfere with her fiancé's dreams or to cause problems in their relationship. She should be encouraged to explain the adverse effects of the drugs to her fiancé, pointing out that he is already experiencing some of them. Adverse effects associated with the drugs can ultimately interfere with, not enhance, his athletic performance. She might be encouraged to practice what she will tell her fiancé and to seek other support as needed.

The sale or distribution of anabolic steroids without a prescription is illegal, and this fact further complicates the situation for K. S. Because she is planning to become a health care provider, she may be obligated by state law to report this information to the authorities. K. S. should research these issues and discuss them further with her clinical instructor and other resource people.

DRUGS IN FOCUS
Anabolic Steroids

Drug Name	Usual Dosage	Usual Indications
oxandrolone (*Oxandrin*)	Adult: 2.5 mg PO b.i.d.–q.i.d. Pediatric: <0.1 mg/kg PO per day, monitor closely, may be repeated intermittently	Promotion of weight gain in debilitated patients; treatment of certain cancers
oxymetholone (*Anadrol-50*)	1–5 mg/kg per day PO	Treatment of anemias in adults
Ⓟ stanozolol (*Winstrol*)	2 mg PO t.i.d. after favorable response, titrate to 2 mg/d PO over 1–3 mo	Treatment of angioedema in adults

Clinically Important Drug–Drug Interactions

Because the anabolic steroids affect the liver, there is a potential for interaction with oral anticoagulants and a potentially decreased need for antidiabetic agents, which may not be metabolized normally. Patients should be monitored closely and appropriate dosage adjustments made.

Nursing Considerations for Patients Receiving Anabolic Steroids

Assessment: History and Examination

Screen for the following conditions, which could be cautions or contraindications to use of the drug: history of allergy to any androgens or anabolic steroids; pregnancy or lactation (because of masculinization of the neonate); prostrate or breast cancer; coronary disease; and hepatic dysfunction.

Include screening for baseline status before beginning therapy and for any potential adverse effects: skin color, texture, hair distribution; affect, orientation; abdominal examination; liver evaluation; serum electrolytes, cholesterol levels; and radiographs of the long bones in children.

Nursing Diagnoses

The patient receiving an anabolic steroid may have the following nursing diagnoses related to drug therapy:

- Disturbed Body Image related to systemic effects
- Acute Pain related to gastrointestinal (GI), central nervous system effects
- Deficient Knowledge regarding drug therapy

Implementation

- Administer with food if GI effects are severe, *to relieve GI distress.*
- Monitor endocrine function, hepatic function, and serum electrolytes before and periodically during therapy, *so that dosage can be adjusted appropriately and severe adverse effects can be avoided.*
- Arrange for radiographs of the long bones of children every 3 to 6 months, *so that the drug can be discontinued if bone growth reaches the norm for the child's age.*
- Provide thorough patient teaching, including measures to avoid adverse effects and warning signs of problems, as well as the need for regular evaluation including blood tests, *to enhance patient knowledge about drug therapy and to promote compliance with drug regimen.* (See Patient Teaching Checklist: Androgens, Anabolic Steroids.)

Evaluation

- Monitor patient response to the drug (increase in hematocrit, protein anabolism).
- Monitor for adverse effects (androgenic effects, serum electrolyte disturbances, epiphyseal closure, hepatic dysfunction, personality changes, cardiac effects).
- Evaluate the effectiveness of the teaching plan (patient can

PATIENT TEACHING CHECKLIST
Androgens, Anabolic Steroids

Create customized patient teaching materials for a specific androgen or anabolic steroid from the CD-ROM. Patient teaching should stress the following points for drugs within this class:

- Androgens or anabolic steroids have properties similar to those of the male sex hormones. Because the drug has widespread effects, there are often many adverse effects associated with its use.

Some of the following adverse effects may occur:

- *Gastrointestinal upset, nausea, vomiting*—Taking the drug with food usually helps this.
- *Acne*—This is a hormone effect; washing your face regularly and avoiding oily foods may help.
- *Increased facial hair, decreased head hair*—These are hormonal effects; if they become bothersome, consult with your health care provider.
- *Menstrual irregularities (women)*—This is a normal effect of the androgens; if you suspect that you might be pregnant, consult with your health care provider immediately.
- *Weight gain, increased muscle development*—These are common hormone effects.
- *Change in sex drive*—This can be distressing and difficult to deal with; consult with your health care provider if this is a serious concern.

Tell any doctor, nurse, or other health care provider that you are taking this drug.

Report any of the following to your health care provider: swelling in fingers or legs; continual erection; uncontrollable sex drive; yellowing skin; fever, chills, or rash; chest pain or difficulty breathing; hoarseness, loss of hair or growth of facial hair (women).

It is important to have regular medical follow-up, including blood tests, to monitor your response to this drug.

Keep this drug and all medications out of the reach of children.

Take this medicine only as directed. Do not give this medication to anyone else or take any similar medication that has not been prescribed for you.

This Teaching Checklist reflects general patient teaching guidelines. It is not meant to be a substitute for drug-specific teaching information, which is available in nursing drug guides.

name drug, dosage, adverse effects to watch for, specific measures to avoid adverse effects).
- Monitor the effectiveness of comfort measures and compliance to the regimen (see Nursing Care Guide: Androgens, Anabolic Steroids).

DRUGS FOR TREATING PENILE ERECTILE DYSFUNCTION

Two very different drugs are approved for the treatment of **penile erectile dysfunction,** a condition in which the corpus

NURSING CARE GUIDE

Androgens, Anabolic Steroids

Assessment	Nursing Diagnoses	Implementation	Evaluation
HISTORY Allergies to any steroids, pregnancy, lactation, breast or prostate cancer in men; hepatic dysfunction; CAD	Disturbed Body Image related to drug effects Sexual Dysfunction Acute Pain related to injections Deficient Knowledge regarding drug therapy	Administer as prescribed. Monitor liver function prior to and periodically during therapy. Monitor patient response and adjust dose as appropriate. Discontinue in children if bone age reaches norm. Provide support and reassurance to deal with drug therapy. Provide patient teaching regarding drug name, dosage, adverse effects, precautions, warnings to report, and safe administration.	Evaluate drug effects: onset of puberty, maintenance of male sex characteristics, suppression of lactation. Monitor for adverse effects: androgenic effects, hypoestrogenic effects, hepatic dysfunction, electrolyte imbalance, endocrine changes. Monitor for drug–drug interactions: as indicated for each drug. Evaluate effectiveness of patient teaching program. Evaluate effectiveness of comfort and safety measures.
PHYSICAL EXAMINATION Neurological: orientation, reflexes, affect Skin: color, lesions, hair CV: P, cardiac auscultation, BP, edema GI: abdominal exam, liver exam Lab tests: serum electrolytes, hepatic function tests, long bone x-rays			

cavernosum does not fill with blood to allow for penile erection. Penile erection can be compromised by the aging process and by vascular and neurological conditions. Alprostadil (*Caverject, MUSE*) is a prostaglandin that relaxes vascular smooth muscle and allows filling of the corpus cavernosum when it is injected directly into the cavernosum. Sildenafil (*Viagra*) selectively inhibits receptors and increases nitrous oxide levels, allowing blood flow into the corpus cavernosum. This drug has the advantage of being an oral drug that is taken 1 hour before erection is desired.

Therapeutic Actions and Indications

The prostaglandin alprostadil is injected and acts locally to relax vascular smooth muscle and promote blood flow into the corpus cavernosum, causing penile erection. Alprostadil is metabolized to inactive compounds in the lungs and excreted in the urine. The drug is not indicated for use in women and is not classified for use in pregnancy or lactation. Because the effects on pregnancy are not known, if alprostadil is be-

ing used, condoms should be used during intercourse with a pregnant woman. Sildenafil is taken orally and acts to increase nitrous oxide levels in the corpus cavernosum. Nitrous oxide activates the enzyme cGMP, which causes smooth muscle relaxation, allowing the flow of blood into the corpus cavernosum. Sildenafil prevents the breakdown of cGMP by phosphodiesterase, leading to increased cGMP levels and prolonged smooth muscle relaxation and promoting the flow of blood into the corpus cavernosum, resulting in penile erection. Sildenafil is well absorbed from the GI tract, undergoes metabolism in the liver, and is excreted in the feces. It is not indicated for use in women, so no adequate studies have been done during pregnancy and lactation. These drugs are both indicated for the treatment of penile erectile dysfunction.

Contraindications and Cautions

These drugs are contraindicated in the presence of any anatomical obstruction or condition that might predispose to priapism; they cannot be used with penile implants; neither

DRUGS IN FOCUS
Drugs Used to Treat Penile Erectile Dysfunction

Drug Name	Usual Dosage	Usual Indications
alprostadil (*Caverject, MUSE*)	0.2–140 μg injected intracavernously, titrate the dose to one that will allow a satisfactory erection that is maintained no longer than 1h	Penile erectile dysfunction
Ⓟ sildenafil (*Viagra*)	25–100 mg PO taken 1 h before sexual stimulation	Penile erectile dysfunction

is indicated for use in women (although sildenafil is being studied for the treatment of sexual dysfunction in women). Caution should be used in patients with bleeding disorders. Sildenafil should also be used cautiously in those patients with coronary artery disease, active peptic ulcer, or retinitis pigmentosa, because of risks of exacerbation of these diseases.

Adverse Effects

Adverse effects associated with alprostadil are local effects such as pain at the injection site, infection, priapism, fibrosis, and rash. Sildenafil is associated with more systemic effects, including headache, flushing (related to relaxation of vascular smooth muscle), dyspepsia, urinary tract infection, diarrhea, dizziness, and rash.

Clinically Important Drug–Drug Interactions

Sildenafil cannot be taken in combination with any organic nitrates; serious cardiovascular effects, including death, have occurred.

Nursing Considerations for Patients Receiving Drugs to Treat Penile Erectile Dysfunction
Assessment: History and Examination

Screen for the following conditions, which could be cautions or contraindications to the use of the drug: history of allergy to either preparation, penile structural abnormalities, penile implants, bleeding disorders, active peptic ulcer, and coronary artery disease.

CULTURAL CONSIDERATIONS
Viagra—Wonder Drug?

The release of the drug *Viagra* to treat penile erectile dysfunction caused a tremendous stir in American society. This was the first oral drug developed to treat a disorder that was common in aging men but was seldom mentioned or discussed. *Viagra*, which facilitates penile erection approximately 1 hour after it is taken, brought the return of sexual function to many of these men.

For many months after its release, the drug was the center of controversy, news coverage, and debate. Stand-up comedians, television situation comedies, and Internet joke networks were buzzing with the latest *Viagra* jokes for months after the drug's release. Insurance companies debated covering the cost of this drug. Was it like cosmetic surgery, and not a necessary treatment, or was it a necessary part of human physiology? Most insurance companies ended up covering the cost of this drug. Women's rights groups became concerned because there was no drug approved and covered to help facilitate a woman's sexual response.

Viagra has proved to be very effective at increasing sexual functioning for many men. It is in trial stages for the treatment of sexual dysfunction in women; early reports seem to indicate that it is not effective.

The use of the drug is not without risks. Deaths have occurred when the drug was combined with nitrates (e.g., nitroglycerin). Headache, flushing, stomach upset, and urinary tract infections often occur. The drug can be used only once per day, and it does not work in the absence of sexual stimulation. Its absorption is delayed if it is taken with a high-fat meal, and patients need to plan accordingly. Patients also should be reminded that they need to use protection against sexually transmitted diseases.

When *Viagra* was the hot, new drug, there was tremendous demand for it from the public. This demand put health care providers in the position of ensuring that the drug was right for the patient's actual needs. The cause of penile erectile dysfunction should be determined, if at all possible. If this is a problem that the patient has never discussed with the health care provider before, there could be an underlying medical condition that should be addressed. The adverse effects, timing of administration, and drug combinations to avoid should be discussed with the patient before giving the drug.

With pharmaceutical companies now advertising in magazines, on television, and over the Internet, health care providers are often asked for specific prescription drugs based on media advertising. This relatively new phenomenon in health care presents new challenges to the health care provider to ensure quality patient teaching to help the patient understand the actual uses, effects, and rationales for a specific drug therapy.

Include screening for baseline status before beginning therapy and for any potential adverse effects: skin, lesions; orientation, affect, reflexes; blood pressure, pulse; respiration, adventitious sounds; local inspection of penis; and bleeding time and liver function tests.

Nursing Diagnoses

The patient receiving drugs for treating penile dysfunction may have the following nursing diagnoses related to drug therapy:

• Disturbed Body Image related to drug effects and indication
• Acute Pain related to injection of alprostadil
• Sexual Dysfunction
• Deficient Knowledge regarding drug therapy

Implementation

• Assess the cause of dysfunction before beginning therapy, *to ensure appropriate use of these drugs.*
• Monitor patients with vascular disease for any sign of exacerbation, *so that the drug can be discontinued before severe adverse effects occur.*
• Instruct the patient in the injection of alprostadil, storage of the drug, filling of the syringe, sterile technique, site rotation, and proper disposal of needles, *to ensure safe and proper administration of the drug.*
• Monitor patients who are taking sildenafil for use of nitrates, *to avert potentially serious drug–drug interactions.*
• Provide thorough patient teaching, including measures to avoid adverse effects and warning signs of problems, as well as the need for regular evaluation, *to enhance patient knowledge about drug therapy and to promote compliance with the drug regimen.*

Evaluation

• Monitor patient response to the drug (improvement in penile erection).
• Monitor for adverse effects (dizziness, flushing, local inflammation or infection, fibrosis, diarrhea, dyspepsia).
• Evaluate the effectiveness of the teaching plan (patient can name drug, dosage, adverse effects to watch for, specific measures to avoid adverse effects; patient can demonstrate proper administration of injected drug).
• Monitor the effectiveness of comfort measures and compliance to the regimen.

▢▣●▢ WEB LINKS
Health care providers and patients may want to consult the following Internet sources:

Information on male fertility—research, explanations, related information, endocrinology research:
http://www.maleinfertilitymds.com
Information on testosterone and testosterone replacement:
http://www.aace.com

Information on erectile dysfunction—overview, teaching aids, patient information, support groups:
http://www.urologychannel.com
Information for professionals, research, new drugs:
http://www.ama-assn.org
Information on benign prostatic hypertrophy—overview, teaching aids, questions, and answers:
http://www.bphpartners.com
Information on current research, professional issues:
http://www.uro.com

CHAPTER SUMMARY

• Androgens are male sex hormones, specifically testosterone or testosterone-like compounds.
• Androgens are responsible for the development and maintenance of male sex characteristics and secondary sex characteristics or androgenic effects.
• Side effects related to androgen use involve excess of the desired effects as well as potentially deadly hepatocellular carcinoma.
• Androgens can be used for replacement therapy or to block other hormone effects, as is seen with their use in the treatment of specific breast cancers.
• Anabolic steroids are analogs of testosterone that have been developed to have more anabolic or protein-building effects than androgenic effects.
• Anabolic steroids have been abused to enhance muscle development and athletic performance, often with deadly effects.
• Anabolic steroids are used to increase hematocrit and improve protein anabolism in certain depleted states.
• Penile erectile dysfunction can inhibit erection and male sexual function.
• Alprostadil, a prostaglandin, can be injected into the penis to stimulate erection.
• Sildenafil is an oral agent that acts quickly to promote vascular filling of the corpus cavernosum and promote penile erection.

Review Questions

1. Testosterone is approved for use in
   a. treatment of breast cancers.
   b. increasing muscle strength in athletes.
   c. oral contraceptives.
   d. increasing hair distribution in male pattern baldness.
2. Androgenic effects would include all of the following except
   a. hirsutism.
   b. deepening of the voice.
   c. testicular enlargement.
   d. acne.
3. Illegal use of large quantities of unprescribed anabolic steroids to enhance athletic performance has been associated with

a. increased sexual prowess.

b. muscle rupture from overexpansion.

c. development of COPD.

d. cardiomyopathy and liver cancers.

4. Anabolic steroids are not indicated for the treatment of

a. anemia.

b. angioedema.

c. debilitation and severe weight loss.

d. breast cancers in males.

5. A child treated with anabolic steroids because of anemia associated with renal disease will not need

a. early sex education classes because of the effects of the drug.

b. radiographs of the long bones every 3 to 6 months, so the drug can be stopped when the bone age size is appropriate to the child's age.

c. to learn to shave.

d. to learn to cope with an altered body image.

6. Erectile penile dysfunction is a condition in which

a. problems with childhood authority figures prevents a male erection.

b. the corpus cavernosum does not fill with blood to allow for penile erection.

c. the sympathetic nervous system fails to function.

d. past exposure to sexually transmitted disease causes physical damage within the penis.

7. A potentially deadly drug–drug interaction can occur if sildenafil (*Viagra*) is combined with

a. corticosteroids.

b. oral contraceptives.

c. organic nitrates.

d. halothane anesthetics.

8. To achieve erection, patients taking sildenafil (*Viagra*) require

a. sexual stimulation of the penis.

b. no additional stimulation.

c. privacy.

d. 10 to 15 minutes after taking the oral drug.

9. Men taking alprostadil for treatment of erectile dysfunction must

a. take the drug orally about 1 hour before anticipated intercourse.

b. arrange for sexual stimulation to promote erection.

c. learn to inject the drug directly into the penis.

d. avoid the use of nitrates for cardiovascular disorders.

10. *Viagra* is known to

a. cause unexpected and enlarged erections.

b. make a person young and agile.

c. promote interpersonal relationships between partners.

d. increase nitrous oxide levels in the corpus cavernosum, causing vascular relaxation and promoting blood flow into the corpus cavernosum.

BIBLIOGRAPHY

Bullock, B. L. (2000). *Focus on pathophysiology*. Philadelphia: Lippincott Williams & Wilkins.

Davis, S. R., & Burger, H. G. (1996). Androgens and postmenopausal women. *Journal of Endocrinology and Metabolism, 81*(8), 2759–2763.

Gilman, A., Hardman, J. G., & Limbird, L. E. (Eds.) (2002). *Goodman and Gilman's the pharmacological basis of therapeutics* (10th ed.). New York: McGraw-Hill.

Karch, A. M. (2002). *2003 Lippincott's nursing drug guide*. Philadelphia: Lippincott Williams & Wilkins.

Miller, K. L. (1996). Hormone replacement therapy in the elderly. *Annals of Pharmacotherapy, 31*(7–8), 915–917.

Drug facts and comparisons. (2002). St. Louis: Facts and Comparisons.

The medical letter on drugs and therapeutics. (2002). New Rochelle, NY: Medical Letter.

Walsh, P. C., et al. (Eds.) (2002). *Campbell's urology* (8th ed.). Philadelphia: W. B. Saunders.

PART

VIII

Drugs Acting on the Cardiovascular System

C H A P T E R

42

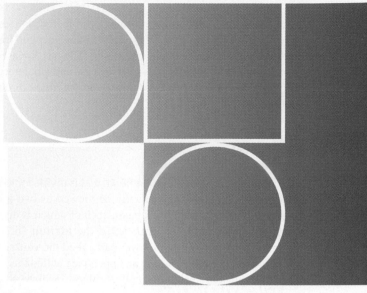

Introduction to the Cardiovascular System

Key Terms

actin
arrhythmia
arteries
atrium
auricle
automaticity
capillary
capacitance system
cardiac cycle
conductivity
diastole
dysrhythmia
electrocardiogram (ECG)
fibrillation
myocardium
myosin
oncotic pressure
pulse pressure
resistance system
sarcomere
sinoatrial (SA) node
Starling's law of the heart
syncytia
systole
troponin
veins
ventricle

555

The cardiovascular system is responsible for delivering oxygen and nutrients to all of the cells of the body and for removing waste products for excretion. The cardiovascular system consists of a pump—the heart—and an interconnected series of tubes that continually move blood throughout the body.

THE HEART

The heart is a hollow, muscular organ that is divided into four chambers. The heart may actually be viewed as two joined hearts: a right heart and a left heart, each of which is divided into two parts, an upper part called the **atrium** (literally "porch" or entryway) and a lower part called the **ventricle.**

Attached to each atrium is an appendage called the **auricle.** The auricle serves to collect blood, which is then pumped into the ventricles by atrial contraction. The ventricles pump blood out of the heart to the lungs or the body. The right auricle is quite large; the left is very small.

Between the atria and ventricles are two cardiac valves, thin tissues that are anchored to an annulus, or fibrous ring, which also gives the hollow organ some structure and helps to keep the organ open and divided into distinct chambers.

A partition called a septum separates the right half of the heart from the left. The right half receives deoxygenated blood from everywhere in the body through the **veins** (vessels that carry blood toward the heart) and directs that blood into the lungs. The left half receives the now oxygenated blood from the lungs and directs it into the aorta. The aorta delivers blood into the systemic circulation by way of **arteries** (vessels that carry blood away from the heart) (Figure 42–1). The heart is the pump that keeps blood flowing through 60,000 miles of tubes, constituting the cardiovascular system, to deliver oxygen and nutrients to all the cells of the body and to remove metabolic waste products from the tissues.

⬛⬛⬤⬛ WEB LINKS

To explore the virtual cardiovascular system, consult the following Internet source:

http://www.InnerBody.com

The Cardiac Cycle

The heart, which contracts thousands of millions of times in a lifetime, possesses structural and functional properties that are different from those of other muscles. The fibers of the cardiac muscle, or **myocardium,** form two intertwining networks called the atrial and ventricular **syncytia.** These interlacing structures enable first the atria and then the ventricles to contract synchronously when excited by the same stimulus. Simultaneous contraction is a necessary property for a muscle that acts as a pump. A hollow pumping mechanism must also pause long enough in the pumping cycle to allow

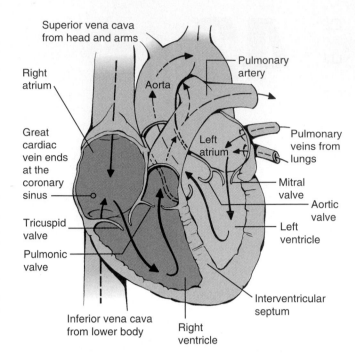

FIGURE 42–1. Blood flow into and out of the heart. Deoxygenated blood enters the right atrium from the great cardiac vein, and the superior and inferior venae cavae and falls through the tricuspid valve into the right ventricle, which contracts and sends the blood through the pulmonic valve into the pulmonary artery and to the lungs. Oxygenated blood from the lungs enters the left atrium through the pulmonary veins and passes through the mitral valve into the left ventricle, which contracts and ejects the blood through the aortic valve into the aorta and out to the systemic circulation.

the chambers to fill with fluid. Heart muscle relaxes long enough to ensure adequate filling; the more completely it fills, the stronger the subsequent contraction. This occurs because the muscle fibers of the heart, stretched by the increased volume of blood that has returned to them, spring back to normal size. This is similar to stretching a rubber band, which returns to its normal size after it is stretched—the further it is stretched, the stronger the spring back to normal. This property is defined in **Starling's law of the heart** (see p. 559).

During **diastole,** the period of cardiac muscle relaxation, blood returns to the heart from the systemic and pulmonic veins, which flow into the right and left atria, respectively. When the pressure generated by the blood volume in the atria is greater than the pressure in the ventricle, blood flows through the atrioventricular (AV) valves into the ventricles. The valve on the right side of the heart is called the tricuspid valve because it is composed of three leaflets or cusps (see Figure 42–1). The valve on the left side of the heart, called the mitral or bicuspid valve, is composed of two leaflets or cusps (see Figure 42–1). Just before the ventricles are stimulated to contract, the atria contract, pushing about 1 more tablespoon of blood into each ventricle. The much more powerful ventricles then contract, pumping blood out to the lungs through the pulmonary valve or out to the aorta through the aortic valve and into the systemic circulation. The contraction of the ventricles is referred to as **systole.**

Each period of systole followed by a period of diastole is called a **cardiac cycle.**

The heart's series of one-way valves keeps the blood flowing in the correct direction, as follows (see Figure 42–1):

Deoxygenated blood—right atrium, through tricuspid valve to right ventricle, through pulmonary valve to the lungs
Oxygenated blood—through the pulmonary veins to the left atrium, through the mitral valve to the left ventricle, through the aortic valve to the aorta

The AV valves close very tightly when the ventricles contract, preventing blood from flowing backward into the atria and keeping it moving forward through the system. The pulmonary and aortic valves open with the pressure of ventricular contraction and close tightly during diastole, keeping blood from flowing backward into the ventricles. These valves operate much like one-way automatic doors: you can go through in the intended direction, but if you try to go the wrong way, the doors close and stop your movement. The proper functioning of the cardiac valves is important in maintaining the functioning of the cardiovascular system.

Conduction System of the Heart

Each cycle of cardiac contraction and relaxation is controlled by impulses that arise spontaneously in certain pacemaker cells of the **sinoatrial (SA) node** of the heart. These impulses are conducted from the pacemaker cells by a specialized conducting system that activates all of the parts of the heart muscle almost simultaneously. These continuous, rhythmic contractions are controlled by the heart itself; the brain does not stimulate the heart to beat. This safety feature allows the heart to beat as long as it has enough nutrients and oxygen to survive, regardless of the status of the rest of the body. This property protects the vital cardiovascular function in many disease states; it is the same property that allows the heart to continue functioning in a patient who is "brain dead."

The conduction system of the heart consists of the SA node, atrial bundles, AV node, bundle of His, bundle branches, and Purkinje fibers (Figure 42–2). The SA node, located in the top of the right atria, acts as the pacemaker of the heart. Atrial bundles conduct the impulse through the atrial muscle. The AV node slows the impulse, allowing for the delay needed for ventricular filling, and sends it from the atria into the ventricles by way of the bundle of His, which enters the septum then divides into three bundle branches. These bundle branches, which conduct the impulses through the ventricles, break into a fine network of conducting fibers called the Purkinje fibers, which deliver the impulse to the ventricular cells.

Automaticity

The cells of the impulse-forming and conducting system are rather primitive, uncomplicated cells called pale or P cells. Because of their simple cell membrane, these cells possess a special property that differentiates them from other cells: they can generate action potentials or electrical impulses

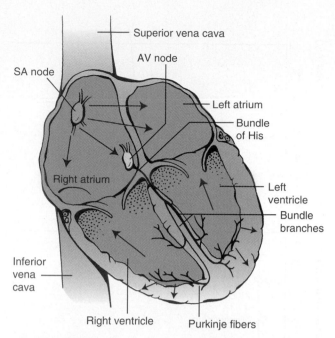

FIGURE 42–2. The conducting system of the heart. Impulses originating in the sinatrial (SA) node are transmitted through the atrial bundles to the atrioventricular (AV) node and down the bundle of His and the bundle branches by way of the Purkinje fibers through the ventricles.

without being excited to do so by external stimuli. This property is called **automaticity.**

All cardiac cells possess some degree of automaticity. During diastole or rest, these cells undergo a spontaneous depolarization because they decrease the flow of potassium ions out of the cell and probably leak sodium into the cell, causing an action potential. This action potential is basically the same as the action potential of the neuron (see Chapter 19). The action potential of the cardiac muscle cell consists of five phases:

- Phase 0 occurs when the cell reaches a point of stimulation. The sodium gates open along the cell membrane, and sodium rushes into the cell, resulting in a positive flow of electrons into the cell—an electrical potential. This is called depolarization.
- Phase 1 is the very short period when the sodium ion concentrations are equal inside and outside the cell.
- Phase 2, or the plateau stage, occurs as the cell membrane becomes less permeable to sodium. Calcium slowly enters the cell, and potassium begins to leave the cell. The cell membrane is trying to return to its resting state, a process called repolarization.
- Phase 3 is a period of rapid repolarization as the gates are closed and potassium rapidly moves out of the cell.
- Phase 4 occurs when the cell comes to rest as the sodium-potassium pump returns the membrane to its previous state, with sodium outside and potassium inside the cell, and spontaneous depolarization begins again.

Each area of the heart has an action potential that appears slightly different from the other action potentials, reflecting

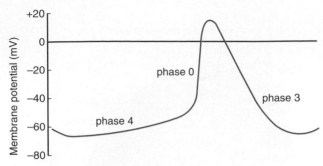

A SA node action potential

B Ventricular muscle cell action potential

FIGURE 42–3. Action potentials recorded from a cell in the sinoatrial (SA) node (**A**), showing diastolic depolarization in phase 4, and recorded from a ventricular muscle cell (**B**). In *phase 0,* the cell is stimulated, sodium rushes into the cell, and the cell is depolarized. In *phase 1,* sodium levels equalize. In *phase 2,* the plateau phase, calcium enters the cell (the slow current), and potassium and sodium leave. In *phase 3,* the slow *current stops, and sodium and potassium leave the cell.* In *phase 4,* the resting membrane potential returns and the pacemaker potential begins in the SA node cell.

the complexity of the cells in that particular area. Because of these differences in the action potential, each area of the heart has a slightly different rate of rhythmicity. The SA node generates an impulse about 90 to 100 times a minute, the AV node about 40 to 50 times a minute, and the complex ventricular muscle cells, only about 10 to 20 times a minute (Figure 42–3).

Conductivity

Normally, the SA node sets the pace for the heart rate because it depolarizes faster than any cell in the heart. However, the other cells in the heart are capable of generating an impulse if anything happens to the SA node, another protective feature of the heart. As mentioned earlier, the SA node is said to be the pacemaker of the heart because it acts to stimulate the rest of the cells to depolarize at its rate. When the SA node sets the pace for the heart rate, the person is said to be in sinus rhythm.

The specialized cells of the heart can conduct an impulse rapidly through the system so that the muscle cells of the heart are stimulated at approximately the same time. This property of cardiac cells is called **conductivity.**

The conduction velocity, or the speed at which the cells can pass on the impulse, is slowest in the AV node and fastest in the Purkinje fibers.

This delay in conduction at the AV node, right between the atria and the ventricles, accounts for the fact that the atria contract a fraction of a second before the ventricles contract. This allows extra time for the ventricles to fill completely before they contract. The almost simultaneous spread of the impulse through the Purkinje fibers permits a simultaneous and powerful contraction of the ventricle muscles, making them an effective pump.

After a cell membrane has conducted an action potential, there is a period of time, called the absolute refractory period, in which it is impossible to stimulate that area of membrane. The absolute refractory period is the minimal amount of time that must elapse between two stimuli applied at one site in the heart for each of these stimuli to cause an action potential. This time reflects the responsiveness of the heart cells to stimuli. Cardiac drugs may affect the refractory period of the cells to make the heart more or less responsive.

Autonomic Influences

The heart can generate action potentials on its own and could function without connection to the rest of the body. The autonomic nervous system (see Chapter 29) can influence the heart rate and rhythm and the strength of contraction. The parasympathetic nerves, primarily the vagus or tenth cranial nerve, can slow the heart rate and decrease the speed of conduction through the AV node. This allows the heart to rest and conserve its strength. The parasympathetic influence on the SA node is the dominant influence most of the time, keeping the resting heart rate at 70 to 80 beats per minute.

The sympathetic nervous system stimulates the heart to beat faster, speeds conduction through the AV node, and causes the heart muscle to contract harder. This action is important during exercise or stress, when the body's cells need to have more oxygen delivered. These two branches of the autonomic nervous system work together to help the heart meet the body's demands. Drugs that influence either of these branches of the autonomic nervous system have autonomic effects on the heart.

Mechanical Activity

The end result of the electrical stimulation of the heart cells is the unified contraction of the atria and ventricles, which moves the blood throughout the vascular system. The basic unit of the cardiac muscle is the **sarcomere.** A sarcomere is made up of two contractile proteins: **actin,** a thin filament, and **myosin,** a thick filament with small projections on it. These proteins readily react with each other, but at rest they are kept apart by the protein **troponin.**

When a cardiac muscle cell is stimulated, calcium enters the cell though channels in the cell membrane and also from storage sites within the cell. This occurs during phase 3 of the action potential, when the cell is starting to repolarize. The calcium reacts with the troponin and inactivates it. This action allows the actin and myosin proteins to react with each other, forming actomyosin bridges. These bridges then break quickly, and the myosin slides along to form new bridges.

As long as calcium is present, the actomyosin bridges continue to form. This action slides the proteins together, shortening or contracting the sarcomere. Cardiac muscle cells are linked together, so when one cell is stimulated to contract, they are all stimulated to contract.

The shortening of numerous sarcomeres causes the contraction and pumping action of the heart muscle. As the cell reaches its repolarized state, calcium is removed from the cell by a sodium–calcium pump, and calcium released from storage sites within the cell returns to the storage sites. The contraction process requires energy and oxygen for the chemical reaction that allows the formation of the actomyosin bridges, and calcium to allow the bridge formation to occur.

The degree of shortening (the strength of contraction) is determined by the amount of calcium present—the more calcium is present, the more bridges will be formed—and by the stretch of the sarcomere before contraction begins. The further apart the actin and myosin proteins are before the cell is stimulated, the more bridges will be formed and the stronger the contraction will be. This correlates with Starling's law of the heart. The more the cardiac muscle is stretched, the greater the contraction will be. The more blood you put into the heart, the greater the contraction will be to empty the heart, up to a point. However, if the bridges are stretched too far apart, they will not be able to reach each other to form the actomyosin bridges, and no contraction will occur (Figure 42–4).

Cardiac Arrhythmias

Various factors—drugs, acidosis, decreased oxygen levels, changes in the electrolytes in the area, buildup of waste products—can change the cardiac rate and rhythm. A disruption in cardiac rate or rhythm is called an **arrhythmia** or a **dysrhythmia.** Arrhythmias interfere with the work of the heart and can disrupt cardiac output, which affects every cell in the body. Arrhythmias can arise because of changes in the automaticity or conductivity of the heart cells. Some arrhythmias occur when there is a shift in the pacemaker of the heart from the SA node to some other site, called an ectopic focus. This occurs most frequently with damage to the heart

muscle and can be seen in the form of premature contractions or extrasystoles. These premature beats may be unimportant and sporadic, but in some cases they can be the prelude to more serious or even fatal arrhythmias if the coordinated pumping action of the muscle is lost.

A lack of or decrease in conductivity through the AV node produces a condition called heart block. In first-degree heart block, all of the impulses from the SA node arrive in the ventricles, but it takes a longer time than normal. In second-degree heart block, some of the impulses are lost and do not get through, resulting in a slow rate of ventricular contraction. In third-degree or complete heart block, no impulses from the SA node get through to the ventricles, and the much slower ventricular automaticity takes over. Very serious arrhythmias arise when the combination of ectopic foci and altered conduction set off an irregular, uncoordinated twitching of the atrial or ventricular muscle, called **fibrillation.** In this situation, the pumping action of the heart is lost, and the cardiac output falls. Individuals can live quite normally with atrial fibrillation, but if the ventricles fibrillate, there is total loss of cardiac output, and death can occur if treatment is not initiated quickly

THE ELECTROCARDIOGRAM

Electrocardiography is a process of recording the patterns of electrical impulses as they move through the heart. It has become a very important diagnostic tool in the care of the cardiac patient. The electrocardiography machine detects the patterns of electrical impulse generation and conduction through the heart and translates that information to a recorded pattern, which is displayed on a cardiac monitor or printed out on calibrated paper as a wave form. It must be remembered that an **electrocardiogram (ECG)** is a measure of electrical activity; it provides no information about the mechanical activity of the heart. The very important aspect of cardiac output—the degree to which the heart is doing its job of pumping blood out to all of the tissues—needs to be carefully assessed by looking at and evaluating the patient.

Normal Sinus Rhythm

The normal ECG pattern is made up of five main waves: the P wave, which is formed as impulses originating in the SA node or pacemaker pass through the atrial tissues; the QRS complex, which represents depolarization of the bundle of His (Q) and the ventricles (RS); and the T wave, which represents repolarization of the ventricles.

The P wave immediately precedes the contraction of the atria. The QRS complex immediately precedes the contraction of the ventricles and then relaxation of the ventricles during the T wave. The repolarization of the atria, the Ta wave, occurs during the QRS complex and usually is not seen on an ECG. In certain conditions of atrial hypertrophy, the Ta wave may appear around the QRS complex (Figure 42–5).

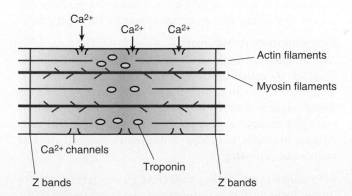

FIGURE 42–4. A sarcomere, the functional unit of cardiac muscle.

Time

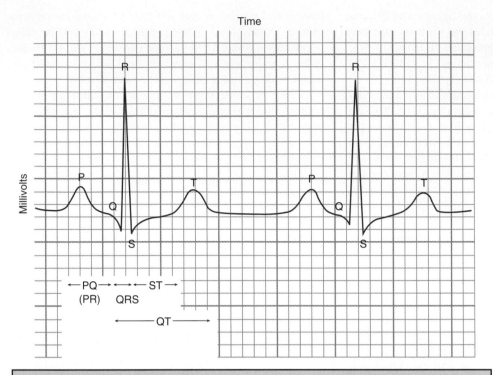

Millivolts

←PQ→ ←→ ←— ST —→
(PR)   QRS

←——— QT ———→

Key:

Each vertical square represents one tenth of a milli-
volt of electrical charge

Each horizontal square equals 0.04 seconds of time.

Approximate values for normal intervals:

PQ(PR) interval—0.16 sec
QT interval—0.3 sec
QRS interval—0.08 sec
P wave—0.08 sec
ST interval—0.1 sec

P wave = Electrical changes associated with atrial depolarization
QRS complex = Electrical changes associated with ventricular depolarization
T wave = Electrical changes associated with ventricular repolarization
The electrical changes associated with atrial repolarization normally coincide with the QRS complex
and are obscured by it.

FIGURE 42-5. The normal electrocardiogram pattern.

The critical points of the ECG are as follows:

P–R interval—reflects the normal delay of conduction at the AV node

Q–T interval—reflects the critical timing of repolarization of the ventricles

S–T segment—reflects important information about the repolarization of the ventricles

Abnormalities in the shape or timing of each part of an ECG tracing reveal the presence of particular cardiac disorders. A person with a normal ECG pattern and a heart rate within the normal range for that person's age group is said to be in normal sinus rhythm.

Types of Arrhythmias

A disruption in cardiac rate or rhythm is called an arrhythmia (or dysrhythmia). Arrhythmias are significant because they interfere with the work of the heart and can disrupt the cardiac output, which eventually will affect every cell in the body.

Sinus Arrhythmias

The SA node is influenced by the autonomic nervous system to change the rate of firing in order to meet the body's demands for oxygen. A faster-than-normal heart rate, usually anything faster than 100 beats/min in an adult, with a normal-appearing ECG pattern is called sinus tachycardia. Sinus bradycardia is a slower-than-normal heart rate (usually less than 60 beats/min) with a normal-appearing ECG pattern.

Supraventricular Arrhythmias

Arrhythmias that originate above the ventricles but not in the SA node are called supraventricular arrhythmias. These arrhythmias feature an abnormally shaped P wave, because the site of origin is not the sinus node; however, they show normal QRS complexes, because the ventricles are still conducting impulses normally. Supraventricular arrhythmias include the following:

• *Premature atrial contractions* (*PACs*), which reflect an ectopic focus in the atria generating an impulse out of the normal rhythm

• *Paroxysmal atrial tachycardia (PAT)*, sporadically occurring runs of rapid heart rate originating in the atria
• *Atrial flutter*, characterized by sawtooth-shaped P waves reflecting a single ectopic focus generating a regular, fast atrial depolarization
• *Atrial fibrillation*, with irregular P waves representing many ectopic foci firing in an uncoordinated manner through the atria

With atrial flutter, often one of every two or one of every three impulses is transmitted to the ventricles. The person may have a 2:1 or 3:1 ratio of P waves to QRS complexes. The ventricles beat faster than normal, losing some efficiency. With atrial fibrillation, so many impulses are bombarding the AV node that an unpredictable number of impulses are transmitted to the ventricles. The ventricles are stimulated to beat in a fast, irregular, and often inefficient manner.

Atrioventricular Block

AV block, also called heart block, reflects a slowing or lack of conduction at the AV node. This can occur because of structural damage, hypoxia, or injury to the heart muscle. First-degree heart block is characterized by a lengthening of the P–R interval beyond the normal 0.16 to 0. 20 seconds. Each P wave is followed by a QRS complex. In second-degree heart block, a QRS complex may follow one, two, three, or four P waves. Third-degree heart block, or complete heart block, shows a total dissociation of P waves from QRS complexes and T waves. Because the P waves can come at any time, the P–R interval is not constant. The QRS complexes appear at a very slow rate and may not be sufficient to meet the body's needs.

Ventricular Arrhythmias

Impulses that originate below the AV node originate from ectopic foci that do not use the normal conduction pathways. The QRS complexes appear wide and prolonged, and the T waves are inverted, reflecting the slower conduction across cardiac tissue that is not part of the rapid conduction system. Premature ventricular contractions (PVCs) can arise from a single ectopic focus in the ventricles, all having the same shape, or from many ectopic foci, which produces PVCs having different shapes. Runs or bursts of PVCs from many different foci are more ominous because they can reflect extensive damage or hypoxia in the myocardium. Runs of several PVCs at a rapid rate are called ventricular tachycardia. Ventricular fibrillation is seen as a bizarre, irregular, distorted wave. It is potentially fatal because it reflects a lack of any coordinated stimulation of the ventricles, which leads to inability to contract in a coordinated fashion, with no blood being pumped to the body or the brain.

THE CARDIOVASCULAR SYSTEM

The purpose of the heart's continual pumping action is to keep blood flowing to and from all of the body's tissues. Blood delivers oxygen and much-needed nutrients to the cells for producing energy, and it carries away carbon dioxide and other waste products of metabolism. The steady circulation of blood is essential for the proper functioning of all of the body's organs, including the heart itself.

Circulation

The circulation of the blood follows two courses:

Heart–lung or pulmonary circulation—the right side of the heart sends blood to the lungs, where carbon dioxide and some waste products are removed from the blood and oxygen is picked up by the red blood cells.
Systemic circulation—the left side of the heart sends oxygenated blood out to all of the cells in the body.

The blood moves through the circulatory system from areas of high pressure to areas of lower pressure. The system is a "closed" system; that is, it has no openings or holes that would allow blood to leak out. The closed nature of the system is what keeps the pressure differences in the proper relationship so that blood always flows in the direction it is intended to flow (Figure 42–6).

Veins—distensible, thin walls

Pulmonary vessels—distensible, thin walls

Arteries—elastic, thick walls

Capillaries

FIGURE 42–6. Blood flow through the systemic and pulmonary vasculature circuits. (From Bullock, B. L. [2000]. *Focus on pathophysiology*. Philadelphia: Lippincott Williams & Wilkins.)

Pulmonary and Systemic Circulation

The right atrium is a very-low-pressure area in the cardiovascular system. All of the deoxygenated blood from the body flows into the right atrium from the inferior and superior venae cavae (see Figure 42–1), and from the great cardiac vein, which returns deoxygenated blood from the heart muscle. As the blood flows into the atria, the pressure increases. When the pressure becomes greater than the pressure in the right ventricle, most of the blood flows into the right ventricle. At this point in the cardiac cycle, the atrium is stimulated to contract and pushes the remaining blood into the right ventricle. The ventricle is then stimulated to contract; it generates pressure that pushes open the pulmonic valve (see Figure 42–1) and sends blood into the pulmonary artery, which takes the blood into the lungs, a very-low-pressure area. The blood then circulates around the alveoli of the lungs, picking up oxygen and getting rid of carbon dioxide, flows through pulmonary capillaries (the tiny blood vessels that connect arteries and veins) into the pulmonary veins, and then flows into the left atrium. When the pressure of blood volume in the left atrium is greater than the pressure in the large left ventricle, this oxygenated blood flows into the left ventricle. The left atrium contracts and pushes any remaining blood into the left ventricle, which is stimulated to contract and generates tremendous pressure to push the blood out the aorta, carrying it throughout the body.

Arteries, Capillaries, and Veins

The aorta and other large arteries have thick, muscular walls. The entire arterial system contains muscles in the walls of the vessels all the way to the terminal branches or arterioles, which consist of fragments of muscle and endothelial cells. These muscles offer resistance to the blood that is sent pumping into the arterial system by the left ventricle, generating pressure. The arterial system is referred to as a **resistance system.** The vessels can either constrict or dilate, increasing or decreasing resistance, based on the needs of the body. The arterioles are able to completely shut off blood flow to some areas of the body; that is, they can shunt blood to another area where it is needed more. The arterioles, because of their ability to increase or decrease resistance in the system, are one of the main regulators of blood pressure.

Blood from the tiny arterioles flows into the **capillary** system, which connects the arterial and venous systems. These microscopic vessels are composed of loosely connected endothelial cells. Oxygen, fluid, and nutrients are able to pass through the arterial end of the capillaries and enter the interstitial area between tissue cells. Fluid at the venous end of the capillary is drawn back into the vessel and contains carbon dioxide and other waste products. This shifting of fluid in the capillaries, called the capillary fluid shift, is carefully regulated by a balance between hydrostatic (fluid pressure) forces on the arterial end of the capillary and **oncotic pressure** (the pulling pressure of the large, vascular proteins) on the venous end of the capillary. In a normal situation, the higher pressure at the arterial end of a capillary forces fluid out of the vessel and into the tissue, and the now-concentrated proteins (which are too large to leave the capillary) exert a pull on the fluid at the venous end of the capillary to pull it back in. A disruption in the hydrostatic pressure or in the concentration of proteins in the capillary can lead to fluid's being left in the tissue, a condition referred to as edema. The capillaries merge into venules, which merge into veins, which are responsible for returning the blood to the heart (Figure 42–7).

The veins are thin-walled, very elastic, low-pressure vessels that can hold large quantities of blood if necessary. The venous system is referred to as a **capacitance system** because the veins have the capacity to hold large quantities of fluid as they distend with fluid volume. These capacitance vessels have a great deal of influence on the venous return to the heart, the amount of blood that is delivered to the right atrium.

	Arterial end		Venous end
Hydrostatic pressure (HP) Driving force of heart tends to push fluid out of capillary	36 mm Hg		21 mm Hg
Oncotic pressure (OP) Pressure exerted by plasma proteins tends to pull fluid into capillary	28 mm Hg		28 mm Hg
Filtration pressure Net force on fluid, determined by the balance between HP and OP	8 mm Hg		–7 mm Hg
	HP > OP Fluid leaves capillary		HP < OP Fluid enters capillary

FIGURE 42–7. The net shift of fluid out of and into the capillary is determined by the balance between the hydrostatic pressure (*HP*) and the oncotic pressure (*OP*). HP tends to push fluid out of the capillary, and OP tends to pull it back into the capillary. At the arterial end of the capillary bed, the blood pressure (*HP*) is higher than at the venous end. At the arterial end, HP exceeds OP, and fluid filters out. At the venous end, HP has fallen and HP is less than OP; fluid is pulled back into the capillary from the surrounding tissue. The lymphatic system also returns fluids and substances from the tissues to the circulation.

Coronary Circulation

The heart muscle itself requires a constant supply of oxygenated blood to keep contracting. The myocardium receives its blood through two main coronary arteries that branch off the base of the aorta from an area called the sinuses of Valsalva. These arteries encircle the heart in a pattern resembling a crown, which is why they are called coronary arteries.

The artery arising from the left side of the aorta bifurcates, or divides, into two large vessels called the left circumflex artery (which travels down the left side of the heart and feeds most of the left ventricle) and the left anterior descending coronary artery (which travels down the front of the heart and feeds the septum and anterior areas, including much of the conduction system). The artery arising from the right side of the aorta feeds most of the right side of the heart, including the sinoatrial node.

The coronary arteries receive blood during diastole, when the muscle is at rest and relaxed so that blood can flow freely down into the muscle. When the ventricle contracts, it forces the aortic valve open, and the leaflets of the valve cover the openings of the coronary arteries. When the ventricles relax, the blood is no longer pumped forward and starts to flow back toward the ventricle. The blood flowing down the sides of the aorta closes the aortic valve and fills up the coronary arteries. The pressure that fills the coronary arteries is the difference between the systolic ejection pressure and the diastolic resting pressure. This is called the **pulse pressure** (systolic minus diastolic blood pressure readings). The pulse pressure is monitored clinically to evaluate the filling pressure of the coronary arteries. The oxygenated blood that is fed into the heart by the coronary circulation reaches every cardiac muscle fiber as the vessels divide and subdivide throughout the myocardium.

The heart has a pattern of circulation, called end-artery circulation. The arteries go into the muscle and end without a great deal of backup or collateral circulation. Normally this is an efficient system and is able to meet the needs of the heart muscle. The heart's supply of and demand for oxygen is met by changes in the delivery of oxygen through the coronary system. Problems can arise, however, when an imbalance develops between the supply of oxygen delivered to the heart muscle and the myocardial demand for oxygen. The main forces that determine the heart's use of oxygen or oxygen consumption are as follows:

- *Heart rate*—The more the heart has to pump, the more oxygen it will require to do that.
- *Preload* (amount of blood that is brought back to the heart to be pumped around)—The more blood that is returned to the heart, the harder it will have to work to pump the blood around. The volume of blood in the system is a determinant of preload.
- *Afterload* (resistance against which the heart has to beat)—The higher the resistance in the system, the harder the heart will have to contract to force open the valves and pump the blood along. Blood pressure is a measure of afterload.

- *Stretch on the ventricles*—If the ventricular muscle is stretched before it is stimulated to contract, more actomyosin bridges will be formed (which will take more energy); or, if the muscle is stimulated to contract harder than usual (which happens with sympathetic stimulation), more bridges will be formed, which will require more energy.

The muscle can be stretched with ventricular hypertrophy related to chronic hypertension or cardiac muscle damage, or with heart failure when the ventricle does not empty completely and blood backs up in the system.

The supply of blood to the myocardium can be altered when the heart fails to pump effectively and cannot deliver blood to the coronary arteries. This happens in congestive heart failure and cases of hypotension. The supply is most frequently altered, however, when the coronary vessels become narrowed and unresponsive to stimuli to dilate and deliver more blood. This happens in atherosclerosis or coronary artery disease. The end result of this narrowing can be total blockage of a coronary artery, leading to hypoxia and eventual death of the cells that depend on that vessel for oxygen. This is called a myocardial infarction (MI), and it is the leading cause of death in the United States (Figure 42–8).

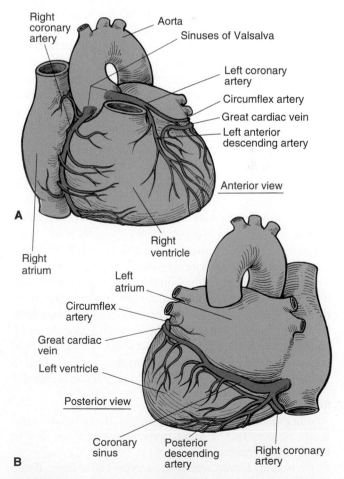

FIGURE 42-8. Coronary arteries and veins. (**A**) Anterior view; (**B**) posterior view. (From Bullock, B. L. [2000]. *Focus on pathophysiology.* Philadelphia: Lippincott Williams & Wilkins.)

Systemic Arterial Pressure

The contraction of the left ventricle, which sends blood surging out into the aorta, creates a pressure that continues to force blood into all of the branches of the aorta. This pressure against arterial walls is greatest during systole (cardiac contraction), and falls to its lowest level during diastole. The measurement of both the systolic and diastolic pressure indicates the pumping pressure of the ventricle and the generalized pressure in the system, or the pressure the ventricle has to overcome to pump blood out of the heart.

Hypotension

The pressure in the arteries needs to remain relatively high to ensure that blood is delivered to every cell in the body and to keep the blood flowing from high-pressure to low-pressure areas. Hypotension can occur if the blood pressure falls dramatically, either from loss of blood volume or from failure of the heart muscle to pump effectively. Severe hypotension can progress to shock and even death as cells are cut off from their oxygen supply.

Hypertension

Constant, excessive high blood pressure, called hypertension, can damage the fragile inner lining of blood vessels and cause a disruption of blood flow to the tissues. It also puts a tremendous strain on the heart muscle, increasing myocardial oxygen consumption and putting the heart muscle itself at risk. Hypertension can be caused by neurostimulation of the blood vessels that causes them to constrict and to raise pressure, or by increased volume in the system. In most cases, the cause of hypertension is not known, and drug therapy to correct it is aimed at changing one or more of the normal reflexes that control vascular resistance or the force of cardiac muscle contraction.

Vasomotor Tone

The smooth muscles in the walls of the arteries receive constant input from nerve fibers of the sympathetic nervous system. These impulses work to dilate the vessels if more blood flow is needed in an area; to constrict vessels if increased pressure is needed in the system; and to maintain muscle tone so that the vessel remains patent and responsive.

The coordination of these impulses is regulated through the medulla in an area called the cardiovascular center. If increased pressure is needed, this center increases sympathetic flow to the vessels. If pressure rises too high, this is sensed by baroreceptors or pressure receptors and the sympathetic flow is decreased. Chapter 43 discusses the drugs that are used to influence the stimulation of vessels to alter blood pressure.

Renin–Angiotensin System

Another determinant of blood pressure is the renin–angiotensin system. This system is activated when blood flow to the kidneys is decreased.

Cells in the kidney release an enzyme called renin. Renin is transported to the liver, where it converts angiotensinogen (produced in the liver) to angiotensin I. Angiotensin I travels

FIGURE 42–9. The renin–angiotensin system for reflex maintenance of blood pressure control.

to the lungs, where it is converted by angiotensin-converting enzyme (ACE) to angiotensin II. Angiotensin II travels through the body and reacts with angiotensin II receptor sites on blood vessels to cause a severe vasoconstriction. This increases blood pressure and should increase blood flow to the kidneys to decrease the release of renin. Angiotensin II also causes the release of aldosterone from the adrenal cortex, which causes retention of sodium and water, leading to the release of antidiuretic hormone (ADH) to retain water and increase blood volume. Increasing blood volume increases blood flow to the kidney. This system works constantly, whenever a position change alters flow to the kidney or blood volume or pressure changes, to help maintain the blood pressure within a range that ensures perfusion (delivery of blood to all of the tissues) (Figure 42–9).

Venous Pressure

Pressure in the veins may also sometimes rise above normal. This can happen when the heart is not pumping effectively and cannot pump out all of the blood that is trying to return to it. This results in a backup or congestion of blood waiting to enter the heart. Pressure rises in the right atrium and then in the veins that are trying to return blood to the heart as they encounter resistance. The venous system begins to back up, or become congested with blood.

Congestive Heart Failure and Edema

When the heart muscle fails to do its job of effectively pumping blood through the system, blood backs up and the system becomes congested. This is called congestive heart failure (CHF). The rise in venous pressure that results from this backup of blood increases the hydrostatic pressure on the venous end of the capillaries. Hydrostatic pressure pushing fluid out of the capillary is soon higher than the oncotic pressure that is trying to pull the fluid back into the vessel, causing fluid to be lost into the tissues. This shift of fluid accounts for the edema seen with CHF. Pulmonary edema results when the left side of the heart is failing; peripheral, abdominal, and liver edema occur when the right side of the heart is failing.

Other factors that can contribute to this loss of fluid in the tissues include protein loss and fluid retention. Protein loss can lead to a fall in oncotic pressure and an inability to pull fluid back into the vascular system. Protein levels fall in renal failure, when protein is lost in the urine, and in liver failure, when the liver is no longer able to produce plasma proteins. Fluid retention, which often is stimulated by aldosterone and ADH as described above, can increase the hydrostatic pressure so much that fluid is pushed out under higher pressure and the balancing pressure to pull it back into the vessel is not sufficient. Drugs that are used to treat CHF may affect the vascular system at any of these areas in an attempt to return a balance to the pressures in the system.

CHAPTER SUMMARY

- The heart is a hollow muscle that is divided into a right and left side by a thick septum, and into four chambers—the two upper atria and the two lower ventricles.
- The heart is responsible for pumping oxygenated blood to every cell in the body and for picking up waste products from the tissues.
- The cardiac cycle consists of a period of rest, or diastole, when blood is returned to the heart by veins, and a period of contraction, or systole, when the blood is pumped out of the heart.
- The right side of the heart receives all of the deoxygenated blood from the body through the veins and directs it into the lungs.
- The left side of the heart receives oxygenated blood from the lungs and pumps it out to every cell in the body through the arteries.
- The heart muscle possesses the properties of automaticity (the ability to generate an action potential in the absence of stimulation) and conductivity (the ability to rapidly transmit an action potential).
- The heart muscle is stimulated to contract by impulses generated in the heart, not by stimuli from the brain. The autonomic nervous system can affect the heart to increase (sympathetic) or decrease (parasympathetic) activity.
- The normal conduction or stimulatory system of the heart consists of the SA node, the atrial bundles, the AV node, the bundle of His, the bundle branches, and the Purkinje fibers.
- In normal sinus rhythm, cells in the SA node generate an impulse that is transmitted through the atrial bundles and delayed slightly at the AV node before being sent down the bundle of His into the ventricles. When cardiac muscle cells are stimulated, they contract.
- Alterations in the generation of conduction of impulses in the heart cause arrhythmias (dysrhythmias), which can upset the normal balance in the cardiovascular system and lead to a decrease in cardiac output, affecting all of the cells of the body.
- Heart muscle contracts by the sliding of actin and myosin filaments in a functioning unit called a sarcomere. Contraction requires energy and calcium to allow the filaments to react with each other and slide together.
- The heart muscle needs a constant supply of blood, which is furnished by the coronary arteries. Increase in demand for oxygen can occur with changes in heart rate, preload, afterload, or stretch on the muscle.
- The cardiovascular system is a closed pressure system that uses arteries (muscular, pressure or resistance tubes) to carry blood from the heart, veins (flexible, distensible capacitance vessels) to return blood to the heart, and capillaries (which connect arteries to veins) to keep blood flowing from areas of high pressure to areas of low pressure.
- Blood pressure is maintained by stimulus from the sympathetic system and reflex control of blood volume and pressure by the renin–angiotensin system and the aldosterone–ADH system. Alterations in blood pressure (hypotension or hypertension) can upset the balance of the cardiovascular system and lead to problems in blood delivery.
- Fluid shifts out of the blood at the arterial ends of capillaries to deliver oxygen and nutrients to the tissues. It is pushed out of the vessel by the hydrostatic or fluid pressure in the arterial side of the system. Fluid returns to the system at the venous end of the capillaries because of the oncotic pull of proteins in the vessels. Disruptions in these pressures can lead to edema or loss of fluid in the tissues.

Review Questions

1. When referring to the heart valves,
   a. the closing of the AV valves is what is responsible for heart sounds.
   b. small muscles attached to the AV valves are responsible for opening and closing the valves with each cycle contraction.
   c. the aortic valve opens when the pressure in the left ventricle become slightly greater than the pressure in the aorta.
   d. the valves leading to the great vessels are called cuspid valves.
2. In the heart,
   a. the ventricles will not contract unless they are stimulated by action potentials arising from the SA node in the right atrium.

b. fibrillation of the atria will cause the blood pressure to fall to zero.

c. spontaneous depolarization of the muscle membrane can occur in the absence of nerve stimulation.

d. the muscle can continue to contract for a long period of time in the absence of oxygen through the use of anaerobic glycolysis to synthesize ATP.

3. The activity of the heart depends on both the inherent properties of the cardiac muscle cells and the activity of the autonomic nerves to the heart. Therefore,

a. cutting all of the autonomic nerves to the heart will produce a decrease in heart rate.

b. blocking the parasympathetic nerves to the heart decreases the heart rate.

c. stimulating the sympathetic nerves to the heart increases the time available to fill the ventricles during diastole.

d. dehydration leads to an increase in heart rate.

4. A heart transplantation patient has no nerve connections to the transplanted heart. In such an individual, one would expect to find

a. a slower than normal resting heart rate.

b. atria that contract at a different rate than ventricles.

c. an increase in heart rate during emotional stress.

d. inability to exercise because there is no way to increase heart rate or force of contraction to increase cardiac output.

5. The baroreceptors in the carotid sinus and aortic arch

a. are in appropriate position to protect the brain from sudden changes in blood pressure and thus blood flow.

b. decrease the frequency of impulses sent to the cardiovascular center when arterial blood pressure is increased.

c. monitor the magnitude of concentration of oxygen in the vessels.

d. react to high levels of carbon dioxide.

6. During diastole, the following would not occur:

a. the atrioventricular valves would open.

b. the myocardial muscle would relax.

c. blood would flow from the atria to the ventricles.

d. the ventricles would contract.

7. Cardiac cells differ from skeletal muscle cells in that

a. they contain actin and myosin.

b. they possess automaticity and conductivity.

c. calcium must be present for muscle contraction to occur.

d. they do not require oxygen to survive.

8. The sympathetic nervous system would not be expected to

a. stimulate the heart to beat faster.

b. speed conduction through the AV node.

c. cause the heart muscle to contract harder.

d. slow conduction through the AV node.

9. Clinically, dysrhythmias or arrhythmias cause

a. alterations in cardiac output that could affect all cells.

b. changes in capillary filling pressures.

c. alterations in osmotic pressure.

d. valvular dysfunction.

10. A patient is brought to the emergency room with a suspected MI. The patient is very upset because he had just had an ECG in his doctor's office and it was fine. The explanation of this common phenomenon would include the fact that

a. the ECG only reflects changes in cardiac output.

b. the ECG is not a very accurate test.

c. the ECG only measures the flow of electrical current through the heart and does not indicate mechanical activity or blood flow to the muscle.

d. the ECG is not related to the heart problems.

11. Blood flow to the myocardium differs from blood flow to the rest of the cells of the body in that

a. blood perfuses the myocardium during systole.

b. blood flow is determined by many local factors including buildup of acid.

c. blood perfuses the myocardium during diastole.

d. oxygenated blood flows to the myocardium via veins.

BIBLIOGRAPHY

Bullock, B. L. (2000). *Focus on pathophysiology.* Philadelphia: Lippincott Williams & Wilkins.

Ganong, W. (1999). *Review of medical physiology* (19th ed.). Norwalk, CT: Appleton & Lange.

Guyton, A., & Hall, J. (2000). *Textbook of medical physiology.* Philadelphia: W. B. Saunders.

Gilman, A., Hardman, J. G., & Limbird, L. E. (Eds.) (2002). *Goodman and Gilman's the pharmacological basis of therapeutics* (10th ed.). New York: McGraw-Hill.

Karch, A. M. (2002). *2003 Lippincott's nursing drug guide.* Philadelphia: Lippincott Williams & Wilkins.

Porth, C. M. (2002). *Pathophysiology: Concepts of altered health states* (6th ed.). Philadelphia: Lippincott Williams & Wilkins.

CHAPTER 43

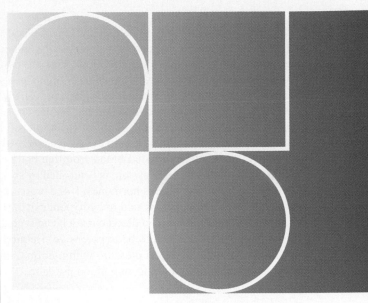

Drugs Affecting Blood Pressure

Key Terms
ACE inhibitor
angiotensin II receptors
baroreceptor
cardiovascular center
essential hypertension
hypotension
peripheral resistance
renin–angiotensin system
shock
stroke volume

Antihypertensive Agents

Angiotensin-Converting Enzyme (ACE) Inhibitors
benazepril
P captopril
enalapril
fosinopril
lisinopril
moexipril
perindopril
quinapril
ramipril
trandolapril

Angiotensin II Receptor Blockers
candesartan
eprosartan
irbesartan
P losartan
telmisartan
valsartan

Calcium Channel Blockers
amlodipine
P diltiazem
felodipine
isradipine
nicardipine
nifedipine
nisoldipine
verapamil

Vasodilators
diazoxide
hydralazine
minoxidil
P nitroprusside
tolazoline

Ganglionic Blocker
mecamylamine

Antihypotensive Agent
midodrine

The cardiovascular system is a closed system of blood vessels that is responsible for delivering oxygenated blood to the tissues and removing waste products from the tissues. The blood in this system flows from areas of higher pressure to areas of lower pressure. The area of highest pressure in the system is always the left ventricle during systole. The pressure in this area propels the blood out of the aorta and into the system. The lowest pressure is in the right atrium, which collects all of the deoxygenated blood from the body. The maintenance of this pressure system is controlled by specific areas of the brain and various hormones. If the pressure becomes too high, the person is said to be hypertensive. If the pressure becomes too low and blood cannot be delivered effectively, the person is said to be hypotensive. Helping the patient to maintain the blood pressure within normal limits is the goal of drug therapy affecting blood pressure.

BLOOD PRESSURE CONTROL

The pressure in the cardiovascular system is determined by three elements: (1) the heart rate; (2) the **stroke volume,** or the amount of blood that is pumped out of the ventricle with each heart beat (primarily determined by the volume of blood in the system); and (3) total **peripheral resistance,** or the resistance of the muscular arteries to the blood being pumped through.

The small arterioles are thought to be the most important factors in determining peripheral resistance. Because they have the smallest diameter, they are able to almost stop blood flow into capillary beds when they constrict, building up tremendous pressure in the arteries behind them as they prevent the blood from flowing through. The arterioles are very responsive to stimulation from the sympathetic nervous system; they constrict when the sympathetic system is stimulated, increasing total peripheral resistance and blood pressure. The body uses this responsiveness to regulate blood pressure on a minute-to-minute basis, to ensure that there is enough pressure in the system to deliver sufficient blood to the brain.

Baroreceptors

As the blood leaves the left ventricle through the aorta, it influences specialized cells in the arch of the aorta called **baroreceptors** (pressure receptors). Similar cells are located in the carotid arteries, which deliver blood to the brain. If there is sufficient pressure in these vessels, the baroreceptors are stimulated, sending that information to the brain. If the pressure falls, the stimulation of the baroreceptors falls off. That information is also sent up to the brain.

The sensory input from the baroreceptors is received in the medulla, in an area called the **cardiovascular center** or vasomotor center. If the pressure is high, the medulla stimulates vasodilation and a decrease in cardiac rate and output, causing the pressure in the system to drop. If the pressure is

low, the medulla directly stimulates an increase in cardiac rate and output and vasoconstriction; this increases total peripheral resistance and raises the blood pressure. The medulla mediates these effects through the autonomic nervous system (see Chapter 29).

The baroreceptor reflex functions continually to maintain blood pressure within a predetermined range of normal. For example, if you have been lying down flat and suddenly stand up, the blood will rush to your feet (an effect of gravity). You may even feel lightheaded or dizzy for a short time. When you stand and the blood flow drops, the baroreceptors are not stretched. The medulla senses this drop in stimulation of the baroreceptors and stimulates a rise in heart rate and cardiac output and a generalized vasoconstriction, which increases total peripheral resistance and blood pressure. These increases should raise pressure in the system, which restores blood flow to the brain and stimulates the baroreceptors. The stimulation of the baroreceptors leads to a decrease in stimulatory impulses from the medulla, and the blood pressure falls back within normal limits (Figure 43–1).

Renin–Angiotensin System

Another compensatory system is activated when the blood pressure within the kidneys falls. Because the kidneys require a constant perfusion to function properly, they have a compensatory mechanism to help ensure that blood flow is maintained. This mechanism is called the **renin–angiotensin system.** (It is also sometimes referred to as the renin–angiotensin–aldosterone system.)

Low blood pressure or poor oxygenation of a nephron causes the release of renin from the juxtaglomerular cells, a group of cells that monitor blood pressure and flow into the glomerulus. Renin is released into the bloodstream and arrives in the liver to convert the compound angiotensinogen (produced in the liver) to angiotensin I. Angiotensin I travels in the bloodstream to the lungs, where the metabolic cells of the alveoli convert it, using angiotensin-converting enzyme (ACE), to angiotensin II. Angiotensin II reacts with specific angiotensin II receptor sites on blood vessels to cause intense vasoconstriction. This effect raises the total peripheral resistance and raises the blood pressure, restoring blood flow to the kidneys and decreasing the release of renin.

Angiotensin II, probably after conversion to angiotensin III, also stimulates the adrenal cortex to release aldosterone. Aldosterone acts on the nephrons to cause the retention of sodium and water. This effect increases blood volume, which should also contribute to increasing blood pressure. The sodium-rich blood stimulates the osmoreceptors in the hypothalamus to cause the release of antidiuretic hormone (ADH), which in turn causes retention of water in the nephrons, further increasing the blood volume. This increase in blood volume increases the blood pressure, which should increase blood flow to the kidneys. This should lead to a decrease in the release of renin, thus causing the compensatory mechanisms to stop (Figure 43–2).

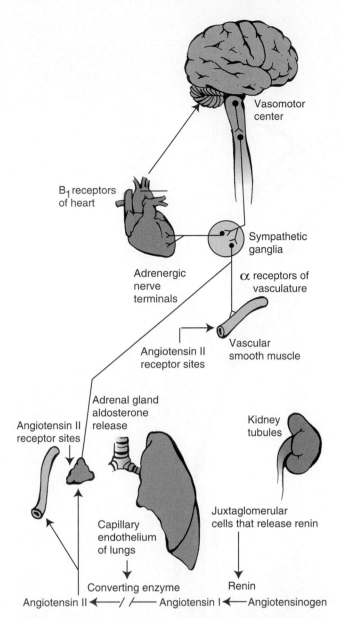

FIGURE 43-1. Control of blood pressure. The vasomotor center in the medulla responds to stimuli from aortic and carotid baroreceptors to cause sympathetic stimulation. The kidneys release renin to activate the renin–angiotensin system, causing vasoconstriction and increased blood volume.

Hypertension

When a person's blood pressure is above normal limits for a sustained period, a diagnosis of hypertension is made (Box 43–1). It is estimated that at least 20% of the people in the United States have hypertension, many of whom are not even aware of it. Ninety percent of the people with hypertension have what is called **essential hypertension,** or hypertension with no known underlying cause. People with essential hypertension usually have an elevated total peripheral resistance. Their organs are being perfused effectively, and they usually display no symptoms. A few people develop secondary hypertension, or high blood

pressure resulting from a known cause. For instance, a tumor in the adrenal medulla, called a pheochromocytoma, can cause hypertension that resolves after the tumor is removed.

The underlying danger of hypertension of any type is the prolonged force on the vessels of the vascular system. The muscles in the arterial system eventually become thickened, leading to a loss of responsiveness in the system. The left ventricle thickens because the muscle must constantly work hard to pump blood out at a greater force. The thickening of the heart muscle and the increased pressure that the muscle has to generate every time it contracts lead to an increased workload on the heart and increased risk of coronary artery disease (CAD). The inner linings of the arteries become damaged from the force of the blood being propelled against them, making these vessels susceptible to atherosclerosis and to narrowing of the lumen of the vessels (Chapter 46). Tiny vessels can become damaged and destroyed, leading to loss of vision (if the vessels are in the retina), kidney function (if the vessels include the glomeruli in the nephrons), or cerebral function (if the vessels are small and fragile vessels in the brain).

Untreated hypertension increases a person's risk for the following conditions: CAD and cardiac death, stroke, renal failure, and loss of vision. Because hypertension has no symptoms, it is difficult to diagnose and treat; it is often called a "silent killer." All of the drugs used to treat hypertension have adverse effects, many of which are seen as unacceptable by otherwise healthy people. Nurses face a difficult challenge trying to convince patients to comply with their drug regimens when they experience adverse effects and do not see any positive effects on their bodies. Research into the cause of hypertension is ongoing. Many theories have been proposed for the cause of the disorder, and it may well be a mosaic of many contributing factors. Factors that have been shown to increase blood pressure in some people include high levels of psychological stress, exposure to high-frequency noise, a high-salt diet, lack of rest, and genetic predisposition.

Hypotension

If blood pressure becomes too low, the vital centers in the brain as well as the rest of the tissues of the body may not receive sufficient oxygenated blood to continue functioning. **Hypotension** can progress to **shock,** when the body is in serious jeopardy as waste products accumulate and cells die from lack of oxygen. Hypotensive states can occur in the following situations:

- When the heart muscle is damaged and unable to pump effectively
- With severe blood loss, when volume drops dramatically
- When there is extreme stress and the body's levels of norepinephrine are depleted, leaving the body unable to respond to stimuli to raise blood pressure

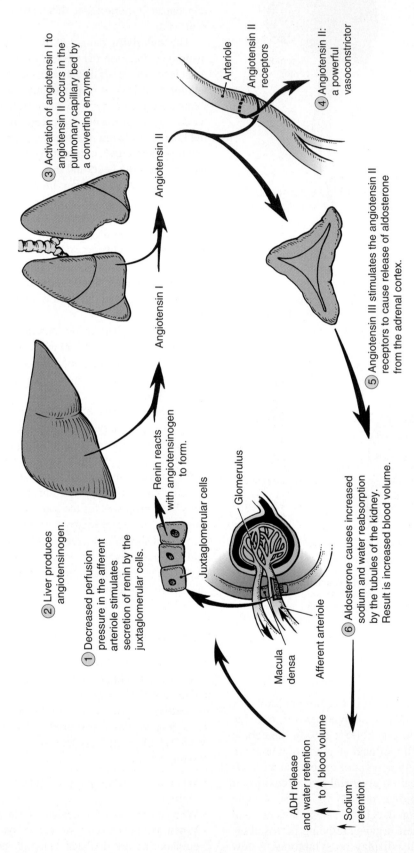

① Decreased perfusion pressure in the afferent arteriole stimulates secretion of renin by the juxtaglomerular cells.

② Liver produces angiotensinogen.

③ Activation of angiotensin I to angiotensin II occurs in the pulmonary capillary bed by a converting enzyme.

④ Angiotensin II: a powerful vasoconstrictor

Arteriole

Angiotensin II receptors

Angiotensin II

Angiotensin I

Renin reacts with angiotensinogen to form.

Juxtaglomerular cells

Glomerulus

Macula densa

Afferent arteriole

⑤ Angiotensin III stimulates the angiotensin II receptors to cause release of aldosterone from the adrenal cortex.

⑥ Aldosterone causes increased sodium and water reabsorption by the tubules of the kidney. Result is increased blood volume.

ADH release and water retention to ↑ blood volume

Sodium retention

FIGURE 43–2. The renin–angiotensin system.

BOX 43-1

Categories Rating the Severity of Hypertension*

Blood Pressure Range (mm Hg)		
Systolic	**Diastolic**	**Category**
<130	<85	Normal
130–139	85–89	High normal
140–159	90–99	Stage 1 (mild)
160–179	100–109	Stage 2 (moderate)
180–209	110–119	Stage 3 (severe)
≥210	≥120	Stage 4 (very severe)

*The risk of developing complications increases as severity increases. If systolic and diastolic pressure are noted to be in different categories, the blood pressure category is identified at the higher level.

ANTIHYPERTENSIVE AGENTS

Because an underlying cause of hypertension is not usually known, altering the body's regulatory mechanisms is the best treatment currently available. Drugs used to treat hypertension work to alter the normal reflexes that control blood pressure. Treatment for essential hypertension does not cure the disease but is aimed at maintaining the blood pressure within normal limits to prevent the damage that hypertension can cause. Not all patients respond the same way to antihypertensive drugs, because different factors may be contributing to each person's hypertension. Patients may have complicating conditions, such as diabetes or acute myocardial infarction (MI), that make it unwise to use certain drugs. Several different types of drugs, which affect different areas of blood pressure control, may need to be used in combination to actually maintain a patient's blood pressure within normal limits. Trials of drugs and combinations of drugs are often needed to develop an individual regimen that is effective yet does not have adverse effects that are unacceptable to the patient.

DRUG THERAPY ACROSS THE LIFESPAN

Drugs Affecting Blood Pressure

Children	Adults	Older Adults
National standards for determining normal levels of blood pressure in children are quite new. It has been determined that hypertension may start as a childhood disease, and more screening studies are being done to establish normal values for each age group. Children are thought to be more likely to have secondary hypertension, caused by renal disease or congenital problems such as coarctation of the aorta. Treatment of childhood hypertension should be done very cautiously, because the long-term effects of the antihypertensive agents are not known. Lifestyle changes should be instituted before drug therapy if at all possible. Weight loss and increased activity may bring an elevated blood pressure back to normal in many children. If drug therapy is used, a mild diuretic may be tried first, with monitoring of blood glucose and electrolyte levels on a regular basis. β-blockers have been used with success in some children; adverse effects may limit their usefulness in others. The safety and efficacy of the angiotensin-converting enzyme (ACE) inhibitors and the angiotensin receptor blockers (ARBs) have not been established in children. Calcium channel blockers have been used to treat hypertension in children and may be a first consideration if drug therapy is needed. Careful follow-up of the growing child is essential to monitor for changes in blood pressure as well as adverse effects.	Adults receiving any of these drugs need to be instructed about adverse reactions that should be reported immediately. They need to be reminded of safety precautions that may be needed in hot weather or with conditions that cause fluid depletion (e.g., diarrhea, vomiting). If they are taking any other drugs, the interacting effects of the various drugs should be evaluated. The importance of other measures to help lower blood pressure—weight loss, smoking cessation, increased activity—should be stressed. The safety for the use of these drugs during pregnancy has not been established. ACE inhibitors and ARBs should not be used during pregnancy, and women of child-bearing age should be advised to use barrier contraceptives to prevent pregnancy while taking these drugs. Calcium channel blockers and vasodilators should not be used in pregnancy unless the benefit to the mother clearly outweighs the potential risk to the fetus. The drugs do enter breast milk and can cause serious adverse effects in the baby. Caution should be used or another method of feeding the baby should be used if one of these drugs is needed during lactation.	Older adults frequently are prescribed one of these drugs. They are more susceptible to the toxic effects of the drugs and are more likely to have underlying conditions that could interfere with their metabolism and excretion. Renal or hepatic impairment can lead to accumulation of the drugs in the body. If renal or hepatic dysfunction is present, the dosage should be reduced and the patient monitored very closely. The total drug regimen of the older patient should be coordinated, with careful attention to interactions among drugs and alternative therapies. Older adults need to use special caution in any situation that could lead to a fall in blood pressure, such as loss of fluids from diarrhea or vomiting, lack of fluid intake, or excessive heat with decreased sweating that comes with age. Dizziness, falls, or syncope can occur if the blood pressure falls too far in these situations. The blood pressure should always be taken immediately before an antihypertensive is administered to an older adult in an institutional setting, to avoid excessive lowering of blood pressure. Older patients should be especially cautioned about sustained-release antihypertensives that cannot be cut, crushed, or chewed, to avoid the potential for excessive dosing if these drugs are inappropriately cut.

NURSING CHALLENGE

"White Coat" Hypertension

The diagnosis of hypertension is accompanied by the impact of serious ramifications, such as increased risk for numerous diseases and cardiovascular death, the potential need for significant lifestyle changes, and the potential need for drug therapy, which may include many unpleasant adverse effects. Consequently, it is important that a patient be properly diagnosed before being labeled hypertensive.

Researchers in the 1990s discovered that some patients were hypertensive only when they were in their doctor's office having their blood pressure measured. This was correlated to a sympathetic stress reaction (which elevates systolic blood pressure) and a tendency to tighten the muscles (isometric exercise, which elevates diastolic blood pressure) while waiting to be seen and during the blood pressure measurement. The researchers labeled this phenomenon "white coat" hypertension.

The American Heart Association has put forth new guidelines for the diagnosis of hypertension. A patient should have three consecutive blood pressure readings above normal, when taken by a nurse, over a period of 2 to 3 weeks. (It was assumed that nurses were not as threatening or stress provoking as doctors). These guidelines point out the importance of using the correct technique when taking a patient's blood pressure, especially because the results can have such a tremendous impact on a patient. It is good practice to periodically review the process for performing this routine task. For example, the nurse should

- Select a cuff that is the correct size for the patient's arm (a cuff that is too small may give a high reading; a cuff that is too large may give a lower reading).
- Try to put the patient at ease; remember that waiting alone in a cold room can be stressful to the body and mind and can increase the blood pressure.
- Ensure that the arm that will be used for the cuff is supported.
- Make sure the rest of the patient's muscles are not tensed while the blood pressure is being taken.
- Place both the cuff and the stethoscope directly on the patient instead of on clothing.
- Listen carefully and record the first sound heard, the muffling of sounds, and the absence of sound (the actual diastolic pressure is thought to be between these two sounds).

Blood pressure machines found in grocery stores and pharmacies often give higher readings than the actual blood pressure, so patients should not be encouraged to use these machines for follow-up readings. The American Heart Association offers many good guidelines for accurate blood pressure measurement. Nurses are often the health care providers most likely to be taking and recording patient blood pressure, so it is important to always use proper technique and to make accurate records.

Stepped Care Approach to Treating Hypertension

The importance of treating hypertension has been proven in numerous research studies. When hypertension is controlled, the patient's risk of cardiovascular death and disease is reduced. The risk of developing cardiovascular complica-

tions is directly related to the patient's degree of hypertension (see Box 43–1). Lowering the degree of hypertension lowers the risk.

The Joint National Committee on Detection, Evaluation and Treatment of Hypertension, from the National Institutes of Health, has established a stepped-care approach to treating hypertension that has proved effective in national studies (Box 43–2). Four steps are involved.

Step 1: Lifestyle modifications are instituted. These include weight reduction, smoking cessation, reduction in the use of alcohol and salt in the diet (all of which have been shown to increase blood pressure), and an increase in physical exercise (which has been shown to decrease blood pressure and improve cardiovascular tone and reserve).

Step 2: If the measures in step 1 are not sufficient to lower the blood pressure to an acceptable level, drug therapy is added. The drug of choice may be a diuretic, which decreases serum sodium levels and blood volume; a β-blocker, which leads to a decrease in heart rate and strength of contraction as well as vasodilation; an **ACE inhibitor,** which blocks the conversion of angiotensin I to angiotensin II; an angiotensin II receptor blocker (ARB), which blocks the effects of angiotensin on the blood vessel; a calcium channel blocker, which relaxes muscle contraction; or other autonomic blockers.

BOX 43-2

Stepped-Care Management of Hypertension from the Joint National Committee on Detection, Evaluation and Treatment of Hypertension

STEP 1: LIFESTYLE MODIFICATIONS
- Weight reduction
- Reduction of sodium intake
- Moderation of alcohol intake
- Smoking cessation
- Physical activity increase

STEP 2: INADEQUATE RESPONSE
- Continue lifestyle modifications
- Initial drug selection:
  1. Diuretic or β-blocker
  2. ACE inhibitor, calcium channel blocker, α-blocker, α- and β-blocker

STEP 3: INADEQUATE RESPONSE
1. Increase drug dose, or
2. Substitute another drug, or
3. Add a second drug from another class

STEP 4: INADEQUATE RESPONSE
Add a second or third agent or diuretic if not already prescribed

Step 3: If the patient's response to step 2 is inadequate, the drug dose or class may be changed or another drug may be added for a combined effect.

Step 4: This step includes all of the above measures with the addition of more antihypertensive agents until the desired level of blood pressure control is achieved.

Hypertensive treatment is further complicated by the presence of other chronic conditions. The Joint National Committee published an algorithm for the treatment of hypertension to help prescribers select an antihypertensive agent in light of complicating conditions (Figure 43–3). The actual patient's response to an antihypertensive is very individual, so the drug of choice for one patient may have little to no effect on another patient.

Diuretics

Diuretics are drugs that increase the excretion of sodium and water from the kidney (see Chapter 51) (Figure 43–4). These drugs are often the first agents tried in mild hypertension and affect blood sodium levels and blood volume. Although these drugs cause increased urination and can cause electrolyte and acid–base disturbances, they are usually tolerated well by most patients (Box 43–3).

Sympathetic Nervous System Blockers

Drugs that block the effects of the sympathetic nervous system (see Chapter 31) are useful in blocking many of the compensatory effects of the sympathetic nervous system (see Figure 43–4).

- β-Blockers block vasoconstriction, increase heart rate, increase cardiac muscle contraction, and tend to increase blood flow to the kidney, leading to a decrease in the release of renin. These drugs have many adverse effects and are not recommended for all people. They are often used as monotherapy in step 2 treatment, and in some patients they control blood pressure adequately.
- α- and β-Blockers are useful in conjunction with other agents and tend to be somewhat more powerful, blocking all of the receptors in the sympathetic system. Patients often complain of fatigue, loss of libido, inability to sleep, and gastrointestinal (GI) and genitourinary disturbances, and they may not be willing to continue taking these drugs.
- α-Adrenergic blockers inhibit the postsynaptic α_1-adrenergic receptors, decreasing sympathetic tone in the vasculature and causing vasodilation, leading to a lowering of blood pressure. However, these drugs also block presynaptic α_2-receptors, preventing the feedback control of norepinephrine release. The result is an increase in the reflex tachycardia that occurs when blood pressure is lowered. These drugs are used to diagnose and manage episodes of pheochromocytoma, but they have limited usefulness in essential hypertension because of the associated adverse effects.
- α_1-Blockers are used to treat hypertension because of their ability to block the postsynaptic α_1-receptor sites. This

causes a decrease in vascular tone and a vasodilation that leads to a fall in blood pressure. These drugs do not block the presynaptic α_2-receptor sites, and therefore the reflex tachycardia that accompanies a fall in blood pressure does not occur.

- α_2-Agonists stimulate the α_2-receptors in the central nervous system (CNS) and inhibit the cardiovascular centers, leading to a decrease in sympathetic outflow from the CNS and a resultant drop in blood pressure. These drugs are associated with many adverse CNS and GI effects as well as cardiac arrhythmias (see Box 43–3).

ANGIOTENSIN-CONVERTING ENZYME INHIBITORS

The ACE inhibitors block the conversion of angiotensin I to angiotensin II in the lungs (see Figure 43–4). This stops that phase of the renin–angiotensin system before vasoconstriction or aldosterone release can occur. The ACE inhibitors may be used as monotherapy in step 2 of hypertension management, or they may be combined with diuretics. ACE inhibitors that are used include the following:

- Benazepril (*Lotensin*), a frequently used oral drug, is approved only for use in treating hypertension; it is usually well tolerated but has been associated with an unrelenting cough.
- Captopril (*Capoten*) is indicated for use in hypertension and in treating congestive heart failure (CHF), diabetic nephropathy, and left ventricular dysfunction after MI; it has been associated with a sometimes fatal pancytopenia, cough, and unpleasant GI distress.
- Enalapril (*Vasotec*), an oral drug, is used for the treatment of hypertension, CHF, and left ventricular dysfunction; it has the advantage of parenteral use (enalaprilat [*Vasotec IV*]) if oral use is not feasible or rapid onset is desirable.
- Fosinopril (*Monopril*) is a well-tolerated oral drug used for the treatment of hypertension and for adjunctive therapy in CHF; it is also associated with a cough.
- Lisinopril (*Prinivil, Zestril*) is an oral drug used in treating hypertension and CHF and in the treatment of stable patients within 24 hours after acute MI to improve the likelihood of survival.
- Moexipril (*Univasc*) is a less well-tolerated oral drug used in the treatment of hypertension; it is associated with many unpleasant GI and skin effects, cough, and cardiac arrhythmias; fatal MI and pancytopenia have sometimes been associated with this drug.
- Perindopril (*Aceon*) is an oral drug that is used alone or in combination with other antihypertensives to control blood pressure. It is associated with a sometimes fatal pancytopenia as well as a serious to fatal airway obstruction (found to occur more frequently in African American patients).
- Quinapril (*Accupril*) is used orally for the treatment of hypertension and as an adjunct treatment of CHF; it is not associated with as many adverse effects as some of the other agents.

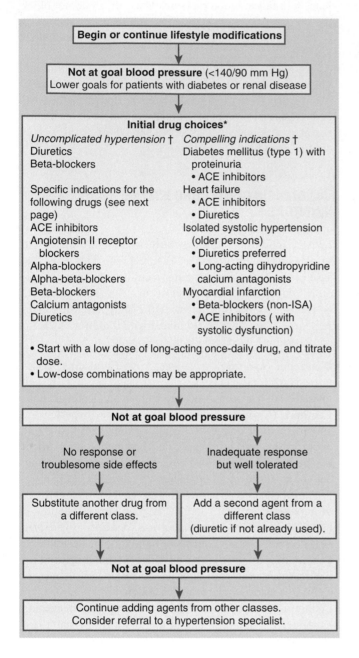

Considerations for individualizing antihypertensive drug therapy*

Indication	Drug Therapy
Compelling indications unless contraindicated	
Diabetes mellitus (type 1) with proteinuria	ACE I
Heart failure	ACE I, diuretics
Isolated systolic hypertension (older patients)	Diuretics (preferred), CA (long-acting DHP)
Myocardial infarction	Beta-blockers (non-ISA), ACE I (with systolic dysfunction)
May have favorable effects on comorbid conditions†	
Angina	Beta-blockers, CA
Atrial tachycardia and fibrillation	Beta-blockers, CA (non-DHP)
Cyclosporine-induced hypertension (caution with the dose of cyclosporine)	CA
Diabetes mellitus (types 1 and 2) with proteinuria	ACE I (preferred), CA
Diabetes mellitus (type 2)	Low-dose diuretics
Dyslipidemia	Alpha-blockers
Essential tremor	Beta-blockers (non-CS)
Heart failure	Carvedilol, losartan potassium
Hyperthyroidism	Beta-blockers
Migraine	Beta-blockers (non-CS), CA (non-DHP)
Myocardial infarction	Diltiazem hydrochloride, verapamil hydrochloride
Osteoporosis	Thiazides
Preoperative hypertension	Beta-blockers
Prostatism (BPH)	Alpha-blockers
Renal insuffiency (caution in renovascular hypertension and creatinine ≥265.2 mmol/L [3 mg/dL])	ACE I
May have unfavorable effects on comorbid conditions†‡	
Bronchospastic disease	Beta-blockers§
Depression	Beta-blockers, central alpha-agonists, reserpine§
Diabetes mellitus (types 1 and 2)	Beta-blockers, high-dose diuretics
Dyslipidemia	Beta-blockers (non-ISA), diuretics (high dose)
Gout	Diuretics
2° to 3° heart block	Beta-blockers,§ CA (non-DHP)§
Heart failure	Beta-blockers (except carvedilol), CA (except amlodipine besylate, felodipine)
Liver disease	Labetalol hydrochloride, methyldopa§
Peripheral vascular disease	Beta-blockers
Pregnancy	ACE I,§ angiotensin II receptor blockers§
Renal insuffiency	Potassium-sparing agents
Renovascular disease	ACE I, angiotensin II receptor blockers

*For initial drug therapy recommendations, see preceding page. ACE I indicates angiotensin-converting enzyme inhibitors; BPH, benign prostatic hyperplasia; CA, calcium antagonists; DHP, dihydropyridine; ISA, intrinsic sympathomimetic activity; MI, myocardial infarction; and non-CS, noncardioselective.
†Conditions and drugs are listed in alphabetical order.
‡These drugs may be used with special monitoring unless contraindicated.
§Contraindicated.

FIGURE 43–3. Algorithm for the treatment of hypertension. (From the Sixth Report of the Joint National Committee on Prevention, Detection, Evaluation, and Treatment of High Blood Pressure. National Institutes of Health Publication No. 98-4080, November 1997.)

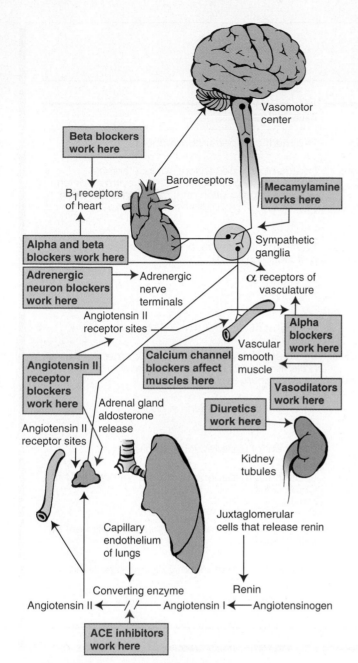

BOX 43-3
Other Drug Classes Used to Treat Hypertension

DIURETICS (CHAPTER 51)

Thiazide and thiazide-like diuretics: bendroflumethiazide, benzthiazide, chlorothiazide, hydrochlorothiazide, hydroflumethiazide, methyclothiazide, polythiazide, trichlormethiazide, chlorthalidone, indapamide, metolazone, quinethazone

Loop diuretics: bumetanide, ethacrynic acid, furosemide torsemide

Carbonic anhydrase inhibitors: acetazolamide, methazolamide

Potassium-sparing diuretics: amiloride, spironolactone, triamterene

SYMPATHETIC NERVOUS SYSTEM DRUGS (CHAPTER 31)

β-Blockers: acebutolol, atenolol, betaxolol, bisoprolol, carteolol, metoprolol, nadolol, penbutolol, pindolol, propranolol, timolol

α- and β-blockers: carvedilol, labetalol, guanabenz, guanadrel, guanethidine

α-Adrenergic blockers: phenoxybenzamine, phentolamine

α₁-Blockers: doxazosin, prazosin, terazosin

α₂-Agonists: clonidine, guanfacine, methyldopa

FIGURE 43–4. Sites of action of antihypertensive drugs.

- Ramipril (*Altace*) is used orally for the treatment of hypertension and as an adjunct treatment of CHF; it is not associated with as many adverse effects as some of the other agents.
- Trandolapril (*Mavik*), used orally for the treatment of hypertension and for CHF after an acute MI, is a fairly well-tolerated drug.

Therapeutic Actions and Indications

ACE inhibitors prevent ACE from converting angiotensin I to angiotensin II, a powerful vasoconstrictor and stimulator of aldosterone release. This action leads to a decrease in blood pressure and in aldosterone secretion with a resultant slight increase in serum potassium and a loss of serum sodium and fluid. These drugs are indicated for the treatment of hypertension, alone or in combination with other drugs. They are also used in conjunction with digoxin and diuretics for the treatment of CHF and left ventricular dysfunction. Their therapeutic effect in these cases is thought to be related to a decrease in cardiac workload associated with the decrease in peripheral resistance and blood volume.

Pharmacokinetics

These drugs are well absorbed, widely distributed, metabolized in the liver, and excreted in the urine and feces. They are known to cross the placenta and have been associated with serious fetal abnormalities. These drugs should not be used during pregnancy. Women of child-bearing age who choose to use one of these drugs should be encouraged to use barrier contraceptives to avoid pregnancy while taking the drug. Several of these drugs have been detected in breast milk. Because of the potential for serious adverse effects in the neonate, another method of feeding the baby should be used during lactation, or another antihypertensive should be chosen.

Contraindications and Cautions

ACE inhibitors are contraindicated in the presence of allergy to any of the ACE inhibitors; with impaired renal function, which could be exacerbated by the effects of this drug in decreasing renal blood flow; with pregnancy, because of the potential for adverse effects on the fetus; and during lactation, because of potential decrease in milk production and effects on the neonate. Caution should be used in patients

DRUGS IN FOCUS
Angiotensin-Converting Enzyme Inhibitors

Drug Name	Usual Dosage	Usual Indications
benazepril (*Lotensin*)	20–40 mg/d PO; reduce dosage with older patients and renal impairment	Treatment of hypertension in adults
Ⓟ captopril (*Capoten*)	25–150 mg PO b.i.d.–t.i.d. for hypertension; 6.25–12.5 mg PO t.i.d. for CHF; 50 mg PO t.i.d. for ventricular dysfunction; 25 mg PO t.i.d. for diabetic nephropathy; reduce dosage with renal impairment and in geriatric patients	Treatment of hypertension; adjunct therapy for congestive heart failure (CHF); treatment of left ventricular dysfunction after myocardial infarction (MI), diabetic nephropathy; for use in adults
enalapril (*Vasotec*)	10–40 mg/d PO; reduce dosage in geriatric patients and those with renal impairment; 2.5 mg PO b.i.d. for CHF or left ventricular dysfunction	Treatment of hypertension, CHF, left ventricular dysfunction in adults
enalaprilat (*Vasotec IV*)	1.25 mg q6h IV over 5 min	
fosinopril (*Monopril*)	20–40 mg/d PO	Treatment of hypertension, CHF in adults
lisinopril (*Prinivil, Zestril*)	20–40 mg/d PO for hypertension; 5–20 mg/d PO for CHF; 5–10 mg/d PO after MI; decrease dosage in geriatric patients and those with renal impairment	Treatment of hypertension, CHF; treatment of stable patients within 24 hours after acute MI to increase survival; for use in adults
moexipril (*Univasc*)	7.5–30 mg/d PO, based on response; reduce dosage with renal impairment and in geriatric patients	Treatment of hypertension in adults
perindopril (*Aceon*)	4 mg/d PO; reduce dosage in geriatric patients and those with renal impairment	Treatment of hypertension in adults
quinapril (*Accupril*)	20–80 mg/d PO, based on response for hypertension; 10–20 mg PO b.i.d. for CHF; reduce dosage with renal impairment and in geriatric patients	Treatment of hypertension; adjunctive treatment of CHF in adults
ramipril (*Altace*)	2.5–20 mg/d PO for hypertension; 5 mg po b.i.d. for CHF; reduce dosage in geriatric patients and those with renal impairment	Treatment of hypertension; adjunctive treatment of CHF in adults
trandolapril (*Mavik*)	1–2 mg PO q.i.d. for hypertension; 4 mg/d PO, titrate slowly to that level for CHF; reduce dosage with renal or hepatic impairment	Treatment of hypertension, CHF, and after MI, in adults

with CHF, because the change in hemodynamics could be detrimental in some cases; and in those with salt/volume depletion, which could be exacerbated by the drug effects.

Adverse Effects

The adverse effects most commonly associated with the ACE inhibitors are related to the effects of vasodilation and alterations in blood flow. Such effects include reflex tachycardia, chest pain, angina, CHF, and cardiac arrhythmias; GI irritation, ulcers, constipation, and liver injury; renal insufficiency, renal failure, proteinuria; and rash, alopecia, dermatitis, and photosensitivity. Many of these drugs cause an unrelenting cough, possibly related to effects in the lungs where the ACE is inhibited, which may lead patients to discontinue the drug. Some of these drugs have been associated with fatal pancytopenia and MI.

Clinically Important Drug–Drug Interactions

There is an increased risk of hypersensitivity reactions if these drugs are taken with allopurinol.

Clinically Important Drug–Food Interactions

There is decreased absorption of oral ACE inhibitors if they are taken with food. They should be taken on an empty stomach, 1 hour before or 2 hours after meals.

Nursing Considerations for Patients Receiving ACE Inhibitors
Assessment: History and Examination

Screen for the following conditions, which could be cautions or contraindications to use of the drug: any known allergies to these drugs; impaired kidney function, which could be exacerbated by these drugs; pregnancy or lactation, because of the potential adverse effects on the fetus or neonate; salt/volume depletion, which could be exacerbated by these drugs; and CHF.

Include screening for baseline status before beginning therapy and for any potential adverse effects. Assess the following: body temperature, weight; skin color, lesions, temperature; pulse, blood pressure, baseline electrocardiogram (ECG), perfusion; respirations, adventitious breath sounds; bowel sounds, abdominal examination; and renal function tests, complete blood count with differential, and serum electrolytes.

Nursing Diagnoses

The patient receiving an ACE inhibitor may have the following nursing diagnoses related to drug therapy:

- Ineffective Tissue Perfusion (Total Body) related to changes in cardiac output
- Impaired Skin Integrity related to dermatologic effects
- Acute Pain related to GI distress, cough
- Deficient Knowledge regarding drug therapy

Implementation

- Encourage the patient to implement lifestyle changes, including weight loss, smoking cessation, decreased alcohol and salt in the diet, and increased exercise, *to increase the effectiveness of antihypertensive therapy.*
- Administer on an empty stomach, 1 hour before or 2 hours after meals, *to ensure proper absorption of drug.*
- Alert the surgeon and mark the patient's chart prominently

BOX 43-4
Endothelin Receptor Antagonist

In late 2001, bosentan (*Tracleer*) became the first endothelin receptor antagonist to be approved for use in the treatment of pulmonary arterial hypertension. This drug specifically blocks receptor sites for endothelin (ET_A and ET_B) in the endothelium and vascular smooth muscles; these endothelins are chemicals that are elevated in the plasma and lung tissues of patients with pulmonary arterial hypertension. Blockade of these receptor sites allows the vessels to relax and dilate, relieving the pressure in the arteries. *Tracleer* is an oral drug that is given to adults, initially as 62.5 mg PO b.i.d. for 4 wk, and then increased to 125 mg PO b.i.d. if the patient's exercise tolerance improves on the drug. Patients need to be monitored closely for any change in their respiratory function, signs of liver toxicity, or signs of peripheral vasodilation, including flushing, headache, hypotension, and palpitations. The drug is pregnancy category X and is known to interact with other drugs, including ketoconzaole, the statins, glyburide, and oral contraceptives. Other drugs that react with the endothelin receptors specifically are under investigation for treatment of hypertension.

---

if the patient is to undergo surgery, *to alert medical personnel that the blockage of compensatory angiotensin II could result in hypotension after surgery that would need to be reversed with volume expansion.*
- Give parenteral forms only if an oral form is not feasible; transfer to an oral form as soon as possible, *to avert an increased risk of adverse effects.*
- Consult with the prescriber to reduce dosage in patients with renal failure, *to account for their decreased production of renin and lower-than-normal levels of angiotensin II.*
- Monitor the patient carefully in any situation that might lead to a drop in fluid volume (e.g., excessive sweating, vomiting, diarrhea, dehydration), *to detect and treat excessive hypotension that may occur.*
- Provide comfort measures *to help the patient tolerate drug effects.* These include small, frequent meals; access to bathroom facilities; bowel program as needed; environmental controls; safety precautions; and appropriate skin care as needed.
- Provide thorough patient teaching, including the name of the drug, dosage prescribed, measures to avoid adverse effects, warning signs of problems, and the need for periodic monitoring and evaluation *to enhance patient knowledge about drug therapy and to promote compliance.* (See Patient Teaching Checklist: ACE Inhibitors.)
- Offer support and encouragement *to help the patient deal with the diagnosis and the drug regimen.*

Evaluation

- Monitor patient response to the drug (maintenance of blood pressure within normal limits).
- Monitor for adverse effects (hypotension, cardiac arrhythmias, renal dysfunction, skin reactions, cough, pancytopenia, CHF).
- Evaluate the effectiveness of the teaching plan (patient can name drug, dosage, adverse effects to watch for, specific measures to avoid adverse effects, importance of continued follow-up).
- Monitor the effectiveness of comfort measures and compliance to the regimen (see Nursing Care Guide: ACE Inhibitors).

ANGIOTENSIN II RECEPTOR BLOCKERS

The ARBs selectively bind the **angiotensin II receptors** in blood vessels to prevent vasoconstriction and in the adrenal cortex to prevent the release of aldosterone that is caused by reaction of these receptors with angiotensin II. These actions lead to a decrease in blood pressure caused by a decrease in total peripheral resistance and blood volume. The ARBs include the following drugs:

- Candesartan (*Atacand*), which is used alone or as part of combination therapy to treat hypertension

PATIENT TEACHING CHECKLIST
ACE Inhibitors

Create customized patient teaching materials for a specific ACE inhibitor from the CD-ROM. Patient teaching should stress the following points for drugs within this class:

• An ACE inhibitor is an antihypertensive drug that is used to treat high blood pressure. High blood pressure is a disorder that may have no symptoms but that can cause serious problems, such as heart attack, stroke, or kidney problems, if left untreated.
• It is very important to take your medication every day, as prescribed, even if you feel perfectly well without the medication. It is possible that you may feel worse because of the adverse effects associated with the medication when you take it. Even if this happens, it is crucial that you take your medication.
• If you find that the adverse effects of this drug are too uncomfortable, discuss the possibility of taking a different antihypertensive medication with your health care provider.

Common effects of these drugs include

• *Dizziness, drowsiness, lightheadedness*—These effects often pass after the first few days. Until they do, avoid driving or performing hazardous or delicate tasks that require concentration. If these effects occur, change positions slowly to decrease the lightheadedness.
• *Nausea, vomiting, change in taste perception*—Small, frequent meals may help ease these effects, which may pass with time. If they persist and become too uncomfortable, consult with your health care provider.
• *Skin rash, mouth sores*—Frequent mouth care may help. Keep the skin dry and use prescribed skin care (lotions, coverings, medication) if needed.
• *Cough*—Although this can be very irritating, do not try to treat the cough with over-the-counter medications. Consult with your health care provider if this occurs and persists.

Report any of the following to your health care provider: difficulty breathing; mouth sores; swelling of the feet, hands, or face; chest pain; palpitations; sore throat; fever or chills.

Do not stop taking this drug for any reason. Consult with your health care provider if you have problems taking this medication.

Tell any doctor, nurse, or other health care provider that you are taking this drug.

Keep this drug, and all medications, out of the reach of children.

Avoid the use of over-the-counter medications while you are taking this drug. If you feel that you need one of these, consult with your health care provider for the best choice. Many of these drugs may interfere with the antihypertensive effect that usually occurs with this drug.

Be extremely careful in any situation that might lead to a drop in blood pressure (e.g., excessive sweating, vomiting, diarrhea, dehydration). If you experience lightheadedness or dizziness in any of these situations, consult your health care provider immediately.

This Teaching Checklist reflects general patient teaching guidelines. It is not meant to be a substitute for drug specific teaching information, which is available in nursing drug guides.

• Eprosartan (*Teveten*) which is used alone or as part of combination therapy to treat hypertension in adults
• Irbesartan (*Avapro*), which is used as monotherapy in the treatment of hypertension
• Losartan (*Cozaar*), which can be used alone or as part of combination therapy for hypertension
• Telmisartan (*Micardis*), which is used alone or as part of combination therapy to treat hypertension
• Valsartan (*Diovan*), which can be used alone or as part of combination therapy for hypertension

Therapeutic Actions and Indications
The ARBs selectively bind with angiotensin II receptor sites in vascular smooth muscle and in the adrenal gland to block vasoconstriction and the release of aldosterone. These actions block the blood pressure–raising effects of the renin—angiotensin system and lower blood pressure. They are indicated to be used alone or in combination therapy for the treatment of hypertension.

Pharmacokinetics
These agents are well absorbed and undergo metabolism in the liver by the cytochrome P450 system. They are excreted in the feces and in the urine. Known to cross the placenta, the ARBs have been associated with serious fetal abnormalities and even death when given in the second or third trimester. Women of child-bearing age should be advised to use barrier contraceptives to avoid pregnancy; if a pregnancy does occur, the ARB should be discontinued immediately. Candesartan, eprosartan, irbesartan, and telmisartan should not be used during the second or third trimester of pregnancy because of associated fetal abnormalities and death. Losartan and valsartan should not be used at any time during pregnancy. It is not known whether the ARBs enter breast milk during lactation. Because of the potential for serious adverse effects in the neonate, these drugs should not be used during lactation.

Contraindications and Cautions
The ARBs are contraindicated in the presence of allergy to any of these drugs; during pregnancy, because of associated fetal death and severe abnormalities; and during lactation, because of potential adverse effects on the neonate. Caution should be used in the presence of hepatic or renal dysfunction, which could alter the metabolism and excretion of these drugs, and with hypovolemia, because of the blocking of potentially life-saving compensatory mechanisms.

Adverse Effects
The adverse effects most commonly associated with ARBs include the following: headache, dizziness, syncope, and weakness, which could be associated with drops in blood pressure; hypotension; GI complaints including diarrhea, abdominal pain, nausea, dry mouth, and tooth pain; symptoms of upper respiratory tract infections and cough; and rash, dry skin, and alopecia. In preclinical trials, these drugs have been associated with the development of cancers.

Clinically Important Drug–Drug Interactions
There is an increased risk of decreased serum levels and loss of effectiveness if the ARB is taken in combination with

NURSING CARE GUIDE

ACE Inhibitors

Assessment	Nursing Diagnoses	Implementation	Evaluation
HISTORY Allergies to any of these drugs, renal dysfunction, pregnancy, salt/volume depletion, sedation, sleep shock, CHF, hypotension	Ineffective Tissue Perfusion related to changes in cardiac output Impaired Skin Integrity related to skin effects Acute Pain related to GI effects, cough Deficient Knowledge regarding drug therapy	Encourage lifestyle changes to increase drug effectiveness. Administer on an empty stomach. Provide comfort and safety measures: Reduce dosage in renal failure; Clearly mark chart before surgery; Use parenteral form only if PO not possible; Monitor for any situation that might lead to a drop in blood pressure. Provide support and reassurance to deal with drug effects. Provide patient teaching regarding drug, dosage, adverse effects, what to report, and safety precautions.	Evaluate drug effects: maintenance of blood pressure within normal limits. Monitor for adverse effects: sedation, dizziness; hypotension, CHF, arrhythmias; skin reactions; renal dysfunction; cough; pancytopenia. Monitor for drug–drug interactions as indicated for each drug. Evaluate effectiveness of patient teaching program. Evaluate effectiveness of comfort and safety measures.
PHYSICAL EXAMINATION CV: BP, P, perfusion, baseline ECG CNS: orientation, affect Skin: color, lesions, texture, temperature Resp: R, adventitious sounds GI: abdominal exam, bowel sounds Lab tests: renal function tests, CBC, electrolytes			

phenobarbital. If this combination is used, the patient should be monitored closely and dosage adjustments made.

Nursing Considerations or Patients Receiving Angiotensin II Receptor Blockers

Assessment: History and Examination

Screen for the following conditions, which could be cautions or contraindications to use of the drug: any known allergies to these drugs; impaired kidney or liver function, which could be exacerbated by these drugs; pregnancy and lactation, because of the potential adverse effects on the fetus and neonate; and hypovolemia.

Include screening for baseline status before beginning therapy and for any potential adverse effects. Assess the following: body temperature, weight; skin color, lesions, temperature; pulse, blood pressure, baseline ECG, perfusion; respirations, adventitious breath sounds; bowel sounds, abdominal examination; and renal and liver function tests.

Nursing Diagnoses

The patient receiving an ARB may have the following nursing diagnoses related to drug therapy:

- Ineffective Tissue Perfusion (Total Body) related to changes in cardiac output
- Impaired Skin Integrity related to dermatological effects
- Acute Pain related to GI distress, cough, skin effects, headache
- Deficient Knowledge regarding drug therapy

Implementation

- Encourage the patient to implement lifestyle changes, including weight loss, smoking cessation, decreased alcohol and salt in the diet, and increased exercise, *to increase the effectiveness of antihypertensive therapy.*
- Administer without regard to meals; give with food, *to decrease GI distress if needed.*

CULTURAL CONSIDERATIONS
Hypertension and Antihypertensive Therapy

In the United States, African Americans are at highest risk for developing hypertension, with men more likely than women to develop the disease. African Americans have documented differences in response to antihypertensive therapy. For example, African Americans are

• Most responsive to single-drug therapy (as opposed to combination drug regimens)
• More responsive to diuretics, calcium channel blockers, and α-adrenergic blockers
• Less responsive to angiotensin-converting enzyme inhibitors and β-blockers

Increased adverse effects (depression, fatigue, drowsiness) often occur when using thiazide and thiazide-like diuretics, potentially requiring the use of different diuretics or lower doses of the thiazide diuretics.

Screening for hypertension among African Americans is very important in order to detect hypertension early and to prevent the organ damage that occurs with prolonged hypertension. Because African Americans are more responsive to diuretics, the stepped-care approach should include the first-line use of a diuretic in combination with diet and other lifestyle changes. The use of calcium channel blockers or α-adrenergic blockers should follow.

tives while she is taking this drug, *to avert potential fetal abnormalities and fetal death, which have been associated with these drugs.*

• Find an alternative method of feeding the baby if the patient is nursing, *to prevent the potentially dangerous blockade of the renin–angiotensin system in the neonate.*

• Monitor the patient carefully in any situation that might lead to a drop in fluid volume (e.g., excessive sweating, vomiting, diarrhea, dehydration), *to detect and treat excessive hypotension that may occur.*

• Provide comfort measures, *to help the patient tolerate drug effects,* including small, frequent meals; access to bathroom facilities; safety precautions if CNS effects occur; environmental controls; appropriate skin care as needed; and analgesics as needed.

• Provide thorough patient teaching, including the name of the drug, dosage prescribed, measures to avoid adverse effects, warning signs of problems, and the need for periodic monitoring and evaluation, *to enhance patient knowledge about drug therapy and to promote compliance.*

• Offer support and encouragement, *to help the patient deal with the diagnosis and the drug regimen.*

Evaluation

• Monitor patient response to the drug (maintenance of blood pressure within normal limits).

• Monitor for adverse effects (hypotension, GI distress, skin reactions, cough, headache, dizziness).

• Evaluate effectiveness of the teaching plan (patient can name drug, dosage, adverse effects to watch for, measures to avoid adverse effects, importance of continued follow-up).

• Monitor the effectiveness of comfort measures and compliance to the regimen.

• Alert the surgeon and mark the patient's chart prominently if the patient is to undergo surgery, *to notify medical personnel that the blockage of compensatory angiotensin II could result in hypotension after surgery that would need to be reversed with volume expansion.*

• Ensure that the female patient is not pregnant before beginning therapy, and suggest the use of barrier contracep-

DRUGS IN FOCUS
Angiotensin II Receptor Blockers

Drug Name	Usual Dosage	Usual Indications
candesartan (*Atacand*)	16–32 mg/d PO	Alone or as part of combination therapy to treat hypertension in adults
eprosartan (*Teveten*)	400–800 mg/d PO	Alone or as part of combination therapy to treat hypertension in adults
irbesartan (*Avapro*)	150–300 mg/d PO	Monotherapy in the treatment of hypertension in adults
P losartan (*Cozaar*)	25–100 mg/d PO	Alone or as part of combination therapy to treat hypertension in adults
telmisartan (*Micardis*)	40–80 mg/d PO	Alone or as part of combination therapy to treat hypertension in adults
valsartan (*Diovan*)	80–320 mg/d PO based on response	Alone or as part of combination therapy to treat hypertension in adults

CALCIUM CHANNEL BLOCKERS

The calcium channel blockers prevent the movement of calcium into the cardiac and smooth muscle cells when the cells are stimulated. This blocking of calcium interferes with the muscle cell's ability to contract, leading to a loss of smooth muscle tone, vasodilation, and a decrease in peripheral resistance. These effects decrease blood pressure, cardiac workload, and myocardial oxygen consumption. Calcium channel blockers are very effective in the treatment of angina (see Chapter 46) because they decrease the cardiac workload.

Not all calcium channel blockers are used to treat hypertension. Some are considered safe and effective in treating hypertension only if they are given as sustained-release or extended-release preparations. The calcium channel blockers used in the treatment of hypertension include the following:

- Amlodipine (*Norvasc*), an oral drug that may be used alone or in combination with other agents to treat hypertension and is used for angina
- Diltiazem (*Cardizem, Tiamate*), a sustained-release preparation only, which is recommended for the treatment of hypertension
- Felodipine (*Plendil*), which is not used for angina but is indicated alone or in combination with other agents for the treatment of hypertension
- Isradipine (*DynaCirc*), which is not used for angina but is indicated alone or in combination with thiazide diuretics for the treatment of hypertension.
- Nicardipine (*Cardene*), which is used alone or in combination with other agents to treat hypertension and angina; also available in intravenous form for short-term use when oral administration is not feasible
- Nifedipine (*Procardia XL*), a sustained-release preparation only, which is indicated for the treatment of hypertension
- Nisoldipine (*Sular*), extended-release tablets, which are indicated for the treatment of hypertension as monotherapy or as part of combination therapy
- Verapamil (*Calan* SR), extended-release tablets, which are indicated for the treatment of essential hypertension

Therapeutic Actions and Indications

Calcium channel blockers inhibit the movement of calcium ions across the membranes of myocardial and arterial muscle cells, altering the action potential and blocking muscle cell contraction. This effect depresses myocardial contractility, slows cardiac impulse formation in the conductive tissues, and relaxes and dilates arteries, causing a fall in blood pressure and a decrease in venous return.

Pharmacokinetics

These drugs are generally well absorbed, metabolized in the liver, and excreted in the urine. These drugs cross the placenta and enter breast milk. Fetal toxicity has been reported in animal studies, and, although there are no well defined studies about effects during pregnancy, they should not be used during pregnancy unless the benefit to the mother clearly outweighs any potential risk to the fetus. Because of the potential for serious adverse effects on the baby, another method of feeding the infant should be used if these drugs are required during lactation.

Contraindications and Cautions

These drugs are contraindicated in the presence of allergy to any of these drugs; with heart block or sick sinus syndrome, which could be exacerbated by the conduction-slowing effects of these drugs; with renal or hepatic dysfunction, which could alter the metabolism and excretion of these drugs; and with pregnancy or lactation, because of the potential for adverse effects on the fetus and neonate.

Adverse Effects

The adverse effects associated with these drugs relate to their effects on cardiac output and on smooth muscle. CNS effects include dizziness, lightheadedness, headache, and fatigue. GI problems include nausea and hepatic injury related to direct toxic effects on hepatic cells. Cardiovascular effects include hypotension, bradycardia, peripheral edema, and heart block. Skin flushing and rash may also occur.

Clinically Important Drug–Drug Interactions

Drug–drug interactions vary with each of the calcium channel blockers used to treat hypertension.

A potentially serious effect to note is an increase in serum levels and toxicity of cyclosporine if taken with diltiazem.

Nursing Considerations for Patients Receiving Calcium Channel Blockers

The main use of calcium channel blockers is for the treatment of angina. See Chapter 46 for the nursing considerations of calcium channel blockers.

VASODILATORS

If other drug therapies do not achieve the desired reduction in blood pressure, it is sometimes necessary to use a direct vasodilator. Vasodilators produce relaxation of the vascular smooth muscle, decreasing peripheral resistance and reducing blood pressure. They do not block the reflex tachycardia that occurs when blood pressure drops. Most of the vasodilators are reserved for use in severe hypertension or hypertensive emergencies. The vasodilators that might be used to treat severe hypertension include the following:

- Diazoxide (*Hyperstat*), which is used as an intravenous drug in hospitalized patients with severe hypertension; this drug also increases blood glucose levels by blocking insulin release, so it must be used with extreme caution with functional hypoglycemia.
- Hydralazine (*Apresoline*), which is available for oral, intravenous, and intramuscular use for the treatment of severe hypertension; it is thought to maintain or increase renal blood flow while relaxing smooth muscle.
- Minoxidil (*Loniten*), which is an oral agent used only for the treatment of severe and unresponsive hypertension; it is associated with reflex tachycardia and increased renin re-

DRUGS IN FOCUS
Calcium Channel Blockers Used in Hypertension

Drug Name	Usual Dosage	Usual Indications
amlodipine (*Norvasc*)	5–10 mg/d PO, reduce dosage with hepatic impairment and in geriatric patients	Alone or in combination with other agents for the treatment of hypertension in adults
ⓟ diltiazem (*Cardizem, Dilacor CR*)	60–120 mg PO b.i.d.	Extended release preparation used to treat hypertension in adults
felodipine (*Plendil*)	10–15 mg/d PO; do not exceed 10 mg/d in geriatric patients or in those with hepatic impairment	Alone or in combination with other agents for the treatment of hypertension in adults
isradipine (*DynaCirc*)	2.5–10 mg PO b.i.d.; 5–10 mg/d PO— controlled release	Alone or in combination with other agents for the treatment of hypertension in adults
nicardipine (*Cardene*)	20–40 mg PO t.i.d.; 0.5–2.2 mg/h IV based on response, switch to oral form as soon as feasible; reduce dosage in geriatric patients and in those with hepatic or renal impairment; 30–60 mg PO b.i.d.— sustained release	Alone or in combination with other agents to treat hypertension and angina; IV form for short-term use when oral route is not feasible; for use in adults
nifedipine (*Procardia XL*)	30–60 mg/d PO	Sustained-release preparation only; indicated for the treatment of hypertension in adults
nisoldipine (*Sular*)	20–40 mg/d PO; reduce dosage in geriatric patients and in those with hepatic impairment	Extended-release tablets for the treatment of hypertension as monotherapy or as part of combination therapy in adults
verapamil (*Calan* SR)	120–240/d PO, reduce dosage in elderly or those with renal impairment	Extended-release tablets for the treatment of essential hypertension

lease leading to volume increase. (The oral drug is associated with changes in body hair growth and distribution, which led to a topical preparation [*Rogaine*] for the treatment of baldness.)

- Nitroprusside (*Nitropress*), which is used intravenously for the treatment of hypertensive crisis and to maintain controlled hypotension during surgery; toxic levels cause cyanide toxicity.
- Tolazoline (*Priscoline*), which is used only intravenously to treat persistent pulmonary hypertension of the newborn; it increases cardiac output and GI activity.

Therapeutic Actions and Indications
The vasodilators act directly on vascular smooth muscle to cause muscle relaxation, leading to vasodilation and drop in blood pressure. They are indicated for the treatment of severe hypertension that has not responded to other therapy.

Pharmacokinetics
These drugs are rapidly absorbed and widely distributed. They are metabolized in the liver and primarily excreted in the urine. They cross the placenta and enter breast milk. They should not be used during pregnancy unless the benefit to the mother clearly outweighs the potential risk to the fetus. If they are needed by a nursing mother, another

method of feeding the baby should be selected. Do not use these drugs during lactation.

Contraindications and Cautions
The vasodilators are contraindicated in the presence of known allergy to the drug; with pregnancy and lactation, because of the potential for adverse effects on the fetus and neonate; and with any condition that could be exacerbated by a sudden fall in blood pressure, such as cerebral insufficiency. Caution should be used in patients with peripheral vascular disease, CAD, CHF, or tachycardia, all of which could be exacerbated by the fall in blood pressure.

Adverse Effects
The adverse effects most frequently seen with these drugs are related to the changes in blood pressure. These include dizziness, anxiety, headache; reflex tachycardia, CHF, chest pain, edema; skin rash, lesions (abnormal hair growth with minoxidil); and GI upset, nausea, and vomiting. Cyanide toxicity (dyspnea, headache, vomiting, dizziness, ataxia, loss of consciousness, imperceptible pulse, absent reflexes, dilated pupils, pink color, distant heart sounds, shallow breathing) may occur with nitroprusside, which is metabolized to cyanide and which also suppresses iodine uptake and can cause hypothyroidism.

Clinically Important Drug–Drug Interactions

Each of these drugs works differently in the body, so each drug should be checked for potential drug–drug interactions before use.

Nursing Considerations for Patients Receiving Vasodilators

Assessment: History and Examination

Screen for the following conditions, which could be cautions or contraindications to use of the drug: any known allergies to these drugs; impaired kidney or liver function; pregnancy or lactation, because of the potential adverse effects on the fetus and neonate; and cardiovascular dysfunction, which could be exacerbated by a fall in blood pressure.

Include screening for baseline status before beginning therapy and for any potential adverse effects. Assess the following: body temperature, weight; skin color, lesions, temperature; pulse, blood pressure, baseline ECG, perfusion; respirations, adventitious breath sounds; bowel sounds, abdominal examination; renal and liver function tests; and blood glucose.

Nursing Diagnoses

The patient receiving a vasodilator may have the following nursing diagnoses related to drug therapy:

- Ineffective Tissue Perfusion (Total Body) related to changes in cardiac output
- Impaired Skin Integrity related to dermatologic effects
- Acute Pain related to GI distress, skin effects, headache
- Deficient Knowledge regarding drug therapy

Implementation

- Encourage the patient to implement lifestyle changes, including weight loss, smoking cessation, decreased alcohol and salt in the diet, and increased exercise, *to increase the effectiveness of antihypertensive therapy.*
- Monitor blood pressure closely during administration, *to evaluate for effectiveness and to ensure quick response if blood pressure falls rapidly or too much.*
- Monitor blood glucose and serum electrolytes, *to avoid potentially serious adverse effects.*
- Monitor the patient carefully in any situation that might lead to a drop in fluid volume (e.g., excessive sweating, vomiting, diarrhea, dehydration), *to detect and treat excessive hypotension that may occur.*
- Provide comfort measures *to help the patient tolerate drug effects,* including small, frequent meals; access to bathroom facilities; safety precautions if CNS effects occur; environmental controls; appropriate skin care as needed; and analgesics as needed.
- Provide thorough patient teaching, including the name of the drug, dosage prescribed, measures to avoid adverse effects, warning signs of problems, and the need for periodic monitoring and evaluation, *to enhance patient knowledge about drug therapy and to promote compliance.*
- Offer support and encouragement, *to help the patient deal with the diagnosis and the drug regimen.*

Evaluation

- Monitor patient response to the drug (maintenance of blood pressure within normal limits).

DRUGS IN FOCUS
Vasodilators

Drug Name	Usual Dosage	Usual Indications
diazoxide (*Hyperstat*)	1–3 mg/kg IV, by rapid bolus over 30 sec; may be repeated q5–15 min as needed	IV use for the treatment of severe hypertension in hospitalized adults
hydralazine (*Apresoline*)	Adult: 20–40 mg IM or IV repeated as necessary Pediatric: 0.1–0.2 mg/kg per 24 h IV or IM in four to six divided doses	Treatment of severe hypertension
minoxidil (*Loniten*)	Adult: 10–40 mg/d PO in divided doses Pediatric (<12 y): 0.25–1 mg/kg per day PO as a single dose	Treatment of severe hypertension unresponsive to other therapy
nitroprusside (*Nitropress*)	All patients: 3 μg/kg per minute, do not exceed 10 μg/kg per minute	IV use for the treatment of hypertensive crisis; to maintain controlled hypotension during surgery
tolazoline (*Priscoline*)	1–2 mg/kg IV through a scalp needle over 10 min, followed by an infusion of 1–2 mg/kg per hour for no longer than 36–48 h	Treatment of persistent pulmonary hypertension of the newborn

- Monitor for adverse effects (hypotension, GI distress, skin reactions, tachycardia, headache, dizziness).
- Evaluate the effectiveness of the teaching plan (patient can name drug, dosage, adverse effects to watch for, specific measures to avoid adverse effects, importance of continued follow-up).
- Monitor the effectiveness of comfort measures and compliance to the regimen.

OTHER ANTIHYPERTENSIVE AGENTS

One other drug that has proven useful in the treatment of severe hypertension is mecamylamine (*Inversine*). Mecamylamine is a ganglionic blocker that occupies cholinergic receptor sites of autonomic neurons, blocking the effects of acetylcholine at both sympathetic and parasympathetic ganglia. It decreases the effectiveness of both of these branches of the autonomic system. Blocking the sympathetic system leads to vasodilation, decreased blood pressure, and a blocking of reflex tachycardia as well as the release of catecholamines from the adrenal gland. It can cause severe hypotension, CHF, and CNS symptoms of dizziness, syncope, weakness, and vision changes; parasympathetic blocking symptoms of dry mouth, glossitis, nausea, vomiting, constipation, and urinary retention; and impotence. It is reserved for use in severe or malignant hypertension when other drugs have not proved successful. The patient receiving this drug must be monitored very closely because of the loss of autonomic reflexes.

▢▮● WEB LINKS
Health care providers and patients may want to consult the following Internet sources:

Information on research, alternative methods of therapy, pharmacology from the National Heart, Lung and Blood Institute:
http://www.heartinfo.org
Patient information on hypertension, treatments, lifestyle adjustments:
http://www.ash-us.org
Patient information, support groups, diet, exercise, research information on hypertension and other cardiovascular diseases:
http://www.americanheart.org
Specific information on the care of the pediatric hypertensive patient:
http://www.medscape.com

ANTIHYPOTENSIVE AGENTS

As mentioned earlier, if blood pressure becomes too low (hypotension), the vital centers in the brain and the rest of the tissues of the body may not receive sufficient oxygenated blood to continue functioning. Severe hypotension or shock puts the body in serious jeopardy; it is often an acute emergency situation, with treatment required to save the patient's life. The first-choice drug for treating shock is usually a sympathomimetic drug.

Sympathetic Adrenergic Agonists

Sympathomimetic drugs react with sympathetic adrenergic receptors to cause the effects of a sympathetic stress response: increased blood pressure, increased blood volume, and increased strength of cardiac muscle contraction. These actions increase blood pressure and may restore balance to the cardiovascular system while the underlying cause of the shock (e.g., volume depletion, blood loss) is treated. The sympathomimetic drugs are discussed in Chapter 30. Box 43–5 lists the sympathomimetics used in the treatment of severe hypotension and shock.

Midodrine

Midodrine (*ProAmatine*) is a drug that is used to treat orthostatic hypotension—hypotension that occurs with position change—that interferes with a person's ability to function and has not responded to any other therapy.

Therapeutic Actions and Indications
Midodrine activates α-receptors in arteries and veins to produce an increase in vascular tone and an increase in blood pressure. It is indicated for the symptomatic treatment of orthostatic hypotension in patients whose lives are impaired by the disorder and who have not had a response to any other therapy.

Pharmacokinetics
Midodrine is rapidly absorbed from the GI tract, reaching peak levels within 1 to 2 hours. It is metabolized in the liver and excreted in the urine with a half-life of 3 to 4 hours. It should be reserved in pregnancy for cases in which the benefit to the mother clearly outweighs the potential risk to the fetus. It is not known whether midodrine enters breast milk, so caution should be used during lactation.

Contraindications and Cautions
Midodrine is contraindicated in the presence of supine hypertension, CAD, or pheochromocytoma because of the risk of precipitating a hypertensive emergency; with acute renal disease, which might interfere with excretion of the drug; with urinary retention, because the stimulation of α-receptors can exacerbate this problem; and with thyrotoxicosis, which could further increase blood pressure. Caution should be used with pregnancy and lactation, because of the potential for adverse effects on the fetus or neonate; with visual problems, which could be exacerbated by vasoconstriction; and with renal or hepatic impairment, which could alter the metabolism and excretion of the drug.

Adverse Effects
The most common adverse effects associated with this drug are related to the stimulation of α-receptors and include piloerection, chills, and rash; hypertension and bradycardia; dizziness, vision changes, vertigo, and headache; and problems with urination.

CASE STUDY

Initiating Antihypertensive Therapy

THE SITUATION

B. R., a 46-year-old African American male business executive, was seen for a routine insurance physical. His examination was negative except for a blood pressure reading of 164/102 mm Hg. He also was approximately 20 lb overweight. Urinalysis and blood work all came back within normal limits. He was given a 1200-calorie-per-day diet to follow and was encouraged to cut down on salt and alcohol intake, start exercising, and stop smoking. He was asked to return in 3 weeks for a follow-up appointment (step 1). Three weeks later, B. R. returned with a 7-pound weight loss and an average blood pressure reading (of three) of 145/92 mm Hg. Discussion was held about starting B. R. on a diuretic (step 2) in addition to the lifestyle changes that B. R. was undertaking. B. R. was reluctant to take a diuretic and asked to be given more time to bring his pressure to a normal range without drug therapy.

CRITICAL THINKING

- What nursing interventions should be done at this point? *Consider the risk factors that B. R. has for hypertension and the damage that hypertension can cause.*
- What are the chances that B. R. can bring his blood pressure within a normal range?
- What additional teaching points should be covered with B. R. before a treatment decision is made?
- What implication does the diagnosis of hypertension have for B. R.'s insurance and job security?
- What effects could diuretic therapy have on B. R.'s busy business day?

DISCUSSION

B. R. was asked to change many things in his life over the last 3 weeks. These changes themselves can be stressful and can increase a person's blood pressure. B. R.'s reluctance to take a diuretic is understandable for a business executive who might not want his day interrupted by many bathroom stops. African Americans often show a

good response to diuretic therapy and a return to normal blood pressure, but they also tend to have more adverse central nervous system effects with the most commonly used diuretics, the thiazides. This may have an impact on B. R.'s business and home life. B. R. should receive a complete teaching program outlining what is known about hypertension and all of the risk factors involved with the disease. The good effects of weight loss, exercise, and other lifestyle changes should be stressed, and B. R. should be praised for his success over the last 3 weeks.

B. R. may benefit from trying for a couple more weeks to make lifestyle changes that will help bring his blood pressure into normal range. He will then feel that he has some control and input into the situation, so if drug therapy is needed, he may be more willing to comply with the prescribed treatment. The diagnosis of hypertension may be delayed for these 2 weeks while B. R. changes his lifestyle. Such a diagnosis should be made only after three consecutive blood pressure readings in the high range are recorded. B. R. may be able to have his blood pressure checked at work in a comfortable environment, which will improve the accuracy of the reading.

Many insurance companies, and some employers, see hypertension as an increased risk. This could have a tremendous impact on B. R.'s ability to get health and life insurance, and even on any future promotions or job changes. As a business executive, B. R. may be well aware of these possibilities—another reason to give him a little more time. He may wish to look into biofeedback for relaxation, a fitness program, smoking cessation programs (if appropriate), and stress reduction. As long as B. R. receives regular follow-up and frequent blood pressure checks, it may be a good idea to allow him to take some control and continue lifestyle changes. If at the end of the 2 weeks no further progress has been made or B. R.'s blood pressure has gone up, drug therapy should be considered. Teaching should be aimed at helping B. R. to incorporate the drug effects into his lifestyle, to improve his compliance and tolerance of the therapy.

Clinically Important Drug–Drug Interactions

There is a risk of increased effects and toxicity of cardiac glycosides, β-blockers, α-adrenergic agents, and cortico-steroids if they are taken with midodrine. Patients who are receiving any of these combinations should be monitored carefully for the need for a dosage adjustment.

BOX 43-5

Drugs Used to Treat Severe Hypotension and Shock States

SYMPATHOMIMETIC DRUGS (CHAPTER 30) dobutamine, dopamine, ephedrine, epinephrine, isoproterenol, metaraminol

Nursing Considerations for Patients Receiving Midodrine
Assessment: History and Examination

Screen for the following conditions, which could be con-traindications or cautions to use of the drug: any known allergy to midodrine; impaired kidney or liver function; pregnancy or lactation because of the potential adverse effects on the fetus and neonate; cardiovascular dysfunction; visual problems; urinary retention; and pheochromocytoma.

Include screening for baseline status before beginning therapy and for any potential adverse effects. Assess the following: body temperature, weight; skin color, lesions, temperature; pulse, blood pressure, orthostatic blood pressure, perfusion; respiration, adventitious sounds; bowel sounds, abdominal examination; and renal and liver function tests.

DRUGS IN FOCUS
Antihypotensive—Midodrine

Drug Name	Usual Dosage	Usual Indications
midodrine (*ProAmatine*)	10 mg PO t.i.d.	Treatment of orthostatic hypotension in adults

Nursing Diagnoses

The patient receiving midodrine may have the following nursing diagnoses related to drug therapy:

- Ineffective Tissue Perfusion (Total Body) related to changes in cardiac output
- Disturbed Sensory Perception (Visual, Kinesthetic, Tactile) related to CNS effects
- Acute Pain related to GI distress, piloerection, chills, headache
- Deficient Knowledge regarding drug therapy

Implementation

- Monitor blood pressure carefully, *to monitor effectiveness and blood pressure changes.*
- Do not administer the drug to patients who are bedridden, but only to patients who are up and mobile, *to ensure therapeutic effects and decrease the risk of severe hypertension.*
- Monitor heart rate regularly when beginning therapy, *to monitor for bradycardia, which commonly occurs at the beginning of therapy; if bradycardia persists, it may indicate a need to discontinue the drug.*
- Monitor patients with known visual problems carefully, *to ensure that the drug is discontinued if visual fields change.*
- Encourage patients to void before taking a dose of the drug, *to decrease the risk of urinary retention problems.*
- Provide comfort measures *to help the patient tolerate drug effects,* including small, frequent meals; access to bathroom facilities; safety precautions if CNS effects occur; environmental controls; appropriate skin care as needed; and analgesics as needed.
- Provide thorough patient teaching, including the name of the drug, dosage prescribed, measures to avoid adverse effects, warning signs of problems, and the need for periodic monitoring and evaluation, *to enhance patient knowledge about drug therapy and to promote compliance.*
- Offer support and encouragement, *to help the patient deal with the diagnosis and the drug regimen.*

Evaluation

- Monitor patient response to the drug (maintenance of blood pressure within normal limits).

- Monitor for adverse effects (hypertension, dizziness, visual changes, piloerection, chills, urinary problems).
- Evaluate the effectiveness of the teaching plan (patient can name drug, dosage, adverse effects to watch for, specific measures to avoid adverse effects, importance of continued follow-up).
- Monitor the effectiveness of comfort measures and compliance to the regimen.

CHAPTER SUMMARY

- The cardiovascular system is a closed system that depends on pressure differences to ensure the delivery of blood to the tissues and the return of that blood to the heart.
- Blood pressure is related to heart rate, stroke volume, and the total peripheral resistance against which the heart has to push the blood.
- Peripheral resistance is primarily controlled by constriction or relaxation of the arterioles. Constricted arterioles raise pressure; dilated arterioles lower pressure.
- Control of blood pressure involves baroreceptor (pressure receptor) stimulation of the medulla to activate the sympathetic nervous system, which causes vasoconstriction and increased fluid retention when pressure is low in the aorta and carotid arteries, and vasodilation and loss of fluid when pressure is too high.
- The kidneys activate the renin–angiotensin system when blood flow to the kidneys is decreased.
- Renin activates conversion of angiotensinogen to angiotensin I in the liver; angiotensin I is converted by angiotensin-converting enzyme (ACE) to angiotensin II in the lungs; angiotensin II then reacts with specific receptor sites on blood vessels to cause vasoconstriction to raise blood pressure and in the adrenal gland to cause release of aldosterone, which leads to retention of fluid and increased blood volume.
- Hypertension is a sustained state of higher-than-normal blood pressure that can lead to damage to blood vessels, increased risk of atherosclerosis, and damage to small vessels in end organs. Because hypertension often has no signs or symptoms, it is called the silent killer.
- Essential hypertension has no underlying cause, and treatment can vary widely from individual to individual. A stepped-care approach is recommended; lifestyle changes

Handwritten notes: Exam 1 #1, #2 (baroreceptors)? #3 #4 #5 ?, #10

are t...
of va...

• Drug...
more...
ureti...
nerv...
lead...
the h...
tensi...
(ARI...
calci...
cles...
direc...

• Hypo...
sure...
cell...
most...
stimu...
strict...

Revie...

1. Pres...
   of tl...
   a. p...
   b. s...
   c. s...
   d. h...

2. The...
   min...
   cept...
   a. a...
   pressure in the system.
   b. sense pressure and immediately send that information to the medulla in the brain.
   c. are directly connected to the sympathetic nervous system.
   d. are as sensitive to oxygen levels as to pressure changes.

3. The renin–angiotensin system is not associated with
   a. intense vasoconstriction and blood pressure elevation.
   b. blood flow through the kidneys.
   c. production of surfactant in the lungs.
   d. release of aldosterone from adrenal cortex.

4. Essential hypertension is the most commonly diagnosed form of high blood pressure. Essential hypertension is
   a. caused by a tumor in the adrenal gland.
   b. associated with no known cause.
   c. related to renal disease.
   d. caused by liver dysfunction.

5. Hypertension is not associated with
   a. loss of vision.
   b. strokes.
   c. atherosclerosis.
   d. many early signs and symptoms.

6. The stepped-care approach to the treatment of hypertension would not include

...modification—including exercise, diet, and
...ed smoking and alcohol.
...diuretic, β-blocker, or ACE inhibitor to sup-
...lifestyle changes.
...ination of antihypertensive drug classes to
...desired control.
...igitalis or another cardiotonic drug.
...tors work on the renin–angiotensin system to
...conversion of angiotensin I to angiotensin II.
...is blocking occurs in the cells in the lung,
...conversion usually occurs, use of ACE in-
...en results in
...ous pneumothorax.
...nia.
...ing cough.
...ry depression.
...taking an ACE inhibitor is scheduled for sur-
...nurse should
...e drug.
...e surgeon and mark the patient's chart promi-
...because the blockage of compensatory angio-
...I could result in hypotension after surgery that
...eed to be reversed with volume expansion.
...the surgery and consult with the prescriber.
...r fluid levels and make the sure the patient is
...stricted before surgery.
...who is hypertensive becomes pregnant. The
...oice for this patient would be
...otensin II receptor blocker.
...E inhibitor.
...ic.
   d. a calcium channel blocker.

10. Midodrine, an antihypotensive drug, should be used
    a. only with patients who are confined to bed.
    b. in the treatment of acute shock.
    c. in patients with known pheochromocytoma.
    d. to treat orthostatic hypotension in patients whose lives are impaired by the disorder.

BIBLIOGRAPHY

Andrews, M., & Boyle, J. (1999). *Transcultural concepts in nursing care*. Philadelphia: Lippincott Williams & Wilkins.

Bullock, B. L. (2000). *Focus on pathophysiology*. Philadelphia: Lippincott Williams & Wilkins.

Drug facts and comparisons. (2002). St. Louis: Facts and Comparisons.

Gilman, A., Hardman, J. G., & Limbird, L. E. (Eds.) (2002). *Goodman and Gilman's the pharmacological basis of therapeutics* (10th ed.). New York: McGraw-Hill.

Karch, A. M. (2002). *2003 Lippincott's nursing drug guide*. Philadelphia: Lippincott Williams & Wilkins.

The medical letter on drugs and therapeutics. (2002). New Rochelle, NY: Medical Letter.

Porth, C. M. (2002). *Pathophysiology: Concepts of altered health states* (6th ed.). Philadelphia: Lippincott Williams & Wilkins.

elsevieradvantage.com

Cardiotonic Agents

Congestive heart failure (CHF) is a condition in which the heart *fails* to effectively pump blood around the body. Because the cardiac cycle normally involves a tight balance between the pumping of the right and left sides of the heart, any failure of the muscle to pump blood out of either side of the heart can result in a backup of blood cells. If this happens, the blood vessels become congested; eventually, the body's cells are deprived of oxygen and nutrients, and waste products build up in the tissues. The primary treatment for CHF involves helping the heart muscle to contract more efficiently to bring the system back into balance.

REVIEW OF CARDIAC MUSCLE FUNCTION

The underlying problem in CHF usually involves muscle function: (1) the muscle could be damaged by atherosclerosis or **cardiomyopathy** (a disease of the heart muscle leading to an enlarged heart and eventually to complete muscle failure and death); (2) the muscle could be forced to work too hard to maintain an efficient output, as with hypertension or valvular disease; or (3) the structure of the heart could be abnormal, as with congenital cardiac defects.

The basic unit of the heart muscle, the sarcomere, contains two contractile proteins, actin and myosin, which are highly reactive with each other but at rest are kept apart by troponin. When a cardiac muscle cell is stimulated, calcium enters the cell and inactivates the troponin, allowing the

actin and myosin to form actomyosin bridges. The formation of these bridges allows the muscle fibers to slide together or contract (Figure 44–1). (See Chapter 42 for a review of heart muscle contraction processes.)

The contraction process requires energy, oxygen, and calcium to allow the formation of the actomyosin bridges. The degree of shortening, or the strength of contraction, is determined by the amount of calcium present (the more calcium that is present, the more bridges will be formed) and by the stretch of the sarcomere before contraction begins (the farther apart the actin and myosin proteins are before the cell is stimulated, the more bridges will be formed and the stronger the contraction will be). This correlates with Starling's law of the heart. The more the cardiac muscle is stretched, the greater the contraction will be. The more blood you put into the heart, the greater the contraction will be to empty the heart, up to a point. If the bridges are stretched too far apart, they will not be able to reach each other to form the actomyosin bridges, and no contraction will occur. This extreme response can be seen with severe cardiomyopathy when the muscle cells are stretched and distorted and eventually stop contracting because they can no longer respond.

CONGESTIVE HEART FAILURE

CHF, a condition that was once called "dropsy" or decompensation, is a syndrome that can occur with any of the disorders that damage or overwork the heart muscle.

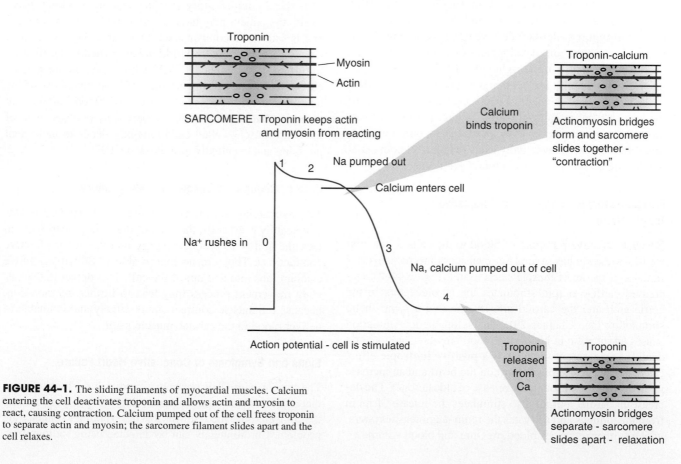

FIGURE 44–1. The sliding filaments of myocardial muscles. Calcium entering the cell deactivates troponin and allows actin and myosin to react, causing contraction. Calcium pumped out of the cell frees troponin to separate actin and myosin; the sarcomere filament slides apart and the cell relaxes.

- Coronary artery disease (CAD) is the leading cause of CHF, accounting for approximately 95% of the cases diagnosed (see Chapter 47 for a discussion of CAD). CAD results in an insufficient supply of blood to meet the oxygen demands of the myocardium. Consequently, the muscles become hypoxic and can no longer function efficiently. When CAD evolves into a myocardial infarction (MI), muscle cells die or are damaged, leading to an inefficient pumping effort.
- Cardiomyopathy can occur as a result of a viral infection, alcoholism, anabolic steroid abuse, or a collagen disorder. It causes muscle alterations and ineffective contraction and pumping.
- Hypertension eventually leads to an enlarged cardiac muscle because the heart has to work harder than normal to pump against the high pressure in the arteries. Hypertension puts constant, increased demands for oxygen on the system because the heart is pumping so hard all of the time.
- Valvular heart disease leads to an overload of the ventricles because the valves do not close tightly, which allows blood to leak backward into the ventricles. This overloading causes muscle stretching and increased demand for oxygen and energy as the heart muscle has to constantly contract harder. (Valvular heart disease is rarely seen today owing to the success of cardiac surgery and effective treatment for rheumatic fever.)

The end result of all of these conditions is that the heart muscle cannot pump blood effectively throughout the vascular system. When the left ventricle pumps inefficiently, blood backs up into the lungs, causing pulmonary vessel congestion and fluid leakage into the alveoli and lung tissue. In severe cases, **pulmonary edema** (rales, wheezes, blood-tinged sputum, low oxygenation, development of a third heart sound [S_3]) can occur. When the right side of the heart is the primary problem, blood backs up in the venous system leading to the right side of the heart. Liver congestion and edema of the legs and feet reflect right-sided failure. Because the cardiovascular system works as a closed system, one-sided failure, if left untreated, eventually leads to failure of both sides, and the signs and symptoms of total CHF occur.

Compensatory Mechanisms in Congestive Heart Failure

Because effective pumping of blood to the cells is essential for life, the body has several compensatory mechanisms that function if the heart muscle starts to fail (Figure 44–2). Decreased cardiac output stimulates the baroreceptors in the aortic arch and the carotid arteries, causing a sympathetic stimulation (see Chapter 29). This sympathetic stimulation causes an increase in heart rate, blood pressure, and rate and depth of respirations, as well as a **positive inotropic** effect (increased force of contraction) on the heart and an increase in blood volume (through the release of aldosterone). The decrease in cardiac output also stimulates the release of renin from the kidneys and activates the renin–angiotensin system, which further increases blood pressure and blood volume.

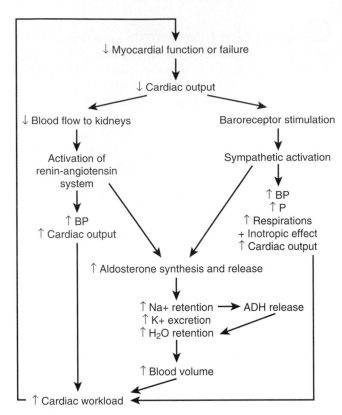

FIGURE 44–2. Compensatory mechanisms in congestive heart failure (CHF), which lead to increased cardiac workload and further CHF.

If these compensatory mechanisms are working effectively, the patient may have no signs or symptoms of CHF and is said to be compensated. Over time, however, all of these effects increase the workload of the heart, contributing to further development of CHF. Eventually, the heart muscle stretches out from overwork, and the chambers of the heart dilate secondary to the increased blood volume that they have had to handle. This hypertrophy (enlargement) of the heart muscle, called **cardiomegaly,** leads to inefficient pumping and eventually to increased CHF.

Cellular Changes in Congestive Heart Failure

The myocardial cells are changed with prolonged CHF. Unlike healthy heart cells, the cells of the failing heart seem to lack the ability to produce energy and use it for effective contractions. They are no longer able to effectively move calcium ions into and out of the cell. This defect in the calcium movement process may lead to further deterioration, because the muscle contracts ineffectively and is unable to deliver blood to the cardiac muscle itself.

Signs and Symptoms of Congestive Heart Failure

The patient with CHF presents a predictable clinical picture that reflects not only the problems with heart pumping but also the compensatory mechanisms that are working to balance the problem. Cardiomegaly can be detected using radiography, electrocardiography (ECG), or direct percussion and palpation. Heart rate will be rapid secondary to sympathetic stimulation, and the patient may develop atrial flutter or fibrillation as atrial cells are stretched and damaged. Anxiety often occurs as the body stimulates the sympathetic stress reaction. Heart murmurs may develop when the muscle is no longer able to support the papillary muscles or the annuli supporting the cardiac valves. Peripheral congestion and edema occur as the blood starts to engorge vessels as it waits to be pumped through the heart. Enlarged liver (hepatomegaly); enlarged spleen (splenomegaly); decreased blood flow to the gastrointestinal (GI) tract causing feelings of nausea and abdominal pain; swollen legs and feet; dependent edema in the coccyx or other dependent areas, with decreased peripheral pulses and hypoxia of those tissues; and, with left-sided failure, edema of the lungs reflected in engorged vessels and increased hydrostatic pressure throughout the cardiovascular system (Figure 44–3).

Left-Sided Congestive Heart Failure

Left-sided CHF reflects engorgement of the pulmonary veins, which eventually leads to difficulty in breathing. Patients complain of **tachypnea** (rapid, shallow respirations); **dyspnea** (discomfort with breathing often accompanied by a panicked feeling of being unable to breathe); and **orthopnea** (increased difficulty breathing when lying down). Orthopnea occurs in the supine position when the pattern of blood flow changes because of the effects of gravity, which causes increased pressure and perfusion in the lungs. Orthopnea is usually relieved when the patient sits up, thereby reducing the blood flow through the lungs. The degree of CHF is often calculated by the number of pillows required to get relief (eg, one-pillow, two-pillow, or three-pillow orthopnea).

The patient with left-sided CHF may also experience coughing and **hemoptysis** (coughing up of blood). Rales may be present, signaling the presence of fluid in the lung tissue. In severe cases, the patient may develop pulmonary edema; this can be life-threatening because, as the spaces in the lungs fill up with fluid, there is no place for gas exchange to occur (Figure 44–4).

Right-Sided Congestive Heart Failure

Right-sided CHF usually occurs as a result of chronic obstructive pulmonary disease (COPD) or other lung diseases that elevate the pulmonary pressure. It often results when the right side of the heart, normally a very low pressure system, must generate more and more force to move the blood into the lungs (Figure 44–5).

In right-sided CHF, venous return to the heart is decreased because of the increased pressure in the right side of the heart. This causes a congestion and backup of blood in the systemic system. An elevated jugular venous pressure (JVP) is seen, with distended neck veins, reflecting increased central venous pressure (CVP). The liver enlarges and becomes congested with blood, which leads initially to pain and tenderness and eventually to liver dysfunction and jaundice.

Dependent areas develop edema or swelling of the tissues as fluid leaves the congested blood vessels and pools in the tissues. Pitting edema in the legs is a common finding of CHF, reflecting a pool of fluid in the tissues. When the patient with right-sided CHF changes position and the legs are no longer dependent, for example, the fluid will be pulled back into circulation and returned to the heart. This increase in cardiovascular volume increases blood flow to the kidneys, causing increased urine output. This is often seen as **nocturia** (excessive voiding during the night) in a person who is up and around during the day and supine at night. The person may need to get up during the night to eliminate all of the urine that has been produced as a result of the fluid shift.

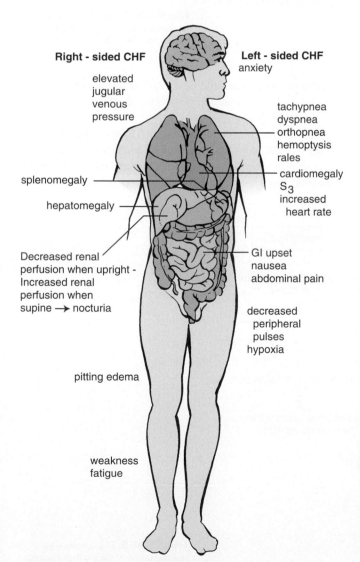

Right - sided CHF
- elevated jugular venous pressure
- splenomegaly
- hepatomegaly
- Decreased renal perfusion when upright - Increased renal perfusion when supine → nocturia
- pitting edema
- weakness fatigue

Left - sided CHF
- anxiety
- tachypnea
- dyspnea
- orthopnea
- hemoptysis
- rales
- cardiomegaly
- S3
- increased heart rate
- GI upset
- nausea
- abdominal pain
- decreased peripheral pulses
- hypoxia

FIGURE 44–3. Signs and symptoms of congestive heart failure.

TREATMENTS FOR CONGESTIVE HEART FAILURE

Several different approaches are used to treat CHF. This chapter focuses on the cardiotonic drugs (also called inotropic drugs) that work to directly increase the force of cardiac muscle contraction. Other drug therapies used to treat CHF are discussed in other chapters and are mentioned only briefly here.

FIGURE 44–4. Highly schematic representation of the pathophysiology of left-sided heart failure.

Vasodilators

Vasodilators (ACE inhibitors and nitrates) are used to treat CHF because they can decrease the workload of the overworked cardiac muscle. By relaxing vascular smooth muscle, these drugs decrease the pressure the heart has to pump against (afterload). They also cause a pooling of blood in

stretchable veins when the vessels relax, decreasing the venous return to the heart and decreasing the preload the heart muscle has to deal with.

Angiotensin-converting enzyme (ACE) inhibitors block the enzyme that converts angiotensin I to angiotensin II in the lungs, thus blocking the vasoconstriction and the release of aldosterone from the adrenal gland caused by angiotensin II

FIGURE 44–5. Highly schematic representation of the pathophysiology of right-sided heart failure.

DRUG THERAPY ACROSS THE LIFESPAN

Cardiotonic Agents

Children	Adults	Older Adults
Digoxin is used widely in children with heart defects and related cardiac problems. The margin of safety for the dosage of the drug is very small with children. The dosage needs to be very carefully calculated and should be double-checked by another nurse before administration. Children should be monitored closely for any sign of impending digitalis toxicity and should have serum digoxin levels monitored The phosphodiesterase inhibitors are not recommended for use in children.	Adults receiving any of these drugs need to be instructed as to what adverse reactions to report immediately. They should learn to take their own pulse and should be encouraged to keep track of rate and regularity on a calendar. They may be asked to weigh themselves in the same clothing and at the same time of the day to monitor for fluid retention. Any changes in diet, gastrointestinal activity, or medications should be reported to the health care provider because of the potential for altering serum levels and causing toxic reactions or ineffective dosing. Patients should also be advised against switching between brands of digoxin, because there have been reports of different bioavailabilities, leading to toxic reactions. The safety for the use of these drugs during pregnancy has not been established. They should not be used in pregnancy unless the benefit to the mother clearly outweighs the potential risk to the fetus. The drugs do enter breast milk, but they have not been associated with any adverse effects in the neonate. Caution should be used, however, if one of these drugs is needed during lactation.	Older adults frequently are prescribed one of these drugs. They, like children at the other end of the life spectrum, are more susceptible to the toxic effects of the drugs and are more likely to have underlying conditions that could interfere with their metabolism and excretion. Renal impairment can lead to accumulation of digoxin in the body. If renal dysfunction is present, the dosage needs to be reduced and the patient monitored very closely for signs of digoxin toxicity. Inamrinone is metabolized in the liver, and patients with liver dysfunction may be at increased risk for toxicity. The dosage needs to be reduced and the patient monitored continually. The total drug regimen of the older patient should be coordinated, with careful attention to interacting drugs or alternative therapies. For backup in situations of stress or illness, a significant other should be instructed in how to take the patient's pulse and the adverse effects to watch for while the patient is taking this drug.

(Figure 44–6). This in turn decreases the afterload by relieving vasoconstriction and by decreasing blood volume through its effects on decreasing the release of aldosterone, which also decreases the afterload. ACE inhibitors are the vasodilators of choice in treating CHF. They are most effective in mild CHF and in patients who are at high risk for development of CHF or who have only beginning signs and symptoms.

Nitrates directly relax vascular muscle and cause a decrease in blood pressure and a pooling of blood in the veins (see Figure 44–6). These two actions also decrease preload and afterload. Nitrates are often used to treat more severe CHF. (See Chapters 43 and 46 for additional information.)

Diuretics

Diuretics are used to decrease blood volume, which decreases venous return and blood pressure (see Figure 44–6). The end result is a decrease in afterload and preload and a decrease in the heart's workload. Diuretics are available in mild to potent compounds and are frequently used as adjunctive therapy in the treatment of all degrees of CHF. (See Chapter 51 for additional information.)

β-Adrenergic Agonists

β-Adrenergic agonists stimulate the β-receptors in the sympathetic nervous system, increasing calcium flow into the myocardial cells and causing increased contraction, a positively inotropic effect (see Figure 44–6). Other sympathetic stimulation effects can cause increased CHF, because the heart's workload is increased by most sympathetic activity. Dobutamine is the β-agonist most frequently used to treat CHF. Because it must be given by intravenous infusion in an acute care setting, it is usually reserved for treatment of acute CHF. (See Chapter 30 for additional information.)

CARDIOTONIC DRUGS

Cardiotonic (inotropic) drugs affect the intracellular calcium levels in the heart muscle, leading to increased contractility. This increase in contraction strength leads to increased cardiac output, which causes increased renal blood flow and increased urine production. Increased renal blood flow decreases renin release, breaking the effects of the renin–angiotensin system,

FIGURE 44-6. Sites of action of drugs used to treat congestive heart failure (CHF).

and increases urine output, leading to decreased blood volume. Together, these effects decrease the heart's workload and help to relieve CHF. Two types of cardiotonic drugs are used: the classic cardiac glycosides, which have been used for hundreds of years, and the newer phosphodiesterase inhibitors.

CARDIAC GLYCOSIDES

The cardiac glycosides were originally derived from the foxglove or digitalis plant. These plants were once ground up to make digitalis leaf. Today, digoxin (*Lanoxin, Lanoxicaps*) is the drug most often used to treat CHF; it has a very rapid onset of action and is available for parenteral and oral use. It is excreted unchanged in the urine, making it a safe drug for patients with liver dysfunction. Digoxin has a very narrow margin of safety (meaning that the therapeutic dose is very close to the toxic dose), so extreme care must be taken when using this drug. Digoxin toxicity is a real possibility in clinical practice because of the narrow margin of safety. A digoxin antidote, digoxin immune Fab, has been developed to rapidly treat digoxin toxicity (Box 44–1).

Therapeutic Actions and Indications
The cardiac glycosides increase intracellular calcium and allow more calcium to enter myocardial cells during depolarization (see Figure 44–6), causing the following effects:

- Increased force of myocardial contraction (a positive inotropic effect)
- Increased cardiac output and renal perfusion (which has a diuretic effect, increasing urine output and decreasing blood volume while decreasing renin release and activation of the renin–angiotensin system)
- Slowed heart rate, owing to slowing of the rate of cellular repolarization (a negative chronotropic effect)
- Decreased conduction velocity through the atrioventricular node

The overall effect is a decrease in the myocardial workload and relief of CHF (Table 44–1). The cardiac glycosides are indicated for the treatment of CHF, atrial flutter, atrial fibrillation, and paroxysmal atrial tachycardia.

Pharmacokinetics
Digoxin is rapidly absorbed and widely distributed throughout the body. Digoxin is primarily excreted unchanged in the urine. Because of this, caution should be used in the presence of renal impairment, because the drug may not be excreted and could accumulate, causing toxicity. It is not known whether digoxin causes fetal toxicity; it should be given during pregnancy only if the benefit to the mother clearly outweighs the risk to the fetus. Digoxin does enter breast milk, but it has not been shown to cause problems for the neonate. Caution should be used, however, during lactation.

BOX 44-1

Digoxin Antidote: Digoxin Immune Fab

Digoxin immune Fab (*Digibind, Digifab*) is an antigen-binding fragment (Fab) derived from specific anti-digoxin antibodies. These antibodies bind molecules of digoxin, making them unavailable at their site of action. The digoxin antibody–antigen complexes accumulate in the blood and are excreted through the kidney. Digoxin immune Fab is used for the treatment of life-threatening digoxin intoxication (serum levels >10 ng/mL with serum potassium >5 mEq/L in a setting of digoxin intoxication) and potential life-threatening digoxin overdose.

The amount of digoxin immune Fab that is infused intravenously is determined by the amount of digoxin ingested or by the serum digoxin level if the ingested amount is unknown. The patient's cardiac status should be monitored continually while the drug is given and for several hours after the infusion is finished. Because there is a risk of hypersensitivity reaction to the infused protein, life-support equipment should be on standby.

Serum digoxin levels will be very high and unreliable for about 3 days after the digoxin immune Fab infusion because of the high levels of digoxin in the blood. The patient should not be redigitalized for several days to 1 week after digoxin immune Fab has been used, because of the potential of remaining fragments in the blood. The drug comes in two preparations: *Digibind* and *Digifab*. The dosing of the two preparations is subtly different, and care must be taken to check the brand name before administering the drug.

Contraindications and Cautions

Cardiac glycosides are contraindicated in the presence of allergy to any digitalis preparation. These drugs also are contraindicated in the following conditions: ventricular tachycardia or fibrillation, which are potentially fatal arrhythmias and should be treated with other drugs; heart block or sick sinus syndrome, which could be made worse by slowing of conduction through the atrioventricular node; idiopathic hypertrophic subaortic stenosis (IHSS), because the increase in force of contraction could obstruct the outflow tract to the aorta and cause severe problems; acute MI, because the increase in force of contraction could cause more muscle damage and infarct; renal insufficiency, because the drug is excreted through the kidneys and toxic levels could develop; and electrolyte abnormalities (eg, increased calcium, decreased potassium, decreased magnesium), which could alter the action potential and change the effects of the drug.

Cardiac glycosides should be used cautiously in patients who are pregnant or lactating because of the potential for adverse effects on the fetus or neonate.

Adverse Effects

The adverse effects most frequently seen with the cardiac glycosides include headache, weakness, drowsiness, and vision changes (a yellow halo around objects is often reported with digoxin toxicity). GI upset and anorexia also commonly occur. A risk of arrhythmia development exists because the glycosides affect the action potential and conduction system of the heart.

Clinically Important Drug–Drug Interactions

There is a risk of increased therapeutic effects and toxic effects of digoxin if it is taken with verapamil, amiodarone, quinidine, quinine, erythromycin, tetracycline, or cyclosporine. If digoxin is combined with any of these drugs, it may be necessary to decrease the digoxin dose to prevent toxicity. If one of these drugs has been part of a medical regimen with digoxin and it is discontinued, the digoxin dose may need to be increased.

An increased risk of cardiac arrhythmias exists if these drugs are taken with potassium-losing diuretics. If this combination is used, the patient's potassium levels should be checked regularly and appropriate replacement done.

Digoxin may be less effective if it is combined with thyroid hormones, metoclopramide, or penicillamine, and increased digoxin dosage may be needed.

TABLE 44-1   Congestive Heart Failure and Response to Cardiac Glycosides

Signs and Symptoms*	Response During Congestive Heart Failure	Response After Full Digitalization†
Heart rate, rhythm, and size	Heart hypertrophied, dilated; rate rapid, irregular; "palpitations"; auscultation—S_3	Dilatation decreased, hypertrophy remains; rate, 70–80, may be regular; auscultation—no S_3
Lungs	Dyspnea on exertion; orthopnea; tachypnea; paroxysmal nocturnal dyspnea; wheezing, rales, cough, hemoptysis (pulmonary edema)	↓ Rate of respiration; wheezes, rales gone
Peripheral congestion	Pitting edema of dependent parts; hepatomegaly; ↑ jugular venous pressure; cyanosis; oliguria; nocturia	↑ Cardiac output and renal blood flow leads to ↑ urine flow, ↓ edema, ↓ signs and symptoms of poor perfusion
Other	Weakness, fatigue, anorexia, insomnia, nausea, vomiting, abdominal pain	↑ Appetite: ↑ strength, energy

*Because the clinical picture in heart failure varies with the stage and degree of severity, the signs and symptoms may vary considerably in different patients.

†Digitalization will not overcome similar symptoms when they are caused by conditions other than heart failure. Overdosage may actually cause symptoms similar to those of heart failure (e.g., anorexia, nausea, and vomiting, cardiac arrhythmias, peripheral congestion).

NURSING CHALLENGE
Lanoxin versus *Lanoxicaps*

Digoxin comes in two similar-sounding, brand-name preparations: *Lanoxin* and *Lanoxicaps*. These drugs both provide digoxin, but the bioavailability of these two drugs is dramatically different. *Lanoxicaps* are absorbed much more effectively—a 0.2-mg dose of *Lanoxicaps* is the equivalent of a 0.25-mg dose of *Lanoxin*, and the 0.1-mg capsule of *Lanoxicaps* is equivalent to the 0.125-mg tablet of *Lanoxin*. Digoxin has a very small margin of safety to begin with, and the room for error is much smaller with *Lanoxicaps*.

Extreme care must be taken when administering either of these drugs to ensure that the right dose goes with the right brand name. Patient education should clearly identify the drug and dose being ordered. Patients should be warned not to trade or share medication because of the potential for serious problems. Here is an example of what can happen: A patient on vacation ran out of his *Lanoxin* tablets, which were ordered at 0.25 mg/day, and borrowed 0.1 mg *Lanoxicaps* from a friend. He took two and a half *Lanoxicaps* each day because he knew he should have 0.25 mg. As a result, the patient became digoxin toxic and required hospitalization to regulate his arrhythmias.

The names of these two drugs are so close that it is easy to make a similar mistake in a patient care setting. By being alert to the possibility of a problem, the nurse may avert adverse consequences for the patient.

Absorption of oral digoxin may be decreased if it is taken with cholestyramine, charcoal, colestipol, bleomycin, cyclophosphamide, or methotrexate. If it is used in combination with any of these agents, the drugs should not be taken at the same time, but should be administered 2 to 4 hours apart.

St. John's wort and psyllium have been shown to decrease the effectiveness of digoxin; this combination should be avoided.

Increased digoxin toxicity has been reported with ginseng, hawthorn and licorice. Patients should be advised to avoid these combinations.

Nursing Considerations for Patients Receiving Cardiac Glycosides
Assessment: History and Examination

Screen for the following conditions, which could be cautions or contraindications to use of the drug: known allergies to any digitalis product; impaired kidney function, which could alter the excretion of the drug; ventricular tachycardia or fibrillation; heart block or sick sinus syndrome; IHSS; acute MI; electrolyte abnormalities (increased calcium, decreased potassium, or decreased magnesium); and pregnancy or lactation, because of the potential adverse effects on the fetus or neonate.

Include screening for baseline status before beginning therapy and for any potential adverse effects. Assess the following: weight, skin color, lesions; affect, orientation, reflexes; pulse, blood pressure, perfusion, baseline ECG, cardiac auscultation; respirations, adventitious sounds; abdominal examination, bowel sounds; renal function tests; and serum electrolyte levels.

Nursing Diagnoses

The patient receiving a cardiac glycoside may have the following nursing diagnoses related to drug therapy:

- Risk for Deficient Fluid Volume related to diuresis
- Ineffective Tissue Perfusion (Total Body) related to change in cardiac output
- Impaired Gas Exchange related to changes in cardiac output
- Deficient Knowledge regarding drug therapy

Implementation

- Consult with the prescriber about the need for a loading dose when beginning therapy, *to achieve desired results as soon as possible.*
- Monitor apical pulse for 1 full minute before administering the drug, *to monitor for adverse effects.* Hold the dose if the pulse is less than 60 beats/min in an adult or less than 90 beats/min in an infant; retake pulse in 1 hour. If pulse remains low, document pulse, withhold the drug, and notify the prescriber, *because the pulse rate could indicate digoxin toxicity.*

DRUGS IN FOCUS
Cardiac Glycosides

Drug Name	Usual Dosage	Usual Indications
℗ digoxin (*Lanoxin, Lanoxicaps*)	Adult: loading dose 0.75–1.25 mg PO or 0.125–0.25 mg IV, then maintenance dose of 0.125–0.25 mg/d PO; decrease dosage with renal impairment Pediatric (dosage based on age): 10–60 µg/kg PO or 8–50 µg/kg IV loading dose, maintenance is 25%–30% of loading dose	Treatment of acute congestive heart failure, atrial arrhythmias

NURSING CHALLENGE
Preventing Digoxin Toxicity in Children and the Elderly

Pediatric and geriatric patients are at increased risk for the development of digoxin toxicity. Individuals in both of these groups have body masses that are smaller than the average adult body mass, and they may have immature or aging kidneys. Digoxin is excreted unchanged in the kidney, so any change in kidney function can result in increased serum digoxin levels and subsequent digoxin toxicity. Extreme care should be taken when administering digoxin to patients in either of these age groups.

Many institutions require that pediatric digoxin doses be checked by a second nurse before administration. This practice provides an extra check to help prevent the toxicity of this potentially dangerous drug. The patient should then be assessed before the drug is given, including careful cardiac auscultation and apical pulse measurement to monitor heart rate and rhythm to detect any possible toxic effects.

Geriatric patients may not receive the same kind of attention as a policy, but they should be monitored for any factor that might affect digoxin levels when the drug is administered. Such factors may include

- Renal function (Is the blood urea nitrogen concentration elevated?)
- Low body mass (Is the patient underweight, undernourished, taking laxatives?)
- Current pulse, including quality and rhythm
- Hydration (Is the skin loose? Are the mucous membranes dry? The presence of these conditions could signal potential electrolyte disturbances.)

Many geriatric patients eventually need a decrease in dose, from 0.25 mg once a day to 0.125 mg once a day or 0.25 mg every other day. The nurse administering the drug is often in the best position to detect any changes in the patient's condition that might indicate a need for further evaluation.

- Monitor pulse for any change in quality or rhythm, *to detect arrhythmias or early signs of toxicity.*
- Check the dosage and preparation carefully, *because digoxin has a very small margin of safety, and inadvertent drug errors can cause serious problems.*
- Check pediatric dosage with extreme care, *because children are more apt to develop digoxin toxicity.* Have the dosage double-checked by another nurse before administration.
- Follow dilution instructions carefully for intravenous use; use promptly *to avoid drug degradation.*
- Administer intravenous doses very slowly over at least 5 minutes, *to avoid cardiac arrhythmias and adverse effects.*
- Avoid intramuscular administration, *which could be quite painful.*
- Arrange for the patient to be weighed at the same time each day, in the same clothes, *to monitor for fluid retention and CHF.*
- Avoid administering the oral drug with food or antacids, *to avoid delays in absorption.*
- Maintain emergency equipment on standby: potassium salts,

PATIENT TEACHING CHECKLIST
Digoxin

Create customized patient teaching materials for digoxin from the CD-ROM. Patient teaching should stress the following points for drugs within this class:

- Digoxin is a digitalis preparation. Digitalis has many helpful effects on the heart; for example, it helps the heart to beat more slowly and efficiently. These effects lead to better circulation and should help to reduce the swelling in your ankles or legs. It also should increase the amount of urine that you produce every day.
- Digoxin is a very powerful drug and must be taken exactly as prescribed. It is important to have regular medical checkups to ensure that the dosage of the drug is correct for you and that it is having the desired effect on your heart.
- Do not stop taking this drug without consulting your health care provider. Never skip doses and never try to "catch up" any missed doses, because serious adverse effects could occur.
- You should learn to take your own pulse. Take it each morning before engaging in any activity. Write your pulse rate on a calendar so you will be aware of any changes and can notify your health care provider if the rate or rhythm of your pulse shows a consistent change. Your normal pulse rate is _____.
- You should monitor your weight fairly closely. Weigh yourself every other day, at the same time of the day and in the same amount of clothing. Record your weight on your calendar for easy reference. If you gain or lose 3 lb or more in 1 day, it may indicate a problem with your drug. Consult your health care provider.

Some of the following adverse effects may occur:

- *Dizziness, drowsiness, headache*—Avoid driving or performing hazardous tasks or delicate tasks that require concentration if these occur. Consult your health care provider for an appropriate analgesic if the headache is a problem.
- *Nausea, gastrointestinal upset, loss of appetite*—Small, frequent meals may help; monitor your weight loss; if it becomes severe, consult your health care provider.
- *Vision changes, "yellow" halos around objects*—These effects may pass with time. Take extra care in your activities for the first few days. If these reactions do not go away after 3 to 4 days, consult with your health care provider.

Report any of the following to your health care provider: unusually slow or irregular pulse; rapid weight gain; "yellow vision"; unusual tiredness or weakness; skin rash or hives; swelling of the ankles, legs, or fingers; difficulty breathing.

Tell any doctor, nurse, dentist, or other health care provider that you are taking this drug.

Keep this drug, and all medications, out of the reach of children.

Avoid the use of over-the-counter medications while you are taking this drug. If you feel that you need one of these, consult with your health care provider for the best choice. Many of these drugs contain ingredients that could interfere with your digoxin.

It might be helpful to wear or carry a Medic-Alert tag to alert any medical personnel who might take care of you in an emergency that you are taking this drug.

Patient Teaching Checklist continues on page 598

PATIENT TEACHING CHECKLIST
(CONTINUED)

Digoxin

Regular medical follow-up is important to evaluate the actions of the drug and to adjust the dosage if necessary.

This Teaching Checklist reflects general patient teaching guidelines. It is not meant to be a substitute for drug-specific teaching information, which is available in nursing drug guides.

lidocaine (*for treatment of arrhythmias*), phenytoin (*for treatment of seizures*), atropine (*to increase heart rate*), and a cardiac monitor *in case severe toxicity should occur.*

- Monitor the patient for therapeutic digoxin level (0.5 to 2 ng/mL), *to evaluate therapeutic dosing and to monitor for the development of toxicity.*
- Provide comfort measures *to help the patient tolerate drug effects.* These include small, frequent meals, access to bathroom facilities if GI upset is severe, environmental controls, safety precautions, adequate lighting if vision changes occur, positioning for comfort, and frequent rest periods to balance supply and demand of oxygen.
- Provide thorough patient teaching, including the name of the

NURSING CARE GUIDE

Digoxin

Assessment	Nursing Diagnoses	Implementation	Evaluation
HISTORY Allergies to any digitalis product, renal dysfunction, IHSS, pregnancy, lactation, arrhythmias, heart block, electrolyte abnormalities	Decreased Cardiac Output related to cardiac effect Deficient Fluid Volume related to diuretic effects Ineffective Tissue Perfusion related to changes in cardiac output Impaired Gas Exchange related to changes in cardiac output Deficient Knowledge regarding drug therapy	Administer a loading dose to provide rapid therapeutic effects. Monitor apical pulse for 1 full minute before administering to assess for adverse and therapeutic effects. Check dosage very carefully. Provide comfort and safety measures: give small, frequent meals; ensure access to bathroom facilities; avoid IM injection; administer IV over 5 min; keep emergency equipment on standby. Provide support and reassurance to deal with drug effects. Provide patient teaching regarding drug, dosage, adverse effects, what to report, safety precautions.	Evaluate drug effects: relief of signs and symptoms of CHF, resolution of atrial arrhythmias, serum digoxin levels 0.5–2 ng/mL. Monitor for adverse effects: -arrhythmias -vision changes (yellow halo) -GI upset -headache, drowsiness Monitor for drug–drug interactions as indicated for each drug. Evaluate effectiveness of patient teaching program. Evaluate effectiveness of comfort and safety measures.
PHYSICAL EXAMINATION CV: BP, P, perfusion, ECG CNS: orientation, affect, reflexes, vision Skin: color, lesions, texture, perfusion Resp: R, adventitious sounds GI: abdominal exam, bowel sounds Lab tests: serum electrolytes, body weight			

drug, dosage prescribed, proper administration, measures to avoid adverse effects, warning signs of problems, and the need for periodic monitoring and evaluation, *to enhance patient knowledge about drug therapy and to promote compliance.* (See Patient Teaching Checklist: Digoxin.)

- Offer support and encouragement, *to help the patient deal with the diagnosis and the drug regimen.*

Evaluation

- Monitor patient response to the drug (improvement in signs and symptoms of CHF, resolution of atrial arrhythmias, serum digoxin level of 0.5 to 2 ng/mL).
- Monitor for adverse effects (vision changes, arrhythmias, CHF, headache, dizziness, drowsiness, GI upset, nausea).
- Evaluate the effectiveness of the teaching plan (patient can name drug, dosage, proper administration, adverse effects to watch for, specific measures to avoid adverse effects, importance of continued follow-up).
- Monitor the effectiveness of comfort measures and compliance to the regimen (see Nursing Care Guide: Digoxin).

PHOSPHODIESTERASE INHIBITORS

The phosphodiesterase inhibitors belong to a second class of drugs that act as cardiotonic (inotropic) agents. Inamrinone (*Inocor*) is available only for intravenous use and is approved only for use in patients with CHF that has not responded to digoxin, diuretics, or vasodilators. Milrinone (*Primacor*) is available only for intravenous use for the short-term management of CHF in patients who are receiving digoxin and diuretics. Because these drugs have been associated with the development of potentially fatal ventricular arrhythmias, their use is limited to severe situations.

Therapeutic Actions and Indications

The phosphodiesterase inhibitors block the enzyme phosphodiesterase. This blocking effect leads to an increase in myocardial cell cyclic adenosine monophosphate (cAMP), which increases calcium levels in the cell (see Figure 44–6). Increased cellular calcium causes a stronger contraction and prolongs the effects of sympathetic stimulation, which can lead to vasodilation, increased oxygen consumption, and arrhythmias. These drugs are indicated for the short-term treatment of CHF that has not responded to digoxin or diuretics alone or that has had a poor response to digoxin, diuretics, and vasodilators.

Pharmacokinetics

These drugs are widely distributed after injection. They are metabolized in the liver and excreted primarily in the urine. There are no adequate studies about the effects of these drugs during pregnancy, and their use should be reserved for situations in which the benefit to the mother clearly outweighs the potential risk to the fetus. It is not known whether these drug enter breast milk, so caution should be used during lactation.

Contraindications and Cautions

Phosphodiesterase inhibitors are contraindicated in the presence of allergy to either of these drugs or to bisulfites. They also are contraindicated in the following conditions: severe aortic or pulmonic valvular disease, which could be exacerbated by increased contraction; acute MI, which could be exacerbated by increased oxygen consumption and increased force of contraction; fluid volume deficit, which could be made worse by increased renal perfusion; and ventricular arrhythmias, which could be exacerbated by these drugs.

Caution should be used in the elderly, who are more likely to develop adverse effects, and in pregnant or lactating women, because of potential adverse effects on the fetus or neonate.

Adverse Effects

The adverse effects most frequently seen with these drugs are ventricular arrhythmias (which can progress to fatal ventricular fibrillation), hypotension, and chest pain. GI effects include nausea, vomiting, anorexia, and abdominal pain. Thrombocytopenia occurs frequently with inamrinone, and it also can occur with milrinone. Hypersensitivity reactions associated with these drugs include vasculitis, pericarditis, pleuritis, and ascites. Burning at the injection site is also a frequent adverse effect.

Clinically Important Drug–Drug Interactions

Precipitates form when these drugs are given in solution with furosemide. Avoid this combination in solution. Use alternate lines if both of these drugs are being given intravenously.

Nursing Considerations for Patients Receiving Phosphodiesterase Inhibitors

Assessment: History and Examination

Screen for the following conditions, which could be cautions or contraindications to use of the drug: any known allergies to these drugs or to bisulfites; acute aortic or pulmonic valvular disease, acute MI or fluid volume deficit, and ventricular arrhythmias, which could be exacerbated by these drugs; and pregnancy and lactation, because of the potential adverse effects on the fetus and neonate.

Include screening for baseline status before beginning therapy and for any potential adverse effects. Assess the following: skin color, lesions, temperature; affect, orientation, reflexes; pulse, blood pressure, perfusion, baseline ECG; respirations, adventitious sounds; abdominal examination; and serum electrolytes and complete blood count.

Nursing Diagnoses

The patient receiving a phosphodiesterase inhibitor may have the following nursing diagnoses related to drug therapy:

- Decreased Cardiac Output related to arrhythmias, hypotension
- Risk for Injury related to CNS, cardiovascular effects
- Ineffective Tissue Perfusion (Total Body) related to hypotension, thrombocytopenia, arrhythmias
- Deficient Knowledge regarding drug therapy

Inadequate Digoxin Absorption

THE SITUATION

G. J. is an 82-year-old white woman with a 50-year history of rheumatic mitral valve disease. G. J. has been stabilized on digoxin for 10 years in a compensated state of congestive heart failure (CHF). G. J. recently moved into an extended care facility, having had difficulty caring for herself independently. She was examined by the admitting facility physician and was found to be stable. Note was made of an irregular pulse of 76 beats/min with electrocardiographic documentation of her chronic atrial fibrillation.

Three weeks after her arrival at the nursing home, G. J. began to develop progressive weakness, dyspnea on exertion, two-pillow orthopnea, and peripheral 2+ pitting edema. These signs and symptoms became progressively worse, and 5 days after the first indication that her CHF was returning, G. J. was admitted to the hospital with a diagnosis of CHF. Physical examination revealed a heart rate of 96 beats/min with atrial fibrillation, third heart sound, rales, wheezes, 2+ pitting edema bilaterally up to the knees, elevated jugular venous pressure, cardiomegaly, weak pulses, and poor peripheral perfusion. G. J.'s serum digoxin level was 0.12 ng/mL (therapeutic range, 0.5–2 ng/mL). G. J. was treated with diuretics and was redigitalized in the hospital with close cardiac monitoring. After she was stabilized, G. J. reported that she knew she had been taking her digoxin every day because she recognized the pill. The only difference she could identify was that she was given the pill in the afternoon with a dish of ice cream, while at home she always took it on an empty stomach first thing in the morning. The nursing home staff confirmed that G. J. had received the drug daily in the afternoon and that it was the same brand name she had used at home.

CRITICAL THINKING

• What nursing interventions should be done at this point? *Think about the signs and symptoms of CHF and how they show the progression of the heart failure.*
• How could the change in the timing of drug administration be related to the decreased serum digoxin levels noted on G. J.'s admission?
• Consider the factors that affect absorption of a drug. What alterations in dosing could be suggested that would prevent this from happening to G. J. again?
• What potential problems with trust could develop for G. J. on her return to the nursing home? Suggest an explanation for what happened to G. J. and possible ways that this problem could have been averted.

DISCUSSION

G. J.'s immediate needs involve trying to alleviate the alteration to her cardiac output that occurred when she lost the therapeutic effects of digoxin. Positioning, cool environment, small and frequent meals, and rest periods can help to decrease the workload on her heart. Digoxin has a small margin of safety and requires an adequate serum level to be therapeutic. G. J. was not absorbing enough digoxin to achieve a therapeutic serum level; consequently, her body began to go through the progression of congestive heart failure, first right-sided and then left-sided.

Consultation with a clinical pharmacologist determined that ice cream, which is cold and causes a vasoconstriction in the stomach and slowing of muscle contraction, contains protein and calcium, two things that increase acid production in the stomach. Taking the digoxin with the ice cream exposed the drug to increased acid levels in the stomach for a longer period than normal. This effect destroyed much of the digoxin, leaving only a small amount to be absorbed. This change was enough to lower G. J.'s digoxin level below a therapeutic range, leading to the development of CHF over the 3-week period.

G. J. should receive extensive patient teaching about her disease, her drugs, and the adverse effects that may signal the development of drug toxicity or lack of therapeutic effectiveness. G. J. should receive this information in writing to take back to the facility with her. To avoid friction when teaching the facility staff about G. J.'s situation, the hospital staff might explain the kind of research that was needed to determine what happened, then discuss how much the nurses learned about the drug and drug mechanics from this process. Working together, both staffs can establish a better timing of G. J.'s digoxin dose that can successfully be incorporated into the routine at the extended care facility. G. J. should have serum digoxin levels drawn in 1 week to determine the effectiveness of the dosing and the drug.

Many factors can change the way that a drug is absorbed or biotransformed in the body, including diet, brand of the drug, environmental stresses, disease states, and interactions with other drugs. Because digoxin must be maintained within a limited range to be effective, any of these factors could greatly influence its bioavailability and effectiveness. Careful patient monitoring is very important with the use of digoxin to ensure a therapeutic effect and to prevent adverse effects.

Implementation

• Protect the drug from light, *to prevent drug degradation.*
• Monitor pulse and blood pressure periodically during administration, *to monitor for adverse effects so that dosage can be altered if needed to avoid toxicity.*
• Monitor input and output and record daily weights, *to evaluate resolution of CHF.*
• Monitor platelet counts before and regularly during therapy, *to ensure that the dose is appropriate;* consult with the prescriber about the need to decrease the dose at the first sign of thrombocytopenia.
• Monitor injection sites and provide comfort measures *if infusion is painful.*
• Provide life support equipment on standby *in case of severe reaction to the drug or development of ventricular arrhythmias.*

DRUGS IN FOCUS
Phosphodiesterase Inhibitors

Drug Name	Usual Dosage	Usual Indications
P inamrinone (*Inocor*)	0.75 mg/kg IV bolus over 2–3 min; may be repeated in 30 min as needed; then 5–10 µg/kg per minute IV; do not exceed 10 mg/kg per day	Treatment of adults with congestive heart failure (CHF) not responsive to digoxin, diuretics, or vasodilators
milrinone (*Primacor*)	50 µg/kg IV bolus over 10 min; then 0.375–0.75 µg/kg per minute IV infusion, do not exceed 1.13 mg/kg per day; reduce dosage in renal impairment	Short-term management of CHF in adults receiving digoxin and diuretics

• Provide comfort measures *to help the patient tolerate drug effects.* These include small, frequent meals, access to bathroom facilities if GI upset is severe and if diuresis occurs, environmental controls, safety precautions, and orientation to surroundings.

• Provide thorough patient teaching, including the name of the drug, dosage prescribed, proper administration, measures to avoid adverse effects, warning signs of problems, and the need for periodic monitoring and evaluation, *to enhance patient knowledge about drug therapy and to promote compliance.*

• Offer support and encouragement, *to help the patient deal with the diagnosis and the drug regimen.*

Evaluation

• Monitor patient response to the drug (alleviation of signs and symptoms of CHF).

• Monitor for adverse effects (hypotension, cardiac arrhythmias, GI upset, thrombocytopenia).

• Evaluate the effectiveness of the teaching plan (patient can name drug, dosage, adverse effects to watch for, specific measures to avoid adverse effects, importance of continued follow-up).

• Monitor the effectiveness of comfort measures and compliance to the regimen.

▢▢◑● WEB LINKS
Health care providers and patients may want to consult the following Internet sources:

Information on diet, exercise, drug therapy, cardiac rehabilitation:
    http://www.jhbmc.jhu.edu/cardiology
Patient information on latest resources, diets, programs:
    http://www.jhbmc.jhu.edu/cardiology/rehab/patientinfo.html
Patient information, support groups, diet, exercise, research information on heart disease and CHF:
    http://www.americanheart.org

Specific information on the acute care of CHF from the American Association of Critical Care Nurses:
    http://www.aacn.org

CHAPTER SUMMARY

• Congestive heart failure (CHF) is a condition in which the heart muscle fails to effectively pump blood through the cardiovascular system, leading to a buildup of blood or congestion in the system.

• CHF can be the result of a damaged heart muscle and increased demand to work harder secondary to coronary artery disease, hypertension, cardiomyopathy, valvular disease, or congenital heart abnormalities.

• The sarcomere, the functioning unit of the heart muscle, is made up of protein fibers—thin actin fibers and thick myosin fibers.

• Actin and myosin fibers react with each other and slide together, contracting the sarcomere, when calcium is present to inactivate troponin, an inhibitory compound that prevents this reaction. This sliding action requires the use of energy.

• Calcium enters the cell during the action potential after the cell has been stimulated. It gains entrance to the cell through calcium channels in the cell membrane and from storage sites within the cell.

• Failing cardiac muscle cells lose the ability to effectively use energy to move calcium into the cell, and contractions become weak and ineffective.

• Treatment for CHF can include the use of vasodilators (to reduce the heart's workload); diuretics (to reduce blood volume and the heart's workload); β-blockers (which decrease the heart's workload precipitated by the activation of the sympathetic reaction); and cardiotonic (inotropic) agents (which directly stimulate the muscle to contract more effectively).

• Signs and symptoms of CHF reflect the backup of blood in the vascular system and the loss of fluid in the tissues. Edema, liver congestion, elevated jugular venous pressure, and nocturia reflect right-sided CHF. Tachypnea, dyspnea, orthopnea, hemoptysis, anxiety, and low blood oxygenation reflect left-sided CHF.

• Cardiac glycosides increase the movement of calcium into the heart muscle. This results in increased force of contraction, which increases blood flow to the kidneys (causing a diuretic effect), slows the heart rate, and slows conduction through the atrioventricular node. All of these effects decrease the heart's workload, helping to bring the system back into balance or compensation.

• Phosphodiesterase inhibitors block the breakdown of cAMP in the cardiac muscle. This allows more calcium to enter the cell (leading to more intense contraction) and increases the effects of sympathetic stimulation (which can lead to vasodilation but also can increase pulse, blood pressure, and workload on the heart). Because these drugs are associated with severe effects, they are reserved for use in extreme situations.

Review Questions

1. Patients with CHF present clinically with
   a. cardiac arrest.
   b. congestion of blood vessels with slowing in delivery of nutrients and removal of waste products.
   c. a myocardial infarction.
   d. a pulmonary embolism.

2. Calcium is needed in the cardiac muscle
   a. to break apart actinomyosin bridges.
   b. to activate troponin.
   c. to allow actinomyosin bridges to form, causing contraction.
   d. to maintain the electrical rhythm.

3. CHF occurs when the heart fails to pump effectively. Causes of CHF would not include
   a. coronary artery disease.
   b. chronic hypertension.
   c. cardiomyopathy.
   d. fluid overload.

4. A patient with left-sided CHF after an MI might present with all of the following except
   a. orthopnea.
   b. polyuria.
   c. tachypnea.
   d. dyspnea.

5. A patient with right-sided CHF might exhibit edema
   a. in any gravity-dependent areas.
   b. in the hands and fingers.
   c. around the eyes.
   d. when lying down.

6. ACE inhibitors and other vasodilators are used in the early treatment of CHF. They act to

   a. cause loss of volume.
   b. increase arterial pressure and perfusion.
   c. cause pooling of the blood and decreased venous return to the heart, decreasing the workload of the muscle.
   d. increase the release of aldosterone and improve fluid balance.

7. Cardiotonic drugs are drugs that
   a. block the sympathetic nervous system.
   b. block the renin–angiotensin system.
   c. block the parasympathetic influence on the heart muscle.
   d. affect the intracellular calcium levels in the heart muscle, leading to increased contractility.

8. A patient taking *Lanoxin* (digoxin) for the treatment of CHF would be advised to
   a. make up any missed doses the next day.
   b. report changes in vision or in heart rate.
   c. avoid exposure to the sun.
   d. switch to generic tablets if they are cheaper.

9. A nurse is about to administer *Lanoxin* to a patient whose apical pulse is 48 beats/min. She should
   a. give the drug and notify the prescriber.
   b. retake the pulse in 15 minutes and give the drug if pulse has not changed.
   c. retake the pulse in 1 hour and withhold the drug if the pulse is still less than 60 beats/min.
   d. withhold the drug and notify the prescriber.

10. Before giving digoxin to an infant, the nurse would
    a. notify the prescriber that the dose is about to be given.
    b. check the apical pulse and have another nurse double-check the dose.
    c. make sure the infant has eaten and has a full stomach.
    d. check the apical pulse and give the drug very slowly.

BIBLIOGRAPHY

Abramowicz, M. (1996). Drugs for chronic heart failure. *Medical Letter, 38*(985).

Bullock, B. L. (2000). *Focus on pathophysiology*. Philadelphia: Lippincott Williams & Wilkins.

Drug facts and comparisons. (2002). St. Louis: Facts and Comparisons.

Gilman, A., Hardman, J. G., & Limbird, L. E. (Eds.) (2002). *Goodman and Gilman's the pharmacological basis of therapeutics* (10th ed.). New York: McGraw-Hill.

Karch, A. M. (2002). *2003 Lippincott's nursing drug guide*. Philadelphia: Lippincott Williams & Wilkins.

The medical letter on drugs and therapeutics. (2002). New Rochelle, NY: Medical Letter.

Porth, C. M. (2002). *Pathophysiology: Concepts of altered health states* (6th ed.). Philadelphia: Lippincott Williams & Wilkins.

CHAPTER

45

Antiarrhythmic Agents

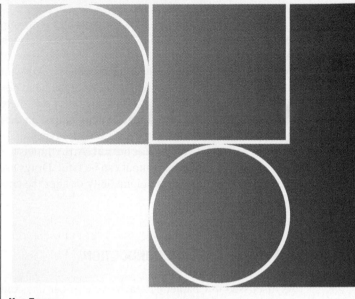

Key Terms

antiarrhythmics

bradycardia

cardiac output

Cardiac Arrhythmia Suppression Trial (CAST)

heart blocks

hemodynamics

premature ventricular contraction (PVC)

premature atrial contraction (PAC)

proarrhythmic

tachycardia

603

Class Ia Antiarrhythmics

disopyramide

moricizine

procainamide

🅟 quinidine

Class Ib Antiarrhythmics

🅟 lidocaine

mexiletine

tocainide

Class Ic Antiarrhythmics

🅟 flecainide

propafenone

Class II Antiarrhythmics

acebutolol

esmolol

🅟 propranolol

Class III Antiarrhythmics

amiodarone

🅟 bretylium

dofetilide

ibutilide

sotalol

Class IV Antiarrhythmics

🅟 diltiazem

verapamil

Other

adenosine

digoxin

As discussed in earlier chapters, disruptions in impulse formation and in the conduction of impulses through the myocardium are called arrhythmias. (They also are called dysrhythmias by some health care providers.) Arrhythmias occur in the heart because all of the cells of the heart possess the property of automaticity (discussed later) and therefore can generate an excitatory impulse. Disruptions in the normal rhythm of the heart can interfere with myocardial contractions and affect the **cardiac output.** Arrhythmias that seriously disrupt the cardiac output can be fatal. Drugs used to treat arrhythmias suppress automaticity or alter the conductivity of the heart.

REVIEW OF CARDIAC CONDUCTION

As discussed in Chapter 42, each cycle of cardiac contraction and relaxation is controlled by impulses that arise spontaneously in the sinoatrial (SA) node of the heart. These impulses are conducted from the pacemaker cells by a specialized conducting system that activates all parts of the heart muscle almost simultaneously. These continuous, rhythmic contractions are controlled by the heart itself. This property allows the heart to beat as long as it has enough nutrients and oxygen to survive, regardless of the status of the rest of the body.

The conduction system of the heart is composed of the following:

The SA node, located in the top of the right atrium, which acts as the pacemaker of the heart

Atrial bundles that conduct the impulse through the atrial muscle

The atrioventricular (AV) node, which slows the impulse and sends it from the atria into the ventricles by way of the bundle of His

The bundle of His, which enters the septum and then divides into three bundle branches

The bundle branches, which conduct the impulses through the ventricles; these branches break into a fine network of conducting fibers called the Purkinje fibers

The Purkinje fibers, which deliver the impulse to the ventricular cells (Figure 45–1).

AUTOMATICITY OF THE HEART

All cardiac cells possess some degree of automaticity, as described in Chapter 42. These cells undergo a spontaneous depolarization during diastole or rest because they decrease the flow of potassium ions out of the cell and probably leak sodium into the cell, causing an action potential. This action potential is basically the same as the action potential of the neuron (described in Chapter 19).

The action potential of the cardiac muscle cell consists of five phases:

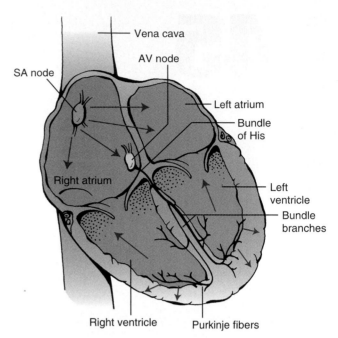

FIGURE 45–1. The conducting system of the heart. Impulses originating in the sinoatrial (SA) node are transmitted through the atrial bundles to the atrioventricular (AV) node and down the bundle of His and the bundle branches by way of the Purkinje fibers through the ventricles.

Phase 0 occurs when the cell reaches a point of stimulation. The sodium gates open along the cell membrane, and sodium rushes into the cell; this positive flow of electrons into the cell results in an electrical potential. This is called depolarization.

Phase 1 is a very short period during which the sodium ion concentration equalize inside and outside of the cell.

Phase 2, or the plateau stage, occurs as the cell membrane becomes less permeable to sodium, calcium slowly enters the cell, and potassium begins to leave the cell. The cell membrane is trying to return to its resting state, a process called repolarization.

Phase 3 is a time of rapid repolarization as the sodium gates are closed and potassium flows out of the cell.

Phase 4 occurs when the cell comes to rest; the sodium–potassium pump returns the membrane to its resting membrane potential, and spontaneous depolarization begins again.

Each area of the heart has a slightly different-appearing action potential that reflects the complexity of the cells in that area. Because of these differences in the action potential, each area of the heart has a slightly different rate of rhythmicity. The SA node generates an impulse about 80 to 90 times a minute; the AV node about 40 to 50 times a minute; and the complex ventricular muscle cells about 10 to 20 times a minute.

CARDIAC ARRHYTHMIAS

As noted earlier, various factors can change the cardiac rate and rhythm. Arrhythmias can be caused by changes in rate (**tachycardia,** which is a faster-than-normal heart rate, or

FIGURE 45–2. Normal sinus rhythm. Rhythm: regular. Rate: 60 to 100 beats/min. P-R interval: 0.12 to 0.20 seconds. QRS: 0.06 to 0.10 seconds. (From Hudak, C. M., & Gallo, B. M. [1998]. *Critical care nursing* [7th ed.]. Philadelphia: Lippincott-Raven.)

bradycardia, which is a slower-than-normal heart rate); by stimulation from an ectopic focus (such as **premature atrial contractions [PACs]** or **premature ventricular contractions [PVCs],** atrial flutter, atrial fibrillation, or ventricular fibrillation); or by alterations in conduction through the muscle (such as **heart blocks** and bundle branch blocks). Figure 45–2 displays an electrocardiogram (ECG) strip showing normal sinus rhythm; Figures 45–3 through 45–6 display ECG strips showing various arrhythmias.

Causes

The underlying causes of arrhythmias can arise from changes to the automaticity or conductivity of the heart cells. These changes can be caused by several factors, including

- Electrolyte disturbances that alter the action potential
- Decreases in oxygen delivered to the cells, which lead to hypoxia or anoxia and which change the cell's action potential and ability to maintain a membrane potential
- Structural damage that changes the conduction pathway through the heart
- Acidosis or accumulation of waste products that alters the action potential in that area

In some cases, changes to the heart's automaticity or conductivity may result from drugs that alter the action potential or cardiac conduction.

Hemodynamics

The study of the forces moving blood throughout the cardiovascular system is called **hemodynamics.** The ability of the heart to effectively pump blood depends on the coordinated contraction of the atrial and ventricular muscles. The muscular walls of these chambers are activated to contract by impulses that arise at the SA node, travel through the atria, are delayed slightly at the AV node, and then stimulate the His–Purkinje system through the ventricles. The conduction system is designed so that atrial stimulation is followed by total atrial contraction and ventricular stimulation is followed by total ventricular contraction.

To be an effective pump, these muscles need to contract together. When this orderly initiation and conduction of impulses is altered, the result can be a poorly coordinated contraction of the ventricles that is unable to deliver an adequate supply of oxygenated blood to the brain and other organs, including the heart muscle itself. If these hemodynamic alterations are severe, serious complications can occur. For example, lack of sufficient blood flow to the brain can cause syncope or precipitate stroke; lack of sufficient blood flow to the myocardium can exacerbate atherosclerosis and cause angina or myocardial infarction (MI).

ANTIARRHYTHMIC DRUGS

Antiarrhythmics affect the action potential of the cardiac cells, altering their automaticity, conductivity, or both. Because of this effect, antiarrhythmic drugs can also produce new arrhythmias—that is, they are **proarrhythmic.** Antiarrhythmics are used in emergency situations when the hemodynamics arising from the patient's arrhythmia are severe and could potentially be fatal.

Antiarrhythmics were widely used on a long-term basis to suppress any abnormal arrhythmia until the publication of

FIGURE 45–3. Premature atrial contractions (PACs). Rhythm: irregular due to the origination of a beat outside the normal conduction system (ectopic). Rate: normal sinus rate, except for the PACs. P-R interval: P wave is abnormal and interval may be slightly shortened in ectopic beat. QRS: normal. (From Hudak, C. M., & Gallo, B. M. [1998]. *Critical care nursing* [7th ed.]. Philadelphia: Lippincott-Raven.)

A

Ventricular premature contraction.

B

Ventricular bigeminy. (Every other beat is a PVC.)

C

Multiformed PVCs.

D

FIGURE 45-4. Premature ventricular contractions (PVCs) or ventricular premature beats (VPBs). Rhythm: irregular. Rate: variable; only interrupts the cycle of the ectopic, ventricular contraction. P-R: normal in sinus beats, not measurable in PVCs. QRS: wide, bizarre, greater than 0.12 seconds. (From Hudak, C. M., & Gallo, B. M. [1998]. *Critical care nursing* [7th ed.]. Philadelphia: Lippincott-Raven.)

FIGURE 45-5. Atrial fibrillation. Rhythm: irregularly irregular. Rate: variable; usually rapid on initiation of rhythm; decreases when controlled by medication. P-R interval: no P waves are seen, replaced by an irregular wavy baseline. The atria are fibrillating because impulses are arising at a rate greater than 350 per minute. The ventricles respond when the atrioventricular (AV) node is stimulated to threshold and can receive the impulse. QRS: normal. (From Hudak, C. M., & Gallo, B. M. [1998]. *Critical care nursing* [7th ed.]. Philadelphia: Lippincott-Raven.)

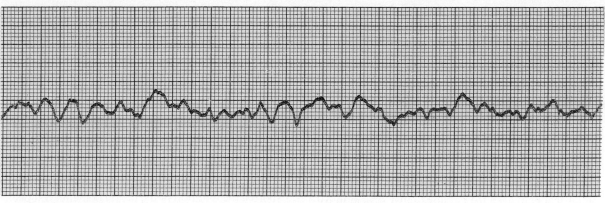

FIGURE 45–6. Ventricular fibrillation. Rhythm: irregular. Rate: not measurable. P-R interval: not measurable. QRS: not measurable, replaced by an irregular wavy baseline. No coordinated electrical or mechanical activity in the ventricle, no cardiac output. (From Hudak, C. M., & Gallo, B. M. [1998]. *Critical care nursing* [7th ed.]. Philadelphia: Lippincott-Raven.)

DRUG THERAPY ACROSS THE LIFESPAN

Antiarrhythmic Agents

Children	Adults	Older Adults
Antiarrhythmic agents are not used as often in children as they are in adults. Children who do require these drugs, after cardiac surgery or because of congenital heart problems, need to be monitored very closely to deal with the related adverse effects that can occur with these drugs. Digoxin is approved for use in children to treat arrhythmias and has an established recommended dosage. If other antiarrhythmics are used, the dosage should be carefully calculated using weight and age and should be double-checked by another nurse before administration. Adenosine, propranolol, procainamide, and digoxin have been successfully used to treat supraventricular arrhythmias, with propranolol and digoxin being the drugs of choice for long-term management. Verapamil should be avoided in children. Many arrhythmias in children are now treated by ablation techniques to destroy the arrhythmia-producing cells. This has been very successful in treating Wolff–Parkinson–White and related syndromes in children. If lidocaine is used for ventricular arrhythmias related to cardiac surgery or digoxin toxicity, serum levels should be monitored regularly to determine the appropriate dosage and to avoid the potential for serious proarrhythmias and other adverse effects. The child should have continual cardiac monitoring.	Adults receive these drugs most often as emergency measures. Patient monitoring and careful evaluation of the total drug regimen should be a routine procedure to ensure the most effective treatment with the least chance of adverse effects. Frequent monitoring and medical follow-up is very important for these patients. The safety for the use of these drugs during pregnancy has not been established. They should not be used in pregnancy unless the benefit to the mother clearly outweighs the potential risk to the fetus. The drugs do enter breast milk, and some have been associated with adverse effects on the neonate. Class I, III, and IV agents should not be used during lactation; if they are needed, another method of feeding the baby should be used.	Older adults frequently are prescribed one of these drugs. Older adults are more likely to develop adverse effects associated with the use of these drugs, including arrhythmias, hypotension, and congestive heart failure. They are also more likely to have renal and/or hepatic impairment related to underlying medical conditions, which could interfere with the metabolism and excretion of these drugs. The dosage for older adults should be started at a lower level than recommended for other adults. The patient should be monitored very closely and the dosage adjusted based on patient response. If other drugs are added or removed from the drug regimen, appropriate dosage adjustments may need to be made.

the **Cardiac Arrhythmia Suppression Trial (CAST)** in the early 1990s. This multicenter, randomized, long-term study, conducted by the National Heart and Lung Institute, looked at the mortality rate of patients with asymptomatic, non–life-threatening arrhythmias who were treated with antiarrhythmics. The results showed that long-term use of some antiarrhythmics was associated with an increased risk of death. In fact, some patients were at two to three times greater risk of death than untreated patients were. These results prompted more clinical trials to look at the effectiveness of long-term use of antiarrhythmics.

It was found that antiarrhythmics may block some reflex arrhythmias that help keep the cardiovascular system in balance, or they may precipitate new, deadly arrhythmias. Therefore, it is important to document the arrhythmia being treated and the rationale for treatment, and to monitor a patient regularly, when using these drugs.

CLASS I ANTIARRHYTHMICS

Class I antiarrhythmics are drugs that block the sodium channels in the cell membrane during an action potential (Figure 45–7). The class I drugs are local anesthetics or membrane-stabilizing agents. They bind more quickly to sodium channels that are open or inactive—ones that have been stimulated and are not yet repolarized. This makes these drugs preferable in conditions such as tachycardia, when the sodium gates are open frequently. The class I antiarrhythmics are further broken down into three subclasses, reflecting the manner in which their blockage of sodium channels affects the action potential.

- *Class Ia drugs* depress phase 0 of the action potential and prolong the action potential duration. Disopyramide (*Norpace*) is an oral drug that is available for adults and children and is recommended for the treatment of life-threatening ventricular arrhythmias. Moricizine (*Ethmozine*) is one of

the drugs found to increase cardiac death because of its proarrhythmic effects. It is available in oral form, for adults only, and should be used only if the benefit clearly outweighs the risk. Procainamide (*Pronestyl*) is available in intramuscular, intravenous, and oral forms, making it a good drug with which to start treatment and then switch to oral therapy if possible. It is used for the treatment of documented life-threatening ventricular arrhythmias. Quinidine (*Quinaglute, Cardioquin*) is available for oral, intramuscular, or intravenous administration and is especially effective in the treatment of atrial arrhythmias.

- *Class Ib drugs* depress phase 0 somewhat and actually shorten the duration of the action potential. Lidocaine (*Xylocaine*), the most frequently used antiarrhythmic, is used intramuscularly or intravenously to manage acute ventricular arrhythmias in patients with MI or during cardiac surgery. It is also used as a bolus injection in emergencies when monitoring is not available to document the exact arrhythmia. Mexiletine (*Mexitil*) is an oral drug that is approved only for use in life-threatening arrhythmias. The CAST showed that its use may not affect mortality. Tocainide (*Tonocard*) is an oral drug that is also approved for use only in the treatment of potentially life-threatening ventricular arrhythmias. This drug is being studied for the treatment of myotonic dystrophy and trigeminal neuralgia because of its effects on action potentials.

- *Class Ic drugs* markedly depress phase 0, with a resultant extreme slowing of conduction. They have little effect on the duration of the action potential. Flecainide (*Tambocor*) is a class Ic drug that was found to increase the risk of death in the CAST study. It is available as an oral drug for use in the treatment of life-threatening ventricular arrhythmias and for the prevention of paroxysmal atrial tachycardia (PAT) in symptomatic patients without structural heart disease. Propafenone (*Rhythmol*) is another oral class Ic drug that can be used to treat potentially life-threatening ventricular arrhythmias as well as for prevention of PAT in symptomatic patients who are without structural heart defects.

Therapeutic Actions and Indications

The class I antiarrhythmics stabilize the cell membrane by binding to sodium channels, depressing phase 0 of the action potential, and changing the duration of the action potential. They have a local anesthetic effect. These drugs are indicated for the treatment of potentially life-threatening ventricular arrhythmias and should not be used to treat other arrhythmias because of the risk of a proarrhythmic effect. Quinidine is especially effective in the treatment of atrial arrhythmias. Flecainide and propafenone are also used to prevent PAT in symptomatic patients who do not have structural heart defects.

Pharmacokinetics

These drugs are widely distributed after injection or after rapid absorption through the GI tract. They undergo extensive hepatic metabolism and are excreted in the urine. These drugs cross the placenta; although no specific adverse ef-

FIGURE 45–7. The cardiac action potentials, showing the effects of class Ia, Ib, and Ic antiarrhythmics.

fects have been associated with their use, it is suggested that they be used in pregnancy only if the benefits to the mother clearly outweigh the potential risks to the fetus. These drugs enter breast milk and, because of the potential for adverse effects on the neonate, they should not be used during lactation. Another method of feeding the baby should be chosen.

Contraindications and Cautions

These drugs are contraindicated in the presence of allergy to any of these drugs; with bradycardia or heart block unless an artificial pacemaker is in place, because changes in conduction could lead to complete heart block; with congestive heart failure (CHF), hypotension, or shock, which could be exacerbated by effects on the action potential; with lactation, because of the potential for adverse effects on the neonate; and with electrolyte disturbances, which could alter the effectiveness of these drugs. Caution should be used with renal or hepatic dysfunction, which could interfere with the biotransformation and excretion of these drugs, and during pregnancy, because of the potential for adverse effects on the fetus.

Adverse Effects

The adverse effects of the class I antiarrhythmics are associated with their membrane-stabilizing effects and effects on action potentials. Central nervous system (CNS) effects can include dizziness, drowsiness, fatigue, twitching, mouth numbness, slurred speech, vision changes, and tremors that can progress to convulsions. Gastrointestinal (GI) symptoms include changes in taste, nausea, and vomiting. Cardiovascular effects include the development of arrhythmias (including heart blocks), hypotension, vasodilation, and the potential for cardiac arrest. Respiratory depression progressing to respiratory arrest can also occur. Other adverse effects include rash, hypersensitivity reactions, loss of hair, and potential bone marrow depression.

Clinically Important Drug–Drug Interactions

Several drug–drug interactions have been reported with these drugs, so the possibility of an interaction should always be considered before any drug is added to a drug regimen containing an antiarrhythmic.

There is increased risk for arrhythmia development if these drugs are combined with other drugs that are known to cause arrhythmias, such as digoxin and the β-blockers.

Because quinidine competes for renal transport sites with digoxin, the combination of these two drugs can lead to increased digoxin levels and digoxin toxicity. If these drugs are used in combination, the patient's digoxin level should be monitored and appropriate dosage adjustment made.

Serum levels and toxicity of the class I antiarrhythmics are increased if they are combined with cimetidine; extreme caution should be used if patients are receiving this combination.

There is increased risk of bleeding effects if these drugs are combined with oral anticoagulants; patients receiving this combination should be monitored closely and have their anticoagulant dose reduced as needed.

Check individual drug monographs for specific interactions associated with each drug.

Clinically Important Drug–Food Interactions

Quinidine requires a slightly acidic urine (normal state) for excretion. Patients receiving quinidine should avoid foods that alkalinize the urine (e.g., citrus juices, vegetables, antacids, milk products), which could lead to increased quinidine levels and toxicity.

Nursing Considerations for Patients Receiving Class I Antiarrhythmics

Assessment: History and Examination

Screen for the following conditions, which could be cautions or contraindications to use of the drug: any known allergies to these drugs; impaired liver or kidney function, which could alter the metabolism and excretion of the drug; and any condition that could be exacerbated by the depressive effects of the drugs (eg, heart block, CHF, hypotension, shock, respiratory dysfunction, electrolyte disturbances); pregnancy and lactation, because of the potential for adverse effects on the fetus or neonate.

Include screening for baseline status before beginning therapy and for any potential adverse effects. Assess the following: body temperature, weight; skin color, lesions, temperature; affect, orientation, reflexes, speech; pulse, blood pressure, perfusion, baseline ECG; respirations, adventitious sounds; bowel sounds, abdominal examination; and renal and liver function tests.

Nursing Diagnoses

The patient receiving an antiarrhythmic may have the following nursing diagnoses related to drug therapy:

- Disturbed Sensory Perception (Visual, Auditory, Kinesthetic, Gustatory, Tactile) related to CNS effects
- Risk for Injury related to CNS effects
- Decreased Cardiac Output related to cardiac effects
- Deficient Knowledge regarding drug therapy

Implementation

- Continually monitor cardiac rhythm when initiating or changing dose, *to detect potentially serious adverse effects and to evaluate drug effectiveness.*
- Maintain life support equipment on standby, *to treat severe adverse reactions that might occur.*
- Give parenteral forms only if the oral form is not feasible; transfer to the oral form as soon as possible, *to decrease the potential for severe adverse effects.*
- Titrate the dose to the smallest amount needed to achieve control of the arrhythmia, *to decrease the risk of severe adverse effects.*
- Consult with the prescriber to reduce the dosage in patients with renal or hepatic dysfunction; reduced dosage may be needed *to ensure therapeutic effects without increased risk of toxic effects.*
- Establish safety precautions, including siderails, lighting, and noise control, if CNS effects occur, *to ensure patient safety.*

DRUGS IN FOCUS
Class I Antiarrhythmics

Drug Name	Usual Dosage	Usual Indications
Class Ia		
disopyramide (*Norpace*)	Adult: 400–800 mg/d PO in divided doses q6–12h; use lower doses with older patients Pediatric: 6–30 mg/kg per day PO in divided doses q6h, base dosage on age	Treatment of life-threatening ventricular arrhythmias
moricizine (*Ethmozine*)	600–900 mg/d PO in divided doses q8h; start with <600 mg/d in older patients and those with hepatic impairment	Treatment of life-threatening ventricular arrhythmias **Special Considerations:** Do not use in patients <18 y of age
procainamide (*Pronestyl*)	Adult: 50 mg/kg per day PO in divided doses q3h; 0.5–1 g IM q4–8h; 500–600 mg IV over 25–30 min, then 2–6 mg/min IV Pediatric: 15–50 mg/kg per day PO in divided doses q3–6h; 20–30 mg/kg per day IM in divided doses q4–6h; 3–6 mg/kg IV over 5 min then 20–80 µg/kg per minute IV	Treatment of life-threatening ventricular arrhythmias
P quinidine (*Quinaglute, Cardioquin*)	400–600 mg PO q2–3h; 600 mg IM, then 400 mg IM q2h as needed; 330 mg IV at a rate of 1 mL/min	Treatment of atrial arrhythmias in adults
Class Ib		
P lidocaine (*Xylocaine*)	Adult: 300 mg of 10% solution IM; 50–100 mg IV bolus at the rate of 20–50 mg/min; 1–4 mg/min IV infusion Pediatric: safety and efficacy not established; 1 mg/kg IV followed by 30 µg/kg per minute IV infusion has been recommended	Treatment of life-threatening ventricular arrhythmias during myocardial infarction or cardiac surgery; emergency treatment of ventricular arrhythmias when diagnostic tests are not available
mexiletine (*Mexitil*)	200 mg PO q8h up to 1200 mg/d PO may be needed	Treatment of life-threatening ventricular arrhythmias in adults
tocainide (*Tonocard*)	1200–1800 mg/d in divided doses q8h; reduce dosage in older patients and with renal or hepatic impairment	Treatment of life-threatening ventricular arrhythmias in adults; studied for the treatment of myotonic dystrophy, trigeminal neuralgia
Class Ic		
P flecainide (*Tambocor*)	50–100 mg PO q12h; reduce dosage as needed with older patients or renal impairment	Treatment of life-threatening ventricular arrhythmias in adults; prevention of paroxysmal atrial tachycardia (PAT) in symptomatic patients with no structural heart defect
propafenone (*Rhythmol*)	150–300 mg PO q8h based on patient response; start with lower dose and increase slowly with older patients	Treatment of life-threatening ventricular arrhythmias in adults; prevention of PAT in symptomatic patients with no structural heart defect

- Arrange for periodic monitoring of cardiac rhythm when the patient is receiving long-term therapy, *to evaluate effects on cardiac status.*
- Provide comfort measures, *to help the patient tolerate drug effects.* These include small, frequent meals; access to bathroom facilities; bowel program as needed; food with drug if GI upset is severe; environmental controls; orientation; and appropriate skin care as needed.
- Provide thorough patient teaching, including the name of the drug, dosage prescribed, measures to avoid adverse effects, and warning signs of problems as well as the need for periodic monitoring and evaluation, *to enhance patient knowledge about drug therapy and promote compliance with the drug regimen.* (See Patient Teaching Checklist: Antiarrhythmics.)
- Offer support and encouragement, *to help the patient deal with the diagnosis and the drug regimen.*

Evaluation

- Monitor patient response to the drug (stabilization of cardiac rhythm and output).

PATIENT TEACHING CHECKLIST
Antiarrhythmics

Create customized patient teaching materials for a specific antiarrhythmic from the CD-ROM. Patient teaching should stress the following points for drugs within this class:

• An antiarrhythmic acts to stop irregular rhythm in the heart, helping it to beat more regularly and therefore more efficiently. The drug may work by making the heart less irritable and by slowing it down to a more effective rate.
• Procainamide must be taken around the clock. You will need to have an alarm clock at night to awaken you to take your medication. It should be taken on an empty stomach. The best times for you to take procainamide are ____, ____, ____, ____.
• Quinidine and disopyramide may be taken with food if gastrointestinal upset occurs.
• Verapamil should be taken on an empty stomach, 1 hour before or 2 hours after a meal. If quinidine has been prescribed for you, plan to limit your intake of certain foods (e.g., citrus juices, milk, vegetables) and avoid over-the-counter drugs (e.g., antacids) that make your urine alkaline. If your urine become alkaline, you may develop signs of an overdose of quinidine. It is helpful to take your pulse on a regular basis. You should count the number of beats in 1 minute and determine whether your pulse is regular or irregular. Your usual resting heart rate is ____. Record your pulse on your calendar for easy reference.

Some of the following adverse effects may occur:

• *Tiredness, weakness*—Space your activities throughout the day and take periodic rest periods to help conserve your energy and rest your heart.
• *Nausea, vomiting, loss of appetite*—These problems may pass over time; taking the drug with meals, if appropriate, or eating small, frequent meals may help.
• *Sensitivity to light* (more pronounced with disopyramide)—Avoid prolonged exposure to ultraviolet light or sunlight.
• *Constipation or diarrhea*—These reactions are very common; if either occurs and becomes too uncomfortable, consult your health care provider.

Report any of the following to your health care provider: chest pain, difficulty breathing, ringing in the ears, swelling in the ankles or legs, unusually slow pulse (<35 beats/min), unusually fast pulse (>15 beats/min above your normal rate), suddenly irregular pulse, fever, rash.

Tell any doctor, nurse, or other health care provider that you are taking this drug.

Keep this drug, and all medications, out of the reach of children.

Avoid the use of over-the-counter medications while you are taking this drug. If you feel that you need one of these, consult with your health care provider for the best choice. Many of these drugs can interfere with your benzodiazepine.

It is important to get regular medical follow-up while you are on this drug, to evaluate your heart rhythm and your response to the drug.

Do not stop taking this medication. If you have to stop the medication for any reason, contact your health care provider immediately.

This Teaching Checklist reflects general patient teaching guidelines. It is not meant to be a substitute for drug-specific teaching information, which is available in nursing drug guides.

• Monitor for adverse effects (sedation, hypotension, cardiac arrhythmias, respiratory depression, CNS effects).
• Evaluate the effectiveness of the teaching plan (patient can name drug, dosage, adverse effects to watch for, specific measures to avoid adverse effects, importance of continued follow-up).
• Monitor the effectiveness of comfort measures and compliance to the regimen (see Nursing Care Guide: Antiarrhythmics).

CLASS II ANTIARRHYTHMICS

The class II antiarrhythmics are β-adrenergic blockers that block β-receptors, causing a depression of phase 4 of the action potential (Figure 45–8). In this way, these drugs slow the recovery of the cells, leading to a slowing of conduction and decreased automaticity. Several β-adrenergic blockers are used as antiarrhythmics.

Acebutolol (*Sectral*), an oral drug also used as an antihypertensive, is especially effective in the treatment of prema-ture ventricular contractions (PVCs). Esmolol (*Brevibloc*), an intravenous drug, is used for the short-term management of supraventricular tachycardia and tachycardia that is not responding to other measures. Propranolol (*Inderal*) is used as an antihypertensive, antianginal, and antimigraine headache drug and as an antiarrhythmic to treat supraventricular tachycardias caused by digoxin or catecholamines.

Therapeutic Actions and Indications
The class II antiarrhythmics competitively block β-receptor sites in the heart and kidneys, thereby decreasing heart rate, cardiac excitability, and cardiac output; slowing conduction through the AV node; and decreasing the release of renin. These effects stabilize excitable cardiac tissue and decrease blood pressure, which decreases the heart's workload and may further stabilize hypoxic cardiac tissue. These drugs are indicated for the treatment of supraventricular tachycardias and PVCs.

Pharmacokinetics
These drugs are absorbed from the GI tract and undergo hepatic metabolism. Food has been found to increase the bioavailability of propranolol, although this effect has not been

NURSING CARE GUIDE

Antiarrhythmics

Assessment	Nursing Diagnoses	Implementation	Evaluation
HISTORY Allergies to any of these drugs, renal or hepatic dysfunction, pregnancy, lactation, heart block, CHF, shock, hypotension, electrolyte disturbances	Disturbed Sensory Perception related to CNS effects High Risk for Injury related to CNS effects Decreased Cardiac Output related to CV effects Deficient Knowledge regarding drug therapy	Continually monitor cardiac rhythm when initiating or changing doses. Provide comfort and safety measures: have life support equipment on standby; use parenteral form only if oral form cannot be used; titrate dose to smallest needed for therapeutic effects; reduce dosage with renal or hepatic dysfunction; lower dose with renal, hepatic impairment; use side rails, environmental control as needed for safety; provide small frequent meals, access to bathroom facilities, skin care. Provide support and reassurance to deal with drug effects. Provide patient teaching regarding drug, dosage, adverse effects, what to report, and safety precautions.	Evaluate drug effects: stabilization of cardiac rhythm and output. Monitor for adverse effects: sedation, dizziness, insomnia; cardiac arrhythmias; GI upset; respiratory depression. Monitor for drug–drug interactions as indicated for each drug. Evaluate effectiveness of patient teaching program. Evaluate effectiveness of comfort and safety measures.
PHYSICAL EXAMINATION CV: BP, P, perfusion CNS: orientation, affect, reflexes, vision Skin: color, lesions, texture Resp: R, adventitious sounds GI: abdominal exam, bowel sounds Lab tests: liver and renal function tests, CBC			

found with other β-adrenergic blocking agents. Propranolol also crosses the blood–brain barrier but carteolol, nadolol, and sotalol do not, making them a better choice if CNS effects occur with propranolol. Because these drugs are excreted in the urine, caution is required in patients with renal impairment. Teratogenic effects have occurred in animal studies with all of these drugs except sotalol. The use of any β-adrenergic blocker during pregnancy should be reserved for situations in which the benefit to the mother outweighs the risk to the fetus. In general, they should not be used during lactation because of the potential for adverse effects on the baby. The safety and efficacy for use of these drugs in children has not been established.

Contraindications and Cautions

The use of these drugs is contraindicated in the presence of sinus bradycardia (rate less than 45 beats/min) and AV block, which could be exacerbated by the effects of these drugs; with cardiogenic shock, CHF, asthma, or respiratory depression, which could be made worse by the blocking of β-receptors; and with pregnancy and lactation, because of the potential for adverse effects on the neonate. Caution should be used in patients with diabetes and thyroid dysfunction, which could be altered by the blockade of the β-receptors, and with renal and hepatic dysfunction, which could alter the metabolism and excretion of these drugs.

CASE STUDY

Recognizing Quinidine Toxicity

THE SITUATION

R. A., a 56-year-old post–myocardial infarction patient with a documented duodenal ulcer, has felt highly "stressed" lately. He called the nurse with complaints of dizziness, confusion, headaches, nausea, vomiting, and a very slow pulse. The nurse requested that R. A. come in immediately to be evaluated. On examination, his pulse was 52 beats/min, and an electrocardiogram (ECG) showed second-degree heart block with occasional escape beats. His blood pressure was 82/60 mm Hg. R. A. reported that he was still taking quinidine, which had been started after the myocardial infarction, to regulate arrhythmias. He stated that he had been taking *Mylanta* (an antacid) for ulcer pain, about 12 tablets a day, and that he has been drinking a lot of orange juice to treat a cold.

CRITICAL THINKING

- Based on your knowledge of the drug quinidine and the symptoms reported by R. A., what do you think happened?
- If R. A. is found to be quinidine toxic, what should be done to alleviate his signs and symptoms and to return him to his normal cardiac rhythm?
- What teaching points will be essential to convey to R. A. before he goes home?
- Should any other problems be addressed while R. A. is being evaluated at this time?

DISCUSSION

R. A. has many of the signs and symptoms of quinidine toxicity—slow pulse, atrioventricular heart block, hypotension, nausea, vomiting, dizziness, headache, confusion. The initial treatment for this condition includes withholding all medications, ordering blood drawn for a serum quinidine level determination, and careful monitoring of R. A., with emergency life support

equipment on standby in case his condition deteriorates. (This equipment should include sodium lactate, which blocks the drug's effects on the myocardium, and adrenergic stimulants, which can increase blood pressure, pulse, and cardiac output.)

R. A. stabilized rapidly, and patient teaching on the current drug therapy was initiated. The effects of foods and drugs on urine pH and on quinidine excretion were stressed, and R. A. received a written list of foods and antacids that cause an alkaline urine (e.g., citrus juices, milk, vegetables). The alkaline urine prevents quinidine excretion, leading to buildup of toxic levels. The combination of the orange juice and the numerous doses of antacid probably made R. A.'s urine quite alkaline, leading to increased serum levels of quinidine and a toxic response to the drug. The signs and symptoms of quinidine toxicity should be reviewed with R. A., as well as precautionary measures that he should take. He should be told that he did the correct thing in calling and should be encouraged to do so again if he has further problems. The teaching program should be directed at preventing future problems.

While R. A. is within the health care system, it is important to offer him support and encouragement. His ulcer can be evaluated at this time, as well as his feelings of stress. R. A. may need to ventilate his feelings and explore new ways of coping with or avoiding stressful situations. The effects of stress on the heart can be reviewed with R. A. to help him realize the importance of stress management. It would also be helpful to review the problems of self-medication for various complaints while taking a prescription drug. R. A. should receive all information in writing for future reference. Eventually, he may be re-evaluated to determine the actual need for continuing this medication. In the meantime, good patient education can help prevent serious complications while he is using the drug.

FIGURE 45–8. The cardiac action potential, showing the effects of class II, III, and IV antiarrhythmics.

Adverse Effects

The adverse effects associated with class II antiarrhythmics are related to the effects of blocking β-receptors in the sympathetic nervous system. CNS effects include dizziness, insomnia, dreams, and fatigue. Cardiovascular symptoms can include hypotension, bradycardia, AV block, arrhythmias, and alterations in peripheral perfusion. Respiratory effects can include bronchospasm and dyspnea. GI problems frequently include nausea, vomiting, anorexia, constipation, and diarrhea. Other effects to anticipate include a loss of libido, decreased exercise tolerance, and alterations in blood glucose levels.

Clinically Important Drug–Drug Interactions

There is a risk of increased effects if these drugs are taken with verapamil; if this combination is used, dosage adjustment will be needed.

There is a possibility of increased hypoglycemia if these drugs are combined with insulin; patients should be monitored closely.

Other specific drug interactions may occur with each drug; check a drug reference before combining these drugs with any others.

Nursing Considerations for Patients Receiving Class II Antiarrhythmics

The nursing considerations for patients taking any antiarrhythmic drug are outlined in the section on class I antiarrhythmics.

CLASS III ANTIARRHYTHMICS

The class III antiarrhythmics block potassium channels, prolonging phase 3 of the action potential, which prolongs repolarization and slows the rate and conduction of the heart (see Figure 45–3). Class III antiarrhythmics include a number of agents.

Amiodarone (*Cordarone*) is available as an oral or an intravenous drug. It should be used only to treat documented life-threatening arrhythmias, because it has been associated with serious and even fatal toxic reactions; other drugs should always be tried first. Bretylium (generic), which is used intravenously or intramuscularly, is indicated for the short-term treatment of ventricular fibrillation or ventricular arrhythmias that do not respond to other drugs. Ibutilide (*Corvert*) is used intravenously to rapidly convert atrial fibrillation or atrial flutter of recent onset; it is most effective if the duration of atrial fibrillation/flutter is less than 90 days. A newer drug, dofetilide (*Tikosyn*), which is used orally to convert atrial fibrillation or flutter to normal sinus rhythm and to maintain normal sinus rhythm after conversion. Sotalol (*Betapace, Betapace AF*) is an oral drug that is indicated for the treatment of documented life-threatening arrhythmias and for the maintenance of normal sinus rhythm after conversion of atrial arrhythmias. Because it is known to be proarrhythmic, patients should be monitored very closely at the initiation of therapy and periodically during therapy.

Therapeutic Actions and Indications

The class III antiarrhythmics block potassium channels and slow the outward movement of potassium during phase 3 of the action potential. This action prolongs the action potential. All of these drugs are proarrhythmic and have the potential of inducing arrhythmias. These drugs are indicated for the treatment of life-threatening ventricular arrhythmias (amiodarone, bretylium, and sotalol), for the conversion of recent-onset atrial fibrillation or atrial flutter to normal sinus rhythm (ibutilide, dofetilide), and for maintenance of sinus rhythm after conversion of atrial arrhythmias (dofetilide sotalol).

Pharmacokinetics

These drugs are well absorbed and widely distributed. Absorption of sotalol is decreased by the presence of food. They are metabolized in the liver and excreted in the urine.

DRUGS IN FOCUS
Class II Antiarrhythmics

Drug Name	Usual Dosage	Usual Indications
acebutolol (*Sectral*)	200–600 mg PO b.i.d., based on patient response; use lower doses with older patients; decrease dose by 50% with renal or hepatic impairment	Management of premature ventricular contractions in adults
esmolol (*Brevibloc*)	Loading dose of 500 μg/kg per minute IV, then 50 μg/kg per minute for 4 min, maintain with 100 μg/kg per minute IV infusion	Short-term management of supraventricular tachycardia in adults
P propranolol (*Inderal*)	10–30 mg PO t.i.d.–q.i.d.; 1–3 mg IV for life-threatening arrhythmias, may repeat in 2 min, then do not repeat for 4 h	Treatment of supraventricular tachycardias caused by digoxin or catecholamines in adults; treatment of hypertension, angina, migraine, situational anxiety

NURSING CHALLENGE
Atrial Fibrillation

Atrial fibrillation (AF) is a relatively common arrhythmia of the atria. It has been associated with coronary artery disease (CAD), myocardial inflammation, valvular disease, cardiomegaly, and rheumatic heart disease. The cells of the atria are connected side to side and top to bottom and are relatively simple cells. In contrast, the cells of the ventricles are connected only from top to bottom, with one cell connected only to one or two other cells. It is much easier, therefore, for an ectopic focus in the atria to spread that impulse throughout the entire atria, setting up a cycle of chaotic depolarization and repolarization. It is more difficult to stimulate fibrillation in the ventricles, because one ectopic site cannot rapidly spread impulses to many other cells, only to the cells connected in its two- or three-cell set.

Fibrillation results in lack of any coordinated pumping action, because the muscles are not stimulated to contract and pump out blood. In the ventricles, this is a life-threatening situation. If the ventricles do not pump blood, no blood is delivered to the brain, the tissues of the body, or the heart muscle itself. However, loss of pumping action in the atria per se does not usually cause much of a problem. The atrial contraction is like an extra kick of blood into the ventricles; it provides a nice backup to the system, but the blood will still flow normally without that kick.

One of the problems with AF occurs when it is present for longer than 1 week. The auricles (those appendages hanging on the atria to collect blood; see Chapter 42) fill with blood that is not effectively pumped into the ventricles. Over time, this somewhat stagnant blood tends to clot. Because the auricles are sacks of striated muscle fibers, blood clots form around these fibers. In this situation, if the atria were to contract in a coordinated manner, there is a substantial risk that those clots or emboli would be pumped into the ventricles and then into the lungs (from the right auricle), which could lead to pulmonary emboli, or to the brain or periphery (from the left auricle), which could cause a stroke or occlusion of peripheral vessels.

Treatment of AF can be complicated if the length of time the patient has been in AF is not known. If a patient goes into AF acutely, drug therapy is available for rapid conversion. For example, ibutilide is often very effective when given intravenously for rapid conversion of the AF. Intramuscular quinidine also may convert AF effectively. In some situations, digoxin has been effective in converting AF. Electrocardioversion, a DC current shock to the chest, may break the cycle of fibrillation and convert a patient to sinus rhythm, after which the rhythm will need to be stabilized with drug therapy. Quinidine is often the drug of choice for long-term stabilization.

If the onset of AF is not known and it is suspected that the atria may have been fibrillating for longer than a week, the patient is better off staying in AF without drug therapy or electrocardioversion. Prophylactic oral anticoagulants are given to decrease the risk of clot formation and emboli being pumped into the system. Conversion in this case could result in potentially life-threatening embolization of the lungs, brain, or other tissues.

The other danger of AF is rapid ventricular response to the atrial stimuli, a condition called supraventricular tachycardia (SVT). With the atria firing impulses, possibly 200 to 300 a minute, the number of stimuli conducted into the ventricles is erratic and irregular. If the ventricle is responding too rapidly—more than 120 times a minute—the filling time of the ventricles is greatly reduced, causing cardiac output to fall dramatically. In these situations, and when AF is anticipated (such as with atrial flutter or paroxysmal atrial tachycardia), drugs may be given to slow conduction and protect the ventricles from rapid rates. Flecainide, propafenone, and propranolol are often used to convert rapid SVT. Esmolol, diltiazem, and verapamil are used intravenously to convert SVT with rapid ventricular response, which could progress to AF.

Careful patient assessment is essential before beginning treatment for AF. If a history cannot be established from patient information and medical records are not available, it is usually recommended that AF be left untreated and anticoagulant therapy be started. This can pose a real challenge for the nurse in trying to teach patients about why their rapid and irregular heart rate will not be treated and explaining all of the factors involved in the long-term use of oral anticoagulants.

There are no well-controlled studies of effects during pregnancy, so use during pregnancy should be limited to those situations in which the benefit to the mother far outweighs any potential risk to the fetus. There is little good information about use during lactation. Because of the potential for adverse effects on the neonate, another method of feeding the baby should be used if the mother requires one of these drugs during lactation.

Contraindications and Cautions

When these drugs are used to treat life-threatening arrhythmias for which no other drug has been effective, there are no contraindications. Ibutilide and dofetilide should not be used in the presence of AV block, which could be exacerbated by the drug. Caution should be used with all of these drugs in the presence of shock, hypotension, or respiratory depres-

sion; with a prolonged QTc interval, which could be made worse by the depressive effects on action potentials; and with renal or hepatic disease, which could alter the biotransformation and excretion of these drugs.

Adverse Effects

The adverse effects associated with these drugs are related to the changes they cause in action potentials. Nausea, vomiting, and GI distress; weakness and dizziness; and hypotension, CHF, and arrhythmia are common. Amiodarone has been associated with a potentially fatal liver toxicity, ocular abnormalities, and the development of very serious cardiac arrhythmias.

Clinically Important Drug–Drug Interactions

These drugs can cause serious toxic effects if they are combined with digoxin or quinidine.

DRUGS IN FOCUS
Class III Antiarrhythmics

Drug Name	Usual Dosage	Usual Indications
amiodarone (*Cordarone*)	800–1600 mg/d PO in divided doses for 1–3 wk, then 600–800 mg/d PO for 1 mo, reduce to 400 mg/d PO if rhythm is stable; 1000 mg IV over 24 h; then 540 mg IV at 0.5 mg/min for 18–96 h	Treatment of life-threatening ventricular arrhythmias not responding to any other drug; for use in adults only
Ⓟ bretylium (generic)	Adult: 5 mg/kg IV bolus, then 1–2 mg/min by continuous IV infusion; 5–10 mg/kg IM repeated at intervals of 6–8 h Pediatric: 5 mg/kg per dose IV followed by 10 mg/kg at intervals of 15–30 min, maintain at 5–10 mg/kg per dose IV q6h	Treatment of ventricular fibrillation and ventricular tachycardias not responsive to other drugs
dofetilide (*Tikosyn*)	125–500 µg PO b.i.d. based on creatinine clearance	Conversion of atrial fibrillation/flutter to normal sinus rhythm, maintenance of normal sinus rhythm after conversion for adults
ibutilide (*Corvert*)	1 mg infused IV over 1 min, may be repeated in 10 min if needed	Conversion of recent-onset atrial fibrillation/flutter in adults
sotalol (*Betapace*)	80 mg/d PO, may be titrated to 240–320 mg/d PO, reduce dosage with renal impairment	Treatment of life-threatening ventricular arrhythmias not responding to any other drug; for use with adults
(*Betapace AF*)	80–120 mg PO q.d.–b.i.d. based on patient response	Maintenance of sinus rhythm after conversion in adults

Other specific drug–drug interactions have been reported with individual drugs; a drug reference should always be consulted when adding a new drug to a regimen containing any of these drugs.

Nursing Considerations for Patients Receiving Class III Antiarrhythmics
The nursing considerations for patients taking any antiarrhythmic agent are outlined in the section on class I antiarrhythmics.

CLASS IV ANTIARRHYTHMICS

The class IV antiarrhythmics act to block calcium channels in the cell membrane, leading to a depression of depolarization and a prolongation of phases 1 and 2 of repolarization, which slows automaticity and conduction (see Figure 45–3). The calcium channel blockers are used as antihypertensives (see Chapter 43) and to treat angina (see Chapter 46). The two calcium channel blockers that seem to have special effects on the heart muscle are diltiazem (*Cardizem*), which is used intravenously to treat paroxysmal supraventricular tachycardia, and verapamil (*Calan, Covera-HS*), which is used parenterally to treat supraventricular tachycardia and to temporarily control the rapid ventricular response to atrial flutter or fibrillation.

Therapeutic Actions and Indications
The class IV antiarrhythmics block the movement of calcium ions across the cell membrane, depressing the genera-

tion of action potentials, delaying phase 1 and 2 of repolarization, and slowing conduction through the AV node. They are indicated for the treatment of supraventricular tachycardia and to control the ventricle response to rapid atrial rates. They are given intravenously for these purposes.

Pharmacokinetics
These drugs are well absorbed, highly protein bound, and metabolized in the liver. They are excreted in the urine. They cross the placenta and have been associated with fetal abnormalities in animal studies. They should not be used in pregnancy unless the benefit to the mother clearly outweighs the risk to the fetus. They enter breast milk, and if they are needed by a lactating mother, another method of feeding the baby should be used because of the risk of adverse effects on the neonate.

Contraindications and Cautions
These drugs are contraindicated with known allergy to any calcium channel blocker; with sick sinus syndrome or heart block (unless an artificial pacemaker is in place), because the block could be exacerbated by these drugs; with pregnancy or lactation, because of the potential for adverse effects on the fetus or neonate; and with CHF or hypotension, because of the hypotensive effects of these drugs. Caution should be used with idiopathic hypertrophic subaortic stenosis (IHSS), which could be exacerbated, or with impaired renal or liver function, which could affect the metabolism or excretion of these drugs.

DRUGS IN FOCUS
Class IV Antiarrhythmics

Drug Name	Usual Dosage	Usual Indications
ⓟ diltiazem (*Cardizem*)	0.25 mg/kg IV bolus then a second bolus of 0.35 mg/kg IV if needed; maintain with continuous infusion of 5–10 mg/h for up to 24 h	IV to treat paroxysmal supraventricular tachycardia in adults
verapamil (*Calan, Covera-HS*)	Adult: 5–10 mg IV over 2 min, may repeat with 10 mg in 30 min if needed
Pediatric: 0.1–0.3 mg/kg IV over 2 min, do not exceed 5 mg/dose; may repeat in 30 min if needed	IV to treat paroxysmal supraventricular tachycardia; slow the ventricular response to rapid atrial rates

Adverse Effects
The adverse effects associated with these drugs are related to their vasodilation of blood vessels throughout the body. CNS effects include dizziness, weakness, fatigue, depression, and headache. GI upset, nausea, and vomiting can occur. Hypotension, CHF, shock, arrhythmias, and edema have also been reported.

Clinically Important Drug–Drug Interactions
Verapamil has been associated with many drug–drug interactions, including increased risk of cardiac depression with β-blockers; additive AV slowing with digoxin; increased serum levels and toxicity of digoxin, carbamazepine, prazosin, and quinidine; increased respiratory depression with atracurium, gallamine, metocurine, pancuronium, rocuronium, tubocurarine, and vecuronium; and decreased effects if combined with calcium products or rifampin.

There is a risk of severe cardiac effects if these drugs are given intravenously within 48 hours of intervenous β-adrenergic drugs. This combination should be avoided.

Diltiazem can increase the serum levels and toxicity of cyclosporine if they are taken concurrently.

Nursing Considerations for Patients Receiving Class IV Antiarrhythmics
The nursing considerations for patients taking any antiarrhythmic are outlined in the section on class I antiarrhythmics.

▄■◉● WEB LINKS
Patients and health care providers may want to consult the following Internet sources:

Information on arrhythmias, drug therapy, and current research, from the National Heart, Lung and Blood Institute:
http://www.nscardiology.com/factsarrhythmia.htm
Patient information on patient teaching, therapy, research, supports, and other educational programs:
http://www.nhlbi.nih.gov

Patient information, support groups, research information on heart disease, scientific programs:
http://www.americanheart.org

OTHER DRUGS USED TO TREAT ARRHYTHMIAS

Adenosine (*Adenocard*) is another antiarrhythmic agent that is used to convert supraventricular tachycardia to sinus rhythm when vagal maneuvers have been ineffective. It is often the drug of choice for terminating supraventricular tachycardias, including those associated with the use of alternative conduction pathways around the AV node (eg, Wolff–Parkinson–White syndrome), for two reasons: (1) it has a very short duration of action (about 15 seconds) and is picked up by circulating red blood cells and cleared through the liver; and (2) it is associated with very few adverse effects (headache, flushing, and dyspnea of short duration). This drug slows conduction through the AV node, prolongs the refractory period, and decreases automaticity in the AV node. It is given intravenously with continuous monitoring of the patient.

Digoxin (see Chapter 44) is also used at times to treat arrhythmias. This drug slows calcium from leaving the cell, prolonging the action potential and slowing conduction and heart rate. Digoxin is effective in the treatment of atrial arrhythmias. The drug is also positively inotropic, leading to increased cardiac output, which increases perfusion of the coronary arteries and may eliminate the cause of some arrhythmias as hypoxia is resolved and waste products are removed more effectively.

Table 45–1 provides a summary of the types of arrhythmias and the specific drugs used to treat each type.

Nursing Considerations for Patients Receiving Other Antiarrhythmics
The nursing considerations for patients taking any of these antiarrhythmics are outlined in the section on class I antiarrhythmics.

TABLE 45-1 | Types of Arrhythmias and Drugs of Choice for Treatment

Arrhythmia	Antiarrhythmic Drugs
ATRIAL	
Flutter or fibrillation	Class Ia: quinidine* (long-term) Class III: ibutilide* (conversion of recent onset), dofetilide (conversion and maintenance) Other: digoxin
Paroxysmal atrial tachycardia (PAT) Supraventricular tachycardia (SVT)	Class Ic: flecainide, propafenone* Class II: esmolol* (short-term), propranolol Class IV: diltiazem (IV), verapamil (IV) Other: adenosine* (SVT, including those caused by using alternate conduction pathways)
VENTRICULAR	
Premature ventricular contractions (PVCs)	Class Ib: lidocaine* Class II: acebutolol
Tachycardia or fibrillation	Class Ib: lidocaine* Class III: bretylium
Life-threatening ventricular arrhythmias	Class Ia: disopyramide, moricizine (X), procainamide Class Ib: mexiletine, tocainide Class Ic: flecainide (X), propafenone Class III: amiodarone (X), sotalol (X)

*drug of choice

(X) not drug of choice; proarrhythmic

CHAPTER SUMMARY

- Disruptions in the normal rate or rhythm of the heart are called arrhythmias (also known as dysrhythmias).
- Cardiac rate and rhythm are normally determined by the heart's specialized conduction system starting with the SA node, progressing through the atria to the AV node, through the bundle of His into the ventricles, and down bundle branches to the fibers of the Purkinje system.
- The cardiac cells possess the property of automaticity, which allows them to generate an action potential and to stimulate the cardiac muscle without stimulation from external sources.
- Disruptions in the automaticity of the cells or in the con-duction of the impulse that result in arrhythmias can be caused by changes in heart rate (tachycardias or bradycardias); stimulation from ectopic foci in the atria or ventricles that cause an uncoordinated muscle contraction; or blocks in the conduction system (eg, AV heart block, bundle branch blocks) that alter the normal movement of the impulse through the system.
- Arrhythmias can arise because of changes to the automaticity or the conductivity of the heart cells caused by electrolyte disturbances; decreases in the oxygen delivered to the cells, leading to hypoxia or anoxia; structural damage that changes the conduction pathway; acidosis or the accumulation of waste products; or drug effects.
- Arrhythmias cause problems because they alter the hemo-

DRUGS IN FOCUS
Other Antiarrhythmics

Drug Name	Usual Dosage	Usual Indications
adenosine (Adenocard)	6 mg IV as a rapid bolus over 1–2 sec; may repeat with 12 mg IV bolus after 1–2 min if needed, may be repeated a second time if needed	Treatment of supraventricular tachycardias, including those caused by the use of alternate conduction pathways in adults
digoxin (Lanoxin, Lanoxicaps)	Adult: 0.75–1.25 mg PO loading dose, then 0.125–0.25 mg/d PO or 0.125–0.25 mg IV loading dose and then 0.125–0.25 mg/d PO Pediatric: 10–50 μg/kg loading dose PO or 8–50 μg/kg loading dose IV, based on age; then maintenance dose of 25%–35% of loading dose	Treatment of atrial flutter, atrial fibrillation, paroxysmal atrial tachycardia

dynamics of the cardiovascular system. They can cause a decrease in cardiac output related to the uncoordinated pumping action of the irregular rhythm, leading to lack of filling time for the ventricles. Any of these effects can interfere with the delivery to blood to the brain, to other tissues, or to the heart muscle itself.

- Antiarrhythmics are drugs that alter the action potential of the heart cells and interrupt arrhythmias. The CAST study found that the long-term treatment of arrhythmias may actually cause cardiac death, so these drugs are now indicated only for the short-term treatment of potentially life-threatening ventricular arrhythmias.
- Class I antiarrhythmics block sodium channels, depress phase 0 of the action potential, and generally prolong the action potential, leading to a slowing of conduction and automaticity.
- Class II antiarrhythmics are β-adrenergic receptor blockers that prevent sympathetic stimulation.
- Class III antiarrhythmics block potassium channels and prolong phase 3 of the action potential.
- Class IV antiarrhythmics are calcium channel blockers that shorten the action potential, disrupting ineffective rhythms and rates.
- A patient receiving an antiarrhythmic drug needs to be constantly monitored while being stabilized and during the use of the drug to detect the development of arrhythmias or other adverse effects associated with alteration of the action potentials of other muscles or nerves.

Review Questions

1. Cardiac contraction and relaxation are controlled by
   a. the brain.
   b. the sympathetic nervous system.
   c. the autonomic nervous system.
   d. impulses that arise spontaneously with the heart itself.
2. The conduction system of the heart does not include
   a. the sinoatrial node.
   b. the sinuses of Valsalva.
   c. the atrial bundles.
   d. the Purkinje fibers.
3. Arrhythmias or dysrhythmias are not usually caused by
   a. lack of oxygen to the heart muscle cells.
   b. acidosis near a cell.
   c. structural damage in the conduction pathway through the heart.
   d. vasodilation in the myocardial vascular bed.
4. Antiarrhythmic drugs act to alter the action potential of the cardiac cells. Because they alter the action potential, antiarrhythmic drugs often
   a. cause congestive heart failure.
   b. alter blood flow to the kidney.
   c. cause new arrhythmias.
   d. cause electrolyte disturbances.
5. Because of the results of the CAST study,
   a. antiarrhythmics are now more widely used.

   b. antiarrhythmics are used as prophylactic measures in situations that might lead to an arrhythmia.
   c. antiarrhythmics are no longer used in the United States.
   d. antiarrhythmics are reserved for use in cases of life-threatening arrhythmias.
6. Ibutilide (Corvert) is a class III antiarrhythmic drug that is used for
   a. sedation during electrocardioversion.
   b. conversion of recent-onset atrial fibrillation and flutter.
   c. treatment of life-threatening ventricular arrhythmias.
   d. treatment of arrhythmias complicated by CHF.
7. The drug of choice for the treatment of a supraventricular tachycardia associated with Wolff–Parkinson–White syndrome is
   a. digoxin.
   b. verapamil.
   c. lidocaine.
   d. adenosine.
8. A patient who is receiving an antiarrhythmic drug needs
   a. constant cardiac monitoring until stabilized.
   b. frequent blood tests including drug levels.
   c. an antidepressant drug to deal with the psychological depression.
   d. changes in diet and exercise programs to prevent irritation of the heart muscle.
9. A patient is brought into the emergency room with a potentially life-threatening ventricular arrhythmia. Immediate treatment would include
   a. a loading dose of digoxin.
   b. injection of quinidine.
   c. bolus and titrated intravenous doses of lidocaine.
   d. loading dose of propafenone.
10. A patient stabilized on quinidine for the regulation of atrial fibrillation would be cautioned to
    a. avoid foods high in potassium.
    b. avoid foods high in tyrosine.
    c. avoid foods high in sodium content.
    d. avoid foods that alkalinize the urine.

BIBLIOGRAPHY

Bullock, B. L. (2000). Focus on pathophysiology. Philadelphia: Lippincott Williams & Wilkins.

Epstein, A. E., et al. (1993). Mortality following ventricular arrhythmic suppression: The original design concept of the CAST study. Journal of the American Medical Association, 270(20).

Gilman, A., Hardman, J. G., & Limbird, L. E. (Eds.) (2002). Goodman and Gilman's the pharmacological basis of therapeutics (10th ed.). New York: McGraw-Hill.

Karch, A. M. (2002). 2003 Lippincott's nursing drug guide. Philadelphia: Lippincott Williams & Wilkins.

McEvoy, B. R. (2002). Facts and comparisons 2002. St. Louis: Facts and Comparisons.

The medical letter on drugs and therapeutics. (2002). New Rochelle, NY: Medical Letter.

Porth, C. M. (2002). Pathophysiology: Concepts of altered health states (6th ed.). Philadelphia: Lippincott Williams & Wilkins.

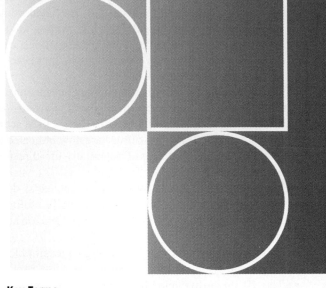

Key Terms
angina pectoris
atheromas
atherosclerosis
coronary artery disease (CAD)
myocardial infarction
nitrates
Prinzmetal's angina
pulse pressure

Antianginal Agents

620

Nitrates
amyl nitrate
isosorbide dinitrate
isosorbide mononitrate
Ⓟ nitroglycerin
β-Blockers
Ⓟ metoprolol
nadolol
propranolol
Calcium Channel Blockers
amlodipine
bepridil

Ⓟ diltiazem
nicardipine
nifedipine
verapamil

Coronary artery disease (CAD) has for many years been the leading cause of death in the United States and most Western nations. Despite great strides in the understanding of the contributing causes of this disease and ways to prevent it, CAD claims more lives than any other disease. The drugs discussed in this chapter are used to prevent myocardial death when the coronary vessels are already seriously damaged and are having trouble maintaining the blood flow to the heart muscle. Chapters 47 and 48 discuss drugs that are used to prevent the blocking of the coronary arteries before they become narrowed and damaged or to restore blood flow through narrowed vessels.

CORONARY ARTERY DISEASE

The myocardium, or heart muscle, must receive a constant supply of blood in order to have the oxygen and nutrients needed to maintain a constant pumping action. The myocardium receives all of its blood from two coronary arteries that exit the sinuses of Valsalva at the base of the aorta. These vessels divide and subdivide to form the capillaries that deliver oxygen to heart muscle fibers.

Unlike other tissues in the body, the heart muscle receives its blood supply during diastole, while it is at rest. This is important because when the heart muscle contracts, it becomes tight and clamps the blood vessels closed, rendering them unable to receive blood during systole, which is when all other tissues receive fresh blood. The openings in the sinuses of Valsalva, which are the beginnings of the coronary arteries, are positioned so that they can be filled when the blood flows back against the aortic valve when the heart is at rest. The pressure that fills these vessels is the **pulse pressure** (the systolic minus the diastolic pressure)— the pressure of the column of blood falling back onto the closed aortic valve. The heart has just finished contracting and using energy and oxygen. The acid and carbon dioxide built up in the muscle causes a local vasodilation, and the blood flows freely through the coronary arteries and into the muscle cells.

In CAD, the lumens of the blood vessels become narrowed so that blood is no longer able to flow freely to the muscle cells. The narrowing of the vessels is caused by the development of **atheromas,** or fatty tumors in the intima of the vessels (Figure 46–1). This is a process called **atherosclerosis.** These fatty deposits cause damage to the intimal lining of the vessels, attracting platelets and immune factors and causing swelling and the development of a larger deposit. Over time, these deposits severely decrease the size of the vessel. While the vessel is being narrowed by the deposits in the intima, the vessels are also losing their natural elasticity and becoming unable to respond to the normal stimuli to dilate or constrict to meet the needs of the tissues.

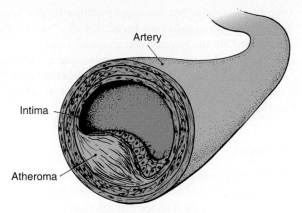

FIGURE 46–1. Schematic illustration of an atheromatous plaque. (From Bullock, B. L. [2000]. *Focus on pathophysiology.* Philadelphia: Lippincott Williams & Wilkins.)

The person with atherosclerosis has a classic supply and demand problem. The heart may do just fine until there is increased activity or other stresses that put a demand on it to beat faster or harder. The normal heart would stimulate the vessels to deliver more blood when this occurs, but the narrowed vessels are not able to respond and cannot supply the blood needed by the working heart (Figure 46–2). The heart muscle then becomes hypoxic. As a result, the heart demands increased blood supply in order

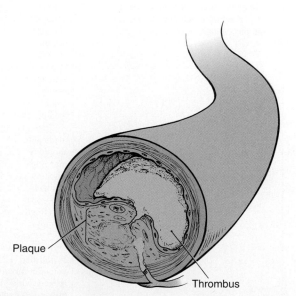

Plaque

Thrombus

FIGURE 46–2. Thrombosis of an atherosclerotic plaque. It may partially or completely occlude the lumen of the vessel. (From Bullock, B. L. [2000]. *Focus on pathophysiology.* Philadelphia: Lippincott Williams & Wilkins.)

to function properly, but the supply cannot be delivered. This happens with **angina pectoris,** literally "suffocation of the chest." If the supply and demand issue becomes worse, or if a vessel becomes so narrow that it occludes, the cells in the myocardium may actually become necrotic and die from lack of oxygen. This is called a **myocardial infarction.**

Stable Angina

The body's response to a lack of oxygen in the heart muscle is pain. Although the heart muscle does not have any pain fibers, a substance called factor P is released from ischemic myocardial cells, and pain is felt wherever substance P reacts with a pain receptor. For many people this is the chest, for others it is the left arm, and still others have pain in the jaw and teeth. The basic response to this type of pain is to stop whatever one is doing and to wait for the pain to go away. In cases of minor limitations to the blood flow through vessels, stopping activity may bring the supply and demand for blood back into balance. This condition is called stable angina. There is no damage to heart muscle, and the basic reflexes surrounding the pain restore blood flow to the heart muscle.

Unstable Angina

When the narrowing of the coronary arteries becomes more pronounced, the heart may experience episodes of ischemia even when the patient is at rest. This condition is called unstable angina. Though there is still no damage to heart muscle, the person is at great risk of a complete cutting off of the

DRUG THERAPY ACROSS THE LIFESPAN

Antianginal Agents

Children	Adults	Older Adults
The antianginals are not indicated for any condition commonly found in children. In some situations, particularly congenital heart defects or cardiac surgery, nitroglycerin may be used. The dosage of the drug should be determined considering age and weight. The child should be very carefully monitored for adverse reactions, including potentially dangerous changes in blood pressure.	Adults who receive these drugs should be instructed in their proper administration, particularly if varying forms of nitroglycerin are used. Patients should also be encouraged to determine what activities or situations tend to precipitate an anginal attack so that they can take measures to avoid those particular circumstances or take an antianginal agent before the event occurs. With nitroglycerin use, it is important that the patient know how to store the drug, how to determine whether it is still effective, and how much to take before seeking emergency medical care. Patients should know that regular medical follow-up is important and should be instructed in nonpharmacological measures—weight loss, smoking cessation, activity changes, diet changes—that could decrease their risk of coronary artery disease and improve the effectiveness of the antianginal therapy. The safety for the use of these drugs during pregnancy has not been established. There is a significant potential for adverse effects on the fetus related to blood flow changes and direct drug effects when the drugs cross the placenta. The drugs do enter breast milk, and it is advised that another method of feeding the baby be used if one of these drugs is prescribed during lactation.	Older adults frequently are prescribed one of these drugs. Older adults are more likely to develop adverse effects associated with the use of these drugs—arrhythmias, hypotenstion, and congestive heart disease. Safety measures may be needed if these effects occur and interfere with the patient's mobility and balance. The older adults are also more likely to have renal and/or hepatic impairment related to underlying medical conditions, which could interfere with the metabolism and excretion of these drugs. The dosage for older adults should be started at a lower level than recommended for younger adults. The patient should be monitored very closely and dosage adjustment based on patient response. If other drugs are added or removed from the drug regimen, appropriate dosage adjustments may need to be made. If the patient is using a different form of nitroglycerin, special care should be taken to make sure that the proper administration, storage, and timing of use is understood.

blood supply to the heart muscle if the heart should have to work hard or increase demand.

Prinzmetal's Angina

Prinzmetal's angina is an unusual form of angina because it seems to be caused by spasm of the blood vessels and not just by vessel narrowing. The person with this type of angina has angina at rest, often at the same time each day, and usually with an associated electrocardiogram (ECG) pattern change.

Acute Myocardial Infarction

When a coronary vessel becomes completely occluded and is unable to deliver blood to the cardiac muscle, the area of muscle that depends on that vessel for oxygen becomes ischemic, then necrotic. This is called a myocardial infarction (MI). The pain associated with this event can be excruciating; the person may also have nausea and a severe sympathetic stress reaction. A serious danger of an MI is that arrhythmias can develop in nearby tissue that is ischemic and very irritable. Most of the deaths caused by MI occur as a result of fatal arrhythmias. If the heart muscle has a chance to heal, within 6 to 10 weeks the dead area will be replaced with a scar and the muscle will compensate for the injury. When the area of the muscle that is damaged is very large, however, the muscle may not be able to compensate for the loss, and congestive heart failure and even cardiogenic shock may occur. These conditions can be fatal or can leave a person severely limited by the weakened heart muscle.

ANTIANGINAL DRUGS

In early cases of angina, avoidance of exertion or stressful situations may be sufficient to prevent anginal pain. Antianginal drugs are used to help restore the supply-and-demand ratio in oxygen delivery to the myocardium when rest is not enough. These drugs can work to improve the blood delivery to the heart muscle in one of two ways: (1) by dilating blood vessels (ie, by increasing the supply of oxygen) or (2) by decreasing the work of the heart (ie, by decreasing the demand for oxygen). Nitrates, β-adrenergic blockers, and calcium channel blockers are used to treat angina (Figure 46–3). They are all effective and are sometimes used in combination to achieve good control of the anginal pain. The type of drug that is best for a patient is determined by tolerance of adverse effects and response to the drug.

NITRATES

Nitrates are drugs that act directly on smooth muscle to cause relaxation and to depress muscle tone. Because the action is direct, it does not have to influence any nerve or other activity. The response to this type of drug is usually quite

FIGURE 46–3. Factors affecting myocardial oxygen demand and points where antianginal drugs have their effects.

fast. The nitrates relax and dilate veins, arteries, and capillaries, allowing increased blood flow through these vessels and lowering systemic blood pressure because of a drop in resistance. Because CAD causes a stiffening and lack of responsiveness in the coronary arteries, the nitrates probably have very little effect on increasing blood flow through these arteries. They do increase blood flow through healthy coronary arteries, so there will be an increased supply of blood through any healthy vessels in the heart, which could help the heart to compensate somewhat.

The main effect of nitrates, however, seems to be related to the drop in blood pressure that occurs. The vasodilation pools blood in veins and capillaries, decreasing the volume of blood that the heart has to pump around (the preload), while the relaxation of the vessels decreases the resistance the heart has to pump against (the afterload). The combination of these effects greatly reduces the cardiac workload and the demand for oxygen, thus bringing the supply and demand ratio back into balance.

Nitroglycerin (*Nitro-Bid, Nitrostat,* and others) is the nitrate of choice in an acute anginal attack. It can be given sublingually, as a translingual spray, intravenously, transdermally, topically, or as a transmucosal agent. It is rapidly absorbed and has an onset of action within minutes. It can be carried with the patient, who can use it when the need arises. It can also be used for prevention of anginal attacks in the slow-release forms. Other nitrates also are available for treating angina. Amyl nitrate (generic) is inhaled and has an onset of action of about 30 seconds. It comes as a capsule that has to be broken and waved under the patient's nose. The administration is somewhat awkward and usually requires a person other than the patient to give it properly. Isosorbide dinitrate (*Isordil* and others) and isosorbide mononitrate (*Imdur, Monoket*), both oral drugs, have a slower onset of action but may last up to 4 hours. They are taken before chest pain begins in situations in which exertion or stress can be anticipated. They are not drugs of choice during an acute attack.

Therapeutic Actions and Indications

The nitrates cause direct relaxation of smooth muscle with a resultant decrease in venous return and decrease in arterial pressure, which reduces cardiac workload and decreases myocardial oxygen consumption. They are indicated for the prevention and treatment of attacks of angina pectoris.

Pharmacokinetics

These drugs are very rapidly absorbed, metabolized in the liver, and excreted in the urine. They cross the placenta and enter breast milk. Because of the potential for serious adverse effects on the fetus and neonate, they are not recommended for use during pregnancy or lactation.

Contraindications and Cautions

Nitrates are contraindicated in the presence of any allergy to nitrates. These drugs also are contraindicated in the following conditions: severe anemia, because the decrease in cardiac output could be detrimental; head trauma or cerebral hemorrhage, because the relaxation of cerebral vessels could cause intracranial bleeding; and pregnancy or lactation, because of potential adverse effects on the neonate and ineffective blood flow to the fetus.

Caution should be used in patients with hepatic or renal disease, which could alter the metabolism and excretion of these drugs. Caution also is required with hypotension, hypovolemia, and conditions limiting cardiac output (e.g., tamponade, low ventricular filling pressure, low pulmonary capillary wedge pressure), because these conditions could be exacerbated, resulting in serious adverse effects.

Adverse Effects

The adverse effects associated with these drugs are related to the vasodilation and decrease in blood flow that occurs. Central nervous system (CNS) effects include headache, dizziness, and weakness. Gastrointestinal (GI) symptoms can include nausea, vomiting, and incontinence. Cardiovascular problems include hypotension, which can be severe and must be monitored; reflex tachycardia that occurs when blood pressure falls; syncope; and angina. Skin-related effects include flushing, pallor, sweating, and increased perspiration. When using the transdermal preparation, there is a risk of contact dermatitis and local hypersensitivity reactions.

Clinically Important Drug–Drug Interactions

There is a risk of hypertension and decreased antianginal effects if these drugs are given with ergot derivatives.

There is also a risk of decreased therapeutic effects of heparin if these drugs are given together; if this combination is used, the patient should be monitored and appropriate dosage adjustments made.

Nursing Considerations for Patients Receiving Nitrates

Assessment: History and Examination

Screen for the following conditions, which could be cautions or contraindications to use of the drug: any known allergies

---

DRUGS IN FOCUS
Nitrates

Drug Name	Usual Dosage	Usual Indications
amyl nitrate (generic)	0.3 mL by inhalation of vapor, may repeat in 3–5 min	Relief of acute anginal pain in adults
isosorbide dinitrate (Isordil)	2.5–5 mg SL; 5-mg chewable tablet; 5–20 mg PO; maintenance 10–40 mg PO q6h or 40–80 mg PO sustained release q8–12h Acute prophylaxis: 5–10 mg SL or chewable tablets q2–3h	Prevention and treatment of angina in adults
isosorbide mononitrate (Ismo, Imdur)	20 mg PO b.i.d., given at least 7h apart; ER tablets 30–60 mg/d PO Acute prophylaxis: 5–10 mg SL or chewable tablets q2–3h	Prevention and treatment of angina in adults
P nitroglycerin (Nitro-Bid, Nitrostat, others)	5 µg/min via IV infusion pump every 3–5 min; one tablet SL every 5 min for acute attack, up to three tablets in 15 min; 0.4-mg metered dose translingual, up to three doses in 15 min for acute attacks Prevention: one tablet SL 5–10 min before activities that might precipitate an attack; 2.5–2.6 mg PO t.i.d.–q.i.d.; sustained release tablets, doses as high as 26 mg PO q.i.d. have been used; 0.5 in q8h for topical application, up to 4–5 in (60–75 mg) have been used; one pad transdermal system per day; 1 mg q3–5h while awake for transmucosal system	Treatment of acute angina attack; prevention of anginal attacks

to nitrates; impaired liver or kidney function, which could alter the metabolism and excretion of the drug; any condition that could be exacerbated by the hypotension and change in blood flow caused by these drugs (eg, early MI, head trauma, cerebral hemorrhage, hypotension, hypovolemia, anemia, low cardiac output states); and pregnancy or lactation, because of the potential adverse effects on the fetus or neonate.

Include screening for baseline status before beginning therapy and for any potential adverse effects. Assess the following: skin color, lesions, temperature; affect, orientation, reflexes; pulse, blood pressure, perfusion, baseline ECG; respirations, adventitious sounds; liver and renal function tests; complete blood count; and hemoglobin level.

Nursing Diagnoses

The patient receiving a nitrate may have the following nursing diagnoses related to drug therapy:

- Decreased Cardiac Output related to hypotensive effects
- Risk for Injury related to CNS, cardiovascular effects
- Ineffective Tissue Perfusion (Total Body) related to hypotension, change in cardiac output
- Deficient Knowledge regarding drug therapy

Implementation

- Give sublingual preparations under the tongue or in the buccal pouch, and encourage the patient not to swallow, *to ensure that therapeutic effectiveness is achieved.* Ask the patient if the tablet "fizzles" or burns, which indicates potency. Always check the expiration date on the bottle and protect the medication from heat and light, *because these drugs are volatile and lose their potency.*
- Give sustained-release forms with water, and caution the patient not to chew or crush them, *because these preparations need to reach the GI tract intact.*
- Rotate the sites of topical forms, *to decrease the risk of skin abrasion and breakdown;* monitor for signs of skin breakdown *and arrange for appropriate skin care as needed.*
- Make sure that translingual spray is used under the tongue and not inhaled, *to ensure that the therapeutic effects can be achieved.*
- Break an amyl nitrate capsule and wave it under the nose of the angina patient *to provide rapid relief using the inhalation form of the drug;* this may be repeated with another capsule in 3 to 5 minutes if needed.
- Provide life support equipment on a standby basis, *in case of severe reaction to the drug or myocardial infarction.*
- Taper the dosage gradually (over 4 to 6 weeks) after long-term therapy, *because abrupt withdrawal could cause a severe reaction, including MI.*
- Provide comfort measures *to help the patient tolerate drug effects.* These include small, frequent meals; access to bathroom facilities if GI upset is severe; environmental controls; safety precautions; orientation; and appropriate skin care as needed.

- Provide thorough patient teaching, including the name of the drug, dosage prescribed, proper administration, measures to avoid adverse effects, warning signs of problems, and the importance of periodic monitoring and evaluation, *to enhance patient knowledge about drug therapy and promote compliance to the drug regimen.* (See Patient Teaching Checklist: Antianginal Nitrates.)
- Offer support and encouragement, *to help the patient deal with the diagnosis and the drug regimen.*

PATIENT TEACHING CHECKLIST
Antianginal Nitrates

Create customized patient teaching materials for a specific antianginal nitrate from the CD-ROM. Patient teaching should stress the following points for drugs within this class:

- A nitrate is given to patients with chest pain that occurs because the heart muscle is not receiving enough oxygen. The nitrates act by decreasing the heart's workload, and thus its need for oxygen, which it uses for energy. This relieves the pain of angina.

Besides taking the drug as prescribed, you can also help your heart by decreasing the work that it must do. For example, you can

- Reduce weight, if necessary.
- Decrease or avoid the use of coffee, cigarettes, or alcoholic beverages.
- Avoid going outside in very cold weather; if this can't be avoided, dress warmly and avoid exertion while outside.
- Avoid stressful activities, especially in combination. For example, if you eat a big meal, do not drink coffee or alcoholic beverages with that meal. If you have just eaten a big meal, do not climb stairs; rest for a while.
- Determine which social interactions cause you to feel stressed or anxious; then find ways to limit or avoid these situations.
- Determine ways to ventilate your feelings (e.g., throwing things, screaming, diversions).
- Learn to slow down, rest periodically, and schedule your activities to allow your heart to pace its use of energy throughout the day and to help you to maintain your activities without pain.

Nitroglycerin tablets are taken sublingually. Place one tablet under your tongue. Do not swallow until the tablet has dissolved. The tablet should burn slightly or "fizzle" under your tongue; if this does not occur, the tablet is not effective and you should get a fresh supply of tablets. Ideally, take the nitroglycerin before your chest pain begins. If you know that a certain activity usually causes pain (e.g., eating a big meal, attending a business meeting, engaging in sexual intercourse), take the tablet before undertaking the particular activity.

Dermal patches should be applied daily. They may be placed on the chest, upper arm, upper thigh, or back. They should be placed on an area that is free of body hair. The site of the application should be changed slightly each day to avoid excess irritation to the skin.

Patient Teaching Checklist continues on page 626

PATIENT TEACHING CHECKLIST
(CONTINUED)

Antianginal Nitrates

Sublingual nitroglycerin is a very unstable compound. Do not buy large quantities at a time, because it does not store well. Keep the drug in a dark, dry place and in a dark-colored glass container, not a plastic bottle, with a tight lid. Leave it in its own bottle. Do not combine it with other drugs.

Some of the following adverse effects may occur:

• *Dizziness, lightheadedness*—This will often pass as you adjust to the drug. Use great care if you are taking sublingual or transmucosal forms of the drug. Sit or lie down to avoid dizziness or falls. Change position slowly to help decrease the dizziness.
• *Headache*—This is a common problem. Over-the-counter headache remedies often provide no relief for the pain. Lying down in a cool environment and resting may help alleviate some of the discomfort.
• *Flushing of the face and neck*—This is usually a very minor problem that passes as the drug's effects pass.

Report any of the following to your health care provider: blurred vision, persistent or severe headache, skin rash, more frequent or more severe angina attacks, fainting.

Sublingual nitroglycerin usually relieves chest pain within 3 to 5 minutes. If pain is not relieved within 5 minutes, take another tablet. If pain continues, take another tablet in 5 minutes. A total of _____ tablets may be used, spaced every 5 minutes. If the pain is not relieved after that time, call your health care provider or go to a hospital emergency room as soon as possible.

Tell any doctor, nurse, or other health care provider that you are taking this drug.

Keep this drug, and all medications, out of the reach of children.

Avoid the use of over-the-counter medications while you are taking this drug. If you feel that you need one of these, consult with your health care provider for the best choice. Many of these drugs can change the effects of this drug and cause problems.

Avoid alcohol while you are taking this drug because the combination can cause serious problems.

If you are taking this drug for a prolonged period of time, do not stop taking it suddenly. Your body will need time to adjust to the loss of the drug. The dosage must be gradually reduced to prevent serious problems from developing.

This Teaching Checklist reflects general patient teaching guidelines. It is not meant to be a substitute for drug-specific teaching information which is available in nursing drug guides.

Evaluation

• Monitor patient response to the drug (alleviation of signs and symptoms of angina, prevention of angina).
• Monitor for adverse effects (hypotension, cardiac arrhythmias, GI upset, skin reactions, headache).
• Evaluate the effectiveness of the teaching plan (patient can name drug, dosage, proper administration, adverse effects

to watch for, specific measures to avoid adverse effects, importance of continued follow-up).
• Monitor the effectiveness of comfort measures and compliance to the regimen (see Nursing Care Guide: Antianginal Nitrates).

β-BLOCKERS

As discussed in Chapter 31, β-adrenergic blockers are used to block the stimulatory effects of the sympathetic nervous system. These drugs block β-adrenergic receptors and vasoconstriction (thereby stopping an increase in blood pressure) and prevent the increase in heart rate and increased intensity of myocardial contraction that occurs with sympathetic stimulation such as exertion or stress. These effects decrease the cardiac workload and the demand for oxygen.

These drugs are sometimes used in combination with nitrates to increase exercise tolerance. β-Blockers have many adverse effects associated with the blockade of the sympathetic nervous system. The dose that is used to prevent angina is lower than doses used to treat hypertension, so there is a decreased incidence of adverse effects associated with this specific use of β-blockers. These drugs are not recommended for use in patients with diabetes, peripheral vascular disease, or chronic obstructive pulmonary disease (COPD), because the effects on the sympathetic nervous system could exacerbate these problems. The β-blockers that are recommended for use in angina are metoprolol (*Toprol, Toprol XL*), propranolol (*Inderal*), and nadolol (*Corgard*).

Therapeutic Actions and Indications

The β-blockers competitively block β-adrenergic receptors in the heart and juxtaglomerular apparatus, decreasing the influence of the sympathetic nervous system on these tissues and thereby decreasing the excitability of the heart, decreasing cardiac output, decreasing cardiac oxygen compensation, and lowering blood pressure. They are indicated for the long-term management of angina pectoris caused by atherosclerosis. They are not indicated for the treatment of Prinzmetal's angina because they could cause vasospasm when they block β-receptor sites. Propranolol is also used to prevent reinfarction in stable patients 1 to 4 weeks after an MI. This effect is thought to be caused by the suppression of myocardial oxygen demand for a prolonged period.

Pharmacokinetics

These drugs are absorbed from the GI tract and undergo hepatic metabolism. Food has been found to increase the bioavailability of propranolol, but this effect has not been found with other β-adrenergic blocking agents. These drugs are excreted in the urine, necessitating caution in patients with renal impairment. Teratogenic effects have occurred in animal studies with all of these drugs except sotalol. The use of any β-adrenergic blocker during pregnancy should be reserved for situations in which the benefit to the mother outweighs the risk to the fetus. In general, they should not be

NURSING CARE GUIDE

Antianginal Nitrates

Assessment	Nursing Diagnoses	Implementation	Evaluation
HISTORY	Decreased Cardiac Output related to hypotension	Ensure proper administration of drug.	Evaluate drug effects: relief of signs and symptoms of angina, prevention of angina.
Allergies to any nitrates, renal or hepatic dysfunction, pregnancy, lactation, early MI, head trauma, hypotension, hypovolemia	Risk for injury related to CNS, CV effects	Provide comfort and safety measures:	Monitor for adverse effects:
	Ineffective Tissue Perfusion (Total Body) related to CV effects	-Protect drug from heat and light.	-headache, dizziness; arrhythmias;
	Deficient Knowledge regarding drug therapy	-Rotate transdermal sites.	-GI upset;
		-Offer environmental control for headaches.	-skin reactions;
		-Give drug with food if GI upset occurs.	-hypotension, CV effects.
		-Provide skin care as needed.	Monitor for drug-drug interactions as indicated for each drug.
		-Taper dosage after long-term use.	Evaluate effectiveness of patient teaching program.
		Provide support and reassurance to deal with drug effects.	Evaluate effectiveness of comfort and safety measures.
		Provide patient teaching regarding drug, dosage, adverse effects, what to report, safety precautions.	
PHYSICAL EXAMINATION			
CV: BP, P, perfusion, ECG			
CNS: orientation, affect, reflexes, vision			
Skin: color, lesions, texture			
Resp: R, adventitious sounds			
GI: abdominal exam, bowel sounds			
Lab tests: liver and renal function tests, CBC Hgb			

used during lactation because of the potential for adverse effects on the baby. The safety and efficacy for use of these drugs in children has not been established.

Contraindications and Cautions

The β-blockers are contraindicated in the presence of bradycardia, heart block, cardiogenic shock, asthma, and COPD because their blocking of the sympathetic response could exacerbate these diseases. They also are contraindicated with pregnancy and lactation, because of the potential for adverse effects on the fetus or neonate. Caution should be used in the presence of diabetes, peripheral vascular disease, and thyrotoxicosis, because the blockade of the sympathetic response blocks normal reflexes that are necessary for maintaining homeostasis in patients with these diseases.

Adverse Effects

The adverse effects associated with these drugs are related to their blockade of the sympathetic nervous system. CNS effects include dizziness, fatigue, emotional depression, and sleep disturbances. GI problems include gastric pain, nausea, vomiting, colitis, and diarrhea. Cardiovascular effects can include congestive heart failure, reduced cardiac output, and arrhythmias. Respiratory symptoms can include bronchospasm, dyspnea, and cough. Decreased exercise tolerance and malaise are also common complaints.

Clinically Important Drug–Drug Interactions

A paradoxical hypertension occurs when clonidine is given with β-blockers, and an increased rebound hypertension with clonidine withdrawal may also occur; it is best to avoid this combination.

CASE STUDY

Handling an Angina Attack

THE SITUATION

S. W. is a 50-year-old white woman with a 2-year history of angina pectoris. She was given sublingual nitroglycerin to use in case of chest pain. For the past 6 months, she has been stable, experiencing little chest pain. This morning after her exercise class, S. W. had an argument with her daughter and experienced severe chest pain that was unrelieved by four nitroglycerin tablets taken over a 20-minute period. S. W.'s daughter rushed her to the hospital, where she was given oxygen through nasal prongs and placed on a cardiac monitor, which showed a sinus tachycardia of 110 beats/min. A 12-lead electro-cardiogram (ECG) showed no changes from her previous ECG of 7 months ago. She did not have elevated troponin levels. The chest pain subsided within 3 minutes after she received another sublingual nitroglycerin. It was decided that S. W. should stay in the emergency room for a few hours for observation. The diagnosis of angina attack was made.

CRITICAL THINKING

• What nursing interventions should be done with S. W. while she is still in the ER? Consider the progression of coronary artery disease (CAD) and the ways in which that progression can be delayed and chest pain avoided. What teaching points should be stressed with this patient?
• What type of guilt may the daughter experience after the fight with S. W.? What interventions would be useful in dealing with mother and daughter during this crisis?
• Should any further tests or treatments be addressed with S. W. when discussing her heart disease?

DISCUSSION

S. W.'s vital signs should be monitored closely while she is in the ER. If her attack subsides, she will be discharged with review of her teaching for CAD. It would be a good time to discuss angina with S. W. and her daughter, reviewing the pathophysiology of the disease and ways to avoid upsetting the supply-and-demand ratio in the heart muscle.

Because S. W. took four nitroglycerin tablets with no effect before coming to the ER, it would be important to find out the age and potency of her drug. Review the storage requirements for the drug, ways to tell if it is potent, and the importance of replacing the pills at least every 6 months.

S. W. and her daughter should be encouraged to ventilate their feelings about this episode; for example, guilt or anger may be precipitated by this scare. They should have the opportunity to explore other ways of handling their problems, how to space activities to avoid excessive demand for oxygen, and what to do if this happens again. They should both receive support and encouragement to cope with the angina and its implications.

Written information should be given to S. W., including drug information. Once S. W. is stabilized, further studies may be indicated to monitor the progress of S. W.'s disease. The use of hormone therapy in this patient may be explored, as well as dietary implications, avoidance of smoking as appropriate, and the need to control blood pressure and monitor activities.

A decreased antihypertensive effect occurs when β-blockers are given with nonsteroidal anti-inflammatory drugs; if this combination is used, the patient should be monitored closely and a dosage adjustment made.

An initial hypertensive episode followed by bradycardia occurs if these drugs are given with epinephrine.

A possibility of peripheral ischemia exists if β-blockers are taken in combination with ergot alkaloids.

DRUGS IN FOCUS
β-Blockers

Drug Name	Usual Dosage	Usual Indications
Ⓟ metoprolol (*Toprol, Toprol XL*)	100 mg/d PO as single dose, extended release tablet; 100–400 mg/d PO in two divided doses regular release	Treatment of angina in adults; prevention of reinfarction within 3–10 d after myocardial infarction (MI)
nadolol (*Corgard*)	40–80 mg/d PO	Long-term management of angina in adults
propranolol (*Inderal*)	10–20 mg PO t.i.d.–q.i.d., titrate based on patient response, 160 mg/d is often needed for maintenance	Long-term management of angina and prevention of reinfarction in patients 1 to 4 wk after MI in adults

There also is a potential for a change in blood glucose levels if these drugs are given with insulin or antidiabetic agents, and the patient will not have the usual signs and symptoms of hypoglycemia or hyperglycemia to alert him or her to potential problems. If this combination is used, the patient should monitor blood glucose frequently throughout the day and should be alert to new warnings about glucose imbalance.

Nursing Considerations for Patients Receiving β-Blockers
See Chapter 31 for the nursing considerations associated with β-blockers.

◻◼◉◼ WEB LINKS
Patients and health care providers may want to explore information from the following Internet sources:

National Heart, Lung and Blood Institute information on angina, drug therapy, current research.
http://www.nscardiology.com/4factsarrhythmia.htm
Patient information on patient teaching, supports, other educational programs.
http://www.cardioassoc.com
Patient information, support groups, research information on heart disease, scientific programs:
http://www.americanheart.org
Information on diet, exercise, drug therapy, cardiac rehabilitation, and prevention of CAD:
http://heartdisease.miningco.com/mbody.htm? PID-2370& COB-home

CALCIUM CHANNEL BLOCKERS

The calcium channel blockers prevent the movement of calcium into the cardiac and smooth muscle cells when the cells are stimulated, interfering with the muscle cell's ability to contract. This leads to a loss of smooth muscle tone, vasodilation, and decreased peripheral resistance. These effects decrease venous return (preload) and the resistance the heart muscle has to pump against (afterload), which in turn decrease cardiac workload and oxygen consumption. The drug of choice depends on the patient's diagnosis and ability to tolerate adverse drug effects.

Therapeutic Actions and Indications
Calcium channel blockers inhibit the movement of calcium ions across the membranes of myocardial and arterial muscle cells, altering the action potential and blocking muscle cell contraction. These effects depress myocardial contractility; slow cardiac impulse formation in the conductive tissues and relax and dilate arteries, causing a fall in blood pressure and a decrease in venous return. These effects decrease the workload of the heart and myocardial oxygen consumption and, in Prinzmetal's angina, relieve the vasospasm of the coronary artery, increasing blood flow to the muscle cells. Research also indicates that these drugs block the proliferation of cells in the endothelial layer of the blood vessel, slowing the progress of the atherosclerosis. These drugs are indicated for the treatment of Prinzmetal's angina, chronic angina, effort-associated angina, and hypertension. Verapamil is also used to treat rapid cardiac arrhythmias, because it slows conduction more than the other calcium channel blockers do.

Pharmacokinetics
These drugs are generally well absorbed, metabolized in the liver, and excreted in the urine. These drugs cross the placenta and enter breast milk. Fetal toxicity has been reported in animal studies. Although there are no well-defined studies about effects during pregnancy, these drugs should not be used during pregnancy unless the benefit to the mother clearly outweighs any potential risk to the fetus. Because of the potential for serious adverse effects on the baby, another method of feeding the infant should be used if these drugs are required during lactation.

Contraindications and Cautions
These drugs are contraindicated in the presence of allergy to any of these drugs; with heart block or sick sinus syndrome, which could be exacerbated by the conduction-slowing effects of these drugs; with renal or hepatic dysfunction, which could alter the metabolism and excretion of these drugs; and with pregnancy or lactation, because of the potential for adverse effects on the fetus or neonate.

Adverse Effects
The adverse effects associated with these drugs are related to their effects on cardiac output and on smooth muscle. CNS effects include dizziness, lightheadedness, headache, and fatigue. GI effects can include nausea and hepatic injury related to direct toxic effects on hepatic cells. Cardiovascular effects include hypotension, bradycardia, peripheral edema, and heart block. Skin effects include flushing and rash.

Clinically Important Drug–Drug Interactions
Drug–drug interactions vary with each of the calcium channel blockers. Potentially serious effects to keep in mind include increased serum levels and toxicity of cyclosporine if taken with diltiazem and increased risk of heart block and digoxin toxicity if combined with verapamil because verapamil increases digoxin serum levels. Both drugs depress myocardial conduction. If any combinations of these drugs must be used, the patient should be monitored very closely and appropriate dosage adjustments made.

Verapamil has also been associated with serious respiratory depression when given with general anesthetics and as an adjunct to anesthesia.

Nursing Considerations for Patients Receiving Calcium Channel Blockers
Assessment: History and Examination

Screen for the following conditions, which could be cautions or contraindications to use of the drug: known allergies to any of these drugs; impaired liver or kidney function, which could alter the metabolism and excretion of the drug; heart block, which could be exacerbated by the conduction de-

DRUGS IN FOCUS
Calcium Channel Blockers Used to Treat Angina

Drug Name	Usual Dosage	Usual Indications
amlodipine (Norvasc)	5 mg/d PO; reduce dosage with hepatic impairment or with geriatric patients	Treatment of chronic, stable angina and of Prinzmetal's angina in adults
bepridil (Vascor)	200–300 mg/d PO	Treatment of chronic stable angina not responsive to other therapies
P diltiazem (Cardizem, Cardizem SR)	180–360 mg/d PO in three or four divided doses; 120–180 mg PO b.i.d. sustained release	Treatment of angina in adults
nicardipine (Cardene)	20–40 mg PO t.i.d.; use immediate release only	Treatment of angina in adults
nifedipine (Adalat, Procardia)	10–20 mg PO t.i.d.	Treatment of angina in adults
verapamil (Calan, Isoptin)	320–480 mg/d PO	Treatment of angina in adults

pression of these drugs; and pregnancy or lactation, because of the potential adverse effects on the fetus or neonate.

Include screening for baseline status before beginning therapy and for any potential adverse effects. Assess the following: skin color, lesions, temperature; affect, orientation, reflexes; pulse, auscultation, blood pressure, perfusion, baseline ECG; respirations, adventitious sounds; and liver and renal function tests.

Nursing Diagnoses

The patient receiving a calcium channel blocker may have the following nursing diagnoses related to drug therapy:

- Decreased Cardiac Output related to hypotension
- Risk for injury related to CNS, cardiovascular effects
- Ineffective Tissue Perfusion (Total Body) related to hypotension, change in cardiac output
- Deficient Knowledge regarding drug therapy

Implementation

- Monitor the patient carefully (blood pressure, cardiac rhythm, cardiac output) while the drug is being titrated or dosage is being changed, *to ensure early detection of potentially serious adverse effects.*
- Monitor blood pressure very carefully if the patient is also taking nitrates, *because there is an increased risk of hypotensive episodes.*
- Periodically monitor blood pressure and cardiac rhythm while the patient is using these drugs, *because of the potential for adverse cardiovascular effects.*
- Provide comfort measures *to help the patient tolerate drug effects.* These include small, frequent meals; access to bathroom facilities if GI upset is severe; environmental controls; and safety precautions.

- Provide thorough patient teaching, including the name of the drug, dosage prescribed, proper administration, measures to avoid adverse effects, warning signs of problems, and the need for periodic monitoring and evaluation, *to enhance patient knowledge about drug therapy and to promote compliance with the drug regimen.*
- Offer support and encouragement, *to help the patient deal with the diagnosis and the drug regimen.*

Evaluation

- Monitor patient response to the drug (alleviation of signs and symptoms of angina, prevention of angina).
- Monitor for adverse effects (hypotension, cardiac arrhythmias, GI upset, skin reactions, headache).
- Evaluate the effectiveness of the teaching plan (patient can name drug, dosage, proper administration, adverse effects to watch for, specific measures to avoid adverse effects, importance of continued follow-up).
- Monitor the effectiveness of comfort measures and compliance to the regimen.

CHAPTER SUMMARY

- Coronary artery disease (CAD) is the leading cause of death in the United States and most western nations.
- CAD develops when changes in the intima of coronary vessels leads to the development of atheromas or fatty tumors, accumulation of platelets and debris, and a thickening of arterial muscles, resulting in a loss of elasticity and responsiveness to normal stimuli.
- Narrowing of the coronary arteries secondary to the atheroma buildup is called atherosclerosis.
- Narrowed coronary arteries eventually become unable to

deliver all the blood that is needed by the myocardial cells, causing a problem of supply and demand.

- Angina pectoris, or "suffocation of the chest," occurs when the myocardial demand for oxygen cannot be met by the narrowed vessels. Pain, anxiety, and fatigue develop when the supply-and-demand ratio is upset.
- Stable angina occurs when the heart muscle is perfused adequately except during exertion or increased demand. People usually respond to the pain of angina by stopping all activity and resting, which decreases the demand for oxygen and restores the supply-and-demand balance.
- Unstable or preinfarction angina occurs when the vessels are so narrowed that the myocardial cells are low on oxygen even at rest.
- Prinzmetal's angina occurs as a result of a spasm of a coronary vessel, leading to decreased blood flow through the narrowed lumen.
- Myocardial infarction occurs when a coronary vessel is completely occluded and the cells that depend on that vessel for oxygen become ischemic, then necrotic, and die.
- Angina can be treated by drugs that either increase the supply of oxygen or decrease the heart's workload, which decreases the demand for oxygen.
- Nitrates and β-blockers are used to cause vasodilation and to decrease venous return and arterial resistance, effects that decrease cardiac workload and oxygen consumption.
- Calcium channel blockers block muscle contraction in smooth muscle and decrease the heart's workload, relax spasm in Prinzmetal's angina, and possibly block the proliferation of the damaged endothelium in coronary vessels.

Review Questions

1. Coronary artery disease results in
   a. an imbalance in the supply and the demand for oxygen in the heart muscle.
   b. delivery of blood to the heart muscle during systole.
   c. increased pulse pressure.
   d. a decreased workload on the heart.
2. Risk factors for the development of atherosclerosis would not include
   a. a high-fat diet.
   b. increasing age.
   c. female gender.
   d. a sedentary lifestyle.
3. Angina
   a. causes death of heart muscle cells.
   b. is pain associated with lack of oxygen to heart muscle cells.
   c. only occurs with vigorous exercise.
   d. is not treatable.
4. An acute myocardial infarction is not usually associated with
   a. permanent injury to the heart muscle.
   b. potentially serious arrhythmias.
   c. pain, nausea, sympathetic stress reaction.
   d. the development of hypertension.
5. Antianginal drugs work to do all of the following except

a. decrease the workload on the heart.
b. increase the supply of oxygen to the heart.
c. change the metabolic pathway in the heart muscle to remove the need for oxygen.
d. restore the supply-and-demand balance of oxygen in the heart.

6. Nitrates are commonly used antianginal drugs that act to
   a. increase the preload on the heart.
   b. increase the afterload on the heart.
   c. dilate coronary vessels to increase the delivery of oxygen through those vessels.
   d. decrease venous return to the heart, thereby decreasing the myocardial workload.
7. A patient who has nitroglycerin to avert an acute anginal attack would need to be taught
   a. to take five or six tablets and then seek medical help if no relief occurs.
   b. to buy the tablets in bulk to decrease the cost.
   c. to protect tablets from light and to discard them if they do not fizzle when placed under the tongue.
   d. to store the tablets in a clearly marked, clear container in open view, where they can easily be found if they are needed.
8. Calcium channel blockers are effective in treating angina because they
   a. prevent any cardiovascular exercise, preventing strain on the heart.
   b. block strong muscle contractions and cause vasodilation, decreasing the work of the heart.
   c. alter the electrolyte balance of the heart and prevent arrhythmias.
   d. increase the heart rate, making it more efficient.
9. Verapamil has been associated with potentially serious adverse effects if given with
   a. oral contraceptives.
   b. cyclosporine.
   c. digoxin.
   d. barbiturate anesthetics.
10. Prinzmetal's angina occurs as a result of
    a. electrolyte imbalance.
    b. a spasm of a coronary vessel.
    c. decreased venous return to the heart.
    d. a ventricular arrhythmia.

BIBLIOGRAPHY

Bullock, B. L. (2000). *Focus on pathophysiology*. Philadelphia: Lippincott Williams & Wilkins.
Drug facts and comparisons. (2002). St. Louis: Facts and Comparisons.
Gilman, A., Hardman, J. G., & Limbird, L. E. (Eds.) (2002). *Goodman and Gilman's the pharmacological basis of therapeutics* (10th ed.). New York: McGraw-Hill.
Karch, A. M. (2002). *2003 Lippincott's nursing drug guide*. Philadelphia: Lippincott Williams & Wilkins.
The medical letter on drugs and therapeutics. (2002). New Rochelle, NY: Medical Letter.
Porth, C. M. (2002). *Pathophysiology: Concepts of altered health states* (6th ed.). Philadelphia: Lippincott Williams & Wilkins.

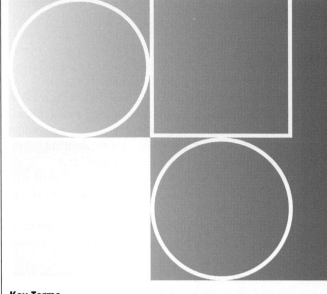

Lipid-Lowering Agents

632

The drugs discussed in this chapter lower serum levels of cholesterol and lipids. There is mounting evidence that the incidence of coronary artery disease (CAD), the leading killer of adults in the Western world, is higher among people with high serum lipid levels. The cause of CAD is poorly understood, but some evidence indicates that cholesterol and fat play a major role in disease development.

CORONARY ARTERY DISEASE

As explained in Chapter 46, CAD is characterized by the progressive growth of atheromatous plaques, or atheromas, in the coronary arteries. These plaques, which begin as fatty streaks in the endothelium, eventually injure the endothelial lining of the artery, causing an inflammatory reaction. This inflammatory process triggers the development of characteristic foam cells, containing fats and white blood cells that further injure the endothelial lining. Over time, platelets, fibrin, other fats, and remnants collect on the injured vessel lining and cause the atheroma to grow, further narrowing the interior of the blood vessel and limiting blood flow.

The injury to the vessel also causes scarring and a thickening of the vessel wall. As the vessel thickens, it becomes less distensible and less reactive to many neurological and chemical stimuli that would ordinarily dilate or constrict it. As a result, the coronary vessels no longer are able to balance the myocardial demand for oxygen with increased blood supply. Even more recent evidence indicates that the makeup of the core of the atheroma may be a primary determinant of which atheromas might rupture and cause acute blockage of a vessel. The softer, more lipid-filled atheromas appear to be more likely to rupture than stable, harder cores.

Strong evidence exists that atheroma development occurs more quickly in patients with elevated cholesterol and lipid levels. Patients who consume high-fat diets are more likely to develop high lipid levels. However, patients without increased lipid levels can also develop atheromas leading to CAD, so other factors evidently contribute to this process. Although the exact mechanism of atherogenesis (atheroma development) is not understood, certain **risk factors** increase the likelihood that a person will develop CAD. The following is a list of untreatable and treatable risk factors:

Unmodifiable Risk Factors

Genetic predispositions: CAD is more likely to occur in people who have a family history of the disease.

Age: The incidence of CAD increases with age.

Gender: Men are more likely to have CAD than premenopausal women; however, the incidence is almost equal in men and postmenopausal women, a possible link to a protective effect of estrogens.

Modifiable Risk Factors

Gout: Increased uric acid levels seem to injure vessel walls.

Cigarette smoking: Nicotine causes vasoconstriction and may have an effect on the endothelium of blood vessels; over time, smoking can lower oxygen levels in the blood.

Sedentary lifestyle: Exercise increases the levels of chemicals that seem to protect the coronary arteries.

High stress levels: Constant sympathetic reactions increase the myocardial oxygen demand while causing vasoconstriction and may contribute to a remodeling of the blood vessel endothelium, leading to an increased susceptibility to atheroma development.

Hypertension: High pressure in the arteries causes endothelial injury and increases afterload and myocardial oxygen demand.

Obesity: This may reflect altered fat metabolism, which increases the heart's workload.

Diabetes: Diabetics have a capillary membrane thickening, which accelerates the effects of atherosclerosis, and an abnormal fat metabolism.

Other factors that, if untreated, may contribute to CAD include bacterial infections (*Chlamydia* infections have been correlated with onset of CAD, and treatment with tetracycline and fluororoentgenography has been associated with decreased incidence of CAD, indicating a possible bacterial link) and an autoimmune process (some plaques contain antibodies and other products of immune reactions, making autoimmune reactions a possibility).

Because an exact cause of CAD is not known, successful treatment involves manipulating a number of these risk factors (Table 47–1). Overall treatment and prevention of CAD should include the following measures: decreasing dietary fats (a decrease in total fat intake and limiting saturated fats seems to have the most impact on serum lipid levels); losing weight; eliminating smoking; increasing exercise levels; decreasing stress; and treating hypertension, diabetes, gout, and estrogen deficiency in women.

METABOLISM OF FATS

Fats are taken into the body as dietary animal fats, then broken down in the stomach to fatty acids, lipids, and cholesterol (Figure 47–1). The presence of these products in the duodenum stimulates contraction of the gall bladder and the release of bile. **Bile acids,** which contain high levels of **cholesterol** (fat), act like a detergent in the small intestine, breaking up fats. (Imagine ads for dishwashing detergents that break up the grease and fats in the dishwashing water; bile acids do much the same thing.)

Bile acids break down the fats into small units, called micelles, that can be absorbed into the wall of the small intestine. The bile acids are then reabsorbed and recycled to the gall bladder, where they remain until the gall bladder is again stimulated to release them to facilitate fat absorption.

Because fats and water do not mix, the fats cannot be absorbed directly into the plasma but need to be transported on a plasma protein. To allow absorption, micelles are carried on **chylomicron,** a package of fats and proteins. The chy-

TABLE 47-1 | Risk Factors for the Development of Coronary Artery Disease

Unmodifiable Risks	Modifiable Risks	Suggested Modifications
Family history	Sedentary lifestyle	Exercise
Age	High-fat diet	Low-fat diet (polyunsaturated and monounsaturated fats)
Gender	Smoking	Smoking cessation
	Obesity	Weight loss
	High stress levels	Stress management
	Bacterial infections	Antibiotic treatment
	Diabetes	Control of blood glucose levels
	Hypertension	Control of blood pressure
	Gout	Control of uric acid levels
	Menopause	Hormone replacement therapy

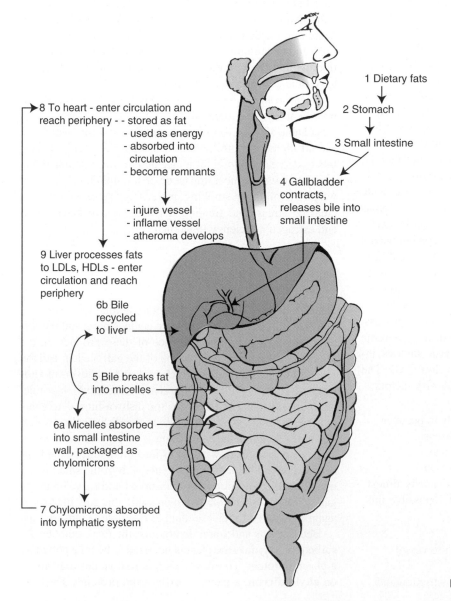

FIGURE 47-1. Metabolism of fats in the body.

GENDER CONSIDERATIONS
Women and Heart Disease

Until the late 1990s, heart disease was considered to be a condition that primarily affected men. Because of that belief, women were seldom screened for heart disease, and when they did experience acute cardiac events, they were not treated promptly or adequately. However, recent research has shown that heart disease is the leading cause of death among women, surpassing such diseases as breast and colon cancers. This finding has led to further research, still ongoing, about women and heart disease.

Women enjoy a protective hormone effect against the development of coronary artery disease (CAD) until menopause, when estrogen loss seems to rapidly increase the production of atheromas and the development of CAD. In several studies, women who received hormone replacement therapy (HRT) at menopause had a significantly reduced risk of CAD and myocardial infarction (MI). Convincing women of a certain age group to use HRT has been a challenge for health care professionals, possibly because many of those women recall that early HRT was associated with an increased risk of breast cancer—a disease that scares women more than heart disease does.

Women should be encouraged to consider HRT if they do not have risk factors that predispose them to breast cancer. They also should be advised to reduce other cardiac risk factors by eating a diet low in saturated fats, exercising regularly, not smoking, controlling weight, managing stress, and seeking treatment for gout, hypertension, and diabetes.

Clearly, heart disease is not just a disease of men. Research will continue to offer health care professionals new information on preventing and treating heart disease in women.

CULTURAL CONSIDERATIONS
Variations in Coronary Artery Disease Risk Among Cultures

Despite the fact that white Americans have the highest incidence of coronary artery disease, certain known risk factors may place other ethnic groups at greater risk. For example, hypertension and diabetes occur more frequently among African Americans and Native Americans than among whites. Regardless of race, all adults should be screened both for risk factors and for signs and symptoms of coronary artery disease.

Cultural variations in key parameters:

• Serum cholesterol levels—Whites > African Americans, Native Americans
• High-density lipoprotein (HDL) levels—African Americans, Asian Americans > Whites; Mexican Americans < Whites

Whites

• Low-density lipoprotein (LDL) levels—African Americans < Whites
• HDL:cholesterol ratio—African Americans < Whites

lomicrons pass through the wall of the small intestine, where they are picked up by the lymphatic system surrounding the intestines. The chylomicrons travel through the lymphatic system to the heart and then are sent out into circulation. The proteins that are exposed on the chylomicron, called apoproteins, determine the fate of the lipids or fats being carried. For example, some of these packages are broken down in the tissues to be used for energy, some are stored in fat deposits for future use as energy, and some continue to the liver, where they are further processed into lipoproteins.

The lipoproteins produced in the liver that have known clinical implications are the **low-density lipoproteins (LDL)** and the **high-density lipoproteins (HDL).** LDLs enter circulation as tightly packed cholesterol, triglycerides, and lipids—all of which are carried by proteins that enter circulation to be broken down for energy or stored for future use as energy. When an LDL package is broken down, many remnants or leftovers need to be returned to the liver for recycling. If a person has many of these remnants in the blood vessels, it is thought that the inflammatory process is initiated to help remove this debris. Some experts believe that this is the underlying process involved in atherogenesis.

HDLs enter circulation as loosely packed lipids that are used for energy and to pick up remnants of fats and cholesterol that are left in the periphery by LDL breakdown. HDLs serve a protective role in cleaning up remnants in blood vessels. It is known that HDL levels increase during exercise, which could explain why people who exercise regularly lower their risk of CAD. HDL levels also increase in response to estrogen, which could explain some of the protective effect of estrogen before menopause and of hormone replacement therapy (HRT) after menopause.

Cholesterol

The body needs fats, particularly cholesterol, to maintain normal function. Cholesterol is the base unit for the formation of the steroid hormones (the sex hormones as well as the adrenal cortical hormones). It is also a basic unit in the formation and maintenance of cell membranes. Cholesterol is usually provided through the diet and the fat metabolism process just described. If dietary cholesterol falls off, the body is prepared to produce cholesterol to ensure that the cell membranes and the endocrine system are intact. Every cell in the body has the metabolic capability of producing cholesterol. The enzyme hydroxymethylglutaryl–coenzyme A reductase (**HMG-CoA reductase**) regulates the early, rate-limiting step in the cellular synthesis of cholesterol. If dietary cholesterol is severely limited, the cellular synthesis of cholesterol will increase (Figure 47–2).

Hyperlipidemias

Hyperlipidemia, an increase in the level of lipids in the blood, increases a person's risk for the development of CAD. Though the exact role that lipids play is not completely un-

Cell

HMG CoA reductase

— HMG CoA reductase inhibitors work here

Cellular cholesterol

FIGURE 47-2. Cellular production of cholesterol.

derstood, the levels of lipids that contribute to CAD risk have been established (Table 47–2). Hyperlipidemia can result from excessive dietary intake of fats or from genetic alterations in fat metabolism leading to a variety of elevated fats in the blood (eg, hypercholesterolemia, hypertriglyceridemia, alterations in LDL and HDL concentrations). Dietary modifications are often successful in treating hyperlipidemia that is the result of excessive dietary intake of fats. Drug therapy is needed if the cause is genetically linked alterations in lipid levels or if dietary limits do not decrease the serum lipid levels to an acceptable range.

| TABLE 47-2 | Lipid Blood Level Classifications as Determined by the National Cholesterol Education Program Adult Treatment Panel II Report (May, 2001)* |

	Serum Concentration (mg/dL)					
Lipid Type	Low	Optimal	Normal or Desirable	Borderline High	High	Very High
Total cholesterol	—	—	>200	200–239	≥240	—
LDL cholesterol	—	<100	100–129	130–159	160–189	≥190
HDL cholesterol	<40	—	—	—	≥60	—
Triglycerides	—	—	<200	200–400	400–1000	>1000

*The low-density lipoprotein (LDL) goal should be determined by the presence of major risk factors: cigarette smoking, hypertension, low high-density lipoprotein (HDL) concentration, family history of premature coronary heart disease (CHD), age ≥45 y (men) or ≥55 y (women). If 0–1 risk factors are present, the goal is <160 mg/dL; if 2 or more risk factors, <130 mg/dL. If CHD and/or diabetes is present, the goal is <100 mg/dL.

DRUG THERAPY ACROSS THE LIFESPAN

Hyperlipidemic Agents

Children

Familial hypercholesterolemia may be seen in children. Because of the importance of lipids in the developing nervous system, treatment is usually restricted to tight dietary restrictions to limit fats and calories.

None of the hyperlipidemic drugs is recommended for use in children; clofibrate has been used to treat genetic hypercholesterolemia that is unresponsive to dietary restrictions.

Adults

Lifestyle changes including dietary restrictions, exercise, smoking cessation, and stress reduction should be tried before any antihyperlipidemic drug is used.

HMG-CoA reductase inhibitors are the first drug of choice in the treatment of hypercholesterolemia in patients who are at risk for, or who have already developed, coronary artery disease. The drugs are well tolerated and less expensive than some of the other antihyperlipidemic drugs. Combination therapy with a bile acid sequestrant, a fibrate, or niacin may be necessary if lipid levels still cannot be reduced.

Women of child-bearing age should not take HMG-CoA reductase inhibitors, which are pregnancy category X. Bile acid sequestrants are the drug of choice for these women if a lipid-lowering agent is needed.

Older Adults

No outcome data are available to prove the impact of lipid-lowering agents in decreasing the incidence of myocardial infarction or cardiac death in the older population.

Lifestyle changes including dietary restrictions, exercise, smoking cessation, and stress reduction should be tried before any antihyperlipidemic drug is used.

Lower doses of HMG-CoA reductase inhibitors should be used in elderly patients and in any patient with renal dysfunction. Care must be taken with those drugs that cannot be cut, crushed, or chewed. Alert patients about these restrictions.

Menopausal women may respond best to the use of hormone replacement therapy (HRT) to replace the protective effect of estrogen lost at menopause. Adverse effects associated with HRT are markedly less than those associated with antihyperlipidemic drugs.

ANTIHYPERLIPIDEMIC AGENTS

Drugs that are used to treat hyperlipidemia include bile acid sequestrants, HMG-CoA inhibitors, fibrates, niacin, and HRT in women. These drugs are often used in combination and should be part of an overall health care regimen that includes exercise, dietary restrictions, and lifestyle changes to decrease the risk of CAD.

BILE ACID SEQUESTRANTS

Bile acid sequestrants bind with bile acids, leading to their excretion in the feces. The resulting low levels of bile acids reentering hepatic circulation stimulate the production of more bile acids in the liver. Bile acids contain cholesterol. Because the liver must use cholesterol to manufacture bile acids, the hepatic intracellular cholesterol level falls, leading to an increased absorption of cholesterol-containing LDL segments from circulation to replenish the cell's cholesterol. The end result is a decrease in plasma cholesterol levels. Three bile acid sequestrants are currently in use. Cholestyramine (*Questran*) is a powder that must be mixed with liquids and taken up to six times a day. Colestipol (*Colestid*), available in both powder and tablet form, is only taken four times a day. Colesevelam (*Welchol*) is available in tablet form and is taken once or twice a day.

Pharmacokinetics

The bile acid sequestrants are resins that bind with bile acids in the intestine to form an insoluble complex which is then excreted in the feces. These drugs are not absorbed systemically. Their action is limited to their effects while they are present in the intestine.

Therapeutic Actions and Indications

Bile acid sequestrants bind with bile acids in the intestine to form a complex that is excreted in the feces (Figure 47–3). As

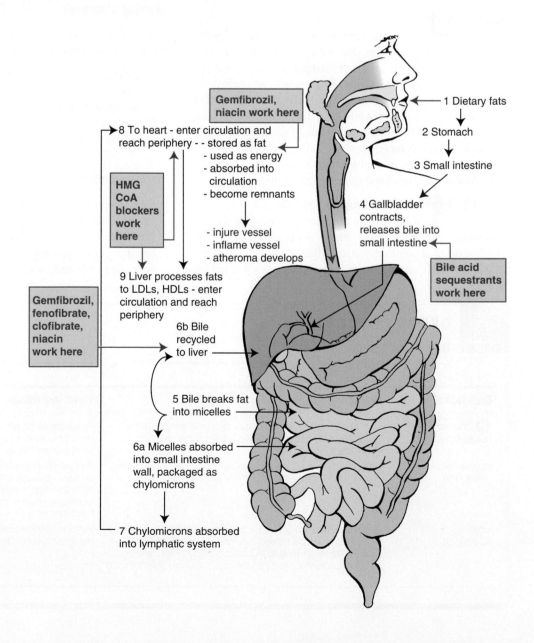

FIGURE 47-3. Sites of action of lipid-lowering agents.

a result, the liver must use cholesterol to make more bile acids. The serum levels of cholesterol and LDL decrease as the circulating cholesterol is used to provide the cholesterol the liver needs to make bile acids. These drugs are used to reduce serum cholesterol in patients with primary hypercholesterolemia (manifested by high cholesterol and high LDLs) as an adjunct to diet and exercise. Cholestyramine is also used to treat pruritus associated with partial biliary obstruction.

Contraindications and Cautions

Bile acid sequestrants are contraindicated in the presence of allergy to any bile acid sequestrant. These drugs also are contraindicated in the following conditions: complete biliary obstruction, which would prevent bile from being secreted into the intestine; abnormal intestinal function, which could be aggravated by the presence of these drugs; and pregnancy or lactation, because the potential decrease in the absorption of fat and fat-soluble vitamins could have a detrimental effect on the fetus or neonate.

Adverse Effects

Adverse effects associated with the use of these drugs include headache, anxiety, fatigue, and drowsiness, which could be related to changes in serum cholesterol levels. Direct gastrointestinal (GI) irritation, including nausea and constipation that may progress to fecal impaction, and aggravation of hemorrhoids may occur. Other effects include increased bleeding times related to a decreased absorption of vitamin K and consequent decreased production of clotting factors; vitamin A and D deficiencies related to decreased absorption of fat-soluble vitamins; rash; and muscle aches and pains.

Clinically Important Drug–Drug Interactions

Malabsorption of fat-soluble vitamins occurs when they are combined with these drugs. There is decreased or delayed absorption of thiazide diuretics, digoxin, warfarin, thyroid hormones, and corticosteroids if they taken with bile acid sequestrants. Consequently, any of these drugs should be taken 1 hour before or 4 to 6 hours after the bile acid sequestrant.

Nursing Considerations for Patients Receiving Bile Acid Sequestrants
Assessment: History and Examination

Screen for the following conditions: known allergies to these drugs; impaired intestinal function, which could be exacerbated by these drugs; biliary obstruction, which could block the effectiveness of these drugs; and pregnancy and lactation, which are contraindications.

Include screening for baseline status before beginning therapy and for any potential adverse effects. Assess the following: body temperature, weight; skin color, lesions, temperature; pulse, blood pressure; affect, orientation, reflexes; bowel sounds, abdominal examination; and serum cholesterol and lipid levels.

Nursing Diagnoses

The patient receiving a bile acid sequestrant may have the following nursing diagnoses related to drug therapy:

- Acute Pain related to central nervous system (CNS) and GI effects
- Constipation related to GI effects
- Decreased Cardiac Output related to increased bleeding
- Deficient Knowledge regarding drug therapy

Implementation

- Do not administer powder in dry form; *the drug must be mixed in fluids to be effective.* They may be mixed with fruit juices, soups, liquids, cereals, pulpy fruits; colestipol, but not cholestyramine, may be mixed with carbonated beverages. Stir and swallow all of the dose.

DRUGS IN FOCUS
Bile Acid Sequestrants

Drug Name	Usual Dosage	Usual Indications
℗ cholestyramine (*Questran*)	4 g PO one to two times per day, maximum dose 24 g/d; must be mixed with water or other noncarbonated fluids	Adjunctive treatment of primary hypercholesterolemia; pruritus associated with partial biliary obstruction
colesevelam (*Welchol*)	Three 625-mg tablets taken twice a day with meals, or six tablets taken once daily with a meal	Adjunctive therapy with diet and exercise to reduce low-density lipoproteins in patients with familial hypercholesterolemia; may be combined with an HMG-CoA reductase inhibitor
colestipol (*Colestid*)	Granule form: 5–30 g/d PO; may be taken in divided doses; must be mixed in water or other liquid Tablet form: 2–16 g/d PO taken once or in divided doses; tablets must not be cut, crushed, or chewed	Adjunctive treatment of primary hypercholesterolemia

- If the patient is taking tablets, ensure that tablets are not cut, chewed, or crushed, *because they are designed to be broken down in the GI tract; if they crushed, the active ingredients will not be effective.* Tablets should be swallowed whole with plenty of fluid.
- Give the drug before meals, *to ensure that the drug is in the GI tract with food.*
- Administer other oral medications 1 hour before or 4 to 6 hours after the bile sequestrant, *to avoid drug–drug interactions.*
- *Arrange for a bowel program as appropriate* if constipation occurs.
- Provide comfort measures *to help the patient tolerate the drug effects.* These include small, frequent meals; access to bathroom facilities; safety precautions to prevent injury if bleeding is a problem; replacement of fat-soluble vitamins; skin care as needed; and analgesics for headache.
- Provide thorough patient teaching, including the name of the drug, dosage prescribed, proper administration, measures to avoid adverse effects, warning signs of problems, the importance of periodic monitoring and evaluation, and the need to avoid overdose and poisoning, *to enhance patient knowledge about drug therapy and promote compliance with the drug regimen.*
- Offer support and encouragement, *to help the patient deal with the diagnosis and the drug regimen and lifestyle changes that may be necessary;* refer the patient to services that might help with the high cost of these drugs.

Evaluation

- Monitor patient response to the drug as appropriate (reduction in serum cholesterol levels, relief of rash).
- Monitor for adverse effects (headache, vitamin deficiency, increased bleeding times, constipation, nausea, rash).
- Evaluate the effectiveness of the teaching plan (patient can name drug, dosage, adverse effects to watch for, specific measures to avoid adverse effects; patient understands importance of continued follow-up).
- Monitor the effectiveness of comfort measures and compliance to the regimen.

HMG-COA REDUCTASE INHIBITORS

The early rate-limiting step in the synthesis of cellular cholesterol involves the enzyme HMG-CoA reductase. If this enzyme is blocked, serum cholesterol and LDL levels decrease, because more LDLs are absorbed by the cells for processing into cholesterol. In contrast, HDL levels increase slightly with this alteration in fat metabolism. HMG-CoA reductase inhibitors block HMG-CoA reductase from completing the synthesis of cholesterol. Most of these drugs are chemical modifications of compounds produced by fungi. As a group, they are frequently referred to as statins.

Pharmacokinetics

The statins are all absorbed from the GI tract and undergo first-pass metabolism in the liver. They are excreted through the feces and urine. Atorvastatin levels are not affected by renal disease, but with other statins patients with renal impairment must be monitored closely. The peak effect of these drugs is usually seen within 2 to 4 weeks. These drugs cross the placenta and have been associated with skeletal malformations of the fetus. The effects of these drugs on cholesterol pathways can cause serious harm to the developing fetus, and they should be avoided by women of child-bearing age who might become pregnant. Most of these drugs have been found to cross into breast milk, and, because of their effect on cholesterol synthesis, they could pose a threat to the neonate. Nursing mothers who need this drug should find another way to feed the baby.

The HMG-CoA reductase inhibitors include the following:

- Atorvastatin (*Lipitor*), which is associated with severe liver complications
- Fluvastatin (*Lescol*), which is actually a fungal product and should not be used with any known allergies to fungal byproducts
- Lovastatin (*Mevacor*), one of the oldest HMG-CoA drugs available, is very long-acting and is not associated with some of the severe liver toxicity that is seen with the other agents; the risk of rhabdomyolysis (an acute, sometimes fatal disease characterized by destruction of the muscles, often associated with renal failure as myoglobin builds up in the kidney) seems to be greater with this agent.
- Pravastatin (*Pravachol*), which is the only statin with outcome data to show that it is effective in decreasing CAD and the incidence of MI. It is used to prevent a first MI even in patients who do not have a documented increased cholesterol concentration, an effect that may be related to blocking of the formation of foam cells in injured arteries, which can decrease the risk of MI. This drug is not associated with the severe liver toxicities of some of the other statins.
- Simvastatin (*Zocor*), which is indicated for lowering cholesterol and preventing MI in patients with known hypercholesterolemia and CAD; this drug is not associated with the severe liver toxicities of some of the other statins.

Therapeutic Actions and Indications

HMG-CoA reductase inhibitors block the formation of cellular cholesterol, leading to a decrease in serum cholesterol and a decrease in serum LDLs, with a slight increase or no change in the levels of HDLs (see Figure 47–2). Because these drugs undergo a marked first-pass effect in the liver, most of their effects are seen in the liver. These drugs may also have some effects on the process that generates atheromas in vessel walls. That exact mechanism of action is not understood. These drugs are indicated as adjuncts with diet and exercise for the treatment of increased cholesterol and LDL levels that are unresponsive to dietary restrictions alone; to slow the progression of CAD in patients with documented CAD (pravastatin and simvastatin); and to prevent first MI in patients who are at risk for MI (pravastatin).

Contraindications and Cautions

These drugs are contraindicated in the presence of allergy to any of the statins or to fungal byproducts or compounds. They also are contraindicated with active liver disease or a history of alcoholic liver disease, which could be exacerbated, leading to severe liver failure, and with pregnancy or lactation, because of the potential for adverse effects on the fetus and neonate. Caution should be used in patients with impaired endocrine function because of the potential alteration in formation of steroid hormones.

Adverse Effects

The most common adverse effects associated with these drugs reflect their effects on the GI system: flatulence, abdominal pain, cramps, nausea, vomiting, and constipation. CNS effects can include headache, dizziness, blurred vision, insomnia, fatigue, and cataract development and may reflect changes in the cell membrane and synthesis of cholesterol. Increased concentrations of liver enzymes commonly occur, and acute liver failure has been reported with the use of atorvastatin and fluvastatin. Rhabdomyolysis (an acute, sometimes fatal disease characterized by destruction of the muscles, often associated with renal failure as myoglobin builds up in the kidney) with acute renal failure has also occurred with the use of lovastatin, atorvastatin, and fluvastatin.

Clinically Important Drug–Drug Interactions

There is an increased risk of rhabdomyolysis if any of these drugs is combined with erythromycin, cyclosporine, gemfibrozil, niacin, or antifungal drugs; such combinations should be avoided.

Increased serum levels and resultant toxicity can occur if these drugs are combined with digoxin or warfarin; if this combination is used, serum digoxin levels and/or clotting times should be monitored carefully and the prescriber consulted for appropriate dosage changes.

Increased estrogen levels can occur if these drugs are taken with oral contraceptives; the patient should be monitored carefully if this combination is used.

Nursing Considerations for Patients Receiving HMG-CoA Reductase Inhibitors
Assessment: History and Examination

Screen for the following conditions, which could be cautions or contraindications to use of the drug: any known allergies to these drugs or to fungal byproducts; active liver disease or history of alcoholic liver disease, which could be exacerbated by the effects of these drugs; pregnancy or lactation, because of potential adverse effects on the fetus or neonate; and impaired endocrine function, which could be exacerbated by effects on steroid hormones.

Include screening for baseline status before beginning therapy and for any potential adverse effects. Assess the following: body temperature, weight; skin color, lesions, temperature; affect, orientation, reflexes; pulse, blood pressure, perfusion; respirations, adventitious sounds; bowel sounds, abdominal examination; renal and liver function tests; and serum lipid levels.

DRUGS IN FOCUS
HMG-CoA Reductase Inhibitors

Drug Name	Usual Dosage	Usual Indications
(P) atorvastatin (*Lipitor*)	10 mg/d PO with a possible dosage range of 10–80 mg/d; may be taken at any time of day	Adjunctive therapy for reduction of increased cholesterol and low-density lipoprotein (LDL) levels, triglycerides
fluvastatin (*Lescol*)	20–80 mg PO, taken at bedtime; >2 h after a bile acid sequestrant, if this combination is being used	Adjunctive therapy for reduction of increased cholesterol and LDL levels; to slow the progression of coronary artery disease (CAD) in patients with known CAD
lovastatin (*Mevacor*)	20 mg/d PO taken with the evening meal; maximum dose 80 mg/d; do not exceed 20 mg/d if patient is taking immunosuppressives or has renal impairment	Adjunctive therapy for reduction of increased cholesterol and LDL levels
pravastatin (*Pravachol*)	10–40 mg/d PO taken at bedtime; start with 10 mg/d in elderly patients and those with hepatic or renal impairment	Prevention of first myocardial infarction (MI) even in patients who do not have a documented increased cholesterol level, slowing of the progression of CAD; adjunctive therapy for reduction of increased cholesterol and LDL levels
simvastatin (*Zocor*)	5–80 mg/d PO taken once a day in the evening; start with 5 mg/d in elderly patients and those with hepatic or renal impairment	Prevention of first MI in patients with known hypercholesterolemia and CAD; adjunctive therapy for reduction of increased cholesterol and LDL levels

Nursing Diagnoses

The patient receiving an HMG-CoA reductase inhibitor may have the following nursing diagnoses related to drug therapy:

- Disturbed Sensory Perception (Visual, Kinesthetic, Gustatory) related to CNS effects
- Risk for Injury related to CNS, liver, and renal effects
- Acute Pain related to headache, myalgia, and GI effects
- Deficient Knowledge regarding drug therapy

Implementation

- Administer the drug at bedtime, because the highest rates of cholesterol synthesis occur between midnight and 5 AM (atorvastatin can be taken at any time during the day), and the *drug should be taken when it will be most effective.*
- Monitor serum cholesterol and LDL levels before and periodically during therapy, *to evaluate the effectiveness of this drug.*
- Arrange for periodic ophthalmic examinations, *to monitor for cataract development.*
- Monitor liver function tests before and periodically during therapy, *to monitor for liver damage;* consult with the prescriber to discontinue drug if the aspartate aminotransferase (AST) or alanine aminotransferase (ALT) level increases to three times normal.
- Ensure that the patient has attempted a cholesterol-lowering diet and exercise program for at least 3 to 6 months before beginning therapy, *to ensure the need for drug therapy.*
- Encourage the patient to make the lifestyle changes necessary *to decrease the risk of CAD and to increase the effectiveness of drug therapy.*
- Withhold lovastatin, atorvastatin, or fluvastatin in any acute, serious medical condition (e.g., infection, hypotension, major surgery or trauma, metabolic endocrine disorders, seizures) *that might suggest myopathy or serve as a risk factor for the development of renal failure.*
- Suggest the use of barrier contraceptives for women of child-bearing age, *because there is a risk of severe fetal abnormalities if these drugs are taken during pregnancy.*
- Provide comfort measures *to help the patient tolerate drug effects.* These include small, frequent meals; access to bathroom facilities; bowel program as needed; food with drug if GI upset is severe; environmental controls; safety precautions; and orientation as needed.
- Provide thorough patient teaching, including the name of the drug, dosage prescribed, measures to avoid adverse effects, warning signs of problems, and the need for periodic monitoring and evaluation, *to enhance the patient's knowledge of drug therapy and to promote compliance with the drug regimen.* (See Patient Teaching Checklist: HMG-CoA Reductase Inhibitors.)
- Offer support and encouragement, *to help the patient deal with the diagnosis, needed lifestyle changes, and the drug regimen.*

PATIENT TEACHING CHECKLIST
HMG-CoA Reductase Inhibitors

Create customized patient teaching materials for a specific HMG-CoA reductase inhibitor from the CD-ROM. Patient teaching should stress the following points for drugs within this class:

- An HMG-CoA reductase inhibitor, or statin, is an antihyperlipidemic agent, which means it works to decrease the levels of certain lipids, or fats, in your blood. An increase in serum lipid levels has been associated with the development of many blood vessel disorders, including coronary artery disease, which can lead to a heart attack. This drug must be used in conjunction with a low-calorie, low-saturated-fat diet and an exercise program.

Some of the following adverse effects may occur:

- *Headache, blurred vision, nervousness, insomnia*—Avoid driving or performing hazardous or delicate tasks that require concentration; these effects may pass with time.
- *Nausea, vomiting, flatulence, constipation*—Small, frequent meals may help. If constipation becomes a problem, consult with your health care provider for appropriate interventions.

Report any of the following to your health care provider: severe GI upset, vision changes, unusual bleeding, dark urine, or light-colored stools.

You will need to have regular medical examinations to monitor the effectiveness of this drug on your lipid levels and to detect any adverse effects. These examinations will include blood tests and eye examinations.

Tell any doctor, nurse, or other health care provider that you are taking this drug.

Keep this drug, and all medications, out of the reach of children.

To help decrease your risk of heart disease, follow these guidelines; adhere to a diet that is low in calories and saturated fat, exercise regularly, stop smoking, and reduce stress.

This Teaching Checklist reflects general patient teaching guidelines. It is not meant to be a substitute for drug-specific teaching information, which is available in nursing drug guides.

Evaluation

- Monitor patient response to the drug (lowering of serum cholesterol and LDL levels, prevention of first MI, slowing of progression of CAD).
- Monitor for adverse effects (headache, dizziness, blurred vision, cataracts, GI upset, liver failure, rhabdomyolysis).
- Evaluate the effectiveness of the teaching plan (patient can name drug, dosage, adverse effects to watch for, specific measures to avoid adverse effects; patient understands importance of continued follow-up).
- Monitor the effectiveness of comfort measures and compliance to the regimen (see Nursing Care Guide: HMG-CoA Reductase Inhibitors).

NURSING CARE GUIDE

HMG-CoA Reductase Inhibitors

Assessment	Nursing Diagnoses	Implementation	Evaluation
HISTORY Allergies to any of these drugs or fungal byproducts; hepatic dysfunction, pregnancy, lactation, endocrine disorders	Disturbed Sensory Perception related to CNS effects Risk for Injury related to CNS, liver, renal effects Acute Pain related to headache, myalgia, and GI effects Deficient Knowledge regarding drug therapy	Administer drug at bedtime. Monitor serum lipids prior to therapy. Provide comfort and safety measures: Give small meals. Arrange for periodic ophthalmic exams to screen for cataracts. Give drug with food if GI upset occurs Institute bowel program as needed Provide safety measures if needed Monitor liver function and arrange to stop drug if liver impairment occurs. Provide support and reassurance to deal with drug effects and need to make lifestyle, diet, and exercise changes. Provider patient teaching regarding drug, dosage, adverse effects, what to report, safety precautions.	Evaluate drug effects: lowering of serum cholesterol and lipid levels, prevention of first MI, slowed progression of CAD. Monitor for adverse effects: sedation, dizziness, headache, cataracts, GI upset; hepatic or renal dysfunction; rhabdomyolysis. Monitor for drug–drug interactions as indicated for each drug. Evaluate effectiveness of patient teaching program. Evaluate effectiveness of comfort and safety measures.
PHYSICAL EXAMINATION CV: BP, P, perfusion CNS: orientation, affect, reflexes, vision Skin: color, lesions, texture Resp: R, adventitious sounds GI: abdominal exam, bowel sounds Lab tests: liver and renal function tests, serum lipids			

OTHER DRUGS USED TO AFFECT LIPID LEVELS

Other drugs that are used to affect lipid levels do not fall into any of the classes discussed previously. They include the fibrates (derivatives of fibric acid), the vitamin niacin, and HRT in postmenopausal women (see Figure 47–3).

The fibrates stimulate the breakdown of lipoproteins from the tissues and their removal from the plasma. They lead to a decrease in lipoprotein and triglyceride synthesis and se-

cretion. The fibrates are absorbed from the GI tract and are metabolized in the liver and excreted in the urine.

Fibrates in use today include the following agents:

• Clofibrate (*Atromid-S*), which also inhibits liver synthesis of LDL and cholesterol, lowers serum lipids and has an antiplatelet effect. It is used to treat genetic hyperlipidemia that does not respond to diet and for adults who have very high triglycerides with abdominal pain and pancreatitis.

The effect on LDL levels starts to been seen in 2 to 5 days, and the peak effect is seen in 4 weeks.

- Fenofibrate (*Tricor*), which inhibits triglyceride synthesis in the liver, resulting in reduction of LDL levels, increases uric acid secretion and may stimulate triglyceride breakdown. It is used for adults with very high triglyceride levels not responsive to strict dietary measures who are at risk for pancreatitis. Peak effects are usually seen within 4 weeks, and the patient's serum lipid levels should be re-evaluated at that time.
- Gemfibrozil (*Lopid*) inhibits peripheral breakdown of lipids, reduces production of triglycerides and LDLs, and increases HDL concentrations. It is associated with GI and muscle discomfort. This drug should not be combined with statins. There is an increased risk of rhabdomyolysis from 3 weeks to several months after therapy when this combination is used. If this combination cannot be avoided, the patient should be monitored very closely.

The vitamin niacin (*Niaspan*) inhibits release of free fatty acids from adipose tissue, increases the rate of triglyceride removal from plasma, and generally reduces LDL and triglyceride levels and increases HDL levels. It may also decrease levels of apoproteins needed to form chylomicrons. The initial effect on lipid levels is usually seen within 5 to 7 days, with the maximum effect occurring in 3 to 5 weeks. Niacin is associated with intense cutaneous flushing, nausea, and abdominal pain, making its use somewhat limited. It also increases serum levels of uric acid and may predispose patients to the development of gout. Niacin is often combined with bile acid sequestrants for increased effect. It is given at bedtime to make maximum use of nighttime cholesterol synthesis, and it must be given 4 to 6 hours after the bile sequestrant to ensure absorption.

HRT is discussed in Chapter 40. The use of estrogens or combinations of estrogen and progesterone to replace the hormones lost in menopause has been shown to significantly decrease the incidence of CAD and MI in postmenopausal women. This therapy should also be combined with a diet and exercise program, and other measures to decrease risk factors should also be considered.

COMBINATION THERAPY

Frequently, if there has been no response to strict dietary modification, exercise, and lifestyle changes and the use of one lipid-lowering agent, combination therapy is used to achieve desirable serum LDL and cholesterol levels. For example, a bile acid sequestrant might be combined with niacin; the combination would decrease the synthesis of LDLs while lowering the serum levels of LDLs. This combination is thought to help slow the progression of CAD. Box 47–1 discusses a drug that combines niacin and lovastatin. However, care must be taken not to combine agents that increase the risk of rhabdomyolysis. For example, HMG-CoA reductase inhibitors should not be combined with niacin or gemfibrozil.

WEB LINKS
Patients and health care providers may want to consult the following Internet sources:

Information on diet, exercise, drug therapy, cardiac rehabilitation:
http://www.heartcenteronline.com
Patient information on latest resources, diets, programs:
http://www.my.webmd.com
Patient information, support groups, diet, exercise, research information on heart disease:
http://www.americanheart.org

DRUGS IN FOCUS
Other Antihyperlipidemic Drugs

Drug Name	Usual Dosage/Route	Usual Indications
clofibrate (*Atromid-S*)	2 g/d PO; monitor patient, dosage may be decreased	Genetic hyperlipidemia; severely elevated triglyceride levels
fenofibrate (*Tricor*)	67 mg/d PO given with a meal; may be increased up to 67 mg PO t.i.d. as needed; monitor patients with impaired renal function and the elderly very carefully	Treatment of very high triglyceride levels in adults who are at risk for pancreatitis if not responsive to dietary measures
gemfibrozil (*Lopid*)	1200 mg/d PO divided into two doses and taken before the morning and evening meals	Treatment of very high triglyceride levels with abdominal pain and potential pancreatitis in adults
niacin (*Niaspan*)	1.5–2 g/d PO in divided doses for tablets; 500–2000 mg/d PO for ER tablets taken at bedtime	Treatment of hyperlipidemia not responding to diet and weight loss; to slow progression of coronary artery disease when combined with a bile acid sequestrant

CASE STUDY

Treating Hyperlipidemia

THE SITUATION

M. M., a 55-year-old white businessman, was seen for a routine insurance physical examination. He was found to be obese and borderline hypertensive, with a nonfasting low-density lipoprotein (LDL) level of 325 mg/dL (very high). M. M. reported smoking two packs of cigarettes a day and noted in his family history that both of his parents died of heart attacks before 50 y of age. He described himself as a "workaholic" with no time to exercise and a tendency to eat most of his meals in restaurants. The primary medical regimen suggested for M. M. included decreased smoking, weight loss, dietary changes to eliminate saturated fats, and decreased stress. On a return visit after 4 weeks, M. M. had lost 7 pounds and reported a decrease in smoking, but his LDL levels were unchanged. The use of an antihyperlipidemic drug was discussed.

CRITICAL THINKING

What nursing interventions are appropriate at this point? *Consider all of the known risk factors for coronary artery disease (CAD), then rank M. M's risk based on those factors.*

What lifestyle changes can help M. M. reduce his risk of heart disease?
What support services should be consulted to help M. M.?
Should other tests be done before considering any drug therapy for M. M.? *Think about the kind of patient teaching that would help M. M. cope with the overwhelming lifestyle changes that have been suggested, yet remain compliant to his medical regimen.*

DISCUSSION

M. M.'s description of himself as a workaholic should alert the nurse to the possibility that he will have trouble adapting to any prescribed lifestyle changes. (Workaholics tend to be very organized, goal-driven, and somewhat controlling individuals). M. M. should first receive extensive teaching about CAD, his risk factors, and his options. The benefits of decreasing or eliminating risk factors should be discussed. M. M. may be more compliant if he exercises some control over his situation, so he should be invited to suggest possible lifestyle changes or adaptations. M. M. also should be encouraged to set short-range goals that are achievable, to help him feel successful.

Referral to a dietician and to an exercise program may help M. M. select foods and exercises that fit into his lifestyle. A stress test, angiogram, or both may be ordered to evaluate the actual state of M. M.'s coronary arteries. The results of these tests could serve as powerful teaching tools and motivators.

M. M. needs to understand that antihyperlipidemic drugs can cause dizziness, headaches, gastrointestinal upset, and constipation. Because of his busy lifestyle, M. M. may have trouble coping with these adverse effects. M. M.'s health care provider may need to try a variety of different drugs or combinations of drugs to find ones that are effective but do not cause unacceptable adverse effects.

The American Heart Association (AHA) has numerous booklets, diets, support groups, and counselors who can help M. M. as he tries to adapt to his medical regimen. He can contact the AHA online at http://www.americanheart.org for a quick reference and referrals to other sources. M. M. will benefit from having a consistent health care provider who can offer him encouragement, answer any questions, and allow him to vent his feelings. This health care provider can help to coordinate all of his various referrals and activities and act as a consistent base for reassurance and questions. Many times, lifestyle changes are the most difficult part of this medical regimen, so M. M. will need constant support.

BOX 47-1

Fixed-Combination Therapy for Lowering Cholesterol Levels

In 2002, the U.S. Food and Drug Administration approved *Advicor,* a fixed combination of extended-release niacin and lovastatin, for reduction of the risk of atherosclerosis in patients with multiple risk factors. The drug is not intended to be used as an initial therapy; it should be used only after the patient has been stabilized on lovastatin and extended-release niacin and found to tolerate the combination and to have good results at lowering cholesterol levels. The drug is available in three strengths: 500 mg niacin/20 mg lovastatin; 750 mg niacin/20 mg lovastatin; and 1000 mg niacin/20 mg lovastatin. The contraindications and cautions for both niacin and lovastatin apply to this drug, and patient teaching should incorporate the same warnings about adverse effects that are used with both agents. It is thought that the convenience of taking one tablet each day in the evening will improve patient compliance with lipid-lowering regimens.

Specific information on exercise programs and safety:
http://www.nhlbi.nih.gov/health

CHAPTER SUMMARY

- Coronary artery disease (CAD) is the leading cause of death in the Western world. It is associated with the development of atheromas or plaques in arterial linings that lead to narrowing of the lumen of the artery and hardening of the artery wall, with loss of distensibility and responsiveness to stimuli for contraction or dilation.
- The cause of CAD is not known, but many contributing risk factors have been identified, including increasing age, male gender, genetic predisposition, high-fat diet, sedentary lifestyle, smoking, obesity, high stress levels, bacterial infections, diabetes, hypertension, gout, and menopause.
- Treatment and prevention of CAD is aimed at manipulating the known risk factors to decrease CAD development and progression.

- Fats are metabolized with the aid of bile acids, which act as a detergent to break fats into small molecules called micelles. Micelles are absorbed into the intestinal wall and combined with proteins to become chylomicrons, which can be transported throughout the circulatory system.
- Some fats are used immediately for energy or are stored in adipose tissue; others are processed in the liver to low-density lipoproteins (LDLs), which are associated with the development of CAD. LDLs are broken down in the periphery and leave many remnants (e.g., fats) that must be removed from blood vessels. This process involves the inflammatory reaction and may initiate or contribute to atheroma production.
- Some fats are processed into high-density lipoproteins (HDLs), which are able to absorb fats and remnants from the periphery and offer a protective effect against the development of CAD.
- Cholesterol is an important fat that is used to make bile acids. It is the base for steroid hormones and provides necessary structure for cell membranes. All cells can produce cholesterol.
- HMG-CoA reductase is an enzyme that controls the final step in production of cellular cholesterol. Blocking this enzyme results in lower serum cholesterol levels, a resultant breakdown of LDLs, and a slight increase in HDLs.
- Bile acid sequestrants bind with bile acids in the intestine and lead to their excretion in the feces. This results in low bile acid levels as the liver uses cholesterol to produce more bile acids. The end result is a decrease in serum cholesterol and LDL levels as the liver changes its metabolism of these fats to meet the need for more bile acids.
- Overall treatment of patients taking lipid-lowering drugs should include diet, exercise, and lifestyle changes to reduce the risk of CAD. Such lifestyle changes include stopping smoking; managing stress; and treating hypertension, gout, diabetes, estrogen deficiencies, and bacterial infections (particularly chlamydial infections).

Review Questions

1. The body uses cholesterol in many ways, including
   a. the production of water-soluble vitamins.
   b. the formation of steroid hormones.
   c. the mineralization of bones.
   d. the development of dental plaques.
2. The formation of atheromas in blood vessels precedes the signs and symptoms of
   a. hepatitis.
   b. coronary artery disease.
   c. diabetes mellitus.
   d. COPD.
3. High cholesterol levels are considered to be
   a. a normal finding in adult males.
   b. related to stress levels.
   c. a treatable risk factor for the development of heart disease.

   d. a side effect of cigarette smoking.
4. The bile acid sequestrants
   a. are absorbed into the liver.
   b. take several weeks to show an effect.
   c. have no associated adverse effects.
   d. work in the small intestine to prevent bile salts from being reabsorbed.
5. Bile acid sequestrants would not be a drug of choice for a patient who has
   a. a high LDL concentration.
   b. a high triglyceride concentration.
   c. intestinal obstruction.
   d. vitamin K deficiency.
6. HMG-CoA reductase works in the
   a. process of bile secretion.
   b. process of formation of cholesterol within the cell.
   c. intestinal wall to block fat absorption.
   d. kidney to block fat excretion.
7. Patients taking HMG-CoA reductase inhibitors
   a. will not have a heart attack.
   b. will not develop CAD.
   c. may develop cataracts as a result.
   d. may stop absorbing fat-soluble vitamins.
8. A patient who has high lipid levels and cannot take fibrates or HMG-CoA reductase inhibitors may be able to take
   a. nicotine.
   b. vitamin C.
   c. niacin.
   d. bran fiber products.
9. Rhabdomyolysis is a very serious adverse effect that can be seen with HMG-CoA reductase inhibitors; to detect it, patients taking these drugs would be monitored for
   a. flatulence and abdominal bloating.
   b. increased bleeding.
   c. the development of cataracts.
   d. muscle pain and weakness.

BIBLIOGRAPHY

Abramowicz, M. (1996). Choice of lipid-lowering drugs. *Medical Letter, 38*(980), 67–70.
Bullock, B. L. (2000). *Focus on pathophysiology.* Philadelphia: Lippincott Williams & Wilkins.
Drug facts and comparisons. (2002). St. Louis: Facts and Comparisons.
Gilman, A., Hardman, J. G., & Limbird, L. E. (Eds.) (2002). *Goodman and Gilman's the pharmacological basis of therapeutics* (10th ed.). New York: McGraw-Hill.
Karch, A. M. (2002). *2003 Lippincott's nursing drug guide.* Philadelphia: Lippincott Williams & Wilkins.
Knopp, R. H. (1999) Drug treatment of lipid disorders. *New England Journal of Medicine, 341,* 498–511.
The medical letter on drugs and therapeutics. (2002). New Rochelle, NY: Medical Letter.
Porth, C. M. (2002). *Pathophysiology: Concepts of altered health states* (6th ed.). Philadelphia: Lippincott Williams & Wilkins.

CHAPTER

48

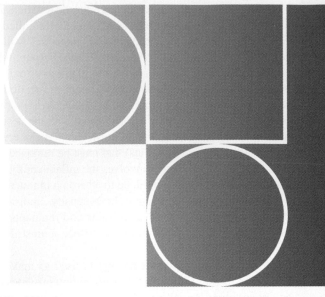

Drugs Affecting Blood Coagulation

Key Terms

anticoagulants
clotting factors
coagulation
extrinsic pathway
Hageman factor
hemorrhagic disorders
hemostatic drugs
intrinsic pathway
plasminogen
platelet aggregation
thromboembolic disorders
thrombolytic drugs

646

Anticoagulants

Antiplatelet Drugs
abciximab
anagrelide
asp **Ⓟ**
cilostazol
clopidogrel
dipyridamole
eptifibatide
sulfinpyrazone
ticlopidine
tirofiban

Anticoagulants
antithrombin
argatroban
bivalirudin
Ⓟ heparin
warfarin
Low-Molecular-Weight Heparins
dalteparin
danaparoid
Ⓟ enoxaparin
tinzaparin
Anticoagulant Adjunctive Therapy
lepirudin

Ⓟ protamine sulfate
vitamin K
Hemorheologic Agent
pentoxifylline
Thrombolytic Agents
alteplase
anistreplase
reteplase
Ⓟ streptokinase
tenecteplase
urokinase

Drugs Used to Control Bleeding

Antihemophilic Agents
Ⓟ antihemophilic factor
coagulation factor VIIa
factor IX complex
Systemic Hemostatic Agents
Ⓟ aminocaproic acid
aprotinin
Topical Hemostatic Agents
Ⓟ absorbable gelatin
microfibrillar collagen
thrombin

The cardiovascular system is a closed system, and blood remains in a fluid state while in it. Because the blood is trapped in a closed space, it maintains the difference in pressures required to keep the system moving along. If the vascular system is injured—from a cut, a puncture, or capillary destruction—the fluid blood could leak out, causing the system to lose pressure and potentially to shut down entirely.

To deal with the problem of blood leaking and potentially shutting down the system, blood that is exposed to an injury in a vessel almost immediately forms into a solid state, or clot, which plugs the hole in the system and keeps the required pressure differences intact. These little injuries to the blood vessels occur all the time (eg, coughing too hard with a cold, knocking into the corner of the desk when sitting down). Consequently, the system must maintain an intricate balance between the tendency to clot or form a solid state, called **coagulation,** and the need to "unclot" or reverse coagulation to keep the vessels open and the blood flowing. When a great deal of vascular damage occurs, such as with a major cut or incision, the balance in the area shifts to a procoagulation mode and a large clot is formed. At the same time, the enzymes in the plasma work to dissolve this clot before blood flow to tissues is lost, with resultant hypoxia and potential cell death.

Drugs that affect blood coagulation work at various steps in the blood clotting and clot-dissolving processes to restore the balance that is needed to maintain the cardiovascular system.

BLOOD COAGULATION

Blood coagulation is a complex process that involves vasoconstriction, platelet clumping or aggregation, and a cascade

of **clotting factors** produced in the liver that eventually react to break down fibrinogen (a protein also produced in the liver) into fibrin threads. When a clot is formed, plasmin (another blood protein) acts to break it down. Blood coagulation can be affected at any step in this complicated process to alter the way that blood clotting occurs.

Vasoconstriction

The first reaction to a blood vessel injury is local vasoconstriction (Figure 48–1). If the injury to the blood vessel is very small, this vasoconstriction can seal off any break and allow the area to heal.

Platelet Aggregation

Injury to a blood vessel exposes blood to the collagen and other substances under the endothelial lining of the vessel. This exposure causes platelets in the circulating blood to stick or adhere to the site of the injury. Once they stick, the platelets release adenosine diphosphate (ADP) and other chemicals that attract other platelets, causing them to gather or aggregate and to stick as well. ADP is also a precursor of the prostaglandins, from which thromboxane A_2 is formed. Thromboxane A_2 causes local vasoconstriction and further **platelet aggregation** and adhesion. This series of events forms a platelet plug at the site of the vessel injury. In many injuries, the combination of vasoconstriction and platelet aggregation is enough to seal off the injury and keep the cardiovascular system intact (Figure 48–2).

Intrinsic Pathway

As blood comes in contact with the exposed collagen of the injured blood vessel, one of the clotting factors, **Hageman**

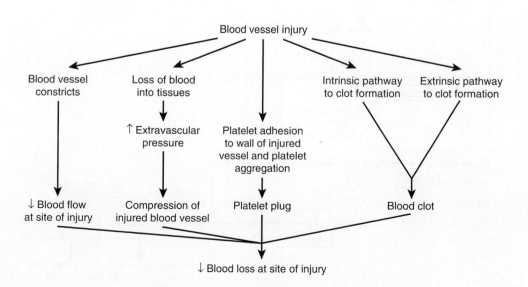

FIGURE 48-1. Process of blood coagulation.

FIGURE 48-2. *A.* Damaged vessel endothelium is a stimulus to circulating platelets, causing platelet adhesion. Platelets release mediators (*B*) and platelet aggregation results. (From Bullock, B. L. [2000]. *Focus on pathophysiology*. Philadelphia: Lippincott Williams & Wilkins.)

factor (also called factor XII), a chemical substance that is found circulating in the blood, is activated. (Clotting factors are often known by a name and by a Roman numeral. When one of these factors becomes activated, the lower-case letter a is added. Activated Hageman factor would also be called factor XIIa.) The activation of Hageman factor starts a number of reactions in the area: the clot formation process is activated, the clot-dissolving process is activated, and the inflammatory response is started (see Chapter 15). The activation of Hageman factor first activates clotting factor XI, then activates a cascading series of coagulant substances, called the **intrinsic pathway** (Figure 48–3), that ends with the conversion of prothrombin to thrombin. Activated thrombin breaks down fibrinogen to form fibrin threads, which form a clot inside the blood vessel. The clot, called a thrombus, acts to plug the injury and seal the system.

Extrinsic Pathway

While that coagulation process is going on inside the blood vessel, the blood that has leaked out of the vascular system and into the surrounding tissues is caused to clot by the **extrinsic pathway.** Injured cells release a substance called tissue thromboplastin, which activates clotting factors in the blood and starts the clotting cascade to form a clot on the outside of the blood vessel. The injured vessel is now vasoconstricted and has a platelet plug as well as a clot both on the inside and the outside of the blood vessel in the area of the injury. These actions maintain the closed nature of the cardiovascular system (see Figure 48–3).

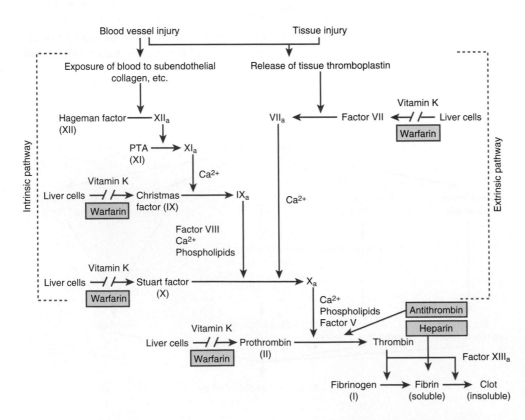

FIGURE 48-3. Details of the intrinsic and extrinsic clotting pathways. The sites of action of some of the drugs that can influence these processes are shown in blue.

CLOT RESOLUTION AND ANTICLOTTING

Blood plasma also contains anticlotting substances that inhibit clotting reactions that might otherwise lead to an obstruction of blood vessels by blood clots. For example, antithrombin III prevents the formation of thrombin, thus stopping the breakdown of the fibrin threads.

Another substance in the plasma, called plasmin or fibrinolysin, dissolves clots to ensure free movement of blood through the system. Plasmin is a protein-dissolving substance that breaks down the fibrin framework of blood clots and opens up vessels. Its precursor, called **plasminogen,** is found in the plasma. The conversion of plasminogen to plasmin begins with the activation of Hageman factor and is facilitated by a number of other factors, including antidiuretic hormone (ADH), epinephrine, pyrogens, emotional stress, physical activity, and the chemicals urokinase and streptokinase. Plasmin helps keep blood vessels open and functional. Very high levels of plasmin are found in the lungs (which contain millions of tiny, easily injured capillaries) and in the uterus (which in pregnancy must maintain a constant blood flow for the developing fetus). The action of plasmin is evident in the female menstrual flow in that clots do not form rapidly when the lining of the uterus is shed; the blood oozes slowly over a period of days (Figure 48–4).

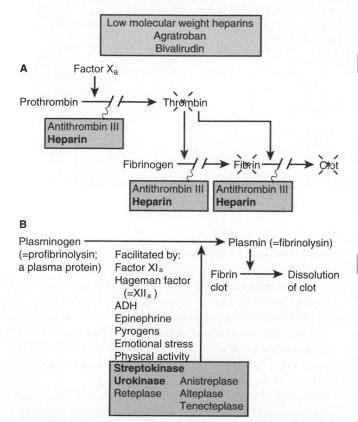

FIGURE 48–4. *A.* Anticlotting process: prevents clotting. Antithrombin III (in plasma) inhibits the activity of Stuart factor (factor Xa) and thrombin; the drug, heparin, enhances the activity of antithrombin III. Steps in clot formation that are inhibited by heparin are shown in red. *B.* Fibrinolytic process: clots are dissolved. The step that is facilitated by the clot-dissolving drugs and by other agents is shown in blue.

THROMBOEMBOLIC DISORDERS

Medical conditions that involve the formation of thrombi result in decreased blood flow through or total occlusion of a blood vessel. These conditions are marked by the signs and symptoms of hypoxia, anoxia, or even necrosis in areas affected by the decreased blood flow. In some of these disorders, pieces of the thrombus, called emboli, can break off and travel through the cardiovascular system until they become lodged in a tiny vessel, plugging it up.

Conditions that predispose a person to the formation of clots and emboli are called **thromboembolic disorders.** Coronary artery disease (CAD) involves a narrowing of the coronary arteries caused by damage to the endothelial lining of these vessels. Thrombi tend to form along the damaged endothelial lining. As the damage builds up, the lumen of the vessels become narrower and narrower. Over time, the coronary arteries are unable to deliver enough blood to meet the needs of the heart muscle, and hypoxia develops. If a vessel becomes so narrow that a tiny clot occludes it completely, the blood supply to that area is cut off and anoxia followed by infarction and necrosis occurs. With age, many of the vessels in the body can be damaged and develop similar problems with narrowing and blood delivery. These disorders are treated with drugs that interfere with the normal coagulation process to prevent the formation of clots in the system.

HEMORRHAGIC DISORDERS

Hemorrhagic disorders, in which excess bleeding occurs, are less common than thromboembolic disorders. These disorders include hemophilia, in which there is a genetic lack of clotting factors; liver disease, in which clotting factors and proteins needed for clotting are not produced; and bone marrow disorders, in which platelets are not formed in sufficient quantity to be effective. These disorders are treated with clotting factors and drugs that promote the coagulation process.

ANTICOAGULANTS

Anticoagulants are drugs that interfere with the normal coagulation process. They can affect the process at any step to slow or prevent clot formation. Antiplatelet drugs alter the formation of the platelet plug. Anticoagulants interfere with the clotting cascade and thrombin formation. **Thrombolytic drugs** break down the thrombus that has been formed by stimulating the plasmin system.

ANTIPLATELET DRUGS

Antiplatelet drugs decrease the formation of the platelet plug by decreasing the responsiveness of the platelets to stimuli

DRUG THERAPY ACROSS THE LIFESPAN

Drugs Affecting Coagulation

Children	Adults	Older Adults
Little research is available on the use of anticoagulants in children. If they are used, the child needs to be monitored very carefully to avoid excessive bleeding related to drug interactions or alterations in gastrointestinal or liver function. People who interact with the child need to understand the importance of preventing injuries and providing safety precautions and should be aware of what to do if the child is injured and begins to bleed.	Adults receiving these drugs need to be instructed in ways to prevent injury— such as using an electric razor instead of a straight razor, using a soft-bristled toothbrush to protect the gums, avoiding contact sports—and instructed in what to do if bleeding does occur (apply constant, firm pressure and contact a health care provider). They should receive a written list of signs of bleeding to watch for and to report to their health care provider.	Older adults may have many underlying medical conditions that require the need for drugs that alter blood clotting (e.g., coronary artery disease, cerebrovascular accident, peripheral vascular disease, transient ischemic attacks). Statistically, older adults also take more medications, making them more likely to encounter drug–drug interactions associated with these drugs. The older adult is also more likely to have impaired liver and kidney function, conditions that can alter the metabolism and excretion of these drugs.
If heparin is used, the dosage should be carefully calculated based on weight and age and checked by another person before the drug is administered.	Because so many drugs and alternative therapies are known to interact with these agents, it is very important that these patients be urged to report the use of this drug to any other health care provider and to consult with one before using any over-the-counter drugs or alternative therapies.	The older adult should be carefully evaluated for liver and kidney function, use of other medications, and ability to follow through with regular blood testing and medical evaluation before therapy begins. Therapy should be started at the lowest possible level and adjusted accordingly after the patient response has been noted.
Warfarin is used with children who are to undergo cardiac surgery. Again, the dosage must be determined based on weight and age and the child should be monitored closely.	It is prudent to advise any patient using one of these drugs in the home setting to carry or wear a Medic-Alert notification in case of emergency.	Careful attention needs to be given to the patient's total drug regimen. Starting, stopping, or changing the dosage of another drug may alter the body's metabolism of the drug that is being used to affect coagulation, leading to increased risk of bleeding or ineffective anticoagulation.
The safety of low-molecular-weight heparins has not been established in children.	The patient also needs to understand the importance of regular, periodic blood tests to evaluate the effects of the drug.	
At this time, there are no indications for the use of antiplatelet or thrombolytic drugs with children.	Because of the many risks associated with increased bleeding or increased blood clotting during pregnancy, these drugs should not be used during pregnancy unless the benefit to the mother clearly outweighs the potential risk to the fetus and to the mother at delivery. Risks of altered blood clotting in the neonate makes these drugs generally unadvisable for use during lactation.	

that would cause them to stick and aggregate on a vessel wall. These drugs are used effectively to treat cardiovascular diseases that are prone to produce occluded vessels; for the maintenance of venous and arterial grafts; to prevent cerebrovascular occlusion; and as adjuncts to thrombolytic therapy in the treatment of myocardial infarction and the prevention of reinfarction. The prescriber's choice of drug depends on the intended use and the patient's tolerance of the associated adverse effects.

Antiplatelet drugs that are available for use include the following.

- Abciximab (*ReoPro*), an intravenous drug that is used in conjunction with heparin and aspirin to prevent acute cardiac events during transluminal coronary angioplasty
- Anagrelide (*Agrylin*), an oral drug that is used to treat es-

sential thrombocytopenia to reduce elevated platelet counts and decrease the risk of thrombosis. This drug works to decrease the bone marrow production of platelets, so patients need to have their platelet count monitored regularly.
- Aspirin (generic), an oral drug shown to be effective in decreasing the incidence of transient ischemic attacks and strokes in men and in reducing the risk of death or nonfatal myocardial infarction (MI) in patients with a past history of MI or with angina
- Cilostazol (*Pletal*), an oral drug that is indicated for the reduction of symptoms of intermittent claudication, allowing increased walking distance
- Clopidogrel (*Plavix*), an oral drug used in patients who are at risk for ischemic events and in those with a history of MI, peripheral artery disease, or ischemic stroke
- Dipyridamole (*Persantine*), which is used orally in combi-

nation with warfarin to prevent thromboembolism in patients with artificial heart valves, and is used intravenously to aid diagnosis of CAD in patients who cannot exercise. This drug was used for long-term treatment of angina, but was found to be only "possibly effective" by the U. S. Food and Drug Administration.
- Eptifibatide (*Integrilin*), an intravenous drug that is used to treat acute coronary syndrome and to prevent ischemic episodes in patients undergoing percutaneous coronary interventions
- Sulfinpyrazone (*Anturane*), an oral drug that is also an antigout agent, used to prevent reinfarction after MI and to decrease the incidence of systemic emboli in patients with rheumatic mitral stenosis

- Ticlopidine (*Ticlid*), an oral drug used in patients who are intolerant to aspirin therapy to decrease the risk of thrombotic stroke in patients with transient ischemic attacks or history of stroke
- Tirofiban (*Aggrastat*), an intravenous drug, used in combination with heparin to treat acute coronary syndrome and prevent cardiac ischemic events during percutaneous coronary intervention

Therapeutic Actions and Indications
The antiplatelet drugs inhibit platelet adhesion and aggregation by blocking receptor sites on the platelet membrane, preventing platelet–platelet interaction or the interaction of platelets with other clotting chemicals. One drug, anagrelide,

DRUGS IN FOCUS
Antiplatelet Drugs

Drug Name	Usual Dosage	Usual Indications
abciximab (*ReoPro*)	0.25 mg/kg IV bolus 10–60 min before procedure, then continuous infusion of 0.125 μg/kg per minute	In conjunction with heparin and aspirin to prevent acute cardiac events during transluminal coronary angioplasty
Anagrelide (*Agrylin*)	0.5 mg PO q.i.d. or 1 mg PO b.i.d., may increase by 0.5 mg/d each week; maximum dose—10 mg/d or 2.5 mg as a single dose	Treatment of essential thrombocytopenia to reduce elevated platelet count and the risk of thrombosis
aspirin (generic)	1300 mg/d PO to decrease TIAs; 300–325 mg/d PO to reduce MI risk	Reduction of the incidence of transient ischemic attacks (TIAs) and strokes in men and reduction of the risk of death or nonfatal myocardial infarction (MI) in patients with a past history of MI or with angina
cilostazol (*Pletal*)	100 mg PO b.i.d. taken ≥ 30 min before or 2h after breakfast and dinner	Reduction of symptoms of intermittent claudication, allowing increased walking distance in adults
clopidogrel (*Plavix*)	75 mg/d PO	Treatment of patients who are at risk for ischemic events and patients with a history of MI, peripheral artery disease, or ischemic stroke
dipyridamole (*Persantine*)	50 mg PO t.i.d. for angina; 75–100 mg PO q.i.d. for heart valve patients; 0.142 mg/kg per minute IV over 4 min for diagnosis	In combination with warfarin to prevent thromboembolism in patients with artificial heart valves; diagnosis of coronary artery disease in patients who cannot exercise; treatment of angina
eptifibatide (*Integrelin*)	180 μg/kg IV over 1–2 min then 2 μg/kg per minute IV for up to 72 h for acute coronary syndrome; 135 μg/kg IV bolus before procedure, then 0.5 μg/kg/min IV for 20–24 h	Treatment of acute coronary syndrome; prevention of schemic episodes in patients undergoing percutaneous coronary interventions
sulfinpyrazone (*Anturane*)	200 mg PO t.i.d. or q.i.d.	Prevention of reinfarction after MI; reduction of incidence of systemic emboli in patients with rheumatic mitral stenosis
ticlopidine (*Ticlid*)	200–400 mg/d in 2 divided doses	Reduction of the risk of thrombotic stroke in patients with TIAs or history of stroke who are intolerant to aspirin therapy
tirofiban (*Aggrastat*)	0.4 μg/kg per minute IV over 30 min, then continuous infusion of 0.1 μg/kg per minute	In combination with heparin to treat acute coronary syndrome and prevent cardiac ischemic events during percutaneous coronary intervention

blocks the production of platelets in the bone marrow. These drugs are used to decrease the risk of fatal MI, to prevent re-infarction after MI, to prevent thromboembolic stroke, and to maintain the patency of grafts; in addition, an unlabeled use is the treatment of other thromboembolic disorders.

Pharmacokinetics

These drugs are generally well absorbed and highly bound to plasma proteins. They are metabolized in the liver and excreted in the urine. There are no adequate studies of these drugs in pregnancy, but, because of the potential for increased bleeding, they should be used during pregnancy only if the benefits to the mother clearly outweigh the potential risks to the fetus. These drugs tend to enter breast milk. If they are needed by a lactating mother, a decision should be made to find another method of feeding the baby.

Contraindications and Cautions

Antiplatelet drugs are contraindicated in the presence of allergy to the specific drug and also with pregnancy or lactation, because of the potential adverse effects on the fetus or neonate. Caution should be used in the following conditions: the presence of any known bleeding disorder, because of the risk of excessive blood loss; recent surgery, because of the risk of increased bleeding in unhealed vessels; and closed head injuries, because of the risk of bleeding from the injured vessels in the brain.

Adverse Effects

The most common adverse effect seen with these drugs is bleeding, which often occurs as increased bruising and bleeding while brushing the teeth. Other common problems include headache, dizziness, and weakness; the cause of these reactions is not understood. Nausea and gastrointestinal (GI) distress may occur because of direct irritating effects of the oral drug on the GI tract. Skin rash, another common effect, may be related to direct drug effects on the dermis.

Clinically Important Drug–Drug Interactions

There is an increased risk of excessive bleeding if any of these drugs is combined with another drug that affects blood clotting.

Nursing Considerations for Patients Receiving Antiplatelet Drugs

Assessment: History and Examination

Screen for the following conditions, which could be cautions or contraindications to use of the drug: any known allergies to these drugs; pregnancy or lactation, because of the potential adverse effects on the fetus or neonate; and bleeding disorders, recent surgery, or closed head injury, because of the potential for excessive bleeding.

Include screening for baseline status before beginning therapy and for any potential adverse effects: body temperature; skin color, lesions, temperature; affect, orientation, reflexes; pulse, blood pressure, perfusion; respirations, adventitious sounds; complete blood count (CBC) and clotting studies.

Nursing Diagnoses

The patient receiving antiplatelet drugs may have the following nursing diagnoses related to drug therapy

- Risk for Injury related to bleeding effects, CNS effects
- Acute Pain related to GI, CNS effects
- Deficient Knowledge regarding drug therapy

Implementation

- Provide small, frequent meals *to relieve GI discomfort* if GI upset is a problem.
- Provide comfort measures and analgesia for headache, *to relieve pain and improve patient compliance to the drug regimen.*
- Suggest safety measures, including the use of an electric razor and avoidance of contact sports, *to decrease the risk of bleeding.*
- Provide increased precautions against bleeding during invasive procedures; use pressure dressings and ice *to decrease excessive blood loss caused by anticoagulation.*
- Mark the chart of any patient receiving this drug, *to alert medical staff that there is a potential for increased bleeding.*
- Provide thorough patient teaching, including the name of the drug, dosage prescribed, measures to avoid adverse effects, warning signs of problems, the need for periodic monitoring and evaluation, and the need to wear or carry a Medic-Alert notification, *to enhance patient knowledge about drug therapy and to promote compliance with the drug regimen.*
- Offer support and encouragement, *to help the patient deal with the diagnosis and the drug regimen.*

Evaluation

- Monitor patient response to the drug (increased bleeding time, prevention of occlusive events).
- Monitor for adverse effects (bleeding, GI upset, dizziness, headache).
- Evaluate the effectiveness of the teaching plan (patient can name drug, dosage, adverse effects to watch for, specific measures to avoid adverse effects; patient understands importance of continued follow-up).
- Monitor the effectiveness of comfort measures and compliance to the regimen.

ANTICOAGULANTS

Anticoagulants interfere with the coagulation process by interfering with the clotting cascade and thrombin formation. Drugs in this class include warfarin, heparin, and antithrombin. These drugs can be used orally (warfarin) or parenterally (heparin and antithrombin).

- Warfarin (*Coumadin*), an oral drug, is used to maintain a state of anticoagulation in situations in which the patient is susceptible to potentially dangerous clot formation. Warfarin works by interfering with the formation of vitamin K–dependent clotting factors in the liver. The eventual effect is a depletion of these clotting factors and a prolongation of clotting times. Warfarin is readily absorbed through the GI tract, metabolized in the liver, and excreted in urine and feces. Warfarin's onset of action is about 3 days; its effects last for 4 to 5 days. Because of the time delay, warfarin is not the drug of choice in an acute situation, but it is convenient and useful for prolonged effects (Box 48–1). It is used to treat patients with atrial fibrillation, artificial heart valves, or valvular damage that makes them susceptible to thrombus and embolus formation. It also is used to treat and prevent venous thrombosis and embolization after acute MI or pulmonary embolism. It is not used during pregnancy or lactation because of the risk of bleeding complications for the mother and the fetus or baby.
- Heparin (generic) is a naturally occurring substance that inhibits the conversion of prothrombin to thrombin, thus blocking the conversion of fibrinogen to fibrin—the final step in clot formation. It is injected intravenously or subcutaneously and has an almost immediate onset of action. It is excreted in the urine. Heparin does not cross the placenta (although some adverse fetal effects have been reported when it is used during pregnancy) and does not enter breast milk, so it would be the anticoagulant of choice if one is needed during lactation. Its usual indications include acute treatment and prevention of venous thrombosis and pulmonary embolism; treatment of atrial fibrillation with embolization; prevention of clotting in blood samples and in dialysis and venous tubing; and diagnosis and treatment of disseminated intravascular coagulation (DIC). It is also used as an adjunct in the treatment of MI and stroke. Because heparin must be injected, it is often not the drug of choice for outpatients, who would be responsible for injecting the drug several times during the day. Patients may be started on heparin in the acute situation, then switched to the oral drug warfarin (Boxes 48–2 and 48–3).
- Antithrombin (*Thrombate III*) is a naturally occurring anticoagulant. The body handles it like it handles naturally occurring antithrombin. It has been used without reported adverse effects during pregnancy and lactation. It is given intravenously to patients with hereditary antithrombin III deficiencies who are undergoing surgery or obstetrical pro-

BOX 48-2

Protamine Sulfate: Antidote for Heparin Overdose

The antidote for heparin overdose is protamine sulfate (generic). This strongly basic protein drug forms stable salts with heparin as soon as the two drugs come in contact, immediately reversing heparin's anticoagulant effects. Paradoxically, if protamine is given to a patient who has not received heparin, it has anticoagulant effects.

The dosage of protamine that is used is determined by the amount of heparin that has been given and the time that has elapsed since the drug was administered. A dose of 1 mg IV protamine neutralizes 90 USP of heparin derived from lung tissue or 110 USP of heparin derived from intestinal mucosa. The drug must be administered very slowly, not to exceed 50 mg intravenously in any 10-minute period. Care must be taken to calculate the amount of heparin that has been given to the patient. Potentially fatal anaphylactic reactions have been reported with the use of protamine sulfate, so life support equipment should be readily available when it is used.

BOX 48-1

Vitamin K: Reversing Warfarin's Effects

Phytonadione (*AquaMEPHYTON*), a form of vitamin K, is used to reverse the effects of warfarin. Vitamin K is responsible for promoting the liver synthesis of several clotting factors. When these pathways have been inhibited by warfarin, clotting time is increased. If an increased level of vitamin K is provided, more of these factors are produced, and the clotting time can be brought back within a normal range.

Because of the way that vitamin K exerts its effects on clotting, there is at least a 24-hour delay from the time the drug is given until some change can be seen. This occurs because there is no direct effect on the warfarin itself, but rather an increased stimulation of the liver, which must then produce the clotting factors. The usual dosage for the treatment of anticoagulant-induced prothrombin (PT) deficiency is 2.5 to 10 mg IM or SC, or (rarely) 25 mg IM or SC. Oral doses can be used if injection is not feasible. A PT response within 6 to 8 hours after parenteral doses or 12 to 48 hours after oral doses will determine the need for a repeat dose. If a response is not seen and the patient is bleeding excessively, fresh-frozen plasma or an infusion of whole blood may be needed.

BOX 48-3

Lepirudin: Treating Heparin Allergy

Lepirudin (*Refludan*) is an intravenous drug that was developed to treat a rare allergic reaction to heparin. In some patients, an allergy to heparin precipitates a heparin-induced thrombocytopenia with associated thromboembolic disease. Lepirudin directly inhibits thrombin, blocking the thromboembolic effects of this reaction. A 0.4 mg/kg initial IV bolus followed by a continuous infusion of 0.15 mg/kg for 2 to 10 days is the recommended treatment. The patient needs to be monitored closely for bleeding from any sites and for the development of direct hepatic injury.

cedures that might put them at risk for thromboembolism. It also is used for replacement therapy in congenital antithrombin III deficiency.

- Argatroban (*Acova*) is an intravenous thrombin-inhibiting drug that is used to treat thrombosis in heparin-induced thrombocytopenia.
- Bivalirudin (*Angiomax*), an intravenous drug that inhibits thrombin, is used with aspirin to prevent ischemic events in patients undergoing transluminal coronary angioplasty.

Therapeutic Actions and Indications

As noted previously, the anticoagulants interfere with the normal cascade of events involved in the clotting process. Warfarin causes a decrease in the production of vitamin K–dependent clotting factors in the liver. Heparin, argatroban, and bivalirudin block the formation of thrombin from prothrombin. Antithrombin interferes with the formation of thrombin from prothrombin. These drugs are used to treat thromboembolic disorders such as atrial fibrillation, MI, pulmonary embolus, and evolving stroke and to prevent the formation of thrombi in such disorders.

Contraindications and Cautions

The anticoagulants are contraindicated in the presence of known allergy to the drugs. They also should not be used with any conditions that could be compromised by increased bleeding tendencies, including hemorrhagic disorders, recent trauma, spinal puncture, GI ulcers, recent surgery, intrauterine device placement, tuberculosis, presence of indwelling catheters, and threatened abortion. In addition, anticoagulants are contraindicated in pregnancy (fetal injury and death have occurred); lactation (use of heparin is suggested if an anticoagulant is needed during lactation); and renal or hepatic disease, which could interfere with the metabolism and effectiveness of these drugs.

Caution should be used in patients with congestive heart failure (CHF), thyrotoxicosis, senility, or psychosis (because of the potential for unexpected effects), and in those with diarrhea or fever, which could alter the normal clotting process by, respectively, loss of vitamin K from the intestine or activation of plasminogen.

Adverse Effects

The most commonly encountered adverse effect of the anticoagulants is bleeding, ranging from bleeding gums with tooth brushing to severe internal hemorrhage. Clotting times should be monitored closely to avoid these problems. Nausea, GI upset, diarrhea, and hepatic dysfunction also may occur secondary to direct drug toxicity. Warfarin has been associated with alopecia and dermatitis as well as bone marrow depression and, less frequently, prolonged and painful erections.

Clinically Important Drug–Drug Interactions

Increased bleeding can occur if heparin is combined with oral anticoagulants, salicylates, penicillins, or cephalosporins. Decreased anticoagulation can occur if heparin is combined with nitroglycerin.

TABLE 48–1 Clinically Important Drug–Drug Interactions with Warfarin

↑ Bleeding effects	↓ Anticoagulation	↑ Activity and Effects of Other Drug
salicylates	barbiturates	phenytoin
chloral hydrate	griseofulvin	
phenylbutazone	rifampin	
clofibrate	phenytoin	
disulfiram	glutethimide	
chloramphenicol	carbamazepine	
metronidazole	vitamin k	
cimetidine	vitamin e	
ranitidine	cholestyramine	
cotrimoxazole	aminoglutethimide	
sulfinpyrazone	ethchlorvynol	
quinidine		
quinine		
oxyphenbutazone		
thyroid drugs		
glucagon		
danazol		
erythromycin		
androgens		
amiodarone		
cefamandole		
cefoperazone		
cefotetan		
moxalactam		
cefazolin		
cefoxitin		
ceftriaxone		
meclofenamate		
mefenamic acid		
famotidine		
nizatidine		
nalidixic acid		

Warfarin has documented drug–drug interactions with a vast number of other drugs (Table 48–1). It is a wise practice never to add or take away a drug from the drug regimen of a patient receiving warfarin without careful patient monitoring and adjustment of the warfarin dosage to prevent serious adverse effects.

Nursing Considerations for Patients Receiving Anticoagulants

Assessment: History and Examination

Screen for any known allergies to these drugs. Also screen for conditions that could be exacerbated by increased bleeding tendencies, including hemorrhagic disorders, recent trauma, spinal puncture, GI ulcers, recent surgery, intrauterine device placement, tuberculosis, presence of indwelling catheters,

DRUGS IN FOCUS
Anticoagulants

Drug Name	Usual Dosage	Usual Indications
antithrombin (*Thrombate III*)	Dosage must be calculated from body weight and baseline levels, given q2–8d	Replacement in antithrombin III deficiency; treatment of patients with this deficiency who are to undergo surgery or obstetrical procedures
argatroban (*Acova*)	2 µg/kg per minute IV until the desired effect is seen, then adjust dosage	Treatment of thrombosis in heparin-induced thrombocytopenia
bivalirudin (*Angiomax*)	1 mg/kg IV bolus, then 2.5 mg/kg per hour IV for 4 h and 0.2 mg/kg per hour IV as a low-dose infusion	With aspirin to prevent ischemic events in patients undergoing transluminal coronary angioplasty
Ⓟ heparin (generic)	10,000–20,000 U SC, then 8,000–10,000 U q8h; 5,000–10,000 U IV q4–6h Pediatric: 50 U/kg IV bolus, then 100 U/kg IV q4h	Prevention and treatment of venous thrombosis, pulmonary embolus, clotting in blood samples and venous lines; diagnosis and treatment of disseminated intravascular coagulation
warfarin (*Coumadin*)	2–5 mg/d PO, then 2–10 mg/d PO based on prothrombin time (PT) or PT/INR ratio, use lower doses with geriatric patients	Prevention and treatment of venous thrombosis, pulmonary embolus, embolus with atrial fibrillation, systemic emboli after myocardial infarction

threatened abortion, pregnancy (fetal injury and death have occurred); lactation (use of heparin is suggested if an anticoagulant is needed during lactation); renal or hepatic disease, which could interfere with the metabolism and effectiveness of these drugs; CHF; thyrotoxicosis; senility or psychosis, because of the potential for unexpected effects; and diarrhea or fever, which could alter the normal clotting process.

Include screening for baseline status before beginning therapy and for any potential adverse effects. Assess the following: body temperature; skin color, lesions, temperature; affect, orientation, reflexes; pulse, blood pressure, perfusion; respirations, adventitious sounds; clotting studies, renal and hepatic function tests, CBC, and stool guaiac; electrocardiogram (ECG) if appropriate.

Nursing Diagnoses

The patient receiving an anticoagulant may have the following nursing diagnoses related to drug therapy:

- Risk for Injury related to bleeding effects, bone marrow depression
- Disturbed Body Image related to alopecia, skin rash
- Ineffective Tissue Perfusion (Total Body) related to blood loss
- Deficient Knowledge regarding drug therapy

Implementation

- Evaluate for therapeutic effects of warfarin—prothrombin time (PT) 1.5 to 2.5 times the control value or ratio of PT to INR (international normalized ratio) of 2 to 3—*to evaluate the effectiveness of the drug dose.*

- Evaluate for therapeutic effects of heparin—whole blood clotting time (WBCT) 2.5 to 3 times control or activated partial thromboplastin time (APTT) 1.5 to 3 times control value—*to evaluate the effectiveness of the drug dose.*
- Evaluate the patient regularly for any sign of blood loss—petechiae, bleeding gums, bruises, dark-colored stools, dark-colored urine—*to evaluate the effectiveness of the drug dose and to consult with the prescriber if bleeding becomes apparent.*
- Establish safety precautions, *to protect the patient from injury.*
- Provide safety measures, such as use of an electric razor and avoidance of contact sports, *to decrease the risk of bleeding.*
- Provide increased precautions against bleeding during invasive procedures; use pressure dressings; avoid intramuscular injections; and do not rub subcutaneous injection sites, *because the state of anticoagulation increases the risk of blood loss.*
- Mark the chart of any patient receiving this drug, *to alert the medical staff that there is a potential for increased bleeding.*
- Maintain antidotes on standby (protamine sulfate for heparin, vitamin K for warfarin), *in case of overdose.*
- Monitor the patient carefully when any drug is added to or withdrawn from the drug regimen of a patient taking warfarin, *because of the risk of drug–drug interactions that would change the effectiveness of the anticoagulant.*
- Make sure that the patient receives regular follow-up and monitoring, including measurement of clotting times, *to ensure maximum therapeutic effects.*

- Provide thorough patient teaching, including the name of the drug, dosage prescribed, measures to avoid adverse effects, warning signs of problems, the need for periodic monitoring and evaluation, and the need to wear or carry a Medic-Alert notification, *to enhance patient knowledge about drug therapy and to promote compliance with the drug regimen.* (See Patient Teaching Checklist: Oral Anticoagulants.)
- Offer support and encouragement, *to help the patient deal with the diagnosis and the drug regimen.*

PATIENT TEACHING CHECKLIST
Oral Anticoagulants

Create customized patient teaching materials for a specific oral anticoagulant from the CD-ROM. Patient teaching should stress the following points for drugs within this class:

- An anticoagulant slows the body's normal blood clotting processes to prevent harmful blood clots from forming. This type of drug is often called a "blood thinner"; however, it cannot dissolve any clots that have already formed.
- *Never* change any medication that you are taking—such as adding or stopping another drug, taking a new over-the-counter medication, or stopping one that you have been taking regularly—without consulting with your health care provider. Many other drugs affect the way that your anticoagulant works; starting or stopping another drug can cause excessive bleeding or interfere with the desired effects of the drug.

Some of the following adverse effects may occur:

- *Stomach bloating, cramps*—These problems often pass with time; consult your health care provider if they persist or become too uncomfortable.
- *Loss of hair, skin rash*—These problems can be very frustrating; you may wish to discuss these with your health care provider.
- *Orange-yellow discoloration of the urine*—This can be frightening, but it may just be an effect of the drug. If you are concerned that this might be blood, simply add vinegar to your urine; the color should disappear. If the color does not disappear, it may be caused by blood and you should contact your health care provider.

Report any of the following to your health care provider: unusual bleeding (when brushing your teeth, excessive bleeding from an injury, excessive bruising); black or tarry stools; cloudy or dark urine; sore throat, fever, or chills; severe headache or dizziness.

Tell any doctor, nurse, or other health care provider that you are taking this drug. You should carry or wear a Medic-Alert bracelet stating that you are taking this drug, to alert emergency medical personnel that you are at increased risk for bleeding.

It is important to avoid situations in which you could be easily injured—for example, engaging in contact sports or using a straight razor.

Keep this drug, and all medications, out of the reach of children.

Avoid the use of over-the-counter medications while you are taking this drug. If you feel that you need one of these, consult with your health care provider for the best choice. Many of these drugs can interfere with your anticoagulant.

PATIENT TEACHING CHECKLIST
(CONTINUED)
Oral Anticoagulants

You will need to have regular, periodic blood tests while you are taking this drug to monitor the effects of the drug on your body and adjust your dosage as needed.

This Teaching Checklist reflects general patient teaching guidelines. It is not meant to be a substitute for drug-specific teaching information, which is available in nursing drug guides.

Evaluation

- Monitor patient response to the drug: increased bleeding time (warfarin, PT 1.5 to 2.5 times the control value or PT/INR ratio of 2 to 3; heparin, WBCT of 2.5 to 3 times the control value or APTT of 1.5 to 3 times control).
- Monitor for adverse effects (bleeding, bone marrow depression, alopecia, GI upset, rash).
- Evaluate the effectiveness of the teaching plan (patient can name drug, dosage, adverse effects to watch for, specific measures to avoid adverse effects; patient understands importance of continued follow-up).
- Monitor the effectiveness of comfort measures and compliance to the regimen (see Nursing Care Guide: Oral Anticoagulants).

LOW-MOLECULAR-WEIGHT HEPARINS

In the late 1990s, a series of low-molecular-weight heparins were developed. These drugs inhibit thrombus and clot formation by blocking factors Xa and IIa. Because of the size and nature of their molecules, these drugs do not greatly affect thrombin, clotting, or prothrombin times. Therefore, they cause fewer systemic adverse effects. These drugs are indicated for very specific uses in the prevention of clots and emboli formation after certain surgeries or prolonged bed rest; however, each of these drugs is being studied for use after additional types of surgery (Box 48–4). The nursing care of a patient receiving one of these drugs is similar to the care of a patient receiving heparin. The drug is given just before (or just after) the surgery, then is continued for 7 to 10 days during the postoperative recovery process. Caution must be used to avoid combining these drugs with standard heparin therapy, serious bleeding episodes and deaths have been reported when this combination was inadvertently used.

THROMBOLYTIC AGENTS

If a thrombus has already formed in a vessel (eg, during an acute MI), it may be necessary to dissolve that clot to open

NURSING CARE GUIDE

Oral Anticoagulants

Assessment	Nursing Diagnoses	Implementation	Evaluation
HISTORY Allergies to any of these drugs, renal or hepatic dysfunction, pregnancy, lactation, gastric ulcers, tuberculosis, indwelling catheters	Ineffective Tissue Perfusion (Total Body) related to alteration in clotting effects Risk for Injury related to anticoagulant effects Disturbed Body Image related to alopecia, skin rash Deficient Knowledge regarding drug therapy	Ensure proper administration of drug. Provide comfort and safety measures: - Give small meals - Provide protection from injury - Provide safety measures with invasive procedures - Institute bowel program as needed - Have antidote on standby (vitamin K) - Provide skin care Provide support and reassurance to deal with drug effects. Provide patient teaching regarding drug, dosage, adverse effects, what to report, safety precautions.	Evaluate drug effects: increased bleeding times, PT 1.5–2.5 times control or PT/INF ratio of 2–3. Monitor for adverse effects: bleeding, alopecia, rash, GI upset, excessive bleeding. Monitor for drug–drug interactions (numerous). Evaluate effectiveness of patient teaching program. Evaluate effectiveness of comfort and safety measures.
PHYSICAL EXAMINATION CV: BP, P, perfusion, baseline ECG CNS: orientation, affect, reflexes, vision Skin: color, lesions, texture Resp: R, adventitious sounds GI: abdominal exam, stool guaiac Lab tests: liver and renal function tests, prothrombin time (PT), INF ratio			

up the vessel and restore blood flow to the dependent tissue. All of the drugs that are available for this purpose work to activate the natural anticlotting system, conversion of plasminogen to plasmin. The activation of this system breaks down fibrin threads and dissolves any formed clot. The thrombolytic drugs are effective only if the patient has plasminogen in the plasma. Thrombolytic agents include the following:

- Alteplase (*Activase*), used for treatment of MI, acute pulmonary embolism, and acute ischemic stroke. It is given intravenously, and the patient needs to be monitored closely for bleeding.
- Anistreplase (*Eminase*), used in the management of acute MI to reduce infarct size and complications. It is given intravenously, and the patient needs to be monitored closely for cardiac arrhythmias.

- Reteplase (*Retavase*), given intravenously the treatment of coronary artery thrombosis associated with an acute MI
- Streptokinase (*Streptase, Kabikinase*), used intravenously to treat coronary artery thrombosis, pulmonary embolism, deep venous thrombosis, and arterial thrombosis or embolism, and to open an occluded atrioventricular cannula.
- Tenecteplase (*TNKase*), given intravenously to reduce mortality associated with acute MI. Timing of administration is critical to success of therapy.
- Urokinase (*Abbokinase*), used intravenously to lyse pulmonary emboli, to treat coronary thrombosis, and to clear occluded intravenous catheters.

Box 48–5 discusses pentoxifylline, a hemorheologic agent. Box 48–6 discusses drotrecogin alfa, a drug that affects coagulation and was recently approved for the treatment of severe sepsis.

BOX 48-4

Specific Factor Xa Inhibitor to Prevent Deep Venous Thrombosis

Fondaparinux (*Arixtra*), a specific blocker of factor Xa, was approved in 2002 for the prevention of venous thromboembolic events in patients undergoing surgery for hip fracture, hip replacement, or knee replacement. The usual dosage of fondaparinux is 2.5 mg/d SC starting 6–8 h after surgical closure and continuing for 5–9 d. It is supplied in prefilled syringes, making it convenient for patients who will be self-administering the drug at home. As with other drugs that affect coagulation, bleeding is the most common and potentially the most serious adverse effect that can occur with the use of this drug. Patients need teaching about administration, disposal of the syringes and signs of bleeding to watch for. Periodic blood tests will be needed to assess the effects of the drug on the body.

Therapeutic Actions and Indications

The thrombolytic agents work by activating plasminogen to plasmin, which in turn breaks down fibrin threads in a clot to dissolve a formed clot. They are indicated for the treatment of acute MI (to dissolve the clot and prevent further tissue damage, if used within 6 hours after the onset of symptoms); to treat pulmonary emboli and ischemic stroke; and to open clotted intravenous catheters.

Pharmacokinetics

These drugs must be injected and are cleared from the body after liver metabolism. They cross the placenta and have been associated with adverse fetal effects. These drugs should not be used during pregnancy unless the benefits to the mother clearly outweigh the potential risks to the fetus. It is not known whether these drugs enter breast milk. Caution should be used during lactation because of the potential risk for bleeding effects.

Contraindications and Cautions

The use of thrombolytic agents is contraindicated in the presence of allergy to any of these drugs. They also should not be used with any condition that could be worsened by the dissolution of clots, including recent surgery, active internal bleeding, cerebrovascular accident (CVA) within the last 2 months, aneurysm, obstetrical delivery, organ biopsy, recent serious GI bleeding, rupture of a noncompressible blood vessel, recent major trauma (including cardiopulmonary resuscitation), known blood clotting defects, cerebrovascular disease, uncontrolled hypertension, liver disease (which could affect normal clotting factors and the production of plas-

C A S E   S T U D Y

Using Oral Anticoagulants to Protect Against Emboli

THE SITUATION

G. R. is a 68-year-old woman with a history of severe mitral valvular disease. For the last several years, she has been able to manage her condition with digoxin, a diuretic, and a potassium supplement. However, a recent visit to her physician revealed that she had been experiencing periods of breathlessness, palpitations, and dizziness. Tests showed that G. R. was having frequent periods of atrial fibrillation (AF), with a heart rate of up to 140 beats/min. Because of the danger of emboli as a result of her valvular disease and the bouts of AF, warfarin therapy was begun.

CRITICAL THINKING

• What nursing interventions should be done at this point?
• Why do people with mitral valve disease frequently develop AF? *Think about why emboli form when the atria fibrillate.*
• *Stabilizing G. R. on warfarin may take several weeks of blood tests and dosage adjustments.* How can this process be made easier?
• What patient teaching points should be covered with G. R. to ensure that she is protected from emboli and does not experience excessive bleeding?

DISCUSSION

G. R.'s situation is complex. She has a progressive degenerative valve disease that usually leads to

congestive heart failure (CHF), and frequently to other complications such as AF and emboli formation. Her digoxin and potassium levels should be checked to determine whether her CHF is stabilized or the digoxin is causing the AF because of excessive doses or potassium imbalance. If these tests are within normal limits, G. R. may be experiencing AF because of irritation to the atrial cells caused by the damaged mitral valve and associated swelling and scarring. If this is the case, an anticoagulant will help protect G. R. against emboli, which form in the auricles when blood pools there while the atria are fibrillating. There is less chance of emboli formation if clotting is slowed.

G. R. will need extensive teaching about warfarin, including the need for frequent blood tests, the list of potential drug–drug interactions, the importance of being alert to the many factors that can affect dosage needs (including illness and diet), and how to monitor for subtle blood loss. This would be a good opportunity to review teaching about her valve disease and CHF and to answer any questions that she might have about how all of these things interrelate. If possible, it would be useful to teach G. R. or a significant other how to take her pulse so she can be alerted to potential arrhythmias and avert problems before they begin. It also would be a good idea to check on support services for G. R., to ensure that her blood tests can be done and that her response to the drug is monitored carefully.

DRUGS IN FOCUS
Low-Molecular-Weight Heparins

Drug Name	Usual Dosage	Usual Indications
dalteparin (*Fragmin*)	DVT: 2500 IU/d SC starting 1–2 h before surgery and then for 5–10 d Angina: 120 IU/kg SC q12h with aspirin therapy for 5–8 d	Prevention of deep vein thrombosis (DVT) that may lead to pulmonary emboli (PE) after abdominal surgery; treatment of unstable angina and non–Q-wave myocardial infarction (MI)
danaparoid (*Orgaran*)	750 anti-Xa USC b.i.d. started 1–4 h before surgery, then at least 2 h after surgery and then at least 7–10 d postop	Prevention of DVT that may lead to PE after elective hip replacement surgery
Ⓟ enoxaparin (*Lovenox*)	Hip surgery: 30 mg SC q12h for 7–10 d Abdominal surgery: 40 mg/d SC for 7–10 d DVT or PE: 1 mg/kg SC q12h Angina: 1 mg/kg SC q12h	Prevention of DVT that may lead to PE after hip replacement or abdominal surgery; with warfarin to treat acute DVT or PE; prevention of ischemic complications of unstable angina or non–Q-wave MI
tinzaparin (*Innohep*)	175 anti-Xa IU/kg per day SC for ≥6 d	Treatment of acute DVT or PE in conjunction with warfarin

minogen), and pregnancy or lactation (because of the possible adverse effects on the fetus or neonate).

Adverse Effects

The most common adverse effect associated with the use of thrombolytic agents is bleeding. Patients should be monitored closely for the occurrence of cardiac arrhythmias (with coronary reperfusion) and hypotension. Hypersensitivity reactions are not uncommon; they range from rash and flushing to bronchospasm and anaphylactic reaction.

Clinically Important Drug–Drug Interactions

There is an increased risk of hemorrhage if thrombolytic agents are used with any anticoagulant or antiplatelet drug.

BOX 48-5
Pentoxifylline: Hemorrheologic Agent

Pentoxifylline (*Trental*) is known as a hemorrheologic agent, or a drug that can induce hemorrhage. It is a xanthine that, like caffeine and theophylline, decreases platelet aggregation and decreases the fibrinogen concentration in the blood. These effects can decrease blood clot formation and increase blood flow through narrowed or damaged vessels. The mechanism of action by which pentoxifylline does these things is not known. It is one of the very few drugs found to be effective in treating intermittent claudication, a painful vascular problem of the legs.

Because pentoxifylline is a xanthine, it is associated with many cardiovascular stimulatory effects; patients with underlying cardiovascular problems need to be monitored carefully when taking this drug. Pentoxifylline can also cause headache, dizziness, nausea, and upset stomach. It is taken orally three times a day for at least 8 weeks to evaluate its effectiveness.

BOX 48-6
First Drug Approved for the Treatment of Severe Sepsis Alters Coagulation Processes

In late 2001, the U.S. Food and Drug Administration approved the first drug for treatment of severe sepsis. Patients with severe sepsis suffer multiple organ failure and often death. The processes that lead to this state can be caused by infection from a number of sources leading to shock and vascular shut down. Drotrecogin alfa (*Xigris*) is a human activated protein C that exerts an antithrombotic effect by inhibiting factors Va and VIIIa. It may also have indirect profibrinolytic activity, activating fibrinolysin to dissolve clots. It is thought that it also may exert an anti-inflammatory effect in the body by inhibiting human necrosis factor production by monocytes, blocking leukocyte adhesion to cells, and limiting thrombin-induced inflammatory responses within the microvascular endothelium.

The mechanism of action of drotrecogin alfa in severe sepsis is not completely understood, but it is thought to be a combination of all of these effects that leads to lessened swelling and inflammation in blood vessels, decreased clotting within the injured vessels, and improved blood flow to the organs before necrosis and cell death occurs. Overall, this would cause a decrease in the complex organ failure associated with sepsis. The drug is approved for use only in adults at a dose of 24 µg/kg per hour by IV infusion for a total of 96 h, not to exceed 24 µg/kg per hour. Increased risk of bleeding is the most common adverse reaction to the drug, and the patient must be monitored closely for any signs of increased bleeding. As more is learned about the minute, intravascular processes in the body, more drugs of this type may be developed.

DRUGS IN FOCUS
Thrombolytic Agents

Drug Name	Usual Dosage	Usual Indications
alteplase (*Activase*)	100 mg IV given over 2 h	Treatment of myocardial infarction (MI), acute pulmonary embolism (PE) and acute ischemic stroke
anistreplase (*Eminase*)	30 U IV given over 2–5 min	Management of acute MI to reduce infarct size and complications
reteplase (*Retavase*)	10 IU + 10 IU double-bolus IV, each over 2 min, 30 min apart	Treatment of coronary artery thrombosis associated with an acute MI
℗ streptokinase (*Streptase, Kabikinase*)	Total dose of 140,000 IU over 60 min for coronary artery thrombosis; 250,000 IU over 30 min and then 100,000 IU/h IV for 24–72 h for PE, DVT, arterial thrombosis, or emoblism; 250,000 IU in 2-mL IV solution to clear cannula	Treatment of coronary artery thrombosis, PE, deep venous thrombosis (DVT), arterial thrombosis, or embolism, and to open occluded atrioventricular cannula
tenecteplase (*TNKase*)	30–50 mg IV over 5 sec based on weight	Reduction of mortality associated with acute MI
urokinase (*Abbokinase*)	4400–10,000 U/min for up to 2 h, based on clinical response	Lysis of pulmonary emboli, to treat coronary thrombosis, and to clear occluded intravenous catheters

Nursing Considerations for Patients Receiving Thrombolytic Agents

Assessment: History and Examination

Screen for any known allergies to these drugs. Also screen for any conditions that could be worsened by the dissolution of clots, including recent surgery, active internal bleeding, CVA within the last 2 months, aneurysm, obstetrical delivery, organ biopsy, recent serious GI bleeding, rupture of a noncompressible blood vessel, recent major trauma (including cardiopulmonary resuscitation); known blood clotting defects; cerebrovascular disease; uncontrolled hypertension; liver disease (which could affect normal clotting factors and the production of plasminogen); and pregnancy or lactation (because of the possible adverse effects on the neonate).

Include screening for baseline status before beginning therapy and for any potential adverse effects. Assess the following: body temperature; skin color, lesions, temperature; affect, orientation, reflexes; pulse, blood pressure, perfusion; respirations, adventitious sounds; and clotting studies, renal and hepatic function tests, CBC, stool guaiac, and ECG.

Nursing Diagnoses

The patient receiving a thrombolytic drug may have the following nursing diagnoses related to drug therapy:

- Risk for Injury related to clot-dissolving effects
- Ineffective Tissue Perfusion (Total Body) related to possible blood loss
- Decreased Cardiac Output related to bleeding, arrhythmias
- Deficient Knowledge regarding drug therapy

Implementation

- Discontinue heparin if it is being given before administration of a thrombolytic agent, unless specifically ordered for coronary artery infusion, *to prevent excessive loss of blood.*
- Evaluate the patient regularly for any sign of blood loss— petechiae, bleeding gums, bruises, dark-colored stools, dark-colored urine—*to evaluate drug effectiveness and to consult with the prescriber if blood loss becomes apparent.*
- Monitor coagulation studies regularly; *consult with the prescriber to adjust the drug dose appropriately.*
- Institute treatment within 6 hours after the onset of symptoms of acute MI, *to achieve optimum therapeutic effectiveness.*
- Arrange to type and cross match blood, *in case of serious blood loss that will require whole-blood transfusion.*
- Monitor cardiac rhythm continuously if being given for acute MI, *because of the risk of alteration in cardiac function;* have life support equipment on standby as needed.
- Provide increased precautions against bleeding during invasive procedures; use pressure dressings and ice; avoid intramuscular injections; and do not rub subcutaneous injection sites, *because of the risk of increased blood loss in the anticoagulated state.*
- Mark the chart of any patient receiving this drug, *to alert medical staff that there is a potential for increased bleeding.*
- Provide thorough patient teaching, including the name of the drug, dosage prescribed, measures to avoid adverse effects, warning signs of problems, and the need for periodic monitoring and evaluation, *to enhance patient knowledge about drug therapy and to promote compliance with the drug regimen.*

- Offer support and encouragement, *to help the patient deal with the diagnosis and the drug regimen.*

Evaluation

- Monitor patient response to the drug (dissolution of the clot and return of blood flow to the area).
- Monitor for adverse effects (bleeding, arrhythmias, hypotension, hypersensitivity reaction).
- Evaluate the effectiveness of the teaching plan (patient can name drug, adverse effects to watch for, specific measures to avoid adverse effects).
- Monitor the effectiveness of comfort measures and compliance to the regimen.

▢▮●■ WEB LINKS

Health care providers and patients may want to explore the following Internet sources:

Information on thrombosis, process, interventions, pathology:
  http://lef.org/protocols/prtcl-104a.shtml
Information designed for patients and families regarding the home use of warfarin:
  http://www.stjames.ie/nmic/warfarin/warfcoun.html
Information on heparin—use, research, complications:
  http://www-heparin.pharmacy.uiowa.edu

DRUGS USED TO CONTROL BLEEDING

On the other end of the spectrum of coagulation problems are various bleeding disorders. These include the following:

Hemophilia, in which there is a genetic lack of clotting factors that leaves the patient vulnerable to excessive bleeding with any injury
Liver disease, in which clotting factors and proteins needed for clotting are not produced
Bone marrow disorders, in which platelets are not formed in sufficient quantity to be effective

These disorders are treated with clotting factors and drugs that promote the coagulation process.

ANTIHEMOPHILIC AGENTS

The drugs used to treat hemophilia are replacement factors for the specific clotting factors that are genetically missing in that particular type of hemophilia.

- Antihemophilic factor (*Bioclate, Koate-HP,* and others) is factor VIII, the clotting factor that is missing in classic hemophilia (hemophilia A). It is used to correct or prevent bleeding episodes or to allow necessary surgery.
- Coagulation factor VIIa (*NovoSeven*) is a preparation made from mouse, hamster, and bovine proteins that contains vari-

able amounts of preformed clotting factors. It is used to treat bleeding episodes in patients with hemophilia A or B.
- Factor IX complex (*Benefix, Profilnine SD,* and others) contains plasma fractions of many of the clotting factors and increases blood levels of factors II, VII, IX, and X. It is given intravenously to prevent or treat hemophilia B (Christmas disease, a deficiency of factor IX), to control bleeding episodes in hemophilia A, and to control bleeding episodes in cases of factor VII deficiency.

Therapeutic Actions and Indications

The antihemophilic drugs replace clotting factors that are either genetically missing or low in a particular type of hemophilia. They are used to prevent blood loss from injury or surgery and to treat bleeding episodes. The drug of choice depends on the particular hemophilia that is being treated.

Pharmacokinetics

These agents replace normal clotting factors and are processed as such by the body. They should be used during pregnancy only if the benefit to the mother clearly outweighs the potential risk to the fetus. It is recommended that another method of feeding the baby be used if these drugs are needed during lactation because of the potential for adverse effects on the baby.

Contraindications and Cautions

Antihemophilic factor is contraindicated in the presence of known allergy to mouse proteins. Factor IX is contraindicated in the presence of liver disease with signs of intravascular coagulation or fibrinolysis. Coagulation factor VIIa is contraindicated with known allergies to mouse, hamster, or bovine products. These drugs are not recommended for use during lactation, and caution should be used during pregnancy because of the potential for adverse effects on the baby and fetus. Because these drugs are used to prevent serious bleeding problems or to treat bleeding episodes, there are few contraindications to their use.

Adverse Effects

The most common adverse effects associated with antihemophilic agents involve risks associated with the use of blood products (e.g., hepatitis, acquired immunodeficiency syndrome [AIDS]). Headache, flushing, chills, fever, and lethargy may occur as a reaction to the injection of a foreign protein. Nausea and vomiting and stinging, itching, and burning at the site of the injection may also occur.

Nursing Considerations for Patients Receiving Antihemophilic Agents
Assessment: History and Examination

Screen for the following conditions, which could be cautions or contraindications to use of the drug: any known allergies to these drugs or to mouse proteins with antihemophilic factor; liver disease.

Include screening for baseline status before beginning therapy and for any potential adverse effects. Assess the following: body temperature; skin color, lesions, temperature;

DRUGS IN FOCUS
Antihemophilic Agents

Drug Name	Usual Dosage	Usual Indications
(P) antihemophilic factor (*Bioclate, others*)	IV dosage based on level of antihemophilic factor, weight, and patient response	Treatment of hemophilia A; to correct bleeding episodes or to allow surgery
coagulation factor VIIa (*NovoSeven*)	90 μg/kg IV q2h until hemostasis is achieved	Treatment of bleeding episodes in hemophilia A or B patients
factor IX complex (*Benefix, others*)	IV dosage based on factor levels, weight, and desired response	Treatment of hemophilia B; treatment of bleeding episodes in patients with factor VII and factor VIII deficiencies

affect, orientation, reflexes; pulse, blood pressure, perfusion; respirations, adventitious sounds; clotting studies; and hepatic function tests.

Nursing Diagnoses

The patient receiving an antihemophilic drug may have the following nursing diagnoses related to drug therapy:

• Ineffective Tissue Perfusion (Total Body) related to changes in coagulation
• Acute Pain related to GI, CNS, and skin effects
• Fear, Anxiety related to the diagnosis and use of blood-related products
• Deficient Knowledge regarding drug therapy

Implementation

• Administer by the intravenous route only, *to ensure therapeutic effectiveness.*
• Monitor clinical response and clotting factor levels regularly, *in order to arrange to adjust dosage as needed.*
• Monitor the patient for any sign of thrombosis, *to arrange to use comfort and support measures as needed* (eg, support hose, positioning, ambulation, exercise).
• Decrease the rate of infusion if headache, chills, fever, or tingling occurs, *to prevent severe drug reaction;* in some individuals the drug will need to be discontinued.
• Arrange to type and cross match blood *in case of serious blood loss that will require whole-blood transfusion.*
• Mark the chart of any patient receiving this drug, *to alert medical staff that there is a potential for increased bleeding.*
• Provide thorough patient teaching, including the name of the drug, dosage prescribed, measures to avoid adverse effects, warning signs of problems, and the need for periodic monitoring and evaluation, *to enhance patient knowledge about drug therapy and to promote compliance with the drug regimen.*

• Offer support and encouragement, *to help the patient deal with the diagnosis and the drug regimen.*

Evaluation

• Monitor patient response to the drug (control of bleeding episodes, prevention of bleeding episodes).
• Monitor for adverse effects (thrombosis, CNS effects, nausea, hypersensitivity reaction, hepatitis, AIDS).
• Evaluate the effectiveness of the teaching plan (patient can name drug, dosage of drug, adverse effects to watch for, specific measures to avoid adverse effects, warning signs to report).
• Monitor the effectiveness of comfort measures and compliance to the regimen.

SYSTEMIC HEMOSTATIC AGENTS

Some situations result in a fibrinolytic state with excessive plasminogen activity and risk of bleeding from clot dissolution. For example, patients undergoing repeat coronary artery bypass graft (CABG) surgery are especially prone to excessive bleeding and may require blood transfusion. **Hemostatic drugs** are used to stop bleeding. The hemostatic drugs that are used systemically include the following:

• Aprotinin (*Trasylol*), an intravenous drug derived from bovine lung tissue, forms complexes with kinins, plasmin, and other clot-dissolving factors to block the activation of the plasminogen system. It is used during repeat CABG surgery and in certain unusual cases of first-time CABG surgery when the patient is at increased risk of bleeding. Aprotinin is widely distributed after intravenous injection and is excreted primarily by the kidneys. Degradation appears to be accomplished by lysosomal enzymes. Safety for use during pregnancy and lactation has not been established, and it should be used only if the benefits to the mother clearly outweigh the potential risks to the fetus.

• Aminocaproic acid (*Amicar*) inhibits plasminogen-activating substances and has some antiplasmin activity. It is available in oral and intravenous forms and is used to limit excessive bleeding in hyperfibrinolysis states, to prevent recurrence of subarachnoid hemorrhage, and, at times, to treat attacks of hereditary angioedema. When taking the oral form, the patient may need to take 10 tablets in the first hour and then continue taking the drug around the clock. This drug is rapidly absorbed and widely distributed throughout the body. It is excreted largely unchanged in the urine. Safety for use during pregnancy and lactation has not been established, and it should be used only if the benefits to the mother clearly outweigh the potential risks to the fetus.

Therapeutic Actions and Indications

The systemic hemostatic agents stop the natural plasminogen clot-dissolving mechanism by blocking its activation or by directly inhibiting plasmin. These drugs are used to prevent or treat excess bleeding in hyperfibrinolytic states, including repeat CABG surgery.

Contraindications and Cautions

Systemic hemostatic agents are contraindicated in the presence of allergy to these drugs and with acute DIC because of the risk of tissue necrosis. Caution should be used in the following conditions: cardiac disease, because of the risk of arrhythmias; renal and hepatic dysfunction, which could alter the excretion of these drugs and the normal clotting processes; pregnancy and lactation, because of the potential for adverse effects on the neonate.

Adverse Effects

The most common adverse effect associated with systemic hemostatic agents is excessive clotting. CNS effects can include hallucinations, drowsiness, dizziness, headache, and psychotic states, all of which could be related to changes in cerebral blood flow associated with changes in clot dissolution. GI effects, including nausea, cramps, and diarrhea, may be related to excessive clotting in the GI tract, causing reflex GI stimulation. Weakness, fatigue, malaise, and muscle pain can occur as small clots build up in muscles. Intrarenal obstruction and renal dysfunction have also been reported.

Aprotinin has been associated with cardiac arrhythmias, MI, CHF, and hypotension. These effects may be related to the fact that this drug is used during coronary bypass surgery. Anaphylactic and respiratory reactions have also been reported with aprotinin, possibly related to immune reactions to the bovine protein.

Clinically Important Drug–Drug Interactions

There is an increased risk of bleeding if these drugs are given with heparin.

Aminocaproic acid is associated with the development of hypercoagulation states if it is combined with oral contraceptives or estrogens.

Nursing Considerations for Patients Receiving Systemic Hemostatic Agents

Assessment: History and Examination

Screen for the following conditions, which could be cautions or contraindications to use of the drug: any known allergies to these drugs; acute DIC, because of the risk of tissue necrosis; cardiac disease, because of the risk of arrhythmias; renal and hepatic dysfunction, which could alter the excretion of these drugs and the normal clotting processes; and lactation, because of the potential for adverse effects on the neonate.

Include screening for baseline status before beginning therapy and for any potential adverse effects. Assess the following: body temperature; skin color, lesions, temperature; affect, orientation, reflexes; pulse, blood pressure, perfusion; respirations, adventitious sounds; bowel sounds, normal output; urinalysis, clotting studies; and renal and hepatic function tests.

NURSING CHALLENGE

Disseminated Intravascular Coagulation

Disseminated intravascular coagulation (DIC) is a syndrome in which bleeding and thrombosis may be found together. It can occur as a complication of many problems, including severe infection with septic shock, traumatic childbirth or missed abortion, and massive injuries. In these disorders, local tissue damage causes the release of coagulation-stimulating substances into circulation. These substances then stimulate the coagulation process, causing fibrin clot formation in small vessels in the lungs, kidneys, brain, and other organs. This continuing reaction consumes excessive amounts of fibrinogen, other clotting factors, and platelets. The end result is increased bleeding. In essence, the patient clots too much, resulting in the possibility of bleeding to death.

The first step in treating this disorder is to control the problem that initially precipitated it. For example, treating the infection, performing dilation and curettage to clear the uterus, or stabilizing injuries can help stop this continuing process. Whole-blood infusions or the infusion of fibrinogen may be used to buy some time until the patient is stable and can form clotting factors again. There are associated problems with giving whole blood (e.g., development of hepatitis or AIDS), and there is a risk that fibrinogen may set off further intravascular clotting. Paradoxically, the treatment of choice for DIC is the anticoagulant heparin. Heparin prevents the clotting phase from being completed, thus inhibiting the breakdown of fibrinogen. It may also help avoid hemorrhage by preventing the body from depleting its entire store of coagulation factors.

Because heparin is usually administered to prevent blood clotting, and the adverse effects that are monitored with heparin therapy include signs of bleeding, it can be a real challenge for the nursing staff to feel comfortable administering heparin to a patient who is bleeding to death. Understanding of the disease process can help alleviate any doubts about the treatment.

DRUGS IN FOCUS
Systemic Hemostatic Agents

Drug Name	Usual Dosage	Usual Indications
℗ aminocaproic acid (*Amicar*)	4–5 mg PO or IV, then 1 g/h; do not exceed 30 g in 24 h	Treatment of excessive bleeding in hyperfibrinolytic states; prevention of recurrence of bleeding with subarachnoid hemorrhage
aprotinin (*Trasylol*)	1–2 million KIU IV into pump primer volume, then 250,000–500,000 KIU per hour while on the pump	Prevention of blood loss and need for transfusion after repeat coronary artery bypass graft (CABG) surgery; in rare instances, for first CABG surgery in patients prone to bleeding

Nursing Diagnoses

The patient receiving a systemic hemostatic drug may have the following nursing diagnoses related to drug therapy:

- Disturbed Sensory Perception related to CNS effects
- Acute Pain related to GI, CNS, muscle effects
- Risk for Injury related to CNS, blood-clotting effects
- Deficient Knowledge regarding drug therapy

Implementation

- Monitor clinical response and clotting factor levels regularly, *in order to arrange to adjust dosage as needed.*
- Monitor the patient for any sign of thrombosis, *in order to arrange to use comfort and support measures as needed* (eg, support hose, positioning, ambulation, exercise).
- Orient patient and offer support and safety measures if hallucinations or psychoses occur, *to prevent patient injury.*
- Offer comfort measures, *to help the patient deal with the effects of the drug.* These include small, frequent meals; mouth care; environmental controls; and safety measures.

- Provide thorough patient teaching, including the name of the drug, dosage prescribed, measures to avoid adverse effects, warning signs of problems, and the need for periodic monitoring and evaluation, *to enhance patient knowledge about drug therapy and to promote compliance with the drug regimen.*
- Offer support and encouragement, *to help the patient deal with the diagnosis and the drug regimen.*

Evaluation

- Monitor the patient response to the drug (control of bleeding episodes).
- Monitor for adverse effects (thrombosis, CNS effects, nausea, hypersensitivity reaction).
- Evaluate the effectiveness of the teaching plan (patient can name drug, dosage of drug, adverse effects to watch for, specific measures to avoid adverse effects, warning signs to report).
- Monitor the effectiveness of comfort measures and compliance to the regimen.

DRUGS IN FOCUS
Topical Hemostatic Agents

Drug Name	Usual Dosage	Usual Indications
℗ absorbable gelatin (*Gelfoam*)	Smear or press onto surface; do not remove, will be absorbed	Control of bleeding from surface cuts or injury
microfibrillar collagen (*Avitene*)	Use dry; apply to area and apply pressure for 3–5 min	Control of bleeding from surface cuts or injury
thrombin (*Thrombostat, Thrombinar*)	100–1000 u/ML freely mixed with blood	Control of bleeding from surface cuts or injury. **Special considerations:** Use caution with allergy to bovine products

TOPICAL HEMOSTATIC AGENTS

Some surface injuries involve so much damage to the small vessels in the area that clotting does not occur and blood is slowly and continually lost. For these situations, topical or local hemostatic agents are often used.

Absorbable gelatin (*Gelfoam*) and microfibrillar collagen (*Avitene*) are available in sponge form and are applied directly to the injured area until the bleeding stops. Use of these products can pose a risk of infection, because bacteria can become trapped in the vascular area when the sponge is applied. Immediate removal of the sponge and cleaning of the area can help to decrease this risk.

Thrombin (*Thrombinar, Thrombostat*), which is derived from bovine sources, is applied topically and mixed in with the blood. Because this drug comes from animal sources, it may precipitate an allergic response; the patient needs to be carefully monitored for such a reaction.

The use of these drugs is incorporated into the care of the wound or decubitus ulcer as adjunctive therapy. The drug of choice depends on the nature of the injury and the prescriber's personal preference.

CHAPTER SUMMARY

- Coagulation is the transformation of fluid blood into a solid state to plug up breaks in the vascular system.
- Coagulation involves several processes, including vasoconstriction, platelet aggregation to form a plug, and intrinsic and extrinsic clot formation initiated by Hageman factor to plug any breaks in the system.
- The final step of clot formation is the conversion of prothrombin to thrombin, which breaks down fibrinogen to form insoluble fibrin threads.
- Once a clot is formed, it must be dissolved to prevent the occlusion of blood vessels and loss of blood supply to tissues.
- Plasminogen is the basis of the clot-dissolving system. It is converted to plasmin (fibrinolysin) by several factors, including Hageman factor. Plasmin dissolves fibrin threads and resolves the clot.
- Anticoagulants block blood coagulation by interfering with one or more of the steps involved, such as blocking platelet aggregation or inhibiting the intrinsic or extrinsic pathways to clot formation.
- Thrombolytic drugs dissolve clots or thrombi that have formed. They activate the plasminogen system to stimulate natural clot dissolution.
- Hemostatic drugs are used to stop bleeding. They may replace missing clotting factors or prevent the plasminogen system from dissolving formed clots.
- Hemophilia, a genetic lack of essential clotting factors, results in excessive bleeding. It is treated by replacing missing clotting factors.

Review Questions

1. Blood coagulation is a complex reaction that involves
   a. vasoconstriction, platelet aggregation, and plasminogen action.
   b. vasodilation, platelet aggregation, and activation of the clotting cascade.
   c. vasoconstriction, platelet aggregation, and the conversion of prothrombin to thrombin.
   d. vasodilation, platelet inhibition, and the action of the intrinsic and extrinsic clotting cascade.

2. Hageman factor does not activate
   a. the clotting cascade.
   b. the anticlotting process.
   c. the inflammatory response.
   d. platelet aggregation.

3. Plasminogen is converted to plasmin, a clot-dissolving substance, by all of the following except
   a. nicotine.
   b. Hageman factor.
   c. streptokinase.
   d. pyrogens.

4. Antiplatelet drugs block the aggregation of platelets and keep vessels open. These drugs would not be useful in
   a. maintaining the patency of grafts.
   b. decreasing the risk of fatal MI.
   c. preventing reinfarction after an MI.
   d. dissolving a pulmonary embolus and improving oxygenation.

5. Warfarin, an oral anticoagulant, acts
   a. to directly prevent the conversion of prothrombin to thrombin.
   b. to decrease the production of vitamin K clotting factors in the liver.
   c. as a catalyst in the conversion of plasminogen to plasmin.
   d. immediately, so it is the drug of choice in emergency situations.

6. Heparin reacts to prevent the conversion of prothrombin to thrombin. Heparin
   a. is available in oral and parenteral forms.
   b. takes about 72 hours to cause a therapeutic effect.
   c. effects are reversed with the administration of protamine sulfate.
   d. effects are reversed with the injection of vitamin K.

7. Evaluating a patient on an anticoagulant for blood loss would not usually include
   a. the presence of petechiae.
   b. bleeding gums while brushing the teeth.
   c. dark-colored urine.
   d. yellow color to the sclera or skin.

8. The low-molecular-weight heparin of choice for preventing deep venous thrombosis after hip replacement therapy would be
   a. tinzaparin.
   b. dalteparin.

    c. danaparoid.

    d. enoxaparin.

9. All of the following would be contraindications to the use of a thrombolytic agent except

    a. CVA within the last 2 months.

    b. acute MI within the last 3 hours.

    c. recent, serious GI bleed.

    d. obstetrical delivery.

10. Antihemophilic agents are used to replace missing clotting factors to prevent severe blood loss. The most common side effects associated with the use of these drugs are

    a. bleeding.

    b. dark stools and urine.

    c. hepatitis, AIDS.

    d. constipation.

BIBLIOGRAPHY

Bullock, B. L. (2000). *Focus on pathophysiology*. Philadelphia: Lippincott Williams & Wilkins.

Drug facts and comparisons. (2002). St. Louis: Facts and Comparisons.

Gilman, A., Hardman, J. G., & Limbird, L. E. (Eds.) (2002). *Goodman and Gilman's the pharmacological basis of therapeutics* (10th ed.). New York: McGraw-Hill.

Karch, A. M. (2002). *2003 Lippincott's nursing drug guide*. Philadelphia: Lippincott Williams & Wilkins.

The medical letter on drugs and therapeutics. (2002). New Rochelle, NY: Medical Letter.

Porth, C. M. (2002). *Pathophysiology: Concepts of altered health states* (6th ed.). Philadelphia: Lippincott Williams & Wilkins.

49

Drugs Used to Treat Anemias

667

The cardiovascular system exists to pump blood to all of the body's cells. Blood is essential for cell survival because it contains oxygen and nutrients and removes waste products that could be toxic to the tissues. It also contains clotting factors that help maintain the vascular system and keep it sealed. In addition, blood contains the important components of the immune system that protect the body from infection. This chapter discusses drugs that are used to treat anemias, which are disorders that involve too few red blood cells (RBCs) or ineffective RBCs that can alter the blood's ability to carry oxygen.

BLOOD COMPONENTS

Blood is composed of liquid and formed elements. The liquid part of blood is called **plasma.** Plasma is mostly water, but it also contains proteins that are essential for the immune response and for blood clotting. The formed elements of the blood include leukocytes (white blood cells), which are an important part of the immune system (see Chapter 15); **erythrocytes** (RBCs), which carry oxygen to the tissues and remove carbon dioxide for delivery to the lungs; and platelets, which play an important role in coagulation (see Chapter 48).

ERYTHROPOIESIS

Erythropoiesis is the process of RBC production. RBCs are produced in the myeloid tissue of the bone marrow. The rate of RBC production is controlled by the glycoprotein **erythropoietin,** which is released from the kidneys in response to decreased blood flow or decreased oxygen tension in the kidneys. Under the influence of erythropoietin, an undifferentiated cell in the bone marrow becomes a hemocytoblast. This cell uses certain amino acids, lipids, carbohydrates, vitamin B_{12}, folic acid, and iron to turn into an immature RBC. In the last phase of RBC production, the cell loses its nucleus and enters circulation. This cell, called a **reticulocyte,** finishes its maturing process in circulation (Figure 49–1).

Although the mature RBC has no nucleus, it does have a vast surface area to improve its ability to transport oxygen and carbon dioxide. Because it lacks a nucleus, the RBC cannot reproduce or maintain itself, so it will eventually wear out. The average lifespan of an RBC is about 120 days. At that time, the elderly RBC is lysed in the liver, spleen, or bone marrow. The building blocks of the RBC (eg, iron, vitamin B_{12}) are then recycled and returned to the bone marrow for the production of new RBCs (see Figure 49–1). The only part of the RBC that cannot be recycled is the toxic pigment, bilirubin, which is conjugated in the liver, passed into the bile, and excreted from the body in the feces or the urine. Bilirubin is what gives color to both of these excretions. Erythropoiesis is a constant process, wherein about 1% of the body's RBCs are destroyed and replaced each day.

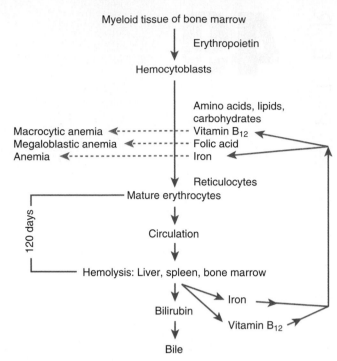

FIGURE 49–1. Erythropoiesis. Red blood cells are produced in the myeloid tissue of the bone marrow in response to the hormone erythropoietin. The hemocytoblasts require various essential factors to produce mature erythrocytes. A lack of any one of these can result in an anemia of the type indicated opposite each factor. Mature erythrocytes survive for about 120 days, and are then lysed in the liver, spleen, or bone marrow.

ANEMIA

Anemia, a decrease in the number of RBCs, can occur when erythropoietin levels are low. This is seen in renal failure, when the kidneys are no longer able to produce erythropoietin. It can also occur if the body does not have enough of the building blocks necessary to form RBCs. To produce healthy RBCs, the bone marrow must have the following:

- Adequate amounts of iron, which is used in forming hemoglobin rings to carry the oxygen.
- Minute amounts of vitamin B_{12} and folic acid, to form a strong supporting structure that can survive being battered through blood vessels for 120 days.
- Essential amino acids and carbohydrates, to complete the hemoglobin rings, cell membrane, and basic structure.

Normally, an individual's diet supplies an adequate amount of all these substances, which are absorbed from the gastrointestinal (GI) tract and transported to the bone marrow. But when the diet cannot supply enough of a nutrient, or enough of the nutrient cannot be absorbed, the person can develop a deficiency anemia. Fewer RBCs are produced, and the ones that are produced are not mature and efficient iron carriers. The person with this type of anemia, a deficiency anemia, may complain of being tired because there is insufficient oxygen delivery to the tissues.

Another type of anemia is **megaloblastic anemia,** a condition in which the bone marrow contains a large number of megaloblasts, or large, immature RBCs. Because these RBCs are so large, they become very crowded in the bone marrow and fewer RBCs are produced. There is an increase in these immature cells in circulation. Overall, fewer RBCs are produced, and those that are produced are ineffective and do not usually survive for the 120 days that is normal for the life of an RBC. Patients with megaloblastic anemia usually have a lack of vitamin B_{12} or folic acid.

Iron Deficiency Anemias

All cells in the body require some amount of iron, but iron can be very toxic to cells, especially neurons. To maintain the needed iron levels and avoid toxic levels, the body has developed a system for controlling the amount of iron that can enter the body through intestinal absorption. Only enough iron is absorbed to replace the amount of iron that is lost each day. Once iron is absorbed, it is carried by a plasma protein called transferrin, a β-globulin. This protein carries iron to various tissues to be stored and transports iron from RBC lysis back to the bone marrow for recycling.

Only about 1 mg of iron is actually lost each day in sweat, in sloughed skin, and from GI and urinary tract linings. Because of the body's efficient iron recycling, very little iron is usually needed in the diet, and most diets quite adequately replace the iron that is lost. However, in situations in which blood is being lost, such as internal bleeding or heavy menstrual flow, a negative iron balance might occur, and the patient could develop **iron deficiency anemia.** This can also occur in certain GI diseases in which the patient is unable to absorb iron from the GI tract. These conditions are usually treated with iron replacement therapy.

Megaloblastic Anemias

Megaloblastic anemias occur when there is not sufficient folic acid or vitamin B_{12} to adequately create the stromal structure needed in a healthy RBC. The lack of these two chemicals causes a slowing of nuclear DNA synthesis in human cells. This effect is seen in other rapidly dividing cells, not just bone marrow cells. For example, cells in the GI tract are often affected, resulting in the appearance of a characteristic red and glossy tongue and diarrhea.

Folic Acid Deficiency

Folic acid is essential for cell division in all types of tissue. Deficiencies in folic acid are noticed first in rapidly growing cells, such as those in cancerous tissues, in the GI tract, and in the bone marrow. Most people can get all of the folic acid they need from their diet. For example, folic acid is found in green leafy vegetables, milk, eggs, and liver. Deficiency in folic acid may occur in certain malabsorption states, such as sprue and celiac diseases. Malnutrition that accompanies alcoholism is also a common cause of folic acid deficiency. Repeated preg-

---

CULTURAL CONSIDERATIONS
Sickle Cell Anemia

Sickle cell anemia is a chronic hemolytic anemia that occurs almost exclusively in blacks. (Hemolytic anemias involve a lysing of red blood cells (RBCs) because of genetic factors or from exposure to toxins.) Sickle cell anemia is characterized by a genetically inherited hemoglobin S, which gives the RBCs a sickle-shaped appearance. The patient with sickle cell anemia produces fewer than normal RBCs, and the RBCs produced are unable to carry oxygen efficiently. The patient may be of short stature with stubby fingers and toes; these characteristics are related to the body's response to the inability to deliver oxygen to the tissues.

The sickle-shaped RBCs can become lodged in tiny blood vessels, where they stack up onto one another and occlude the vessel. This occlusion leads to anoxia and infarction of the tissue in that area, which is characterized by severe pain and an acute inflammatory reaction—a condition often called sickle cell crisis. (The patient may have ulcers on the extremities as a result of such occlusions.) Severe, acute episodes of sickling with vessel occlusion may be associated with acute infections and the body's reactions to the immune and inflammatory responses.

In the past, the only treatment for sickle cell anemia was pain medication and support of the patient. Now hydroxyurea (*Hydrea*) has been found to effectively treat this disease. Hydroxyurea is a cytotoxic antineoplastic agent that is used to treat leukemia, ovarian cancer, and melanoma. It has been shown that it increases the amount of fetal hemoglobin produced in the bone marrow and dilutes the formation of the abnormal hemoglobin S in patients with sickle cell anemia. The process takes several months, but, once effective, it prevents the clogging of small vessels and the painful, anoxic effects of RBC sickling. Because this drug is associated with several uncomfortable adverse effects—including gastrointestinal problems, rash, headache, and possible bone marrow depression—the decision to use it is not made lightly. However, it has been found to be effective in preventing the painful crises of sickle cell anemia.

CULTURAL CONSIDERATIONS
Hematological Laboratory Test Variations

There are racial variations in hematological laboratory test results:

Hemoglobin/hematocrit—African Americans are generally 1 g lower than other groups.

Serum transferrin levels (children age 1–3.5 y)—The mean value for African American children is 22 mg/100 mL higher than for white children. (This may be because African Americans have lower hematocrit and hemoglobin; transferrin levels increase normally in the presence of anemia.)

Because of these variations, the diagnosis and treatment of anemia in African Americans should be based on a different norm than with other groups of patients.

nancies and extended treatment with certain antiepileptic medications can also contribute to folic acid deficiency. This disorder is treated by the administration of folic acid or folate.

Vitamin B$_{12}$ Deficiency

Vitamin B$_{12}$ is used in minute amounts by the body and is stored for use if dietary intake falls. It is necessary not only for the health of the RBCs, but also for the formation and maintenance of the myelin sheath in the central nervous system (CNS). It is found in the diet in meats, seafood, eggs, and cheese. Strict vegetarians who eat nothing but vegetables may develop a vitamin B$_{12}$ deficiency. Such individuals with a dietary insufficiency of vitamin B$_{12}$ typically respond to vitamin B$_{12}$ replacement therapy to reverse their anemia.

DRUG THERAPY ACROSS THE LIFESPAN

Drugs Used to Treat Anemias

Children	Adults	Older Adults
Proper nutrition should be established for children to provide the essential elements needed for formation of red blood cells (RBCs). The cause of the anemia should be determined to avoid prolonged problems. The safety and efficacy of epoetin alfa use has not been established for children. If the drugs is used, careful dosage calculation should be done based on weight and age, and the child should be monitored very closely for response, iron levels, and nutrition. Iron doses for replacement therapy are determined by age. If liquid solutions are being used, the child should drink it through a straw to avoid staining of the teeth. Periodic blood counts should be performed; it may take 4–6 mo of oral therapy to reverse an iron deficiency. Remember that iron can be toxic to children, and iron supplements should be kept out of their reach and administration monitored. Maintenance doses for folic acid have been established for children, based on age. Nutritional means should be used to establish folic acid levels whenever possible. Children with pernicious anemia will require a monthly injection of vitamin B$_{12}$, the nasal form has not been approved for use with children.	The underlying cause of the anemia should be established and appropriate steps taken to reverse the cause if possible. Adults receiving epoetin alfa or darbapoetin alfa should be monitored closely for response and for the need for iron or other RBC building blocks. Advertised heavily in the mass media, epoetin is often requested by adults to help return energy. Careful patient teaching about the drug, and how and why it is administered, may be needed. Adults receiving iron replacement may experience gastrointestinal upset and frequently experience constipation. Appropriate measures to maintain bowel function may be needed. Adults also needs to know that periodic blood tests will be needed to evaluate response. Adults being treated for pernicious anemia may opt for the nasal vitamin B$_{12}$. These patients need to receive careful instructions about the proper administration of the drug and should have nasal mucous membranes evaluated periodically. Proper nutrition during pregnancy and lactation is often still not an adequate way to meet the increased demands of those states. Prenatal vitamins contain iron and folic acid and are usually prescribed for pregnant women. Use of epoetin alfa or darbapoetin alfa is not recommended during pregnancy or lactation because of the potential for adverse effects on the fetus or baby. Iron replacement is frequently needed postpartum to provide the iron lost during delivery. The new mother should be reminded to keep the drug out of the reach of children and not to combine prescribed iron with over-the-counter preparation containing high levels of iron. Women maintained on vitamin B$_{12}$ before pregnancy should continue the treatment during pregnancy. Increased doses may be needed due to changes associated with the pregnancy.	Older adults may have nutritional problems related to age and may lose more iron through cellular sloughing. Older adults should be assessed for anemia, and possible causes should be evaluated. Replacement therapy in the older adult can cause the same adverse effects as are seen in the younger person. Bowel training programs may be needed to prevent severe constipation. Use of nasal vitamin B$_{12}$, may not be practical. If the patient desires to use this administration technique, nasal mucous membranes should be evaluated before and periodically during treatment.

The most common cause of this deficiency, however, is inability of the GI tract to absorb the needed amounts of the vitamin. Gastric mucosal cells produce a substance called intrinsic factor, which is necessary for the absorption of vitamin B_{12} by the upper intestine. **Pernicious anemia** occurs when the gastric mucosa cannot produce intrinsic factor and vitamin B_{12} cannot be absorbed. The person with pernicious anemia will complain of fatigue and lethargy and will also have CNS effects because of damage to the myelin sheath. Patients will complain of numbness, tingling, and eventually lack of coordination and motor activity. Pernicious anemia was once a fatal disease, but it is now treated with injections of vitamin B_{12} to replace the amount that can no longer be absorbed.

ERYTHROPOIETINS

Patients who are no longer able to produce enough erythropoietin in the kidneys may benefit from treatment with erythropoietin (EPO), which is available as the drugs epoetin alfa (*Epogen, Procrit*) and darbopoetin alfa (*Aranesp*).

Epogen is used to treat anemia associated with renal failure (including patients on dialysis). It is also used to decrease the need for blood transfusions in patients undergoing surgery and to treat anemias related to treatment for acquired immunodeficiency syndrome (AIDS). It is not approved to treat severe anemia associated with other causes, and it is not meant to replace whole blood for emergency treatment of anemia. There is a risk of decreasing the normal levels of erythropoietin if this drug is given to patients with normal renal functioning and adequate levels of erythropoietin. A negative feedback occurs with the renal cells, and less endogenous erythropoietin is produced when exogenous erythropoietin is given. Administration of this drug to an anemic patient with normal renal function may actually cause a more severe anemia when the endogenous levels fall and no longer stimulate RBC production.

Procrit is also used to treat severe anemia related to chemotherapy in cancer patients, when bone marrow is depressed and kidneys may be affected by the toxic drugs (Figure 49–2).

Darbopoetin alfa (*Aranesp*) is an erythropoietin-like protein produced in Chinese hamster ovary cells with the use of recombinant DNA technology. It is used to treat anemia associated with chronic renal failure, including patients on dialysis. It has the advantage of having to be given only once a week, instead of two to three times a week, as with epoetin.

Therapeutic Actions and Indications

Epoetin alfa acts like the natural glycoprotein erythropoietin to stimulate the production of RBCs in the bone marrow (Figure 49–3). It is indicated for the treatment of anemia associated with renal failure and for patients on dialysis. It is also used to decrease the need for blood transfusions in patients undergoing surgery, for the treatment of anemia associated with AIDS therapy, and for the treatment of anemia

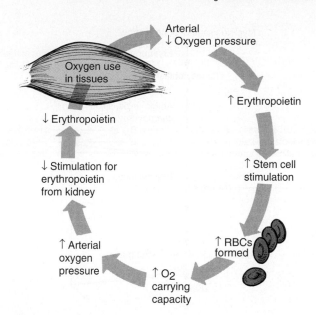

FIGURE 49–2. Erythropoiesis controls the rate of blood cell production. (From Bullock, B. L. [2000]. *Focus on pathophysiology.* Philadelphia: Lippincott Williams & Wilkins.)

associated with cancer chemotherapy (*Procrit* only). Darbopoetin alfa is indicated only for the treatment of anemia associated with chronic renal failure.

Pharmacokinetics

Epoetin alfa is metabolized through the normal kinetic processes, with a half-life of 4 to 13 hours. Darbopoetin alfa has a half-life of 21 hours after intravenous administration or 49 hours after subcutaneous administration. There are no adequate studies in pregnancy, so use should be limited to those situations in which the benefit to the mother clearly outweighs the potential risk to the fetus. It is not known whether epoetin alfa enters into breast milk. Darbopoetin alfa does cross into breast milk. Caution should be used if the drug is needed by a nursing mother.

Contraindications and Cautions

Epoetin alfa and darbopoetin alfa are contraindicated in the presence of uncontrolled hypertension, because of the risk of even further hypertension when RBC numbers increase and the pressure within the vascular system increases; with allergy to mammalian cell–derived products or to human albumin; and with lactation, because of the potential for allergic-type reactions with the neonate.

Adverse Effects

The adverse effects most commonly associated with these drugs include the CNS effects of headache, fatigue, asthenia, and dizziness, and the potential for serious seizures. These effects may be the result of a cellular response to the glycoprotein. Nausea, vomiting, and diarrhea also are common effects. Cardiovascular symptoms can include hypertension, edema, and possible chest pain and may be related to the increase in RBC numbers' changing the balance within the

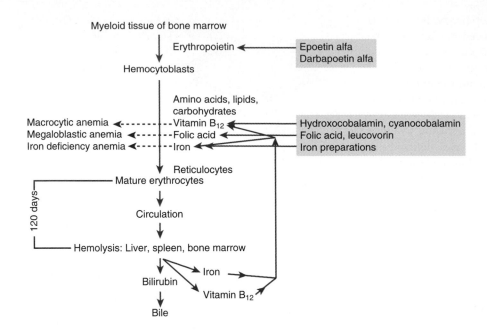

FIGURE 49-3. Sites of action of drugs used to treat anemia.

cardiovascular system. Patients receiving intravenous administration must also be monitored for possible clotting of the access line related to direct cellular effects of the drug.

Nursing Considerations for Patients Receiving Erythropoietins

Assessment: History and Examination

Screen for the following conditions, which could be cautions or contraindications to use of the drug: any known allergies to this drug, to mammalian cell–derived products, or to human albumin; severe hypertension, which could be exacerbated; and lactation, because of potential adverse effects on the neonate.

Include screening for baseline status before beginning therapy and for any potential adverse effects. Assess the following: affect, orientation, reflexes; pulse, blood pressure, perfusion; respirations, adventitious breath sounds; and renal function tests, complete blood count (CBC), hematocrit, iron concentration, and electrolytes.

Nursing Diagnoses

The patient receiving erythropoietins may have the following nursing diagnoses related to drug therapy:

• Nausea, Diarrhea related to GI effects
• Risk for Injury related to CNS effects
• Risk for Imbalanced Fluid Volume related to cardiovascular effects
• Deficient Knowledge regarding drug therapy

Implementation

• Confirm the chronic, renal nature of the patient's anemia before administering the drug, *to ensure proper use of the drug.*
• Give epoetin alfa three times per week, either intravenously or subcutaneously, *to achieve appropriate therapeutic drug levels.* Darbopoetin alfa is given once per week, subcutaneously or intravenously. The patient should receive a cal-

DRUGS IN FOCUS
Erythropoietin

Drug Name	Usual Dosage	Usual Indications
darbapoetin alfa (*Aranesp*)	0.45 mcg/kg IV or SC once per week	Treatment of anemia associated with chronic renal failure, including in dialysis patients
Ⓟ epoetin alfa (*Epogen*)	50–100 U/kg IV or SC three times per week	Treatment of anemia associated with renal failure; reduction in need for transfusions in surgical patients; treatment of anemia associated with AIDS therapy
(*Procrit*)	150 U/kg SC three times per week	Treatment of anemia associated with cancer chemotherapy

endar of marked days *to increase compliance with the drug regimen.*

- Do not give with any other drug solution, *to avoid drug–drug interactions.*
- Monitor access lines for clotting and *arrange to clear line as needed.*
- Arrange for hematocrit reading before drug administration *to determine correct dosage.* If the patient does not respond within 8 weeks, re-evaluate the cause of anemia.
- Evaluate iron stores before and periodically during therapy, *because supplemental iron may be needed as the patient makes more RBCs.*
- Maintain seizure precautions on standby, *in case seizures occur as a reaction to the drug.*
- Provide comfort measures, *to help the patient tolerate the drug effects.* These include small, frequent meals; access to bathroom facilities; and analgesia for headache or arthralgia.
- Provide thorough patient teaching, including the name of the drug, dosage prescribed, measures to avoid adverse effects, warning signs of problems, and the need for periodic monitoring and evaluation, *to enhance patient knowledge about drug therapy and to promote compliance with the drug regimen.*
- Offer support and encouragement, *to help the patient deal with the diagnosis and the drug regimen.*

Evaluation

- Monitor patient response to the drug (alleviation of anemia).
- Monitor for adverse effects (headache, hypertension, nausea, vomiting, seizures, dizziness).
- Evaluate the effectiveness of the teaching plan (patient can name drug, dosage, adverse effects to watch for, specific measures to avoid adverse effects; patient understands importance of continued follow-up).
- Monitor the effectiveness of comfort measures and compliance to the regimen.

IRON PREPARATIONS

Although most people get all the iron they need through diet, there are some situations in which diet alone may not be adequate. Iron deficiency anemia is a relatively common problem in certain groups, including the following:

- Menstruating women who lose RBCs monthly
- Pregnant and nursing women who have increased demands for iron
- Rapidly growing adolescents, especially those who do not have a nutritious diet
- Persons with GI bleeding; even individuals with slow bleeding associated with use of nonsteroidal anti-inflammatory drugs (NSAIDs)

Oral iron preparations are often used to help these patients regain a positive iron balance; these preparations need to be supplemented with adequate dietary intake of iron. Ferrous fumarate (*Feostat*), ferrous gluconate (*Fergon*), ferrous sulfate (*Feosol*), and ferrous sulfate exsiccated (*Ferralyn Lanacaps, Slow FE*) are the oral iron preparations that are available for use. Most of the drug that is taken is lost in the feces, but slowly some of the metal is absorbed into the intestine and transported to the bone marrow. It can take 2 to 3 weeks to see improvement and up to 6 to 10 months to return to a stable iron level once a deficiency exists. The drug of choice depends on the prescriber's personal preference and experience, and often on what kinds of samples are available to give the patient.

Iron dextran (*InFeD*) is a parenteral form of iron that can be used when the oral form cannot be given or cannot be tolerated. Patients with severe GI absorption problems may require this form of iron. If given intramuscularly, it must be given by the Z-track method, because it can stain the tissues brown and can be very painful. Patients should be switched to the oral form if at all possible. Severe hypersensitivity reactions have been associated with the parenteral form of iron. Iron sucrose (*Venofer*) and sodium ferric gluconate complex (*Ferrlecit*) are given intravenously, specifically for patients who are undergoing chronic hemodialysis and who are also receiving supplemental erythropoietin therapy.

Therapeutic Actions and Indications
Iron preparations elevate the serum iron concentration (see Figure 49–3). They are then either converted to hemoglobin or trapped in reticuloendothelial cells for storage and eventual release and conversion into a useable form of iron for RBC production. They are indicated for the treatment of iron deficiency anemias and may also be used as adjunctive therapy in patients receiving epoetin alfa.

Pharmacokinetics
Iron is primarily absorbed from the small intestine by an active transport system. It is transported in the blood, bound to transferrin. Small amounts are lost daily in the sweat, urine, sloughing of skin and mucosal cells, and sloughing of intestinal cells and in the menstrual flow of women. It is used during pregnancy and lactation to help the mother meet the increased demands for iron that occur at those times.

Contraindications and Cautions
These drugs are contraindicated with known allergy to any of these preparations. They also are contraindicated in the following conditions: hemochromatosis (excessive iron); hemolytic anemias, which may increase serum iron levels and cause toxicity; normal iron balance, because the drug will not be absorbed and will just pass through the body; and peptic ulcer, colitis, or regional enteritis, because the drug can be directly irritating to these tissues and can cause exacerbation of the diseases.

Adverse Effects
The most common adverse effects associated with oral iron are related to direct GI irritation; these include GI upset, anorexia, nausea, vomiting, diarrhea, dark stools, and consti-

BOX 49-1
Chelating Agents

Heavy metals, including iron, lead, arsenic, mercury, copper, and gold, can cause toxicity in the body by their ability to tie up chemicals in living tissues that need to be free in order for the cell to function normally. When these vital substances (thiols, sulfurs, carboxyls, and phosphoryls) are bound to the metal, certain cellular enzyme systems become deactivated, resulting in failure of cellular function and eventual cell death. Drugs that have been developed to counteract metal toxicity are called chelating agents (from the Greek word for "claw").

Chelating agents grasp and hold a toxic metal so that it can be carried out of the body before it has time to harm the tissues. The chelating agent binds the molecules of the metal, preventing it from damaging the cells within the body. The complex that is formed by the chelating agent and the metal is nontoxic and is excreted by the kidneys.

Chelating Agent	Toxic Metal	Notes
calcium disodium edetate	lead	Given IM or IV; monitor renal and hepatic function, because serious and even fatal toxicity can occur
deferoxamine mesylate (Desferal)	iron	Given IM, SC, or IV; rash and vision changes are common
dimercaprol (BAL in Oil)	arsenic, gold, mercury	Given IM only for 7–10 days; cardiovascular toxicity may occur; push fluids and alkalinize urine to increase excretion

pation. With increasing serum levels, iron can be directly CNS toxic, causing coma and even death. (Box 49–1 discusses iron toxicity and drugs that are used to counteract this effect.) Parenteral iron is associated with severe anaphylactic reactions, local irritation, staining of the tissues, and phlebitis.

Clinically Important Drug–Drug Interactions

There is decreased iron absorption if iron preparations are taken with antacids, tetracyclines, or cimetidine; if these drugs must be used, they should be spaced at least 2 hours apart.

There can be a decreased anti-infective response to ciprofloxacin, norfloxacin, or ofloxacin if taken with iron, because of a decrease in absorption; these drugs also should be taken at least 2 hours apart.

Increased iron levels occur if iron preparations are taken with chloramphenicol; patients receiving this combination should be monitored closely for any sign of iron toxicity.

There may be decreased effects of levodopa if taken with iron preparations; patients receiving both of these drugs should take them at least 2 hours apart.

Clinically Important Drug–Food Interactions

Iron is not absorbed if taken with antacids, eggs, milk, coffee, or tea. These should not be administered concurrently.

Nursing Considerations for Patients Receiving Iron Preparations
Assessment: History and Examination

Screen for the following conditions, which could be cautions or contraindications to use of the drug: any known allergies to this drug; hyperchromatosis; colitis, enteritis, peptic ulcer, and hemolytic anemias.

Include screening for baseline status before beginning therapy and for any potential adverse effects. Assess the following: skin color, gums, teeth; affect, orientation, reflexes; pulse, blood pressure, perfusion; respirations, adventitious sounds; bowel sounds; CBC, hematocrit, hemoglobin, and serum ferritin assays.

Nursing Diagnoses

The patient receiving iron may have the following nursing diagnoses related to drug therapy:

- Acute Pain related to CNS, GI effects
- Disturbed Body Image related to drug staining
- Risk for Injury related to CNS effects
- Deficient Knowledge regarding drug therapy

Implementation

- Confirm iron deficiency anemia before administering drugs, *to ensure proper use of the drug.*
- Consult with the physician to arrange for treatment of the underlying cause of anemia if possible, *because iron replacement will not correct the cause of the iron loss.*
- Administer with meals (avoiding eggs, milk, coffee, and tea), *to relieve GI irritation* if GI upset is severe. Have patient drink solutions through a straw *to prevent staining of teeth.*
- Caution the patient that stool may be dark or green, *to prevent undue alarm if this occurs.*
- Administer intramuscularly only by Z-track technique, *to ensure proper administration and to avoid staining.*
- Arrange for hematocrit and hemoglobin measurements before administration and periodically during therapy, *to monitor drug effectiveness.*
- Provide comfort measures, *to help the patient tolerate drug effects.* These include small, frequent meals and access to bathroom facilities.
- Provide thorough patient teaching, including the name of the drug, dosage prescribed, measures to avoid adverse effect, warning signs of problems, and the need for periodic monitoring and evaluation, *to enhance patient knowledge about drug therapy and to promote compliance with drug regimen.* (See Patient Teaching Checklist: Iron Preparations.)
- Offer support and encouragement, *to help the patient deal with the diagnosis and the drug regimen.*

DRUGS IN FOCUS
Iron Preparations

Drug Name	Usual Dosage	Usual Indications
ferrous fumarate (*Feostat*)	100–200 mg/d PO 2–12 y: 50–100 mg/d PO 6 mo–2 y: 6 mg/kg per day PO Infants: 10–25 mg/d PO	Treatment of iron deficiency anemia
ferrous gluconate (*Fergon*)	100–200 mg/d PO 2–12 y: 50–100 mg/d PO 6 mo–2 y: 6 mg/kg per day PO Infants: 10–25 mg/d PO	Treatment of iron deficiency anemia
ferrous sulfate (*Feosol*)	100–200 mg/d PO 2–12 y: 50–100 mg/d PO 6 mo–2 y: 6 mg/kg per day PO Infants: 10–25 mg/d PO	Treatment of iron deficiency anemia
ferrous sulfate exsiccated (*Ferralyn Lanacaps, Slow FE*)	100–200 mg/d PO 2–12 y: 50–100 mg/d PO 6 mo–2 y: 6 mg/kg per day PO Infants: 10–25 mg/d PO	Treatment of iron deficiency anemia
iron dextran (*InFeD*)	mg iron = 0.3 × (weight in lb) × {(100 − (hemoglobin in g/dL) × 100) / 14.8} Given IM, using Z-track technique	Parenteral treatment of iron deficiency anemia
iron sucrose (*Venofer*)	100 mg one to three times per week given IV during dialysis sessions, slowly over 1 min	Treatment of iron deficiency in patients undergoing chronic hemodialysis who are also receiving supplemental erythropoietin therapy
sodium ferric gluconate complex (*Ferrlecit*)	10 mL diluted gluconate complex in 100 mL 0.9% sodium chloride for injection over 60 min; initially 8 doses given at separate dialysis sessions, then give periodically to maintain hematocrit	Treatment of iron deficiency in patients undergoing chronic hemodialysis who are also receiving supplemental erythropoietin therapy

---

PATIENT TEACHING CHECKLIST
Iron Preparations

Create customized patient teaching materials for a specific iron preparation from the CD-ROM. Patient teaching should stress the following points for drugs within this class:

• Iron is a naturally occurring mineral found in many foods. It is used by the body to make red blood cells, which carry oxygen to all parts of the body. Supplemental iron needs to be taken when the body does not have enough iron available to make healthy red blood cells, a condition called anemia.
• Iron is a toxic substance if too much is taken. You must avoid self-medicating with over-the-counter preparations containing iron while you are taking this drug.
• You will need to return for regular medical check-ups while taking this drug to determine its effectiveness.

Take your medication as follows, depending on the specific iron preparation that has been prescribed:

• Dissolve *ferrous salts* in orange juice to improve the taste.

PATIENT TEACHING CHECKLIST
(CONTINUED)
Iron Preparations

• Take *liquid iron preparations* with a straw, because this will prevent the iron from staining teeth.
• Place iron drops on the back of the tongue to prevent staining of the teeth.

Some of the following adverse effects may occur:

• *Dark, tarry, or green stools*—The iron preparations stain the stools; the color remains as long as you are taking the drug and should not cause concern.
• *Constipation*—This is a common problem; if it becomes too uncomfortable, consult with your health care provider for an appropriate remedy.
• *Nausea, indigestion, vomiting*—This problem can often be solved by taking the drug with food, making sure to avoid the foods listed earlier.

Patient Teaching Checklist continues on page 676

PATIENT TEACHING CHECKLIST
(CONTINUED)

Iron Preparations

Report any of the following to your health care provider: severe diarrhea, severe abdominal pain or cramping, unusual tiredness or weakness, bluish tint to the lips or fingernail beds.

Tell any doctor, nurse, or other health care provider that you are taking this drug.

Keep this drug, and all medications, out of the reach of children. Because iron can be very toxic, seek emergency medical help immediately if you suspect that a child has taken this preparation unsupervised.

Because iron can interfere with the absorption of some drugs, do not take iron at the same time as *tetracycline* or *antacids*. These drugs must be taken at intervals when iron is not in the stomach.

This Teaching Checklist reflects general patient teaching guidelines. it is not meant to be a substitute for drug-specific teaching information, which is available in nursing drug guides.

Evaluation

- Monitor patient response to the drug (alleviation of anemia).
- Monitor for adverse effects (GI upset and reaction, CNS toxicity, coma).
- Evaluate the effectiveness of the teaching plan (patient can name drug, dosage, adverse effects to watch for, specific measures to avoid adverse effects; patient understands importance of continued follow-up).
- Monitor the effectiveness of comfort measures and compliance to the regimen (see Nursing Care Guide: Iron Preparations).

FOLIC ACID DERIVATIVES AND VITAMIN B₁₂

Megaloblastic anemia is treated with folic acid and vitamin B_{12}. Folate deficiencies usually occur secondary to increased demand (as in pregnancy or growth spurts) as a result of absorption problems in the small intestine; because of drugs that cause folate deficiencies; or secondary to the malnutrition of alcoholism. Vitamin B_{12} deficiencies can result from poor diet or increased demand, but the usual cause is lack of intrinsic factor in the stomach, which is necessary for absorption. The drugs are usually given together to ensure that the problem is addressed and the blood cells can be formed properly.

Folic acid (*Folvite*) can be given in oral, intramuscular, intravenous, and subcutaneous forms. The parenteral drugs are preferred for patients with potential absorption problems; all other patients should be given the oral form if at all possible. Leucovorin (*Wellcovorin*) is a reduced form of folic acid that is available for oral, intramuscular, and intravenous use. (It is used for the "leucovorin rescue" of patients

receiving high doses of methotrexate for osteocarcinoma, allowing noncancerous cells to survive the chemotherapy. It is also used with fluorouracil for palliative treatment of colorectal cancer—see Chapter 14.)

Hydroxocobalamin (*Hydro-Crysti 12*) is the traditional treatment for pernicious anemia and vitamin B_{12} deficiency. It must be given intramuscularly every day for 5 to 10 days to build up levels, then once a month for life. It cannot be taken orally, because the problem with pernicious anemia is the inability to absorb vitamin B_{12} secondary to low levels of intrinsic factor. It can be used in states of increased demand (eg, pregnancy, growth spurts) or dietary deficiency, but oral vitamins are preferred in most of those cases. Cyanocobalamin (*Crystamine, Crysti 100*) is also available for injection. It is not as tightly bound to proteins and does not last in the body as long as hydroxocobalamin. It is also available in a newer preparation as *Nascobal*, an intranasal gel that allows vitamin B_{12} absorption directly through the nasal mucosa. *Nascobal* is used once a week as an intranasal spray in one nostril.

Therapeutic Actions and Indications

Folic acid and vitamin B_{12} are essential for cell growth and division and for the production of a strong stroma in RBCs (see Figure 49–3). Vitamin B_{12} is also necessary for maintenance of the myelin sheath in nerve tissue. Both are given as replacement therapy for dietary deficiencies; as replacement in high-demand states such as pregnancy and lactation; and to treat megaloblastic anemia. Folic acid is used as a rescue drug for cells exposed to some toxic chemotherapeutic agents.

Pharmacokinetics

These vitamins are well absorbed after injection, metabolized mainly in the liver, and excreted in the urine. Much of the hydroxocobalamin is highly protein bound and slowly released for use in the body. Cyanocobalamin is primarily stored in the liver and slowly released as needed for metabolic functions. These vitamins are considered essential during pregnancy and lactation because of the increased demands of the mother's metabolism.

Contraindications and Cautions

These drugs are contraindicated in the presence of known allergies to these drugs or to their components. They should be used cautiously in patients who are pregnant or lactating or who have other anemias. Nasal cyanocobalamin should be used with caution in the presence of nasal erosion or ulcers.

Adverse Effects

These drugs have relatively few adverse effects because they are used as replacement for required chemicals. Pain and discomfort can occur at injection sites. Nasal irritation can occur with the use of intranasal spray.

Nursing Considerations for Patients Receiving Folic Acid Derivatives or Vitamin B₁₂
Assessment: History and Examination

Screen for the following conditions, which could be cautions or contraindications to use of the drug: any known allergies

NURSING CARE GUIDE

Iron Preparations

Assessment	Nursing Diagnoses	Implementation	Evaluation
HISTORY Allergies to any iron preparation, colitis, enteritis, hepatic dysfunction, peptic ulcer	Acute Pain related to GI, CNS effects Risk for Injury related to CNS effects Disturbed Body Image related to drug staining Deficient Knowledge regarding drug therapy	Confirm iron deficiency anemia before administering the drug: Provide comfort and safety measures: - Give small meals - Ensure access to bathroom facilities - Use Z-track method for IM administrations - Give drug with food if GI upset occurs - Institute bowel program as needed Arrange for treatment of underlying cause of anemia. Provide support and reassurance to deal with drug effects. Provide patient teaching regarding drug, dosage, adverse effects, what to report, safety precautions.	Evaluate drug effects: relief of signs and symptoms of anemia, hematocrit within normal limits Monitor for adverse effects: GI upset, CNS toxicity, coma. Monitor hematocrit and hemoglobin periodically. Monitor for drug–drug interactions as indicated for each drug. Evaluate effectiveness of patient teaching program. Evaluate effectiveness of comfort and safety measures.
PHYSICAL EXAMINATION CV: BP, P, perfusion CNS: orientation, affect, reflexes, vision Skin: color, lesions, gums, teeth Resp: R, adventitious sounds GI: abdominal exam, bowel sounds Lab tests: CBC, Hgb, Hct, serum ferritin assays			

to these drugs or drug components, other anemias, pregnancy, lactation, and nasal erosion.

Include screening for baseline status before beginning therapy and for any potential adverse effects. Assess the following: affect, orientation, reflexes; pulse, blood pressure, perfusion; respirations, adventitious sounds; and renal function tests, CBC, hematocrit, iron levels, and electrolytes.

Nursing Diagnoses

The patient receiving folic acid/vitamin B_{12} may have the following nursing diagnoses related to drug therapy:

• Acute Pain related to injection, nasal irritation

• Risk for Fluid Volume Imbalance related to cardiovascular effects

• Deficient Knowledge regarding drug therapy

Implementation

• Confirm the nature of the megaloblastic anemia, *to ensure that the proper drug regimen is being used.*

• Give both types of drugs in cases of pernicious anemia, *to ensure therapeutic effectiveness.*

• Parenteral vitamin B must be given intramuscularly each day for 5 to 10 days and then once a month for life, *if used to treat pernicious anemia.*

CASE STUDY

Iron Preparations and Toxicity

THE SITUATION

L. L., a 28-year-old woman, suffered a miscarriage 6 weeks ago. She lost a great deal of blood during the miscarriage and underwent a dilation and curettage to control the bleeding. On her 6-week routine follow-up visit, she was found to have recovered physically from the event but was still depressed over her loss. Her hematocrit was 31%, and she admitted feeling tired and weak. She was offered emotional support and given a supply of ferrous sulfate tablets, with instructions to take one tablet three times a day.

At home, L. L. transferred the pills to a decorative bottle that had once held vitamins and left it on her table as a reminder to take the tablets. The next day, she discovered her 2-year-old daughter eating the tablets and punished her for getting into them. About 1 hour later, the toddler complained of a really bad "tummy ache" and started vomiting. She then became lethargic and L. L. called the pediatrician, who told them to go immediately to the emergency room and bring the remaining tablets with them. The toddler was found to have a weak, rapid pulse (156 beats/min); rapid, shallow respirations (32 per minute); and a low blood pressure (60/42 mm Hg). When a diagnosis of acute iron toxicity was made, L. L. became distraught. She said she had no idea that iron could be dangerous because it can be bought over the counter (OTC) in so many preparations. She had not read the written information given to her because it was "just iron."

CRITICAL THINKING

- What nursing interventions should be done at this point?
- What sort of crisis intervention would be most appropriate for L. L.? *Think about the combined depression from the miscarriage, fear and anxiety related to this crisis, and L. L.'s iron-depleted state.*
- What kind of reserve does she have for dealing with this crisis? Which measures would be appropriate for helping

the mother cope with this crisis, and for treating the toddler?

DISCUSSION

The first priority is to support and detoxify the child in iron toxicity. In cases of acute iron poisoning, the patient should be induced to vomit and given eggs and milk to bind the iron and prevent absorption. Gastric lavage, using a 1% sodium bicarbonate solution, can be done in a medical facility. This procedure is safe for about the first hour after ingestion. After that time, there is an increased risk of gastric erosion caused by the corrosive iron, making the lavage very dangerous. Because this toddler is well beyond the first hour, other measures will be needed. Supportive measures to deal with shock, dehydration, and gastrointestinal damage will be necessary. In addition, an iron chelating agent such as deferoxamine mesylate may be tried.

During this crisis, L. L. will need a great deal of support, including a significant other who can stay with her. She also will need reassurance and a place to rest. After the situation is stabilized, L. L. will need teaching and additional support. For example, she should be reassured that most people do not take OTC drugs seriously, and many do not even read the labels. However, the nurse can use this opportunity to stress the importance of reading all of the labels and following the directions that come with OTC drugs. L. L. also should be commended for calling the pediatrician and getting medical care for the toddler quickly. Finally, she should receive a review of the iron teaching information and be encouraged to ask questions.

This case is a good example for a staff in-service program, stressing not only the dangers of iron toxicity but also the vital importance of providing good patient education before sending a patient home with a new drug. Simply giving a patient written information is often not enough.

DRUGS IN FOCUS

Folic Acid Derivatives and Vitamin B$_{12}$

Drug Name	Usual Dosage	Usual Indications
Folic acid derivatives		
Ⓟ folic acid (*Folvite*)	1 mg/d PO, IM, SC, or IV	Replacement therapy and treatment of megaloblastic anemia
leucovorin (*Wellcovorin*)	1 mg/d IM for replacement; 12–15 g/m^2 PO, then 10 g/m^2 PO q6h for 72 h for rescue	Replacement therapy and treatment of megaloblastic anemia; rescue after chemotherapy
Vitamin B$_{12}$		
Ⓟ hydroxocobalamin (*Hydro-Crysti 12*)	30 μg/d IM for 5–10 d, then 100–200 μg/mo IM Pediatric: 1–5 mg IM over 2 or more weeks, then 30–50 μg IM every 4 wk	Replacement therapy; treatment of megaloblastic anemia, pernicious anemia
cyanocobalamin (*Crysti100, Crystamine*) (*Nascobal*)	30 μg/d IM or SC for 5–10 d, then 100–200 μg IM or SC every 4 wk One spray (500 μg) in one nostril once a week	Replacement therapy; treatment of megaloblastic anemia (as nasal gel)

- Arrange for nutritional consultation, *to ensure a well-balanced diet.*
- Monitor for the possibility of hypersensitivity reactions; *have life support equipment on standby in case reactions occur.*
- Arrange for hematocrit readings before and periodically during therapy, *to monitor drug effectiveness.*
- Provide comfort measures, *to help the patient tolerate drug effects.* These include small, frequent meals, access to bathroom facilities, and analgesia for muscle or nasal pain.
- Provide thorough patient teaching, including the name of the drug, dosage prescribed, measures to avoid adverse effects, warning signs of problems, and the need for periodic monitoring and evaluation, *to enhance patient knowledge about drug therapy and to promote compliance with drug regimen.*
- Offer support and encouragement, *to help the patient deal with the diagnosis and the drug regimen.*

Evaluation

- Monitor patient response to the drug (alleviation of anemia).
- Monitor for adverse effects (nasal irritation, pain at injection site, nausea).
- Evaluate the effectiveness of the teaching plan (patient can name drug, dosage, adverse effects to watch for, specific measures to avoid adverse effects; patient understands importance of continued follow-up).
- Monitor the effectiveness of comfort measures and compliance to the regimen.

◻◼◉◻ WEB LINKS

Health care providers and patients may want to explore the following Internet sources:

Information on various forms of anemias, causes, characteristics, diagnosis, treatment:
  http://www.aplastic.org
Information designed for patients and families regarding anemias:
  http://www.thedailyapple.com
Information on iron toxicity—treatment, diagnosis, and complications, for patients and health care providers:
  http://www.ansci.cornell.edu
Information on erythropoietin—action, uses:
  http://www.noblood.com/wf/articles/00200545.htm

CHAPTER SUMMARY

- The cardiovascular system exists to pump blood to all of the body's cells.
- Blood contains oxygen and nutrients that are essential for cell survival; it delivers these to the cells and removes waste products from the tissues.
- Blood is composed of a liquid plasma (containing water, proteins, glucose, and electrolytes) and formed components including white blood cells, red blood cells (RBCs), and platelets.

- RBCs are produced in the bone marrow in a process called erythropoiesis, which is controlled by the glycoprotein erythropoietin, produced by the kidneys.
- RBCs do not have a nucleus, and their lifespan is about 120 days, at which time they are lysed and their building blocks are recycled to make new RBCs.
- The bone marrow uses iron, amino acids, carbohydrates, folic acid, and vitamin B_{12} to produce healthy, efficient RBCs.
- An insufficient number or maturity of RBCs results in low oxygen levels in the tissues, with tiredness, fatigue, and loss of reserve.
- Anemia is a state of too few RBCs. Anemia can be caused by a lack of erythropoietin or by a lack of the components needed to produce RBCs.
- Iron deficiency anemia occurs when there is inadequate iron intake in the diet or an inability to absorb iron from the GI tract. Iron is needed to produce hemoglobin, which carries the oxygen. Iron deficiency anemia is treated with iron replacement.
- Iron is a very toxic mineral at high levels. The body controls the absorption of iron and carefully regulates its storage and movement in the body.
- Folic acid and vitamin B_{12} are needed to produce a strong supporting structure in the RBC so that it can survive 120 days of being propelled through the vascular system. These are usually found in adequate amounts in the diet.
- A dietary lack of or inability to absorb folic acid, vitamin B_{12}, or both will produce a megaloblastic anemia, in which the RBCs are large and immature and have a short lifespan.
- Pernicious anemia is a lack of vitamin B_{12}, which is also used by the body to maintain the myelin sheath on nerve axons. If vitamin B_{12} is lacking, these neurons will degenerate and cause many CNS effects.
- Pernicious anemia is caused by the deficient production of intrinsic factor by gastric cells.
- Intrinsic factor is needed to allow the body to absorb vitamin B_{12}. If intrinsic factor is lacking, vitamin B_{12} must be given parenterally or intranasally for life to ensure absorption.

Review Questions

1. The rate of red blood cell production is controlled by
   a. iron.
   b. folic acid.
   c. erythropoietin.
   d. vitamin B_{12}.
2. Red blood cells must be continually produced by the body because
   a. the iron within the RBC wears out.
   b. with no nucleus, the RBC cannot maintain itself and wears out over time.
   c. there is continual loss of RBCs from the gastrointestinal tract of healthy adults.
   d. RBCs are processed into bile salts and must be replaced.
3. Anemia is
   a. a decreased number of red blood cells.
   b. a lack of iron in the body.

c. a lack of vitamin B_{12} in the body.

d. an excessive number of platelets.

4. In a healthy person, very little iron is needed on a daily basis. Loss of iron is associated with all of the following except
   a. heavy menstrual flow.
   b. bile duct obstruction.
   c. internal bleeding.
   d. traumatic injury and loss of blood.

5. Megaloblastic anemia is a result of insufficient folic acid or vitamin B_{12}, and it affects
   a. white blood cell production.
   b. vegetarians.
   c. all cells in the body that are rapidly turning over.
   d. slow-growing cells.

6. *Epogen* (epoetin alfa) would be the drug of choice
   a. for acute blood loss during surgery.
   b. to replace blood loss from traumatic injury.
   c. for treatment of anemia during lactation.
   d. for the treatment of anemia associated with renal failure.

7. A patient with anemia who is given iron salts could expect to show a therapeutic increase in hematocrit
   a. within 72 hours.
   b. within 2 to 3 weeks.
   c. over 6 to 10 months.
   d. within 1 to 2 weeks.

8. Iron is not absorbed from the gastrointestinal tract if it is taken with
   a. protein.
   b. anticoagulants.

c. dairy products.

d. any other drugs.

9. A patient with pernicious anemia would be advised to take vitamin B_{12}
   a. orally with breakfast.
   b. orally at bedtime.
   c. subcutaneously every day.
   d. intramuscularly every 5 to 10 days.

10. Patients are often given iron pills by their clinic. Instructions in giving these pills should include
   a. taking the drug with milk to avoid gastrointestinal problems.
   b. the potential for severe diarrhea.
   c. keeping these potentially toxic pills away from children.
   d. taking the drug with antacids to alleviate the gastrointestinal upset.

BIBLIOGRAPHY

Bullock, B. L. (2000). *Focus on pathophysiology*. Philadelphia: Lippincott Williams & Wilkins.

Drug facts and comparisons. (2002). St. Louis: Facts and Comparisons.

Gilman, A., Hardman, J. G., & Limbird, L. E. (Eds.) (2002). *Goodman and Gilman's the pharmacological basis of therapeutics* (10th ed.). New York: McGraw-Hill.

Karch, A. M. (2002). *2003 Lippincott's nursing drug guide*. Philadelphia: Lippincott Williams & Wilkins.

The medical letter on drugs and therapeutics. (2002). New Rochelle, NY: Medical Letter.

Porth, C. M. (2002). *Pathophysiology: Concepts of altered health states* (6th ed.). Philadelphia: Lippincott Williams & Wilkins.

IX

Drugs Acting on the Renal System

CHAPTER

50

Introduction to the Kidney and the Urinary Tract

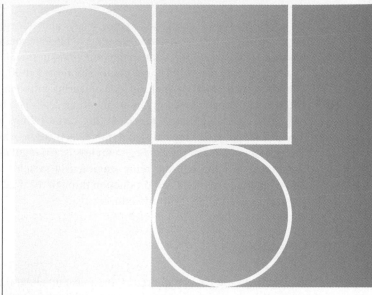

Key Terms

aldosterone

antidiuretic hormone (ADH)

carbonic anhydrase

countercurrent mechanism

filtration

glomerulus

nephron

prostate gland

reabsorption

renin–angiotensin system

secretion

The renal system is composed of the kidneys and the organs of the urinary tract: the ureters, the urinary bladder, and the urethra. This system has four major functions in the body: (1) maintaining the volume and composition of body fluids within normal ranges, which includes clearing nitrogenous wastes from protein metabolism, maintaining acid–base balance and electrolyte levels, and excreting various drugs and drug metabolites; (2) regulating vitamin D activation, which helps to maintain and regulate calcium levels; (3) regulating blood pressure through the renin–angiotensin system; and (4) regulating red blood cell production through the production and secretion of erythropoietin.

THE KIDNEYS

The kidneys are two small organs that make up about 0.5% of total body weight but receive about 25% of the cardiac output. Approximately 1600 L of blood flows through these two small organs each day for cleansing. Most of the fluid that is filtered out by the kidneys is returned to the body, while the waste products that remain are excreted in a relatively small amount of water as urine.

The kidneys are located under the ribs, for protection from injury, and have three protective layers that make up the renal capsule: a fiber layer, a perirenal or brown fat layer, and the renal parietal layer. The capsule contains pain fibers, which are stimulated if the capsule is stretched secondary to an inflammatory process. The kidney has three identifiable regions: the outer cortex, the inner medulla, and the renal pelves. The renal pelves drain the urine into the ureters. The ureters are muscular tubes that lead into the urinary bladder, where urine is stored until it is excreted (Figure 50–1).

The functional unit of the kidney is called the **nephron.** There are approximately 2.4 million nephrons in an adult. All of the nephrons filter fluid and make urine, but only the medullary nephrons can concentrate or dilute urine. It is estimated that only about 25% of the total number of nephrons are necessary to maintain healthy renal function. That means that the renal system is well protected from failure with a large backup system. However, it also means that by the time a patient has signs and symptoms of renal failure, extensive damage to the kidneys has already occurred.

The nephron is basically a tube (Figure 50–2). It begins with Bowman's capsule, which has a fenestrated or "windowed" epithelium that works like a sieve or a strainer to allow fluid to flow through, but keeps large things (such as proteins) from entering. The nephron then curls around in a section called the proximal convoluted tubule. From there, it narrows to form the descending and ascending loop of Henle, widens as the distal convoluted tubule, then flows into the collecting ducts, which meet at the renal pelvis. Each section of the tubule functions in a slightly different manner to maintain fluid and electrolyte balance in the body.

The blood flow to the nephron is unique. The renal arteries come directly off the aorta and enter each kidney. As a

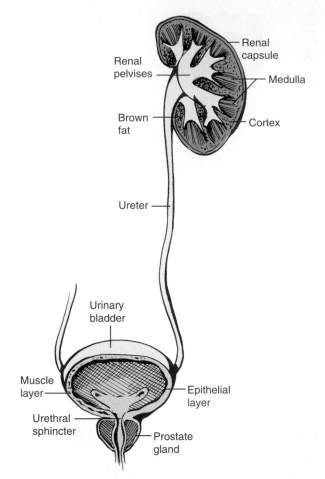

FIGURE 50-1. The kidney and organs of the urinary tract.

renal artery enters each of the kidneys, it divides to form interlobar arteries, which become smaller arcuate (bowed) arteries, then afferent arterioles. The afferent arterioles branch to form the **glomerulus** inside Bowman's capsule. The glomerulus is like a tuft of blood vessels with a capillary-like endothelium that allows easy passage of fluid and waste products. The efferent arteriole exits from the glomerulus and branches into the peritubular capillary system, which returns fluid and electrolytes that have been reabsorbed from the tubules to the bloodstream. These capillaries flow into the vasa recta, which flows into intralobar veins, which in turn drain into the inferior vena cava. The two arterioles around the glomerulus work together to closely regulate the flow of fluid into the glomerulus, increasing or decreasing pressure on either side of the glomerulus as needed.

A small group of cells, called the juxtaglomerular apparatus, connects the afferent arteriole to the distal convoluted tubule; this is where erythropoietin and renin are produced. Because of their proximity to the afferent arteriole, these cells are especially sensitive to the volume and quality of blood flow into the glomerulus.

Surrounding the nephrons is an area called the macula densa, which is full of immune system cells and chemicals that can respond quickly to any cellular damage or injury.

FIGURE 50-2. The nephron, the functional unit of the kidney. Secretion and reabsorption of water, electrolytes, and other solutes in the various segments of the renal tubule, the loop of Henle, and the collecting duct can be influenced by diuretics, other drugs, and endogenous substances, including certain hormones. In the kidney, the distal convoluted tubule wraps around and is actually next to the afferent arteriole.

Renal Processes

The nephrons function by using three basic processes: glomerular **filtration** (straining fluid into the nephron), tubular **secretion** (actively removing components from the capillary system and depositing them into the tubule), and tubular **reabsorption** (removing components from the tubule to return them to the capillary system and circulation).

Glomerular Filtration

The glomerulus acts as an ultrafine filter for all of the blood that flows into it. The semipermeable membrane keeps blood cells, proteins, and lipids inside the vessel, while the hydrostatic pressure from the blood pushes water and smaller components of the plasma into the tubule. A clinical sign of renal damage is the presence of blood cells or protein in the urine. This can happen when the semipermeable membrane is scarred, swollen, or damaged, allowing the larger plasma components to escape into the filtrate. The large size of these components prevents them from being reabsorbed by the tubule, and they are lost in the urine.

Approximately 125 mL of fluid is filtered out each minute, or 180 L/day. About 99% of the filtered fluid is returned to the bloodstream as the filtrate progresses through the renal tubule. Approximately 1% of the filtrate, less than 2 L of fluid, is excreted each day in the form of urine.

Tubular Secretion

The epithelial cells that line the renal tubule can secrete substances from the blood into the tubular fluid. This is an energy-using process that allows active transport systems to remove electrolytes, some drugs and drug metabolites, and uric acid from the surrounding capillaries and secrete them into the filtrate. For instance, the epithelial cells can use tubular secretion to help maintain acid–base levels by secreting hydrogen ions as needed.

Tubular Reabsorption

The cells lining the renal tubule reabsorb water and various essential substances from the filtrate back into the vascular system. About 99% of the water filtered at the glomerulus is reabsorbed. Other filtrate components that are reabsorbed regularly include vitamins, glucose, electrolytes, sodium bicarbonate, and sodium chloride. The reabsorption process uses a series of transport systems that exchange needed ions for unwanted ones (see Chapter 7 for a review of cellular transport systems). Drugs that affect renal function frequently overwhelm one of these transport systems or interfere with its normal activity, leading to an imbalance in acid–base or electrolyte levels. The precision of the reabsorption process allows the body to maintain the correct extracellular fluid volume and composition.

Maintenance of Volume and Composition of Body Fluids

The kidney regulates the composition of body fluids by balancing the levels of the key electrolytes, secreting or absorbing these electrolytes to maintain the desired levels. The volume of body fluids is controlled by diluting or concentrating the urine.

Sodium Regulation

Sodium is one of the body's major cations (positively charged ions). It filters through the glomerulus and enters the renal tubule, then is actively reabsorbed in the proximal convoluted tubule to the peritubular capillaries. As sodium is actively moved out of the filtrate, it takes chloride ions and water with it. This occurs by passive diffusion as the body maintains the osmotic and electrical balances on both sides of the tubule.

Sodium ions are also reabsorbed via a transport system that functions under the influence of the catalyst **carbonic anhydrase**, which allows carbon dioxide and water to combine, forming carbonic acid. The carbonic acid immediately dissociates to form sodium bicarbonate, using a sodium ion from the renal tubule and a free hydrogen ion (an acid). The hydrogen ion is then left in the filtrate, causing the urine to be slightly acidic. The bicarbonate is stored in the renal tubule as the body's alkaline reserve, for use when the body becomes too acidic and a buffer is needed.

The distal convoluted tubule acts to further adjust the sodium levels in the filtrate under the influence of **aldosterone** (a hormone produced by the adrenal gland) and natruretic hormone (probably produced by the hypothalamus). Aldosterone is released into the circulation in response to high potassium levels, sympathetic stimulation, or angiotensin III. Aldosterone stimulates a sodium–potassium exchange pump in the cells of the distal tubule that reabsorbs sodium in exchange for potassium (see Chapter 7 for a review of the sodium pump). As a result of aldosterone stimulation, sodium is reabsorbed into the system and potassium is lost in the filtrate. Natruretic hormone causes a decrease in sodium reabsorption from the distal tubules with a resultant dilute urine or increased volume. Natruretic hormone is released in response to fluid overload or hemodilution.

Countercurrent Mechanism

Sodium is further regulated in the medullary nephrons in what is known as the **countercurrent mechanism** in the loop of Henle. In the descending loop of Henle, the cells are freely permeable to water and sodium. Sodium is actively reabsorbed into the surrounding peritubular tissue, and water flows out of the tubule into this sodium-rich tissue to maintain osmotic balance. The filtrate at the end of the descending loop of Henle is concentrated in comparison to the rest of the filtrate.

In contrast, the ascending loop of Henle is impermeable to water, so water that remains in the tubule is trapped there. Chloride is actively transported out of the tubule using energy in a process that is referred to as the chloride pump; sodium leaves with the chloride to maintain electrical neutrality. As a result, the fluid in the ascending loop of Henle becomes hypotonic in comparison to the hypertonic situation in the peritubular tissue.

Antidiuretic hormone (ADH), which is produced by the hypothalamus and stored in the posterior pituitary gland, is important in maintaining fluid balance. ADH is released in response to falling blood volume, sympathetic stimulation, or rising sodium levels (a concentration that is sensed by the osmotic cells of the hypothalamus).

If ADH is present at the distal convoluted tubule and the collecting duct, the permeability of the membrane to water is increased. Consequently, the water remaining in the tubule rapidly flows into the hypertonic tissue surrounding the loop of Henle, where it is either absorbed by the peritubular capillaries or re-enters the descending loop of Henle in a countercurrent style. The resulting urine is hypertonic and of small volume. If ADH is not present, the tubule remains impermeable to water. The water that has been trapped in the ascending loop of Henle passes into the collection duct, resulting in a hypotonic urine of greater volume. This countercurrent mechanism allows the body to finely regulate fluid volume by regulating the control of sodium and water (Figure 50–3).

Potassium Regulation

Potassium is another cation that is vital to proper functioning of the nervous system, muscles, and cell membranes. About 65% of the potassium that is filtered at the glomerulus is reabsorbed at Bowman's capsule and the proximal convoluted tubule. Another 25% to 30% is reabsorbed in the ascending loop of Henle. The fine tuning of potassium levels occurs in the distal convoluted tubule, where aldosterone activates the sodium–potassium exchange, leading to a loss of potassium. If potassium levels are very high, the retention of sodium in exchange for potassium also leads to a retention of water and a dilution of the blood volume, which further decreases the potassium concentration (see Figure 50–3).

Chloride Regulation

Chloride is an important negatively charged ion that helps to maintain electrical neutrality with the movement of cations across the cell membrane. Chloride is primarily reabsorbed in the loop of Henle, where it promotes the movement of sodium out of the cell.

FIGURE 50-3. Nephron and points of regulation of sodium, chloride, potassium, calcium, and water. ADH, antidiuretic hormone; PTH, parathyroid hormone.

Regulation of Vitamin D Activation

Calcium is another important cation that is regulated by the kidney. The absorption of calcium from the gastrointestinal (GI) tract is regulated by vitamin D. Vitamin D is taken in as part of the diet and then must be activated in the kidney to a form that will promote the absorption of calcium from the GI tract. Once absorbed from the GI tract, calcium levels are maintained within a very tight range by the activity of parathyroid hormone (PTH) and calcitonin.

Calcium Regulation

Calcium is important in muscle function, blood clotting, bone formation, contraction of cell membranes, and muscle movement. Calcium is filtered at the glomerulus and mostly reabsorbed in the proximal convoluted tubule and ascending loop of Henle. Fine tuning of calcium reabsorption occurs in the distal convoluted tubule, where the presence of PTH stimulates reabsorption of calcium to increase serum calcium levels when they are low (see Figure 50-3 and Chapter 37).

Blood Pressure Control: Renin–Angiotensin System

The fragile nephrons require a constant supply of blood and are equipped with a system to ensure that they are perfused. This mechanism, called the **renin–angiotensin system** (sometimes called the renin–angiotensin–aldosterone system), involves a total body reaction to decreased blood flow to the nephrons.

Whenever blood flow or oxygenation to the nephron is decreased (due to hemorrhage, shock, congestive heart failure, or hypotension), renin is released from the juxtaglomerular

cells. (These cells, which are positioned next to the glomerulus, are stimulated by decreased stretch and decreased oxygen levels.) The released renin immediately is absorbed into the capillary system and enters circulation.

The released renin activates angiotensinogen, a substrate produced in the liver, which becomes angiotensin I. Angiotensin I is then converted to angiotensin II by a converting enzyme found in the lungs and some vessels. Angiotensin II is a very powerful vasoconstrictor, reacting with angiotensin II receptor sites in blood vessels to cause vasoconstriction. This powerful vasoconstriction raises blood pressure and should increase blood flow to the kidneys.

Angiotensin II is converted in the adrenal gland to angiotensin III, which stimulates the release of aldosterone from the adrenal gland. Aldosterone acts on the renal tubules to retain sodium and therefore water. This increases blood volume and further increases blood pressure, which should increase blood flow to the kidney. The osmotic center in the brain senses the increased sodium levels and releases ADH, leading to a further retention of water and a further increase in blood volume and pressure, which should again increase blood flow to the kidney.

The renin–angiotensin system constantly works to maintain blood flow to the kidneys. For example, an individual rising from a lying position experiences a drop in blood flow to the kidney as blood pools in the legs because of gravity. This causes a massive release of renin and activation of this system to ensure that blood pressure is maintained and the kidneys are perfused. Blood loss from injury or during surgery also activates this system to increase blood flow through the kidneys.

It is important to note that drugs that interfere with any aspect of this system will cause a reflex response. For instance, taking a drug such as a diuretic to decrease fluid volume can lead to decreased blood flow to the kidney as blood volume drops. This in turn leads to a rebound retention of fluid as part of the renin–angiotensin system's effects (Figure 50–4).

Regulation of Red Blood Cell Production

Whenever blood flow or oxygenation to the nephron is decreased (due to hemorrhage, shock, congestive heart failure, or hypotension), the hormone erythropoietin is also released from the juxtaglomerular cells. This hormone stimulates the bone marrow to increase production of red blood cells, which act to bring oxygen to the kidneys. Erythropoietin is the only known factor that can regulate the rate of red blood cell production. When a patient develops renal failure and the production of erythropoietin drops, the production of red blood cells falls and the patient becomes anemic.

THE URINARY TRACT

As noted previously, the urinary tract is composed of the ureters, urinary bladder, and urethra (see Figure 50–1). One ureter exits each kidney, draining the filtrate from the collecting ducts. The ureters have a smooth endothelial lining and circular muscular layers. Urine entering the ureter stimulates a peristaltic wave that pushes the urine down toward the urinary bladder.

The urinary bladder is a muscular pouch that stretches and holds the urine until it is excreted from the body. Urine is usually a slightly acidic fluid; this acidity helps to maintain the normal transport systems and to destroy bacteria that may enter the bladder.

In the female, the urethra is very short and leads to an area populated by normal flora including *Escherichia coli,* which can cause frequent bladder infections or cystitis. In the male, the urethra is much longer and passes through the **prostate gland,** a small gland that produces an acidic fluid that is important in maintaining the sperm and lubricating the tract. Enlargement and infection in the prostate gland are often problems in older males. Control of bladder emptying is learned control over the urethral sphincter; once it is established, a functioning nervous system is necessary to maintain control.

CHAPTER SUMMARY

- The kidneys are two small organs that receive about 25% of the cardiac output.
- The functional unit of the kidney is called the nephron; it is composed of Bowman's capsule, the proximal convoluted tubule, the loop of Henle, the distal convoluted tubule, and the collecting duct.
- The blood flow to the nephron is unique, allowing autoregulation of blood flow through the glomerulus.
- The nephrons function by using three basic processes: glomerular filtration (straining fluid into the nephron), tubular secretion (actively removing components from the capillary system and depositing them into the tubule), and tubular reabsorption (removing components from the tubule to return them to the capillary system and circulation).
- Sodium levels are regulated throughout the tubule by active and passive movement and are fine-tuned by the presence of aldosterone in the distal tubule.
- The countercurrent mechanism in the medullary nephrons allows for the concentration or dilution of urine under the influence of ADH secreted by the hypothalamus.
- Potassium concentration is regulated throughout the tubule, with aldosterone being the strongest influence for potassium loss.
- The kidneys play a key role in the regulation of calcium by activating vitamin D to allow GI calcium reabsorption and by reabsorbing or excreting calcium from the tubule under the influence of parathyroid hormone (PTH).
- The kidneys influence blood pressure control, releasing renin to activate the renin–angiotensin system, which leads to increased blood pressure and volume and a resultant increased blood flow to the kidney. The balance of this reflex system can lead to water retention or excretion and has an impact on drug therapy that promotes water or sodium loss.

FIGURE 50–4. The renin–angiotensin system for reflex maintenance of blood pressure control.

• The ureters, urinary bladder, and urethra make up the rest of the urinary tract. The longer male urethra passes through the prostate gland, which may enlarge or become infected, a problem often associated with advancing age.

◻◼◆◼ WEB LINKS

To explore the virtual kidney and urinary tract, visit the following Internet source:

http://www.InnerBody.com

Review Questions

1. During severe exertion, a man may lose up to 4 L of hypotonic sweat per hour. This loss would result in
   a. decreased plasma volume.
   b. decreased plasma osmolarity.
   c. decreased circulating levels of ADH.
   d. return of body fluid balance to normal after ingestion of 100 mL of water.
2. Urine passes through the ureter by
   a. osmosis.
   b. air pressure.
   c. filtration.
   d. gravity and peristalsis.
3. Renal reabsorption
   a. is the movement of substances from the renal tubule into the blood.
   b. is the movement of substances from the blood into the renal tubule.
   c. of water is increased in the absence of ADH.
   d. of sodium occurs only in the proximal tubule.
4. During severe diarrhea, there is a loss of water, bicarbonate, and sodium from the gastrointestinal tract. Physiological compensation for this would probably not include
   a. increased alveolar ventilation.
   b. decreased hydrogen ion secretion by the renal tubules.
   c. decreased urinary excretion of sodium and water.
   d. increased renin secretion.
5. The major reason older adults should monitor their intake of fluids is that
   a. older people have decreased levels of ADH.
   b. older people do not exercise, so fluids do not shift between compartments easily.
   c. total body water decreases with age and restoration of homeostasis is slower.
   d. older people lose more fluid through the skin as it becomes thinner.
6. Maintenance of blood pressure is important in maintaining the fragile nephrons. Reflex systems that work to ensure blood flow to the kidney do not include

a. the renin–angiotensin system causing vasoconstriction.
b. baroreceptor monitoring of the renal artery.
c. aldosterone release secondary to angiotensin stimulation.
d. ADH release in response to decreased blood volume or increased osmolarity.
7. Blood flow to the nephron differs from blood flow to other tissues in that
   a. the venous system is not involved.
   b. there are no capillaries in the nephron.
   c. efferent and afferent arterioles allow for autoregulation of blood flow through the glomerulus.
   d. the capillary bed has a fenestrated membrane.
8. Concentration and dilution of the urine is controlled by
   a. afferent arterioles.
   b. the renin–angiotensin system.
   c. aldosterone release.
   d. the countercurrent mechanism in medullary nephrons.
9. Women tend to have more problems with bladder infections than men because
   a. women have E. coli in the urinary tract.
   b. the female has a short urethra, making access to the bladder easier for bacteria.
   c. the prostate gland secretes a substance that protects men from bladder infections.
   d. women are more acidotic, encouraging the growth of bladder bacteria.
10. Considering the metabolic functions of the kidney, renal failure would be expected to cause all of the following except
    a. anemia.
    b. loss of calcium regulation.
    c. urea buildup on the skin.
    d. respiratory alkalosis.

BIBLIOGRAPHY

Bullock, B. L. (2000). *Focus on pathophysiology*. Philadelphia: Lippincott Williams & Wilkins.
Fox, S. (1991). Perspectives on human biology. Dubuque, IA: Wm. C. Brown Publishers.
Ganong, W. (1999). Review of medical physiology (19th ed.). Norwalk, CT: Appleton & Lange.
Gilman, A., Hardman, J. G., & Limbird, L. E. (Eds.) (2002). *Goodman and Gilman's the pharmacological basis of therapeutics* (10th ed.). New York: McGraw-Hill.
Guyton, A. & Hall, J. (2000). Textbook of medical physiology. Philadelphia: W.B. Saunders.

Diuretic Agents

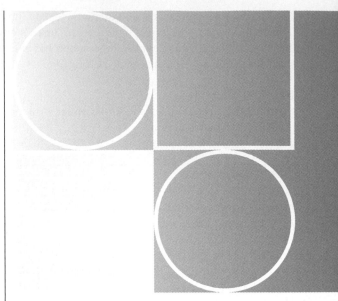

Key Terms

alkalosis

edema

fluid rebound

high-ceiling diuretics

hyperaldosteronism

hypokalemia

osmotic pull

690

Thiazide Diuretics

bendroflumethiazide

benzthiazide

chlorothiazide

ⓟ hydrochlorothiazide

hydroflumethiazide

methyclothiazide

polythiazide

trichlormethiazide

Thiazide-Like Diuretics

ⓟ chlorthalidone

indapamide

metolazone

Loop Diuretics

bumetanide

ethacrynic acid

ⓟ furosemide

torsemide

Carbonic Anhydrase Inhibitors

ⓟ acetazolamide

methazolamide

Potassium-Sparing Diuretics

amiloride

ⓟ spironolactone

triamterene

Osmotic Diuretics

glycerin

isosorbide

ⓟ mannitol

urea

There are five classes of diuretics, each working at a slightly different site in the nephron or using a different mechanism. Diuretic classes include the thiazide and thiazide-like diuretics, the loop diuretics, the carbonic anhydrase inhibitors, the potassium-sparing diuretics, and the osmotic diuretics. The overall nursing care of a patient receiving any diuretic is similar. The diuretics classes are discussed in this chapter, starting with the most frequently used drugs.

DIURETIC AGENTS

Diuretic agents are commonly thought of simply as drugs that increase the amount of urine produced by the kidneys. Most diuretics do increase the volume of urine produced to some extent, but the greater clinical significance of diuretics is their ability to increase sodium excretion.

Therapeutic Actions and Indications

Diuretics prevent the cells lining the renal tubules from reabsorbing an excessive proportion of the sodium ions in the glomerular filtrate. As a result, sodium and other ions (and the water in which they are dissolved) are lost in the urine instead of being returned to the blood, where they would cause increased intravascular volume and therefore hydrostatic pressure, which could result in a leaking of fluids at the capillary level.

Diuretics are indicated for the treatment of **edema** associated with congestive heart failure, acute pulmonary edema, liver disease (including cirrhosis), renal disease, and for the treatment of hypertension. They are also used to decrease

DRUG THERAPY ACROSS THE LIFESPAN

Diuretic Agents

Children	Adults	Older Adults
Diuretics are often used in children to treat edema associated with heart defects, to control hypertension, and to treat edema associated with renal and pulmonary disorders. Hydrochlorothiazide and chlorothiazide have established pediatric dosing guidelines. Furosemide is often used when a stronger diuretic is needed; care should be taken not to exceed 6 mg/kg per day when using this drug. Ethacrynic acid may be used orally in some situations but should not be used in infants. Bumetanide, although not recommended for use in children, may be used for children who are taking other ototoxic drugs, including antibiotics, and may cause less hypokalemia, making it preferable to furosemide for children also taking digoxin. Spironolactone is the only potassium-sparing diuretic that is recommended for use in children, but, as with adults, it should not be used in the presence of severe renal impairment. Because of the size and rapid metabolism of children, the effects of diuretics may be rapid and adverse effects may occur suddenly. The child receiving a diuretic should be monitored for serum electrolyte changes; for evidence of fluid volume changes; for rapid weight gain or loss, which could reflect fluid volume; and for signs of ototoxicity.	Adults may be taking diuretics for prolonged periods and need to be aware of the signs and symptoms of fluid imbalance to report to their health care provider. Adults receiving chronic diuretic therapy should weigh themselves on the same scale, in the same clothes, and at the same time each day to monitor for fluid retention or sudden fluid loss. They should be alerted to situations that could aggravate fluid loss, such as diarrhea, vomiting, or excessive heat and sweating, which could change their need for the diuretic. They should also be urged to maintain their fluid intake to help balance their body's compensatory mechanisms and to prevent fluid rebound. Patients taking potassium-losing diuretics should be encouraged to eat foods that are high in potassium and to have their serum potassium levels checked periodically. Patients taking potassium-sparing diuretics should be cautioned to avoid those same foods. The use of diuretics to change the fluid shifts associated with pregnancy is not appropriate. Women maintained on these drugs for underlying medical reasons should not stop taking the drug, but they need to be aware of the potential for adverse effects on the fetus. Women who are nursing and need a diuretic should find another method of feeding the baby because of the potential for adverse effects on the baby as well as the lactating mother.	Older adults often have conditions that are treated with diuretics. They are also more likely to have renal or hepatic impairment, which requires cautious use of these drugs. Older adults should be started on the lowest possible dose of the drug, and the dosage should titrated slowly based on patient response. Frequent serum electrolyte measurements should be done to monitor for adverse reactions. The intake and activity level of the patient can alter the effectiveness and need for the diuretic. High-salt diets and inactivity can aggravate conditions that lead to edema, and patients should be encouraged to follow activity and dietary guidelines if possible.

fluid pressure in the eye (intraocular pressure), which is useful in treating glaucoma. Diuretics that decrease potassium levels may also be indicated in the treatment of conditions that cause hyperkalemia.

Congestive heart failure (CHF) can cause edema as a result of several factors. The failing heart muscle does not pump sufficient blood to the kidneys, causing activation of the renin–angiotensin system and resulting increases in blood volume and sodium retention. Because the failing heart muscle cannot respond to the usual reflex stimulation, the increased volume is slowly pushed out into the capillary level as venous pressure increases because the blood is not being pumped effectively (see Chapter 44).

Pulmonary edema, or left-sided CHF, develops when the increased volume of fluids backs up into the lungs. The fluid pushed out into the capillaries in the lungs interferes with gas exchange. When this condition develops rapidly, it can be life-threatening.

Patients with liver failure and cirrhosis often present with edema and ascites. This is caused by (1) reduced plasma protein production, resulting in less oncotic pull in the vascular system and fluid loss at the capillary level; and (2) obstructed blood flow through the portal system caused by increased pressure from congested hepatic vessels.

Renal disease produces edema because of the loss of plasma proteins into the urine when there is damage to the glomerular basement membrane. Other types of renal disease produce edema because of activation of the renin–angiotensin system as a result of decreasing volume (associated with the loss of fluid into the urine) which causes a drop in blood pressure or because of failure of the renal tubules to regulate electrolytes effectively.

Hypertension is predominantly an idiopathic disorder; in other words, the underlying pathology is not known. Treatment of hypertension is aimed at reducing the higher-than-normal blood pressure, which can damage end organs and lead to serious cardiovascular disorders. Diuretics were once the key element in antihypertensive therapy, the goal of which was to decrease volume and sodium, which would then decrease pressure in the system. Now several other classes of drugs, including angiotensin-converting enzyme (ACE) inhibitors, angiotensin receptor blockers (ARBs), β-blockers, and calcium channel blockers, are used more frequently for the initial treatment of hypertension. Currently, diuretics are often used as an adjunct to improve the effectiveness of these other drugs.

Glaucoma is an eye disease that is characterized by increased pressure in the eye (intraocular pressure, IOP), which can cause optic nerve atrophy and blindness. Diuretics are used to provide osmotic pull to remove some of the fluid from the eye, which decreases the IOP, or as adjunctive therapy to reduce fluid volume and pressure in the cardiovascular system, which also decreases pressure in the eye somewhat.

Contraindications and Cautions

Diuretic use is contraindicated in the presence of allergy to any of the drugs given. Other conditions in which diuretics are contraindicated include fluid and electrolyte imbalances, which can be potentiated by the fluid and electrolyte changes caused by the diuretics, and severe renal disease, which may prevent the diuretic from working or could be pushed into a crisis stage by the blood flow changes brought about by the diuretic.

Caution should be used with the following conditions: systemic lupus erythematosus, which frequently causes glomerular changes and renal dysfunction that could precipitate renal failure in some cases; glucose tolerance abnormalities or diabetes mellitus, which is worsened by the glucose-elevating effects of many diuretics; gout, which reflects an abnormality in normal tubule reabsorption and secretion; liver disease, which could interfere with the normal metabolism of the drugs, leading to an accumulation of the drug or toxicity; and pregnancy and lactation, which are conditions that could be jeopardized by changes in fluid and electrolyte balance.

Adverse Effects

Adverse effects associated with diuretics are specific to the particular class used. For details, see the section on adverse effects for each class of diuretics discussed in this chapter and refer to Table 51–1. The most common adverse effects seen with diuretics include gastrointestinal (GI) upset, fluid and electrolyte imbalances, hypotension, and electrolyte disturbances.

Clinically Important Drug–Drug Interactions

When diuretics are used, there is a potential for interactions with drugs that depend on a particular electrolyte balance for their therapeutic effects (eg, antiarrhythmics such as digoxin), with drugs that depend on urine alkalinity for proper excretion (eg, quinidine), and with drugs that depend on normal reflexes to balance their effects (eg, antihypertensives, antidiabetic agents), because these factors are altered by the action of diuretics.

Other specific drug–drug interactions that might relate to the chemical makeup of a particular diuretic are noted later.

THIAZIDE AND THIAZIDE-LIKE DIURETICS

Hydrochlorothiazide (*HydroDIURIL*), the most frequently used of the thiazide diuretics, is often used in combination with other drugs for the treatment of hypertension. It can be used in a smaller doses because it is more potent than chlorothiazide (*Diuril*), which is the oldest drug of this class, and it is considered the prototype. Other thiazides include bendroflumethiazide (*Naturetin*), benzthiazide (*Exna*), hydroflumethiazide (*Diucardin*), methyclothiazide (*Aquatensen*), polythiazide (*Renese*), and trichlormethiazide (*Diurese*).

The thiazide-like diuretics include chlorthalidone (*Hygroton*), indapamide (*Lozol*), and metolazone (*Mykrox*). All of these drugs are used less often than hydrochlorothiazide and are typically chosen according to the prescriber's personal preference.

TABLE 51-1	Comparison of Diuretics

Diuretic Class	Major Site of Action	Usual Indications	Major Adverse Effects
Thiazide, thiazide-like	Distal convoluted tubule	Edema of CHF, liver and renal disease Adjunct for hypertension	GI upset, CNS complications, hypovolemia
Loop	Loop of Henle	Acute CHF Acute pulmonary edema Hypertension Edema of CHF, renal and liver disease	Hypokalemia, volume depletion, hypotension, CNS effects, GI upset, hyperglycemia
Carbonic anhydrase inhibitors	Proximal tubule	Glaucoma Diuresis in CHF Mountain sickness Epilepsy	GI upset, urinary frequency
Potassium-sparing	Distal tubule and collecting duct	Adjunct for edema of CHF, liver and renal disease Treatment of hypokalemia Adjunct for hypertension Hyperaldosteronism	Hyperkalemia, CNS effects, diarrhea
Osmotic	Glomerulus, tubule	Reduction of intracranial pressure Prevention of oliguric phase of renal failure Reduction of intraocular pressure Renal clearance of toxic substances	Hypotension, GI upset, fluid and electrolyte imbalances

Therapeutic Actions and Indications

The thiazide diuretics belong to a chemical class of drugs called the sulfonamides. Thiazide-like diuretics have a slightly different chemical structure but work in the same way that thiazide diuretics do. Their action is to block the chloride

NURSING CHALLENGE
Avoiding Fluid Rebound

Care must be taken when using diuretics to avoid **fluid rebound,** which is associated with fluid loss. If patient stops taking in water and takes the diuretic, the result will be a concentrated plasma of smaller volume. The decreased volume is sensed by the nephrons, which activate the renin–angiotensin cycle. When the concentrated blood is sensed by the osmotic center in the brain, antidiuretic hormone (ADH) is released to hold water and dilute the blood. The result can be a "rebound" edema as fluid is retained.

Many patients who are taking a diuretic markedly decrease their fluid intake so as to decrease the number of trips to the bathroom. The result is a rebound of water retention after the diuretic effect. This effect can also be seen in many diets that promise "immediate result"; they frequently contain a key provision to increase fluid intake to 8 to 10 full glasses of water daily. The reflex result of diluting the system with so much water is a drop in ADH release and fluid loss. Some people can lose 5 lb in a few days by doing this. However, the body's reflexes soon kick in, causing rebound retention of fluid to re-establish fluid and electrolyte balance. Most people get frustrated at this point and give up the fad diet. It is important to be able to explain this effect. Balancing the desired diuretic effect with the actions of the normal reflexes is a clinical challenge.

pump. Chloride is actively pumped out of the tubule by cells lining the ascending limb of the loop of Henle and the distal tubule. Sodium passively moves with the chloride to maintain an electrical neutrality. (Chloride is a negative ion and sodium is a positive ion.) Blocking of the chloride pump keeps the chloride and the sodium in the tubule to be excreted in the urine, thus preventing the reabsorption of both chloride and sodium in the vascular system (Figure 51–1). Because these segments of the tubule are impermeable to water, there is little increase in the volume of urine produced, but it will be sodium rich, a saluretic effect. Thiazides are considered to be mild diuretics compared to the more potent loop diuretics.

Thiazide and thiazide-like diuretics are usually indicated for the treatment of edema associated with CHF or with liver or renal disease. These drugs also are used as adjuncts for the treatment of hypertension.

Pharmacokinetics

These drugs are well absorbed from the GI tract, with onset of action ranging from 1 to 3 hours. They are metabolized in the liver and excreted in the urine. These diuretics cross the placenta and enter breast milk. Routine use during pregnancy is not appropriate and should be saved for situations in which the mother has pathological reasons for use, not pregnancy manifestations or complications, and when the benefit to the mother clearly outweighs the risk to the fetus. If one of these drugs is needed during lactation, another method of feeding the baby should be used, because of the potential of adverse effects on fluid and electrolyte changes in the baby.

Adverse Effects

Adverse effects of thiazide use are related to the interference with the normal regulatory mechanisms of the nephron. Potassium is lost at the distal tubule because of the actions

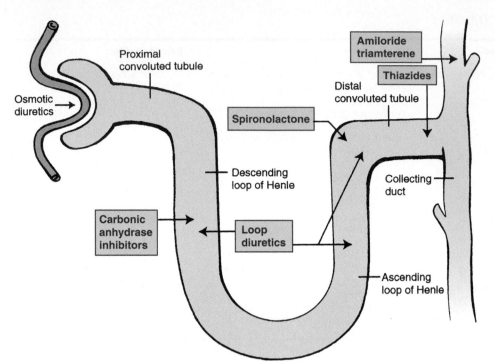

FIGURE 51–1. Sites of action of diuretics in the nephron.

on the pumping mechanism, and hypokalemia (low blood levels of potassium) may result. Signs and symptoms of **hypokalemia** include weakness, muscle cramps, and arrhythmias. Another adverse effect is decreased calcium excretion, which leads to increased calcium levels. Uric acid excretion also is decreased, because the thiazides interfere with its secretory mechanism. High levels of uric acid can result in a condition called gout.

When these drugs are used over a prolonged period, blood glucose levels may be increased. This may result from the changes in potassium levels (which keep glucose out of the cells), or it may relate to some other mechanism of glucose control.

Urine will be slightly alkalinized when the thiazides are used, because they block the reabsorption of bicarbonate. This effect can cause problems for patients who are susceptible to bladder infections and for those taking quinidine, which requires an acid urine for excretion.

Clinically Important Drug–Drug Interactions

Decreased absorption of these drugs may occur if they are combined with cholestyramine or colestipol. If this combination is used, the drugs should be separated by at least 2 hours.

There is an increased risk of digoxin toxicity related to potential changes in potassium levels; serum potassium should be monitored if this combination is used.

Decreased effectiveness of antidiabetic agents may occur related to the changes in glucose metabolism; dosage adjustment of those agents may be needed.

There is an increased risk of lithium toxicity if these drugs are combined. Serum lithium levels should be monitored and appropriate dosage adjustment made as needed.

LOOP DIURETICS

Loop diuretics are so named because they work in the loop of Henle. Four loop diuretics are currently available. Furosemide (*Lasix*), the most commonly used loop diuretic, is less powerful than the new loop diuretics, bumetanide (*Bumex*) and torsemide (*Demadex*), so it has a larger margin of safety for home use. Ethacrynic acid (*Edecrin*), the first loop diuretic introduced, is used less frequently in the clinical setting because of the improved potency and reliability of the newer drugs.

Therapeutic Actions and Indications

Loop diuretics are also referred to as **high-ceiling diuretics** because they cause a greater degree of diuresis than other diuretics do. These drugs block the chloride pump in the ascending loop of Henle, where normally 30% of all filtered sodium is reabsorbed. This action decreases the reabsorption of sodium and chloride. The loop diuretics have a similar effect in the descending loop of Henle and in the distal convoluted tubule, resulting in the production of a copious amount of sodium-rich urine. These drugs work even in the presence of acid–base disturbances, renal failure, electrolyte imbalances, or nitrogen retention.

Because they can produce a loss of fluid of up to 20 lb/day, loop diuretics are the drugs of choice when a rapid and extensive diuresis is needed. In cases of severe edema or acute pulmonary edema, it is important to remember that these drugs can have an effect only on the blood that reaches the nephrons. A rapid diuresis occurs, producing a more hypertonic intravascular fluid. In pulmonary edema, this fluid then circulates back to the lungs, pulls fluid out of the interstitial spaces by its oncotic pull, and delivers this fluid to the kidneys, where

DRUGS IN FOCUS
Thiazide Diuretics

Drug Name	Usual Dosage	Usual Indications
Thiazide diuretics		
bendroflumethiazide (*Naturetin*)	2.5–5 mg/d PO for edema; 2.5–15 mg/d PO for hypertension	All of the thiazide diuretics are indicated for the treatment of edema caused by congestive heart failure (CHF), liver disease, or renal disease, and for adjunctive treatment of hypertension
benzthiazide (*Exna*)	50–150 mg/d PO for edema; 50–200 mg/d PO, in two divided doses for hypertension	
chlorothiazide (*Diuril*)	Adult: 0.5–2 g PO or IV, q.d.–b.i.d. for edema; 0.5–2 g/d PO for hypertension Pediatric (< 6 mo): up to 33 mg/kg per day PO Pediatric (>6 mo): 22 mg/kg per day PO in two divided doses	
(P) hydrochlorothiazide (*HydroDIURIL*)	Adult: 25–100 mg/d PO or intermittently, up to 200 mg/d maximum for edema, 25–100 mg/d PO for hypertension Pediatric (< 6 mo): up to 3.3 mg/kg per day PO in two divided doses Pediatric (6 mo–2 y): 12.5–37.5 mg/d PO in two divided doses Pediatric (2–12 y): 37.6–100 mg/d PO in two divided doses	
hydroflumethiazide (*Diucardin*)	25–200 mg PO b.i.d. for edema; 50–100 mg/d PO for hypertension	
methyclothiazide (*Aquatensen*)	2.5–10 mg/d PO for edema; 2.5–5 mg/d PO for hypertension	
polythiazide (*Renese*)	1–4 mg/d PO for edema; 2–4 mg/d PO for hypertension	
trichlormethiazide (*Diurese*)	2–4 mg/d PO for edema or hypertension	
Thiazide-like diuretics		
(P) chlorthalidone (*Hygroton*)	50–100 mg/d PO for edema; 25–100 mg/d PO for hypertension	All of the thiazide-like diuretics are indicated for the treatment of edema caused by CHF or by liver or renal disease, and for adjunctive treatment of hypertension
indapamide (*Lozol*)	1.25–5 mg/d PO for edema or hypertension, based on patient response	
metolazone (*Mykrox, Zaroxolyn*)	*Mykrox:* 0.5–1 mg/d PO for mild hypertension *Zaroxolyn:* 2.5–5 mg/d PO for hypertension; 5–20 mg/d PO for edema, based on patient response	

the water is pulled out, completing the cycle. In the treatment of pulmonary edema, it may sometimes take hours to move all of the fluid out of the lungs, because the fluid must be pulled out of the interstitial spaces in the lungs before it can be circulated to the kidneys for removal. Remembering how the drugs work and the way fluid moves in the vascular system will make it easier to understand the effects to anticipate.

Loop diuretics are commonly indicated for the treatment of acute CHF, acute pulmonary edema, edema associated with CHF or with renal or liver disease, and hypertension.

Box 51–1 describes nesiritide, a recombinant form of natriuretic peptide that was recently approved for the treatment of CHF.

Pharmacokinetics

These drugs are metabolized and excreted primarily through the urine. There are no well-controlled studies of the effects of these drugs during pregnancy. They have been associated with fetal and maternal death in animal studies and they should not be used during pregnancy unless the benefit to the

BOX 51-1

First New Treatment for Congestive Heart Failure in More Than a Decade

The U.S. Food and Drug Administration recently approved nesiritide (*Natrecor*), a recombinant form of natriuretic peptide. This drug acts like natriuretic hormone, a natural substance, probably produced by the hypothalamus, which causes a decrease in sodium reabsorption from the distal renal tubules with a resultant dilute urine or increased volume. Natriuretic hormone is normally released in response to fluid overload or hemodilution. In studies, this drug was effective in the treatment congestive heart failure (CHF), reducing volume and cardiac workload.

Nesiritide is given as an IV bolus of 2 μg/kg followed by a continuous infusion of 0.01 μg/kg/min for up to 48 h. It was approved in late 2001 for the treatment of patients with acutely decompensated CHF who have dyspnea at rest or with minimal activity. After therapy with nesiritide, patients reported increased activity tolerance and easier breathing at rest.

mother far outweighs the potential risk. These drugs enter breast milk; if one of these drugs is needed during lactation, a decision should be made about whether to discontinue nursing or to discontinue the drug. Safety for use in children younger than 18 years of age has not been established. If one of these drugs is used with a child, careful monitoring of the child's fluid and electrolyte balance is needed, and emergency support measures should be on standby.

Adverse Effects

Adverse effects are related to the imbalance in electrolytes and fluid that these drugs cause. Hypokalemia is a very common adverse effect, because potassium is lost when the transport systems in the tubule try to save some of the sodium being lost. **Alkalosis,** or a drop in serum pH to an alkaline state, may occur as bicarbonate is lost in the urine. Calcium is also lost in the tubules along with the bicarbonate, which may result in hypocalcemia and tetany. The fast loss of fluid can result in hypotension and dizziness if it causes a rapid imbalance in fluid levels. Long-term use of these drugs may also result in hyperglycemia because of the diuretic effect on blood glucose levels, so susceptible patients need to be monitored for this effect. Ototoxicity and even deafness have been reported with these drugs, but the loss of hearing is usually reversible when the drug is stopped. This may be an effect of electrolyte changes on the conduction of fragile nerves in the central nervous system.

Clinically Important Drug–Drug Interactions

There is an increased risk of ototoxicity if loop diuretics are combined with aminoglycosides or cisplatin.

C A S E   S T U D Y

Using Furosemide (*Lasix*) in Congestive Heart Failure

THE SITUATION

M. R. is a 68-year-old woman with rheumatic mitral valve heart disease. She has refused any surgical intervention and has developed progressively worsening congestive heart failure (CHF). M. R. recently received a prescription for furosemide (*Lasix*), 40 mg PO q.d., along with digoxin. After 10 days with the new prescription, M. R. calls to tell you that she is allergic to the new medicine and can't take it any more. She reports extensive ankle swelling and difficulty breathing and is referred to a cardiologist for immediate review.

CRITICAL THINKING

• Think about the physiology of mitral valve disease and the progression of CHF in this patient. How does furosemide work in the body?
• What additional activities will be important to help maintain some balance in this patient's cardiac status?
• What is the nature of M. R.'s reported allergy, and what other options could be tried?

DISCUSSION

Over time, an incompetent mitral valve leads to an enlarged and overworked left ventricle as the backup of blood "waiting to be pumped" continues to progress. Drug therapy for a patient with this disorder is usually aimed at decreasing the workload of the heart as much as possible to maintain cardiac output. Digoxin increases the contractility of the heart muscle, which should lead to better perfusion of the kidneys. Furosemide, a loop diuretic, acts on the loop of Henle to block the reabsorption of sodium and water and lead to a diuresis, which decreases the volume of blood the heart needs to pump and makes the blood that is pumped more efficient. This blood then has an oncotic pull to move fluid from the tissue into circulation, where it can be acted on by the kidney, leading to further diuresis.

M. R. should be encouraged to maintain fluid intake and to engage in activity as much as possible, but to take frequent rest periods. Her potassium should be monitored regularly (this is especially important because she is also taking digoxin, which is very sensitive to potassium levels), her edematous limbs should be elevated periodically during the day, and she should monitor her sodium intake.

When M. R. was questioned about her reported allergy, it was discovered that her "allergic reaction" was actually increased urination (a therapeutic effect). M. R. requires teaching about the actions of the drug. She also needs information about the timing of administration so that the resultant diuresis will not interfere with rest or with her daily activities. CHF is a progressive, incurable disease, so patient education is a very important part of the overall management regimen.

DRUGS IN FOCUS
Loop Diuretics

Drug Name	Usual Dosage	Usual Indications
bumetanide (*Bumex*)	0.5–2 mg/d PO as a single dose repeated to a maximum of 10 mg; 0.5–1 mg IM or IV given over 1–2 min, may be repeated in 2–3 h, do not exceed 10 mg/d Geriatric or renal-impaired patient: 12 mg by continuous IV infusion over 12 h may be most effective and least toxic	All of the loop diuretics are indicated for the treatment of acute congestive heart failure (CHF); acute pulmonary edema; hypertension; and edema of CHF, renal disease, or liver disease
ethacrynic acid (*Edecrin*)	50–200 mg/d PO based on patient response; 0.5–1 mg/kg IV slowly Pediatric: 25 mg PO with slow titration up as needed; do not use with infants	
Ⓟ furosemide (*Lasix*)	20–80 mg/d PO, up to 600 mg/d may be given; 20–40 mg IM or IV given slowly; 40 mg IV over 1–2 min for acute pulmonary edema, increase to 80 mg after 1 h if response is not adequate; 40 mg PO b.i.d. for hypertension Geriatric or renal-impaired patient: 2–2.5 g/d PO Pediatric: 2 mg/kg per day PO for hypertension, do not exceed 6 mg/kg per day; 1 mg/kg IV or IM for edema, increase by 1 mg/kg as needed; do not exceed 6 mg/kg	
torsemide (*Demadex*)	10–20 mg/d PO for IV for CHF or chronic renal failure; 5–10 mg/d PO for hypertension	

There may be an increase in anticoagulation effects if these drugs given with anticoagulants.

There may also be a decreased loss of sodium and decreased antihypertensive effects if these drugs are combined with indomethacin, ibuprofen, salicylates, or other nonsteroidal anti-inflammatory agents. The patient receiving this combination should be monitored closely and appropriate dosage adjustments made.

CARBONIC ANHYDRASE INHIBITORS

The carbonic anhydrase inhibitors are relatively mild diuretics. Most often, they are used to treat glaucoma, because the inhibition of carbonic anhydrase results in decreased secretion of aqueous humor of the eye. Available agents include acetazolamide (*Diamox*) and methazolamide (*Neptazane*).

Therapeutic Actions and Indications
The enzyme carbonic anhydrase is a catalyst for the formation of sodium bicarbonate, which is stored as the alkaline reserve in the renal tubule, and the excretion of hydrogen, which results in a slightly acidic urine. Diuretics that block the effects of carbonic anhydrase slow down the movement of hydrogen ions; as a result, more sodium and bicarbonate are lost in the urine.

These drugs are used as adjuncts to other diuretics when a more intense diuresis is needed. Acetazolamide is used to treat glaucoma, in conjunction with other drugs to treat epilepsy,

DRUGS IN FOCUS
Carbonic Anhydrase Inhibitors

Drug Name	Usual Dosage	Usual Indications
Ⓟ acetazolamide (*Diamox*)	500 mg IV repeated in 2–4h, then 250 mg–1 g per day in divided doses q6–8h for glaucoma; 8–30 mg/kg per day in divided doses for epilepsy	Treatment of glaucoma; adjunctive treatment of epilepsy, mountain sickness
methazolamide (*Neptazane*)	50–100 mg PO b.i.d.–t.i.d.	Treatment of glaucoma

and to treat mountain sickness. Methazolamide (*Neptazane*) is used primarily for the treatment of glaucoma.

Pharmacokinetics

These drugs are rapidly absorbed and widely distributed. They are excreted in the urine. Some of these agents have been associated with fetal abnormalities, and they should not be used during pregnancy. Because of the potential for adverse effects on the baby, another method of feeding the infant should be used if one of these drugs is needed during lactation.

Adverse Effects

Adverse effects of carbonic anhydrase inhibitors are related to the disturbances in acid–base and electrolyte balance. Metabolic acidosis is a relatively common and potentially dangerous effect that occurs when bicarbonate is lost. Hypokalemia is also common, because potassium excretion is increased as the tubule loses potassium in an attempt to retain some of the sodium that is being excreted. Patients also complain of paresthesias (tingling) of the extremities, confusion, and drowsiness, all of which are probably related to the neural effect of the electrolyte changes.

Clinically Important Drug–Drug Interactions

There may be an increased excretion of salicylates and lithium if combined with these drugs. Caution should be used to monitor serum levels of patients taking lithium.

POTASSIUM-SPARING DIURETICS

The potassium-sparing diuretics include amiloride (*Midamor*), spironolactone (*Aldactone*), and triamterene (*Dyrenium*). These diuretics are used for patients in whom a high risk of hypokalemia associated with diuretic use exists (eg, patients receiving digitalis, patients with cardiac arrhythmias). They are not as powerful as the loop diuretics, but they retain potassium instead of wasting it.

Therapeutic Actions and Indications

Certain diuretics act to cause loss of sodium while retaining potassium. Spironolactone acts as an aldosterone antagonist, blocking the actions of aldosterone in the distal tubule. Amiloride and triamterene act to block potassium secretion through the tubule. The diuretic effect of these drugs comes from the balance achieved in losing sodium to offset potassium retained.

Potassium-sparing diuretics are often used as adjuncts with thiazide or loop diuretics or in patients who are especially at risk if hypokalemia develops, such as patients taking certain antiarrhythmics or digoxin and those who have particular neurological conditions. Spironolactone, the most frequently prescribed of these drugs, is the drug of choice for treating **hyperaldosteronism,** a condition seen in cirrhosis of the liver and nephrotic syndrome.

Pharmacokinetics

These drugs are well absorbed, protein bound, and widely distributed. They are metabolized in the liver and primarily excreted in the urine. These diuretics cross the placenta and enter breast milk. Routine use during pregnancy is not appropriate and should be saved for situations in which the mother has pathological reasons for use, not pregnancy manifestations or complications, and the benefit to the mother clearly outweighs the risk to the fetus. If one of these drugs is needed during lactation, another method of feeding the baby should be used, because of the potential for adverse effects on fluid and electrolyte changes in the baby.

Adverse Effects

The most common adverse effect of potassium-sparing diuretics is hyperkalemia, which can cause lethargy, confusion, ataxia, muscle cramps, and cardiac arrhythmias. Patients taking these drugs need to be evaluated regularly for signs of increased potassium and informed about the signs and symptoms to watch for. They also should be advised to avoid foods that are high in potassium (Box 51–2).

Clinically Important Drug–Drug Interactions

There is a decreased diuretic effect if potassium-sparing diuretics are combined with salicylates. Dosage adjustment may be necessary to achieve therapeutic effects.

OSMOTIC DIURETICS

Osmotic diuretics pull water into the renal tubule without sodium loss. They are the diuretics of choice in cases of increased cranial pressure or acute renal failure due to shock, drug overdose, or trauma. The osmotic diuretics include two mild agents—glycerin (*Osmoglyn*) and isosorbide (*Ismotic*)—and two powerful ones—mannitol (*Osmitrol*) and urea (*Ureaphil*). Glycerin can be given intravenously to treat elevated intracranial pressure and is used orally to treat glau-

---

BOX 51-2

Potassium-Rich Foods (Important to Eat With Potassium-Wasting Diuretics)

avocados	bananas	broccoli	cantaloupe	dried fruits
grapefruit	lima beans	nuts	navy beans	oranges
peaches	potatoes	prunes	rhubarb	*Sanka* coffee
sunflower seeds	spinach	tomatoes		

DRUGS IN FOCUS
Potassium-Sparing Diuretics

Drug Name	Usual Dosage	Usual Indications
amiloride (*Midamor*)	15–20 mg/d PO with monitoring of electrolytes	All of the potassium-sparing diuretics are indicated for the adjunctive treatment of edema caused by congestive heart failure, liver disease, or renal disease; hypertension; hyperkalemia; and hyperaldosteronism **Special considerations:** Not for use in children
Ⓟ spironolactone (*Aldactone*)	100–200 mg/d PO for edema; 100–400 mg/d PO for hyperaldosteronism; 50–100 mg/d PO for hypertension Pediatric: 3.3 mg/kg per day PO	**Special considerations:** Can be used in children with careful monitoring of electrolytes
triamterene (*Dyrenium*)	100 mg/d PO b.i.d.	**Special considerations:** Not for use in children

coma. Isosorbide is available only in oral form and is a preferred drug for the treatment of glaucoma. Mannitol, which is available only for intravenous use, is the mainstay for treatment of elevated intracranial pressure and acute renal failure. Urea also is available only for intravenous use; it is indicated for reduction of intracranial pressure and in the treatment of acute glaucoma.

Therapeutic Actions and Indications

Some nonelectrolytes are used intravenously to increase the volume of fluid produced by the kidneys. Mannitol, for example, is a sugar that is not well reabsorbed by the tubules; it acts to pull large amounts of fluid into the urine by the **osmotic pull** of the large sugar molecule. Because the tubule is not able to reabsorb all of the sugar pulled into it, large amounts of fluid are lost in the urine. The effects of these osmotic drugs are not limited to the kidney, because the injected substance pulls fluid into the vascular system from extravascular spaces, including the aqueous humor. Therefore, these drugs are often used in acute situations when it is necessary to decrease intraocular pressure before eye surgery or during acute attacks of glaucoma. Mannitol is also used to decrease intracranial pressure, to prevent the oliguric phase of renal failure, and to promote the movement of toxic substances through the kidneys.

Pharmacokinetics

These drugs are freely filtered at the renal glomerulus, poorly reabsorbed by the renal tubule, not secreted by the tubule, and resistant to metabolism. Their action depends on the concentration of the osmotic activity in the solution. It is not known whether these drugs can cause fetal harm, and their use during pregnancy should be limited to situations in which the benefit to the mother outweighs the potential risk

DRUGS IN FOCUS
Osmotic Diuretics

Drug Name	Usual Dosage	Usual Indications
glycerin (*Osmoglyn*)	1–2 g/kg PO for glaucoma	Treatment of elevated intraocular pressure; glaucoma
isosorbide (*Ismotic*)	1.5 g/kg PO b.i.d.–q.i.d.	Treatment of glaucoma
Ⓟ mannitol (*Osmitrol*)	50–100 g IV for oliguria; 1.5–2 g/kg IV to reduce intracranial pressure; dosage not established for children <12 y old	Treatment of elevated intracranial pressure; renal failure; acute glaucoma
urea (*Ureaphil*)	1–1.5 g/kg IV, do not exceed 120 g/d Pediatric: 0.5–1.5 mg/kg IV; as little as 0.1 mg/kg may be sufficient in children <2 y	Treatment of elevated intracranial pressure; acute glaucoma

to the fetus. Effects of these drugs during lactation are not well understood; because of the potential for risk to the fetus or changes in the fluid balance of the mother, caution should be used if one of these drugs is needed during lactation.

Adverse Effects

The most common and potentially dangerous adverse effect related to osmotic diuretics is the sudden drop in fluid levels. Nausea, vomiting, hypotension, lightheadedness, confusion, and headache can be accompanied by cardiac decompensation and even shock. Patients receiving these drugs should be closely monitored for fluid and electrolyte imbalance.

Nursing Considerations for Patients Receiving Diuretics

Assessment: History and Examination

Screen for the following conditions, which could be cautions or contraindications to use of the drug: any known allergies to diuretics; fluid or electrolyte disturbances, which could be exacerbated by the diuretic or render the diuretic ineffective; gout, which reflects an abnormal tubule function and could be worsened by the diuretic or reflect a condition that would render the diuretic ineffective; glucose tolerance abnormalities, which may be exacerbated by the glucose-elevating effects of some diuretics; liver disease, which could alter the metabolism of the diuretic leading to toxic levels; systemic lupus erythematosus, which frequently affects the glomerulus and could be exacerbated by the use of a diuretic; and pregnancy or lactation, which could be affected by the change in fluid and electrolyte balance.

Physical assessment should include the following: thorough skin examination (including color, texture, and the presence of edema), to provide a baseline as a reference for drug effectiveness; assessment of blood pressure, pulse, and cardiac auscultation, to provide a baseline for effects on blood pressure and volume; body weight, to provide a baseline to monitor fluid load; liver evaluation, to determine potential problems in drug metabolism; check of urinary output, to establish a baseline of renal function; and evaluation of blood tests, to provide a baseline reference for electrolyte balance, glucose levels, uric acid levels, and liver function tests.

Nursing Diagnoses

The patient receiving a diuretic may have the following nursing diagnoses related to drug therapy:

- Risk for Deficient Fluid Volume, related to diuretic effect
- Impaired Urinary Elimination, related to diuretic effect
- Imbalanced Nutrition: Less than Body Requirements, related to GI upset and metabolic changes
- Deficient Knowledge regarding drug therapy

Implementation

- Administer oral drug with food or milk, *to buffer the drug effect on the stomach lining if GI upset is a problem.*
- Administer intravenous drug slowly, *to prevent severe changes in fluid and electrolytes;* protect the drug from light, *because disintegration can occur;* discard diluted drug after 24 hours, *to prevent contamination or ineffective drug use.*
- Continuously monitor urinary output, cardiac response, and heart rhythm of patients receiving intravenous diuretics, *to monitor for rapid fluid switch and potential electrolyte disturbances leading to cardiac arrhythmia.* Switch to the oral form, *which is less potent and easier to monitor,* as soon as possible.
- Administer early in the day, *so that increased urination will not interfere with sleep.*
- Monitor the dose carefully and reduce the dosage of one or both drugs if given with antihypertensive agents; *loss of fluid volume can precipitate hypotension.*
- Monitor the patient response to the drug (eg, blood pressure, urinary output, weight, serum electrolytes, hydration, periodic blood glucose monitoring), *to evaluate the effectiveness of the drug and monitor for adverse effects.*
- Provide comfort measures, including skin care and nutrition consultation, *to increase compliance to drug therapy and decrease severity of adverse effects;* provide safety measures if dizziness and weakness are a problem.
- Provide potassium-rich or potassium-poor diet as appropriate for drug being given, *to maintain electrolyte balance and replace lost potassium.*
- Provide thorough patient teaching, including measures to avoid adverse effects and warning signs of problems and ways to incorporate diuretic effect in planning the day's activities, *to enhance patient knowledge about drug therapy and to promote compliance.* (See Patient Teaching Checklist: Diuretic Agents.)

PATIENT TEACHING CHECKLIST
Diuretic Agents

Create customized patient teaching materials for a specific diuretic agent from the CD-ROM. Patient teaching should stress the following points for drugs within this class:

- A diuretic, or "water pill," will help to reduce the amount of fluid that is in your body by causing the kidneys to pass larger amounts of water and salt into your urine. By removing this fluid, the diuretic helps to decrease the work of the heart, lower blood pressure, and get rid of edema or swelling in your tissues.
- This drug can be taken with food, which may eliminate any stomach upset. When taking a diuretic, you should maintain your usual fluid intake and try to avoid excessive intake of salt.
- If your diuretic is one that causes potassium loss, you should eat foods that are high in potassium (e.g., orange juice, raisins, bananas). You also may be asked to take a potassium substitute, if appropriate. If your diuretic is one that causes potassium retention, you should avoid foods high in potassium as well as salt substitutes, as appropriate.
- Weigh yourself each day, at the same time of day and in the same clothing. Record these weights on a calendar. Report any loss or gain of 3 lb or more in 1 day.

PATIENT TEACHING CHECKLIST
(CONTINUED)

Diuretic Agents

Common effects of this drug include

• *Increased volume and frequency of urination*—Have ready access to bathroom facilities. Once you are used to the drug, you will know how long the effects last for you.
• *Dizziness, feeling faint on arising, drowsiness*—Loss of fluid can lower blood pressure and cause these feelings. Change positions slowly; if you feel drowsy, avoid driving or other dangerous activities. These feelings are often increased if alcohol is consumed; avoid this combination or take special precautions if you combine them.
• *Increased thirst*—As fluid is lost, you may experience a feeling of thirst. Sucking on sugarless lozenges and frequent mouth care might help alleviate this feeling. Do not drink an excessive amount of fluid while taking a diuretic. Try to maintain your usual fluid intake.

Report any of the following to your health care provider: muscle cramps or pain, loss or gain of more than 3 lb in one day, swelling in your fingers or ankles, nausea or vomiting, unusual bleeding or bruising, trembling or weakness.
Avoid the use of any over-the-counter medication without first checking with your health care provider. Several of these medications can interfere with the effectiveness of this drug.
Tell any doctor, nurse, or other health care provider that you are taking this drug.
Keep this drug, and all medications, out of the reach of children.

This Teaching Checklist reflects general patient teaching guidelines. It is not meant to be a substitute for drug-specific teaching information, which is available in nursing drug guides.

Evaluation

• Monitor patient response to the drug (weight, urinary output, edema changes, blood pressure).
• Monitor for adverse effects (electrolyte imbalance, orthostatic hypotension, rebound edema, hyperglycemia, increased uric acid levels, acid–base disturbances, dizziness).
• Evaluate the effectiveness of the teaching plan (patient can name drug, dosage, adverse effects to watch for, specific measures to avoid adverse effects).
• Monitor the effectiveness of comfort measures and compliance to the regimen (see Nursing Care Guide: Diuretic Agents).

▢▣◕◔ WEB LINKS

Health care providers and patients may want to consult the following Internet sources:

Information on diuretics, good teaching guides and aids:
http://www.med.virginia.edu/med-ed/handouts/physiology/renal/diuretic.html

Information on congestive heart failure, pathophysiology, treatment, research:
http://www.americanheart.org
http://www.nhlbi.nih.gov
Information on liver disease and related treatment:
http://cpmcnet.columbia.edu/dept/gi/other.html

CHAPTER SUMMARY

• Diuretics are drugs that increase the excretion of sodium, and therefore water, from the kidneys.
• Diuretics are used in the treatment of edema associated with congestive heart failure and pulmonary edema, liver failure and cirrhosis, and various types of renal disease, and as adjuncts in the treatment of hypertension.
• Diuretics must be used cautiously in any condition that would be exacerbated by changes in fluid and electrolyte balance.
• Adverse effects associated with diuretics include electrolyte imbalance (potassium, sodium, chloride); hypotension and hypovolemia; hypoglycemia; and metabolic alkalosis.
• Classes of diuretics differ in their site of action and intensity of effects. Thiazide diuretics work to block the chloride pump in the distal convoluted tubule. This effect leads to a loss of sodium and potassium and a minor loss of water. Thiazides are frequently used in combination with other drugs to treat hypertension. They are considered to be mild diuretics.
• Loop diuretics work in the loop of Henle and have a powerful diuretic effect, leading to the loss of water, sodium, and potassium. These drugs are the most potent diuretics and are used in acute situations as well as chronic conditions not responsive to milder diuretics.
• Carbonic anhydrase inhibitors work to block the formation of carbonic acid and bicarbonate in the renal tubule. These drugs can cause an alkaline urine and loss of the bicarbonate buffer. Carbonic anhydrase inhibitors are used in combination with other diuretics when a stronger diuresis is needed, and they are frequently used to treat glaucoma because they decrease the amount of aqueous humor produced in the eye.
• Potassium-sparing diuretics are mild diuretics that act to spare potassium in exchange for the loss of sodium and water in the urine. These diuretics are preferable if potassium loss could be detrimental to a patient's cardiac or neuromuscular condition. Patients must be careful not to become hyperkalemic while taking these drugs.
• Osmotic diuretics use hypertonic pull to remove fluid from the intravascular spaces and to deliver large amounts of water into the renal tubule. There is a danger of sudden change of fluid volume and massive fluid loss with some of these drugs. These drugs are used to decrease intracranial pressure, to treat glaucoma, and to help push toxic substances through the kidney.
• Patients receiving diuretics need to be monitored for fluid loss and retention (daily weights, blood pressure, skin eval-

NURSING CARE GUIDE

Diuretic Agents

Assessment	Nursing Diagnoses	Implementation	Evaluation
HISTORY Allergies to diuretics, fluid or electrolyte disturbances, gout, glucose tolerance abnormalities, liver disease, SLE, pregnancy and lactation.	Risk for Deficient Fluid Volume related to diuretic effect Impaired Urinary Elimination Imbalanced Nutrition: Less than Body Requirements, related to GI upset and metabolic changes Deficient Knowledge regarding drug therapy	Obtain daily weights, monitor output. Provide comfort and safety measures: sugarless lozenges, mouth care, safety precautions, skin care, nutrition. Administer with food, early in day. Provide support and reassurance to deal with drug effects and lifestyle changes. Provide patient teaching regarding drug name, dosage, side effects, precautions, warnings to report, daily weighing, and recording dietary changes as needed.	Evaluate drug effects: urinary output, weight changes, status of edema, BP changes. Monitor for adverse effects: hypotension, hypokalemia hyperkalemia, hypocalcemia, hypercalcemia, hyperglycemia, increased uric acid levels. Monitor for drug–drug interactions as indicated for each drug. Evaluate effectiveness of patient teaching program. Evaluate effectiveness of comfort/safety measures.
PHYSICAL EXAMINATION Neurological: orientation, reflexes, strength Skin: color, texture, edema CV: BP, P, cardiac auscultation GI: liver evaluation GU: urinary output Lab tests: hematologic; serum electrolytes, glucose, uric acid; liver function tests			

uation, urinary output); have periodic electrolyte evaluations and blood glucose determinations; and have evaluations of the effectiveness of their teaching program.

Review Questions

1. Diuretics are not currently recommended for the treatment of
   a. hypertension.
   b. renal disease.
   c. obesity.
   d. severe liver disease.
2. Most diuretics act in the body to cause
   a. loss of water.
   b. loss of sodium.
   c. retention of potassium.
   d. retention of chloride.
3. Diuretics cause a loss of blood volume in the body. The

drop in volume activates compensatory mechanisms to restore the volume, including
   a. suppression of ADH release.
   b. suppression of aldosterone release.
   c. activation of the renin–angiotensin system with increased ADH and aldosterone.
   d. stimulation of the countercurrent mechanism.
4. Thiazide diuretics are considered mild diuretics because
   a. they block the sodium pump in the loop of Henle.
   b. they block the chloride pump, which causes loss of sodium and chloride but little water.
   c. they do not cause a fluid rebound when they work in the kidney.
   d. they have no effect on electrolytes.
5. A loop diuretic would be the drug of choice in treating
   a. hypertension.
   b. shock.

c. pulmonary edema.

d. fluid retention of pregnancy.

6. Any patient receiving a loop diuretic needs to have regular monitoring of

a. sodium levels.

b. bone marrow function.

c. calcium levels.

d. potassium levels.

7. The diuretic of choice for treating hyperaldosteronism would be

a. spironolactone.

b. furosemide.

c. hydrochlorothiazide.

d. acetazolamide.

8. A patient with severe glaucoma who is about to undergo eye surgery would benefit from a decrease in intraocular fluid. This is often best accomplished by giving the patient

a. a loop diuretic.

b. a thiazide diuretic.

c. a carbonic anhydrase inhibitor.

d. an osmotic diuretic.

9. Routine nursing care of a patient receiving a diuretic would not include

a. daily weights.

b. tight fluid restrictions.

c. periodic electrolyte evaluations.

d. monitoring of urinary output.

10. Patients receiving diuretics should be taught to report

a. yellow vision.

b. weight loss of 1 lb/day.

c. muscle pain or cramping.

d. increased urination.

BIBLIOGRAPHY

Bullock, B. L. (2000). *Focus on pathophysiology*. Philadelphia: Lippincott Williams & Wilkins.

Drug facts and comparisons. (2002). St. Louis: Facts and Comparisons.

Gilman, A., Hardman, J. G., & Limbird, L. E. (Eds.) (2002). *Goodman and Gilman's the pharmacological basis of therapeutics* (10th ed.). New York: McGraw-Hill.

Karch, A. M. (2002). *2003 Lippincott's nursing drug guide*. Philadelphia: Lippincott Williams & Wilkins.

Professional's guide to patient drug facts. (2002). St. Louis: Facts and Comparisons.

CHAPTER 52

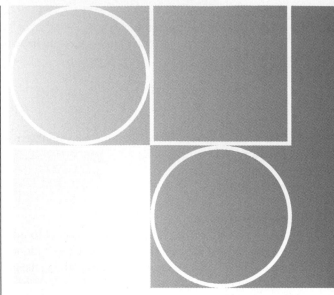

Drugs Affecting the Urinary Tract and the Bladder

Key Terms

acidification

antispasmodics

benign prostatic hyperplasia (BPH)

cystitis

dysuria

interstitial cystitis

nocturia

pyelonephritis

urgency

urinary frequency

704

Urinary Tract Anti-infectives

cinoxacin

fosfomycin

methenamine

methylene blue

nalidixic acid

nitrofurantoin

Ⓟ norfloxacin

Urinary Tract Antispasmodics

flavoxate

Ⓟ oxybutynin

tolterodine

Urinary Tract Analgesic

phenazopyridine

Bladder Protectant

pentosan polysulfate sodium

**Drugs Used to Treat Benign Prostatic
   Hyperplasia**

Ⓟ doxazosin

dutasteride

finasteride

tamsulosin

terazosin

Acute urinary tract infections (UTIs) occur second in frequency only to respiratory tract infections in the American population. Females, with shorter urethras, are particularly vulnerable to repeated bladder and even kidney infections. Patients with indwelling catheters or intermittent catheterizations often are affected by bladder infections or **cystitis,** which can result from bacteria introduced into the bladder by these devices. Blockage anywhere in the urinary tract can lead to backflow problems and the spread of bladder infections into the kidney.

The signs and symptoms of a UTI are uncomfortable and include **urinary frequency; urgency;** burning on urination (associated with cystitis); and chills, fever, flank pain, and tenderness (associated with acute **pyelonephritis**). To treat these infections, clinicians use antibiotics (see Chapter 9) as well as specific agents that reach antibacterial levels only in the kidney and bladder and are thought to sterilize the urinary tract.

Drugs also are available to block spasms of the urinary tract muscles, decrease urinary tract pain, protect the cells of the bladder from irritation, and treat enlargement of the prostate gland in men. All of these agents are discussed in this chapter. Table 52–1 provides a summary of urinary tract problems and the drugs of choice to treat them.

URINARY TRACT ANTI-INFECTIVES

Urinary tract anti-infectives are of two types. One type is the antibiotics. These include

- Cinoxacin (*Cinobac*), which interferes with DNA replication in gram-negative bacteria. This drug is rapidly absorbed, undergoes hepatic metabolism, and is excreted in the urine. It is used in lower doses in the presence of renal impairment, because it is not excreted properly. It should be used with caution during pregnancy and lactation, because it does cross the placenta and enter breast milk.
- Norfloxacin (*Noroxin*), a newer and more broad-spectrum drug that is effective against even more gram-negative strains than is cinoxacin. This drug is rapidly absorbed and undergoes hepatic metabolism and renal excretion. Dosage

must be reduced in the presence of renal impairment. This drug crosses the placenta and enters breast milk and should not be used during pregnancy or lactation unless the benefit to the mother clearly outweighs the potential risk to the fetus.
- Fosfomycin (*Monurol*), a drug that has the convenience of only one dose. It is not recommended for children younger than 18 years of age. It is rapidly absorbed, undergoes slow hepatic metabolism, and is excreted in the urine and feces. It might be a drug of choice for cystitis during pregnancy or lactation because of the short exposure to the drug. Unpleasant gastrointestinal (GI) effects limited its usefulness in some patients.
- Nalidixic acid (*NegGram*), an older drug that is not effective against as many strains of gram-negative bacteria as the other antibiotics used for UTIs. This drug is rapidly absorbed, metabolized in the liver, and excreted in the urine. It has a short half-life—1 to 2.5 hours. It is known to cross the placenta and to enter breast milk, so it should not be used during pregnancy or lactation. It is available in a suspension form and has an established dosage for children ages 3 months to 12 years.
- Nitrofurantoin (*Furadantin*), another older drug with a very short half-life (20 to 60 minutes). It is not effective against as many gram-negative bacteria as the newer drugs are, but it has been successfully used for suppression therapy in adults and children with chronic UTIs. It is metabolized in the liver and excreted in the urine. It is not recommended during pregnancy or lactation because of the potential for adverse effects on the neonate or baby.

The other type of urinary tract anti-infectives work to acidify the urine, killing bacteria that might be in the bladder. This group includes two drugs:

- Methenamine (*Hiprex*), which undergoes metabolism in the liver and is excreted in the urine. It crosses the placenta and enters breast milk and should not be used during pregnancy or lactation. Methenamine has established dosage guidelines for children and comes in a suspension form.
- Methylene blue (*Urolene Blue*), which is widely distributed, metabolized in the tissues, and excreted in the urine, bile, and feces. This drug stains the tissues and can cause GI upset. It is not recommended during pregnancy or lactation.

| **TABLE 52-1** | Drugs Used to Treat Urinary Tract Problems |

Urinary Tract Problem	Drugs of Choice
Infection	Urinary tract anti-infectives: fosfomycin, cinoxacin, methenamine, nalidixic acid, methylene blue, nitrofurantoin, norfloxacin
Spasm	Antispasmodics: fluvoxate, oxybutynin, tolterodine
Pain	Urinary tract analgesic: phenazopyridine Bladder protectant for interstitial cystitis: pentosan
Benign prostatic hyperplasia	α-Adrenergic blockers: doxazosin, tamsulosin, terazosin Testosterone inhibitor: finasteride

DRUG THERAPY ACROSS THE LIFESPAN

Urinary Tract Agents

Children	Adults	Older Adults
Children often have cystitis and need to be treated with a urinary tract agent. Some children, because of congenital problems or indwelling catheters, require other urinary tract agents. The older anti-infectives—nalidixic acid, nitrofurantoin and methenamine—have established pediatric guidelines. Children need to be instructed in proper hygiene and should not be given bubble baths if urinary tract infections occur. They should be encouraged to avoid the alkaline ash juices and urged to drink lots of water. If an anti-spasmodic is needed, oxybutynin is indicated for children >5 y of age, and flavoxate can be used in children >12 y. Phenazopyridine is indicated as a urinary tract analgesic for children 6–12 y of age. The child should be cautioned about the change in urine color, which might be frightening if the child is not expecting it.	Adults need to be cautioned about the various measures that can be used to decrease the likelihood of urinary tract infections. They should be encouraged to drink plenty of fluids to maintain bladder health. If taking an anticholinergic to block spasm, adult patients need to be advised of other precautions to take when the parasympathetic system is blocked. Adult men being treated for benign prostatic hyperplasia need to be aware of the possibility of decreased sexual function, as well as fatigue, lethargy, and the potential for dizziness, which could interfere with working or activities of daily living. The use of urinary tract agents during pregnancy should be approached with caution. If an antibiotic is needed, the one-dose fosfomycin might be a drug of choice because of the limited exposure to the drug. Women who are nursing should use these agents with caution because of the potential for adverse effects on the baby, or they should find another method of feeding the baby.	Older adults often have conditions that are treated with the urinary tract agents. They are also more likely to have renal or hepatic impairment, which requires caution in the use of these drugs. Older adults should be started on the lowest possible dose of the drug, and it should titrated slowly based on patient response. Special precautions to monitor cardiac function, intraocular pressure, blood pressure, and bladder emptying need to be taken when using α-adrenergic blockers with these patients. Older patients may have a difficult time maintaining fluid intake and might benefit from extra encouragement to drink fluids, including cranberry juice, and to avoid alkaline ash drinks.

Therapeutic Actions and Indications

Urinary tract anti-infectives act specifically within the urinary tract to destroy bacteria, either through a direct antibiotic effect or through **acidification** of the urine. They do not generally have an antibiotic effect systemically, being activated or effective only in the urinary tract (Figure 52–1). They are used to treat chronic UTIs, as adjunctive therapy in acute cystitis and pyelonephritis, and as prophylaxis with urinary tract anatomical abnormalities and residual urine disorders. Fosfomycin, a relatively new agent, is a one-dose-only antibacterial. Ease of treatment makes this a very desirable agent; however, many patients experience unpleasant adverse effects, especially GI effects, with this drug.

Contraindications and Cautions

These drugs are contraindicated in the presence of any known allergy to any of these drugs. They should be used with caution in the presence of renal dysfunction, which could interfere with the excretion and action of these drugs; and with pregnancy and lactation, because of the potential for adverse effects on the fetus or neonate.

Adverse Effects

Adverse effects associated with these drugs include nausea, vomiting, diarrhea, anorexia, bladder irritation, and dysuria.

Infrequent symptoms include pruritus, urticaria, headache, dizziness, nervousness, and confusion. These effects may result from GI irritation caused by the agent, which may be somewhat alleviated if the drug is taken with food, or from a systemic reaction to the urinary tract irritation.

Clinically Important Drug–Drug Interactions

Because these drugs are from several different chemical classes, the drug–drug interactions that can occur are very specific to the drug being used. Consult a nursing drug guide for specific interactions.

Nursing Considerations for Patients Receiving Urinary Tract Anti-infectives

Assessment: History and Examination

Screen for the following conditions, which could be cautions or contraindications to use of the drug: any history of allergy to antibacterials; liver or renal dysfunction that might interfere with the drug's metabolism and excretion; and pregnancy and lactation, which are contraindications to the use of these drugs.

Physical assessment should be done to establish baseline data for assessing the effectiveness of the drug and the occurrence of any adverse effects associated with drug therapy. Assess for the following: skin, to evaluate for the de-

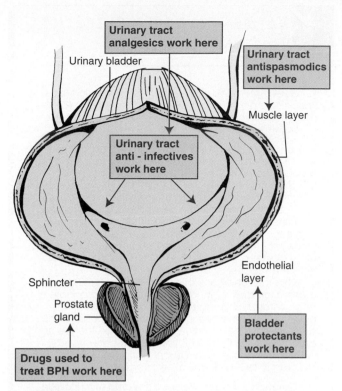

FIGURE 52-1. Sites of action of drugs acting on the urinary tract.

velopment of rash or hypersensitivity reactions; orientation and reflexes, to evaluate any central nervous system (CNS) effects of the drug; and renal and hepatic function tests, to determine baseline function of these organs.

Nursing Diagnoses

The patient receiving a urinary tract anti-infective may have the following nursing diagnoses related to drug therapy:

- Acute Pain related to GI, CNS, skin effects of drug
- Disturbed Sensory Perception (Kinesthetic, Tactile, Visual) related to CNS effects
- Deficient Knowledge regarding drug therapy

Implementation

- Ensure that culture and sensitivity tests are performed before therapy begins and repeated if the response is not as expected, *to ensure appropriate treatment of the infection.*
- Administer the drugs with food, *to decrease GI adverse effects if they occur.*
- Institute safety precautions if the patient experiences CNS effects, *to prevent patient injury.*
- Advise patients to continue the full course of the drug ordered and not to stop taking it as soon as the uncomfortable

DRUGS IN FOCUS
Urinary Tract Anti-Infectives

Drug Name	Usual Dosage	Usual Indications
cinoxacin (*Cinobac*)	1 g/d PO for 7–14 d; 250 mg/d PO at h.s. for prevention; reduce dosage with impaired renal function	Treatment of urinary tract infections caused susceptible bacteria in patients >12 y
fosfomycin (*Monurol*)	1 packet (3 g) dissolved in water PO	Treatment of urinary tract infections caused by susceptible bacteria (one-dose drug) in patients > 18 y
methenamine (*Hiprex*)	1 g b.i.d.–q.i.d. PO Pediatric (6–12 y): 0.5–1 g PO b.i.d.–q.i.d. Pediatric (<6 y): 0.25–0.5 mg/kg per day PO in divided doses	Suppression or elimination of bacteriuria associated with urinary tract infections and anatomical abnormalities
methylene blue (*Urolene Blue*)	65–130 mg PO t.i.d.	Suppression or elimination of bacteriuria associated with urinary tract infections and anatomical abnormalities
nalidixic acid (*NegGram*)	1 g PO q.i.d. for 1–2 wk, reduce to 2 g/d for prolonged use Pediatric (<12 y) 55 mg/kg per day PO in four divided doses, for prolonged therapy reduce to 33 mg/kg per day	Treatment of urinary tract infections caused by susceptible bacteria
nitrofurantoin (*Furadantin*)	50–100 mg PO q.i.d. for 10–14 d; 50–100 mg PO h.s. for chronic suppressive therapy Pediatric: 5–7 mg/kg per day in four divided doses; 1 mg/kg per day PO h.s. for chronic suppressive therapy	Treatment of urinary tract infections caused by susceptible bacteria
Ⓟ norfloxacin (*Noroxin*)	400 mg q12h PO, length of therapy dependent on site and intensity of infection	Treatment of urinary tract infections caused by susceptible bacteria (broad-spectrum agent)

signs and symptoms pass, *to ensure eradication of the infection and prevent the emergence of resistant strains of bacteria.*

- Encourage the patient to push fluids (unless contraindicated by other conditions), *to flush the bladder and urinary tract frequently and decrease the opportunity for bacteria growth.*
- Educate patients with chronic UTIs about additional activities that can facilitate an acidic urine, *to increase the effectiveness of urinary tract anti-infectives.* For example, all patients should

Avoid foods that cause an alkaline ash and produce an alkaline urine (eg, citrus juices, fruits, antacids).
Drink high-acid cranberry juice.
Void immediately after sexual intercourse, to help clear any invading organisms.

In addition, women should

Avoid baths if possible, especially bubble baths (because the bubbles act as transport agents to deliver bacteria through the short urethra).
Wipe front to back and never back to front, which introduces *Escherichia coli* and other agents to the urethra.

Provide thorough patient teaching, including the drug name and prescribed dosage, measures to help avoid adverse effects, warning signs that may indicate problems, and the need for periodic monitoring and evaluation, *to enhance patient knowledge about drug therapy and to promote compliance.* (See Patient Teaching Checklist: Urinary Tract Anti-infectives.)

Evaluation

- Monitor patient response to the drug (resolution of UTI and relief of signs and symptoms); repeat culture and sensitivity tests are recommended for evaluation of the effectiveness of all of these drugs.
- Monitor for adverse effects (skin evaluation, orientation and reflexes, GI effects).
- Evaluate the effectiveness of the teaching plan (patient can name drug, dosage, adverse effects to watch for, specific measures to avoid adverse effects, and measures to take to increase the effectiveness of the drug).
- Monitor the effectiveness of comfort and safety measures and compliance to the regimen (see Nursing Care Guide: Urinary Tract Anti-infectives).

URINARY TRACT ANTISPASMODICS

Urinary tract **antispasmodics** block the spasms of urinary tract muscles caused by various conditions. Flavoxate (*Urispas*) prevents smooth muscle spasm specifically in the urinary tract, but it is associated with CNS effects (blurred vision,

PATIENT TEACHING CHECKLIST
Urinary Tract Anti-Infectives

Create customized patient teaching materials for a specific urinary tract anti-infective from the CD-ROM. Patient teaching should stress the following points for drugs within this class:

- A urinary tract anti-infective works to treat urinary tract infections by destroying bacteria and by helping produce an environment that is not conducive to bacterial growth.
- If this drug causes stomach upset, it can be taken with food. It is important to avoid foods that alkalinize the urine, such as citrus fruits and milk, because they decrease the effectiveness of the drug. Cranberry juice is one juice that can be used. As much fluid as possible (8–10 glasses of water a day) should be taken to help treat the infection.
- Avoid the use of any over-the-counter (OTC) medication that might contain sodium bicarbonate (e.g., antacids, baking soda), because these drugs alkalinize the urine and interfere with the ability of the drugs to treat the infection. If you question the use of any OTC drug, check with your health care provider.
- Take the full course of your prescription. Do not use this drug to self-treat any other infection.

Common adverse effects of this drug may include

- *Stomach upset, nausea*—Taking the drug with food or eating small, frequent meals may help.
- *Painful urination*—If this occurs, report it to your health care provider. A dosage adjustment may be needed.

The following activities can help to decrease urinary tract infections:

- Avoid bubble baths.
- Void whenever you feel the urge; try not to wait.
- Always try to void after sexual intercourse to flush the urethra.
- *For women:* Always wipe from front to back, never from back to front.

Report any of the following to your health care provider: skin rash or itching, severe GI upset, GI upset that prevents adequate fluid intake, very painful urination, pregnancy.

Tell any doctor, nurse, or other health care provider that you are taking this drug.

Keep this drug, and all medications, out of the reach of children.

This Teaching Checklist reflects general patient teaching guidelines. It is not meant to be a substitute for drug-specific teaching information, which is available in nursing drug guides.

dizziness, confusion) that make it less desirable to use in certain patients. Oxybutynin (*Ditropan*) is a potent urinary antispasmodic, but it has numerous anticholinergic effects, making it undesirable in certain conditions or situations that might be aggravated by decreased sweating, urinary retention, tachycardia, and changes in GI activity. Tolterodine (*Detrol, Detrol LA*) is a newer agent that blocks muscarinic

NURSING CARE GUIDE

Urinary Tract Anti-infectives

Assessment	Nursing Diagnoses	Implementation	Evaluation
HISTORY Allergies to antibacterials, liver or renal dysfunction, pregnancy and lactation	Acute Pain related to GI, CNS, skin effects of drug Disturbed Sensory Perception related to CNS effects Deficient Knowledge regarding drug therapy	Obtain culture and sensitivity test of urine. Provide comfort and safety measures: safety precautions, skin care, nutrition. Encourage acidifying foods. Push fluids. Teach hygiene measures. Administer with food if GI upset is a problem. Provide support and reassurance to deal with drug effects and lifestyle changes. Provide patient teaching regarding drug name, dosage, adverse effects, precautions, warnings to report, hygiene measures, and dietary changes as needed.	Evaluate drug effects: relief of symptoms, resolution of infection. Monitor for adverse effects: GI upset, headache, dizziness, confusion, dysuria, pruritus, urticaria. Monitor for drug–drug interactions as indicated for each drug. Evaluate effectiveness of patient teaching program. Evaluate effectiveness of comfort and safety measures.
PHYSICAL EXAMINATION Neurological: orientation, reflexes, strength Skin: color, texture, edema GI: liver evaluation GU: urinary output Lab tests: liver function tests, urinalysis, urine for culture & sensitivity			

receptors, preventing bladder contraction and spasm. It is indicated for the treatment of overactive bladder in patients who exhibit urinary frequency, urgency, or incontinence. It has been widely marketed directly to the consumer.

Therapeutic Actions and Indications
Inflammation in the urinary tract, such as cystitis, prostatitis, urethritis, and urethrocystitis/urethrotrigonitis, causes smooth muscle spasms along the urinary tract. Irritation of the urinary tract leading to muscle spasm also occurs in patients who have uninhibited neurogenic and neurogenic bladders. These spasms lead to the uncomfortable effects of dysuria (pain or discomfort with urination), urgency, incontinence, nocturia (recurrent nighttime urination), and suprapubic pain. The urinary tract antispasmodics act to relieve these spasms by blocking parasympathetic activity and relaxing the detrusor and other urinary tract muscles (see Figure 52–1).

Pharmacokinetics
These drugs are rapidly absorbed, widely distributed, metabolized in the liver, and excreted in the urine. Caution should be used in the presence of hepatic or renal impairment because of the potential of alterations in metabolism or excretion of the drugs. They cross the placenta and are found in breast milk. They should be used during pregnancy and lactation only if the benefit to the mother clearly outweighs the potential risk to the fetus or neonate.

Contraindications and Cautions
These drugs are contraindicated in the presence of known allergy to the drugs; with pyloric or duodenal obstruction or recent surgery, because the anticholinergic effects can cause serious complications; with obstructive urinary tract problems, which could be further aggravated by the blocking of muscle activity; and with glaucoma, myasthenia gravis, or acute hem-

CASE STUDY

Teaching Plan for Treating Cystitis

THE SITUATION

J. K. is a 6-year-old girl with a history of repeated urinary tract infections. She is seen with complaints of dysuria, frequency, urgency, and a low-grade fever. A urine sample is sent for culture and sensitivity testing. J. K. is started on methenamine, 500 mg q.i.d., and is referred to the nurse for teaching.

CRITICAL THINKING

• What is the best approach for this patient?
• What key teaching points (at least five) should be emphasized to assist the pharmacological therapy in treating this infection? *Think about the following points: what the drug is doing, how does it work, and how does it work best.*

DISCUSSION

Cystitis is very difficult to treat in young girls and can become a chronic problem. Patient and parent education is very important for trying to block the growth of bacteria and cure the infection. Teaching points should emphasize activities that will decrease the number of

bacteria introduced into the bladder, acidify the urine to make the bladder an unpleasant environment for bacterial growth, and flush the bladder to prevent stagnant urine from encouraging bacterial growth.

To decrease the number of bacteria introduced into the bladder, patient education should cover the following hygiene measures: always wipe from front to back and never from back to front, to avoid the introduction of intestinal bacteria into the urethra; avoid baths, particularly bubble baths, which facilitate the entry of bacteria into the urethra on the bubbles; and wear dry, cotton underwear to discourage bacterial growth.

Patient education also should stress the importance of avoiding alkaline ash foods (e.g., citrus fruits, certain vegetables) and encouraging foods that acidify the urine. Cranberry juice is often recommended as a choice for fruit juice, because it helps to acidify the bladder and destroy bacteria. Fluid, especially water, should be pushed as much as possible to keep the bladder flushed out. Finally, the patient should be encouraged to complete the full course of medication prescribed and not to stop taking the drug when symptoms disappear.

---

orrhage, which could all be exacerbated by the anticholinergic effects of these drugs. Caution should be used in the presence of renal or hepatic dysfunction, which could alter the metabolism and excretion of the drugs; and with pregnancy and lactation, because of potential adverse effects on the neonate secondary to the anticholinergic effects of the drugs.

Adverse Effects

Adverse effects of urinary tract antispasmodics are related to the blocking of the parasympathetic system and include nausea, vomiting, dry mouth, nervousness, tachycardia, and vision changes.

Clinically Important Drug–Drug Interactions

Decreased effectiveness of phenothiazines and haloperidol has been associated with the combination of these drugs with oxybutynin. If any such combinations must be used, the patient should be monitored closely and appropriate dosage adjustments made.

Nursing Considerations for Patients Receiving Urinary Tract Antispasmodics
Assessment: History and Examination

Screen for the following conditions, which could be cautions or contraindications to use of the drug: any history of allergy

---

DRUGS IN FOCUS
Urinary Tract Antispasmodics

Drug Name	Usual Dosage	Usual Indications
flavoxate (*Urispas*)	100–200 mg PO t.i.d.–q.i.d.; reduce dosage when patient improves	Symptomatic relief of urinary bladder spasm in patients >12 y
(P) oxybutynin (*Ditropan*)	5 mg PO t.i.d.–q.i.d.; ER tablets—5 mg/d PO up to a maximum 30 mg/d Pediatric (>5 y): 5 mg PO b.i.d. up to a maximum 5 mg PO t.i.d.	Symptomatic relief of urinary bladder spasm
tolterodine (*Detrol, Detrol LA*)	1–2 mg PO b.i.d. or 4 mg/d for ER capsules; reduce dosage with hepatic impairment to 1 mg PO b.i.d.	Treatment of overactive bladder in patients with urinary urgency, frequency, or incontinence

to these drugs; pyloric or duodenal obstruction or other GI lesions or obstructions, which could be dangerously exacerbated by these drugs; obstructions of the lower urinary tract, which also could be exacerbated by these drugs; glaucoma, which requires caution because of the blockage of the parasympathetic nervous system and the potential for increased intraocular pressure; and pregnancy or lactation, which require caution if using these drugs.

Physical assessment should be done to establish baseline data for assessing the effectiveness of the drug and the occurrence of any adverse effects associated with drug therapy. Assess the following: skin, to evaluate for the development of rash or hypersensitivity reactions; orientation and reflexes, to evaluate any CNS effects of the drug; ophthalmological examination including intraocular pressure, to assess for any developing glaucoma; and pulse, to establish a baseline for evaluating the extent of parasympathetic blockade.

Nursing Diagnoses

The patient receiving a urinary tract antispasmodic may have the following nursing diagnoses related to drug therapy:

- Acute Pain related to GI, CNS, ophthalmological effects of drug
- Disturbed Sensory Perception (Visual) related to CNS, ophthalmological effects
- Deficient Knowledge regarding drug therapy

Implementation

- Arrange for appropriate treatment of any underlying UTI, *which may be causing the spasm.*
- Arrange for an ophthalmological examination at the beginning of therapy and periodically during long-term treatment, *to evaluate drug effects on intraocular pressure so that the drug can be stopped if intraocular pressure increases.*
- Institute safety precautions if the patient experiences CNS effects, *to prevent patient injury.*
- Encourage the patient to continue treatment for the underlying cause of the spasm, *to treat the cause and prevent the return of the signs and symptoms.*

- Provide thorough patient teaching, including the drug name and prescribed dosage, measures to help avoid adverse effects, warning signs that may indicate problems, and the need for periodic monitoring and evaluation, *to enhance patient knowledge about drug therapy and to promote compliance.*
- Offer support and encouragement, *to help the patient deal with the discomfort of the drug therapy.*

Evaluation

- Monitor patient response to the drug (resolution of urinary tract spasms and relief of signs and symptoms); repeat culture and sensitivity tests are recommended for evaluation of the effectiveness of all of these drugs.
- Monitor for adverse effects (skin evaluation, orientation and reflexes, intraocular pressure).
- Evaluate the effectiveness of the teaching plan (patient can name drug, dosage, adverse effects to watch for, specific measures to avoid adverse effects).
- Monitor the effectiveness of comfort and safety measures and compliance to the regimen.

URINARY TRACT ANALGESIC

Urinary tract pain can be very uncomfortable and lead to urinary retention and increased risk of infection. The agent phenazopyridine (*Azo-Standard, Baridium,* and others) is a dye that is used to relieve that pain.

Therapeutic Actions and Indications
When phenazopyridine is excreted in the urine, it exerts a direct, topical analgesic effect on the urinary tract mucosa (see Figure 52–1). It is used to relieve symptoms (burning, urgency, frequency, pain, discomfort) related to urinary tract irritation from infection, trauma, or surgery.

Pharmacokinetics
Phenazopyridine is rapidly absorbed and has a very rapid onset of action. It is widely distributed, crossing the placenta and entering breast milk. It is metabolized in the liver and excreted in the urine. Effects during pregnancy and lactation

DRUGS IN FOCUS
Urinary Tract Analgesic

Drug Name	Usual Dosage	Usual Indications
phenazopyridine (*Azo-Standard, Baridium, Pyridium*)	200 mg PO t.i.d. for up to 2 days Pediatric (6–12 y): 12 mg/kg per day or 350 mg/m² per day PO, divided into three doses, do not exceed 2 d	Symptomatic relief of the discomforts associated with urinary tract trauma or infection

are not well documented, so use during pregnancy and lactation should be reserved for those situations in which the benefit to the mother clearly outweighs any potential risk to the fetus or neonate.

Contraindications and Cautions

Phenazopyridine is contraindicated in the presence of known allergy to the drug and with serious renal dysfunction, which would interfere with the excretion and effectiveness of the drug. Caution should be used with pregnancy and lactation because of the potential for adverse effects on the neonate.

Adverse Effects
Adverse effects associated with this drug include GI upset, headache, rash, and a reddish-orange coloring of the urine, all of which are related to the drug's chemical actions in the system. There also is a potential for renal or hepatic toxicity. This drug should not be used for longer than 2 days because the toxic effects may be increased.

Clinically Important Drug–Drug Interactions
There is an increased risk of toxic effects of this drug if it is combined with antibacterial agents used for treating UTIs. If this combination is used, the phenazopyridine should not be used longer than 2 days.

Nursing Considerations for Patients Receiving a Urinary Tract Analgesic
Assessment: History and Examination

Screen for the following conditions, which could be cautions or contraindications to use of the drug: history of allergy to these drugs or renal insufficiency, which are contraindications to the use of this drug; pregnancy or lactation, which require caution if using this drug.

Physical assessment should be done to establish baseline data for assessing the effectiveness of the drug and the occurrence of any adverse effects associated with drug therapy. Assess for the following: skin, to evaluate for the development of rash or hypersensitivity reactions; normal GI function and liver evaluation, to establish baseline data to assess adverse effects of the drug; renal and hepatic function tests, to assess for any underlying condition that might affect the metabolism or excretion of this drug; urinalysis, to assess for underlying infection or renal problems.

Nursing Diagnoses

The patient receiving a urinary tract analgesic may have the following nursing diagnoses related to drug therapy:

• Acute Pain related to GI effects of drug and headache
• Deficient Knowledge regarding drug therapy

Implementation

• Arrange for appropriate treatment of any underlying UTI, *which may be causing the pain.*

• Caution the patient that urine may be reddish-brown and may stain fabrics, *to prevent undue anxiety when this adverse effect occurs.*
• Administer the drug with food, *to alleviate GI irritation if GI upset is a problem.*
• Teach the patient to discontinue the drug and contact the health care provider if sclera or skin become yellowish—*a sign of drug accumulation in the body and a possible sign of hepatic toxicity.*
• Provide thorough patient teaching, including the drug name and prescribed dosage, measures to help avoid adverse effects, warning signs that may indicate problems, and the need for periodic monitoring and evaluation, *to enhance patient knowledge about drug therapy and to promote compliance.*

Evaluation

• Monitor patient response to the drug (resolution of urinary tract pain).
• Monitor for adverse effects (skin evaluation, GI upset and complaints, headache).
• Evaluate the effectiveness of the teaching plan (patient can name drug, dosage, adverse effects to watch for, specific measures to avoid adverse effects).
• Monitor the effectiveness of comfort measures and compliance to the regimen.

BLADDER PROTECTANT

The bladder protectant pentosan polysulfate sodium (*Elmiron*) is used to coat or adhere to the bladder mucosal wall and protect it from irritation related to solutes in the urine.

Therapeutic Actions and Indications
Pentosan polysulfate sodium is a heparin-like compound that has anticoagulant and fibrinolytic effects. This drug adheres to the bladder wall mucosal membrane and acts as a buffer to control cell permeability, preventing irritating solutes in the urine from reaching the bladder wall cells (see Figure 52–1). It is used specifically to decrease the pain and discomfort associated with **interstitial cystitis.**

Pharmacokinetics
Very little of this drug is absorbed (3%). It is distributed to the GI tract, liver, spleen, skin, bone marrow and periosteum. It undergoes metabolism in the liver and spleen and is excreted in the urine. There are no adequate studies of the effects of pentosan during pregnancy or lactation. Use should be limited to those situations in which the benefit to the mother outweighs the potential risk to the fetus or neonate.

Contraindications and Cautions
Because of its heparin-like effects, pentosan should not be used with any condition that involves an increased risk of bleeding (surgery, pregnancy, anticoagulation, hemophilia). It is also contraindicated in the presence of a history of heparin-

DRUGS IN FOCUS
Bladder Protectant

Drug Name	Usual Dosage	Usual Indications
pentosan polysulfate sodium (*Elmiron*)	100 mg PO t.i.d.	Relief of bladder pain or discomfort associated with interstitial cystitis

induced thrombocytopenia, which could recur with use of this drug. Caution should be used in patients with hepatic or splenic dysfunction, which could be affected by the heparin-like actions of the drug, and in pregnant or lactating women, because of the potential for adverse effects on the fetus.

Adverse Effects

Adverse effects associated with pentosan use include bleeding that may progress to hemorrhage (related to the drug's heparin effects), headache, alopecia (seen with heparin-type drugs), and GI disturbances related to local irritation of the GI tract with administration.

Clinically Important Drug–Drug Interactions

There is a potential for increased bleeding risks if this drug is combined with anticoagulants, aspirin, or nonsteroidal anti-inflammatory drugs. If such a combination is used, the patient should be monitored very closely for any signs of bleeding, and appropriate dosage adjustments should be made.

Nursing Considerations for Patients Receiving a Bladder Protectant
Assessment: History and Examination

Screen for the following conditions, which could be cautions or contraindications to use of the drug: history of allergy to this drug; history of bleeding abnormalities, splenic disorders, or hepatic dysfunction, which could result in bleeding when combined with the heparin-like effect of this drug; and pregnancy and lactation, which require cautious use of this drug.

Physical assessment should be done to establish baseline data for assessing the effectiveness of the drug and the occurrence of any adverse effects associated with drug therapy. Assess the following: skin, to evaluate for the development of rash or hypersensitivity reactions; orientation, affect, and reflexes, to establish a baseline to evaluate CNS effects of the drug; and liver function tests and bleeding times, to establish a baseline to monitor safe use of the drug and the occurrence of adverse effects.

Nursing Diagnoses

The patient receiving a bladder protectant may have the following nursing diagnoses related to drug therapy:

- Ineffective Tissue Perfusion related to bleeding secondary to heparin effects of the drug
- Acute Pain related to headache, CNS effects, and GI effects of the drug
- Risk for Injury related to bleeding and CNS effects
- Deficient Knowledge regarding drug therapy

Implementation

- Establish the presence of interstitial cystitis by biopsy or cytoscopy before beginning therapy, *to ensure that appropriate therapy is being used.*
- Administer the drug on an empty stomach, 1 hour before or 2 hours after meals, *to relieve GI discomfort and improve absorption.*
- Monitor bleeding times periodically during therapy, *to assess for excessive heparin effect.*
- Arrange for a wig or appropriate head covering *if alopecia develops as a result of drug therapy.*
- Provide thorough patient teaching, including the drug name and prescribed dosage, measures to help avoid adverse effects, warning signs that may indicate problems, and the need for periodic monitoring and evaluation, *to enhance patient knowledge about drug therapy and to promote compliance.*

Evaluation

- Monitor patient response to the drug (relief of bladder pain and discomfort).
- Monitor for adverse effects (skin evaluation, GI upset and complaints, headache, bleeding time).
- Evaluate the effectiveness of the teaching plan (patient can name drug, dosage, adverse effects to watch for, specific measures to avoid adverse effects).
- Monitor the effectiveness of comfort measures and compliance with the regimen.

☐☐●● WEB LINKS
Health care providers and patients may want to consult the following Internet sources:

Information on benign prostatic hyperplasia (BPH), support groups, research, treatment for patients:

http://www.pslgroup.com/ENLARGPROST.HTM
Information on BPH research and medical information:
http://www.uro.com/bph.htm
Information on neurogenic bladder:
http://www.nlm.nih.gov/medlineplus/ency/article/000754.htm
Information on interstitial cystitis:
http://www.ichelp.org
Information on cystitis—research, prevention, treatment, pathology:
http://www.nlm.nih.gov

DRUGS FOR TREATING BENIGN PROSTATIC HYPERPLASIA

Two types of drugs are currently used to relieve the symptoms of **benign prostatic hyperplasia (BPH)** in men. α-Adrenergic blockers doxazosin (*Cardura*), tamsulosin (*Flomax*), and terazosin (*Hytrin*) are used to block the dilation of arterioles in the bladder and urinary tract. Tamsulosin was developed specifically for the treatment of BPH and is not associated with as many adverse adrenergic blocking effects as the other two drugs are. Finasteride (*Proscar*) and dutasteride (*Duagen*) are specifically used to treat BPH by blocking testosterone production and are associated with more androgen-blocking effects than the other drugs are.

Therapeutic Actions and Indications
BPH is a common problem in men, and it increases in incidence with age. This enlargement of the gland surrounding the urethra leads to discomfort, difficulty in initiating a stream of urine, feelings of bloating, and an increased incidence of cystitis. α-Adrenergic blockers are indicated for the treatment of symptomatic BPH. These drugs block postsy-

naptic α₁-adrenergic receptors, which results in a dilation of arterioles and veins and a relaxation of sympathetic effects on the bladder and urinary tract. These drugs are also indicated for the treatment of hypertension (see Chapter 43).

Finasteride and dutasteride inhibit the intracellular enzyme that converts testosterone to a potent androgen (DHT), which the prostate gland depends on for its development and maintenance (see Figure 52–1). These drugs are used for long-term therapy to shrink the prostate and relieve the symptoms of hyperplasia. Finasteride (*Propecia*) is also used to prevent male-pattern baldness in patients with a strong family history.

When any of these drugs are used, it is important to make sure that the prostate enlargement is benign and not caused by cancer, infection, stricture, or hypotonic bladder. Patients receiving long-term therapy need to be reassessed periodically.

Pharmacokinetics
The α₁-selective adrenergic blocking agents are well absorbed and undergo extensive hepatic metabolism. Therefore, they must be used with caution in patients with hepatic impairment. They are excreted in the urine. Finasteride and dutasteride are rapidly absorbed from the GI tract, undergo hepatic metabolism, and are excreted in the feces and urine. They have no indications for women and are rated pregnancy category X because of androgen effects. Women must be cautioned not to touch finasteride or dutasteride because of the risk of absorption through the skin.

Contraindications and Cautions
These drugs are contraindicated in the presence of allergy to the drugs. Caution should be used in the presence of hepatic or renal dysfunction, which could alter the metabolism and excretion of the drugs. The adrenergic blockers should be used with caution in the presence of congestive heart failure or known coronary disease.

DRUGS IN FOCUS
Drugs Used to Treat Benign Prostatic Hyperplasia (BPH)

Drug Name	Usual Dosage	Usual Indications
P doxazosin (*Cardura*)	1 mg PO q.d. with titration up to 8 mg/d if needed; not for use in children	Relief of symptoms of BPH; hypertension
dutasteride (*Duagen*)	0.5 mg/d PO	Treatment of symptoms of BPH
finasteride (*Proscar, Propecia*)	5 mg/d PO for BPH, 1 mg/d PO for male pattern baldness (*Propecia*)	Relief of symptoms of BPH; prevention of male-pattern baldness
tamsulosin (*Flomax*)	0.4–0.8 mg/d PO, 30 min after the same meal each day	Treatment of BPH
terazosin (*Hytrin*)	1–10 mg/d PO based on patient response	Relief of symptoms of BPH; hypertension

Adverse Effects

Adverse effects of α-adrenergic blockers include headache, fatigue, dizziness, postural dizziness, lethargy, tachycardia, hypotension, GI upset, and sexual dysfunction, all of which are effects seen with blockade of the α-receptors. Finasteride and dutasteride are associated with decreased libido, impotence, and sexual dysfunction, all of which are related to decreased levels of DHT.

Clinically Important Drug–Drug Interactions

There is a possibility of decreased theophylline levels if combined with these drugs. The patient should be monitored and appropriate dosage adjustment made if this combination is used.

Nursing Considerations for Patients Receiving Drugs to Treat Benign Prostatic Hypertrophy

Assessment

Screen for the following conditions, which could be cautions or contraindications to the use of the drug: history of allergy to this drug; history of congestive heart failure; and renal or hepatic failure, which would require caution when using these drugs.

Physical assessment should be done to establish baseline data for assessing the effectiveness of the drug and the occurrence of any adverse effects associated with drug therapy. Assess the following: skin, to evaluate for the development of rash or hypersensitivity reactions; blood pressure, pulse, auscultation, and perfusion, to evaluate the cardiovascular effects of α-adrenergic blockade; urinalysis and normal urinary function; prostate palpation, and appropriate tests, including prostate-specific antigen (PSA) levels, to evaluate prostate problems.

Nursing Diagnoses

The patient receiving a drug to treat BPH may have the following nursing diagnoses related to drug therapy:

- Sexual Dysfunction related to drug effects
- Acute Pain related to headache, CNS effects, and GI effects of the drug
- Deficient Knowledge regarding drug therapy

Implementation

- Determine the presence of BPH and periodically evaluate, *to reconfirm that no other problem is occurring through prostate examination and measurement of PSA levels.*
- Administer the drug without regard to meals, but give with meals *if GI upset is a problem.*
- Provide thorough patient teaching, including the drug name and prescribed dosage, measures to help avoid adverse effects, warning signs that may indicate problems, and the need for periodic monitoring and evaluation, *to enhance patient knowledge about drug therapy and to promote compliance.*

- Offer support and encouragement, *to help the patient cope with potential decreases in sexual functioning.*

Evaluation

- Monitor patient response to the drug (relief of signs and symptoms of BPH, improved urine flow, decrease in discomfort).
- Monitor for adverse effects (skin evaluation, GI upset and complaints, headache, cardiovascular effects).
- Evaluate the effectiveness of the teaching plan (patient can name drug, dosage, adverse effects to watch for, specific measures to avoid adverse effects).
- Monitor the effectiveness of comfort measures and compliance with the regimen.

CHAPTER SUMMARY

- Acute urinary tract infections (UTIs) are second in frequency to respiratory tract infections in the American population.
- Urinary tract anti-infectives are drugs used to kill bacteria in the urinary tract by producing an acidic urine, which is undesirable to bacteria growth, or by acting to destroy bacteria in the urinary tract.
- Many activities are necessary to help decrease the bacteria in the urinary tract (eg, hygiene measures, proper diet, forcing fluids), to facilitate the treatment of UTIs and help the urinary tract anti-infectives be more effective.
- Inflammation and irritation of the urinary tract can cause smooth muscle spasms along the urinary tract. These spasms lead to the uncomfortable effects of dysuria, urgency, incontinence, nocturia, and suprapubic pain.
- The urinary tract antispasmodics act to relieve spasms of the urinary tract muscles by blocking parasympathetic activity and relaxing the detrusor and other urinary tract muscles.
- The urinary tract analgesic, phenazopyridine, is used to provide relief of symptoms (burning, urgency, frequency, pain, discomfort) related to urinary tract irritation resulting from infection, trauma, or surgery.
- Pentosan polysulfate sodium is a heparin-like compound that has anticoagulant and fibrinolytic effects and adheres to the bladder wall mucosal membrane to act as a buffer to control cell permeability. This action prevents irritating solutes in the urine from reaching the cells of the bladder wall. It is used specifically to decrease the pain and discomfort associated with interstitial cystitis.
- Benign prostatic hyperplasia (BPH) is a common enlargement of the prostate gland in older men.
- Drugs frequently used to relieve the signs and symptoms of prostate enlargement include α-adrenergic blockers, which relax the sympathetic effects on the bladder and sphincters, and finasteride and dutasteride, which block the body's production of a powerful androgen. The prostate is dependent on testosterone for its maintenance and develop-

ment; blocking the androgen leads to shrinkage of the gland and relief of symptoms.

Review Questions

1. In evaluating a patient for the presence of a bladder infection, one would not expect to find reports of
   a. frequency of urination.
   b. painful urination.
   c. edema of the fingers and hands.
   d. urgency of urination.

2. Methylene blue is a urinary tract anti-infective that acts by
   a. interfering with bacterial cell wall formation.
   b. interfering with bacterial cell division.
   c. alkalinizing the urine, which kills bacteria.
   d. acidifying the urine, which kills bacteria.

3. The antibiotic of choice for a patient with a cystitis who has great difficulty following medical regimens would be
   a. cinoxacin.
   b. fosfomycin.
   c. nitrofurantoin.
   d. norfloxacin.

4. Important educational points for patients with cystitis would not include
   a. avoidance of bubble baths.
   b. voiding immediately after sexual intercourse.
   c. always wiping back to front.
   d. avoidance of foods high in alkaline ash.

5. Urinary tract antispasmodics block the pain and discomfort associated with spasm in the smooth muscle of the urinary tract. The numerous adverse effects associated with these drugs are related to
   a. their blockade of sympathetic β-receptors.
   b. their stimulation of cholinergic receptors.
   c. their stimulation of sympathetic receptors.
   d. their blockade of cholinergic receptors.

6. BPH is a very common diagnosis in older men. Two types of drugs have been developed to treat the signs and symptoms of this disorder:
   a. α-adrenergic blockers and anticholinergic drugs.
   b. α-adrenergic blockers and testosterone production blockers.
   c. anticholinergic drugs and adrenergic stimulators.
   d. testosterone production blockers and adrenal androgens.

7. The drug of choice for treatment of BPH in a man with known hypotension might be
   a. doxazosin.
   b. terazosin.
   c. tamsulosin.
   d. propranolol.

8. Before administering a drug for the treatment of BPH, the nurse should ensure that
   a. the patient has had a prostate examination and measurement of the PSA level.
   b. the patient has not had a vasectomy.
   c. the patient is still sexually active.
   d. the patient is hypertensive and will tolerate the blood pressure–lowering effects.

9. A male who is very concerned about his hair loss and who is being treated for BPH might prefer treatment with
   a. doxazosin.
   b. finasteride.
   c. tamsulosin.
   d. terazosin.

10. After bladder surgery, many patients experience burning, urgency, frequency, and pain related to the urinary tract irritation. Such patients would benefit from treatment with
    a. methylene blue.
    b. fosfomycin.
    c. phenazopyridine.
    d. flavoxate.

BIBLIOGRAPHY

Bullock, B. L. (2000). *Focus on pathophysiology.* Philadelphia: Lippincott Williams & Wilkins.

Drug facts and comparisons. (2002). St. Louis: Facts and Comparisons.

Gilman, A., Hardman, J. G., & Limbird, L. E. (Eds.) (2002). *Goodman and Gilman's the pharmacological basis of therapeutics* (10th ed.). New York: McGraw-Hill.

Karch, A. M. (2002). *2003 Lippincott's nursing drug guide.* Philadelphia: Lippincott Williams & Wilkins.

The medical letter on drugs and therapeutics. (2002). New Rochelle, NY: Medical Letter.

Porth, C. M. (2002). *Pathophysiology: Concepts of altered health states* (6th ed.). Philadelphia: Lippincott Williams & Wilkins.

Professional's guide to patient drug facts. (2002). St. Louis: Facts and Comparisons.

P A R T

X

Drugs Acting on the Respiratory System

717

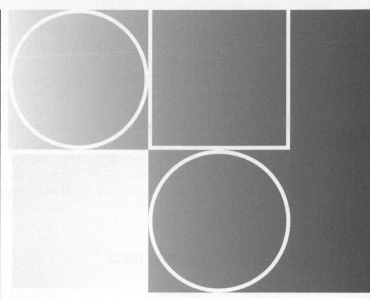

CHAPTER 53

Introduction to the Respiratory System

Key Terms

alveoli

asthma

bronchial tree

chronic obstructive pulmonary disease (COPD)

cilia

common cold

cough

larynx

lower respiratory tract

pneumonia

respiration

respiratory membrane

seasonal rhinitis

sinuses

sinusitis

sneeze

surfactant

trachea

upper respiratory tract

ventilation

The respiratory system is essential for survival. It brings oxygen into the body, allowing for the exchange of gases and expelling carbon dioxide and other waste products. The normal functioning of the respiratory system depends on an intricate balance of the nervous, cardiovascular, and musculoskeletal systems. The respiratory system consists of two parts: the **upper respiratory tract** and the **lower respiratory tract.** The upper portion, or conducting airways, is composed of the nose, mouth, pharynx, larynx, trachea, and the upper **bronchial tree** (Figure 53–1). The lower portion is made up of the smallest bronchi and the **alveoli** (respiratory sacs), which make up the lungs.

THE UPPER RESPIRATORY TRACT

Air usually moves into the body through the nose and into the nasal cavity. The nasal hairs catch and filter foreign substances that may be present in the inhaled air. The air is warmed and humidified as it passes by blood vessels close to the surface of the epithelial lining in the nasal cavity. The epithelial lining contains goblet cells that produce mucus, which traps dust, microorganisms, pollen, and any other foreign substances. The epithelial cells of this lining contain **cilia**—microscopic, hair-like projections of the cell membrane—which are constantly moving and directing the mucus and any trapped substances down toward the throat (Figure 53–2).

Pairs of **sinuses** (air-filled passages through the skull) open into the nasal cavity. Because the epithelial lining of the nasal passage is continuous with the lining of the sinuses, the mucus produced in the sinuses drains into the nasal cavity. From there, the mucus drains into the throat and is swallowed into the gastrointestinal tract, where stomach acid destroys foreign materials.

Air moves from the nasal cavity into the pharynx and **larynx.** The larynx contains the vocal chords and the epiglottis, which close during swallowing to protect the lower respiratory tract from any foreign particles. From the larynx, air proceeds to the **trachea,** the main conducting airway into the lungs. The trachea bifurcates, or divides, into two main bronchi, which further divide into smaller and smaller branches. All of these tubes contain mucus-producing goblet cells and cilia to entrap any particles that may have escaped the upper protective mechanisms. The cilia in these tubes move the mucus up the trachea and into the throat, where again it is swallowed.

The bronchial tubes are composed of three layers: cartilage, muscle, and epithelial cells. The cartilage keeps the tube open and becomes progressively less abundant as the bronchi divide and get smaller. The muscles keep the bronchi open; the muscles in the bronchi become smaller and less abundant, with only a few muscle fibers remaining in the terminal bronchi and alveoli. The epithelial cells are very similar in structure and function to the epithelial cells in the nasal passage.

The walls of the trachea and conducting bronchi are highly sensitive to irritation. When receptors in the walls are stimulated, a central nervous system reflex is initiated and a

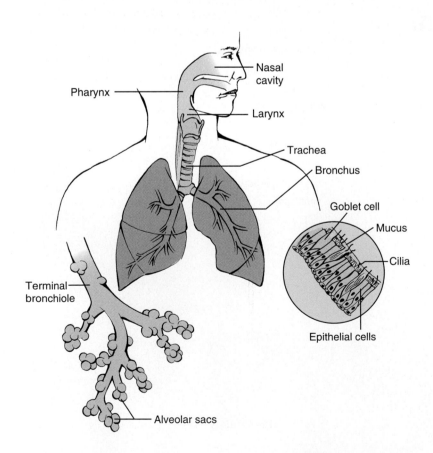

Pharynx

Nasal cavity

Larynx

Trachea

Bronchus

Goblet cell

Mucus

Cilia

Terminal bronchiole

Epithelial cells

Alveolar sacs

FIGURE 53-1. The respiratory tract.

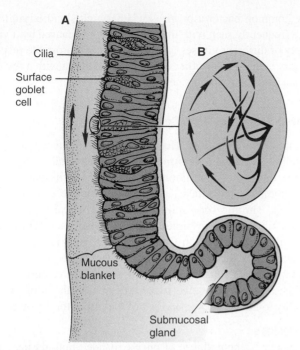

FIGURE 53-2. *A.* The mucociliary escalator. *B.* Conceptual scheme of ciliary movement, which allows forward motion to move the viscous gel layer and backward motion to occur entirely within the more fluid sol layer. (From Bullock, B. L. [2000]. *Focus on pathophysiology.* Philadelphia: Lippincott Williams & Wilkins.)

cough results. The cough causes air to be pushed through the bronchial tree under tremendous pressure, cleaning out any foreign irritant. This reflex, along with the similar **sneeze** reflex (which is initiated by receptors in the nasal cavity), forces foreign materials directly out of the system, opening it for more efficient flow of gas.

Throughout the airways, many macrophage scavengers freely move about the epithelium and destroy invaders. Mast cells are present in abundance and release histamine, serotonin, adenosine triphosphate (ATP), and other chemicals to ensure a rapid and intense inflammatory reaction to any cell injury. The end result of these various defense mechanisms is that the lower respiratory tract is virtually sterile—an important protection against respiratory infection that could interfere with essential gas exchange.

THE LOWER RESPIRATORY TRACT

The lower respiratory tract (ie, the respiratory airways) comprises the smallest bronchioles and the alveoli (see Figure 53–1). These structures are the functional units of the lungs. Within the lungs are a network of bronchi, alveoli, and blood vessels. The lung tissue receives its blood supply from the bronchial artery, which branches directly off the aorta. The alveoli receive unoxygenated blood from the right ventricle via the pulmonary artery. The delivery of this blood to the alveoli is referred to as perfusion.

Gas exchange occurs in the alveoli. In this process, carbon dioxide is lost from the blood and oxygen is transferred to the blood. The exchange of gases at the alveolar level is called **ventilation.** The alveolar sac holds the gas, allowing needed oxygen to diffuse across the **respiratory membrane** into the capillary while carbon dioxide, which is more abundant in the capillary blood, diffuses across the membrane and enters the alveolar sac to be expired.

The respiratory membrane is made up of the capillary endothelium, the capillary basement membrane, the interstitial space, the alveolar basement membrane, the alveolar epithelium, and the surfactant layer (Figure 53–3). The sac is able to stay open because the surface tension of the cells is decreased by the lipoprotein **surfactant.** Absence of surfactant leads to alveolar collapse. Surfactant is produced by the type II cells in the alveoli. These cells have other metabolic functions, including the conversion of angiotensin I to angiotensin II, the degradation of serotonin, and possibly the metabolism of various hormones. The oxygenated blood is returned to the left atrium via the pulmonary veins; from there it is pumped throughout the body to deliver oxygen to the cells and to pick up waste products.

Respiration

Respiration, or the act of breathing, is controlled by the central nervous system. The inspiratory muscles—diaphragm, external intercostals, and abdominal muscles—are stimulated to contract by the respiratory center in the medulla. The medulla receives input from chemoreceptors (neuroreceptors sensitive to carbon dioxide and acid levels) and increases the rate and/or depth of respiration to maintain homeostasis in the body.

The vagus nerve, a predominantly parasympathetic nerve, plays a key role in stimulating diaphragm contraction and inspiration. Vagal stimulation also leads to a bronchoconstric-

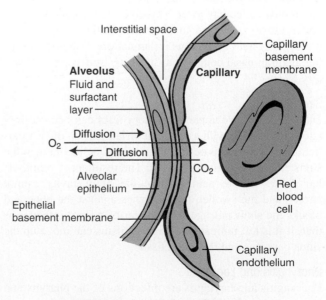

FIGURE 53-3. The respiratory membrane.

tion or tightening. The sympathetic system also innervates the respiratory system. Stimulation of the sympathetic system leads to increased rate and depth of respiration and dilation of the bronchi to allow freer flow of air through the system.

◼◼◼◼ WEB LINKS

To explore the virtual respiratory tract, refer to the following Internet source:

http://www.InnerBody.com

RESPIRATORY PATHOLOGY

Upper Respiratory Tract Conditions

The most common conditions that affect the upper respiratory tract involve the inflammatory response.

The Common Cold

A number of viruses cause the **common cold.** These viruses invade the tissues of the upper respiratory tract, initiating the release of histamine and prostaglandins and causing an inflammatory response. As a result of the inflammatory response, the mucous membranes become engorged with blood, the tissues swell, and the goblet cells increase the production of mucus. These effects cause the person with a common cold to complain of sinus pain, nasal congestion, runny nose, sneezing, watery eyes, scratchy throat, and headache. In susceptible people, this swelling can block the outlet of the eustachian tube, which drains the inner ear and equalizes pressure across the tympanic membrane. If this outlet becomes blocked, feelings of ear stuffiness and pain can occur, and the individual is more likely to develop an ear infection (otitis media).

Seasonal Rhinitis

A similar condition that afflicts many people is allergic or **seasonal rhinitis** (an inflammation of the nasal cavity), commonly called hay fever. This condition occurs when the upper airways respond to a specific antigen (eg, pollen, mold, dust) with a vigorous inflammatory response, resulting again in nasal congestion, sneezing, stuffiness, and watery eyes.

Sinusitis

Other areas of the upper respiratory tract can become irritated or infected, with a resultant inflammation of that particular area. **Sinusitis** occurs when the epithelial lining of the sinus cavities becomes inflamed. The resultant swelling often causes severe pain because the bony cavity cannot stretch and the swollen tissue pushes against the bone and blocks the sinus passage. The danger of a sinus infection is that, if it is left untreated, microorganisms can move up the sinus passages and into brain tissue.

Pharyngitis and Laryngitis

Pharyngitis and laryngitis are infections of the pharynx and larynx, respectively. These infections are frequently caused by common bacteria or viruses. Pharyngitis and laryngitis are frequently seen with influenza, which is caused by a variety of different viruses and produces uncomfortable respiratory symptoms or other inflammations along with a fever, muscle aches and pains, and malaise.

Lower Respiratory Tract Conditions

A number of disorders affect the lower respiratory tract, including atelectasis, **pneumonia** (bacterial, viral, or aspiration), bronchitis or inflammation of the bronchi (acute and chronic), bronchiectasis, and the obstructive disorders—asthma, chronic obstructive pulmonary disease (COPD), cystic fibrosis, and respiratory distress syndrome (RDS). Tuberculosis, discussed in Chapter 9, is a bacterial infection. Once known as consumption, this disease has been responsible for many respiratory deaths throughout the centuries. All of these disorders involve, to some degree, an alteration in the ability to move gases in and out of the respiratory system.

Atelectasis

Atelectasis, the collapse of once-expanded lung tissue, can occur as a result of outside pressure against the alveoli—for example, from a pulmonary tumor, a pneumothorax (air in the pleural space exerting high pressure against the alveoli), or a pleural effusion. Atelectasis most commonly occurs as a result of blockage of the airway, which prevents air from entering the alveoli and keeping it expanded. This occurs when a mucous plug, edema of the bronchioles, or a collection of pus or secretions occludes the airway and prevents the movement of air. Patients may experience atelectasis after surgery, when the effects of anesthesia on the lungs, pain, and decreased coughing reflexes can lead to a decreased tidal volume and accumulation of secretions in the lower airways. Patients may present with rales, dyspnea, fever, cough, hypoxia, and changes in chest wall movement. Treatment may involve clearing the airways, delivery of oxygen, and assisted ventilation.

Pneumonia

Pneumonia is an inflammation of the lungs caused either by bacterial or viral invasion of the tissue or by aspiration of foreign substances into the lower respiratory tract. The rapid inflammatory response to any foreign presence in the lower respiratory tract leads to a localized swelling, engorgement, and exudation of protective sera. The respiratory membrane is affected, resulting in decreased gas exchange. Patients complain of difficulty breathing and fatigue, and they present with fever, noisy breath sounds, and poor oxygenation.

Bronchitis

Acute bronchitis occurs when bacteria, viruses, or foreign materials infect the inner layer of the bronchi. The person with bronchitis may have a narrowed airway during the inflammation; this condition can be very serious in a person with obstructed or narrowed airflow. Chronic bronchitis is an inflammation of the bronchi that does not clear.

Bronchiectasis

Bronchiectasis is a chronic disease that involves the bronchi and bronchioles. It is characterized by dilation of the bronchial tree and chronic infection and inflammation of the bronchial passages. With chronic inflammation, the bronchial epithelial cells are replaced by a fibrous scar tissue. The loss of the protective mucous and ciliary movement of the epithelial cell membranes, combined with the dilation of the bronchial tree, leads to chronic infections in the now unprotected lower areas of the lung tissue. Patients with bronchiectasis often have an underlying medical condition that makes them more susceptible to infections (eg, immune suppression, acquired immunodeficiency syndrome, chronic inflammatory conditions). Patients present with the signs and symptoms of acute infection, including fever, malaise, myalgia, arthralgia, and a purulent, productive cough.

OBSTRUCTIVE PULMONARY DISEASES

As noted previously, the obstructive pulmonary diseases include asthma, cystic fibrosis, COPD, and RDS.

Asthma is characterized by reversible bronchospasm, inflammation, and hyperactive airways (Figure 53–4). The hyperactivity is triggered by allergens or nonallergic inhaled irritants or by factors such as exercise and emotions. The triggers cause an immediate release of histamine, which re-

sults in bronchospasm in about 10 minutes. The later response (3 to 5 hours) is cytokine-mediated inflammation, mucus production, and edema contributing to obstruction. Appropriate treatment depends on understanding the early and late responses. The extreme case of asthma is called status asthmaticus; this is a life-threatening bronchospasm that does not respond to usual treatment and occludes air flow into the lungs.

Chronic obstructive pulmonary disease (COPD) is a permanent, chronic obstruction of airways, often related to cigarette smoking. It is caused by two related disorders, emphysema and chronic bronchitis, both of which result in airflow obstruction on expiration; and by overinflated lungs and poor gas exchange. Emphysema is characterized by loss of the elastic tissue of the lungs, destruction of alveolar walls, and a resultant hyperinflation and tendency to collapse with expiration. Chronic bronchitis is a permanent inflammation of the airways with mucus secretion, edema, and poor inflammatory defenses. Characteristics of both disorders often are present in the person with COPD (Figure 53–5).

Cystic fibrosis is a hereditary disease that results in the accumulation of copious amounts of very thick secretions in the lungs. Eventually, the secretions obstruct the airways, leading to destruction of the lung tissue. Treatment is aimed at keeping the secretions fluid and moving and maintaining airway patency as much as possible.

Respiratory distress syndrome (RDS) is frequently seen in premature babies who are delivered before their lungs have fully developed and while surfactant levels are still very low. Surfactant is necessary for lowering the surface tension in the alveoli so that they can stay open to allow the flow of gases. Treatment is aimed at instilling surfactant to prevent atelectasis and to allow the lungs to expand. Adult respiratory distress syndrome (ARDS) is characterized by progressive loss of lung compliance and increasing hypoxia. This syndrome occurs as a result of a severe insult to the body, such as cardiovascular collapse, major burns, severe trauma, or rapid depressurization. Treatment of ARDS in-

FIGURE 53–4. Asthma. The bronchiole is obstructed on expiration, particularly by muscle spasm, edema of the mucosa, and thick secretions. (From Bullock, B. L. [2000]. *Focus on pathophysiology*. Philadelphia: Lippincott Williams & Wilkins.)

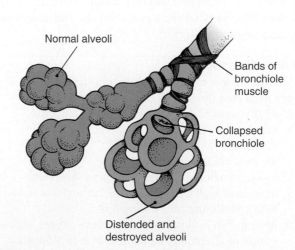

FIGURE 53–5. Distended and destroyed alveoli versus normal alveoli. (From Bullock, B. L. [2000]. *Focus on pathophysiology*. Philadelphia: Lippincott Williams & Wilkins.)

volves reversal of the underlying cause of the problem combined with ventilatory support.

CHAPTER SUMMARY

- The respiratory system is composed of the upper respiratory tract, or conducting airways (nose, mouth, pharynx, larynx, trachea, and the bronchial tree), and the lower respiratory tract, made up of alveoli (respiratory sacs), which make up the lungs.
- The respiratory system is essential for survival; it brings oxygen into the body, allowing for the exchange of gases (ventilation) and the expelling of carbon dioxide and other waste products.
- The upper airways have many features to protect the fragile alveoli: hairs filter the air; goblet cells produce mucus to trap material; cilia move the trapped material toward the throat for swallowing; the blood supply close to the surface warms the air and adds humidity to improve gas movement and gas exchange; and the cough and sneeze reflexes clear the airways.
- The alveolar sac is where gas exchange occurs across the respiratory membrane. The alveoli produce surfactant to decrease surface tension within the sac and have other metabolic functions.
- Respiration is controlled through the medulla in the central nervous system and depends on a balance between the sympathetic and parasympathetic systems and a functioning muscular system.
- Inflammation of the upper respiratory tract results in many uncomfortable disorders, including the common cold, seasonal rhinitis, sinusitis, pharyngitis, and laryngitis.
- Inflammation of the lower respiratory tract can result in serious disorders that interfere with gas exchange, including bronchitis and pneumonia.
- Obstructive disorders interfere with the ability to deliver gases to the alveoli because of obstructions in the conducting airways and eventually in the respiratory airways. These disorders include asthma, chronic obstructive pulmonary disease (COPD), cystic fibrosis, and respiratory distress syndrome (RDS).

Review Questions

1. In order for gas exchange to occur in the lungs, the oxygen must pass through all of the following except
   a. 47 divisions of conducting airways.
   b. the alveolar epithelium.
   c. the pleural fluid.
   d. the interstitial alveolar wall.
2. The oxyhemoglobin dissociation curve shows that
   a. in areas of high temperature, the hemoglobin holds on to O_2, protecting cells during fever.
   b. hemoglobin is almost saturated at an oxygen concentration of 70, protecting humans at high altitudes.
   c. in an acid environment, the hemoglobin holds on to O_2, a protection during exercise.

   d. in early lung disease, the hemoglobin cannot carry oxygen, making COPD an early diagnosed disease.
3. Diffusion of CO_2 from the tissues into the capillary blood
   a. occurs if the concentration of CO_2 in the tissues is greater than in the blood.
   b. decreases as blood acidity increases.
   c. increases in the absence of carbonic anhydrase.
   d. is accompanied by a decrease in plasma bicarbonate.
4. The walls of the alveoli are composed of type I and type II cells. The function of the type II cells is
   a. to replace mucous in the alveoli.
   b. production of serotonin.
   c. secretion of surfactant.
   d. protection of the lungs from bacterial invasion.
5. The pleurae are vital to the integrity of the lungs because they
   a. contain the cilia that protect the lungs.
   b. regulate the lung volume.
   c. maintain the proper temperature of the lungs during sleep.
   d. secrete a lubricating secretion that allows the lungs to glide over the thorax wall during breathing.
6. The nose performs all but which of the following functions in the respiratory system:
   a. serves as a passageway for air movement.
   b. warms and humidifies the air.
   c. cleanses the air using hair fibers.
   d. stimulates surfactant release from the alveoli.
7. For respiration to occur, a person must have
   a. low levels of oxygen.
   b. low levels of CO_2.
   c. functioning inspiratory muscles.
   d. an actively functioning autonomic system.
8. The common cold is caused by
   a. bacteria that grow best in the cold.
   b. allergens in the environment.
   c. irritation of the delicate mucous membrane.
   d. a number of different viruses.
9. A patient with COPD would have
   a. a viral infection.
   b. loss of the protective respiratory mechanisms after prolonged irritation or damage.
   c. localized swelling and inflammation within the lungs.
   d. inflammation or swelling of the sinus membranes over a prolonged period.
10. Inflammation of the upper respiratory tracts does not usually cause
    a. a runny nose.
    b. laryngitis.
    c. sneezing.
    d. hypoxia.

BIBLIOGRAPHY

Bullock, B. L. (2000). *Focus on pathophysiology*. Philadelphia: Lippincott Williams & Wilkins.

Fox, S. (1991). *Perspectives on human biology*. Dubuque, IA: Wm. C. Brown Publishers.

Ganong, W. (1999). *Review of medical physiology* (19th ed.). Norwalk, CT: Appleton & Lange.

Gilman, A., Hardman, J. G., & Limbird, L. E. (Eds.) (2002). *Goodman and Gilman's the pharmacological basis of therapeutics* (10th ed.). New York: McGraw-Hill.

Guyton, A., & Hall, J. (2000). *Textbook of medical physiology*. Philadelphia: W. B. Saunders.

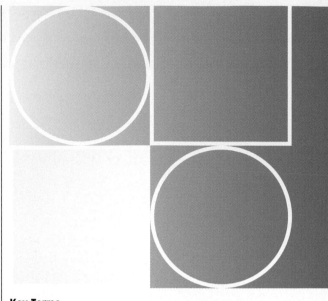

CHAPTER

54

Drugs Acting on the Upper Respiratory Tract

Key Terms
antihistamines
antitussives
decongestants
expectorants
mucolytics
rebound congestion
rhinitis medicamentosa

726

Antitussives
benzonatate
codeine
Ⓟ dextromethorphan
hydrocodone
terpin hydrate

Decongestants
Topical Nasal Decongestants
Ⓟ ephedrine
oxymetazoline
phenylephrine
tetrahydrozoline
xylometazoline

Oral Decongestants
Ⓟ pseudoephedrine
Topical Nasal Steroid Decongestants
beclomethasone
budesonide
dexamethasone
Ⓟ flunisolide
fluticasone
triamcinolone

Antihistamines
azatadine
azelastine
brompheniramine

buclizine
cetirizine
chlorpheniramine
clemastine
cyclizine
cyproheptadine
desloratadine
dexchlorpheniramine
dimenhydrinate
Ⓟ diphenhydramine
fexofenadine
hydroxyzine
loratadine

meclizine
promethazine
tripelennamine

Expectorants
Ⓟ guaifenesin
terpin hydrate

Mucolytics
Ⓟ acetylcysteine
dornase alfa

Drugs that affect the respiratory system work to keep the airways open and gases moving efficiently. The classes discussed in this chapter mainly act on the upper respiratory tract and include the following:

- **Antitussives**—which block the cough reflex
- **Decongestants**—which decrease the blood flow to the upper respiratory tract and decrease the overproduction of secretions
- **Antihistamines**—which block the release or action of histamine, a chemical released during inflammation that increases secretions and narrows airways
- **Expectorants**—which increase productive cough to clear the airways
- **Mucolytics**—which increase or liquefy respiratory secretions to aid the clearing of the airways

Figure 54–1 displays the sites of action of these drugs.

ANTITUSSIVES

Antitussives are drugs that suppress the cough reflex. Many disorders of the respiratory tract, including the common cold,

sinusitis, pharyngitis, and pneumonia, are accompanied by an uncomfortable, unproductive cough. Persistent coughing can be exhausting and can cause muscle strain and further irritation of the respiratory tract. A cough that occurs without the presence of any active disease process or persists after treatment may be a symptom of another disease process and should be investigated before any medication is given to alleviate it.

Therapeutic Actions and Indications

The traditional antitussives, including codeine (generic only), hydrocodone (*Hycodan*), and dextromethorphan (*Benylin* and many others), act directly on the medullary cough center of the brain to depress the cough reflex. Because they are centrally acting, they are not the drugs of choice for anyone who has a head injury or who could be impaired by central nervous system (CNS) depression. These drugs are rapidly absorbed, metabolized in the liver, and excreted in the urine. They cross the placenta and enter breast milk and should not be used during pregnancy or lactation because of the potential for CNS depressive effects on the fetus or neonate.

Other antitussives have a direct effect on the respiratory tract. Terpin hydrate (generic only) stimulates the secretory cells in the respiratory tract lining, leading to more copious secretions, which buffer the irritation in the respiratory tract

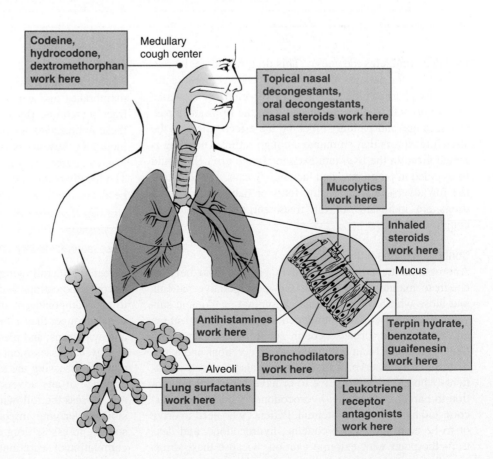

FIGURE 54–1. Sites of action of drugs acting on the upper respiratory tract.

DRUG THERAPY ACROSS THE LIFESPAN

Upper Respiratory Tract Agents

Children	Adults	Older Adults
These drugs are used frequently with children. Most of these agents have established pediatric guidelines. Care must be taken when these drugs are used with children because the risk of adverse effects—including sedation, confusion, and dizziness—are more common with children. Because many of these agents are available in over-the-counter (OTC) cold, flu, and allergy remedies, it is very important to educate parents about reading labels and following dosing guidelines to avoid potentially serious accidental overdose. Parents should always be asked specifically whether they are giving the child an OTC or herbal remedy. Parents should also be encouraged to implement nondrug measures to help the child cope with the upper respiratory problem—drink plenty of fluids, use a humidifier, avoid smoke-filled areas, avoid contact with known allergens or irritants, and wash hands frequently during the cold and flu season.	Adults may inadvertently overdose on these agents when taking multiple OTC preparations to help them get through the misery of a cold or flu.. They need to be questioned specifically about the use of OTC or herbal remedies before any of these drugs are advised or administered. Adults can also be encouraged to use nondrug measures to help them cope with the signs and symptoms. The safety for the use of these drugs during pregnancy and lactation has not been established. There is a potential for adverse effects on the fetus related to blood flow changes and direct drug effects when the drugs cross the placenta. The drugs may enter breast milk and also may alter fluid balance and milk production. It is advised that caution be used if one of these drugs is prescribed during lactation.	Older adults frequently are prescribed one of these drugs. Older adults are more likely to develop adverse effects associated with the use of these drugs, including sedation, confusion, and dizziness. Safety measures may be needed if these effects occur and interfere with the patient's mobility and balance. Older adults are also more likely to have renal and/or hepatic impairment related to underlying medical conditions, which could interfere with the meta-bolism and excretion of these drugs. The dosage for older adults should be started at a lower level than recommended for younger adults. The patient should be monitored very closely and dosage adjustment should be based on the patient's response. These patients also need to be alerted to the potential for toxic effects when using OTC preparations and should be advised to check with their health care provider before beginning any OTC drug regimen.

wall that stimulates the cough. This drug would not be rec-ommended for patients already impaired by copious secre-tions. Its pharmacokinetics are not reported. Benzonatate (*Tessalon*) acts as a local anesthetic on the respiratory pas-sages, lungs, and pleurae, blocking the effectiveness of the stretch receptors that stimulate a cough reflex. This drug is metabolized in the liver and excreted in the urine. It should be avoided in pregnancy and lactation because of the poten-tial for adverse effects on the fetus or baby. All of these drugs are indicated for the treatment of nonproductive cough.

Contraindications and Cautions

Antitussives are contraindicated in patients who need to cough to maintain the airways (eg, postoperative patients and those who have undergone abdominal or thoracic sur-gery). Careful use is recommended for patients with asthma and emphysema, because cough suppression in these pa-tients could lead to an accumulation of secretions and a loss of respiratory reserve. Caution should also be used in pa-tients who are hypersensitive to or have a history of addic-tion to narcotics (codeine, hydrocodone). Codeine is a nar-cotic and has addiction potential. Patients who need to drive or to be alert should use codeine, hydrocodone, and dex-tromethorphan with extreme caution, because these drugs can cause sedation and drowsiness.

Adverse Effects

Traditional antitussives have a drying effect on the mucous membranes and can increase the viscosity of respiratory tract secretions. Because they affect centers in the brain, these antitussives are associated with CNS adverse effects including drowsiness and sedation. Their drying effect can lead to nausea, constipation, and complaints of dry mouth. The locally acting antitussives are associated with GI upset, headache, feelings of congestion, and sometimes dizziness.

Nursing Considerations for Patients Receiving Antitussives

Assessment: History and Examination

Screen for the following conditions, which could be cautions or contraindications to use of the drug: any history of allergy to any component of the drug or drug vehicle; cough that persists longer than 1 week or is accompanied by other signs and symptoms; and pregnancy or lactation.

Physical assessment should be done to establish baseline data for assessing the effectiveness of the drug and the oc-currence of any adverse effects associated with drug ther-apy. Assess the following: temperature, to evaluate for pos-sible underlying infection; respirations and adventitious sounds, to assess drug effectiveness and to monitor for ac-cumulation of secretions; and orientation and affect, to mon-itor for CNS effects of the drug.

DRUGS IN FOCUS
Antitussives

Drug Name	Usual Dosage	Usual Indications
benzonatate (*Tessalon*)	Adult and pediatric (>10 y): 100 mg PO t.i.d.	All of the antitussives are indicated for treatment of nonproductive cough
codeine (generic)	Adult: 10–20 mg PO q4–6h Pediatric (6–12 y): 5–10 mg PO q4–6h Pediatric (2–6 y): 2.5–5 mg PO q4–6h	
ⓟ dextromethorphan (*Benylin* and others)	Adult: 10–30 mg PO q4–8h; 60 mg PO b.i.d. for sustained action products Pediatric (6–12 y): 5–10 mg PO q4h; 30 mg PO b.i.d. for sustained action products Pediatric (2–6 y): 2.5–7.5 mg PO q4–8h; 15 mg PO b.i.d. for sustained action products	
hydrocodone (*Hycodan*)	Adult: 5–10 mg PO q4–6h Pediatric (2–12 y): 1.25–5 mg PO q4–6h	
terpin hydrate (generic)	Adult: 85–170 mg PO t.i.d.–q.i.d. Pediatric (1–4 y): 20 mg PO t.i.d.–q.i.d. Pediatric (5–9 y): 40 mg PO t.i.d.–q.i.d. Pediatric (10–12 y): 85 mg PO t.i.d.–q.i.d.	

Nursing Diagnoses

The patient receiving an antitussive may have the following nursing diagnoses related to drug therapy:

- Ineffective Airway Clearance related to excessive drug effects
- Disturbed Sensory Perception related to CNS effects
- Deficient Knowledge regarding drug therapy

Implementation

- Ensure that the drug is not taken any longer than recommended, *to prevent serious adverse effects and increased respiratory tract problems.*
- Arrange for further medical evaluation for coughs that persist or are accompanied by high fever, rash, or excessive secretions, *to detect the underlying cause of the cough and to arrange for appropriate treatment of the underlying problem.*
- Provide other measures *to help relieve cough* (eg, humidity, cool temperatures, fluids, use of topical lozenges) as appropriate.
- Provide thorough patient teaching, including the drug name and prescribed dosage, measures to help avoid adverse effects, warning signs that may indicate problems, and the need for periodic monitoring and evaluation, *to enhance patient knowledge about drug therapy and to promote compliance.*
- Offer support and encouragement, *to help the patient cope with the disease and the drug regimen.*

Evaluation

- Monitor patient response to the drug (control of nonproductive cough).
- Monitor for adverse effects (respiratory depression, dizziness, sedation).
- Evaluate the effectiveness of the teaching plan (patient can name drug, dosage, adverse effects to watch for, specific measures to avoid adverse effects, measures to take to increase the effectiveness of the drug).
- Monitor effectiveness of other measures to relieve cough.

DECONGESTANTS

Decongestants are drugs, usually adrenergics or sympathomimetics, that cause local vasoconstriction and therefore decrease the blood flow to the irritated and dilated capillaries of the mucous membranes lining the nasal passages and sinus cavities. This vasoconstriction leads to a shrinking of swollen membranes and tends to open up clogged nasal passages, providing relief from the discomfort of a blocked nose and promoting drainage of secretions and improved air flow. An adverse effect that accompanies frequent or prolonged use of these drugs is a rebound congestion, officially called **rhinitis medicamentosa.** The reflex reaction to vasoconstriction is a rebound vasodilation, which often leads to prolonged overuse of decongestants.

Topical steroids are also used as decongestants. Topical steroids act to directly block the effects of inflammation on the nasal mucous membranes. This blocks the swelling, congestion, and increased secretions that accompany inflammation. The end result is an opening of the nasal passages and an increase in air flow. These drugs take several weeks to be really effective and are more often used in cases of chronic rhinitis.

TOPICAL NASAL DECONGESTANTS

The topical nasal decongestants include ephedrine (*Kondon's Nasal*), oxymetazoline (*Afrin, Allerest,* and others), phenylephrine (*Coricidin,* many others), tetrahydrozoline (*Tyzine*), and xylometazoline (*Otrivin*). Many of these are available as over-the-counter (OTC) preparations. The choice of a topical nasal decongestant is individual. Some patients may have no response to one and respond very well to another.

Therapeutic Actions and Indications

Topical decongestants are sympathomimetics, meaning that they imitate the effects of the sympathetic nervous system to cause vasoconstriction, leading to decreased edema and inflammation of the nasal membranes. Because these drugs are applied topically, the onset of action is almost immediate and there is less chance of systemic effects. They are available as nasal sprays that are used to relieve the discomfort of nasal congestion that accompanies the common cold, sinusitis, and allergic rhinitis. These drugs can also be used when dilation of the nares is desired to facilitate medical examination or to relieve the pain and congestion of otitis media. Opening the nasal passage allows better drainage of the eustachian tube, relieving pressure in the middle ear.

Pharmacokinetics

Although they are not generally absorbed systemically, any portion of these topical decongestants that is absorbed is metabolized in the liver and excreted in the urine. There are no studies regarding the effects of these topical drugs in pregnancy or lactation. As with any drug used during pregnancy or lactation, caution should be used.

Contraindications and Cautions

Caution should be used when there is any lesion or erosion in the mucous membranes that could lead to systemic absorption. Because these agents have adrenergic properties, caution should also be used in patients with any condition that might be exacerbated by sympathetic activity, such as glaucoma, hypertension, diabetes, thyroid disease, coronary disease, or prostate problems.

Adverse Effects

Adverse effects associated with topical decongestants include local stinging and burning, which may occur the first few times the drug is used. If the sensation does not pass, the drug should be discontinued, because it may indicate lesions or erosion of the mucous membranes. Use for longer than 3 to 5 days can lead to a rebound congestion. (**Rebound congestion** occurs when the nasal passages become congested as the drug effect wears off. As a result, patients tend to use more drug to decrease the congestion, thus initiating a vicious cycle of congestion–drug–congestion, which leads to abuse of the decongestant.) Sympathomimetic effects (eg, increased pulse, blood pressure; urinary retention) should be monitored because some systemic absorption may occur, al-

DRUGS IN FOCUS
Topical Nasal Decongestants

Drug Name	Usual Dosage	Usual Indications
Ⓟ ephedrine (*Kondon's Nasal*)	Instill solution in each nostril q4h, do not use for children <6 y unless advised by physician	Relief of the discomfort of nasal congestion associated with the common cold, sinusitis, allergic rhinitis; relief of pressure of otitis media
oxymetazoline (*Afrin, Allerest*)	Adult and pediatric (>6 y): two to three spray or drops in each nostril b.i.d. Pediatric (2–5 y): two to three drops of 0.25% solution in each nostril b.i.d.	Relief of the discomfort of nasal congestion associated with the common cold, sinusitis, allergic rhinitis
phenylephrine (*Coricidin*)	Adult and pediatric (>6 y): one to two sprays in each nostril q3–4h	Relief of the discomfort of nasal congestion associated with the common cold, sinusitis, allergic rhinitis
tetrahydrozoline (*Tyzine*)	Adult and pediatric (>6 y): two to four drops in each nostril t.i.d.–q.i.d. Pediatric (2–6 y): two to three drops of 0.05% solution in each nostril q4–6h	Relief of the discomfort of nasal congestion associated with the common cold, sinusitis, allergic rhinitis; relief of pressure of otitis media
xylometazoline (*Otrivin*)	Adult: two to three sprays or two to three drops in each nostril q8–10h Pediatric (2–12 y): two to three drops of 0.05% solution q8–12h	Relief of the discomfort of nasal congestion associated with the common cold, sinusitis, allergic rhinitis; relief of pressure of otitis media

though these effects are less likely with topical administration than with other routes.

Clinically Important Drug–Drug Interactions

The use of the topical nasal decongestants is contraindicated with concurrent use of cyclopropane or halothane anesthesia, because serious cardiovascular effects could occur. Combined use with any other sympathomimetic drug or sympathetic-blocking drug could result in toxic or noneffective responses. Monitor the use of these combinations carefully.

Nursing Considerations for Patients Receiving Topical Nasal Decongestants

Assessment: History and Examination

Screen for the following conditions, which could be cautions or contraindications to use of the drug: any history of allergy to the drug or a component of the drug vehicle; glaucoma, hypertension, diabetes, thyroid disease, coronary disease, and prostate problems, all of which could be exacerbated by the sympathomimetic effects; and pregnancy or lactation, which require cautious use of the drug.

Physical assessment should be done to establish baseline data for assessing the effectiveness of the drug and the occurrence of any adverse effects associated with drug therapy. Assess the following: skin color and temperature, to assess sympathetic response; orientation and reflexes, to evaluate CNS effects of the drug; pulse, blood pressure, cardiac auscultation, to monitor cardiovascular, sympathomimetic effects; respirations, adventitious breath sounds, to assess effectiveness of drug and potential excess effect; bladder percussion, to monitor for urinary retention related to sympathomimetic effects; and nasal mucous membrane evaluation, to monitor for lesions that could lead to systemic absorption and to evaluate decongestant effect.

Nursing Diagnoses

The patient receiving a topical nasal decongestant may have the following nursing diagnoses related to drug therapy:

- Acute Pain related to GI, CNS, local effects of drug
- Disturbed Sensory Perception (Kinesthetic) related to CNS effects (less likely with this route of administration)
- Deficient Knowledge regarding drug therapy

Implementation

- Teach the patient the proper administration of the drug, *to ensure therapeutic effect.* The patient should be instructed to clear the nasal passages before use, to tilt the head back when applying the drops or spray, and to keep it tilted back for a few seconds after administration. This technique *helps ensure contact with the affected mucous membranes and decreases the chances of letting the drops trickle down the back of throat, which may lead to more systemic effects.*
- Caution patients not to use the drug for longer than 5 days, and to seek medical care if signs and symptoms persist af-

ter that time, *to facilitate detection of underlying medical conditions that may require treatment.*
- Caution patients that these drugs are found in many OTC preparations and that *care should be taken not to inadvertently combine drugs with the same ingredients, leading to overdose.*
- Provide safety measures if dizziness or sedation occur as a result of drug therapy, *to prevent patient injury.*
- Institute other measures *to help relieve the discomfort of congestion* (eg, humidity, increased fluid intake, cool environment, avoidance of smoke-filled areas) as appropriate.
- Provide thorough patient teaching, including the drug name and prescribed dosage, measures to help avoid adverse effects, warning signs that may indicate problems, and the need for periodic monitoring and evaluation, *to enhance patient knowledge about drug therapy and to promote compliance.*
- Offer support and encouragement, *to help the patient cope with the disease and the drug regimen.*

Evaluation

- Monitor patient response to the drug (relief of nasal congestion).
- Monitor for adverse effects (local burning and stinging; adrenergic effects such as increased pulse, blood pressure, urinary retention, cool and clammy skin).
- Evaluate the effectiveness of the teaching plan (patient can name drug, dosage, adverse effects to watch for, specific measures to avoid adverse effects, measures to take to increase the effectiveness of the drug, proper administration technique).
- Monitor the effectiveness of comfort and safety measures and compliance with the regimen.

ORAL DECONGESTANTS

Oral decongestants are drugs that are taken orally to decrease nasal congestion related to the common cold, sinusitis, and allergic rhinitis. They are also used to relieve the pain and congestion of otitis media. Opening of the nasal passage allows better drainage of the eustachian tube, relieving pressure in the middle ear. The only oral decongestant currently available for use is pseudoephedrine (*Dorcol, Decofed,* and others).

Box 54–1 discusses the removal of phenylpropanolamine from the market.

Therapeutic Actions and Indications

Oral decongestants shrink the nasal mucous membrane by stimulating the α-adrenergic receptors in the nasal mucous membranes. This shrinkage results in a decrease in membrane size, promoting drainage of the sinuses and improving air flow. Because this drug is taken systemically, adverse effects related to the sympathomimetic effects (eg, cardiac stimulation, feelings of anxiety) are more likely to occur.

BOX 54-1

Phenylpropanolamine Removed from the Market

In late 2000, the U.S. Food and Drug Administration removed the oral decongestant phenylpropanolamine (PPA) from the market. This drug, which had been the center of controversy for many years, was found to be associated with an increased number of strokes in young women who took the drug. The drug had been an ingredient in many over-the-counter cold, allergy, and flu remedies. After a short absence, most of these products reappeared on the market with the drug pseudoephedrine taking the place of PPA. This drug, a sympathomimetic, is also known to cause sympathetic effects, including increased blood pressure and increased heart rate. Close follow-up of the effects of this drug will be done to monitor for any increased risk associated with its use.

Pharmacokinetics

Pseudoephedrine is generally well absorbed and reaches peak levels quickly—in 20 to 45 minutes. It is widely distributed in the body, metabolized in the liver, and primarily excreted in the urine. There are no adequate studies about its use during pregnancy and lactation, and such use should be reserved for situations in which the benefit to the mother outweighs any potential risk to the neonate.

Contraindications and Cautions

Because pseudoephedrine has adrenergic properties, caution should be used in patients with any condition that might be exacerbated by sympathetic activity, such as glaucoma, hypertension, diabetes, thyroid disease, coronary disease, and prostate problems.

Adverse Effects

Adverse effects associated with pseudoephedrine include rebound congestion. Sympathetic effects include feelings of anxiety, tenseness, restlessness, tremors, hypertension, arrhythmias, sweating, and pallor.

Nursing Considerations for Patients Receiving an Oral Decongestant

Assessment: History and Examination

Screen for the following conditions, which could be cautions or contraindications to use of the drug: any history of allergy to the drug and pregnancy or lactation, which are contraindications to drug use; hypertension or coronary artery disease, which require cautious use; and hyperthyroidism, diabetes mellitus, or prostate enlargement, all of which could be exacerbated by these drugs.

Physical assessment should be done to establish baseline data for assessing the effectiveness of the drug and the occurrence of any adverse effects associated with drug therapy. Assess the following: skin color and lesions, to monitor for adverse reactions; orientation, reflexes, and affect, to monitor CNS effects of the drug; blood pressure, pulse, and auscultation, to monitor cardiovascular stimulations; respiration and adventitious sounds, to monitor drug effectiveness; and urinary output, to evaluate for urinary retention.

Nursing Diagnoses

The patient receiving an oral decongestant may have the following nursing diagnoses related to drug therapy:

- Acute Pain related to GI, CNS, skin effects of drug
- Increased Cardiac Output related to sympathomimetic actions of the drug
- Disturbed Sensory Perception (Kinesthetic) related to CNS effects
- Deficient Knowledge regarding drug therapy

Implementation

- Note that this drug is found in many OTC products, especially combination cold and allergy preparations; *care should be taken to prevent inadvertent overdose or excessive adverse effects.*
- Provide safety measures as needed if CNS effects occur, *to prevent patient injury.*
- Monitor pulse, blood pressure, and cardiac response to the drug, especially in patients who are at risk for cardiac stim-

DRUGS IN FOCUS
Oral Decongestant

Drug Name	Usual Dosage	Usual Indications
pseudoephedrine (*Dorcol, Decofed*)	Adult: 60 mg PO q4–6h Pediatric: 6–12 y—30 mg PO q4–6h; 2–5 y—15 mg PO q4–6h; 1–2 y—0.02 mL/kg PO q4–6h; 3–12 mo—3 drops/kg PO q4–6h	Decrease nasal congestion associated with the common cold, allergic rhinitis; relief of pain and congestion of otitis media

ulation, *to detect adverse effects early and arrange to reduce dosage or discontinue the drug.*

- Encourage the patient not to use this drug for longer than 1 week and to seek medical evaluation if symptoms persist after that time, *to encourage the detection of underlying medical conditions that could be causing these symptoms and to arrange for appropriate treatment.*
- Provide thorough patient teaching, including the drug name and prescribed dosage, measures to help avoid adverse effects, warning signs that may indicate problems, and the need for periodic monitoring and evaluation, *to enhance patient knowledge about drug therapy and to promote compliance.*
- Offer support and encouragement, *to help the patient cope with the disease and the drug regimen.*

Evaluation

- Monitor patient response to the drug (improvement in nasal congestion).
- Monitor for adverse effects (sympathomimetic reactions including increased pulse, blood pressure, pallor, sweating, arrhythmias, feelings of anxiety, tension, dry skin).
- Evaluate the effectiveness of the teaching plan (patient can name drug, dosage, adverse effects to watch for, specific measures to avoid adverse effects, measures to take to increase the effectiveness of the drug).
- Monitor the effectiveness of comfort and safety measures and compliance with the regimen.

TOPICAL NASAL STEROID DECONGESTANTS

Topical nasal steroid decongestants are currently very popular for the treatment of allergic rhinitis. They have been found to be effective in patients who are no longer getting a response with other decongestants. The topical nasal steroid decongestants include beclomethasone (*Beclovent* and others), budesonide (*Rhinocort*), dexamethasone (*Decaderm* and others), flunisolide (*AeroBid* and others), fluticasone (*Flovent*), and triamcinolone (*Kenacort*).

Therapeutic Actions and Indications

The exact mechanism of action of topical steroids is not known. Their anti-inflammatory action results from their ability to produce a direct local effect that blocks many of the complex reactions responsible for the inflammatory response. Because they are applied topically, there is less of a chance of systemic absorption and associated adverse effects. The onset of action is not immediate, and they may actually require up to a week to cause any changes. If no effects are seen after 3 weeks, the drug should be discontinued. Topical nasal steroidal preparations are used to treat seasonal allergic rhinitis for patients who are not getting any response from other decongestant preparations. They are frequently used to relieve inflammation after the removal of nasal polyps.

Pharmacokinetics

Because these drugs are not generally absorbed systemically, their pharmacokinetics are not reported. If they were to be absorbed systemically, they would have the same pharmacokinetics as other steroids (Chapter 36).

Contraindications and Cautions

Because nasal steroids block the inflammatory response, their use is contraindicated in the presence of acute infections. Increased incidence of *Candida albicans* infection has been reported with their use, related to the anti-inflammatory and anti-immune activities associated with steroids. Caution should be used in any patient who has an active infection, including tuberculosis, because systemic absorption would interfere with the inflammatory and immune responses. Patients using nasal steroids should avoid exposure to any airborne infection, such as chickenpox or measles.

Adverse Effects

The most common adverse effects associated with the use of topical nasal steroids are local burning, irritation, stinging, dryness of the mucosa, and headache. Because healing is suppressed by steroids, patients who have recently experienced nasal surgery or trauma should be monitored closely until healing has occurred.

Nursing Considerations for Patients Receiving Topical Steroid Nasal Decongestants
Assessment: History and Examination

Screen for the following conditions, which could be cautions or contraindications to use of the drug: any history of allergy to steroid drugs or any components of the drug vehicle, which would be a contraindication; and acute infection, which would require cautious use.

Physical assessment should be done to establish baseline data for assessing the effectiveness of the drug and the occurrence of any adverse effects associated with drug therapy. Intranasal examination should be performed to determine the presence of any lesions that would increase the risk of systemic absorption of drug. Assess the following: respiration and adventitious sounds, to evaluate drug effectiveness; and temperature, to monitor for the possibility of acute infection.

Nursing Diagnoses

The patient receiving topical nasal steroid nasal decongestants may have the following nursing diagnoses related to drug therapy:

- Acute Pain related to local effects of the drug
- Risk for Injury related to suppression of inflammatory reaction
- Deficient Knowledge regarding drug therapy

Implementation

- Teach the patient the proper administration of these drugs, *which is very important to ensure effectiveness and prevent*

DRUGS IN FOCUS
Topical Steroid Nasal Decongestants

Drug Name	Usual Dosage	Usual Indications
beclomethasone (*Beclovent*)	Adult and pediatric: one inhalation in each nostril b.i.d.–q.i.d.	All of the topical steroid nasal decongestants are indicated for treatment of seasonal allergic rhinitis in patients who are not obtaining a response with other decongestants or preparations and for relief of inflammation after the removal and nasal polyps
budesonide (*Rhinocort*)	Adult and pediatric (>6 y): two sprays in each nostril morning and evening or four sprays in each nostril in the morning	
dexamethasone (*Decaderm*)	Adult: two sprays in each nostril b.i.d.–t.i.d. Pediatric: one to two sprays in each nostril bid	
P flunisolide (*AeroBid*)	Adult: two sprays in each nostril b.i.d. Pediatric (6–15 y): one spray in each nostril t.i.d. to two sprays in each nostril b.i.d.	
fluticasone (*Flovent*)	Adult: 88–440 µg b.i.d.	
triamcinolone (*Kenacort*)	Adult: two sprays in each nostril q.d.	

systemic effects. A variety of preparations are available (eg, sprays, aerosols, powder disks). Advise the patient about the proper administration technique for whichever preparation is recommended.

- Have the patient clear nasal passages before using the drug, *to improve the effectiveness of the drug.*
- Encourage the patient to continue using the drug regularly, even if results are not seen immediately, *because benefits may take 2 to 3 weeks to appear.*
- Monitor the patient for the development of acute infection *that would require medical intervention. Encourage the patient to avoid areas where airborne infections could be a problem, because steroid use decreases the effectiveness of the immune and inflammatory responses.*
- Provide thorough patient teaching, including the drug name and prescribed dosage, measures to help avoid adverse effects, warning signs that may indicate problems, and the need for periodic monitoring and evaluation, *to enhance patient knowledge about drug therapy and to promote compliance.*
- Offer support and encouragement, *to help the patient cope with the disease and the drug regimen.*

Evaluation

- Monitor patient response to the drug (relief of nasal congestion).
- Monitor for adverse effects (local burning and stinging).
- Evaluate the effectiveness of the teaching plan (patient can name drug, dosage, adverse effects to watch for, specific

measures to avoid adverse effects, measures to take to increase the effectiveness of the drug).
- Monitor the effectiveness of comfort and safety measures and compliance with the regimen.

ANTIHISTAMINES

Antihistamines are found in multiple OTC preparations that are designed to relieve respiratory symptoms and to treat allergies. These agents block the effects of histamine, bringing relief to patients suffering from itchy eyes, swelling, congestion, and drippy nose.

Numerous antihistamines are available, including first- and second-generation agents. First-generation antihistamines have greater anticholinergic effects, with resultant drowsiness. These drugs include azatadine (*Optimine*), azelastine (*Astelin*), brompheniramine (*Dimetane* and others), buclizine (*Bucladin-S*), cetirizine (*Reactine*), chlorpheniramine (*Aller-Chlor* and others), clemastine (*Tavist*), cyclizine (*Marezine*), cyproheptadine (*Periactin*), dexchlorpheniramine (*Dexchlor*), dimenhydrinate (*Dimentabs* and others), diphenhydramine (*Benadryl* and others), hydroxyzine (*Vistaril* and others), meclizine (*Bonine*), promethazine (*Phenergan* and others), and tripelennamine (*PBZ*). Second-generation antihistamines, including desloratadine (*Clarinex*), fexofenadine (*Allegra*), and loratadine (*Claritin*), have fewer anticholinergic effects than first-generation agents.

When choosing an antihistamine, the individual patient's reaction to the drug is usually the governing factor. If a person needs to be alert, one of the second-generation, nonse-dating antihistamines would be the drug of choice. Because of their OTC availability, these drugs are often misused to treat colds and influenza.

Therapeutic Actions and Indications

The antihistamines selectively block the effects of histamine at the histamine-1 receptor sites, decreasing the allergic response. They also have anticholinergic (atropine-like) and antipruritic effects. Antihistamines are used for the relief of symptoms associated with seasonal and perennial allergic rhinitis, allergic conjunctivitis, uncomplicated urticaria, and angioedema. They are also used for amelioration of allergic reactions to blood or blood products; for relief of discomfort associated with dermographism; and as adjunctive therapy in anaphylactic reactions. Other uses that are being explored include relief of exercise- and hyperventilation-induced asthma and histamine-induced bronchoconstriction in asthmatics. They are most effective if used before the onset of symptoms.

Pharmacokinetics

The oral antihistamines are well absorbed orally, with an onset of action ranging from 1 to 3 hours. They are generally metabolized in the liver, with excretion in the feces and urine. These drugs cross the placenta and enter breast milk, so their use should be avoided in pregnancy and lactation unless the benefit to the mother outweighs the potential risk to the fetus or baby.

Contraindications and Cautions

Antihistamines are contraindicated during pregnancy or lactation. They should be used with caution in renal or hepatic impairment, which could alter the metabolism and excretion of the drug. Special care should be taken when these drugs are used by any patient with a history of arrhythmias or prolonged Q-T intervals, because fatal cardiac arrhythmias have been associated with the use of certain antihistamines and drugs that increase Q-T intervals, including erythromycin.

Adverse Effects

The adverse effects most often seen with antihistamine use are drowsiness and sedation, although second-generation antihistamines are less sedating in many people. The anticholinergic effects that can be anticipated include drying of the respiratory and GI mucous membranes, GI upset and nausea, arrhythmias, dysuria, urinary hesitancy, and skin eruption and itching associated with dryness.

Nursing Considerations for Patients Receiving Antihistamines
Assessment: History and Examination

Screen for the following conditions, which could be cautions or contraindications to use of the drug: any history of allergy to antihistamines; pregnancy or lactation; and prolonged Q-T interval, which are contraindications to the use of the drug; and renal or hepatic impairment, which requires cautious use of the drug.

Physical assessment should be done to establish baseline data for assessing the effectiveness of the drug and the occurrence of any adverse effects associated with drug therapy. Assess the following: skin color, texture, and lesions, to monitor for anticholinergic effects or allergy; orientation, affect, and reflexes, to monitor for changes due to CNS effects; respirations and adventitious sounds, to monitor drug effects; and serum liver and renal function tests, to monitor for factors that could affect the metabolism or excretion of the drug.

Nursing Diagnoses

The patient receiving antihistamines may have the following nursing diagnoses related to drug therapy:

- Acute Pain related to GI, CNS, skin effects of the drug
- Disturbed Sensory Perception (Kinesthetic) related to CNS effects
- Deficient Knowledge regarding drug therapy

Implementation

- Administer the drug on an empty stomach, 1 hour before or 2 hours after meals, *to increase the absorption of the drug;* the drug may be given with meals if GI upset is a problem.
- Note that a patient may have poor response to one of these agents but a very effective response to another; the prescriber may need to try several different agents *to find the one that is most effective.*
- Because of the drying nature of antihistamines, patients often experience dry mouth, which may lead to nausea and anorexia; *suggest sugarless candies or lozenges to relieve some of this discomfort.*
- Provide safety measures as appropriate, if CNS effects occur, *to prevent patient injury.*
- Increase humidity and push fluids, *to decrease the problem of thickened secretions and dry nasal mucosa.*
- Have the patient void before each dose, *to decrease urinary retention if this is a problem.*
- Provide skin care as needed if skin dryness and lesions become a problem, *to prevent skin breakdown.*
- Caution the patient to avoid excessive dosage and to *check OTC drugs for the presence of antihistamines, which could cause toxicity and which are found in many OTC preparations.*
- Caution the patient to avoid alcohol while taking these drugs, *because serious sedation can occur.*
- Provide thorough patient teaching, including the drug name and prescribed dosage, measures to help avoid adverse effects, warning signs that may indicate problems, and the need for periodic monitoring and evaluation, *to enhance patient knowledge about drug therapy and to promote compliance.* (See Patient Teaching Checklist: Antihistamines.)
- Offer support and encouragement, *to help the patient cope with the disease and the drug regimen.*

of the underlying cough. Prolonged use of the OTC preparations could result in the masking of important symptoms of a serious underlying disorder. These drugs should not be used for more than 1 week; if the cough persists, encourage the patient to seek health care.

Nursing Considerations for Patients Receiving Expectorants

Assessment: History and Examination

Screen for the following conditions, which could be cautions or contraindications to use of the drug: any history of allergy to the drug; persistent cough due to smoking, asthma, or emphysema, which would be cautions to the use of the drug; and very productive cough, which would indicate an underlying problem that should be evaluated.

Physical assessment should be done to establish baseline data for assessing the effectiveness of the drug and the occurrence of any adverse effects associated with drug therapy. Assess the following: skin, for presence of lesions and color (to monitor for any adverse reaction); temperature (to monitor for an underlying infection); respirations and adventitious sounds (to evaluate the respiratory response to the drug effects); and orientation and affect (to monitor CNS effects of the drug).

Nursing Diagnoses

The patient receiving an expectorant may have the following nursing diagnoses related to drug therapy:

- Acute Pain related to GI, CNS, skin effects of the drug
- Disturbed Sensory Perception (Kinesthetic) related to CNS effects
- Deficient Knowledge regarding drug therapy

Implementation

- Caution the patient not to use these drugs for longer than 1 week and to seek medical attention if the cough still persists after that time, *to evaluate for any underlying medical condition and to arrange for appropriate treatment.*

- Advise the use of small, frequent meals, *to alleviate some of the GI discomfort associated with these drugs.*
- Advise the patient to avoid driving or performing dangerous tasks if dizziness and drowsiness occur, *to prevent patient injury.*
- Alert the patient that these drugs may be found in OTC preparations and that *care should be taken to avoid excessive dosage.*
- Provide thorough patient teaching, including the drug name and prescribed dosage, measures to help avoid adverse effects, warning signs that may indicate problems, and the need for periodic monitoring and evaluation, *to enhance patient knowledge about drug therapy and to promote compliance.*
- Offer support and encouragement, *to help the patient cope with the disease and the drug regimen.*

Evaluation

- Monitor patient response to the drug (improved effectiveness of cough).
- Monitor for adverse effects (skin rash, GI upset, CNS effects).
- Evaluate the effectiveness of the teaching plan (patient can name drug, dosage, adverse effects to watch for, specific measures to avoid adverse effects, measures to take to increase the effectiveness of the drug).
- Monitor the effectiveness of comfort and safety measures and compliance with the regimen.

☐■●◆ WEB LINKS

Health care providers and patients may want to consult the following Internet sources:

Information on allergic rhinitis and seasonal rhinitis, including support groups, research, treatment: http://www.rhinitisinfo.com

Information on education programs, research, and other information related to allergies and seasonal rhinitis: http://www.healthy.net

---

DRUGS IN FOCUS
Expectorants

Drug Name	Usual Dosage	Usual Indications
℗ guaifenesin (*Anti-Tuss, others*)	Adult and pediatric (>12 y): 100–400 mg PO q4h Pediatric (6–12 y): 100–200 mg PO q4h Pediatric (2–6 y): 50–100 mg PO q4h	Symptomatic relief of dry, nonproductive cough
terpin hydrate (generic)	Adult and pediatric (>12 y): 85–170 mg PO t.i.d.–q.i.d. Pediatric: 1–4 y—20 mg PO t.i.d.–q.i.d.; 5–9 y—40 mg PO t.i.d.–q.i.d.; 10–12 y: 85 mg PO t.i.d.–q.i.d.	Symptomatic relief of dry, nonproductive cough

Information about allergy research and treatment:
http://www.sickbay.com/healthline
Information for patients, including special pediatric
information on seasonal allergies, hay fever, resources,
references:
http://allergy.mcg.edu/media/rhinit.html
Information on cystic fibrosis, including research,
treatments, resources:
http://www.cff.org

MUCOLYTICS

Mucolytics work to break down mucus in order to aid the high-risk respiratory patient in coughing up thick, tenacious secretions. The medication may be administered by nebulization or by direct instillation into the trachea via an endotracheal tube or tracheostomy. The mucolytics include acetylcysteine (*Mucomyst* and others) and dornase alfa (*Pulmozyme*).

Therapeutic Actions and Indications

Mucolytics are usually reserved for patients who have difficulty mobilizing and coughing up secretions, such as individuals with chronic obstructive pulmonary disease (COPD), cystic fibrosis, pneumonia, or tuberculosis. These drugs are also indicated for patients who develop atelectasis because of thick mucus secretions. They can be used during diagnostic bronchoscopy to clear the airway and to facilitate the removal of secretions, as well as postoperatively and in patients with tracheostomies to facilitate airway clearance and suctioning.

Acetylcysteine is used orally to protect liver cells from being damaged during episodes of acetaminophen toxicity, because it normalizes hepatic glutathione levels and binds with a reactive hepatotoxic metabolite of acetaminophen. Acetylcysteine affects the mucoproteins in the respiratory secretions by splitting apart disulfide bonds that are responsible for holding the mucus material together. The result is a decrease in the tenacity and viscosity of the secretions. Acetylcysteine is metabolized in the liver and excreted

somewhat in the urine. It is not known whether it crosses the placenta or enters breast milk.

Dornase alfa is a mucolytic prepared by recombinant DNA techniques that selectively breaks down respiratory tract mucus by separating extracellular DNA from proteins. It has a long duration of action, and its fate in the body is not known. There are no data on its effects in pregnancy or lactation. This drug is used to relieve the buildup of secretions in cystic fibrosis, to help keep the airways open and functioning longer.

Contraindications and Cautions

Caution should be used in cases of acute bronchospasm, peptic ulcer, and esophageal varices, because the increased secretions could aggravate the problem.

Adverse Effects

Adverse effects most commonly associated with mucolytic drugs include GI upset, stomatitis, rhinorrhea, bronchospasm, and occasionally a rash.

Nursing Considerations for Patients Receiving Mucolytics

Assessment: History and Examination

Screen for the following conditions, which could be cautions or contraindications to use of the drug: any history of allergy to the drug and the presence of acute bronchospasm, which are contraindications to the use of these drugs; and peptic ulcer and esophageal varices, which would require careful monitoring and cautious use.

Physical assessment should be done to establish baseline data for assessing the effectiveness of the drug and the occurrence of any adverse effects associated with drug therapy. Assess the following: skin color and lesions, to monitor for adverse reactions; blood pressure and pulse, to evaluate cardiac response to drug treatment; and respirations and adventitious sounds, to monitor drug effectiveness.

Nursing Diagnoses

The patient receiving a mucolytic may have the following nursing diagnoses related to drug therapy:

DRUGS IN FOCUS
Mucolytics

Drug Name	Usual Dosage	Usual Indications
℗ acetylcysteine (*Mucomyst*)	By nebulization, 2–20 mL of 10% solution q2–6h; by direct instillation, 1–2 mL of 10%–20% solution q1–4h; 140 mg/kg PO loading dose, then 17 doses of 70 mg/kg PO q4h as an antidote	Liquification of secretions in patients who have difficulty moving secretions; clearing of secretions for diagnostic tests; postoperatively to facilitate clearing of secretions; orally to protect liver from acetaminophen toxicity
dornase alfa (*Pulmozyme*)	2.5 mg inhaled through nebulizer, may increase to 2.5 mg b.i.d. if needed	`To relieve the buildup of secretions in cystic fibrosis to keep airways open longer

- Acute Pain related to GI, CNS, skin effects of the drug
- Disturbed Sensory Perception (Kinesthetic) related to CNS effects
- Ineffective Airway Clearance related to bronchospasm
- Deficient Knowledge regarding drug therapy

Implementation

- Avoid combining with other drugs in the nebulizer, *to avoid the formation of precipitates and potential loss of effectiveness of either drug.*
- Dilute the concentrate with sterile water for injection, *if buildup becomes a problem that could impede drug delivery.*
- Note that patients receiving acetylcysteine by face mask should have the residue wiped off the face mask and off their face with plain water, *to prevent skin breakdown.*
- Review the use of the nebulizer with patients receiving dornase alfa at home, *to ensure the most effective use of the drug.* Patients should be cautioned to store the drug in the refrigerator, protected from light.
- Caution cystic fibrosis patients receiving dornase alfa about the need to continue all therapies for their cystic fibrosis, *because dornase alfa is only a palliative therapy that improves respiratory symptoms, and other therapies are still needed.*
- Provide thorough patient teaching, including the drug name and prescribed dosage, measures to help avoid adverse effects, warning signs that may indicate problems, and the need for periodic monitoring and evaluation, *to enhance patient knowledge about drug therapy and to promote compliance.*
- Offer support and encouragement, *to help the patient cope with the disease and the drug regimen.*

Evaluation

- Monitor patient response to the drug (improvement of respiratory symptoms, loosening of secretions).
- Monitor for adverse effects (CNS effects, skin rash, bronchospasm, GI upset).
- Evaluate the effectiveness of the teaching plan (patient can name drug, dosage, adverse effects to watch for, specific measures to avoid adverse effects, measures to take to increase the effectiveness of the drug).
- Monitor the effectiveness of comfort and safety measures and compliance with the regimen.

CHAPTER SUMMARY

- The classes of drugs that affect the upper respiratory system work to keep the airways open and gases moving efficiently.
- Antitussives are drugs that suppress the cough reflex. They can act centrally, to suppress the medullary cough center, or locally, to increase secretion and buffer irritation or to act as local anesthetics. These drugs should not be used longer than 1 week; patients with persistent cough after that time should seek medical evaluation.
- Decongestants are drugs that cause local vasoconstriction and therefore decrease the blood flow to the irritated and dilated capillaries of the mucous membranes lining the nasal passages and sinus cavities.
- An adverse effect that accompanies frequent or prolonged use of decongestants is rebound vasodilation, called rhinitis medicamentosa. The reflex reaction to vasoconstriction is a rebound vasodilation, which often leads to prolonged overuse of decongestants.
- Topical nasal decongestants are preferable in patients who need to avoid systemic adrenergic effects. Oral decongestants are associated with systemic adrenergic effects and require caution in patients with cardiovascular disease, hyperthyroidism, or diabetes mellitus.
- Topical nasal steroid decongestants block the inflammatory response from occurring. These drugs, which take several days to weeks to reach complete effectiveness, are preferred for patients with allergic rhinitis who need to avoid the complications of systemic steroid therapy.
- The antihistamines selectively block the effects of histamine at the histamine-1 receptor sites, decreasing the allergic response. Antihistamines are used for the relief of symptoms associated with seasonal and perennial allergic rhinitis, allergic conjunctivitis, uncomplicated urticaria, or angioedema.
- Patients taking antihistamines may react to dryness of the skin and mucous membranes. The nurse should encourage them to drink plenty of fluids, to use a humidifier if possible, to avoid smoke-filled rooms, and to use good skin care and moisturizers.
- Antihistamines should be avoided with any patient who has a prolonged Q-T interval, because serious cardiac complications and even death have occurred.
- Expectorants are drugs that liquefy the lower respiratory tract secretions. They are used for the symptomatic relief of respiratory conditions characterized by a dry, nonproductive cough.
- Mucolytics work to break down mucus in order to aid high-risk respiratory patients in coughing up thick, tenacious secretions.
- Many of the drugs that act on the upper respiratory tract are found in various OTC cough and allergy preparations. Patients need to be advised to always read the labels carefully to avoid inadvertent overdose and toxicity.

Review Questions

1. A patient with sinus pressure and pain related to a seasonal rhinitis would benefit from taking
   a. an antitussive.
   b. an expectorant.
   c. a mucolytic.
   d. a decongestant.
2. Antitussives are useful in blocking the cough reflex and preserving the energy associated with prolonged, nonproductive coughing. Antitussives are best used with
   a. postoperative patients.
   b. asthma patients.

c. patients with a dry, irritating cough.

d. COPD patients who tire easily.

3. Patients with seasonal rhinitis experience irritation and inflammation of the nasal passages and passages of the upper airways. Treatment for these patients might include
   a. systemic corticosteroids.
   b. mucolytic agents.
   c. an expectorant.
   d. topical nasal steroids.

4. A patient taking an OTC cold medication and an OTC allergy medicine is found to be taking both phenylpropanolamine and pseudoephedrine. As a result, the patient might exhibit
   a. ear pain.
   b. restlessness, tenseness, tremors, palpitations.
   c. sinus pressure.
   d. an irritating cough.

5. Common adverse effects associated with the use of topical nasal steroids would not include
   a. local burning and stinging.
   b. dryness of the mucosa.
   c. headache.
   d. constipation and urinary retention.

6. An antihistamine would not be the drug of choice for treating
   a. itchy eyes.
   b. irritating cough.
   c. nasal congestion.
   d. drippy nose.

7. Antihistamines should be used very cautiously in patients with
   a. a history of arrhythmias or prolonged Q-T intervals, because fatal cardiac arrhythmias can occur.
   b. COPD.
   c. asthma.
   d. angioedema.

8. Additional nursing interventions for patients receiving antihistamines probably would not include
   a. use of a humidifier.
   b. sucking sugarless lozenges to help the dry mouth.
   c. limiting fluid intake to decrease swelling.
   d. provision of safety measures to prevent falls or injury.

9. A patient is not getting a response to the antihistamine that was prescribed. Appropriate action might include
   a. switching to a decongestant.
   b. stopping the drug and increasing fluids.
   c. trying a different antihistamine.
   d. switching to a corticosteroid.

10. Dornase alfa (*Pulmozyme*), because of its mechanism of action, is reserved for use in
    a. clearing secretions before diagnostic tests.
    b. facilitating removal of secretions postoperatively.
    c. protecting the liver from acetaminophen toxicity.
    d. relieving the buildup of secretions in cystic fibrosis.

BIBLIOGRAPHY

Bullock, B. L. (2000). *Focus on pathophysiology*. Philadelphia: Lippincott Williams & Wilkins.

Drug facts and comparisons. (2002). St. Louis: Facts and Comparisons.

Gilman, A., Hardman, J. G., & Limbird, L. E. (Eds.) (2002). *Goodman and Gilman's the pharmacological basis of therapeutics* (10th ed.). New York: McGraw-Hill.

Karch, A. M. (2002). *2003 Lippincott's nursing drug guide*. Philadelphia: Lippincott Williams & Wilkins.

The medical letter on drugs and therapeutics. (2002). New Rochelle, NY: Medical Letter.

Professional's guide to patient drug facts. (2002). St. Louis: Facts and Comparisons.

CHAPTER

55

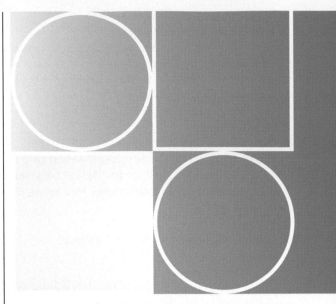

Drugs Used to Treat Obstructive Pulmonary Disorders

744

Pulmonary obstructive diseases include asthma and chronic obstructive pulmonary disease (COPD), which includes emphysema. These diseases cause obstruction of the major airways. The obstruction of asthma, emphysema, and COPD can be related to inflammation that results in narrowing of the interior of the airway and to muscular constriction that results in narrowing of the conducting tube (Figure 55–1). With chronic inflammation, muscular and cilial action is lost, and complications related to the loss of these protective processes can occur, such as infections, pneumonia, and movement of inhaled substances deep into the respiratory system. In severe COPD, air is trapped in the lower respiratory tract, the alveoli degenerate and fuse together, and the exchange of gases is greatly impaired.

Reducing environmental exposure to irritants—stopping smoking, filtering allergens from the air, avoiding exposure to known irritants and allergens—is the first step in treating these conditions. If these efforts are not sufficient to prevent problems, treatment is aimed at either opening the conducting airways through muscular bronchodilation or decreasing the effects of inflammation on the lining of the airway. See Table 55–1 for guidelines for maintenance treatment of asthma.

Another obstructive disease, **respiratory distress syndrome (RDS),** causes obstruction at the alveolar level. The obstruction of RDS in the neonate is related to a lack of the lipoprotein surfactant, which leads to an inability to maintain an open alveolus. Surfactant is essential in decreasing the surface tension in the tiny alveolus, allowing it to expand and remain open. If surfactant is lacking, the alveoli collapse and gas exchange cannot occur. Pharmacological therapy for this condition involves instilling surfactant into the alveoli.

Adult respiratory distress syndrome (ARDS) is characterized by progressive loss of lung compliance and increasing hypoxia. This syndrome occurs as a result of a severe insult to the body, such as cardiovascular collapse, major burns, severe trauma, and rapid depressurization. Treatment of ARDS involves reversal of the underlying cause of the problem combined with ventilatory support.

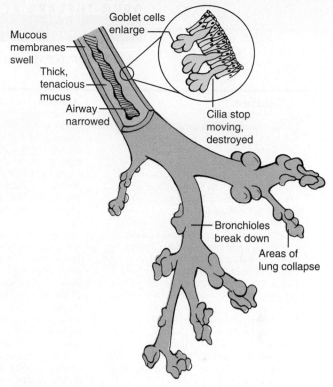

FIGURE 55-1. Changes in the airways with chronic obstructive pulmonary disease.

TABLE 55-1	Guidelines for Maintenance Treatment of Asthma*

Treatment	Intermittent Asthma (symptoms less than once a week, no symptoms between attacks) Prevention	Acute	Mild Persistent Asthma (symptoms at least once a week but less than once a day) Prevention	Acute	Moderate Persistent Asthma (daily symptoms and treatment, attacks affect activities) Prevention	Acute	Severe Asthma (continuous symptoms, limited physical activity, frequent exacerbations) Prevention	Acute
Short-acting inhaled β-agonist[†]	X		X		X			X
Inhaled corticosteroids[†]			X		X		X	
Mast cell stabilizer			X					
Leukotriene receptor agonist			X[†]					
Long-acting bronchodilators Inhaled β-agonists[†] Sustained-release theophylline Long-acting oral β-agonist			X[§]		X		X	
Corticosteriods							X[‖]	

*Effective treatment depends on patient response; a combination of therapies may be required to achieve good control.
[†]Considered drug of choice.
[†]May be preferred treatment in children older than 2 years.
[§]Not a preferred treatment.
[‖]Wean to inhaled preparation as soon as possible.

DRUG THERAPY ACROSS THE LIFESPAN

Lower Respiratory Tract Agents

Children	Adults	Older Adults
Antiasthmatics are frequently used in children. The leukotriene receptor antagonists have been found to be especially effective for long-term prophylaxis in children. Acute episodes are best treated with a β-agonist and then a long-acting inhaled steroid or a mast cell stabilizer. Parents need to be encouraged to take measures to prevent acute attacks, including avoidance of known allergens, smoke-filled rooms, and crowded or dusty areas. Parents should be cautioned about the proper way to measure liquid preparations to avoid inadvertent toxic doses or lack of therapeutic effects. Theophylline has been used in children, but because of its many adverse effects and the better control afforded by newer agents, its use is reserved for cases that do not respond to other therapies. As the child grows and matures, the disease will need to be re-evaluated and dosage adjustments made to meet the needs of the growing child. Teenagers need to learn the proper administration and use of inhaled steroids for prevention of exercise-induced asthma. As with other classes of medications, children may be more susceptible to the adverse effects associated with these drugs and need to be carefully monitored and evaluated. Over-the-counter (OTC) drugs and herbal remedies should be avoided if possible; if they are used, they should be reported to the health care provider so that appropriate dosage adjustments can be made where needed. The parents of premature babies undergoing surfactant therapy will require consistent support and education to help them to cope with the stress of this event.	Adults may be able to manage their asthma quite well with the use of inhalers and avoidance of aggravating situations. Periodic review of the proper use of the various inhalers should be part of routine evaluation of these patients. Periodic telemetry readings should be done to evaluate the effectiveness of the therapy. The safety of these drugs during pregnancy and lactation has not been established. There is a potential for adverse effects of the fetus related to blood flow changes and direct drug effects when the drugs cross the placenta. Use should be reserved for those situations in which the benefit to the mother outweighs the potential risk to the fetus. The drugs may enter breast milk and also may alter fluid balance and milk production. It is advised that caution be used if one of these drugs is prescribed during lactation.	Older adults frequently are prescribed one or more of these drugs. Older adults are more likely to develop adverse effects associated with the use of these drugs, such as sedation, confusion, dizziness, urinary retention, and cardiovascular effects. Safety measures may be needed if these effects occur and interfere with the patient's mobility and balance. Older adults are also more likely to have renal and/or hepatic impairment related to underlying medical conditions, which could interfere with the metabolism and excretion of these drugs. The dosage for older adults should be started at a lower level than recommended for young adults. Patients should be monitored very closely and dosage adjustment based on patient response. These patients also need to be alerted to the potential for toxic effects when using OTC preparations and should be advised to check with their health care provider before beginning any OTC drug regimen. Older adults with progressive chronic obstructive pulmonary disease may be taking many combined drugs to help them maintain effective respirations. These patients should have an overall treatment plan involving complex pulmonary toilet, positioning, fluids, nutrition, humidified air, rest, and activity plans, as well as a complicated drug regimen to deal with the impact of this disease.

BRONCHODILATORS/ANTIASTHMATICS

Bronchodilators, or antiasthmatics, are medications used to facilitate respirations by dilating the airways. They are helpful in symptomatic relief or prevention of bronchial asthma and for bronchospasm associated with COPD. Several of the bronchodilators are administered orally and absorbed systemically, giving them the potential for many systemic adverse effects. Other medications are administered directly into the airways by nebulizers. These medications have the advantage of a decreased number of systemic adverse reactions.

XANTHINES

The **xanthines,** including caffeine and theophylline, come from a variety of naturally occurring sources. These drugs were once the main choice for treatment of asthma and bronchospasm. However, they have a relatively narrow margin of safety, and they interact with many other drugs. Consequently, they are no longer considered the first-choice bronchodilators. Xanthines used to treat respiratory disease include aminophylline (*Truphylline*), caffeine (*Caffedrine* and others), dyphylline (*Dilor* and others), oxtriphylline (*Choledyl-SA*), and theophylline (*Slo-bid, Theo-Dur*).

Therapeutic Actions and Indications

The xanthines have a direct effect on the smooth muscles of the respiratory tract, both in the bronchi and in the blood vessels (Figure 55–2). Although the exact mechanism of action is not known, one theory suggests that xanthines work by directly affecting the mobilization of calcium within the cell. They do this by stimulating two prostaglandins, resulting in smooth muscle relaxation. The effect of smooth muscle relaxation increases the vital capacity that has been impaired by bronchospasm or air trapping. Xanthines also inhibit the release of slow-reacting substance of anaphylaxis (SRSA) and histamine, decreasing the bronchial swelling and narrowing that occurs as a result of these two chemicals.

Xanthines are indicated for the symptomatic relief or prevention of bronchial asthma and for reversal of bronchospasm associated with COPD. Unlabeled uses include stimulation of respirations in **Cheyne–Stokes respiration** and the treatment of apnea and bradycardia in premature infants.

Pharmacokinetics

The xanthines are rapidly absorbed from the gastrointestinal (GI) tract, reaching peak levels within 2 hours. They are widely distributed and metabolized in the liver. Excretion occurs in the urine. Xanthines cross the placenta and enter breast milk. They have been associated with fetal abnormalities and breathing difficulties at birth in animal studies. Although no clear studies are available in human pregnancy, use should be limited to situations in which the benefit to the mother clearly outweighs the potential risk to the fetus. Be-

cause the xanthines enter breast milk and could affect the baby, another method of feeding the baby should be selected if these drugs are needed during lactation.

Contraindications and Cautions

Caution should be taken with any patient with GI problems, coronary disease, respiratory dysfunction, renal or hepatic disease, alcoholism, or hyperthyroidism, because these conditions can be exacerbated by the systemic effects of xanthines. Xanthines are available for oral and parenteral use; the parenteral drug should be switched to the oral form as soon as possible, because the systemic effects of the oral form are less acute and more manageable.

Adverse Effects

Adverse effects associated with xanthines are related to theophylline levels in the blood. Therapeutic theophylline levels are from 10 to 20 μg/mL. With increasing levels, predictable adverse effects are seen, ranging from GI upset, nausea, irritability, and tachycardia to seizures, brain damage, and even death (Table 55–2).

Clinically Important Drug–Drug Interactions

Because of the mechanism of xanthine metabolism in the liver, many drugs interact with xanthines. The list of interacting drugs should be checked any time a drug is added or removed from a drug regimen.

Nicotine increases the metabolism of xanthines in the liver; xanthine dosage must be increased in patients who continue to smoke while using xanthines. In addition, extreme caution

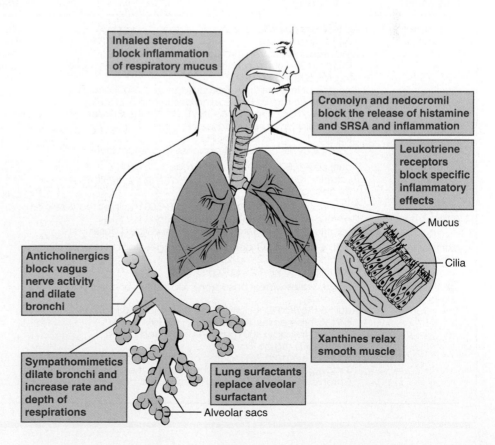

FIGURE 55–2. Sites of action of drugs used to treat obstructive pulmonary disorders.

TABLE 55-2 | Adverse Effects Associated with Various Serum Levels of Theophylline

Serum Level	Adverse Effects
≤20 (μg/mL)	Uncommon
>20–25 (μg/mL)	Nausea, vomiting, diarrhea, insomnia, headache, irritability
>30–35 (μg/mL)	Hyperglycemia, hypotension, cardiac arrhythmias, tachycardia, seizures, brain damage, death

must be used if the patient decides to decrease or discontinue smoking, because severe xanthine toxicity can occur.

Nursing Considerations for Patients Receiving Xanthines

Assessment: History and Examination

Screen for the following conditions, which could be cautions or contraindications to use of the drug: any known allergies; cigarette use which would affect the metabolism of the drug; peptic ulcer, gastritis, renal or hepatic dysfunction, and coronary disease, all of which require cautious use; and pregnancy and lactation, which are contraindications.

Physical assessment should be done to establish baseline data for assessing the effectiveness of the drug and the occurrence of any adverse effects associated with drug therapy. Perform the following assessments: thorough skin examination including color and the presence of lesions, to provide a baseline as a reference for drug effectiveness; blood pressure, pulse, cardiac auscultation, peripheral perfusion, and baseline electrocardiogram (ECG), to provide a baseline for effects on the cardiovascular system; and bowel sounds, liver evaluation, and blood tests, to provide a baseline for renal and hepatic function tests. In addition, evaluate serum theophylline levels, to provide a baseline reference

---

DRUGS IN FOCUS
Xanthine Bronchodilators

Drug Name	Usual Dosage	Usual Indications
aminophylline (*Truphylline*)	Adult: 7.6 mg/kg PO loading dose, then 3.8 mg/kg q4h × three doses Maintenance: 3.8 mg/kg q6h Range: 600–1600 mg/d PO in three to four divided doses Rectal: 500 mg q6–8h Geriatric or impaired: reduce dosage and monitor closely Pediatric: 7.6 mg/kg PO loading dose, then 5.1 mg/kg (6 mo–9 y) or 3.8 mg/kg (9–16 y) q4h for three doses, then maintain at same dose q6h Range: 12 mg/kg per day PO Base all doses on patient response and serum levels	All of the xanthine bronchodilators are indicated for symptomatic relief or prevention of bronchial asthma and reversal of bronchospasm associated with COPD
caffeine (generic)	Adult: 500–1000 mg IM, do not exceed 2.5 g/d Pediatric: 10 mg/kg IV followed by 2.5 mg/kg per day for neonatal apnea	
dyphylline (*Dilor*)	Adult: up to 15 mg/kg PO q.i.d. or 250–500 mg injected slowly IM Geriatric or impaired adult: use caution Pediatric: 4.4–6.6 mg/kg per day PO in divided doses	
oxtriphylline (*Choledyl-SA*)	Adult: 4.7 mg/kg PO q8h or 400–600 mg sustained release q12h Pediatric (1–9 y): 6.2 mg/kg PO q6h Pediatric (9–16 y): 4.7 mg/kg PO q6h	
(P) theophylline (*Slo-bid*, *Theo-Dur*)	Dosage varies widely based on preparation and patient response Adult: 6 mg/kg PO loading dose followed by 3 mg/kg PO q4h × three doses, then 3 mg/kg PO q6h Chronic therapy: 400 mg/d PO in divided doses Rectal: 500 mg q6–8h Pediatric: 6 mg/kg PO loading dose, then 4 mg/kg (6 mo–9 y) or 3 mg/kg (9–16 y) PO q4h × three doses, then the same dose q6h Chronic therapy: 400 mg/d PO in divided doses	

and identify conditions that may require caution in the use of diuretics.

Nursing Diagnoses

The patient receiving a xanthine bronchodilator may have the following nursing diagnoses related to drug therapy:

- Acute Pain related to headache and GI upset
- Decreased Cardiac Output
- Disturbed Sensory Perception (Kinesthetic, Visual) related to central nervous system (CNS) effects
- Deficient Knowledge regarding drug therapy

Implementation

- Administer oral drug with food or milk, *to relieve GI irritation, if GI upset is a problem.*
- Monitor patient response to the drug (eg, relief of respiratory difficulty, improved air flow), *to determine the effectiveness of the drug dosage and to adjust dosage as needed.*
- Provide comfort measures, including rest periods, quiet environment, dietary control of caffeine, and headache therapy as needed, *to help the patient cope with the effects of drug therapy.*
- Provide periodic follow-up including blood tests, *to monitor serum theophylline levels.*
- Provide thorough patient teaching, including the drug name and prescribed dosage, measures to help avoid adverse effects, warning signs that may indicate problems, and the need for periodic monitoring and evaluation, *to enhance patient knowledge about drug therapy and to promote compliance.* (See Patient Teaching Checklist: Xanthines.)

Evaluation

- Monitor patient response to the drug (improved air flow, ease of respirations).
- Monitor for adverse effects (CNS effects, cardiac arrhythmias, GI upset, local irritation).
- Monitor for potential drug–drug interactions; consult with the prescriber to adjust dosages as appropriate.
- Evaluate the effectiveness of the teaching plan (patient can name drug, dosage, adverse effects to watch for, specific measures to avoid adverse effects).
- Monitor effectiveness of comfort measures and compliance with the regimen (see Nursing Care Guide: Xanthines).

SYMPATHOMIMETICS

Sympathomimetics are drugs that mimic the effects of the sympathetic nervous system. One of the actions of the sympathetic nervous system is dilation of the bronchi with increased rate and depth of respiration. This is the desired effect when selecting a sympathomimetic as a bronchodilator.

PATIENT TEACHING CHECKLIST
Xanthines

Create customized patient teaching materials for a specific xanthine from the CD-ROM. Patient teaching should stress the following points for drugs within this class:

- Bronchodilators work by relaxing the airways, helping to make breathing easier and to decrease wheezes and shortness of breath. To be effective, this drug must be taken exactly as prescribed.
- This drug should be taken on an empty stomach with a full glass of water. If gastrointestinal upset is severe, you can take the drug with food. Do not chew the enteric-coated or timed-release capsules or tablets—they must be swallowed whole to be effective.

Common effects of this drug include

- *Gastrointestinal upset, nausea, vomiting, heartburn—*Taking the drug with food may help this problem.
- *Restlessness, nervousness, difficulty in sleeping—*The body often adjusts to these effects over time. Avoiding other stimulants, such as caffeine, may help decrease some of these symptoms.
- *Headache—*This often goes away with time. If headaches persist or become worse, notify your health care provider.

Many foods can change the way that your drug works; if you decide to change your diet, consult with your health care provider.

Adverse effects of the drug can be avoided by avoiding foods that contain caffeine or other xanthine derivatives (coffee, cola, chocolate, tea) or by using them in moderate amounts. This is especially important if you experience nervousness, restlessness or sleeplessness.

Cigarette smoking affects the way your body uses this drug. If you decide to change your smoking habits, such as increasing or decreasing the number of cigarettes you smoke each day, consult with your health care provider regarding the possible need to adjust your dosage.

Report any of the following to your health care provider: vomiting, severe abdominal pain, pounding or fast heartbeat, confusion, unusual tiredness, muscle twitching, skin rash, hives.

Avoid the use of any over-the-counter medication without first checking with your health care provider. Several of these medications can interfere with the effectiveness of this drug.

Tell any doctor, nurse, or other health care provider that you are taking this drug.

Keep this drug, and all medications, out of the reach of children.

This Teaching Checklist reflects general patient teaching guidelines. It is not meant to be a substitute for drug-specific teaching information; which is available in nursing drug guides.

Sympathomimetics that are used as bronchodilators include the following.

- Albuterol (*Proventil* and others) is long-acting and available in inhaled and oral forms for patients older than 2 years of age.

NURSING CARE GUIDE

Xanthines

Assessment	Nursing Diagnoses	Implementation	Evaluation
HISTORY Allergies, peptic ulcer, gastritis, renal or hepatic dysfunction, coronary disease, cigarette use, pregnancy, and lactation.	Acute Pain related to GI effects, dry mouth Decreased Cardiac Output Impaired Sensory Perception (Kinesthetic, Visual) Activity Intolerance Deficient Knowledge regarding drug therapy	Provide comfort and safety measures: 　-Give drug with meals. 　-Allow for rest periods. 　-Provide a quiet environment. 　-Ensure dietary control of caffeine. 　-Provide headache therapy as needed. Provide support and reassurance to deal with drug effects and lifestyle changes. Provide patient teaching regarding, drug name, dosage, adverse effects, precautions, warnings to report, dietary cautions, and need for follow-up.	Evaluate drug effects: relief of respiratory difficulty, improvement of air movement. Monitor for adverse effects: GI upset, CNS effects, cardiac arrhythmias, local irritation (suppositories). Monitor for drug-drug interactions as indicated for each drug. Evaluate effectiveness of patient teaching program. Evaluate effectiveness of comfort and safety measures.
PHYSICAL EXAMINATION Neurological: orientation, reflexes, affect, coordination Skin: color, lesions CV: BP, P, peripheral perfusion, baseline EKG GI: bowel sounds, abdominal exam Lab tests: serum theophylline levels, renal, hepatic function tests			

- Bitolterol (*Tornalate*) is long-acting and inhaled; it is preferred for prophylaxis of bronchospasm in patients older than 12 years of age.
- Ephedrine (generic) is used parenterally for acute bronchospasm in adults and children, although epinephrine is the drug of choice.
- Epinephrine (*Sus-Phrine, EpiPen,* and others) is the drug of choice in adults and children for the treatment of acute bronchospasm, including that caused by anaphylaxis; it is also available for inhalation. Because epinephrine is associated with systemic sympathomimetic effects, it is not the drug of choice for patients with cardiac conditions.
- Formoterol (*Foradil*) is an inhaled drug used for maintenance treatment of asthma and prevention of bronchospasm in patients older than 5 years of age who have reversible obstructive airway disease, and for prevention of exercise-induced bronchospasm in patients older than 12 years of age.
- Isoetharine (*Bronkosol* and others) is an inhaled drug used for prophylaxis and treatment of bronchospasm. Dosage guidelines for children have not been established.
- Isoproterenol (*Isuprel* and others) is used for treatment of bronchospasm during anesthesia and as an inhalant for treatment of bronchospasm in adults and children; it is associated with more cardiac side effects than some other drugs.
- Levalbuterol (*Xopenex*) is an inhaled agent used to treat and prevent bronchospasm in patients older than 6 years of age who have reversible obstructive pulmonary disease.
- Metaproterenol (*Alupent*) is available as an oral or inhaled agent and is used for both treatment and prophylaxis of bronchospasm in patients older than 6 years of age.

CASE STUDY

Toxic Reaction to Theophylline

THE SITUATION
M. K. has a medical diagnosis of chronic bronchitis and has been stabilized on theophylline for the past 3 years. She has been labeled as noncompliant with medical therapy because she continues to smoke cigarettes (more than three packs per day), knowing that she has a progressive pulmonary disease. M. K. was referred to a student nurse for teaching. After several sessions, in which the student presented posters and pictures and gave M. K. a great deal of personal attention and encouragement, it was determined that M. K. had a good understanding of her problem and would stop or at least cut down on her smoking. Three days later, M. K. presented to the emergency department with complaints of dizziness, nausea, vomiting, confusion, grouchiness, and palpitations. Her admission heart rate was 96 beats/min with occasional to frequent premature ventricular contractions.

CRITICAL THINKING
• What probably happened to M. K.?
• What information should the student have known before conducting the teaching program?
• How could that information have been included in the patient teaching program?
• What would the best approach be to this patient now?

DISCUSSION
M. K. probably did cut down on her smoking. However, she was not aware that cigarette smoking increases the metabolism of theophylline and that she had been stabilized on a dose that took that information into account. When she cut down on smoking, theophylline was not metabolized as quickly and began to accumulate, leading to the toxic reaction that brought M. K. into the emergency department. This is a real nursing challenge. By following the teaching program and doing what she was asked to do, M. K. became sicker and felt awful. A careful teaching approach will be necessary to encourage M. K. to continue cutting down on cigarette smoking.

Staff should be educated on the numerous variables that affect drug therapy and encouraged to check drug interactions frequently when making any changes in a patient's regimen. Regular follow-up and support will be important to help M. K. regain trust in her medical care providers and continue her progress in cutting down smoking. Frequent checks of theophylline levels should be done while M. K. is cutting back, and dosage adjustments should be made by her prescriber to maintain therapeutic levels of theophylline and avoid toxic levels.

• Pirbuterol (*Maxair*) is an inhaled drug used for both treatment and prophylaxis of bronchospasm in patients older than 12 years of age.
• Salmeterol (*Serevent*) is an inhaled drug successfully used to prevent exercise-induced asthma and for prophylaxis of bronchospasm in selected patients older than 4 years of age.
• Terbutaline (*Brethaire* and others) can be used orally, parenterally, and by inhalation for both prophylaxis and treatment of bronchospasm in patients older than 12 years of age

Therapeutic Actions and Indications
Most of the sympathomimetics used as bronchodilators are β_2-selective adrenergic agonists. That means that at therapeutic levels their actions are specific to the β_2 receptors found in the bronchi (see Chapter 30). This specificity is lost at higher levels. Other systemic effects of sympathomimetics include increased blood pressure, increased heart rate, vasoconstriction, and decreased renal and GI blood flow—all actions of the sympathetic nervous system. These overall effects limit the systemic usefulness of these drugs in certain patients.

The sympathomimetic epinephrine is given by injection during acute asthma attacks, when the need for bronchodilation outweighs the risk of adverse effects. Other sympathomimetics are used in the treatment of bronchospasm in reversible obstructive airway disease (e.g., acute or chronic asthma, chronic bronchitis). They have also been effective in preventing exercise-induced bronchospasm (see Figure 55–2).

Pharmacokinetics
These drugs are rapidly distributed after injection; they are metabolized in the liver to metabolites that are excreted in the urine. The half-life of these drugs is relatively short, less than 1 hour. These drugs should be used during pregnancy and lactation only if the benefits to the mother clearly outweigh potential risks to the fetus, because they are known to cross the placenta and to enter breast milk. The inhaled drugs are rapidly absorbed into the lung tissue. Any absorbed drug will still be metabolized in the liver and excreted in the urine.

Contraindications and Cautions
These drugs are contraindicated or should be used with caution, depending on the severity of the underlying condition, in conditions that would be aggravated by the sympathetic stimulation, including cardiac disease, vascular disease, arrhythmias, diabetes, hyperthyroidism, pregnancy, and lactation.

Adverse Effects
Adverse effects of these drugs, which can be attributed to sympathomimetic stimulation, include CNS stimulation, GI upset, cardiac arrhythmias, hypertension, bronchospasm, sweating, pallor, and flushing.

Clinically Important Drug–Drug Interactions
Special precautions should be taken to avoid the combination of sympathomimetic bronchodilators with the general anesthetics cyclopropane and halogenated hydrocarbons.

DRUGS IN FOCUS
Sympathomimetic Bronchodilators

Drug Name	Usual Dosage	Usual Indications
albuterol (*Proventil*)	Adult: 2–4 mg PO t.i.d.–q.i.d. *or* two inhalations q4–6h *or* two inhalations 15 min before exercise Pediatric: >12 y—adult dosage; 6–12 y—2 mg t.i.d.–q.i.d. oral tablets; 6–14 y); 2 mg t.i.d.–q.i.d. PO oral syrup; 2–6 y) 0.1 mg/kg PO t.i.d. oral syrup Pediatric (2–12 y inhalation): 1.25–2.5 mg; for prevention of exercise-induced bronchospasm, 200–μg capsule inhaled 15 min before exercise	Treatment and prophylaxis of bronchospasm; prevention of exercise-induced bronchospasm
bitolterol (*Tornalate*)	Adult: two inhalations q8h for prevention, at intervals of 1–3 min for treatment; use special caution if >60 y of age *Pediatric* (>12 y): as adult Pediatric (<12 y): not recommended	Treatment and prophylaxis for bronchospasm
ephedrine (generic)	Adult: 25–50 mg IM, SC, or IV Pediatric: 25–100 mg/m² IM or SC divided into four to six doses	Treatment of acute bronchospasm
P epinephrine (*Sus-Phrine*)	Adult: 0.1–0.3 mL SC q20min for 4 h as needed, may also be given by aerosol inhalation or nebulization Pediatric: 0.01–0.3 mL/m² SC q20min for 4 h as needed	Drug of choice for treatment of acute bronchospasm
formoterol (*Foradil*)	Adult and pediatric >5 y for asthma maintenance: 12–μg capsule q12h, inhaled using the *Aerolizer inhaler* Adult and pediatric >12 y: 12–μg capsule inhaled using the *Aerolizer inhaler,* at least 15 min before exercising, do not use additional doses for 12 h	Maintenance treatment of asthma and prevention of bronchospasm in patients >5 y of age with reversible obstructive airway disease; prevention of exercise-induced bronchospasm in patients >12 y of age **Special considerations:** If taking the drug for asthma maintenance, do not use for additional drug for exercise-induced asthma.
isoetharine (*Bronkosol*)	Adult: four inhalations from handheld nebulizers or 1–2 mL over 15–20 min with oxygen aerosolization; use caution if >60 y of age	Treatment and prophylaxis of bronchospasm
isoproterenol (*Isuprel*)	Adult: 0.01–0.02 mg IV during anesthesia; 1:200 solution with 15 deep inhalations for acute bronchial asthma, or 5–15 inhalations using nebulizer for COPD-related bronchospasm Pediatric: 0.25 mL or the 1:200 solution for each 10–15 min of nebulization	Treatment of bronchospasm during anesthesia and prophylaxis of bronchospasm
levalbuterol (*Xopenex*)	Adult and pediatric (>12 y): 0.63 mg q6–8h by nebulization	Treatment and prevention of bronchospasm
metaproterenol (*Alupent*)	Adult: 20 mg PO t.i.d.–q.i.d. or two to three inhalations q3–4h; use caution if >60 y of age Pediatric: 9 y—20 mg t.i.d.–q.i.d.; 6–9 y—10 mg PO t.i.id.–q.i.d.; <6 y—1.3–2.6 mg/kg per day in divided doses of syrup Inhalation: >12 y, same as adult Nebulizer: 6–12 y, 0.1–0.2 mL in saline	Treatment of prophylaxis of bronchospasm and acute asthma attacks in children <6 yr.
pirbuterol (*Maxair*)	Adult and pediatric (>12 y): 0.4 mg (two inhalations) q4–6h, do not exceed 12 inhalations per day	Treatment and prophylaxis of bronchospasm
salmeterol (*Serevent*)	Adult: two puffs q12h; or 2 puffs 30–60 min before exercise Pediatric: one inhalation b.i.d. at least 12 h apart; one inhalation >30 min before exercising	Prophylaxis of bronchospasm and prevention of exercise-induced asthma
terbutaline (*Brethaire*)	Adult and pediatric (>15 y): 5 mg PO q6h while awake; 0.25 mg SC repeat in 15 min as needed; two inhalations separated by 60 sec q4–6h Pediatric: (12–15 y): 2.5 mg PO t.i.d.; two inhalations separated by 60 sec q4–6h as needed	Treatment and prophylaxis of bronchospasm

Because these drugs sensitize the myocardium to catecholamines, serious cardiac complications could occur.

Nursing Considerations for Patients Receiving Sympathomimetic Bronchodilators

Assessment: History and Examination

Screen for the following conditions, which could be cautions or contraindications to use of the drug: allergy to any sympathomimetic or drug vehicle; pregnancy or lactation, which would require cautious use of the drug; acute asthma attack, which would be a contraindication for use of the drug; cardiac disease, vascular disease, arrhythmias, diabetes, and hyperthyroidism, which may be exacerbated by sympathomimetic effects; and use of the general anesthetics cyclopropane and halogenated hydrocarbons, which sensitize the myocardium to catecholamines and could cause serious cardiac complications if used with these drugs.

Physical assessment should be done to establish baseline data for assessing the effectiveness of the drug and the occurrence of any adverse effects associated with drug therapy. Assess the following: reflexes and orientation, to evaluate CNS effects of the drug; respirations and adventitious sounds, to establish a baseline for drug effectiveness and possible adverse effects; pulse, blood pressure, and, in certain cases, a baseline ECG, to monitor the cardiovascular effects of sympathetic stimulation; and liver function tests, to assess for changes that could interfere with metabolism of the drug and require dosage adjustment.

Nursing Diagnoses

The patient receiving a sympathomimetic bronchodilator may have the following nursing diagnoses related to drug therapy:

- Increased Cardiac Output related to sympathomimetic effects
- Acute Pain related to CNS, GI, cardiac effects of the drug
- Disturbed Thought Processes related to CNS effects
- Deficient Knowledge related to drug therapy

Implementation

- Reassure the patient that the drug of choice will vary with each individual. *These sympathomimetics are slightly different chemicals and are prepared in a variety of delivery systems. A patient may have to try several different sympathomimetics before the most effective one is found.*
- Advise patients to use the minimal amount needed for the shortest period necessary, *to prevent adverse effects and accumulation of drug levels.*
- Teach patients who use one of these drugs for exercise-induced asthma to use it 30 to 60 minutes before exercising *to ensure peak therapeutic effects when they are needed.*
- Provide safety measures as needed if CNS effects become a problem, *to prevent patient injury.*
- Provide small, frequent meals and nutritional consultation if GI effects interfere with eating, *to ensure proper nutrition.*

- Carefully teach the patient about the proper use of the prescribed delivery system. Review that procedure periodically, *because improper use may result in ineffective therapy.*
- Provide thorough patient teaching, including the drug name and prescribed dosage, measures to help avoid adverse effects, warning signs that may indicate problems, and the need for periodic monitoring and evaluation, *to enhance patient knowledge about drug therapy and to promote compliance.*
- Offer support and encouragement, *to help the patient cope with the disease and the drug regimen.*

Evaluation

- Monitor patient response to the drug (improved breathing).
- Monitor for adverse effects (CNS effects, increased pulse and blood pressure, GI upset).
- Evaluate the effectiveness of the teaching plan (patient can name drug, dosage, adverse effects to watch for, specific measures to avoid adverse effects, measures to take to increase the effectiveness of the drug).
- Monitor the effectiveness of other measures to ease breathing.

ANTICHOLINERGIC BRONCHODILATOR

Patients who are not able to tolerate the sympathetic effects of the sympathomimetics might respond to the anticholinergic drug ipratropium (*Atrovent*). This drug is not as effective as the sympathomimetics, but it can provide some relief to those patients who cannot tolerate the other drugs.

Therapeutic Actions and Indications

Anticholinergics are used as bronchodilators because of their effect on the vagus nerve, which is to block or antagonize the action of the neurotransmitter acetylcholine at vagal-mediated receptor sites (see Figure 55–2). Normally, vagal stimulation results in a stimulating effect on smooth muscle, causing contraction. By blocking the vagal effect, relaxation of smooth muscle in the bronchi occurs, leading to bronchodilation. Ipratropium is the only anticholinergic recommended for bronchodilation. It is indicated for the maintenance treatment of patients with COPD, including bronchospasm and emphysema.

Pharmacokinetics

Ipratropium has an onset of action of 15 minutes when inhaled. Its peak effects occur in 1 to 2 hours, and it has a duration of effect of 3 to 4 hours. Little is known about its fate in the body. It is generally not absorbed systemically.

Contraindications and Cautions

Caution should be used in any condition that would be aggravated by the anticholinergic or atropine-like effects of the drug, such as narrow-angle glaucoma (drainage of the vitreous humor can be blocked by smooth muscle relaxation), bladder neck obstruction, or prostatic hypertrophy (relaxed muscle causes decreased bladder tone), and conditions aggravated by dry mouth and throat. The use of ipratropium is contraindicated in the presence of known allergy to the drug.

Adverse Effects

Adverse effects are related to the anticholinergic effects of the drug if it is absorbed systemically. These effects include dizziness, headache, fatigue, nervousness, dry mouth, sore throat, palpitations, and urinary retention.

Nursing Considerations for Patients Receiving an Anticholinergic Bronchodilator

Assessment: History and Examination

Screen for the following conditions, which could be cautions or contraindications to use of the drug: allergy to atropine or other anticholinergics; acute bronchospasm, which would be a contraindication; narrow-angle glaucoma (drainage of the vitreous humor can be blocked by smooth muscle relaxation), bladder neck obstruction or prostatic hypertrophy (relaxed muscle causes decreased bladder tone), and conditions aggravated by dry mouth and throat, all of which could be exacerbated by the use of this drug; and pregnancy and lactation, which would require cautious use.

Physical assessment should be done to establish baseline data for assessing the effectiveness of the drug and the occurrence of any adverse effects associated with drug therapy. Assess the following: skin color and lesions, to assess for dryness or allergic reaction; orientation, affect, and reflexes, to evaluate CNS effects; pulse and blood pressure, to monitor cardiovascular effects of the drug; respirations and adventitious sounds, to monitor drug effectiveness and possible adverse effects; and urinary output and prostate palpation as appropriate, to monitor anticholinergic effects.

Nursing Diagnoses

The patient receiving an anticholinergic bronchodilator may have the following nursing diagnoses related to drug therapy:

- Acute Pain related to CNS, GI, respiratory effects of drug
- Imbalanced Nutrition: Less than Body Requirements, related to dry mouth and GI upset
- Deficient Knowledge regarding drug therapy

Implementation

- Ensure adequate hydration and provide environmental controls, such as the use of a humidifier, *to make the patient more comfortable.*
- Encourage the patient to void before each dose of medication, *to prevent urinary retention related to drug effects.*
- Provide safety measures if CNS effects occur, *to prevent patient injury.*
- Provide small, frequent meals and sugarless lozenges *to relieve dry mouth and GI upset.*
- Review use of the inhalator with the patient; caution the patient not to exceed 12 inhalations in 24 hours, *to prevent serious adverse effects.*
- Advise the patient not to drive or use hazardous machinery if nervousness, dizziness, and drowsiness occur with this drug, *to prevent injury.*
- Provide thorough patient teaching, including the drug name and prescribed dosage, measures to help avoid adverse effects, warning signs that may indicate problems, and the need for periodic monitoring and evaluation, *to enhance patient knowledge about drug therapy and to promote compliance.*
- Offer support and encouragement, *to help the patient cope with the disease and the drug regimen.*

Evaluation

- Monitor patient response to the drug (improved breathing).
- Monitor for adverse effects (CNS effects, increased pulse, blood pressure; GI upset; dry skin and mucous membranes).
- Evaluate the effectiveness of the teaching plan (patient can name drug, dosage, adverse effects to watch for, specific measures to avoid adverse effects, measures to take to increase the effectiveness of the drug).
- Monitor the effectiveness of other measures to ease breathing.

INHALED STEROIDS

Inhaled steroids have been found to be a very effective treatment for bronchospasm. Agents approved for this use include beclomethasone (*Beclovent* and others), budesonide

---

DRUGS IN FOCUS
Anticholinergic Bronchodilator

Drug Name	Usual Dosage	Usual Indications
ipratropium (*Atrovent*)	36 μg (two inhalations) four times per day, up to 12 inhalations if needed	Maintenance treatment of adults with COPD

(*Pulmicort*), flunisolide (*AeroBid*), fluticasone (*Flovent*), and triamcinolone (*Azmacort* and others). The drug of choice depends on the individual patient's response. For example, a patient may have little response to one agent and do very well on another. It is usually useful to try another preparation if one is not effective within 2 to 3 weeks.

Therapeutic Actions and Indications

Inhaled steroids are used to decrease the inflammatory response in the airway. In an airway that is swollen and narrowed by inflammation and swelling, this action will increase air flow and facilitate respiration. Inhaling the steroid tends to decrease the numerous systemic effects that are associated with steroid use. When administered into the lungs by inhalation, steroids decrease the effectiveness of the inflammatory cells. This has two effects: decreased swelling associated with inflammation and promotion of β-adrenergic receptor activity, which may promote smooth muscle relaxation and inhibit bronchoconstriction (see Figure 55–2).

These drugs are used for the prevention and treatment of asthma, to treat chronic steroid-dependent bronchial asthma, and as adjunct therapy for patients whose asthma is not controlled by traditional bronchodilators. These drugs are rapidly absorbed but take from 2 to 3 weeks to reach effective levels.

Pharmacokinetics

These drugs are absorbed well from the respiratory tract. They are metabolized by natural systems, mostly within the liver, and are excreted in the urine. The glucocorticoids are known to cross the placenta and to enter breast milk; they should be used during pregnancy and lactation only if the benefits to the mother clearly outweigh the potential risks to the fetus.

Contraindications and Cautions

Inhaled corticosteroids are not for emergency use and not for use during an acute asthma attack or status asthmaticus. They should not be used during pregnancy or lactation. These preparations should be used with caution in any patient who has an active infection of the respiratory system, because the depression of the inflammatory response could result in serious illness.

Adverse Effects

Adverse effects are limited because of the route of administration. Sore throat, hoarseness, coughing, dry mouth, and pharyngeal and laryngeal fungal infections are the most common side effects encountered. If a patient does not administer the drug appropriately or develops lesions that allow absorption of the drug, the systemic side effects associated with steroids may occur.

Nursing Considerations for Patients Receiving Inhaled Steroids
Assessment: History and Examination

Screen for the following conditions, which could be cautions or contraindications to use of the drug: acute asthmatic attacks, allergy to the drugs, and pregnancy and lactation, which are contraindications; and systemic infections, which require cautious use.

Physical assessment should be done to establish baseline data for assessing the effectiveness of the drug and the occurrence of any adverse effects associated with drug ther-

DRUGS IN FOCUS
Inhaled Steroids

Drug Name	Usual Dosage	Usual Indication
beclomethasone (*Beclovent*)	Adult: 84–168 μg t.i.d.–q.i.d. (two inhalations) Pediatric (6–12 y): one to two inhalations t.i.d.–q.i.d., do not exceed 10 inhalations per day	All of the inhaled steroids are used for the prevention and treatment of asthma; for treatment of chronic steroid-dependent bronchial asthma; and as adjunctive therapy for asthma patients who do not respond to traditional bronchodilators
budesonide (*Pulmicort*)	Adult and pediatric (>6 y): 256 μg/d given as two sprays in each nostril morning and evening	
Ⓟ flunisolide (*AeroBid*)	Adult: two inhalations b.i.d. (500 μg) morning and evening Pediatric (6–15 y): two inhalations bid (500 μg) morning and evening	
fluticasone (*Flovent*)	Adult: 88–440 μg b.i.d. by inhalation Pediatric (4–11 y): 50–100 μg bid by inhalation	
triamcinolone (*Azmacort*)	Adult: two inhalations (200 μg) t.i.d.–q.i.d. Pediatric (6–12 y): one to two inhalations t.i.d.–q.i.d.	

apy. Assess the following: temperature, to monitor for possible infections; blood pressure, pulse, and auscultation, to evaluate cardiovascular response; and respirations and adventitious sounds, to monitor drug effectiveness. In addition, conduct an examination of the nares to evaluate for any lesions that might lead to systemic absorption of the drug.

Nursing Diagnoses

The patient receiving an inhaled steroid may have the following nursing diagnoses related to drug therapy:

- Risk for Injury related to immunosuppression
- Acute Pain related to local effects of the drug
- Deficient Knowledge regarding drug therapy

Implementation

- Do not administer the drug to treat an acute asthma attack or status asthmaticus, *because these drugs are not intended for treatment of acute attack.*
- Taper systemic steroids carefully during the transfer to inhaled steroids; *deaths have occurred from adrenal insufficiency with sudden withdrawal.*
- Have the patient use decongestant drops before using the inhaled steroid, *to facilitate penetration of the drug if nasal congestion is a problem.*
- Have the patient rinse the mouth after using the inhaler, *because this will help to decrease systemic absorption and decrease GI upset and nausea.*
- Monitor the patient for any sign of respiratory infection; *continued use of steroids during an acute infection can lead to serious complications related to the depression of the inflammatory and immune responses.*
- Provide thorough patient teaching, including the drug name and prescribed dosage, measures to help avoid adverse effects, warning signs that may indicate problems, and the need for periodic monitoring and evaluation, *to enhance patient knowledge about drug therapy and to promote compliance.*
- Offer support and encouragement, *to help the patient cope with the disease and the drug regimen.*

Evaluation

- Monitor patient response to the drug (improved breathing).
- Monitor for adverse effects (nasal irritation, fever, GI upset).
- Evaluate the effectiveness of the teaching plan (patient can name drug, dosage, adverse effects to watch for, specific measures to avoid adverse effects, measures to take to increase the effectiveness of the drug).
- Monitor the effectiveness of other measures to ease breathing.

☐☐●☐ WEB LINKS

Health care providers and patients may want to consult the following Internet sources:

Information on living with COPD, aimed at patients and families:
  http://copd.20m.com
Information on support groups, treatment programs, resources, and research involving COPD and asthma:
  http://www.newtechpub.com/health.html
Information on lung diseases, community support groups, getting involved, treatment, research, definitions:
  http://www.lungusa.org/index.html

▮ LEUKOTRIENE RECEPTOR ANTAGONISTS

A newer class of drugs, the **leukotriene receptor antagonists,** was developed to act more specifically at the site of the problem associated with asthma. Zafirlukast (*Accolate*) was the first drug of this class to be developed. Montelukast (*Singulair*) and Zileuton (*Zyflo*) are the other drugs currently available in this class. Because this class is relatively new, long-term effects and the benefits of one drug over another have not yet been determined.

Therapeutic Actions and Indications

Leukotriene receptor antagonists selectively and competitively block (zafirlukast, montelukast) or antagonize (zileuton) receptors for the production of leukotrienes D_4 and E_4, components of SRSA. As a result, these drugs block many of the signs and symptoms of asthma, such as neutrophil and eosinophil migration, neutrophil and monocyte aggregation, leukocyte adhesion, increased capillary permeability, and smooth muscle contraction. These factors contribute to inflammation, edema, mucus secretion, and bronchoconstriction seen in patients with asthma. The leukotriene receptor antagonists are indicated for the prophylaxis and chronic treatment of bronchial asthma in adults and in patients younger than 12 years of age. They are not indicated for the treatment of acute asthmatic attacks (see Figure 55–2).

Pharmacokinetics

These drugs are rapidly absorbed from the GI tract. Zafirlukast and montelukast are extensively metabolized in the liver by the cytochrome P450 system and are primarily excreted in the feces. Zileuton is metabolized and cleared through the liver. These drugs cross the placenta and enter breast milk. Fetal toxicity has been reported in animal studies, so these drugs should be used during pregnancy only if the benefit to the mother clearly outweighs the potential risks to the fetus. No adequate studies have been done on the effects on the baby if these drugs are used during lactation; caution should be used.

Contraindications and Cautions

These drugs should be used cautiously in patients with hepatic or renal impairment, because these conditions can affect the drug's metabolism and excretion, and during pregnancy and lactation, because of the potential for adverse effects on the fetus or neonate.

DRUGS IN FOCUS
Leukotriene Receptor Antagonists

Drug Name	Usual Dosage	Usual Indications
montelukast (*Singulair*)	Adult and pediatric (>15 y): 10 mg PO q.d. in the evening Pediatric (2–5 y): 4 mg chewable tablet PO in the evening Pediatric (6–14 y): 5 mg chewable tablet PO in the evening	Prophylaxis and chronic treatment of bronchial asthma
Ⓟ zafirkulast (*Accolate*)	Adult and pediatric (>12 y): 20 mg PO b.i.d. Pediatric (7–11 y): 10 mg PO b.i.d.	Prophylaxis and chronic treatment of bronchial asthma
zileuton (*Zyflo*)	600 mg PO q.i.d. for a total of 2400 mg/d	Prophylaxis and chronic treatment of bronchial asthma in patients >12 y of age

Adverse Effects

Adverse effects associated with leukotriene receptor antagonists include headache, dizziness, myalgia, nausea, diarrhea, abdominal pain, elevated liver enzyme concentrations, vomiting, generalized pain, fever, and myalgia.

Clinically Important Drug–Drug Interactions

Caution should be used if propranolol, theophylline, terfenadine, or warfarin is taken with these drugs, because increased toxicity can occur.

Toxicity may also occur if these drugs are combined with calcium channel blockers, cyclosporine, or aspirin; decreased dosage of either drug may be necessary.

Nursing Considerations for Patients Receiving Leukotriene Receptor Antagonists
Assessment: History and Examination

Screen for the following conditions, which could be cautions or contraindications to use of the drug: allergy to the drug, pregnancy or lactation, and acute bronchospasm or asthmatic attack, all of which would be contraindications to the use of the drug; and impaired renal or hepatic function, which could alter the metabolism and excretion of the drug and might require a dosage adjustment.

Physical assessment should be done to establish baseline data for assessing the effectiveness of the drug and the occurrence of any adverse effects associated with drug therapy. Assess the following: temperature, to monitor for underlying infection; orientation and affect, to monitor for CNS effects of the drug; respirations and adventitious breath sounds, to monitor the effectiveness of the drug; liver and renal function tests, to assess for impairments; and abdominal evaluation, to monitor GI effects of the drug.

Nursing Diagnoses

The patient receiving a leukotriene receptor antagonist may have the following nursing diagnoses related to drug therapy:

- Acute Pain related to headache, GI upset, myalgia
- Risk for Injury related to CNS effects
- Deficient Knowledge regarding drug therapy

Implementation

- Administer the drug on an empty stomach, 1 hour before or 2 hours after meals; *the bioavailability of these drugs is decreased markedly by the presence of food.*
- Caution the patient that these drugs are not to be used during an acute asthmatic attack or bronchospasm; *instead, regular emergency measures will be needed.*
- Caution the patient to take the drug continuously and not to stop the medication during symptom-free periods, *to ensure that therapeutic levels are maintained.*
- Provide appropriate safety measures if dizziness occurs, *to prevent patient injury.*
- Urge the patient to avoid over-the-counter preparations containing aspirin, *which might interfere with the effectiveness of these drugs.*
- Provide thorough patient teaching, including the drug name and prescribed dosage, measures to help avoid adverse effects, warning signs that may indicate problems, and the need for periodic monitoring and evaluation, *to enhance patient knowledge about drug therapy and to promote compliance.*
- Offer support and encouragement, *to help the patient cope with the disease and the drug regimen.*

Evaluation

- Monitor patient response to the drug (improved breathing).
- Monitor for adverse effects (drowsiness, headache, abdominal pain, myalgia).
- Evaluate the effectiveness of the teaching plan (patient can name drug, dosage, adverse effects to watch for, specific measures to avoid adverse effects, measures to take to increase the effectiveness of the drug).
- Monitor the effectiveness of other measures to ease breathing.

LUNG SURFACTANTS

Lung surfactants are naturally occurring compounds or lipoproteins containing lipids and apoproteins that reduce the surface tension within the alveoli, allowing expansion of the alveoli for gas exchange. Four lung surfactants currently available for use are beractant (*Survanta*), calfactant (*Infasurf*), colfosceril (*Exosurf Neonatal*), and the newest drug, poractant (*Curosurf*). Poractant is being tried in the treatment of adult RDS and with adults after near-drowning.

Therapeutic Actions and Indications

These drugs are used to replace the surfactant that is missing in the lungs of neonates with RDS (see Figure 55–2). They are indicated for the rescue treatment of infants who have developed RDS. They are also used for prophylactic treatment of infants at high risk for RDS—those with a birth weight of less than 1350 g and those with a birth weight greater than 1350 g who have evidence of respiratory immaturity.

Pharmacokinetics

These drugs begin to act immediately on instillation into the trachea. They are metabolized in the lungs by the normal surfactant metabolic pathways. They are not indicated for use in pregnancy or lactation and are not categorized.

Adverse Effects

Adverse effects that are associated with the use of lung surfactants include patent ductus arteriosus, hypotension, intraventricular hemorrhage, pneumothorax, pulmonary air leak, hyperbilirubinemia, and sepsis. These effects may be related to the immaturity of the patient, the invasive procedures used, or reactions to the lipoprotein. Because lung surfactants are used as emergency drugs, there are no contraindications.

Nursing Considerations for Patients Receiving Lung Surfactants

Assessment: History and Examination

Screen for time of birth and exact weight to determine appropriate dosages. Because this drug is used as an emergency treatment, there are no contraindications to screen for.

Physical assessment should be done to establish baseline data for assessing the effectiveness of the drug and the occurrence of any adverse effects associated with drug therapy. Assess the following: skin temperature and color, to evaluate perfusion; respirations, adventitious sounds, endotracheal tube placement and patency, and chest movements, to evaluate the effectiveness of the drug and drug delivery; blood pressure, pulse, and arterial pressure, to monitor the status of the infant; blood gases and oxygen saturation, to monitor drug effectiveness; and temperature and complete blood count, to monitor for sepsis.

Nursing Diagnoses

The patient receiving a lung surfactant may have the following nursing diagnoses related to drug therapy:

- Decreased Cardiac Output related to cardiovascular and respiratory effects of the drug
- Risk for Injury related to prematurity and risk of infection
- Ineffective Airway Clearance related to the possibility of mucous plugs
- Deficient Knowledge regarding drug therapy (for parents)

DRUGS IN FOCUS
Lung Surfactants

Drug Name	Usual Dosage	Usual Indications
(P) beractant (*Survanta*)	4 mL/kg birth weight, instilled intratracheally, may repeat up to four times in 48 h	Rescue treatment of infants who have developed respiratory distress syndrome (RDS); prophylactic treatment of infants at high risk for development of RDS
calfactant (*Infasurf*)	3 mg/kg birth weight as soon as possible for prophylaxis; 3 mg/kg birth weight divided into two doses, repeat up to a total of three doses 12 h apart for rescue	Rescue treatment of infants who have developed RDS; prophylactic treatment of infants at high risk for RDS
colfosceril (*Exosurf Neonatal*)	5 mL/kg birth weight as soon after birth as possible for prophylaxis, repeat at 12 and 24 h; two 5 mL/kg birth weight doses, one at diagnosis and one in 12 h for rescue	Rescue treatment of infants who have developed RDS; prophylactic treatment of infants at high risk for RDS
poractant (*Curosurf*)	2.5 mL/kg birth weight intratracheally, half in each bronchus, may repeat with up to two 1.25-mL/kg doses at 12-h intervals	Rescue treatment of infants who have developed RDS

Implementation

- Monitor the patient continuously during administration and until stable, *to provide life support measures as needed.*
- Ensure proper placement of the endotracheal tube with bilateral chest movement and lung sounds, *to provide adequate delivery of the drug.*
- Have staff view the manufacturer's teaching video before regular use, *to review the specific technical aspects of administration.*
- Suction the infant immediately before administration, but do not suction for 2 hours after administration unless clinically necessary, *to allow the drug time to work.*
- Provide support and encouragement to parents of the patient, explaining the use of the drug in the teaching program, *to help them cope with the diagnosis and treatment of their infant.*
- Continue other supportive measures related to the immaturity of the infant, *because this is only one aspect of medical care needed for premature infants.*

Evaluation

- Monitor patient response to the drug (improved breathing, alveolar expansion).
- Monitor for adverse effects (pneumothorax, patent ductus arteriosus, bradycardia, sepsis).
- Evaluate the effectiveness of the teaching plan and support parents as appropriate.
- Monitor the effectiveness of other measures to support breathing and stabilize the patient.
- Evaluate effectiveness of other supportive measures related to the immaturity of the infant.

MAST CELL STABILIZERS

Two other drugs that are often used in the treatment of asthma and allergy are cromolyn (*Intal*) and nedocromil (*Tilade*).

These drugs are **mast cell stabilizers.** They prevent the release of inflammatory and bronchoconstricting substances when the mast cells are stimulated to release these substances because of irritation or the presence of an antigen.

Therapeutic Actions and Indications

Cromolyn works at the cellular level to inhibit the release of histamine (released from mast cells in response to inflammation or irritation) and inhibits the release of SRSA (see Figure 55–2). By blocking these chemical mediators of the immune reaction, cromolyn prevents the allergic asthmatic response when the respiratory tract is exposed to the offending allergen. It is inhaled from a capsule and may not reach its peak effect for 1 week. It is recommended for the treatment of chronic bronchial asthma, exercise-induced asthma, and allergic rhinitis.

Nedocromil inhibits the mediators of a variety of inflammatory cells, including eosinophils, neutrophils, macrophages, and mast cells (see Figure 55–2). By blocking these effects, nedocromil decreases the release of histamine and blocks the overall inflammatory response. This drug is indicated for the management of patients with mild to moderate bronchial asthma who are older than 12 years of age. This drug should be taken continually for best results and is often used concomitantly with corticosteroids.

Pharmacokinetics

Cromolyn is primarily active in the lungs, and most of the inhaled dose is exhaled or swallowed and excreted in the feces. Nedocromil, when absorbed, is excreted primarily unchanged in the urine. Safety for use in pregnancy and lactation has not been established. Use should be reserved for those situations when the benefit to the mother greatly outweighs any potential risk to the fetus or neonate.

Contraindications and Cautions

Both drugs are contraindicated in the presence of known allergy to the drug. Cromolyn cannot be used during an acute attack, and patients need to be instructed in this precaution. Neither drug is recommended for pregnant or nursing women. Cromolyn is not recommended for children younger than 2

DRUGS IN FOCUS
Mast Cell Stabilizers

Drug Name	Used Dosage	Usual Indications
cromolyn (*Intal*)	Adult and pediatric (>5 y): 20 mg inhaled q.i.d. Adult and pediatric (>2 y): 20 mg q.i.d. via nebulizer Adult and pediatric (>6 y): one spray of nasal solution in each nostril three to six times per day Adult: two ampules PO q.i.d. Pediatric (2–12 y): one ampule PO q.i.d.	Treatment of chronic bronchial asthma, exercise-induced asthma, and allergic rhinitis
nedocromil (*Tilade*)	Adult and pediatric (>12 y): two inhalations q.i.d. at regular intervals	Management of mild to moderate bronchial asthma

years of age, and nedocromil is not recommended before 12 years of age.

Adverse Effects

Few adverse effects have been reported with the use of cromolyn; those that do occur on occasion include swollen eyes, headache, dry mucosa, and nausea. Careful patient management (avoidance of dry or smoky environments, analgesics, use of proper inhalation technique, use of a humidifier, and pushing fluids as appropriate) can help to make drug-related discomfort tolerable. Adverse effects associated with nedocromil include headache, dizziness, fatigue, tearing, GI upset, and cough; this drug should not be discontinued abruptly.

Nursing Considerations for Patients Receiving Mast Cell Stabilizers

Assessment: History and Examination

Screen for the following conditions, which could be cautions or contraindications to use of the drug: allergy to cromolyn or nedocromil; impaired renal or hepatic function, which could interfere with the metabolism or excretion of the drug, leading to a need for dosage adjustment; and pregnancy or lactation, which requires very cautious administration.

Physical assessment should be done to establish baseline data for assessing the effectiveness of the drug and the occurrence of any adverse effects associated with drug therapy. Assess the following: skin color and lesions, to monitor for adverse effects of the drug; respirations and adventitious sounds, to evaluate drug effectiveness; patency of nares, to determine efficacy of inhaled preparations; orientation, to monitor adverse effects and headache; and liver and renal function tests, to assess for potential problems with drug metabolism or excretion.

Nursing Diagnoses

The patient receiving cromolyn may have the following nursing diagnoses related to drug therapy:

- Acute Pain related to local effects, headache, GI effects
- Risk for Injury related to CNS effects
- Deficient Knowledge regarding drug therapy

Implementation

- Review administration procedures with the patient periodically; *proper use of the delivery device is important in maintaining the effectiveness of this drug.*
- Caution the patient not to discontinue use abruptly; *cromolyn and nedocromil should be tapered slowly if discontinuation is necessary, to prevent rebound adverse effects.*
- Caution the patient to continue taking this drug, even during symptom-free periods, *to ensure therapeutic levels of the drug.*
- Administer oral drug 30 minutes before meals and at bedtime, *to promote continual drug levels and relief of asthma.*
- Initiate safety precautions if dizziness and fatigue are problems with nedocromil therapy, *to prevent patient injury.*

- Advise the patient not to wear soft contact lenses; *if cromolyn eye drops (used for allergic reactions) are used, lenses can be stained or warped.*
- Provide thorough patient teaching, including the drug name and prescribed dosage, measures to help avoid adverse effects, warning signs that may indicate problems, and the need for periodic monitoring and evaluation, *to enhance patient knowledge about drug therapy and to promote compliance.*
- Offer support and encouragement, *to help the patient cope with the disease and the drug regimen.*

Evaluation

- Monitor patient response to the drug (improved breathing, relief of signs or allergic disorders).
- Monitor for adverse effects (drowsiness, dizziness, headache, GI upset, local irritation).
- Evaluate the effectiveness of the teaching plan (patient can name drug, dosage, adverse effects to watch for, specific measures to avoid adverse effects, measures to take to increase the effectiveness of the drug).
- Monitor the effectiveness of other measures to ease breathing.

CHAPTER SUMMARY

- Pulmonary obstructive diseases include asthma, emphysema, and chronic obstructive pulmonary disease (COPD), which cause obstruction of the major airways, and respiratory distress syndrome (RDS), which causes obstruction at the alveolar level.
- Drugs used to treat asthma and COPD include drugs to block inflammation and drugs to dilate bronchi.
- The xanthine derivatives have a direct effect on the smooth muscle of the respiratory tract, both in the bronchi and in the blood vessels.
- The adverse effects of the xanthines are directly related to the theophylline concentration in the blood and can progress to coma and death.
- Sympathomimetics are drugs that mimic the effects of the sympathetic nervous system; they are used for dilation of the bronchi and to increase the rate and depth of respiration.
- Anticholinergics can be used as bronchodilators because of their effect on the vagus nerve, resulting in a relaxation of smooth muscle in the bronchi, which leads to bronchodilation.
- Steroids are used to decrease the inflammatory response in the airway. Inhaling the steroid tends to decrease the numerous systemic effects that are associated with steroid use.
- Leukotriene receptor antagonists block or antagonize receptors for the production of leukotrienes D_4 and E_4, thus blocking many of the signs and symptoms of asthma.
- Lung surfactants are instilled into the respiratory system of premature infants who do not have enough surfactant to ensure alveolar expansion.
- The mast cell stabilizers are antiasthmatic drugs that block

mediators of inflammation and help to decrease swelling and blockage in the airways.

Review Questions

1. Treatment of obstructive pulmonary disorders is aimed at
   a. opening the conducting airways through muscular bronchodilation or by decreasing the effects of inflammation on the lining of the airway.
   b. blocking the autonomic reflexes that alter respirations.
   c. blocking the effects of the immune and inflammatory systems.
   d. altering the respiratory membrane to increase flow of oxygen and carbon dioxide.

2. The xanthines
   a. block the sympathetic nervous system.
   b. stimulate the sympathetic nervous system.
   c. directly affect the smooth muscles of the respiratory tract.
   d. act in the CNS to cause bronchodilation.

3. Your patient has been maintained on theophylline for many years and has recently taken up smoking. The theophylline levels in this patient would be expected to
   a. rise, because nicotine prevents the breakdown of theophylline.
   b. stay the same, because smoking has no effect on theophylline.
   c. fall, because the nicotine stimulates liver metabolism of theophylline.
   d. rapidly reach toxic levels.

4. A person with hypertension and known heart disease has frequent bronchospasms and asthma attacks that are most responsive to sympathomimetic drugs. This patient might be best treated with
   a. an inhaled sympathomimetic, to decrease systemic effects.
   b. a xanthine.
   c. no sympathomimetics, because they would be contraindicated.
   d. an anticholinergic.

5. A patient with many adverse reactions to drugs is tried on an inhaled steroid for treatment of bronchospasm. For the first 3 days, the patient does not notice any improvement. You should
   a. switch the patient to a xanthine.
   b. encourage the patient to continue the drug for 2 to 3 weeks; if no response is noted by then, try another inhaled steroid.
   c. switch the patient to a sympathomimetic.
   d. try the patient on surfactant.

6. Leukotriene receptor antagonists act to block production of a component of SRSA. They are most beneficial in treating
   a. seasonal rhinitis.
   b. pneumonia.
   c. COPD.
   d. asthma.

7. Patients who are using inhalers require careful teaching about
   a. avoiding food 1 hour before and 2 hours after dosing.
   b. storage of the drug.
   c. administration techniques to promote therapeutic effects and avoid adverse effects.
   d. lying flat for up to 2 hours after dosing.

8. Respiratory distress syndrome occurs in
   a. babies with frequent colds.
   b. babies with genetic allergies.
   c. premature babies and those with low birth weight.
   d. babies stressed during the pregnancy.

9. Lung surfactants used therapeutically are
   a. injected into a developed muscle.
   b. instilled via a nasogastric tube.
   c. injected into the umbilical artery.
   d. instilled into an endotracheal tube properly placed in the baby's lungs.

BIBLIOGRAPHY

Bullock, B. L. (2000). *Focus on pathophysiology*. Philadelphia: Lippincott Williams & Wilkins.

Drazen, J. (1998). New directions in asthma drug therapy. *Hospital Practice 33*(2).

Drug facts and comparisons. (2002). St. Louis: Facts and Comparisons.

Gilman, A., Hardman, J. G., & Limbird, L. E. (Eds.) (2002). *Goodman and Gilman's the pharmacological basis of therapeutics* (10th ed.). New York: McGraw-Hill.

Karch, A. M. (2002). *2003 Lippincott's nursing drug guide*. Philadelphia: Lippincott Williams & Wilkins.

Professional's guide to patient drug facts. (2002). St. Louis: Facts and Comparisons.

PART

XI

Drugs Acting on the Gastrointestinal System

56

Introduction to the Gastrointestinal System

765

The gastrointestinal (GI) system is the only system in the body that is open to the external environment. The GI system is composed of one continuous tube that begins at the mouth, progresses through the esophagus, stomach, and small and large intestines, and ends at the anus. The pancreas, liver, and gallbladder are accessory organs that support the functions of the GI system (Figure 56–1). The GI system has four major activities:

- *Secretion*—of enzymes, acid, bicarbonate, and mucus
- *Absorption*—of water and almost all of the essential nutrients needed by the body
- *Digestion*—of food into usable and absorbable components
- *Motility*—movement of food and secretions through the system (what is not used is excreted in the form of feces)

The GI system is responsible for only a very small part of waste excretion. The kidneys and lungs are responsible for excreting most of the waste products of normal metabolism.

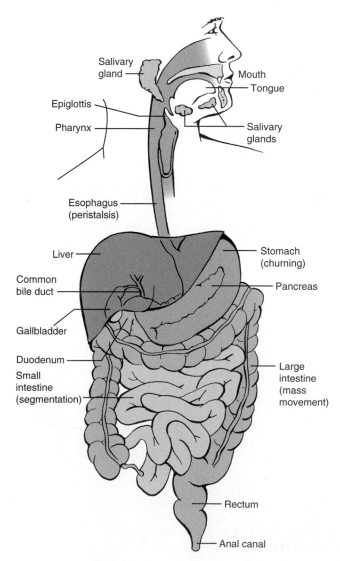

FIGURE 56-1. The gastrointestinal tract.

COMPOSITION OF THE GASTROINTESTINAL TRACT

The tube that comprises the GI tract is continuous with the external environment, opening at the mouth and again at the anus. Because of this, the GI tract contains many foreign agents and bacteria that are not found in the rest of the body. The peritoneum lines the abdominal wall and also the viscera, with a small "free space" between the two layers. It helps keep the GI tract in place and prevents a buildup of friction with movement. The greater and lesser omenta hang from the stomach over the lower GI tract and are full of lymph nodes, lymphocytes, monocytes, and other components of the mononuclear phagocyte system. This barrier provides rapid protection for the rest of the body if any of the bacteria or other foreign agents in the GI tract should be absorbed into the body (see Figure 56–1).

The GI tube is composed of four layers: the mucosa, the muscularis mucosa, the **nerve plexus,** and the adventitia.

- The mucosal layer provides the inner lining of the GI tract. It can be seen in the mouth and is fairly consistent throughout the tube. It is important to remember when assessing a patient that if the mouth is very dry or full of lesions, that is a reflection of the state of the entire GI tract and may indicate that the patient has difficulty digesting or absorbing nutrients. This layer has an epithelial component and a connective tissue component.
- The muscularis mucosa layer is made up of muscles. Most of the GI tract has two muscle layers. One layer runs circularly around the tube, helping keep the tube open and squeezing the tube to aid digestion and motility. The other layer runs horizontally, which helps propel the gastrointestinal contents down the tract. The stomach has a third layer of muscle, which runs obliquely and gives the stomach the ability to move contents in a churning motion.
- The nerve plexus has two layers of nerves, one submucosal layer and one myenteric layer. These nerves give the GI tract local control of movement, secretions, and digestion. The nerves respond to local stimuli and act on the contents of the GI tract accordingly. The GI tract is also innervated by the sympathetic and parasympathetic nervous systems. These systems can slow down or speed up the activity in the GI tract but cannot initiate local activity. The sympathetic system is stimulated during times of stress (eg, "fight or flight" response) when digestion is not a priority. To slow the GI tract, the sympathetic system decreases muscle tone, secretions, and contractions, and increases sphincter tone. By shutting down the GI activity, the body saves energy for other activities. In contrast, the parasympathetic system ("rest and digest" response) stimulates the GI tract, increasing muscle tone, secretions, and contractions and decreasing sphincter tone, allowing easy movement.
- The adventitia, the outer layer of the GI tract, serves as a supportive layer and helps the tube maintain its shape and stay in position (Figure 56–2).

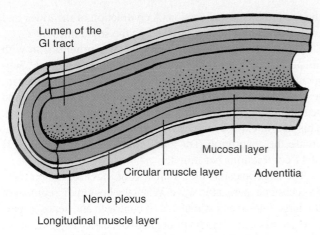

FIGURE 56–2. Layers of the gastrointestinal tract.

Lumen of the GI tract

Mucosal layer

Circular muscle layer

Adventitia

Nerve plexus

Longitudinal muscle layer

GASTROINTESTINAL ACTIVITIES

The GI tract has four functions: secretion, digestion, absorption, and motility. These functions are discussed in detail in the following sections.

Secretion

The GI tract secretes various compounds to aid the movement of the food bolus through the GI tube, to protect the inner layer of the GI tract from injury, and to facilitate the digestion and absorption of nutrients (see Figure 56–1). Secretions begin in the mouth. **Saliva,** which contains water and digestive enzymes, is secreted from the salivary glands to begin the digestive process and to facilitate **swallowing** by making the bolus slippery. Mucus is also produced in the mouth to protect the epithelial lining and to aid swallowing. The esophagus produces mucus to protect the inner lining of the GI tract and to further facilitate the movement of the bolus down the tube.

The stomach produces acid and digestive enzymes. In addition, it generates a large amount of mucus to protect the stomach lining from the acid and the enzymes. In the stomach, secretion begins with what is called the cephalic phase of digestion. The sight, smell, or taste of food stimulates the stomach to begin secreting before any food reaches the stomach. Once the bolus of food arrives at the stomach, **gastrin** is secreted. Gastrin stimulates the stomach muscles to contract, the parietal cells to release **hydrochloric acid,** and the chief cells to release pepsin. Parasympathetic stimulation also leads to acid release. Gastrin and the parasympathetic system stimulate **histamine-2 receptors** near the parietal cells, causing the cells to release hydrochloric acid into the lumen of the stomach. The presence of proteins, calcium, alcohol, and caffeine in the stomach increases gastrin secretion. High levels of acid decrease the secretion of gastrin. Other digestive enzymes are released appropriately, in response to proteins and carbohydrates, to begin digestion.

Peptic ulcers can develop when there is a decrease in the protective mucosal layer or an increase in acid production.

As the now acidic bolus leaves the stomach and enters the small intestine, secretin is released, which stimulates the pancreas to secrete large amounts of sodium bicarbonate (to neutralize the acid bolus), the **pancreatic enzymes** chymotrypsin and trypsin (to break down proteins to smaller amino acids), other lipases (to break down fat), and amylases (to break down sugars). These enzymes are delivered to the GI tract through the common duct, which is shared with the gallbladder.

If fat is present in the bolus, the gallbladder contracts and releases bile into the small intestine. **Bile** contains a detergent-like substance that breaks apart fat molecules so that they can be processed and absorbed. The bile in the gallbladder is produced by the liver during normal metabolism. Once delivered to the gallbladder for storage, it is concentrated; water is removed by the walls of the gallbladder. Some people are prone to develop **gallstones** in the gallbladder when the concentrated bile crystallizes. These stones can move down the duct and cause severe pain or even blockage of the bile duct. See Box 56–1 for information on drugs used to dissolve gallstones.

In response to the presence of food, the small and large intestines may secrete various endocrine hormones, including growth hormone, aldosterone, and glucagon. They also

---

BOX 56-1

Gallstone Solubilizers

Surgery is usually the treatment of choice for the removal of gallstones. Severe pain, nausea, and vomiting usually accompany an acute gall bladder attack, and removal is desirable. Some patients are not candidates for surgery because of other underlying medical conditions and these patients might benefit from the use of gallstone solubilizers to dissolve certain gallstones. Available drugs are

Chenodiol (*Chenix*), which was the first such drug developed and is now available only as an orphan drug. Because this agent causes serious diarrhea and sometimes hepatitis and even colon cancer, its use must be weighed carefully against the dangers of the obstructed gall bladder.

Ursodiol (*Actigall*), another oral gallstone solubilizer, which is not associated with severe adverse effects but may require months of therapy to achieve an outcome. It is best used when the gallstones are small and not obstructing. The drug is given at a dose of 8–10 mg/kg per day PO in two or three divided doses. Up to 50% of the patients who do respond to this drug have a recurrence of stones within 5 years.

Mono-octanoin (*Moctanin*), which is a semisynthetic glycerol that must be delivered by a continuous perfusion pump through a catheter inserted into the common bile duct. Treatment with mono-octanoin must continue for 7 to 21 days. This drug is reserved for postcholecystectomy patients who still have gallstones in the biliary tract.

secrete large amounts of mucus to facilitate the movement of the bolus through the rest of the GI tract.

Digestion

Digestion is the process of breaking food into usable, absorbable nutrients. Digestion begins in the mouth, with the enzymes in the saliva starting the process of breaking down sugars and proteins. The stomach continues the digestion process with muscular churning, breaking down some foodstuffs while mixing them thoroughly with the hydrochloric acid and enzymes. The acid and enzymes further break down sugars and proteins into building blocks and separate vitamins, electrolytes, minerals, and other nutrients from ingested food for absorption. The beginning of the small intestine introduces bile to the food bolus, which is now called **chyme.** Bile breaks down fat molecules for processing and absorption into the bloodstream. Digestion is finished at this point, and absorption of the nutrients begins.

Absorption

Absorption is the active process of removing water, nutrients, and other elements from the GI tract and delivering them to the bloodstream for use by the body. The portal system drains all of the lower GI tract, where absorption occurs, and delivers what is absorbed into the venous system directly to the liver. The liver filters, clears, and further processes most of what is absorbed before it is delivered to the body (see Figure 56–1). Some absorption occurs in the lower end of stomach (eg, water, alcohol). The small intestine absorbs about 8500 mL/day, including nutrients, drugs, and anything that is taken into the GI tract, as well as any secretions. The small intestine mucosal layer is specially designed to facilitate this absorption, with long villi on the epithelial layer providing a vast surface area for absorption. The large intestine absorbs approximately 350 mL/day, mostly sodium and water.

Motility

The GI tract depends on an inherent motility to keep things moving through the system. The nerve plexus maintains a basic electrical rhythm (BER), much like the pacemaker rhythm in the heart. The cells within the plexus are somewhat unstable and leak electrolytes, leading to the regular firing of an action potential. This rhythm maintains the tone of the GI tract muscles and can be affected by local or autonomic stimuli to increase or decrease the rate of firing.

The basic movement seen in the esophagus is **peristalsis,** a constant wave of contraction that moves from the top to the bottom of the esophagus. The act of swallowing, a response to a food bolus in the back of the throat, stimulates the peristaltic movement that directs the food bolus into the stomach. The stomach uses its three muscle layers to produce a churning action. This action mixes the digestive enzymes and acid with the food to increase digestion. A contraction of the lower end of the stomach sends the chyme into the small intestine.

The small intestine uses a process of **segmentation** with an occasional peristaltic wave to clear the segment. Segmentation involves contraction of one segment of small intestine while the next segment is relaxed. The contracted segment then relaxes, and the relaxed segment contracts. This action exposes the chyme to a vast surface area to increase the absorption. The small intestine maintains a BER of 11 contractions per minute.

The large intestine uses a process of mass movement with an occasional peristaltic wave. When the beginning segment of the large intestine is stimulated, it contracts and sends a massive peristaltic movement throughout the entire large intestine. The end result of the mass movement is usually excretion of waste products. Rectal distention after mass movement stimulates a defecation reflex that causes relaxation of the external and internal sphincters. Control of the external sphincter is a learned behavior. The receptors in the external sphincter adopt relatively quickly to stretch and require more and more distention to stimulate the reflex if the reflex is ignored.

▣■●◗ WEB LINKS

To explore the virtual GI system, consult the following Internet sources:

http://www.InnerBody.com
http://www1.biostr.washington.edu/DigitalAnatomist.html

Local Gastrointestinal Reflexes

Stimulation of local nerves within the GI tract causes increased or decreased movement within the system, maintaining homeostasis. Loss of reflexes or stimulation can result in constipation, and the lack of movement of the bolus along the GI tract, or diarrhea, with increased motility and excretion. The longer a fecal bolus remains in the large intestine, the more sodium and water is absorbed from it and the harder and less mobile it can become. There are many **local gastrointestinal reflexes,** and some knowledge of how they operate makes it easier to understand what happens when the reflexes are blocked or overstimulated and how therapeutic measures are often used to cause reflex activity.

- *Gastroenteric reflex*—Stimulation of the stomach by stretching, the presence of food, or cephalic stimulation causes an increase in activity in the small intestine. It is thought that this prepares the small intestine for the coming chyme.
- *Gastrocolic reflex*—Stimulation of the stomach also causes increased activity in the colon, again preparing to empty any contents to provide space for the new chyme.
- *Duodenal–colic reflex*—The presence of food or stretch in the duodenum stimulates colon activity and mass movement, again to empty the colon for the new chyme.

It is important to remember the gastroenteric, gastrocolic, and duodenal reflexes when helping patients to maintain GI movement. Taking advantage of stomach stimulation (eg, having the patient drink prune juice or hot water or eat bran) and providing the opportunity of time and privacy for a bowel movement encourages normal reflexes to keep things in control.

Other local GI reflexes include the following:

- *Ileogastric reflex*—The introduction of chyme or stretch to the large intestine slows stomach activity as well as the introduction of chyme into the small and large intestine, allowing time for absorption. In part, this reflex explains why patients who are constipated often have no appetite: the continued stretch on the ileum that comes with constipation continues to slow stomach activity and makes the introduction of new food into the stomach undesirable.

- *Intestinal–intestinal reflex*—Excessive irritation to one section of the small intestine causes a cessation of activity above that section, to prevent further irritation, and an increase in activity below that section, which leads to a flushing of the irritant. This reflex is active in "Montezuma's revenge" (traveler's diarrhea): local irritation of the intestine causes increased secretions and movement below that section, resulting in watery diarrhea and a cessation of movement above that section. Loss of appetite or even nausea may occur. An extreme reaction to this reflex can be seen after abdominal surgery, when the handling of the intestines causes intense irritation and the reflex can cause the entire intestinal system to cease activity, leading to a paralytic ileus.

- *Peritoneointestinal reflex*—Irritation of the peritoneum as a result of inflammation or injury leads to a cessation of GI activity, preventing continued movement of the GI tract and thus further irritation of the peritoneum.

- *Renointestinal reflex*—Irritation or swelling of the renal capsule causes a cessation of movement in the GI tract, again to prevent further irritation to the capsule.

- *Vesicointestinal reflex*—Irritation or overstretching of the bladder can cause a reflex cessation of movement in the GI tract, again to prevent further irritation to the bladder from the GI movement. Many patients with cystitis or overstretched bladders from occupational constraints or neurological problems complain of constipation, which can be attributable to this reflex.

- *Somatointestinal reflex*—Taut stretching of the skin and muscles over the abdomen irritates the nerve plexus and causes a slowing or cessation of GI activity to prevent further irritation. During the era when tight girdles were commonly worn, this reflex was often seen among women, and constipation was a serious problem for many women who wore such constraining garments. Tight-fitting clothing (eg, jeans) can have the same effect. Patients who complain of chronic constipation may be suffering from overactivity of the somatointestinal reflex.

Central Reflexes

Two centrally mediated reflexes—swallowing and vomiting—are very important to the functioning of the GI tract.

The swallowing reflex is stimulated whenever a food bolus stimulates pressure receptors in the back of the throat and pharynx. These receptors send impulses to the medulla, which stimulates a series of nerves that cause the following actions: the soft palate elevates and seals off the nasal cavity; respirations cease in order to protect the lungs; the larynx rises and the glottis closes to seal off the airway; and the pharyngeal constrictor muscles contract and force the food bolus into the top of the esophagus, where pairs of muscles contract in turn to move the bolus down the esophagus into the stomach. This reflex is complex, involving more than 25 pairs of muscles.

There are a number of ways that this reflex can be facilitated if swallowing (food or medication) is a problem. Icing the tongue by sucking on a popsicle or an ice cube blocks external nerve impulses and allows this more basic reflex to respond. Icing the sternal notch or the back of the neck, although not as appealing, has also proved effective in stimulating the swallowing reflex. In addition, keeping the head straight (not turned to one side) allows the muscle pairs to work together and helps the process. Providing stimulation of the receptors in the mouth through temperature variations and textured foods helps initiate the reflex. Patients who do not produce their own saliva can be given artificial saliva to increase digestion and to lubricate the food bolus, which also help the swallowing reflex.

The **vomiting** reflex is another basic reflex that is centrally mediated and important in protecting the system from unwanted irritants. The vomiting reflex is stimulated by two centers in the medulla. The more primitive center is called the emetic zone. When stimulated, it initiates a projectile vomiting. This type of intense reaction is seen in young children and whenever increased pressure in the brain or brain damage allows the more primitive center to override the more mature chemoreceptor trigger zone (CTZ). The CTZ is stimulated in several ways:

- Tactile stimulation of the back of the throat, a reflex to get rid of something that is too big or too irritating to be swallowed
- Excessive stomach distention
- Increasing intracranial pressure by direct stimulation
- Stimulation of the vestibular receptors in the inner ear (a reaction often seen with dizziness after wild rides in amusement parks)
- Stimulation of stretch receptors in the uterus and bladder (a possible explanation for vomiting in early pregnancy and before delivery)
- Intense pain fiber stimulation
- Direct stimulation by various chemicals, including fumes, certain drugs, and debris from cellular death (a reason for vomiting after chemotherapy or radiation therapy that results in cell death).

Once the CTZ is stimulated, a series of reflexes occurs. Salivation increases, and there is a large increase in the production of mucus in the upper GI tract, which is accompanied by a decrease in gastric acid production. This action protects the lining of the GI tract from potential damage by the acidic stomach contents. (Nauseated patients who start swallowing repeatedly or complain about secretions in their throat are in the process of preparing for vomiting.) The sympathetic system is stimulated, with a resultant increase in sweating, increased heart rate, deeper respirations, and nausea. This prepares the body for fight or flight and the insult of vomiting. The esophagus then relaxes and becomes distended, and the gastric sphincter relaxes. The patient takes one deep respiration; the glottis closes and the palate rises, trapping the air in the lungs and sealing off entry to the lungs. The abdominal and thoracic muscles contract, increasing intra-abdominal pressure. The stomach then relaxes and the lower section of the stomach contracts in waves, approximately six times per minute. With nothing in the stomach, this movement is known as retching, and it can be quite tiring and uncomfortable. This action causes a backward peristalsis and movement of stomach contents up the esophagus and out the mouth. The body thus rids itself of offending irritants.

The vomiting reflex is complex and protective, but it can be undesirable in certain clinical situations, when the stimulant is not something that can be vomited or when the various components of the vomiting reflex could be detrimental to a patient's health status.

CHAPTER SUMMARY

- The gastrointestinal (GI) system is composed of one long tube that starts at the mouth; includes the esophagus, the stomach, the small intestine, and the large intestine; and ends at the anus. The GI system is responsible for digestion and absorption of nutrients.
- Secretion of digestive enzymes, acid, bicarbonate, and mucus facilitates the digestion and absorption of nutrients.
- The GI system is controlled by a nerve plexus, which maintains a basic electrical rhythm and responds to local stimuli to increase or decrease activity. The autonomic system can influence the activity of the GI tract, with the sympathetic system slowing and the parasympathetic system increasing activity. Initiation of activity depends on local reflexes.
- A series of local reflexes within the GI tract helps maintain homeostasis within the system. Overstimulation of any of these reflexes can result in constipation (underactivity) or diarrhea (overactivity).
- Swallowing is a centrally mediated reflex that is important in delivering food to the GI tract for processing. It is controlled by the medulla and involves a complex series of timed reflexes.
- Vomiting is controlled by the chemoreceptor trigger zone (CTZ) in the medulla or by the emetic zone in immature or injured brains. The CTZ is stimulated by several different processes and initiates a complex series of responses that first prepare the system for vomiting and then cause a strong backward peristalsis to rid the stomach of its contents.

Review Questions

1. Constipation
   a. results from increased peristaltic activity in the intestinal tract.
   b. occurs only if one does not have a bowel movement at least once a day.
   c. leads to decreased salt and water absorption from the large intestine.
   d. symptoms can be artificially induced by increasing the volume of the large intestine.
2. The pancreas
   a. is only an endocrine gland.
   b. secretes enzymes in response to an increased plasma glucose concentration.
   c. neutralizes the hydrochloric acid secreted by the stomach.
   d. produces bile.
3. Gastrin
   a. stimulates acid secretion in the stomach.
   b. secretion is blocked by the products of protein digestion in the stomach.
   c. secretion is stimulated by acid in the duodenum.
   d. is responsible for the chemical or gastric phase of intestinal secretion.
4. The chemoreceptor trigger zone in the brain is not activated by
   a. stretch of the uterus.
   b. stretch of the bladder.
   c. decreased GI activity.
   d. radiation.
5. The activities of the GI tract, movement and secretion, are controlled by
   a. the sympathetic nervous system.
   b. the parasympathetic nervous system.
   c. local nerve reflexes initiated in the nerve plexus layer of the GI tract.
   d. the medulla.
6. The presence of fat in the duodenum causes
   a. acid indigestion.
   b. decrease in acid production.
   c. increased gastrin release.
   d. contraction of the gall bladder.
7. Acid production in the stomach is not stimulated by
   a. protein in the stomach.
   b. calcium products in the stomach.
   c. high levels of acid in the stomach.
   d. alcohol in the stomach.
8. Pancreatic digestive enzymes help in the breakdown of all of the following except
   a. gastric acid.
   b. fats.
   c. proteins.
   d. sugars.
9. The basic type of movement that occurs in the small intestine is
   a. peristalsis.

b. mass movement.

c. churning.

d. segmentation.

10. Most of the nutrients absorbed from the GI tract pass immediately into the portal venous system and are processed by the liver. This is possible because almost all absorption occurs through

a. the lower section of the stomach.

b. the top section of the large intestine.

c. the small intestine.

d. the ileum.

BIBLIOGRAPHY

Bullock, B. L. (2000). *Focus on pathophysiology*. Philadelphia: Lippincott Williams & Wilkins.

Fox, S. (1996). Perspectives on human biology. Dubuque, IA: Wm. C. Brown.

Ganong, W. (1999). Review of medical physiology (19th ed.). Norwalk, CT: Appleton & Lange.

Gilman, A., Hardman, J. G., & Limbird, L. E. (Eds.) (2002). *Goodman and Gilman's the pharmacological basis of therapeutics* (10th ed.). New York: McGraw-Hill.

Guyton, A. & Hall, J. (2000). Textbook of medical physiology. Philadelphia: W. B. Saunders.

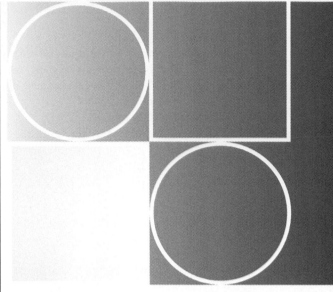

Drugs Affecting Gastrointestinal Secretions

Gastrointestinal (GI) disorders are among the most common complaints seen in clinical practice. Many products are available for the self-treatment of upset stomach, heartburn, and sour stomach. The underlying causes of these disorders can range from dietary excess, stress, hiatal hernia, esophageal reflux, and adverse drug effects to the more serious peptic ulcer disease.

Drugs that affect GI secretions can decrease GI secretory activity, block the action of GI secretions, form protective coverings on the GI lining to prevent erosion from GI secretions, or replace missing GI enzymes that the GI tract or ancillary glands and organs can no longer produce (Figure 57–1).

PEPTIC ULCERS

Erosions in the lining of the stomach and adjacent areas of the GI tract are called **peptic ulcers.** Ulcer patients present with a predictable description of gnawing, burning pain, often occurring a few hours after meals. Many of the drugs that are used to affect GI secretions are designed to prevent, treat, or aid in the healing of these ulcers. The actual cause of chronic peptic ulcers is not completely understood. For many years it was believed that ulcers were caused by excessive acid production, and treatment was aimed at neutralizing acid or blocking the parasympathetic system to decrease normal GI activity and secretions. Further research led many to believe that, because acid production was often normal in ulcer patients, ulcers were caused by a defect in the mucous lining that coats the inner lumen of the stomach to protect it from acid and digestive enzymes. Treatment was aimed at improving the balance between the acid produced and the mucous layer that protects the stomach lining. Currently it is believed that chronic ulcers are the result of bacterial infection by *Helicobacter pylori* bacteria. Combination antibiotics have been found to be quite effective in treating patients with chronic ulcers.

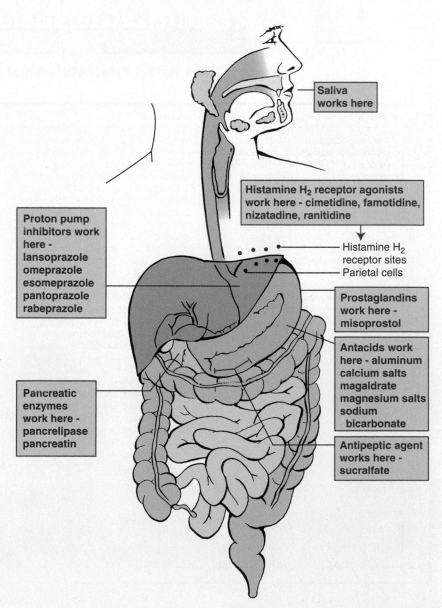

FIGURE 57–1. Sites of action of drugs affecting gastrointestinal secretions.

Acute ulcers, or "stress ulcers," are often seen in situations that involve acute stress, such as trauma, burns, or prolonged illness. The activity of the sympathetic nervous system during stress decreases blood flow to the GI tract, leading to weakening of the mucosal layer of the stomach and erosion by acid in the stomach.

Many of the drugs available for treating various peptic ulcers act to alter acid-producing activities of the stomach. Five types of drugs are used in the treatment of ulcers:

1. **Histamine-2 (H$_2$) antagonists** block the release of hydrochloric acid in response to gastrin.
2. Antacids interact with acids at the chemical level to neutralize them.
3. **Proton pump inhibitors** suppress the secretion of hydrochloric acid into the lumen of the stomach.
4. **Antipeptic agents** coat any injured area in the stomach to prevent further injury from acid.

5. **Prostaglandins** inhibit the secretion of gastrin and increase the secretion of the mucous lining of the stomach, providing a buffer.

DIGESTIVE ENZYME DYSFUNCTION

Some patients require a supplement to the production of digestive enzymes. Patients with strokes, salivary gland disorders, or extreme surgery of the head and neck may not be able to produce saliva. Saliva is important in beginning the digestion of sugars and proteins and is essential in initiating the swallowing reflex. Artificial saliva may be necessary for these patients. Patients with common duct problems, pancreatic disease, or cystic fibrosis may not be able to produce or secrete pancreatic enzymes. These enzymes may need to be administered to allow normal digestion and absorption of nutrients.

DRUG THERAPY ACROSS THE LIFESPAN

Agents That Affect Gastrointestinal Secretions

Children	Adults	Older Adults
Antacids may be used in children who complain of upset stomach or who are receiving therapy known to increase acid production; 5–15 mL q1–3h is usually an effective dose. The proton pump inhibitors, although not specifically indicated for use in children, have been very successfully used to decrease ulcer formation related to stress or drug therapy. Dosage should be determined by the age and weight of the child. Special caution should be used with any of these agents to prevent electrolyte disturbances or any interference with nutrition, which could be especially detrimental to children.	Adults should be cautioned not to overuse these agents and to check with their health care provider if gastrointestinal discomfort continues after repeated use of any of these drugs. Patients should be monitored for any electrolyte disturbances or interference with the absorption or action of other drugs. If antacids are used, they should be spaced 1–2 h before or after the use of other drugs. The safety of these drugs during pregnancy and lactation has not been established. Misoprostol is an abortifacient and should never be used during pregnancy. Women of child-bearing age who use this drug should be advised to use barrier-type contraceptives. Use of these agents should be reserved for those situations in which the benefit to the mother outweighs the potential risk to the fetus. The drugs may enter breast milk and also may alter electrolyte levels or gastric secretions in the neonate. It is advised that caution be used if one of these drugs is prescribed during lactation.	Older adults frequently are prescribed one or more of these drugs. Older adults are more likely to develop adverse effects associated with the use of these drugs, including sedation, confusion, dizziness, urinary retention, and cardiovascular effects. Safety measures may be needed if these effects occur and interfere with the patient's mobility and balance. Older adults are also more likely to have renal and/or hepatic impairment related to underlying medical conditions, which could interfere with the metabolism and excretion of these drugs. The dosage for older adults should be started at a lower level than recommended for younger adults. Patients should be monitored very closely, and dosage adjustment should be made based on patient response. These patients also need to be alerted to the potential for toxic effects when using over-the-counter (OTC) preparations that may contain the same ingredients as many of these agents. They should be advised to check with their health care provider before beginning any OTC drug regimen. Proton pump inhibitors may be the best choice for treating gastroesophageal reflux disease in older patients because of fewer adverse effects and better therapeutic response with these drugs.

HISTAMINE-2 ANTAGONISTS

The H$_2$ antagonists selectively block H$_2$ receptors. These receptors are located on the parietal cells; blocking them prevents gastrin, which causes local release of histamine and stimulation of these receptors, from stimulating the production of hydrochloric acid. This action also decreases pepsin production by the chief cells.

Four H$_2$ antagonists are available:

- Cimetidine (*Tagamet, Tagamet HB*) was the first drug in this class to be developed. It has been associated with antiadrenergic effects, including gynecomastia and galactorrhea. It is metabolized mainly in the liver and can slow the metabolism of many other drugs that use the same metabolizing enzyme system. It is excreted in the urine and is known to cross the placenta and enter breast milk. It should be used with caution during pregnancy, and another method of feeding the baby should be used during lactation. It is available in oral and parenteral forms.
- Ranitidine (*Zantac*), which is longer acting and more potent than cimetidine, is not associated with the antiadrenergic adverse effects or the marked slowing of metabolism in the liver. It is available in oral and parenteral forms. It is also excreted in the urine. It crosses the placenta and enters breast milk; caution should be used during pregnancy and lactation.
- Famotidine (*Pepcid, Pepcid AC*) is similar to ranitidine in terms of its actions and adverse effects, but it is much more potent than either cimetidine or ranitidine. It can be given orally or intravenously. It is metabolized in the liver and excreted in the urine. Famotidine crosses the placenta and enters breast milk; it should be used with caution during pregnancy and lactation.
- Nizatidine (*Axid*), the newest drug in this class, is similar to ranitidine in its effectiveness and adverse effects. It differs from the other three drugs in that it is eliminated by the kidneys, with no first-pass metabolism in the liver. It is the drug of choice for patients with liver dysfunction and for those who are taking other drugs whose metabolism is slowed by the hepatic activity of the other three H$_2$ antagonists. It is available only in an oral form. It too crosses the placenta and enters the breast milk.

Therapeutic Actions and Indications

H$_2$ antagonists selectively block histamine-2 receptor sites. This blocking leads to a reduction in gastric acid secretion and reduction in overall pepsin production (see Figure 57–1). H$_2$ receptor sites are also found in the heart, and high levels of these drugs can produce cardiac arrhythmias.

These drugs are used in the following conditions:

- Short-term treatment of active duodenal ulcer or benign gastric ulcer (reduction in the overall acid level can promote healing and decrease discomfort)
- Treatment of pathological hypersecretory conditions such as Zollinger–Ellison syndrome (blocking the overproduction of hydrochloric acid that is associated with these conditions)
- Prophylaxis of stress-induced ulcers and acute upper GI bleeding in critical patients (blocking the production of acid protects the stomach lining, which is at risk because of decreased mucus production associated with extreme stress)
- Treatment of erosive gastroesophageal reflux (decreasing the acid being regurgitated into the esophagus will promote healing and decrease pain)
- Relief of symptoms of heartburn, acid indigestion, and sour stomach (over-the-counter preparations)

Contraindications and Cautions

The H$_2$ antagonists should not be used with known allergy to any drugs of this class. Caution should be used during pregnancy or lactation, and with hepatic or renal dysfunction that could interfere with drug metabolism and excretion. (Hepatic dysfunction is not as much of a problem with nizatidine.) Care should also be taken if prolonged or continual use of these drugs is necessary, because they may be masking serious underlying conditions.

Adverse Effects

The adverse effects most commonly associated with H$_2$ antagonists include the following: GI effects of diarrhea or constipation; CNS effects of dizziness, headache, somnolence, confusion, or even hallucinations (thought to be related to possible H$_2$ receptor effects in the CNS); cardiac arrhythmias and hypotension (related to H$_2$ cardiac receptor blocking; more commonly seen with intravenous or intramuscular administration or with prolonged use); and gynecomastia (more common with long-term use of cimetidine) and impotence.

Clinically Important Drug–Drug Interactions

The three H$_2$ antagonists that are metabolized in the liver (cimetidine, famotidine, and ranitidine) can slow the metabolism of the following drugs, leading to increased serum levels and possible toxic reactions: warfarin anticoagulants, phenytoin, β-adrenergic blockers, alcohol, quinidine, lidocaine, theophylline, chloroquine, benzodiazepines, nifedipine, pentoxifylline, tricyclic antidepressants, procainamide, and carbamazepine. It is a good idea to review a patient's other medications carefully any time an H$_2$ antagonist is prescribed or a patient reports taking an over-the-counter form.

Nursing Considerations for Patients Receiving Histamine-2 Antagonists
Assessment: History and Examination

Screen for the following conditions, which could be cautions or contraindications to use of the drug: history of allergy to any H$_2$ antagonists; impaired renal or hepatic function; pregnancy or lactation; and a detailed description of the GI problem, including length of time of the disorder and medical evaluation.

Include screening for presence of any skin lesions; orientation and affect; baseline pulse and blood pressure, electrocardiogram (if intravenous use is needed); liver and abdominal examination; and liver and renal function tests.

DRUGS IN FOCUS
Histamine-2 Antagonists

Drug Name	Usual Dosage	Usual Indications
cimetidine (*Tagamet, Tagamet HB*)	300 mg PO q.i.d. at meals and h.s.; or 800 mg PO h.s.; 300 mg IV or IM q6–8h or 200 mg PO for heartburn; reduce dosage with geriatric patients or renal impairment.	Treatment of duodenal ulcer, benign gastric ulcer, pathological hypersecretory syndrome, gastroesophageal reflux disease (GERD); prophylaxis of stress ulcers; relief of symptoms of heartburn, acid indigestion, sour stomach **Special considerations:** Not for children <16 y old
famotidine (*Pepcid, Pepcid AC*)	20–40 mg PO or IV h.s. *or* 20 mg PO b.i.d.; 10 mg PO for prevention or relief of heartburn; reduce dosage in renal impaired or geriatric patients	Treatment of duodenal ulcer, benign gastric ulcer, pathological hypersecretory syndrome, GERD; relief of symptoms of heartburn, acid indigestion, sour stomach **Special considerations:** Not recommended for use in children
nizatidine (*Axid*)	150–300 mg PO h.s. *or* 150 mg PO b.i.d., 75 mg PO 30 min before food to prevent heartburn; reduce dosage in renal impaired or geriatric patients	Treatment of duodenal ulcer, benign gastric ulcer, pathological hypersecretory syndrome, GERD; relief of symptoms of heartburn, acid indigestion, sour stomach in adults
ranitidine (*Zantac*)	150 mg q.d.–b.i.d. PO IM or IV; 75 mg PO as needed for heartburn; reduce dosage in renal impaired or geriatric patients.	Treatment of duodenal ulcer, benign gastric ulcer, pathological hypersecretory syndrome, GERD; relief of symptoms of heartburn, acid indigestion, sour stomach in adults

Nursing Diagnoses

The patient who is receiving any H$_2$ antagonist may have the following nursing diagnoses related to drug therapy:

- Acute Pain related to CNS and GI effects
- Disturbed Sensory Perception (Kinesthetic, Auditory) related to CNS effects
- Decreased Cardiac Output related to cardiac arrhythmias
- Deficient Knowledge regarding drug therapy

Implementation

- Administer oral drug with or before meals and at bedtime (exact timing varies with product), *to ensure therapeutic levels when the drug is most needed.*
- Arrange for decreased dosage in cases of hepatic or renal dysfunction, *to prevent serious toxicity.*
- Monitor patient continually if giving intravenous doses, *to allow early detection of potentially serious adverse effects, including cardiac arrhythmias.*
- Assess patient carefully for any potential drug–drug interactions if giving in combination with other drugs, *because of the drug effects on liver enzyme systems.*
- Provide comfort and safety measures, including analgesics, ready access to bathroom facilities, assistance with ambulation, and periodic orientation if GI or CNS effects occur, *to ensure patient safety and improve patient tolerance of the drug and drug effects.*
- Arrange for regular follow-up, *to evaluate drug effects and the underlying problem.*

- Provide thorough patient teaching, including drug name, prescribed dosage, measures for avoidance of adverse effects, and warning signs that may indicate possible problems. Instruct patients about the need for periodic monitoring and evaluation, *to enhance patient knowledge about drug therapy and to promote compliance.* (See Patient Teaching Checklist: Histamine-2 Antagonists.)
- Offer support and encouragement, *to help patients cope with the disease and the drug regimen.*

PATIENT TEACHING CHECKLIST
Histamine-2 Antagonists

Create customized patient teaching materials for a specific histamine-2 antagonist from the CD-ROM. Patient teaching should stress the following points for drugs within this class:

- A histamine-2 antagonist decreases the amount of acid that is produced in the stomach. It is used to treat conditions that are aggravated by excess acid.

Some of the following adverse effects may occur with this drug:

- *Diarrhea*—Have ready access to bathroom facilities. This usually becomes less severe over time.

PATIENT TEACHING CHECKLIST
(CONTINUED)

Histamine-2 Antagonists

- *Dizziness, feeling faint on arising, headache*—These usually lessen as your body adjusts to the drug. Change positions slowly. If you fell drowsy, avoid driving or dangerous activities.

  Report any of the following to your health care provider: sore throat, unusual bleeding or bruising, confusion, muscle or joint pain, heart palpitations.

  Avoid the use of any over-the-counter medication without first checking with your health care provider. Several of these medications can interfere with the effectiveness of this drug. If an antacid has been ordered for you, take it exactly as prescribed.

  Tell any physician, nurse, or other health care provider that you are taking this drug.

  If you are taking any other medications, do not vary the drug schedules. Consult with your primary health care provider if anything should happen to change any of these drugs or your scheduled doses.

  It is important to have regular medical follow-up while you are taking this drug to evaluate your response to the drug and any possible underlying problems.

  Keep this drug, and all other medications, out of the reach of children.

This Teaching Checklist reflects general patient teaching guidelines. It is not meant to be a substitute for drug-specific teaching information, which is available in nursing drug guides.

Evaluation

- Monitor patient response to the drug (relief of GI symptoms, ulcer healing, prevention of progression of ulcer).
- Monitor for adverse effects (dizziness, confusion, hallucinations, GI alterations, cardiac arrhythmias, hypotension, gynecomastia).
- Evaluate effectiveness of teaching plan (patient can name drug, dosage, adverse effects to watch for, and specific measures to avoid adverse effects).
- Monitor effectiveness of comfort measures and compliance with regimen (see Nursing Care Guide: Histamine-2 Antagonists).

ANTACIDS

The antacids are a group of inorganic chemicals that have long been used to neutralize stomach acid. Antacids are available over the counter, and many patients use them to self-treat a variety of GI symptoms. All antacids have adverse effects, and there is no perfect antacid.

Administering an antacid frequently causes **acid rebound.** Neutralizing the stomach contents to an alkaline level stimulates gastrin production to cause an increase in acid produc-

tion and return the stomach to its normal acidic state. In many cases, the acid rebound causes an increase in symptoms, which results in an increased intake of the antacid. This leads to more acid production, and a cycle develops. When more and more antacid is used, the risk for systemic effects rises.

The choice of an antacid depends on adverse effect and absorption factors. Available agents are the following.

- Sodium bicarbonate (*Bell/Ans*), the oldest drug in this group, is readily available in many preparations, including baking soda. This drug is widely distributed when absorbed, crossing the placenta and entering breast milk. It should be used with caution during pregnancy and lactation because of the potential for adverse effects on the fetus or neonate. It is excreted in the urine and can cause serious electrolyte imbalance in people with renal impairment.
- Calcium carbonate (*Calciday-667, Tums,* and others), the next antacid to be developed, is actually precipitated chalk. The main drawbacks to this agent are constipation and acid rebound. It can be absorbed systemically and cause calcium imbalance. When absorbed, it is metabolized in the liver and excreted in the urine and feces. Known to cross the placenta and enter breast milk, this drug should be used with caution during pregnancy and lactation.
- Magnesium salts (*Milk of Magnesia* and others) are very effective in buffering acid in the stomach but have been known to cause diarrhea. Although these agents are not generally absorbed systemically, absorbed magnesium can lead to nerve damage and even coma. Because they are minimally absorbed systemically, this may be a drug of choice if an antacid is needed during pregnancy or lactation.
- Aluminum salts (*Basaljel, Amphojel,* and others) do not cause acid rebound but are not very effective in neutralizing acid. They are bound in the feces for excretion. They have been related to severe constipation. Aluminum binds dietary phosphates and cause hypophosphatemia, which can then cause calcium imbalance throughout the system. For that reason, this drug should be used with caution during pregnancy and should be avoided during lactation because of the potential for adverse effects on the fetus and neonate.
- Magaldrate (*Lowsium, Riopan*), an aluminum and magnesium salt combination, minimizes the GI effects of constipation and diarrhea by combining these two salts. It may cause a rebound hyperacidity and alkalosis. Magaldrate is not generally absorbed systemically. This drug should be used with caution during pregnancy and lactation because the potential for effects on the fetus or neonate is restricted.

Many of these antacids are available in combination forms to take advantage of the acid-neutralizing effect and block adverse effects. For example, a combination of calcium and aluminum salts (*Maalox*) buffers acid and produces neither constipation nor diarrhea.

Antacids can greatly effect the absorption of drugs from the GI tract. Most drugs are prepared for an acidic environment, and an alkaline environment can prevent them from being broken down for absorption or can actually neutralize

NURSING CARE GUIDE

Histamine-2 Antagonists

Assessment	Nursing Diagnoses	Implementation	Evaluation
HISTORY Allergies to any of these drugs, renal or hepatic failure, pregnancy and lactation, other drugs being taken	Acute Pain related to GI, CNS effects Disturbed Sensory Perception (Kinesthetic, Auditory) related to CNS effects Decreased Cardiac Output related to cardiac effects Deficient Knowledge regarding drug therapy	Administer with meals and at bedtime. Provide comfort and safety measures: analgesics, access to bathroom, safety precautions. Arrange for decreased dose in renal/hepatic disease. Provide support and reassurance to deal with drug effects and life-style changes. Provide patient teaching regarding drug name, dosage, adverse effects, precautions, warnings to report.	Evaluate drug effects: relief of GI symptoms, ulcer healing, prevention of ulcer progression. Monitor for adverse effects: dizziness, confusion; gynecomastia; arrhythmias; GI alterations. Monitor for drug–drug interactions as indicated for each drug. Evaluate effectiveness of patient teaching program. Evaluate effectiveness of comfort and safety measures.
PHYSICAL EXAMINATION Neurological: orientation, affect Skin: color, lesions CV: P, cardiac auscultation GI: liver evaluation Lab tests: CBC, liver, renal function tests			

them so that they cannot be absorbed. Patients taking antacids should be advised to separate them from any other medications by 1 to 2 hours.

Therapeutic Actions and Indications

Antacids neutralize stomach acid by direct chemical reaction (see Figure 57–1). They are recommended for the symptomatic relief of upset stomach associated with hyperacidity as well as the hyperacidity associated with peptic ulcer, gastritis, peptic esophagitis, gastric hyperacidity, and hiatal hernia.

Contraindications and Cautions

The antacids are contraindicated in the presence of any known allergy to antacid products. Caution should be used in the following instances: any condition that can be exacerbated by electrolyte or acid–base imbalance; any electrolyte imbalance; GI obstruction, which could cause systemic absorption; allergy to any component of the drug; renal dysfunction, which could lead to electrolyte disturbance if any absorbed antacid is not neutralized properly; and pregnancy and lactation, because of the potential for adverse effects on the fetus or neonate.

Adverse Effects

The adverse effects associated with these drugs relate to their effects on acid–base levels and electrolytes. Rebound acidity, in which the stomach produces more acid in response to the alkaline environment, is common. Alkalosis with resultant metabolic changes (nausea, vomiting, neuromuscular changes, headache, irritability, muscle twitching, and even coma) may occur. The use of calcium salts may lead to hypercalcemia and milk-alkali syndrome (seen as alkalosis, renal calcium deposits, severe electrolyte disorders). Constipation or diarrhea may result, depending on the antacid being used. Hypophosphatemia can occur with the use of aluminum salts. Finally, fluid retention and congestive heart failure can occur with sodium bicarbonate because of its high sodium content.

Nursing Considerations for Patients Receiving Antacids

Assessment: History and Examination

Screen for the following conditions, which could be cautions or contraindications to use of the drug: any history of allergy

CASE STUDY

Histamine-2 Antagonists

THE SITUATION

W. T., a 48-year old traveling salesman, had experienced increasing epigastric discomfort over a 7-month period. When he finally sought medical care, the diagnosis was a duodenal ulcer. He began taking magaldrate (*Riopan*) for relief of his immediate discomfort as well as cimetidine (*Tagamet*), 300 mg q.i.d.. W. T. was referred to the nurse for patient teaching and given an appointment for a follow-up visit in 3 weeks.

CRITICAL THINKING

• *Think about the physiology of duodenal ulcers and the various factors that can contribute to aggravating the problem.* What patient teaching points should be covered with this patient regarding diet, stress factors, and use of alcohol and tobacco?
• What adverse effects of the drugs should this patient be aware of?
• What lifestyle changes may be necessary to ensure ulcer healing, and how can W. T. be assisted in making these changes fit into the demands of his job?

DISCUSSION

Further examination indicated that W. T. is a healthy man except for the ulcer. Because he is basically healthy and does not seek medical care unless very uncomfortable (7 months of pain), he may find it difficult to comply with his drug therapy and any suggested lifestyle changes.

W. T. needs patient education, which, for purposes of building trust, should preferably be with the same nurse. The instruction should include information on duodenal ulcer disease; ways to decrease acid production (such as avoiding cigarettes, acid-stimulating foods, alcohol, and caffeine); and ways to improve the protective mucous layer of the stomach by decreasing stress and anxiety-causing situations. Cimetidine can cause dizziness and drowsiness, which could be a major problem if W. T. needs

to drive to meet his clients. Because of this adverse effect, another histamine-2 inhibitor may be preferable. Dizziness and drowsiness are more often associated with cimetidine than with some of the newer histamine-2 inhibitors. This effect should be discussed with W. T. If driving is an important part of W. T.'s job demands, he may want to explore other means of dealing with his ulcer pain and healing.

In addition, spacing of the cimetidine and antacid doses should be stressed. Cimetidine should be taken 1 hour before or 2 hours after any antacids, because they can interfere with the absorption of cimetidine and the patient may not receive a therapeutic dose. W. T. should be encouraged to avoid over-the-counter medications and self-medication, because several of these products contain ingredients that could aggravate his ulcer or interfere with the effectiveness of the drugs that have been prescribed. W. T. should be encouraged to return for regular medical evaluation of his drug therapy and his underlying condition.

Finally, W. T. should feel that he has some control over his situation. Because he does not routinely seek medical care, he may be more comfortable with a medical regimen that he has participated in planning. Allow him to suggest ways to decrease stress, ways to cut down on smoking or the use of alcohol without interfering with the demands of his job, and the best times to take the drugs in his schedule. He will learn in time which foods and situations irritate his condition. However, research has not shown that bland or restrictive diets are particularly effective in decreasing ulcer pain or spread, and they may actually increase patient anxiety. W. T. should be encouraged to jot down the situations or times of day that seem to cause him the most problems. This information can help to provide a guide for adjusting lifestyle and/or dietary patterns to aid ulcer healing and prevent further development of ulcers.

to antacids; renal dysfunction that might interfere with the drug's metabolism and excretion; electrolyte disturbances that could be exacerbated by the effects of the drug; and pregnancy or lactation, which would require caution.

Include screening for baseline data for assessing the effectiveness of the drug and the occurrence of any adverse effects associated with drug therapy. Assess the following: abdominal sounds, to ensure GI motility; mucous membrane status, to evaluate potential problems with absorption; and serum electrolytes and renal function tests.

Nursing Diagnoses

The patient receiving antacids may have the following nursing diagnoses related to drug therapy:

• Diarrhea related to GI effects
• Risk for Constipation related to GI effects

• Imbalanced Nutrition: Less Than Body Requirements, related to GI effects
• Risk for Excessive Fluid Volume related to systemic effects
• Deficient Knowledge regarding drug therapy

Implementation

• Administer the drug apart from any other oral medications (1 hour before or 2 hours after), *to ensure adequate absorption of the other medications.*
• Have patients chew tablets thoroughly and follow with water, *to ensure therapeutic levels reach the stomach to decrease acid.*
• Periodically monitor serum electrolytes, *to evaluate drug effects.*
• Assess patients for any signs of acid–base or electrolyte imbalance, *to arrange for appropriate interventions.*

DRUGS IN FOCUS
Antacids

Drug Name	Usual Dosage	Usual Indications
aluminum salts (*Basaljel, Amphojel*)	Adult: 500–1500 mg three to six times per day between meals and h.s. Pediatric: 50–150 mg/kg PO q24h in divided doses q4–6h	Symptomatic relief of gastrointestinal (GI) hyperacidity; treatment of hyperphosphatemia; prevention of formation of phosphate urinary stones
calcium salts (*Calciday, Tums*)	0.5–2 g PO as needed as an antacid	Symptomatic relief of GI hyperacidity, treatment of calcium deficiency, prevention of hypocalcemia
magaldrate (*Lowsium, Riopan*)	480–1080 mg PO 1 and 3 h after meals and h.s.	Symptomatic relief of GI hyperacidity in adults
magnesium salts (*Milk of Magnesia*, others)	280–1500 mg PO q.i.d., dose based on salt used Pediatric: one-half of the adult dose	Symptomatic relief of GI hyperacidity; prophylaxis of stress ulcers; relief of constipation
Ⓟ sodium bicarbonate (*Bell/Ans*)	Adult: 300–2000 mg PO q.d.–q.i.d.	Symptomatic relief of GI hyperacidity, minimization of uric acid crystalluria, adjunctive treatment in severe diarrhea

- Provide thorough patient teaching, including drug name, prescribed dosage, measures for avoidance of adverse effects, and warning signs that may indicate possible problems. Instruct patients about the need for periodic monitoring and evaluation, *to enhance patient knowledge about drug therapy and to promote compliance.*
- Offer support and encouragement, *to help patients cope with the disease and the drug regimen.*

Evaluation

- Monitor patient response to the drug (relief of GI symptoms caused by hyperacidity).
- Monitor for adverse effects (GI effects, serum electrolytes, and acid–base levels).
- Evaluate effectiveness of teaching plan (patient can give the drug and dosage, as well as describe adverse effects to watch for, specific measures to avoid adverse effects, and measures to take to increase the effectiveness of the drug).
- Monitor effectiveness of comfort measures and compliance with regimen.

PROTON PUMP INHIBITORS

The gastric acid pump or proton pump inhibitors suppress gastric acid secretion by specifically inhibiting the hydrogen–potassium adenosine triphosphatase (H^+,K^+-ATPase) enzyme system on the secretory surface of the gastric parietal cells. This action blocks the final step of acid production, lowering the acid levels in the stomach.

Five proton pump inhibitors are currently available.

- Omeprazole (*Prilosec*) is a faster-acting and more quickly excreted drug. It is used in combination therapy to treat ulcers caused by *H. pylori* bacteria. Omeprazole is also recommended for the relief of symptoms of heartburn.
- Esomeprazole (*Nexium*) is a longer-acting drug; it is not broken down as fast in the liver, compared with the parent drug omeprazole. It is indicated for the treatment of gastroesophageal reflux disease (GERD), severe erosive esophagitis, and pathological hypersecretory conditions.
- Lansoprazole (*Prevacid*), available only in a delayed-release form, is used in the treatment of gastric ulcers, GERD, and pathological hypersecretory syndromes; as part of maintenance therapy for healing duodenal ulcers and esophagitis; and in combination therapy for the eradication of *H. pylori* infection.
- Pantoprazole (*Protonix*) is used for the treatment of GERD, peptic ulcer, and Zollinger–Ellison syndrome. This drug is also available in a parenteral form for short-term use when the oral form cannot be tolerated.
- Rabeprazole (*Aciphex*) is available only in a delayed-release form and is used to heal and maintain GERD, for the healing of duodenal ulcers, and for the treatment of pathological hypersecretory conditions.

Therapeutic Actions and Indications

Proton pump inhibitors act at specific secretory surface receptors to prevent the final step of acid production and thereby decrease the level of acid in the stomach (see Figure 57–1). They are recommended for the short-term treatment of active duodenal ulcers, GERD, erosive esophagitis, and benign active gastric ulcer; for the long-term treatment of pathological hypersecretory conditions; as maintenance therapy for healing of erosive esophagitis and ulcers; and in combination with amoxicillin and clarithromycin for the treatment of *H. pylori* infection.

Pharmacokinetics

These drugs are acid labile and are rapidly absorbed from the GI tract. They undergo extensive metabolism in the liver and are excreted in the urine. There are no adequate studies of these drugs during pregnancy and lactation. Caution should be used, however, because of the potential for adverse effects on the fetus or neonate. The safety and efficacy of these drugs has not been established for patients younger than 18 years of age.

Contraindications and Cautions

These drugs are contraindicated in the presence of known allergy to either the drug or the drug components. Caution should be used in pregnant or lactating women.

Adverse Effects

The adverse effects associated with these drugs are related to their effects on the H^+,K^+-ATPase pump on the parietal and other cells. CNS effects of dizziness and headache are commonly seen; asthenia (loss of strength), vertigo, insomnia, apathy, and dream abnormalities may also be observed. GI effects can include diarrhea, abdominal pain, nausea, vomiting, dry mouth, and tongue atrophy. Upper respiratory tract symptoms, including cough, stuffy nose, hoarseness, and epistaxis, are frequently seen. Other, less common adverse effects include rash, alopecia, pruritus, dry skin, back pain, and fever. In preclinical studies, long-term effects of proton pump inhibitors included the development of gastric cancer.

Nursing Considerations for Patients Receiving Proton Pump Inhibitors

Assessment: History and Examination

Screen for any history of allergy to a proton pump inhibitor, pregnancy, or lactation.

Include screening to establish baseline data for assessing the effectiveness of the drug and the occurrence of any adverse effects associated with drug therapy. Assess skin color and lesions as well as reflexes, affect, and orientation. In addition, perform an abdominal and respiratory examination.

Nursing Diagnoses

The patient receiving proton pump inhibitors may have the following nursing diagnoses related to drug therapy:

• Diarrhea related to GI effects
• Risk for Constipation related to GI effects
• Imbalanced Nutrition: Less Than Body Requirements, related to GI effects
• Disturbed Sensory Perception (Kinesthetic, Auditory) related to CNS effects
• Deficient Knowledge regarding drug therapy

Implementation

• Administer drug before meals; ensure that the patient does not open, chew, or crush capsules; they should be swallowed whole *to ensure therapeutic effectiveness of the drug.*
• Provide appropriate safety and comfort measures if CNS effects occur, *to prevent patient injury.*

DRUGS IN FOCUS
Proton Pump Inhibitors

Drug Name	Usual Dosage	Usual Indications
esomeprazole (*Nexium*)	Acute: 20–40 mg/d PO for 4–8 wk; 20–40 mg/d PO for maintenance	Gastroesophageal reflux disease (GERD), severe erosive esophagitis, pathological hypersecretory conditions
lansoprazole (*Prevacid*)	15–30 mg/d PO based on condition and response	Treatment of gastric ulcer, GERD, pathological hypersecretory syndromes; maintenance therapy for healing duodenal ulcers and esophagitis; in combination therapy for the eradication of *Helicobacter pylori* infection
Ⓟ omeprazole (*Prilosec*)	20–40 mg/d PO for 4–8 wk based on condition and response	Treatment of gastric ulcers, GERD, pathological hypersecretory syndromes; maintenance therapy for healing duodenal ulcers and esophagitis; in combination therapy for the eradication of *H. pylori* infection
pantoprazole (*Protonix*)	40 mg PO q.d.–b.i.d. for ≤ 8 wk; 4 mg IV once daily for 7–10 d	Treatment of GERD in adults, healing of erosive esophagitis, treatment of hypersecretory syndromes
rabeprazole (*Aciphex*)	20–60 mg/d PO based on condition and response	Healing and maintenance of GERD, duodenal ulcers, pathological hypersecretory conditions

- Arrange for medical follow-up if symptoms are not resolved after 4 to 8 weeks of therapy, *because serious underlying conditions could be causing the symptoms.*
- Provide thorough patient teaching, including drug name, prescribed dosage, measures for avoidance of adverse effects, and warning signs that may indicate possible problems. Instruct patients about the need for periodic monitoring and evaluation, *to enhance patient knowledge about drug therapy and to promote compliance.*
- Offer support and encouragement, *to help patients cope with the disease and the drug regimen.*

Evaluation

- Monitor patient response to the drug (relief of GI symptoms caused by hyperacidity; healing of erosive GI lesions).
- Monitor for adverse effects (GI effects, CNS changes, dermatological effects, respiratory effects).
- Evaluate effectiveness of teaching plan (patient can give the drug and dosage and describe adverse effects to watch for, specific measures to avoid adverse effects, and measures to take to increase the effectiveness of the drug).
- Monitor effectiveness of comfort and safety measures and compliance with regimen.

ANTIPEPTIC AGENT

The antipeptic agent sucralfate (*Carafate*) is given to protect eroded ulcer sites in the GI tract from further damage by acid and digestive enzymes.

Therapeutic Actions and Indications

Sucralfate forms an ulcer-adherent complex at duodenal ulcer sites, protecting the sites against acid, pepsin, and bile salts. This action prevents further breakdown of the area and promotes ulcer healing. The drug also inhibits pepsin activity in gastric juices, preventing further breakdown of proteins in the stomach, including the protein wall of the stomach (see Figure 57–1).

Sucralfate is recommended for the short-term treatment of duodenal ulcers. It is used at a reduced dose for maintenance of duodenal ulcers after healing. In addition, this agent is undergoing investigation for the treatment of gastric ulcers; gastric damage induced by nonsteroidal anti-inflammatory drugs (NSAIDs); prevention of stress ulcers in acutely ill individuals; and the treatment of oral and esophageal ulcers due to radiation, chemotherapy, or sclerotherapy.

Pharmacokinetics

Sucralfate is rapidly absorbed, metabolized in the liver, and excreted in the feces. It crosses the placenta and may enter breast milk. Because of the potential adverse effects on the fetus or neonate, this drug should not be used during pregnancy or lactation unless the benefit to the mother clearly outweighs the potential adverse effects.

Contraindications and Cautions

Sucralfate should not be given to any person with known allergy to the drug or any of its components. It should not be given to individuals with renal failure or dialysis, because a buildup of aluminum may occur if it is used with aluminum-containing products. Caution should be used in patients who are pregnant or lactating.

Adverse Effects

The adverse effects associated with sucralfate are primarily related to its GI effects. Constipation is the most frequently seen adverse effect. Diarrhea, nausea, indigestion, gastric discomfort, and dry mouth may also occur. Other adverse effects that have been reported with the this drug include dizziness, sleepiness, vertigo, skin rash, and back pain.

Clinically Important Drug–Interactions

If aluminum salts are combined with sucralfate, there is a risk of high aluminum levels and aluminum toxicity. Extreme care should be taken if this combination is used.

In addition, if phenytoin, fluoroquinolone antibiotics (eg, ciprofloxacin, norfloxacin), or penicillamine is combined with sucralfate, decreased serum levels and drug effectiveness may result. In such combinations, the individual agents should be administered separately, with at least 2 hours between drugs.

Nursing Considerations for Patients Receiving an Antipeptic Agent
Assessment: History and Examination

Screen for the following conditions, which could be cautions or contraindications to use of the drug: any history of allergy

---

DRUGS IN FOCUS
Antipeptic Agent

Drug Name	Usual Dosage	Usual Indications
sucralfate (*Carafate*)	1 g PO b.i.d.–q.i.d.	Short-term treatment of duodenal ulcers; maintenance of duodenal ulcers after healing in adults

to sucralfate, renal dysfunction or dialysis, and pregnancy or lactation.

Include screening to establish baseline data for assessing the effectiveness of the drug and the occurrence of any adverse effects associated with drug therapy. Assess the following: skin color and lesions; reflexes, affect, and orientation; abdominal examination; and mucous membranes.

Nursing Diagnoses

The patient receiving sucralfate may have the following nursing diagnoses related to drug therapy:

- Diarrhea related to GI effects
- Risk for Constipation related to GI effects
- Imbalanced Nutrition: Less Than Body Requirements, related to GI effects
- Disturbed Sensory Perception (Kinesthetic) related to CNS effects
- Deficient Knowledge regarding drug therapy

Implementation

- Administer drug on an empty stomach, 1 hour before or 2 hours after meals and at bedtime, *to ensure therapeutic effectiveness of the drug.*
- Monitor patient for GI pain, *and arrange to administer antacids to relieve pain if needed.*
- Administer antacids between doses of sucralfate, not within 30 minutes of a sucralfate dose, *because sucralfate can interfere with the absorption of oral agents.*
- Provide comfort and safety measures if CNS effects occur, *to prevent patient injury.*
- Provide frequent mouth care; sugarless lozenges to suck; bowel training as needed; and small, frequent meals *if GI effects are uncomfortable.*
- Provide thorough patient teaching, including drug name, prescribed dosage, measures for avoidance of adverse effects, and warning signs that may indicate possible problems. Instruct patients about the need for periodic monitoring and evaluation, *to enhance patient knowledge about drug therapy and to promote compliance.*
- Offer support and encouragement, *to help patients cope with the disease and the drug regimen.*

Evaluation

- Monitor patient response to the drug (relief of GI symptoms caused by hyperacidity; healing of erosive GI lesions).
- Monitor for adverse effects (GI effects, CNS changes, dermatological effects).
- Evaluate effectiveness of teaching plan (patient can name drug and dosage and describe adverse effects to watch for, specific measures to avoid adverse effects, and measures to take to increase the effectiveness of the drug).
- Monitor effectiveness of comfort and safety measures and compliance with regimen.

PROSTAGLANDIN

The synthetic prostaglandin E_1 analog, misoprostol (*Cytotec*), is used to protect the lining of the stomach in situations that might lead to serious GI complications.

Therapeutic Actions and Indications

Prostaglandin E_1 inhibits gastric acid secretion and increases bicarbonate and mucous production in the stomach, thus protecting the stomach lining (see Figure 57–1). Misoprostol is used to prevent NSAID-induced gastric ulcers in patients who are at high risk for complications from a gastric ulcer (e.g., elderly or debilitated patients, patients with a past history of ulcer). It has also been found to be effective for treatment of duodenal ulcers in patients who are not responsive to H_2 antagonists, and it is being investigated for that purpose.

Pharmacokinetics

Misoprostol is rapidly absorbed from the GI tract, metabolized in the liver, and excreted in the urine. Caution should be used in the presence of hepatic or renal impairment, which could interfere with the effective metabolism and excretion of the drug. Misoprostol crosses the placenta and enters breast milk. It has been associated with fetal deaths in animal studies and should be given to women of child-bearing age only after a negative pregnancy test and with warnings to use a barrier form of contraceptives while taking this drug. If this drug is needed during lactation, another method of feeding the baby should be used.

Contraindications and Cautions

This drug is contraindicated during pregnancy; it is an abortifacient. Women of child-bearing age should be advised to have a negative serum pregnancy test within 2 weeks of beginning treatment, and they should begin the drug on the second or third day of their next menstrual cycle. In addition, they should be instructed to use barrier contraceptives during therapy. Caution should be used during lactation and with any known allergy to prostaglandins.

Adverse Effects

The adverse effects associated with this drug are primarily related to its GI effects—nausea, diarrhea, abdominal pain, flatulence, vomiting, dyspepsia, and constipation. Genitourinary effects, which are related to the actions of prostaglandins on the uterus, include miscarriages, excessive bleeding, spotting, cramping, hypermenorrhea, dysmenorrhea, and other menstrual disorders. Women taking this drug should be notified, both in writing and verbally, of these potential effects of this drug.

Nursing Considerations for Patients Receiving Prostaglandin

Assessment: History and Examination

Screen for the following contraindications to the use of the drug: any history of allergy to misoprostol, and pregnancy or lactation.

Include screening to establish baseline data for assessing

DRUGS IN FOCUS
Prostaglandin

Drug Name	Usual Dosage	Usual Indications
misoprostol (*Cytotec*)	200 μg PO q.i.d.; reduce dosage with renal impairment	Prevention of NSAID-induced ulcers in adults at high risk for development of these gastric ulcers

the effectiveness of the drug and the occurrence of any adverse effects associated with drug therapy. Assess abdominal examination, pregnancy test, and normal menstrual activity.

Nursing Diagnoses

The patient receiving misoprostol may have the following nursing diagnoses related to drug therapy:

- Diarrhea related to GI effects
- Risk for Constipation related to GI effects
- Imbalanced Nutrition: Less Than Body Requirements, related to GI effects
- Sexual Dysfunction related to genitourinary effects
- Deficient Knowledge regarding drug therapy

Implementation

- Administer to patients at high risk for NSAID-induced ulcers during the full course of NSAID therapy, *to prevent the development of gastric ulcers*. Administer four times a day—with meals and at bedtime.
- Arrange for a serum pregnancy test within 2 weeks before beginning treatment; begin therapy on the second or third day of the menstrual period, *to ensure that women of childbearing age are not pregnant and to prevent abortifacient effects associated with this drug.*
- Provide patient with both written and oral information regarding the associated risks of pregnancy, *to ensure that the patient understands the risks involved;* advise the use of barrier contraceptives during therapy, *to ensure prevention of pregnancy.*
- Assess nutritional status if GI effects are severe, *in order to arrange for appropriate measures to relieve discomfort and ensure nutrition.*
- Provide thorough patient teaching, including drug name, prescribed dosage, measures for avoidance of adverse effects, and warning signs that may indicate possible problems. Instruct patients about the need for periodic monitoring and evaluation, *to enhance patient knowledge about drug therapy and to promote compliance.*
- Offer support and encouragement, *to help patients cope with the disease and the drug regimen.*

Evaluation

- Monitor patient response to the drug (prevention of GI ulcers related to NSAIDs).
- Monitor for adverse effects (GI, genitourinary).
- Evaluate effectiveness of teaching plan (patient can name drug and dosage and describe adverse effects to watch for, specific measures to avoid adverse effects, and measures to take to increase the effectiveness of the drug).
- Monitor effectiveness of comfort and safety measures and compliance with regimen.

▢▮◕ WEB LINKS
Health care providers and patients may want to consult the following Internet sources:

Information on the anatomy and physiology of the GI tract, pathophysiology of various gastrointestinal ulcer disorders, treatments, and research:
http://webmd.lycos.com/content

Information for patients and families on ulcers, including treatments and causes of ulcers and *H. pylori* infection:
http://www.familydoctor.org/handouts/271.html

Information on gastroesophageal reflux disorders:
http://www.gerd.com

Information about *H. pylori* research and treatment:
http://www.cdc.gov

Educational materials on a variety of GI disorders:
http://healthanswers.com

DIGESTIVE ENZYMES

Some patients—those who have suffered strokes, salivary gland disorders, or extreme surgery of the head and neck, and those with cystic fibrosis or pancreatic dysfunction—may require a supplement to the production of digestive enzymes. Three digestive enzymes are available for replacement in conditions that result in lower than normal levels of these enzymes.

- Saliva substitute (*MouthKote, Salivart*) helps in conditions that result in dry mouth—stroke, radiation therapy, chemotherapy, and other illnesses. This drug is not generally absorbed systemically.

• Pancreatin (*Creon Capsules*) is used to aid the digestion and absorption of fats, proteins, and carbohydrates in conditions that result in a lack of this enzyme. This drug is thought to be processed through normal metabolic systems in the body. Little is known about its pharmacokinetics.

• Pancrelipase (*Cotazym, Ilozyme*) is used like pancreatin in conditions that result in a lack of pancrelipase. This drug is thought to be processed through normal metabolic systems in the body. Little is known about its pharmacokinetics.

Therapeutic Actions and Indications

Saliva substitute contains electrolytes and carboxymethylcellulose to act as a thickening agent in dry mouth conditions. This makes the food bolus easier to swallow and begins the early digestion process. The pancreatic enzymes are replacement enzymes that help the digestion and absorption of fats, proteins, and carbohydrates (see Figure 57–1). They are used as replacement therapy in patients with cystic fibrosis, chronic pancreatitis, ductal obstruction, pancreatic insufficiency, steatorrhea, or malabsorption syndrome and after pancreatectomy or gastrectomy.

Contraindications and Cautions

Saliva substitute is contraindicated in the presence of known allergy to parabens or any component of the drug. It should be used cautiously in patients with congestive heart failure, in hypertension, or renal failure, because there may be an abnormal absorption of electrolytes, including sodium, leading to increased cardiovascular load. Pancreatic enzymes should not be used with known allergy to the product or to pork products. In addition, they should be used cautiously in pregnancy and lactation.

Adverse Effects

The adverse effects most commonly seen with saliva substitute involve complications from abnormal electrolyte absorption, such as increased levels of magnesium, sodium, or potassium. The adverse effects that most often occur with pancreatic enzymes are related to GI irritation and include nausea, abdominal cramps, and diarrhea.

Nursing Considerations for Patients Receiving Digestive Enzymes

Assessment: History and Examination

Screen for the following conditions, which could be cautions or contraindications to use of the drug: any history of allergy to any of the drugs or to pork products (pancreatic enzymes); pregnancy or lactation; congestive heart failure or hypertension (saliva substitute).

Include screening for establishment of baseline data for assessing the effectiveness of the drug and the occurrence of any adverse effects associated with drug therapy. Assess the following: abdominal examination, mucous membranes; blood pressure, cardiac evaluation, and pancreatic enzyme levels (pancreatic enzymes).

Nursing Diagnoses

The patient receiving digestive enzymes may have the following nursing diagnoses related to drug therapy:

• Diarrhea related to GI effects
• Imbalanced Nutrition: Less Than Body Requirements, related to GI effects
• Deficient Knowledge regarding drug therapy

DRUGS IN FOCUS
Digestive Enzymes

Drug Name	Usual Dosage	Usual Indications
ⓟ pancreatin (*Creon Capsules*)	Adult: one to two capsules PO with meals or snacks	An aid for digestion and absorption of fats, proteins, and carbohydrates in conditions that result in a lack of this enzyme **Special considerations:** Not recommended for use in children.
pancrelipase (*Cotazym, Ilozyme*)	Adult: 4,000–48,000 U PO with each meal and snacks Pediatric: 6 mo–1 y—2000 U PO per meal; 1–6 y—4000–8000 U PO with meals, 4000 U with snacks; 7–12 y—4,000–12,000 U PO with each meal and snack	An aid for digestion and absorption of fats, proteins, and carbohydrates in conditions that result in a lack of this enzyme
saliva substitute (*MouthKote, Salivart*)	Spray or apply to oral mucosa	An aid in conditions resulting in dry mouth—stroke, radiation therapy, chemotherapy, and other illnesses

Implementation

- Have patient swish a saliva substitute around the mouth as needed for dry mouth and throat, *to coat the mouth and ensure therapeutic effectiveness of the drug.*
- Monitor swallowing, *because it may be impaired and additional therapy may be needed.*
- Administer pancreatic enzymes with meals and snacks, so that enzyme is available when it is needed. Avoid spilling powder on the skin, *because it may be irritating.* Do not crush the capsule or allow the patient to chew it; it must be swallowed whole, *to ensure full therapeutic effects.*
- Assess nutritional status if there are GI effects, *in order to arrange for appropriate measures to relieve discomfort and ensure nutrition.*
- Provide thorough patient teaching, including drug name, prescribed dosage, measures for avoidance of adverse effects, and warning signs that may indicate possible problems. Instruct patients about the need for periodic monitoring and evaluation, *to enhance patient knowledge about drug therapy and to promote compliance.*
- Offer support and encouragement, *to help patients cope with the disease and the drug regimen.*

Evaluation

- Monitor patient response to the drug (eg, relief of dry mouth and throat; digestion of fats, proteins, and carbohydrates).
- Monitor for adverse effects (eg, electrolyte imbalance, GI effects).
- Evaluate effectiveness of teaching plan (patient can name the drug and dosage and describe adverse effects to watch for, specific measures to avoid adverse effects, and measures to take to increase the effectiveness of the drug).
- Monitor effectiveness of comfort/safety measures and compliance with regimen.

CHAPTER SUMMARY

- GI complaints are some of the most common symptoms seen in clinical practice.
- Peptic ulcers may result from increased acid production, decrease in the protective mucous lining of the stomach, infection with *Helicobacter pylori* bacteria, or a combination of these.
- Agents used to decrease the acid content of the stomach include H_2 antagonists, which block the release of acid in response to gastrin or parasympathetic release; antacids, which chemically react with the acid to neutralize it; and proton pump inhibitors, which block the last step of acid production to prevent release.
- Acid rebound occurs when the stomach produces more gastrin and more acid in response to lowered acid levels in the stomach. Balancing the reduction of the stomach acid without increasing acid production is a clinical challenge.

- The antipeptic agent sucralfate forms a protective coating over the eroded stomach lining to protect it from acid and digestive enzymes and to aid healing.
- The prostaglandin misoprostol blocks gastric acid secretion while increasing the production of bicarbonate and mucous lining in the stomach.
- Digestive enzymes such as substitute saliva and pancreatic enzymes may be needed if normal enzyme levels are very low and proper digestion cannot take place.

Review Questions

1. Histamine-2 antagonists
   a. block the release of gastrin.
   b. selectively block histamine receptors reducing swelling and inflammation.
   c. selectively block H_2 receptor sites, leading to a reduction in gastric acid secretion and reduction in overall pepsin production.
   d. are effective only with long-term use.
2. H_2 receptors are found
   a. in the nasal passages, upper airways, and stomach.
   b. in the CNS and upper airways.
   c. in the respiratory tract and the heart.
   d. in the heart, CNS, and stomach.
3. The H_2 receptor blocker of choice for a patient with known liver dysfunction would be
   a. cimetidine.
   b. famotidine.
   c. nizatidine.
   d. ranitidine.
4. A patient receiving intravenous cimetidine for an acute ulcer problem needs to be monitored for
   a. GI upset.
   b. gynecomastia.
   c. cardiac arrhythmias.
   d. constipation.
5. Acid rebound occurs when
   a. lowering gastric acid to an alkaline level stimulates the release of gastric acid.
   b. raising gastric acid levels cause heartburn.
   c. combining protein, calcium, and smoking greatly elevates gastric acid levels.
   d. eating citrus fruit neutralizes gastric acid.
6. Frequent use of antacids is associated with many adverse effects but not
   a. systemic alkalosis.
   b. electrolyte imbalances.
   c. hyperkalemia.
   d. metabolic acidosis.
7. A patient taking a proton pump inhibitor should be instructed
   a. to take the drug after every meal.
   b. to chew or crush tablets to increase their absorption.
   c. to swallow tablets or capsules whole.
   d. to stop taking the drug after 3 weeks of therapy.

8. Misoprostol is a prostaglandin that is used to
   a. prevent uterine contractions.
   b. prevent NSAID-related gastric ulcers in patients at high risk.
   c. decrease hyperacidity with meals.
   d. relieve the burning associated with hiatal hernia at night.

9. Saliva substitute may be useful in all of the following conditions except
   a. cancer radiation therapy.
   b. after stroke.
   c. Parkinson's disease.
   d. brain injury.

10. A patient receiving pancreatic enzymes as replacement therapy, should be assessed for
    a. hypertension.
    b. cardiac arrhythmias.
    c. excessive weight gain.
    d. signs of GI irritation.

BIBLIOGRAPHY

Bullock, B. L. (2000). *Focus on pathophysiology*. Philadelphia: Lippincott Williams & Wilkins.

Drug facts and comparisons. (2002). St. Louis: Facts and Comparisons.

Gilman, A., Hardman, J. G., & Limbird, L. E. (Eds.) (2002). *Goodman and Gilman's the pharmacological basis of therapeutics* (10th ed.). New York: McGraw-Hill.

Karch, A. M. (2002). *2003 Lippincott's nursing drug guide*. Philadelphia: Lippincott Williams & Wilkins.

Professional's guide to patient drug facts. (2002). St. Louis: Facts and Comparisons.

C H A P T E R

58

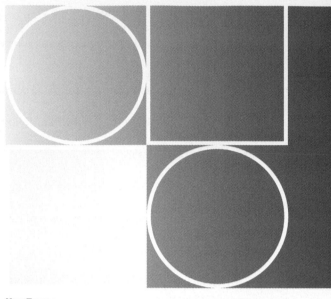

Key Terms

antidiarrheal drug
bulk stimulant
cathartic dependence
chemical stimulant
constipation
diarrhea
lubricant

Laxative and Antidiarrheal Agents

788

Drugs used to affect the motor activity of the gastrointestinal (GI) tract can do so in several different ways. They can be used to speed up or improve the movement of intestinal contents along the GI tract when movement becomes too slow or sluggish to allow for proper absorption of nutrients and excretion of wastes, as in **constipation.** Drugs are also used to increase the tone of the GI tract and to stimulate motility throughout the system. They can also be used to decrease movement along the GI tract when rapid movement decreases the time for absorption of nutrients, leading to a loss of water and nutrients and the discomfort of **diarrhea** (Figure 58–1).

LAXATIVES

Laxative, or cathartic, drugs are used in several ways to speed the passage of the intestinal contents through the GI

tract. Laxatives may be either **chemical stimulants,** which chemically irritate the lining of the GI tract; **bulk stimulants** (also called mechanical stimulants), which cause the fecal matter to increase in bulk; or **lubricants,** which help the intestinal contents move more smoothly (Table 58–1).

Chemical Stimulants

Drugs that act as chemical stimulants directly stimulate the nerve plexus in the intestinal wall, causing increased movement and the stimulation of local reflexes. Such laxatives include the following agents:

- Cascara (generic), a reliable agent that leads to intestinal evacuation; it may have a slow, steady effect or may cause severe cramping and rapid evacuation of the contents of the large intestine.
- Senna (*Senokot*), another reliable drug with effects similar

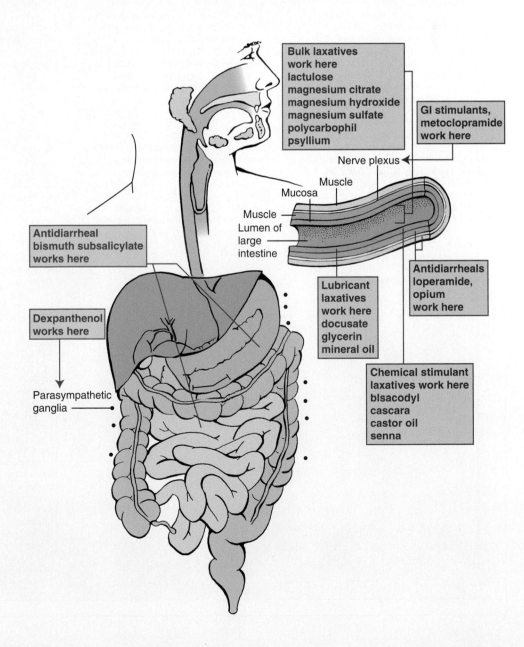

FIGURE 58–1. Sites of action of drugs affecting gastrointestinal motility.

TABLE 58-1 | Laxatives

Type	Names
Chemical stimulants	bisacodyl, cascara, castor oil, senna
Bulk stimulants	lactulose, magnesium citrate, magnesium hydroxide, magnesium sulfate, polycarbophil, psyllium
Lubricants	docusate, glycerin, mineral oil

DRUG THERAPY ACROSS THE LIFESPAN

Laxatives and Antidiarrheal Agents

Children	Adults	Older Adults
Laxatives should not be used in children routinely. Proper diet including roughage, plenty of fluids, and exercise should be tried first if a child has a tendency to become constipated. If a laxative is needed, glycerin suppositories are the best choice for infants and young children. Stool softeners can be used in older children; harsh stimulants should be avoided. Children with encoporesis, however, are often given senna preparations or mineral oil to help them evacuate the massive stool. Children receiving these agents should only use them for a short period and should be evaluated for potential underlying medical or nutritional problems if they are not able to return to normal function. Loperamide may be the antidiarrheal of choice in children >2 years of age if such a drug is needed. Special precautions need to be taken to monitor for electrolyte and fluid disturbances and supportive measures taken as needed.	Adults who use laxatives need to be cautioned not to become dependent. Proper diet, exercise and adequate intake of fluids should be adequate to keep the gastrointestinal tract functioning normally. If an antidiarrheal is needed, adults should be carefully instructed in the proper dosing of the drug and monitoring of their total use to avoid excessive dosage. The safety for the use of these drugs during pregnancy and lactation has not been established. Use should be reserved for those situations in which the benefit to the mother outweighs the potential risk to the fetus. A mild stool softener is often used after delivery. The drugs may enter breast milk and also may affect gastrointestinal activity in the neonate. It is advised that caution be used if one of these drugs is prescribed during lactation.	Older adults are more likely to develop adverse effects associated with the use of these drugs, including sedation, confusion, dizziness, electrolyte disturbances, fluid imbalance, and cardiovascular effects. Safety measures may be needed if these effects occur and interfere with the patient's mobility and balance. Older patients also may be taking other drugs that are associated with constipation and may need help to prevent severe problems from developing. Older adults are more likely to have renal and/or hepatic impairment related to underlying medical conditions, which could interfere with the metabolism and excretion of these drugs. The dosage for older adults should be started at a lower level than recommended for younger adults. The patient should be monitored very closely and dosage adjustment should be made based on patient response. These patients also need to be alerted to the potential for toxic effects when using over-the-counter (OTC) preparations and should be advised to check with their health care provider before beginning any OTC drug regimen. A psyllium product is the agent of choice with older adults because there is less risk of adverse reactions. The patient needs to be cautioned to drink plenty of fluid after taking one of these agents, to prevent problems that can occur if the drug starts to pull in fluid while still in the esophagus. The older adult should be encouraged to drink plenty of fluids, to exercise every day, and to get plenty of roughage in the diet. Many older adults have established routines, such as drinking warm water or prune juice at the same time each morning, that are disrupted with illness or hospitalization. These patients should be encouraged and helped to try to maintain their usual protocol as much as possible.

to cascara; it is found in many over-the-counter (OTC) preparations.

- Castor oil (*Neoloid*), an old standby, is used when a thorough evacuation of the intestine is desirable. This agent begins working at the beginning of the small intestine and increases motility throughout the rest of the GI tract. Because castor oil blocks absorption of fats (including fat-soluble vitamins) and may lead to constipation from GI tract exhaustion when there is no stimulus to movement, its frequent use is not desirable.
- Bisacodyl (*Dulcolax*), chemically related to phenolphthalein, is a very popular OTC laxative that was withdrawn from the market in 2000 because of adverse effects, including central nervous system (CNS) effects. This drug, which causes a slow and steady increase in movement in the large intestine, is often the drug of choice if mild stimulation is needed to prevent constipation and straining after GI surgery or myocardial infarction.

Bulk Stimulants

Bulk stimulants are rapid-acting, aggressive laxatives that increase the motility of the GI tract by increasing the fluid in the intestinal contents, which enlarges bulk, stimulates local stretch receptors, and activates local activity. Available bulk stimulants include the following agents:

- Magnesium sulfate (*Epsom Salts*), a very potent laxative, is used when total evacuation of the GI tract is needed rapidly, as in cases of GI poisoning. This agent acts by exerting a hypertonic pull against the mucosal wall, drawing fluid into the intestinal contents.
- Magnesium citrate (*Citrate of Magnesia*), found in a citrus-flavored base, is often used to stimulate bowel evacuation before many GI tests and examinations.
- Magnesium hydroxide (*Milk of Magnesia*) is used to stimulate bulk and is a milder and slower-acting laxative. It also works by a saline pull, bringing fluids into the lumen of the GI tract.
- Lactulose (*Chronulac*) is the alternative choice for patients with cardiovascular problems. This saltless osmotic laxative pulls fluid out of the venous system and into the lumen of the small intestine.
- Polycarbophil (*FiberCon*) is a natural substance that forms a gelatin-like bulk out of the intestinal contents. This agent stimulates local activity. It is considered milder and less irritating than many other bulk stimulants. Patients must use caution and take polycarbophil with plenty of water. If only a little water is used, it may absorb enough fluid in the esophagus to swell into a gelatin-like mass that can obstruct the esophagus and cause severe problems.
- Psyllium (*Metamucil*), another gelatin-like bulk stimulant, is similar to polycarbophil in action and effect.

Lubricating Laxatives

Sometimes it is desirable to make defecation easier without stimulating the movement of the GI tract by the use of lubri-

cants. Patients with hemorrhoids and those who have recently had rectal surgery may need lubrication of the stool. Some patients who could be harmed by straining might also benefit from this type of laxative.

- Docusate (*Colace*) has a detergent action on the surface of the intestinal bolus, increasing the admixture of fat and water and making a softer stool. This drug is frequently used as prophylaxis for patients who should not strain (such as after surgery, myocardial infarction, or obstetrical delivery).
- Glycerin (*Sani-Supp*) is a hyperosmolar laxative that is used in suppository form to gently evacuate the rectum without systemic effects higher in the GI tract.
- Mineral oil (*Agoral Plain*) is the oldest of these laxatives. It is not absorbed and forms a slippery coat on the contents of the intestinal tract. When the intestinal bolus is coated with mineral oil, less water is absorbed out of the bolus and the bolus is less likely to become hard or impacted. Frequent use of mineral oil can interfere with absorption of the fat-soluble vitamins A, D, E, and K. In addition, leakage and staining may be a problem when mineral oil is used and the stool cannot be retained by the external sphincter.

The type of laxative recommended depends on the condition of the patient, the speed of relief needed, and the possible implication of various adverse effects.

Therapeutic Actions and Indications

Laxatives work in three ways: (1) by direct chemical stimulation of the GI tract; (2) by production of bulk or increased fluid in the lumen of the GI tract, leading to stimulation of local nerve receptors; or (3) by lubrication of the intestinal bolus to promote passage through the GI tract (see Figure 58–1).

Laxatives are indicated for the short-term relief of constipation; to prevent straining when it is clinically undesirable (such as after surgery, myocardial infarction, or obstetrical delivery); to evacuate the bowel for diagnostic procedures; to remove ingested poisons from the lower GI tract; and as an adjunct in anthelmintic therapy when it is desirable to flush helminths from the GI tract. The use of proper diet and exercise, as well as taking advantage of the actions of the intestinal reflexes, has eliminated the need for laxatives in many situations; therefore, these agents are used less frequently than they once were in clinical practice. Most laxatives are available in OTC preparations, and they are often abused by people who then become dependent on them for stimulation of GI movement. Such individuals may develop chronic intestinal disorders as a result.

Pharmacokinetics

Most of these agents are only minimally absorbed and exert their therapeutic effect directly in the GI tract. Changes in absorption, water balance, and electrolytes resulting from GI changes can have adverse effects on patients with underlying medical conditions that are affected by volume and electrolyte changes. Use with caution during pregnancy and lactation, because of the lack of studies regarding the effects of these drugs. Castor oil should not be used during pregnancy, because its irritant effect has been associated with induction of premature labor. Magnesium laxatives can cause a diarrhea effect in the neonate.

Contraindications and Cautions

Laxatives are contraindicated in acute abdominal disorders, including appendicitis, diverticulitis, and ulcerative colitis, when increased motility could lead to rupture or further exacerbation of the inflammation. Laxatives should be used with great caution during pregnancy and lactation. In some cases, stimulation of the GI tract can precipitate labor, and many of these agents cross the placenta and are excreted in breast milk.

Adverse Effects

The adverse effects most commonly associated with laxatives are GI effects such as diarrhea, abdominal cramping, and nausea. CNS effects, including dizziness, headache, and weakness, are not uncommon and may relate to loss of fluid and electrolyte imbalances that may accompany laxative use. Sweating, palpitations, flushing, and even fainting have been reported after laxative use. These effects may be related to a sympathetic stress reaction to intense neurostimulation of the GI tract or to the loss of fluid and electrolyte imbalance.

A very common adverse effect that is seen with frequent laxative use or laxative abuse is **cathartic dependence.** This reaction occurs when patients use laxatives over a long period and the GI tract becomes dependent on the vigorous stimulation of the laxative. Without this stimulation, the GI tract does not move for a period of time (ie, several days), which could lead to constipation and drying of the stool and ultimately to impaction.

Clinically Important Drug–Drug Interactions

Because laxatives increase the motility of the GI tract and some interfere with the timing or process of absorption, it is advisable not to take laxatives with other prescribed med-

DRUGS IN FOCUS
Laxatives

Drug Name	Usual Dosage	Usual Indications
Chemical stimulants		
bisacodyl (Dulcolax)	10–15 mg PO or 2.5 g in water via enema	Prevention of constipation and straining after gastrointestinal (GI) surgery, myocardial infarction (MI), obstetrical delivery; short-term treatment of constipation
cascara (generic)	325–650 mg PO	Short-term treatment of constipation; evacuation of the large intestine for diagnostic examination
P castor oil (Neoloid)	15–30 mL PO	Emptying of the GI tract for diagnostic testing; short-term treatment of constipation
senna (Senokot)	1–8 tablets per day h.s. or 10–25 mL syrup	Short-term treatment of constipation; treatment of encopresis
Bulk laxatives		
lactulose (Chronulac)	15–30 mL PO	Short-term treatment of constipation; especially useful in patients with cardiovascular disorders
P magnesium citrate (Citrate of Magnesia)	1 glassful; 1/2 glass for pediatric patients	Bowel evacuation before GI diagnostic tests and examinations
magnesium hydroxide (Milk of Magnesia)	15–30 mL PO	Short-term treatment of constipation; prevention of straining after GI surgery, delivery, MI
magnesium sulfate (Epsom Salts)	10–25 mg PO	Treatment of GI poisoning; rapid evacuation of the GI tract
polycarbophil (FiberCon)	1 g PO, one to four times per day as needed; do not exceed 6 g/d for adults or 3 g/d for children	Mild laxative; short-term treatment of constipation
psyllium (Metamucil)	1 tsp or packet in cold water, one to three times per day; 1/2 packet for children	Mild laxative; short-term treatment of constipation
Lubricants		
docusate (Colace)	50–240 mg PO	Prevention of straining in postoperative, post-MI, and postpartum patients
glycerin (Sani-Supp)	4 mL liquid suppository	Short-term treatment of constipation
P mineral oil (Agoral Plain)	5–45 mL PO	Short-term treatment of constipation

ications. The administration of laxatives and other medications should be separated by at least 30 minutes.

Nursing Considerations for Patients Receiving Laxatives

Assessment: History and Examination

Screen for the following conditions, which could be cautions or contraindications to use of the drug: history of allergy to laxative, fecal impaction, or intestinal obstruction; acute abdominal pain, nausea, or vomiting; and pregnancy or lactation.

Include screening for the presence of any skin lesions; orientation and affect; baseline pulse; abdominal examination, including bowel sounds; and serum electrolytes.

Nursing Diagnoses

The patient receiving any laxative may have the following nursing diagnoses related to drug therapy:

- Acute Pain related to CNS and GI effects
- Diarrhea related to drug effects
- Deficient Knowledge regarding drug therapy

Implementation

- Administer only as a temporary measure, *to prevent development of cathartic dependence.*
- Arrange for appropriate dietary measures, exercise, and environmental controls, *to encourage return of normal bowel function.*
- Administer with a full glass of water, and caution the patient not to chew tablets, *to ensure that laxative reaches the GI tract to allow for therapeutic effects.* Encourage fluid intake throughout the day as appropriate, *to maintain fluid balance and improve GI movement.*
- Do not administer in the presence of acute abdominal pain, nausea, or vomiting, *which might indicate a serious underlying medical problem that could be exacerbated by laxative use.*
- Monitor bowel function, *to evaluate drug effectiveness.* If diarrhea or cramping occurs, discontinue the drug, *to relieve discomfort and to prevent serious fluid and electrolyte imbalance.*
- Provide comfort and safety measures, *to improve patient compliance and to ensure patient safety,* including ready access to bathroom facilities, assistance with ambulation, and periodic orientation if GI or CNS effects occur.
- Offer support and encouragement, *to help patient deal with the discomfort of the condition and drug therapy.*
- Provide thorough patient teaching, including name of drug, dosage prescribed, proper administration, measures to avoid adverse effects, warning signs of problems, and the importance of periodic monitoring and evaluation, *to enhance patient knowledge about drug therapy and promote compliance with the drug regimen.* (See Patient Teaching Checklist: Laxatives.)
- Offer support and encouragement, *to help patient deal with the diagnosis and the drug regimen.*

PATIENT TEACHING CHECKLIST

Laxatives

Create customized patient teaching materials for a specific laxative from the CD-ROM. Patient teaching should stress the following points for drugs within this class:

- A laxative prevents constipation and helps keep the gastrointestinal tract functioning on a regular basis. It is used when straining could be dangerous or when a situation arises that may result in constipation.
- This drug should be taken only as a temporary measure to relieve constipation.

Common effects of this drug include:

- *Diarrhea*—Have ready access to bathroom facilities. Consult with your health care provider if this becomes a problem.
- *Dizziness, weakness*—Change positions slowly. If you feel drowsy, avoid driving or dangerous activities.

Report any of the following conditions to your health care provider: sweating, flushing, dizziness, muscle cramps, excessive thirst.

Increase your intake of dietary fiber and fluid, and try to maintain daily exercise to encourage bowel regularity.

Tell any doctor, nurse, or other health care provider that you are taking this drug.

Keep this drug and all medications out of the reach of children.

This Teaching Checklist reflects general patient teaching guidelines. It is not meant to be a substitute for drug-specific teaching information, which is available in nursing drug guides.

Evaluation

- Monitor patient response to the drug (relief of GI symptoms, absence of straining, evacuation of GI tract).
- Monitor for adverse effects (dizziness, confusion, GI alterations, sweating, electrolyte imbalance, cathartic dependence).
- Evaluate effectiveness of teaching plan (patient can name the drug and dosage as well as describe adverse effects to watch for and specific measures to use to avoid adverse effects).
- Monitor effectiveness of comfort measures and compliance with regimen (see Nursing Care Guide: Laxatives).

GASTROINTESTINAL STIMULANTS

Some drugs are available for more generalized GI stimulation that results in an overall increase in GI activity and secretions. These drugs stimulate parasympathetic activity or make the GI tissues more sensitive to parasympathetic activity. Such stimulants include

- Dexpanthenol (*Ilopan*), which increases acetylcholine levels and stimulates the parasympathetic system

NURSING CARE GUIDE

Laxatives

Assessment	Nursing Diagnoses	Implementation	Evaluation
HISTORY	Acute Pain related to GI, CNS effects	Administer only as a temporary measure.	Evaluate drug effects:
Allergies to any of these drugs, acute abdominal pain, nausea, vomiting, Pregnancy and lactation	Diarrhea related to GI effects	Provide comfort and safety measures:	-relief of GI symptoms
	Deficient Knowledge regarding drug therapy	-assistance	-ulcer healing
		-access to bathroom	-prevention of ulcer progression
		-safety precautions.	Monitor for adverse effects:
		Do not administer in presence of acute abdominal pain, nausea, or vomiting.	-GI alterations
		Monitor bowel function.	-dizziness, confusion
		Provide support and reassurance for coping with drug effects and discomfort.	-cathartic dependence
			-electrolyte imbalance
		Provide patient teaching regarding	Monitor for drug–drug interactions as indicated for each drug.
		-drug name and dosage	Evaluate effectiveness of patient teaching program.
		-adverse effects and precautions	Evaluate effectiveness of comfort and safety measures.
		-warnings to report	
PHYSICAL EXAMINATION			
Neurological: orientation, affect			
Skin: color, lesions			
CV: P			
GI: abdominal evaluation			
Lab tests: serum electrolytes			

- Metoclopramide (*Reglan*), which blocks dopamine receptors and makes the GI cells more sensitive to acetylcholine, leading to increased GI activity and rapid movement of food through the upper GI tract

Therapeutic Actions and Indications

By stimulating parasympathetic activity within the GI tract, these drugs act to increase GI secretions and motility on a general level throughout the tract (see Figure 58–1). They do not have the local effects of laxatives to increase activity only in the intestines. These drugs are indicated when more rapid movement of GI contents is desirable. Dexpanthenol is indicated in many postoperative situations when intestinal atony or loss of tone could become a problem. Metoclopramide is indicated for relief of symptoms of gastroesophageal reflux disease; for prevention of nausea and vomiting after emetogenic chemotherapy or after surgery; for relief of symptoms of diabetic gastroparesis; and for the promotion of GI movement during small bowel intubation or to promote rapid movement of barium.

Pharmacokinetics

These drugs are rapidly absorbed, metabolized in the liver, and excreted in the urine. They cross the placenta and enter breast milk. No adequate studies are available on their effects during pregnancy and lactation, but they should be used only if the benefit to the mother clearly outweighs the potential risk to the fetus or neonate. Metoclopramide is being studied for improvement of lactation in doses of 30 to 45 mg/d. Its effectiveness in improving lactation may be linked to its dopamine-blocking effect, which is often associated with increased prolactin levels.

Contraindications and Cautions

GI stimulants should not be used in patients with a history of allergy to any of these drugs or with any GI obstruction or perforation. They should be used with caution during pregnancy or lactation.

Adverse Effects

The most common adverse effects seen with GI stimulants involve GI stimulation and include nausea, vomiting, diarrhea, intestinal spasm, and cramping. Other adverse effects, such as declining blood pressure and heart rate, weakness, and fatigue, may be related to parasympathetic stimulation.

Clinically Important Drug–Drug Interactions

Metoclopramide has been associated with decreased absorption of digoxin from the GI tract; patients taking this combination should be monitored carefully.

Decreased immunosuppressive effects and increased toxicity of cyclosporine have occurred when these drugs were combined. This combination should be avoided.

Increased sedation can occur if either of these drugs is combined with alcohol or other CNS sedative drugs.

Nursing Considerations for Patients Receiving Gastrointestinal Stimulants

Assessment: History and Examination

Screen for the following conditions, which could be cautions or contraindications to the use of the drug: any history of allergy to these drugs; intestinal obstruction, bleeding, or perforation; and pregnancy or lactation.

Include screening to establish baseline data for assessing the effectiveness of the drug and the occurrence of any adverse effects associated with drug therapy. Perform an abdominal evaluation, checking bowel sounds to ensure GI motility; assess pulse and blood pressure to monitor for adverse effects; and check skin color and lesions to assess for hypersensitivity reactions.

Nursing Diagnoses

The patient receiving GI stimulants may have the following nursing diagnoses related to drug therapy:

- Diarrhea related to drug effects
- Acute Pain related to GI effects
- Deficient Knowledge regarding drug therapy

Implementation

- Administer at least 15 minutes before each meal and at bedtime, *to ensure therapeutic effectiveness.*
- Monitor blood pressure carefully if giving drug intravenously, *to detect and consult with the prescriber about treatment for sudden drops in blood pressure.*
- Monitor diabetic patients, *in order to arrange for alteration in insulin dose or timing as appropriate.*
- Provide thorough patient teaching, including name of drug, dosage prescribed, proper administration, measures to avoid adverse effects, warning signs of problems, and the importance of periodic monitoring and evaluation, *to enhance patient knowledge about drug therapy and promote compliance with the drug regimen.*
- Offer support and encouragement, *to help the patient deal with the diagnosis and the drug regimen.*

Evaluation

- Monitor patient response to the drug (increased tone and movement of GI tract).
- Monitor for adverse effects (GI effects, parasympathetic activity).
- Evaluate effectiveness of teaching plan (patient can name the drug and dosage, as well as describe adverse effects to watch for and specific measures to take to avoid adverse effects and increase the effectiveness of the drug).
- Monitor effectiveness of comfort measures and compliance with regimen.

◻◼●◼ WEB LINKS

Health care providers and patients may want to consult the following Internet sources:

DRUGS IN FOCUS
Gastrointestinal Stimulants

Drug Name	Usual Dosage	Usual Indications
dexpanthenol (*Ilopan*)	250–500 mg IM, repeat in 2 h and then q6h as needed	Prevention of intestinal atony in postoperative situations in adults
℗ metoclopramide (*Reglan*)	10–20 mg IM, IV, or PO Pediatric (6–14 y): 2.5–5 mg IV over 1–2 min Pediatric (<6 y): 0.1 mg/kg IV over 1–2 min	Relief of symptoms of gastroesophageal reflux disease; prevention of nausea and vomiting after emetogenic chemotherapy or postoperatively; relief of symptoms of diabetic gastroparesis; promotion of gastrointestinal movement during small bowel intubation or promotion of rapid movement of barium

Information for the traveler about causes, treatments, and prevention of traveler's diarrhea:
http://www.cdc.gov/travel

Information on constipation—causes, diagnosis, research, treatment, and prevention across the life span:
http://medlineplus.nlm.nih.gov/medlineplus/constipation.html

Information on diarrhea—guidelines for prevention and treatment:
http://webmd.lycos.com

ANTIDIARRHEAL DRUGS

Antidiarrheal drugs, which block stimulation of the GI tract, are used for symptomatic relief from diarrhea. Available agents include the following:

• Bismuth subsalicylate (*Pepto-Bismol*) acts locally to coat the lining of the GI tract and soothe any irritation that might be stimulating local reflexes to cause excessive GI activity and diarrhea. This agent has been found to be very helpful in treating traveler's diarrhea and in preventing cramping and distention associated with dietary excess and some viral infections. Bismuth subsalicylate is absorbed from the GI tract, metabolized in the liver, and excreted in the urine. It crosses the placenta and should be used in pregnancy only if the benefit to the mother outweighs any potential risk to the fetus. It is not known whether it enters breast milk.

• Loperamide (*Imodium*) has a direct effect on the muscle layers of the GI tract to slow peristalsis and allow increased time for absorption of fluid and electrolytes. Loperamide is slowly absorbed, metabolized in the liver, and excreted in the urine and feces. It may cross the placenta and enter breast milk. It should be used in pregnancy or lactation only if the benefits clearly outweigh any potential risks to the fetus or neonate.

• Opium derivatives (paregoric) act to stimulate spasm within the GI tract, stopping peristalsis and diarrhea and the discomfort associated with it. A category C-III controlled substance, opium is readily absorbed, metabolized in the liver, and excreted in the urine. It crosses the placenta and enters breast milk and can have adverse effects on the fetus or neonate.

Box 58–1 describes combination antidiarrheal products. See Box 58–2 for a discussion of irritable bowel syndrome and its treatment.

BOX 58-1
Combination Antidiarrheal Products

Two very popular antidiarrheal agents combine atropine with a meperidine-like compound. Meperidine (*Demerol*) has a local effect on the gastrointestinal wall, causing a slowing of intestinal motility. Difenoxin and diphenoxylate are chemically related to meperidine and are used at doses that decrease gastrointestinal activity without having analgesic or respiratory effects. These drugs, which are controlled substances—difenoxin is category C-IV and diphenoxylate is category C-V—are combined with atropine to discourage deliberate use of excessive doses to get the euphoric effects associated with meperidine.

difenoxin with atropine (*Motofen*)	Adult: 2 tablets PO, then 1 tablet after each loose stool. Do not exceed 8 tablets in 24 h. Pediatric: not for use in children <12 y
diphenoxylate with atropine (*Lomotil, Logen, Lomanate*)	Adult: 5 mg PO q.i.d. Pediatric (2–12 y): use liquid form only, start with 0.3–0.4 mg/kg per day PO in four divided doses

BOX 58-2
Irritable Bowel Syndrome

Irritable bowel syndrome (IBS) is a very common disorder, striking three times as many women as men, and reportedly accounts for half of all referrals to gastrointestinal (GI) specialists. The disorder is characterized by abdominal distress, bouts of diarrhea or constipation, bloating, nausea, flatulence, headache, fatigue, depression and anxiety. No anatomical cause has been found for this disorder. Underlying causes might be stress related. Patients with this disorder have often suffered for years, not enjoying meals or activities because of their GI pain and discomfort.

Alosetron (*Lotronex*) was the first drug to provide relief to this patient population. This drug, a serotonin 5-HT antagonist, blocks specific serotonin receptors in the enteric nervous system of the GI tract, which leads to decreased perception of abdominal pain and discomfort, decreased GI motility, and increased colon transit time. In late 2000, alosetron was pulled from the market after less than a year of availability. Reports of ischemic colitis, mesenteric colitis and even death in patients who were using the drug led to this decision. In July 2002, after hearing lots of testimony and reading many petitions from patients, the FDA agreed to approve the release of the drug for marketing. This is the first time in the history of the FDA that a drug pulled from the market because of safety concerns has been re-released. Restrictions have been applied to the use of the drug, and patients who use it must read and sign a Patient-Physician Agreement. *Lotronex* should be discontinued immediately if the patient develops constipation or symptoms of ischemic colitis.

Tegaserod (*Zelmac*), a 5-HT$_4$ modulator, was then approved for the treatment of women with IBS; this slightly different serotonin receptor site is thought to help regulate the normal intestinal reflexes while relieving abdominal pain and discomfort. Hyoscyamine (*Nulev*), an anticholinergic agent that was found to decrease GI spasm, was approved in 2001 as an adjunctive therapy for the treatment of IBS. Support and symptomatic relief remain the mainstays of treating this disorder. Stress management and a consistent relationship with a health care provider may help to relieve some of the problems associated with this common, although not entirely understood, disorder.

Therapeutic Actions and Indications

Antidiarrheal agents slow the motility of the GI tract through direct action on the lining of the GI tract to inhibit local reflexes (bismuth subsalicylate); through direct action on the muscles of the GI tract to slow activity (loperamide); or through action on CNS centers that cause GI spasm and slowing (opium derivatives). These drugs are indicated for the relief of symptoms of acute and chronic diarrhea; reduction of volume of discharge from ileostomies; and prevention and treatment of traveler's diarrhea (see Figure 58–1).

Contraindications and Cautions

Antidiarrheal drugs should not be given to anyone with known allergy to the drug or any of its components. Caution should be used in pregnancy and lactation. Care should also be taken in individuals with any history of GI obstruction, acute abdominal conditions, or diarrhea due to poisonings.

Adverse Effects

The adverse effects associated with antidiarrheal drugs, such as constipation, distention, abdominal discomfort, nausea, vomiting, dry mouth, and even toxic megacolon, are related to their effects on the GI tract. Other adverse effects that have been reported include fatigue, weakness, dizziness, and skin rash.

Nursing Considerations for Patients Receiving Antidiarrheals

Assessment: History and Examination

Screen for the following conditions, which could be cautions or contraindications to the use of the drug: any history of allergy to these drugs; acute abdominal conditions; poisoning; and pregnancy or lactation.

Include screening for establishment of baseline data for assessing the effectiveness of the drug and the occurrence of any adverse effects associated with drug therapy. Assess skin color and lesions; abdominal examination; and orientation and affect.

Nursing Diagnoses

The patient receiving antidiarrheal drugs may have the following nursing diagnoses related to drug therapy:

- Constipation related to GI slowing
- Acute Pain related to GI effects
- Disturbed Sensory Perception (Kinesthetic, Gustatory) related to CNS effects
- Deficient Knowledge regarding drug therapy

Implementation

- Monitor response carefully. If no response is seen within 48 hours, *the diarrhea could be related to an underlying medical condition*. Arrange to discontinue the drug and arrange for medical evaluation, *to allow for diagnosis of underlying medical conditions*.
- Provide appropriate safety and comfort measures if CNS effects occur, *to prevent patient injury*.
- Administer drug after each unformed stool, *to ensure therapeutic effectiveness*. Keep track of exact amount given, *to ensure that dosage does not exceed recommended daily maximum dose*.
- Provide thorough patient teaching, including name of drug, dosage prescribed, proper administration, measures to avoid adverse effects, warning signs of problems, and the importance of periodic monitoring and evaluation, *to enhance patient knowledge about drug therapy and promote compliance with the drug regimen*.
- Offer support and encouragement, *to help the patient deal with the diagnosis and the drug regimen*.

Evaluation

- Monitor patient response to the drug (relief of diarrhea).
- Monitor for adverse effects (GI effects, CNS changes, dermatologic effects).

DRUGS IN FOCUS
Antidiarrheals

Drug Name	Usual Dosage	Usual Indications
bismuth subsalicylate (*Pepto-Bismol*)	Adult: 524 mg PO q30–60 min as needed, up to eight doses per day Pediatric: <3 y—not recommended; 3–6 y—⅓ tablet or 5 mL PO; 6–9 y—⅔ tablet or 10 mL PO; 9–12 y—1 tablet or 15 mL PO	Treatment of traveler's diarrhea; prevention of cramping and distention associated with dietary excess and some viral infections
Ⓟ loperamide (*Imodium*)	Adult: 4 mg PO, then 2 mg PO after each loose stool Pediatric (2–12 y): 1–2 mg PO t.i.d. Pediatric (<2 y): not recommended	Short-term treatment of diarrhea associated with dietary problems, viral infections
opium derivatives (paregoric)	Adult: 5–10 mL PO q.d.–q.i.d. Pediatric: 0.25–0.5 mL/kg PO q.d.–q.i.d. as needed	Short-term treatment of cramping and diarrhea

CASE STUDY

Traveler's Diarrhea

THE SITUATION

P. F. had received an all-expenses-paid trip to Mexico in honor of his graduation from college. He was very excited about getting away for a week of sun and fun and had arranged to stay in the same hotel as two college friends who were also celebrating. The three men had a wonderful time visiting the beaches, bars, and nightclubs in the area. On the third day of the trip, P. F. began experiencing nausea, some vomiting, and a low-grade fever. Several hours later he began experiencing intense cramping and diarrhea. For the next 2 days, P. F. felt so ill he was unable to leave his hotel room. The next morning, he called to arrange for an emergency trip home.

CRITICAL THINKING

• What is probably happening to P. F.? *Think about the gastrointestinal reflexes and explain the underlying cause for his signs and symptoms.*
• What treatment should be started now?
• What could have been done to prevent this problem from occurring?
• What possible drug therapy might have been helpful for P. F.?

DISCUSSION

P., F. is probably experiencing the common disorder called traveler's diarrhea. This disorder occurs when pathogens found in the food and water of a foreign environment are ingested. (Because these pathogens are commonly found in the environment, they do not normally cause problems for the people who live in the area.) When the pathogen, usually a strain of *Escherichia coli*, enters a host that is not accustomed to the bacteria, it releases enterotoxins and sets off an intestinal–intestinal reaction in the host.

The intestinal–intestinal reaction results in a slowing of activity above the point of irritation (which causes nausea and in some cases vomiting) and an increase in activity below the point of irritation. The body is trying to flush the invader from the body. A low-grade fever may occur as a reaction to the toxins released by the bacteria. Muscle aches and pains, malaise, and fatigue are often common symptoms. It is important at this stage of the disease to maintain fluid intake to prevent dehydration from occurring.

P. F. may want to fly home, but with intense cramping and diarrhea it might not be a good idea to try. Bismuth subsalicylate (*Pepto-Bismol*), taken four times a day, has been shown to be effective in preventing traveler's diarrhea and associated problems. Taken during a course of traveler's diarrhea, it may relieve the stomach upset and nausea and some of the discomfort of the diarrhea. Some patients respond to the prophylactic antibiotics *Bactrim* and *Septra*, combinations of trimethoprim and sulfamethoxazole that are often prescribed as prophylactic measures for patients who are traveling to areas known to be associated with traveler's diarrhea and for those who are known to be very susceptible to the disorder.

The best course of action, however, is prevention. Several measures can be taken to avoid ingestion of the local bacteria: drinking only bottled or mineral water; avoiding fresh fruits and vegetables that may have been washed in the local water, unless they are peeled; avoiding ice cubes in drinks, because the ice cubes are made from the local water; avoiding any food that might be undercooked or rare, including shellfish; and even being cautious about using water to brush the teeth or gargle. People who have suffered a bout of traveler's diarrhea are very cautious about exposure to local bacteria when they travel again, often combining prophylactic drug therapy with careful avoidance of local pathogens. P. F. can be reassured that in a few days the diarrhea and associated signs and symptoms should pass and he will regain his strength and energy.

• Evaluate effectiveness of teaching plan (patient can name the drug and dosage, as well as describe adverse effects to watch for, specific measures to use to avoid adverse effects, and measures to take to increase the effectiveness of the drug).
• Monitor effectiveness of comfort and safety measures and compliance with regimen.

CHAPTER SUMMARY

• Laxatives are drugs used to stimulate movement along the GI tract and to aid excretion. They may be used to prevent or treat constipation.
• Laxatives can be chemical stimulants, which directly irritate the local nerve plexus; bulk stimulants, which increase the size of the food bolus and stimulate stretch receptors in the wall of the intestine; or lubricants, which facilitate movement of the bolus through the intestines.
• Use of proper diet and exercise, as well as taking advantage of the actions of the intestinal reflexes, has eliminated the need for laxatives in many situations.
• Cathartic dependence can occur with the chronic use of laxatives, leading to a need for external stimuli for normal functioning of the GI tract.
• GI stimulants act to increase parasympathetic stimulation in the GI tract and to increase tone and general movement throughout the GI system.
• Antidiarrheal drugs are used to soothe irritation to the intestinal wall; block GI muscle activity to decrease movement; or affect CNS activity to cause GI spasm and stop movement.

Review Questions

1. Laxatives are drugs that are used to
   a. increase the quantity of wastes excreted.
   b. speed the passage of the intestinal contents through the GI tract.
   c. increase digestion of intestinal contents.
   d. increase the water content of the intestinal contents.
2. A laxative of choice when mild stimulation is needed to prevent straining would be
   a. senna.
   b. castor oil.
   c. bisacodyl.
   d. magnesium citrate.
3. Mineral oil would not be the laxative of choice for a
   a. debilitated patient low on nutrients.
   b. patient with hemorrhoids.
   c. patient with recent rectal surgery.
   d. child with encopresis.
4. Laxatives are not known to work by
   a. acting as chemical stimulants.
   b. acting as lubricants of the intestinal bolus.
   c. act to increase bulk of the intestinal bolus and stimulate movement.
   d. stimulating CNS centers in the medulla to cause GI movement.
5. Cathartic dependence can occur when
   a. patients do not use laxatives and become very constipated.
   b. chronic use of laxatives leads to a reliance on the intense stimulation of laxatives to cause movement.
   c. patients maintain a good diet including roughage.
   d. patients start an exercise program.
6. Drugs that stimulate parasympathetic activity are used to increase GI activity and secretions. This could be therapeutic in the treatment of
   a. duodenal ulcers.
   b. gastric ulcers.
   c. signs and symptoms of gastroesophageal reflux disease.
   d. poisoning, to induce nausea and vomiting.
7. The drug of choice for treating traveler's diarrhea would be
   a. loperamide.
   b. opium.
   c. cisapride.
   d. bismuth subsalicylate.
8. Patient teaching for a patient taking a laxative would not include
   a. the importance of proper diet and fluid intake.
   b. the need to take the drug for several weeks to get the full effect.
   c. the importance of exercise.
   d. taking advantage of natural reflexes by providing privacy and time to allow them to work.

BIBLIOGRAPHY

Bullock, B. L. (2000). *Focus on pathophysiology*. Philadelphia: Lippincott Williams & Wilkins.
Drug facts and comparisons. (2002). St. Louis: Facts and Comparisons.
Gilman, A., Hardman, J. G., & Limbird, L. E. (Eds.) (2002). *Goodman and Gilman's the pharmacological basis of therapeutics* (10th ed.). New York: McGraw-Hill.
Karch, A. M. (2002). *2003 Lippincott's nursing drug guide*. Philadelphia: Lippincott Williams & Wilkins.
The medical letter on drugs and therapeutics. (2002). New Rochelle, NY: Medical Letter.
Porth, C. M. (2002). *Pathophysiology: Concepts of altered health states* (6th ed.). Philadelphia: Lippincott Williams & Wilkins.

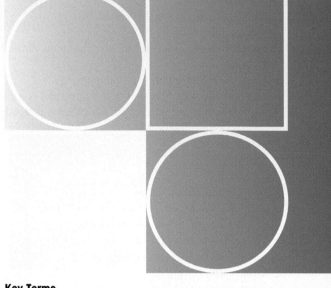

Key Terms
antiemetic
emetic
intractable hiccough
phenothiazine
photosensitivity
vestibular

Emetic and Antiemetic Agents

800

One of the most common and most uncomfortable complaints encountered in clinical practice is that of nausea and vomiting. Vomiting is a complex reflex reaction to various stimuli (see Chapter 56). In some cases of overdose or poisoning, it may be desirable to induce vomiting to rapidly rid the body of a toxin. This can be accomplished by physical stimuli, often to the back of the throat, or by treatment with an **emetic** agent such as syrup of ipecac. In some cases, gastric lavage is used to wash out the contents of the stomach.

In many clinical conditions, the reflex reaction of vomiting is not beneficial in ridding the body of any toxins but is uncomfortable and even clinically hazardous to the patient's condition. In such cases, an **antiemetic** is used to decrease or prevent nausea and vomiting. Antiemetic agents can be centrally acting or locally acting, and they have varying degrees of effectiveness.

EMETIC AGENTS

Ipecac syrup is the standard emetic agent in use today. It can be purchased in prepackaged 1-ounce containers without a prescription to have on hand in case of emergency. Ipecac administration is always followed by water. Drinking the water helps to ensure that the drug is flushed through the gastrointestinal (GI) tract and greatly decreases any absorption.

Therapeutic Actions and Indications
Ipecac syrup irritates the GI mucosa locally (Figure 59–1), which stimulates the chemoreceptor trigger zone (CTZ) in the brain to induce vomiting within 20 minutes. Ipecac syrup is used to induce vomiting as a treatment for drug overdose and certain poisonings.

Pharmacokinetics
Very little ipecac is absorbed systemically when taken as instructed, followed by water. It should be used with caution during pregnancy because of the potential for adverse effects associated with vomiting.

Contraindications and Cautions
The use of ipecac syrup is contraindicated in the following conditions: when caustic alkali or corrosive mineral acids have been ingested, because the potential for serious damage to the upper GI tract and airways overrides any benefit; when a volatile petroleum distillate such as kerosene has

DRUG THERAPY ACROSS THE LIFESPAN

Emetic and Antiemetic Agents

Children	Adults	Older Adults
Children are often given ipecac after accidental ingestion of potentially toxic substances. Parents who keep an emergency ipecac kit in the home should be instructed in the proper use of the drug, the importance of following it with plenty of water, and where to call if the child does not respond. Antiemetics should be used with caution in children who are at higher risk for adverse effects, including central nervous system (CNS) effects, as well as fluid and electrolyte disturbances. Prochlorperazine is often a drug of choice with children, and it has established oral, rectal and parenteral doses. Promethazine often has fewer adverse effects, but it should not be used with children who have liver impairment, Reye's syndrome, or sleep apnea. The serotonin 5-HT$_3$ agents have been very successfully used in children younger than 2 years of age. Care should be used when determining dosage and timing of dosage. Dronabinol does not have established guidelines for children, but if it is used, the child should be constantly supervised and dosage should be calculated very carefully based on age and weight.	Adults who use ipecac should be cautioned to follow the drug with plenty of water to avoid inadvertent absorption. Antiemetics are often used after surgery or chemotherapy, and precautions should be used to ensure that CNS effects do not interfere with mobility or other activities. The safety of these drugs during pregnancy and lactation has not been established. Use should be reserved for those situations in which the benefit to the mother outweighs the potential risk to the fetus. The drugs may enter breast milk and also may cause fluid imbalance that could interfere with milk production. It is advised that caution be used if one of these drugs is prescribed during lactation.	Older adults are more likely to develop adverse effects associated with the use of these drugs including sedation, confusion, dizziness, fluid imbalance, and cardiovascular effects. Safety measures may be needed if these effects occur and interfere with the patient's mobility and balance. Older adults are also more likely to have renal and/or hepatic impairment related to underlying medical conditions, which could interfere with the metabolism and excretion of these drugs. The dosage for older adults should be started at a lower level than recommended for young adults. The patient should be monitored very closely, and dosage adjustment should be made based on patient response. If dronabinol is used with older patients, special safety precautions should be in place, because the older patient is more likely to experience CNS effects and related problems when using this drug.

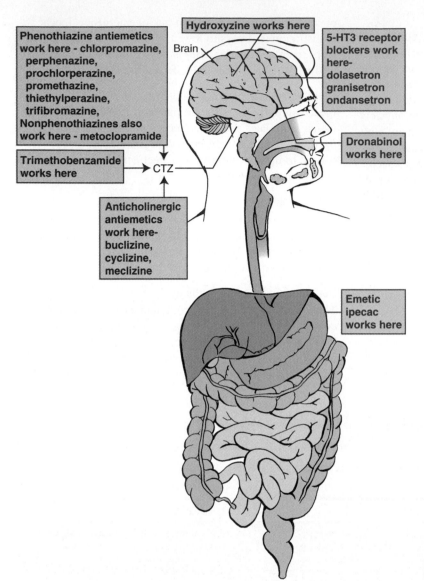

Phenothiazine antiemetics work here - chlorpromazine, perphenazine, prochlorperazine, promethazine, thiethylperazine, trifibromazine, Nonphenothiazines also work here - metoclopramide

Trimethobenzamide works here

Anticholinergic antiemetics work here- buclizine, cyclizine, meclizine

Brain

Hydroxyzine works here

5-HT3 receptor blockers work here- dolasetron granisetron ondansetron

Dronabinol works here

CTZ

Emetic ipecac works here

FIGURE 59–1. Sites of action of emetics/antiemetics. CTZ, chemoreceptor trigger zone.

been swallowed, because the risk of aspiration into the lungs, with a resultant fulminant and untreatable pneumonia, is serious; when a patient is comatose or semicomatose or shows signs of convulsing, again because the risk of aspiration is too great; or when a rapid-acting and specific antidote to the poison is available and that treatment would be the most appropriate. These contraindications are summarized in Box 59–1. Caution should be used during pregnancy.

BOX 59-1

Contraindications to Induced Vomiting

Ingestion of caustic or corrosive mineral acid
Ingestion of a volatile petroleum distillate
Comatose or semicomatose patient
Signs of convulsions

Adverse Effects

The adverse effects associated with the use of ipecac syrup, such as nausea, diarrhea, and GI upset, are related to its irritating effect on the GI mucosa. Its central nervous system (CNS) effects include mild CNS depression. Cardiotoxicity may occur if large amounts of the drug are absorbed, not vomited.

Nursing Considerations for Patients Receiving an Emetic Agent

Assessment: History and Examination

Screen for the exact poison or toxin that might have been swallowed; for a history of convulsions; and for semiconscious state.

Include screening for orientation, affect, baseline pulse, auscultation, and bowel sounds.

Nursing Diagnoses

The patient receiving an emetic agent may have the following nursing diagnoses related to drug therapy:

DRUGS IN FOCUS
Emetic Agent

Drug Name	Usual Dosage	Usual Indications
P ipecac (generic)	Adult: 15–30 mL PO followed by 3–4 glasses of water Pediatric (<1 y): 5–10 mL PO followed by ½–1 glass of water Pediatric (>1 y): 15 mL PO followed by 2–3 glasses of water. Dosage may be repeated if vomiting does not occur within 20–30 min; if vomiting does not occur within 30–45 min after second dose, perform gastric lavage	Induction of vomiting as a treatment for drug overdose or certain poisonings

- Acute Pain related to CNS and GI effects
- Decreased Cardiac Output related to cardiotoxicity
- Deficient Knowledge regarding drug therapy

Implementation

- Administer the drug to conscious patients only, *to prevent aspiration of the liquid.*
- Administer the drug as soon after poisoning or overdose as possible, *to increase effectiveness of induced vomiting and to decrease risk of absorption of the drug or poison.*
- Use caution to differentiate ipecac syrup from ipecac fluid concentrate, *which is 14 times stronger and has caused deaths.*
- Consult with a poison control center, *if in doubt about using ipecac syrup or if vomiting has not occurred within 30 to 45 minutes after a second dose.*
- Administer with a large amount of water to ensure that the drug reaches the GI tract and *to ensure that the stomach contains fluid to vomit, to decrease the incidence of acid burns during vomiting.*
- Maintain emergency equipment on standby, *in case poisoning is not reversed or ipecac does not induce vomiting.*
- Provide comfort and safety measures, including analgesics, ready access to bathroom facilities, assistance with ambulation, and periodic orientation if GI or CNS effects occur, *to prevent patient injury and increase patient comfort.*
- Provide thorough patient teaching, including name of drug, dosage prescribed, proper administration, measures to avoid adverse effects, warning signs of problems, the importance of periodic monitoring and evaluation, and the need to avoid overdose and poisoning, *to enhance patient knowledge about drug therapy and promote compliance with the drug regimen.*
- Offer support and encouragement, *to help the patient deal with the drug effects and the effects of the poison.*

Evaluation

- Monitor patient response to the drug (vomiting within 20 to 30 minutes after the first dose of the drug or within 30 to 45 minutes after a second dose of drug).

- Monitor for adverse effects (dizziness, confusion, GI upset, diarrhea, cardiac arrhythmias).
- Evaluate effectiveness of teaching plan (patient can name the drug and dosage as well as describe the adverse effects to watch for and specific measures to avoid these adverse effects).
- Monitor effectiveness of comfort measures and compliance with regimen.

◻◉◻ WEB LINKS
Health care providers and patients may want to consult the following Internet sources:

Information on nausea and vomiting associated with cancer chemotherapy:
http://www.anzemet.com

Information on nausea and vomiting, including causes, research, and alternative therapies:
http://www.aomc.org/HOD2/general/general-NAUSEA.html

Information on drugs used to treat nausea and vomiting:
http://www.medinfo.co.uk

Information for patients and healthcare workers on ipecac and home treatment of various poisons:
http://www.mgh.org/poison/index.html

ANTIEMETIC AGENTS

Drugs used in the management of nausea and vomiting are called antiemetics. All of them work by reducing the hyperactivity of the vomiting reflex in one of two ways: locally, to decrease the local response to stimuli that are being sent to the medulla to induce vomiting, or centrally, to directly block the CTZ or suppress the vomiting center. The locally acting antiemetics may be antacids, local anesthetics, adsorbents, protective drugs that coat the GI mucosa, or drugs that prevent distention and stretch stimulation of the GI tract. These agents are often reserved for use in mild nausea. Many of these drugs are discussed in Chapter 58.

Centrally acting antiemetics can be divided into several groups: phenothiazines, nonphenothiazines, serotonin (5-HT$_3$) receptor blockers, anticholinergics/antihistamines, and a miscellaneous group (Table 59-1).

The two most commonly used **phenothiazines** are prochlorperazine (*Compazine*) and promethazine (*Phenergan*), both of which have rapid onset and limited adverse effects. Other drugs in this group include chlorpromazine (*Thorazine*), perphenazine (*Trilafon*), thiethylperazine (*Torecan*), and triflupromazine (*Vesprin*). Chapter 22 discusses the phenothiazines in greater detail.

The nonphenothiazine available for use is metoclopramide (*Reglan*), which acts to reduce the responsiveness of the nerve cells in the CTZ to circulating chemicals that induce vomiting. Chapter 58 discusses metoclopramide in greater detail.

Anticholinergics/antihistamines include buclizine (*Bucladin-S*), cyclizine (*Marezine*), and meclizine (*Antivert*). These drugs are anticholinergics that act as antihistamines and block the transmission of impulses to the CTZ. Chapter 33 discusses the anticholinergics in greater detail.

The 5-HT$_3$ receptor blockers are blockers of those receptors associated with nausea and vomiting in the CTZ and locally. They include dolasetron (*Anzemet*), granisetron (*Kytril*), and ondansetron (*Zofran*). These drugs are rapidly absorbed, metabolized in the liver, and excreted in the urine and feces. Because they are known to cross the placenta and enter breast milk, use during pregnancy and lactation should be limited to situations in which the benefit to the mother outweighs the potential risk to the fetus or neonate.

Miscellaneous agents include dronabinol (*Marinol*), which contains the active ingredient of cannabis (marijuana); hydroxyzine (generic), which may suppress cortical areas of the CNS; and trimethobenzamide (*Tigan*), which is similar to the antihistamines but is not an antihistamine and is not as sedating. Trimethobenzamide is often a drug of choice in this group because it is not associated with as much sedation and CNS suppression. It is available in oral, parenteral, and suppository forms. It is rapidly absorbed, metabolized in the liver, and excreted in the urine. It crosses the placenta and enters breast milk, and use should be reserved for situations in which the benefit to the mother outweighs and potential risk to the fetus or neonate.

Hydroxyzine used for nausea and vomiting before or after obstetrical delivery or surgery. It is rapidly absorbed, me-tabolized in the liver, and excreted in the urine. It has not been associated with fetal problems during pregnancy and is not thought to enter breast milk. As with all drugs, caution should be used during pregnancy and lactation.

Dronabinol is approved for use in managing the nausea and vomiting associated with cancer chemotherapy in cases that have not responded to other treatment. Its exact mechanism of action is not understood. This drug, a category C-III controlled substance, must be used under close supervision because of the possibility of altered mental status. It is readily absorbed and metabolized in the liver, with excretion through the bile and in the urine.

Therapeutic Actions and Indications

As stated earlier, the locally active antiemetics are used to relieve mild nausea. The centrally acting antiemetics change the responsiveness or stimulation of the CTZ in the medulla (see Figure 59-1). The phenothiazines are recommended for the treatment of nausea and vomiting, including that specifically associated with anesthesia; severe vomiting; **intractable hiccoughs,** which occur with repetitive stimulation of the diaphragm and lead to persistent diaphragm spasm; and nausea and vomiting. The anticholinergics that act as antihistamines are recommended for the nausea and vomiting associated with motion sickness or **vestibular** (inner ear) problems. Some of these agents are available over the counter in a reduced dose for prevention or self-treatment of motion sickness. The 5-HT$_3$ receptor blockers are specific for the treatment of nausea and vomiting associated with emetogenic chemotherapy. These are relatively new drugs, and the drug of choice depends on personal preference and experience.

Contraindications and Cautions

In general, antiemetics should not be used in patients with coma or severe CNS depression, or in those who have experienced brain damage or injury, because of the risk of further CNS depression. Other contraindications include severe hypotension or hypertension and severe liver dysfunction, which might interfere with the metabolism of the drug. Caution should be used in individuals with renal dysfunction, active peptic ulcer, or pregnancy and lactation.

Adverse Effects

Adverse effects associated with antiemetics are linked to their interference with normal CNS stimulation or response.

TABLE 59-1 Antiemetic Agents

Type	Names
Phenothiazines	chlorpromazine, perphenazine, prochlorperazine, promethazine, thiethylperazine, triflupromazine
Nonphenothiazine	metoclopropamide
Anticholinergics/Antihistamines	buclizine, cyclizine, meclizine, antihistamines
5-HT$_3$ receptor blockers	dolasetron, granisetron, ondansetron
Miscellaneous	dronabinol, hydroxyzine, trimethobenzamide

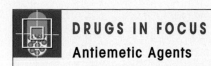

DRUGS IN FOCUS
Antiemetic Agents

Drug Name	Usual Dosage	Usual Indications
Phenothiazines		
chlorpromazine (*Thorazine*)	Adult: 10–25 mg PO q4–6h *or* 50–100 mg PR *or* 25 mg IM Pediatric: 0.55 mg/kg PO q4–6h; 1.1 mg/kg PR q6–8h *or* 0.55 mg/kg IM q6–8h	Treatment of nausea and vomiting, including that specifically associated with anesthesia; severe vomiting, intractable hiccoughs
perphenazine (*Trilafon*)	8–16 mg/d PO in divided doses; 5–10 mg IM for rapid control; 5 mg IV in divided doses, slowly	Treatment of severe nausea and vomiting; intractable hiccoughs
Ⓟ prochlorperazine (*Compazine*)	Adult: 5–10 mg PO t.i.d.–q.i.d.; 25 mg PR b.i.d.; 5–10 mg IM q3–4 h, up to 40 mg/d; 5–10 mg IM 1–2 h before anesthesia or during or after anesthesia, may repeat in 30 min Pediatric: 9.1–13.2 kg—2.5 mg PO or PR q.d.–b.i.d., do not exceed 7.5 mg/d; 13.6–17.7 kg—2.5 mg PO or PR b.i.d.–t.i.d., do not exceed 10 mg/d; 18.2–38.6 kg—2.5 mg PO or PR t.i.d. to 5 mg b.i.d., do not exceed 15 mg/d, *or* 0.132 mg/kg IM as a single dose	Treatment of severe nausea and vomiting, including that specifically associated with anesthesia
promethazine (*Phenergan*)	Adult: 25 mg PO or PR, repeat doses of 12.5–25 mg q4–6h as needed; 12.5–25 mg IM or IV q4–6h Pediatric: 1 mg/kg PO q4–6h as needed	Prevention and control of nausea and vomiting associated with anesthesia and surgery
thiethylperazine (*Torecan*)	10–30 mg/d PO in divided doses; 2 mL IM, one to three times per day	Relief of nausea and vomiting in adults
triflupromazine (*Vesprin*)	Adult: 5–15 mg IM q4h up to 60 mg/d; 1 mg IV, up to 3 mg/d Pediatric: 0.2–0.25 mg/kg IM up to a maximum of 10 mg/d; do not give IV	Control of severe nausea and vomiting
Nonphenothiazine		
Ⓟ metoclopropamide (*Reglan*)	10–20 mg IM at the end of surgery; 2 mg/kg IV over not less than 15 min given 30 min before chemotherapy, then q2h for 2 doses, than q3h for 3 doses	Treatment of nausea and vomiting, especially related to chemical stimulation of the chemoreceptor trigger zone in adults
Anticholinergics/Antihistamines		
buclizine (*Bucladin-S*)	50 mg PO, up to 150 mg/d has been used	Treatment of nausea and vomiting associated with motion sickness in adults
cyclizine (*Marezine*)	Adult: 50 mg PO 30 min before exposure to motion, then q4–6h as needed Pediatric: (6–12 y): 25 mg PO up to three times per day	Treatment of nausea and vomiting associated with motion sickness
Ⓟ meclizine (*Antivert*)	25–50 mg PO 1 h before travel, may repeat q24h during trip	Treatment of nausea and vomiting associated with motion sickness in patients >12 y
5-HT₃ Receptor blockers		
dolasetron (*Anzemet*)	Adult: 100 mg PO within 1 h of procedure; 12.5 mg IV for postoperative vomiting; 1.8 mg/kg IV or 100 mg IV injection before chemotherapy Pediatric (2–16 y): 1.8 mg/kg PO 1 h before chemotherapy, diluted in apple or apple-grape juice; 1.8 mg/kg IV 30 min before chemotherapy; 1.2 mg/kg IV for postoperative vomiting	Treatment of nausea and vomiting associated with emetogenic chemotherapy
granisetron (*Kytril*)	Adult and pediatric (>2 y): 10 µg/kg IV over 5 min starting within 30 min of chemotherapy; *or* 1 mg PO b.i.d. beginning up to 1 h before chemotherapy and giving the second dose 12 h after, use only on days of chemotherapy	Treatment of nausea and vomiting associated with emetogenic chemotherapy

Drugs in Focus continues on page 806

DRUGS IN FOCUS (CONTINUED)
Antiemetic Agents

Drug Name	Usual Dosage	Usual Indications
(P) ondansetron (*Zofran*)	Adult: 8 mg PO t.i.d. or 24 mg PO 30 min before chemotherapy; three 0.15-mg/kg doses IV over 15 min beginning before chemotherapy or one 32-mg dose infused over 30 min, given 30 min before chemotherapy; 4 mg IV *or* 4 mg IM *or* 16 mg PO 1 h before surgery to prevent postoperative vomiting Pediatric (4–12 y): 4 mg PO t.i.d.; use same IV dose as adults	Treatment of severe nausea and vomiting
Miscellaneous drugs dronabinol (*Marinol*)	5 mg/m^2 PO 1–3 h before chemotherapy, repeat q2–4h as needed for a total of 4–6 doses per day	Management of nausea and vomiting associated with cancer chemotherapy in adults
hydroxyzine (generic)	Adult: 25–100 mg IM Pediatric: 1.1 mg/kg IM	Treatment of prepartum and postpartum and postoperative nausea and vomiting
trimethobenzamide (*Tigan*)	Adult: 250 mg PO t.i.d.–q.i.d.; 200 mg PR t.i.d.–q.i.d.; 200 mg IM t.i.d.–q.i.d. Pediatric (≥30 lb): 100–200 mg PO or PR t.i.d.–q.i.d. Pediatric (<30 lb): 100 mg PR t.i.d.–q.i.d.	Treatment of nausea and vomiting (not sedating)

Drowsiness, dizziness, weakness, tremor, and headache are common adverse effects. As previously stated, some of the antiemetics are thought to have fewer CNS effects. Other, not uncommon adverse effects include hypotension, hypertension, and cardiac arrhythmias. When the phenothiazines and antihistamines are used as antiemetics, autonomic effects such as dry mouth, nasal congestion, anorexia, pallor, sweating, and urinary retention often occur. **Photosensitivity** (increased sensitivity to the sun and ultraviolet light) is a common adverse reaction with many of the antiemetics. Patients should be advised to use sunscreens and protective garments if exposure cannot be avoided.

Clinically Important Drug–Drug Interactions
Additive CNS depression can be seen with any of the antiemetics if they are combined with other CNS depressants, including alcohol. Patients should be advised to avoid this combination and any over-the-counter preparation unless they check with their health care provider. Other drug–drug interactions are specific to each drug (refer to a nursing drug guide).

Nursing Considerations for Patients Receiving an Antiemetic
Assessment: History and Examination

Screen for the following conditions, which could be cautions or contraindications to the use of the drug: history of allergy to antiemetic; impaired renal or hepatic function; pregnancy or lactation; coma or semiconscious state, CNS depression;

hypotension or hypertension; active peptic ulcer; and CNS injury.

Include screening for orientation, affect, and reflexes: baseline pulse and blood pressure; skin lesions and color; liver and abdominal examination; and liver and renal function tests.

Nursing Diagnoses

The patient receiving an antiemetic may have the following nursing diagnoses related to drug therapy:

- Acute Pain related to CNS, skin, and GI effects
- Risk for Injury related to CNS effects
- Decreased Cardiac Output related to cardiac effects
- Deficient Knowledge regarding drug therapy

Implementation

- Assess the patient carefully for any potential drug–drug interactions if giving antiemetics in combination with other drugs, *to avert potentially serious drug–drug interactions.*
- Provide comfort and safety measures, including mouth care, ready access to bathroom facilities, assistance with ambulation and periodic orientation, ice chips to suck, protection from sun exposure, and remedial measures to treat dehydration if it occurs, *to protect patient from injury and to increase patient comfort.*
- Provide support and encouragement, as well as other mea-

CASE STUDY

Handling Postoperative Nausea and Vomiting

THE SITUATION

A. J. is a 16-year-old boy who has undergone reconstructive knee surgery after a football injury. After the surgery, A. J. complains of nausea and vomited three times in 2 hours. A. J. becomes increasingly agitated. Rectal prochlorperazine (*Compazine*) is ordered to relieve the nausea, to be followed by an oral order when tolerated. The prochlorperazine is somewhat helpful in relieving the nausea, but A. J. expresses a desire to try cannabis, which he has read is good for the relief of nausea.

CRITICAL THINKING

- What are the important nursing implications in this case?
- What other measures could be taken to relieve A. J.'s nausea?
- What explanation could be given to the request for cannabis?

DISCUSSION

It is often impossible to pinpoint an exact cause of a patient's nausea and vomiting in a hospital setting. For example, the underlying cause may be related to the pain, a reaction to the pain medication being given, or a response to what A. J. described as the "awful hospital smell." A combination of factors should be considered when dealing with nausea and vomiting. A. J., as a teenager, may become increasingly agitated by the discomfort and possible embarrassment of vomiting. The administration of rectal prochlorperazine may "take the edge off" the nausea. A. J. will have to be reminded that the drug he is being given may make him dizzy, weak, or

drowsy and that he should ask for assistance if he needs to move.

When the nausea and vomiting have diminished somewhat, it will be possible to try other interventions to help stop the vomiting reflex. One such intervention is removing the offending odor that A. J. described, if possible, because doing so may relieve a chemical stimulus to the chemoreceptor trigger zone (CTZ). Administration of pain medication, as prescribed, may relieve the CTZ stimulus that comes with intense pain. Other interventions include providing a relaxed, quiet environment and encouraging A. J. to take slow, deep breaths, which stimulate the parasympathetic system (vagus nerve) and partially override the sympathetic activity stimulated by the CTZ to activate vomiting. For many patients, mouth care, ice chips, or small sips of water may also help to relieve the discomfort and ease the sensation of nausea.

After A. J. has relaxed a bit and his nausea has abated, the use of cannabis for treating nausea can be discussed. This may be a good opportunity to explain the many effects of cannabis to A. J. The drug has been shown to relieve nausea and vomiting, especially in chemotherapy patients. It also has been shown to decrease activity in the respiratory tract, to affect the development of sperm in males, and to alter thinking patterns and brain chemistry. The U.S. Food and Drug Administration has approved the use of the active ingredient in cannabis, delta-9-tetrahydracannabinol, in an oral form (dronabinol (*Marinol*)) for the relief of nausea and vomiting in cancer chemotherapy patients who have not responded to other therapies and for the treatment of anorexia associated with acquired immunodeficiency syndrome. It is not approved for use in the postoperative setting.

---

sures (quiet environment, carbonated drinks, deep breathing), *to help the patient cope with the discomfort of nausea and vomiting and drug effects.*

- Provide thorough patient teaching, including name of drug, dosage prescribed, proper administration, measures to avoid adverse effects, warning signs of problems, the importance of periodic monitoring and evaluation, and the need to avoid overdose and poisoning, *to enhance patient knowledge about drug therapy and promote compliance with the drug regimen.* (See Patient Teaching Checklist: Antiemetics.)

Evaluation

- Monitor patient response to the drug (relief of nausea and vomiting).
- Monitor for adverse effects (dizziness, confusion, GI alterations, cardiac arrhythmias, hypotension, gynecomastia).
- Evaluate effectiveness of teaching plan (patient can name the drug and dosage as well as describe adverse effects to watch for and specific measures to avoid these adverse effects).

PATIENT TEACHING CHECKLIST

Antiemetics

Create customized patient teaching materials for a specific antiemetic from the CD-ROM. Patient teaching should stress the following points for drugs within this class:

- An antiemetic helps prevent nausea and vomiting and the discomfort they cause.

Common effects of this drug include

- *Dizziness, weakness*—Change positions slowly. If you feel drowsy, avoid driving or dangerous activities (such as the use of heavy machinery or tasks requiring coordination).
- *Sensitivity to the sun*—Avoid exposure to the sun and ultraviolet light, because serious reactions may occur. If exposure cannot be prevented, use sunscreen and protective clothing to cover the skin.

Patient Teaching Checklist continues on page 808

PATIENT TEACHING CHECKLIST
(CONTINUED)

Antiemetics

• *Dehydration*—Avoid excessive heat exposure and try to drink fluids as much as possible, because you will have an increased risk for heat stroke.

Report any of the following conditions to your health care provider: fever, rash, yellowing of the eyes or skin, dark urine, pale stools, easy bruising, rash, and vision changes.

Avoid over-the-counter medications. If you feel that you need one, check with your health care provider first.

PATIENT TEACHING CHECKLIST
(CONTINUED)

Antiemetics

Tell any doctor, nurse, or other health care provider that you are taking this drug.

Keep this drug and all medications out of the reach of children.

This Teaching Checklist reflects general patient teaching guidelines. It is not meant to be a substitute for drug-specific teaching information, which is available in nursing drug guides.

NURSING CARE GUIDE

Antiemetics

Assessment	Nursing Diagnoses	Implementation	Evaluation
HISTORY	Acute Pain related to GI, skin, CNS effects	Administer only as a temporary measure.	Evaluate drug effects:
Allergies to any of these drugs, Coma, CNS depression, Severe hypotension, Liver dysfunction, Bone marrow depression, Epilepsy, Pregnancy and lactation	Risk for Injury related to CNS, CV effects	Provide comfort and safety measures:	- relief of nausea
	Deficient Knowledge regarding drug therapy	- assistance	- vomiting.
		- access to bathroom	Monitor for adverse effects:
		- safety precautions	GI alterations
		- mouth care	- orthostatic hypotension
		- ice chips.	- dizziness, confusion
		Protect from sun exposure:	- sun sensitivity
		- coverings	- dehydration.
		- sunscreens	Monitor for drug–drug interactions as indicated for each drug.
		Monitor for dehydration; provide remedial measures as needed.	Evaluate effectiveness of patient teaching program.
		Provide support and reassurance for coping with drug effects and discomfort.	Evaluate effectiveness of comfort and safety measures.
		Provide patient teaching regarding drug name, dosage, adverse effects, precautions, warning to report.	
PHYSICAL EXAMINATION			
Neurological: orientation, affect			
Skin: color, lesions			
CV: P, BP, orthostatic BP			
GI: abdominal, liver evaluation			
Lab tests: hematological, CBC, liver function tests			

- Monitor effectiveness of comfort measures and compliance with regimen (see Nursing Care Guide: Antiemetics).

CHAPTER SUMMARY

- Emetic drugs are used to induce vomiting in cases of poisoning or drug overdose.
- Ipecac syrup, the standard emetic agent, can be toxic if absorbed and not vomited. Administration of ipecac syrup is always followed by glasses of water to help decrease any chance of absorption of the drug.
- Antiemetics are used to manage nausea and vomiting in situations in which they are not beneficial and could actually cause harm to the patient.
- Antiemetics act by depressing the hyperactive vomiting reflex, either locally or through alteration of CNS actions.
- The choice of an antiemetic depends on the cause of the nausea and vomiting and the expected actions of the drug.
- Most antiemetics cause some CNS depression with resultant dizziness, drowsiness, and weakness. Care must be taken to protect the patient and advise him or her to avoid dangerous situations.
- Photosensitivity is another common adverse effect with antiemetics. Patients should be protected from exposure to the sun and ultraviolet light. Sunscreens and protective clothing are essential if exposure cannot be prevented.

Review Questions

1. The standard emetic agent in use today, available in pre-dosed packaging for parents to keep at home, is
   a. dronabinol.
   b. cyclizine.
   c. ipecac.
   d. spirits of wintergreen.
2. A second dose of ipecac should be given if a patient does not vomit within
   a. 10 minutes after the first dose.
   b. 1 to 2 minutes after the first dose.
   c. 1 hour after the first dose.
   d. 20 to 30 minutes after the first dose.
3. Ipecac might be the drug of choice for a
   a. patient who has swallowed kerosene.
   b. child who has chewed an entire bottle of baby aspirin.
   c. comatose patient.
   d. convulsing patient who has swallowed poison.

4. Prochlorperazine is the antiemetic of choice for
   a. nausea and vomiting after anesthesia.
   b. nausea and vomiting associated with cancer chemotherapy.
   c. motion sickness.
   d. intractable hiccoughs.
5. Most antiemetics work with the CNS to decrease the activity of
   a. the medulla.
   b. the CTZ.
   c. the respiratory center.
   d. the sympathetic nervous system.
6. Photosensitivity is a common adverse effect associated with the use of antiemetic agents. Patients should be cautioned
   a. to avoid having their picture taken.
   b. to cover the head at extremes of temperature.
   c. to take extra precautions to avoid heat stroke.
   d. to wear protective clothing and use a sunscreen if exposed to the sun or ultraviolet light.
7. The 5-HT$_3$ receptor blockers, including ondansetron and granisetron, are particularly effective in decreasing the nausea and vomiting associated with
   a. vestibular problems.
   b. emetogenic cancer chemotherapy.
   c. pregnancy.
   d. severe pain.
8. Nursing interventions for the patient receiving an antiemetic drug would probably not include
   a. frequent mouth care and ice chips to suck.
   b. bowel program to deal with constipation.
   c. protection from falls or injury.
   d. fluids to guard against dehydration.

BIBLIOGRAPHY

Bullock, B. L. (2000). *Focus on pathophysiology*. Philadelphia: Lippincott Williams & Wilkins.
Drug facts and comparisons. (2002). St. Louis: Facts and Comparisons.
Gilman, A., Hardman, J. G., & Limbird, L. E. (Eds.) (2002). *Goodman and Gilman's the pharmacological basis of therapeutics* (10th ed.). New York: McGraw-Hill.
Karch, A. M. (2002). *2003 Lippincott's nursing drug guide*. Philadelphia: Lippincott Williams & Wilkins.
The medical letter on drugs and therapeutics. (2002). New Rochelle, NY: Medical Letter.
Porth, C. M. (2002). *Pathophysiology: Concepts of altered health states* (6th ed.). Philadelphia: Lippincott Williams & Wilkins.

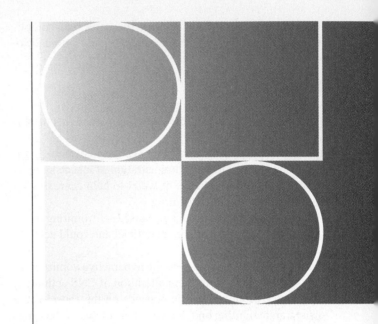

Answers to Review Questions

Chapter 1:
1. b   2. d   3. c   4. d   5. a   6. d   7. a   8. a

Chapter 2:
1. c   2. b   3. d   4. a   5. b   6. c   7. a   8. b

Chapter 3:
1. c   2. d   3. b   4. a   5. d   6. d

Chapter 4:
1. c   2. a   3. d   4. c   5. a   6. d   7. c   8. a

Chapter 5:
1. b   2. c   3. d   4. b   5. b   6. b   7. d   8. b

Chapter 6:
1. c   2. b   3. b   4. a   5. c   6. c   7. b

Chapter 7:
1. d   2. a   3. b   4. c   5. b   6. c   7. b   8. b

Chapter 8:
1. c   2. d   3. c   4. a   5. c   6. b   7. c   8. d

Chapter 9:
1. d   2. c   3. b   4. a   5. c   6. d   7. b   8. c   9. c   10. b
11. b   12. d

Chapter 10:
1. c   2. b   3. c   4. d   5. c   6. b   7. c   8. c   9. b   10. b

Chapter 11:
1. b   2. c   3. d   4. c   5. b   6. c   7. b

Chapter 12:
1. d   2. c   3. d   4. b   5. c   6. d   7. c   8. a   9. c

Chapter 13:
1. c   2. a   3. c   4. d   5. a   6. b   7. d

Chapter 14:
1. c   2. d   3. a   4. c   5. b   6. b   7. d   8. b   9. c   10. c

Chapter 15:
1. d   2. b   3. b   4. b   5. d   6. d   7. c   8. b   9. d   10. b

Chapter 16:
1. d   2. c   3. d   4. b   5. b   6. a   7. d   8. c   9. c   10. c

Chapter 17:
1. d   2. c   3. d   4. a   5. d   6. c   7. d   8. c

Chapter 18:
1. b   2. d   3. a   4. c   5. d   6. b   7. d   8. b   9. a

Chapter 19:
1. d   2. b   3. b   4. c   5. d   6. a   7. b   8. c   9. a   10. b

Chapter 20:
1. d   2. d   3. a   4. d   5. a   6. c   7. c   8. d   9. a

Chapter 21:
1. b   2. c   3. b   4. c   5. d   6. b   7. d   8. b   9. d   10. c

Chapter 22:
1. d   2. c   3. b   4. c   5. c   6. b   7. a   8. d   9. a   10. b

Chapter 23:
1. c   2. d   3. b   4. a   5. d   6. c   7. a   8. b   9. b   10. a

Chapter 24:
1. d   2. c   3. c   4. d   5. a   6. b   7. c   8. b   9. c   10. d

Chapter 25:
1. c   2. d   3. c   4. d   5. c   6. d   7. b   8. c   9. c

Chapter 26:
1. b   2. c   3. a   4. b   5. c   6. c   7. b   8. d   9. b   10. c

Chapter 27:
1. c   2. b   3. c   4. d   5. b   6. c   7. a   8. c

Chapter 28:
1. a   2. b   3. c   4. b   5. c   6. b   7. a   8. d

Chapter 29:
1. c   2. b   3. c   4. d   5. c   6. c   7. d   8. b   9. d   10. a

Chapter 30:
1. c   2. b   3. c   4. d   5. a   6. b   7. c   8. a

Chapter 31:
1. d   2. c   3. a   4. b   5. c   6. a   7. c   8. d   9. c   10. a

Chapter 32:
1. b   2. c   3. c   4. a   5. c   6. b   7. d   8. b   9. c

Chapter 33:
1. a   2. c   3. d   4. a   5. b   6. d

Chapter 34:
1. c   2. d   3. b   4. a   5. c   6. c   7. d   8. c   9. d   10. c

Chapter 35:
1. a   2. c   3. d   4. b   5. b   6. d   7. b   8. c   9. d   10. b

Chapter 36:
1. b   2. c   3. d   4. c   5. c   6. a   7. d   8. a   9. c   10. d

Chapter 37:
1. b   2. c   3. a   4. c   5. b   6. d   7. b   8. c   9. b   10. a

Chapter 38:
1. c   2. d   3. a   4. b   5. d   6. c   7. b   8. c   9. c   10. b

Chapter 39:
1. a   2. b   3. b   4. d   5. c   6. b   7. c   8. d   9. b   10. a

Chapter 40:
1. d   2. b   3. c   4. a   5. b   6. d   7. b   8. c   9. c   10. a

Chapter 41:
1. a   2. c   3. d   4. d   5. a   6. b   7. c   8. a   9. c   10. d

Chapter 42:
1. c   2. c   3. d   4. c   5. a   6. d   7. b   8. d   9. a   10. c
11. c

Chapter 43:
1. c   2. b   3. c   4. b   5. d   6. d   7. c   8. b   9. c   10. d

Chapter 44:
1. b   2. c   3. d   4. b   5. a   6. c   7. d   8. b   9. c   10. b

Chapter 45:
1. d   2. b   3. d   4. c   5. d   6. b   7. d   8. a   9. c   10. d

Chapter 46:
1. a   2. c   3. b   4. d   5. c   6. d   7. c   8. b   9. c   10. b

Chapter 47:
1. b   2. b   3. c   4. d   5. c   6. b   7. c   8. b   9. d

Chapter 48:
1. c   2. d   3. a   4. d   5. b   6. c   7. d   8. d   9. b   10. c

Chapter 49:
1. c   2. b   3. a   4. b   5. c   6. d   7. b   8. c   9. d   10. c

Chapter 50:
1. a   2. d   3. a   4. b   5. c   6. b   7. c   8. d   9. b   10. d

Chapter 51:
1. c   2. b   3. c   4. b   5. c   6. d   7. a   8. d   9. b   10. c

Chapter 52:
1. c   2. d   3. b   4. c   5. d   6. b   7. c   8. a   9. b   10. c

Chapter 53:
1. c   2. b   3. a   4. c   5. d   6. d   7. c   8. d   9. b   10. d

Chapter 54:
1. d   2. c   3. d   4. b   5. d   6. b   7. a   8. c   9. c   10. d

Chapter 55:
1. a   2. c   3. c   4. a   5. b   6. d   7. c   8. c   9. d

Chapter 56:
1. d   2. c   3. a   4. d   5. c   6. d   7. c   8. a   9. d   10. c

Chapter 57:
1. c   2. d   3. c   4. c   5. a   6. d   7. c   8. b   9. c   10. d

Chapter 58:
1. b   2. c   3. a   4. d   5. b   6. c   7. d   8. b

Chapter 59:
1. c   2. d   3. b   4. c   5. b   6. d   7. b   8. b

Glossary

A fibers: large-diameter nerve fibers that carry peripheral impulses associated with touch and temperature to the spinal cord

abortifacients: drugs used to stimulate uterine contractions and promote evacuation of the uterus to cause abortion or to empty the uterus after fetal death

absence seizure: type of generalized seizure that is characterized by sudden, temporary loss of consciousness, sometimes with staring or blinking for 3 to 5 seconds; formerly known as a petit mal seizure

absorption: what happens to a drug from the time it enters the body until it enters the circulating fluid; intravenous administration causes the drug to directly enter the circulating blood, bypassing the many complications of absorption from other routes

ACE inhibitor: drug that blocks the enzyme responsible for converting angiotensin I to angiotensin II in the lungs; this blocking prevents the vasoconstriction and aldosterone release related to angiotensin II

acetylcholine receptor site: area on the muscle cell membrane where acetylcholine (ACh) reacts with a specific receptor site to cause stimulation of the muscle in response to nerve activity

acetylcholinesterase: enzyme responsible for the immediate breakdown of acetylcholine when released from the nerve ending; prevents overstimulation of cholinergic receptor sites

acid rebound: reflex response of the stomach to lower-than-normal acid levels; when acid levels are lowered through the use of antacids, gastrin production and secretion are increased to return the stomach to its normal acidity

acidification: the process of increasing the acid level; used to treat bladder infections, making the bladder an undesirable place for bacteria

acquired immunodeficiency syndrome (AIDS): collection of opportunistic infections and cancers that occurs when the immune system is severely depressed by a decrease in the number of functioning helper T cells; caused by infection with human immunodeficiency virus (HIV)

acromegaly: thickening of bony surfaces in response to excess growth hormone after the epiphyseal plates have closed

actin: thin filament that makes up a sarcomere or muscle unit

action potential: sudden change in electrical charge of a nerve cell membrane; the electrical signal by which neurons send information

active immunity: the formation of antibodies secondary to exposure to a specific antigen; leads to the formation of plasma cells, antibodies, and memory cells to immediately produce anti-bodies if exposed to that antigen in the future; imparts lifelong immunity

A-delta and C fibers: small-diameter nerve fibers that carry peripheral impulses associated with pain to the spinal cord

adrenal cortex: outer layer of the adrenal gland; produces glucocorticoids and mineralocorticoids in response to ACTH stimulation; also responds to sympathetic stimulation

adrenal medulla: inner layer of the adrenal gland; a sympathetic ganglion, it releases norepinephrine and epinephrine into circulation in response to sympathetic stimulation

adrenergic agonist: a drug that stimulates the adrenergic receptors of the sympathetic nervous system, either directly (by reacting with receptor sites) or indirectly (by increasing norepinephrine levels)

adrenergic receptor: receptor sites on effectors that respond to norepinephrine

adrenergic receptor site specificity: a drug's affinity for only adrenergic receptor sites; certain drugs may have specific affinity for only α- or only β-adrenergic receptor sites

adverse effects: drug effects that are not the desired therapeutic effects; may be unpleasant or even dangerous

aerobic: bacteria that depend on oxygen for survival

affect: feeling that a person experiences when he or she responds emotionally to the environment

afferent: neurons or groups of neurons that bring information to the central nervous system; sensory nerve

agonist: a drug that acts like or increases the effects of a specific neurotransmitter or hormone

AIDS-related complex (ARC): collection of less serious opportunistic infections with HIV infection; the decrease in the number of helper T cells is less severe than in fully developed AIDS

aldosterone: hormone produced by the adrenal gland that causes the distal tubule to retain sodium, and therefore water, while losing potassium into the urine

alkalosis: state of not having enough acid to maintain normal homeostatic processes; seen with loop diuretics, which cause loss of bicarbonate in the urine

alopecia: hair loss; a common adverse effect of many antineoplastic drugs, which are more effective against rapidly multiplying cells such as those of hair follicles

α-agonist: specifically stimulating to the α-receptors within the sympathetic nervous system, causing body responses seen when the α-receptors are stimulated

α_1-selective adrenergic blocking agents: drugs that block the postsynaptic α_1-receptor sites, causing a decrease in vascular tone and a vasodilation that leads to a fall in blood pressure; these drugs do not block the presynaptic α_2-receptor sites, and therefore the reflex tachycardia that accompanies a fall in blood pressure does not occur

α-receptors: adrenergic receptors that are found in smooth muscles

alternative therapy: including herbs and other "natural" products as found in ancient records, these products are not controlled or tested by the U. S. Food and Drug Administration, and because of this, the advertising surrounding these products is not as restricted or as accurate as it would be with classic drugs

alveoli: the respiratory sac, the smallest unit of the lungs where gas exchange occurs

Alzheimer's disease: degenerative disease of the cortex with loss of acetylcholine-producing cells and cholinergic receptors; characterized by progressive dementia

amebiasis: amebic dysentery, which is caused by intestinal invasion of the trophozoite stage of the protozoan *Entamoeba histolytica*

amnesia: loss of memory of an event or procedure

anabolic steroids: androgens developed with more anabolic or protein-building effects than androgenic effects

anaerobic: bacteria that survive without oxygen, which are often seen when blood flow is cut off to an area of the body

analgesia: loss of pain sensation

analgesic: compounds with pain-blocking properties, capable of producing analgesia

anaplasia: loss of organization and structure; property of cancer cells

androgenic effects: effects associated with development of male sexual characteristics and secondary characteristics (eg, deepening of voice, hair distribution, genital development, acne)

androgens: male sex hormones, primarily testosterone; produced in the testes and adrenal glands

anemia: a decrease in the number of red blood cells (RBCs), leading to an inability to effectively deliver oxygen to the tissues

angina pectoris: "suffocation of the chest"; pain caused by the imbalance between oxygen being supplied to the heart muscle and demand for oxygen by the heart muscle

angiotensin II receptors: specific receptors found in blood vessels and in the adrenal gland that react with angiotensin II to cause vasoconstriction and release of aldosterone

Anopheles mosquito: type of mosquito that is essential to the life cycle of *Plasmodium;* injects the protozoa into humans for further maturation

anterior pituitary: lobe of the pituitary gland that produces stimulating hormones as well as growth hormone, prolactin, and melanocyte-stimulating hormone

antiarrhythmics: drugs that affect the action potential of cardiac cells and are used to treat arrhythmias and return normal rate and rhythm

antibiotic: chemical that is able to inhibit the growth of specific bacteria or cause the death of susceptible bacteria

antibodies: immunoglobulins; produced by B cell plasma cells in response to a specific protein; react with that protein to cause its destruction directly or through activation of the inflammatory response

anticholinergic: drug that opposes the effects of acetylcholine at acetylcholine receptor sites

anticoagulants: drugs that block or inhibit any step of the coagulation process, preventing or slowing clot formation

antidiarrheal drug: drug that blocks the stimulation of the gastrointestinal (GI) tract, leading to decreased activity and increased time for absorption of needed nutrients and water

antidiuretic hormone (ADH): hormone produced by the hypothalamus and stored in the posterior pituitary gland; important in maintaining fluid balance; causes the distal tubules and collecting ducts of the kidney to become permeable to water, leading to an antidiuretic effect and fluid retention

antiemetic: agent that blocks the hyperactive response of the chemoreceptor trigger zone (CTZ) to various stimuli, the response that produces nonbeneficial nausea and vomiting

antiepileptic: drug used to treat the abnormal and excessive energy bursts in the brain that are characteristic of epilepsy

antigen: foreign protein

antihistamines: drugs that block the release or action of histamine, a chemical released during inflammation that increases secretions and narrows airways

anti-inflammatory: blocking the effects of the inflammatory response

antineoplastic agent: drug used to combat cancer or the growth of neoplasms

antipeptic: drug that coats any injured area in the stomach to prevent further injury from acid or pepsin

antipsychotic: drug used to treat disorders involving thought processes; dopamine receptor blocker that helps affected people organize their thoughts and respond appropriately to stimuli

antipyretic: blocking fever, often by direct effects on the thermoregulatory center in the hypothalamus or by blockade of prostaglandin mediators

antispasmodics: agents that block muscle spasm associated with irritation or neurological stimulation

antitoxins: immune sera that contains antibodies to specific toxins produced by invaders; may prevent the toxin from adhering to body tissues and causing disease

antitussives: drugs that block the cough reflex

anxiety: unpleasant feeling of tension, fear, or nervousness in response to an environmental stimulus, whether real or imaginary

anxiolytic: drug used to depress the central nervous system (CNS); prevents the signs and symptoms of anxiety

apothecary system: a very old system or measure that was specifically developed for use by apothecaries or pharmacists; it uses the minim as the basic unit of liquid measure and the grain as the basic unit of solid measure.

arachidonic acid: released from injured cells to stimulate the inflammatory response through activation of various chemical substances

arrhythmia: a disruption in cardiac rate or rhythm

arteries: vessels that take blood away from the heart; muscular, resistance vessels

assessment: information-gathering regarding the current status of a particular patient, including evaluation of past history and physical examination; provides a baseline of information and clues to effectiveness of therapy

asthma: disorder characterized by recurrent episodes of bronchospasm (ie, bronchial muscle spasm leading to narrowed or obstructed airways)

atheroma: plaque in the endothelial lining of arteries; contains fats, blood cells, lipids, inflammatory agents, platelets; leads to narrowing of the lumen of the artery, stiffening of the artery, and loss of distensibility and responsiveness

atherosclerosis: narrowing of the arteries caused by build up of atheromas, swelling, and accumulation of platelets; leads to a loss of elasticity and responsiveness to normal stimuli

atrium: top chamber of the heart, receives blood from veins

attention-deficit disorder: behavioral syndrome characterized by an inability to concentrate for longer than a few minutes and excessive activity

auricle: appendage on the atria of the heart, holds blood to be pumped out with atrial contraction

autoimmune: having antibodies to self-cells or self-proteins; leads to chronic inflammatory disease and cell destruction

automaticity: property of heart cells to generate an action potential without an external stimulus

autonomic nervous system: portion of the central and peripheral nervous systems that, with the endocrine system, functions to maintain internal homeostasis

autonomy: loss of the normal controls and reactions that inhibit growth and spreading; property of cancer cells

axon: long projection from a neuron that carries information from one nerve to another nerve or effector

B cells: lymphocytes programmed to recognize specific proteins; when activated, these cells cause the production of antibodies to react with that protein

bactericidal: substance that causes the death of bacteria, usually by interfering with cell membrane stability or with proteins or enzymes necessary to maintain the cellular integrity of the bacteria

bacteriostatic: substance that prevents the replication of bacteria, usually by interfering with proteins or enzyme systems necessary for reproduction of the bacteria

balanced anesthesia: use of several different types of drugs to achieve the quickest, most effective anesthesia with the fewest adverse effects

barbiturate: former mainstay drug used for the treatment of anxiety and for sedation and sleep induction; associated with potentially severe adverse effects and many drug–drug interactions, which makes it less desirable than some of the newer agents

baroreceptor: pressure receptor; located in the arch of the aorta and in the carotid artery; responds to changes in pressure and influences the medulla to stimulate the sympathetic system to increase or decrease blood pressure

basal ganglia: lower area of the brain associated with coordination of unconscious muscle movements that involve movement and position

belladonna: a plant that contains atropine as an alkaloid; used to dilate the pupils as a fashion statement in the past; used in herbal medicine much as atropine is used today

benign prostatic hyperplasia (BPH): enlargement of the prostate gland, associated with age and inflammation

benzodiazepine: drug that acts in the limbic system and the reticular activating system to make γ-aminobutyric acid (GABA), an inhibitory neurotransmitter, more effective, causing interference with neuron firing; depresses CNS to block the signs and symptoms of anxiety and may cause sedation and hypnosis (extreme sedation with further CNS depression and sleep) in higher doses

β-adrenergic blocking agents: drugs that, at therapeutic levels, selectively block the β-receptors of the sympathetic nervous system

β-agonist: specifically stimulating to the β-receptors within the sympathetic nervous system, causing body responses seen when the β-receptors are stimulated

β-receptors: adrenergic receptors that are found in the heart, lungs, and vascular smooth muscle

β₁-selective adrenergic blocking agents: drugs that, at therapeutic levels, specifically block the β₁-receptors in the sympathetic nervous system, while not blocking the β₂-receptors and resultant effects on the respiratory system

bile acids: cholesterol-containing acids found in the bile that act like detergents to break up fats in the small intestine

bile: fluid stored in the gall bladder that contains cholesterol and bile salts; essential for the proper breakdown and absorption of fats

biogenic amine: one of the neurotransmitters norepinephrine, serotonin, or dopamine; it is thought that a deficiency of these substances in key areas of the brain results in depression

biotransformation: the alteration of a drug by the body into new chemicals that are less active, less toxic, and more easily excreted by the body; this action usually occurs in the liver

bisphosphonates: drugs used to block bone resorption and lower serum calcium levels in several conditions

blood dyscrasia: bone marrow depression caused by drug effects on the rapidly multiplying cells of the bone marrow; lower than normal levels of blood components can be seen

bone marrow suppression: inhibition of the blood-forming components of the bone marrow; a common adverse effect of many antineoplastic drugs, which are more effective against rapidly multiplying cells such as those in bone marrow; also seen in anemia, thrombocytopenia, and leukopenia

bradycardia: slower than normal heart rate (usually <60 beats/min)

bradykinesia: difficulty in performing intentional movements and extreme slowness and sluggishness; characteristic of Parkinson's disease

brand name: name given to a drug by the pharmaceutical company that developed it; also called trade name

bronchial tree: the conducting airways leading into the alveoli; they branch smaller and smaller, appearing much like a tree

bronchodilation: relaxation of the muscles in the bronchi, resulting in a widening of the bronchi; an effect of sympathetic stimulation

bronchodilator: medication used to facilitate respirations by dilating the airways; helpful in symptomatic relief or prevention of bronchial asthma and bronchospasm associated with chronic obstructive pulmonary disease

bulk stimulant: agent that increases in bulk, frequently by osmotic pull of fluid into the feces; the increased bulk stretches the GI wall, causing stimulation and increased GI movement

calcitonin: hormone produced by the parafollicular cells of the thyroid; counteracts the effects of parathyroid hormone to maintain calcium levels

calor: heat, one of the four cardinal signs of inflammation; caused by activation of the inflammatory response

Candida: fungus that is normally found on mucous membranes; can cause yeast infections or thrush of the GI tract and vagina in immunosuppressed patients

capacitance system: the venous system; distensible, flexible veins that are capable of holding large amounts of blood

capillary: small vessel made up of loosely connected endothelial cells that connect arteries to veins

carbonic anhydrase: a catalyst that speeds up the chemical reaction combining water and carbon dioxide, which react to form carbonic acid and which immediately dissociate to form sodium bicarbonate

carcinoma: tumor that originates in epithelial cells

cardiac cycle: a period of cardiac muscle relaxation (diastole) followed by a period of contraction (systole) in the heart

cardiac output: the amount of drug the heart can pump per beat; influenced by the coordination of cardiac muscle contraction, heart rate, and blood return to the heart

Cardiac Arrhythmia Suppression Test (CAST): a large research study run by the National Heart and Lung Institute that found that long-term treatment of arrhythmias may have a questionable effect on mortality, and in some cases actually lead to increased cardiac death; basis for the current indication for antiarrhythmics (short-term use to treat life-threatening ventricular arrhythmias)

cardiomegaly: enlargement of the heart, seen with chronic hypertension, valvular disease, and congestive heart failure

cardiovascular center: area of the medulla at which stimulation will activate the sympathetic nervous system to increase blood pressure, heart rate, and so forth

cathartic dependence: overuse of laxatives that can lead to the need for strong stimuli to initiate movement in the intestines; local reflexes become resistant to normal stimuli after prolonged use of harsher stimulants, leading to further laxative use

cell membrane: lipoprotein structure that separates the interior of a cell from the external environment; regulates what can enter and leave a cell

cell cycle: life cycle of a cell, which includes the phases G_0, G_1, S, G_2, and M; during the M phase, the cell divides into two identical daughter cells

cerebellum: lower portion of the brain associated with coordination of muscle movements, including voluntary motion, as well as extrapyramidal control of unconscious muscle movements

cestode: tapeworm with a head and segmented body parts that is capable of growing to several yards in the human intestine

chemical name: name that reflects the chemical structure of a drug

chemical stimulant: agent that stimulates the normal GI reflexes by chemically irritating the lining of the GI wall, leading to increased activity in the GI tract

chemotaxis: property of drawing neutrophils to an area

chemotherapeutic agents: synthetic chemicals used to interfere with the functioning of foreign cell populations; this term is frequently used to refer to the drug therapy of neoplasms, but it also refers to drug therapy affecting any foreign cell

Cheyne–Stokes respiration: abnormal pattern of breathing characterized by apneic periods followed by periods of tachypnea; may reflect delayed blood flow through the brain

cholesterol: necessary component of human cells that is produced and processed in the liver, then stored in the bile until

stimulus causes the gall bladder to contract and send the bile into the duodenum via the common bile duct; a fat that is essential for the formation of steroid hormones and cell membranes; it is produced in cells and taken in by dietary sources

cholinergic: responding to acetylcholine; refers to receptor sites stimulated by acetylcholine as well as neurons that release acetylcholine

cholinergic receptor: receptor sites on effectors that respond to acetylcholine

chronic obstructive pulmonary disease (COPD): chronic condition that occurs over time; often the result of chronic bronchitis or repeated and severe asthma attacks; leads to destruction of the respiratory defense mechanisms and physical structure

chrysotherapy: treatment with gold salts; gold is taken up by macrophages, which then inhibit phagocytosis; it is reserved for use in patients who are unresponsive to conventional therapy and can be very toxic

chylomicron: carrier for lipids in the bloodstream, consisting of proteins, lipids, cholesterol, and so forth

chyme: contents of the stomach containing ingested food and secreted enzymes, water, and mucus

cilia: microscopic, hair-like projections of the epithelial cell membrane lining the upper respiratory tract, which are constantly moving and directing the mucus and any trapped substance toward the throat

cinchonism: syndrome of quinine toxicity characterized by nausea, vomiting, tinnitus, and vertigo

Clark's Rule: a method of determining the correct drug dose for a child based on the known adult dose (assumes that the adult dose is based on a 150-lb person); it states

$$\text{child's dose} = \frac{\text{weight of child (lb)}}{150 \text{ lb}} \times \text{average adult dose}$$

clotting factors: substances formed in the liver, many requiring vitamin K, that react in a cascading sequence to cause the formation of thrombin from prothrombin; thrombin then breaks down fibrin threads from fibrinogen to form a clot

coagulation: the process of blood's changing from a fluid state to a solid state to plug injuries to the vascular system

common cold: viral infection of the upper respiratory tract that initiates the release of histamine and prostaglandins and causes an inflammatory response

complement: series of cascading proteins that react with the antigen–antibody complex to destroy the protein or stimulate an inflammatory reaction

conductivity: property of heart cells to rapidly conduct an action potential of electrical impulse

congestive heart failure (CHF): a condition in which the heart muscle fails to adequately pump blood around the cardiovascular system, leading to a backup or congestion of blood in the system

constipation: slower than normal evacuation of the large intestine, which can result in increased water absorption from the feces and can lead to impaction

conversion: finding the equivalent values between two systems of measure

convulsion: tonic–clonic muscular reaction to excessive electrical energy arising from nerve cells in the brain

coronary artery disease (CAD): characterized by progressive narrowing of coronary arteries, leading to a decreased delivery of oxygen to cardiac muscle cells; leading killer of adults in the Western world

corpus luteum: remains of follicle that releases mature ovum at ovulation; becomes an endocrine gland producing estrogen and progesterone

corpus striatum: part of the brain that reacts with the substantia nigra to maintain a balance of suppression and stimulation

corticosteroids: steroid hormones produced by the adrenal cortex; include androgens, glucocorticoids, and mineralocorticoids

cost comparison: a comparison of the relative cost of the same drug provided by different manufacturers to determine the costs to the consumer

cough: reflex response to irritation in the respiratory membrane, results in expelling of forced air through the mouth

countercurrent mechanism: process used by medullary nephrons to concentrate or dilute the urine in response to body stimuli to maintain fluid and electrolyte balance

cretinism: lack of thyroid hormone in an infant; if untreated, leads to mental retardation

critical concentration: the concentration a drug must reach in the tissues that respond to the particular drug to cause the desired effect

culture: sample of the bacteria (eg, from sputum, cell scrapings, urine) to be grown in a laboratory to determine the species of bacteria that is causing an infection

cycloplegia: inability of the lens in the eye to accommodate to near vision, causing blurring and inability to see near objects

cystitis: inflammation of the bladder, caused by infection or irritation

cytomegalovirus (CMV): DNA virus that accounts for many respiratory, ophthalmic, and liver infections

cytoplasm: interior of a cell; contains organelles for producing proteins, energy, and so on

D

decongestants: drugs that decrease the blood flow to the upper respiratory tract and decrease the overproduction of secretions

dendrite: short projection on a neuron that transmits information

depolarization: opening of the sodium channels in a nerve membrane to allow the influx of positive sodium ions, reversing the membrane charge from negative to positive

depolarizing neuromuscular junction (NMJ) blocker: stimulation of a muscle cell, causing it to contract, with no allowance for repolarization and restimulation of the muscle; characterized by contraction and then paralysis

depression: affective disorder in which a person experiences sadness that is much more severe and long-lasting than is warranted by the event that seems to have precipitated it, with a more intense mood; the condition may not even be traceable to a specific event or stressor

dermatological reactions: skin reactions commonly seen as adverse effects of drugs; can range from simple rash to potentially fatal exfoliative dermatitis

diabetes insipidus: lack of ADH, which results in the production of copious amounts of glucose-free urine

diabetes mellitus: a metabolic disorder characterized by high blood glucose levels and altered metabolism of proteins and fats; associated with thickening of the basement membrane, leading to numerous complications

diarrhea: more frequent than normal bowel movements, often characterized as fluid-like and watery because not enough time for absorption is allowed during the passage of food through the intestines

diastole: resting phase of the heart; blood is returned to the heart during this phase

diffusion: movement of solutes from an area of high concentration to an area of low concentration across a concentration gradient

distribution: movement of a drug to body tissues; the places where a drug may be distributed depend on the drug's solubility, perfusion of the area, cardiac output, and binding of the drug to plasma proteins

diurnal rhythm: response of the hypothalamus and then the pituitary and adrenals to wakefulness and sleeping; normally, the hypothalamus begins secretion of corticotropin-releasing factor (CRF) in the evening, peaking at about midnight; adrenocortical peak response is between 6 and 9 AM; levels fall during the day until evening, when the low level is picked up by the hypothalamus and CRF secretion begins again

dolor: pain, one of the four cardinal signs of inflammation; caused by activation of the inflammatory response

dopaminergic: drug that increases the effects of dopamine at receptor sites

drug allergy: formation of antibodies to a drug or drug protein; causes an immune response when the person is next exposed to that drug

drugs: chemicals that are introduced into the body to bring about some sort of change

dwarfism: small stature, resulting from lack of growth hormone in children

dyspnea: discomfort with respirations, often with a feeling of anxiety and inability to breathe, seen with left-sided CHF

dysuria: painful urination

E

edema: movement of fluid into the interstitial spaces; occurs when the balance between osmotic pull (from plasma proteins) and hydrostatic push (from blood pressure) is upset

effector: cell stimulated by a nerve; may be a muscle, a gland, or another nerve

efferent: neurons or groups of neurons that carry information from the central nervous system to an effector; motor neurons

electrocardiogram (ECG): an electrical tracing reflecting the conduction of an electrical impulse through the heart muscle; does not reflect mechanical activity

emetic: agent used to induce vomiting to rid the stomach of toxins or drugs

endocytosis: engulfing substances and moving them into a cell by extending the cell membrane around the substance; pinocytosis and phagocytosis are two kinds of endocytosis

engram: short-term memory made up of a reverberating electrical circuit of action potentials

epilepsy: collection of various syndromes, all of which are characterized by seizures

ergosterol: steroid-type protein found in the cell membrane of fungi; similar in configuration to adrenal hormones and testosterone

ergot derivative: drug that causes a vascular constriction in the brain and the periphery; relieves or prevents migraine headaches but is associated with many adverse effects

erythrocytes: red blood cells (RBCs), responsible for carrying oxygen to the tissues and removing carbon dioxide; have no nucleus and live approximately 120 days

erythropoiesis: process of RBC production and life cycle; formed by megaloblastic cells in the bone marrow, using iron, folic acid, carbohydrates, vitamin B_{12}, and amino acids; they circulate in the vascular system for about 120 days, then are lysed and recycled

erythropoietin: glycoprotein produced by the kidneys, released in response to decreased blood flow or oxygen tension in the kidney; controls the rate of RBC production in the bone marrow

essential hypertension: sustained blood pressure above normal limits with no discernible underlying cause

estrogen: hormone produced by the ovary, placenta, and adrenal gland; stimulates development of female characteristics and prepares the body for pregnancy

excretion: removal of a drug from the body; primarily occurs in the kidneys but can occur through the skin, lungs, bile, or feces

exocytosis: removal of substances from a cell by pushing them through the cell membrane

expectorants: drugs that increase productive cough to clear the airways

extrapyramidal tract: cells from the cortex and subcortical areas, including the basal ganglia and the cerebellum, which coordinate unconsciously controlled muscle activity; allows the body to make automatic adjustments in posture or position and balance

extrinsic pathway: cascade of clotting factors in blood that has escaped the vascular system to form a clot on the outside of the injured vessel

fertility drugs: drugs used to stimulate ovulation and pregnancy in women with functioning ovaries who are having trouble conceiving

fibrillation: rapid, irregular stimulation of the cardiac muscle resulting in lack of pumping activity

filtration: passage of fluid and small components of the blood through the glomerulus into the nephron tubule

first-pass effect: a phenomenon in which drugs given orally are carried directly to the liver after absorption, where they may be largely inactivated by liver enzymes before they can enter the general circulation; oral drugs frequently are given in higher doses than drugs given by other routes because of this early breakdown

fluid rebound: reflex reaction of the body to the loss of fluid or sodium; the hypothalamus causes the release of ADH, which retains water, and stress related to fluid loss combines with decreased blood flow to the kidneys to activate the renin–angiotensin system, leading to further water and sodium retention

focal seizure: seizure that involves one area of the brain and does not spread throughout the entire brain; also known as a partial seizure

follicle: storage site of each ovum in the ovary; allows the ovum to grow and develop, produces estrogen and progesterone

follicles: structural unit of the thyroid gland; cells arranged in a circle

Food and Drug Administration (FDA): federal agency responsible for the regulation and enforcement of drug evaluation and distribution policies

forebrain: upper level of the brain; consists of the two cerebral hemispheres, where thinking and coordination of sensory and motor activity occur

Fried's Rule: a method of determining a pediatric drug dose for a child younger than 1 year of age; based on the child's age and the usual adult dose (assumes that an adult dose would be appropriate for a 12.5-year-old child); it states

$$\text{dose (for child} <1 \text{ y)} = \frac{\text{infant's age (mo)}}{150 \text{ mo}} \times \frac{\text{average adult}}{\text{dose}}$$

fungus: a cellular organism with a hard cell wall that contains chitin and many polysaccharides as well as a cell membrane that contains ergosterols

ganglion: a closely packed group of nerve cell bodies

gastrin: secreted by the stomach in response to many stimuli; stimulates the release of hydrochloric acid from the parietal cells and pepsin from the chief cells; causes histamine release at histamine-2 receptors to effect the release of acid

gate control theory: theory that states that the transmission of a nerve impulse can be modulated at various points along its path by descending fibers from the brain that close the "gate" and block transmission of pain information and by A fibers that are able to block transmission in the dorsal horn by closing the gate for transmission for the A-delta and C fibers

general anesthetic: drug that induces a loss of consciousness, amnesia, analgesia, and loss of reflexes to allow performance of painful surgical procedures

generalized seizure: seizure that begins in one area of the brain and rapidly spreads throughout both hemispheres

generic drugs: drugs sold by their chemical name; not brand (or trade) name products

generic name: the original designation that a drug is given when the drug company that developed it applies for the approval process

genetic engineering: process of altering DNA, usually of bacteria, to produce a chemical to be used as a drug

giardiasis: protozoal intestinal infection that causes severe diarrhea and epigastric distress; may lead to serious malnutrition

gigantism: response to excess levels of growth hormone before the epiphyseal plates close; heights of 7 to 8 feet are not uncommon

glomerulus: the tuft of blood vessel between the afferent and efferent arterioles in the nephron; the fenestrated membrane of the glomerulus allows filtration of fluid from the blood into the nephron tubule

glucocorticoids: steroid hormones released from the adrenal cortex; they increase blood glucose levels, fat deposits, and protein breakdown for energy

glycogen: storage form of glucose; can be broken down for rapid glucose level increases during times of stress

glycogenolysis: breakdown of stored glucose to increase the blood glucose levels

glycosuria: presence of glucose in the urine

gram-negative: bacteria that accept a negative stain and are frequently associated with infections of the genitourinary or GI tract

gram-positive: bacteria that take a positive stain and are frequently associated with infections of the respiratory tract and soft tissues

grand mal seizure: see *tonic-clonic seizure*

Hageman factor: first factor activated when a blood vessel or cell is injured; starts the cascading reaction of the clotting factors, activates the conversion of plasminogen to plasmin to dissolve clots, and activates the kinin system responsible for activation of the inflammatory response

half-life: the time it takes for the amount of drug in the body to decrease to one-half of the peak level it previously achieved

heart blocks: blocks to conduction of an impulse through the cardiac conduction system; can occur at the atrioventricular node, interrupting conduction from the atria into the ventricles, or in the bundle branches within the ventricles, preventing the normal conduction of the impulse

helminth: worm that can cause disease by invading the human body

helper T cell: human lymphocyte that helps initiate immune reactions in response to tissue invasion

hemodynamics: the study of the forces moving blood throughout the cardiovascular system

hemoptysis: blood-tinged sputum, seen in left-sided CHF when blood backs up into the lungs and fluid leaks out into the lung tissue

hemorrhagic disorders: disorders characterized by a lack of clot-forming substances, leading to states of excessive bleeding

hemostatic drugs: drugs that stop blood loss, usually by blocking the plasminogen mechanism and preventing clot dissolution

herpes: DNA virus that accounts for many diseases, including shingles, cold sores, genital herpes, and encephalitis

high-ceiling diuretics: powerful diuretics that work in the loop of Henle to inhibit the reabsorption of sodium and chloride, leading to a sodium-rich diuresis

high-density lipoprotein (HDL): loosely packed chylomicron containing fats, able to absorb fats and fat remnants in the periphery; thought to have a protective effect, decreasing the development of CAD

hindbrain: most primitive area of the brain, the brainstem; consists of the pons and medulla, which control basic, vital functions and arousal, and the cerebellum, which controls motor functions that regulate balance

hirsutism: hair distribution associated with male secondary sex characteristics (eg, increased hair on trunk, arms, legs, face)

histamine-2 (H₂) antagonist: drug that blocks the H_2 receptor sites; used to decrease acid production in the stomach (H_2 sites are stimulated to cause the release of acid in response to gastrin or parasympathetic stimulation)

histamine-2 (H₂) receptors: sites near the parietal cells of the stomach which, when stimulated, cause the release of hydrochloric acid into the lumen of the stomach; also found near cardiac cells

histocompatibility antigens: proteins found on the surface of the cell membrane, which are determined by genetic code; provide cellular identity as self-cell

HMG-CoA reductase: enzyme that regulates the last step in cellular cholesterol synthesis

hormones: chemical messengers working within the endocrine system to communicate within the body

human immunodeficiency virus (HIV): retrovirus that attacks helper T cells, leading to a decrease in immune function and AIDS or ARC

hydrochloric acid: acid released by the parietal cells of the stomach in response to gastrin release or parasympathetic stimulation; makes the stomach contents more acidic to aid digestion and breakdown of food products

hyperaldosteronism: excessive output of aldosterone from the adrenal gland, leading to increased sodium and water retention and loss of potassium

hyperglycemia: elevated blood glucose levels (>110 mg/dL) leading to multiple signs and symptoms and abnormal metabolic pathways

hyperlipidemia: increased levels of lipids in the serum, associated with increased risk of CAD development

hyperparathyroidism: excessive parathormone

hypersensitivity: excessive responsiveness to either the primary or the secondary effects of a drug; may be caused by a pathological or individual condition

hyperthyroidism: excessive levels of thyroid hormone

hypertonia: state of excessive muscle response and activity

hypnotic: drug used to depress the CNS; causes sleep

hypocalcemia: calcium deficiency

hypoglycemia: lower than normal blood sugar (<40 mg/dL); often results from imbalance between insulin or oral agents and patient's eating, activity, and stress

hypogonadism: underdevelopment of the gonads (testes in the male)

hypokalemia: low potassium in the blood, which often occurs after diuretic use; characterized by weakness, muscle cramps, trembling, nausea, vomiting, diarrhea, and cardiac arrhythmias

hypnosis: extreme sedation resulting in CNS depression and sleep

hypoparathyroidism: rare condition of absence of parathormone; may be seen after thyroidectomy

hypopituitarism: lack of adequate function of the pituitary; reflected in many endocrine disorders

hypotension: sustained blood pressure that is lower than that required to adequately perfuse all of the body's tissues

hypothalamic–pituitary axis: interconnection of the hypothalamus and pituitary to regulate the levels of certain endocrine hormones through a complex series of negative feedback systems

hypothalamus: "master gland" of the neuroendocrine system; regulates both nervous and endocrine responses to internal and external stimuli

hypothyroidism: lack of sufficient thyroid hormone to maintain metabolism

immune stimulant: drug used to energize the immune system when it is exhausted from fighting prolonged invasion or needs help fighting a specific pathogen or cancer cell

immune suppressant: drug used to block or suppress the actions of the T cells and antibody production; used to prevent transplant rejection and to treat autoimmune diseases

immune sera: preformed antibodies found in immune globulin from animals or humans who have had a specific disease and developed antibodies to it

immunization: the process of stimulating active immunity by exposing the body to weakened or less toxic proteins associated with specific disease-causing organisms; the goal is to stimulate immunity without causing the full course of a disease

induction: time from the beginning of anesthesia until achievement of surgical anesthesia

influenza A: RNA virus that invades tissues of the respiratory tract, causing the signs and symptoms of the common cold or "flu"

inhibin: estrogen-like substance produced by seminiferous tubules during sperm production; acts as a negative feedback stimulus to decrease release of follicle-stimulating hormone (FSH)

insulin: hormone produced by the beta cells in the pancreas; stimulates insulin receptor sites to move glucose into the cells; promotes storage of fat and glucose in the body

interferon: tissue hormone that is released in response to viral invasion; blocks viral replication

interleukins: chemicals released by WBCs to communicate with other WBCs and to support the inflammatory and immune reactions

Internet: the world-wide digital information system accessed through computer systems

interneuron: neuron in the CNS that communicates with other neurons, not with muscles or glands

interstitial or Leydig cells: part of the testes that produce testosterone in response to stimulation by luteinizing hormone (LH)

interstitial cystitis: chronic inflammation of the interstitial connective tissue of the bladder; may extend into deeper tissue

intractable hiccough: repetitive stimulation of the diaphragm that leads to hiccough, a diaphragmatic spasm that persists over time

intrinsic pathway: cascade of clotting factors leading to the formation of a clot within an injured vessel

iodine: important dietary element used by the thyroid gland to produce thyroid hormone

iron deficiency anemia: low RBC count with low iron available because of high demand, poor diet, or poor absorption; treated with iron replacement

ketosis: breakdown of fats for energy, resulting in an increase in ketones to be excreted from the body

kinin system: system activated by Hageman factor as part of the inflammatory response; includes bradykinin

larynx: the vocal chords and the epiglottis, which close during swallowing to protect the lower respiratory tract from any foreign particles

leishmaniasis: skin, mucous membrane, or visceral infection caused by a protozoan passed to humans by the bites of sand flies

leukocytes: white blood cells (WBCs); can be neutrophils, basophils, or eosinophils

leukotriene receptor antagonists: drugs that selectively and competitively block or antagonize receptors for the production of leukotrienes D_4 and E4, components of slow-reacting substance of anaphylaxis (SRSA)

limbic system: area in the midbrain that is rich in epinephrine, norepinephrine, and serotonin and seems to control emotions

liothyronine (T3): the most potent thyroid hormone, with a short half-life of 12 hours

lipoprotein: structure composed of proteins and lipids; bipolar arrangement of the lipids monitors substances passing in and out of the cell

local gastrointestinal reflex: reflex response to various stimuli that allows the GI tract local control of its secretions and movements based on the contents or activity of the whole GI system

local anesthetic: powerful nerve blocker that prevents depolarization of nerve membranes, blocking the transmission of pain stimuli and, in some cases, motor activity

low-density lipoprotein (LDL): tightly packed fats that are thought to contribute to the development of CAD when remnants left over from the LDL are processed in the arterial lining

lower respiratory tract: the smallest bronchi and the alveoli that make up the lungs; the area where gas exchange takes place

lubricant: agent that increases the viscosity of the feces, making it difficult to absorb water from the bolus and easing movement of the bolus through the intestines

lymphocytes: white blood cells with large, varied nuclei; can be T cells or B cells

lysosomes: encapsulated digestive enzymes found within a cell; they digest old or damaged areas of the cell and are responsible for destroying the cell when the membrane ruptures and the cell dies

macrophages: mature leukocytes that are capable of phagocytizing an antigen (foreign protein); also called monocytes or mononuclear phagocytes

major tranquilizer: former name of antipsychotic drugs; no longer used because it implies that its primary effect is sedation, which is no longer thought to be the desired therapeutic action

malaria: protozoal infection with *Plasmodium*, characterized by cyclic fever and chills as the parasite is released from ruptured red blood cells; causes serious liver, CNS, heart, and lung damage

malignant hyperthermia: reaction to some NMJ drugs in susceptible individuals; characterized by extreme muscle rigidity, severe hyperpyrexia, acidosis, and in some cases death

mania: state of hyperexcitability; one phase of bipolar disorders, which alternate between periods of severe depression and mania

mast cell stabilizer: drug that works at the cellular level to inhibit the release of histamine (released from mast cells in response to inflammation or irritation) and the release of slow-reacting substance of anaphylaxis (SRSA)

megaloblastic anemia: anemia caused by lack of vitamin B_{12} and/or folic acid, in which RBCs are fewer in number and have a weak stroma and a short lifespan; treated by replacement of folic acid and vitamin B_{12}

menopause: depletion of the female ova; results in lack of estrogen and progesterone

menstrual cycle: cycling of female sex hormones in interaction with the hypothalamus and anterior pituitary feedback systems

metabolism: rate at which the cells burn energy

metastasis: ability to enter the circulatory or lymphatic system and travel to other areas of the body that are conducive to growth and survival; property of cancer cells

metric system: the most widely used system of measure, based on the decimal system; all units in the system are determined as multiples of ten

midbrain: the middle area of the brain; it consists of the hypothalamus and thalamus and includes the limbic system

migraine headache: headache characterized by severe, unilateral, pulsating head pain associated with systemic effects, including GI upset and sensitization to light and sound; related to a hyperperfusion of the brain from arterial dilation

mineralocorticoids: steroid hormones released by the adrenal cortex; they cause sodium and water retention and potassium excretion

miosis: constriction of the pupil; relieves intraocular pressure in some types of glaucoma

mitochondria: rod-shaped organelles; they produce adenosine triphosphate (ATP) for energy within the cell

monoamine oxidase (MAO): enzyme that breaks down norepinephrine to make it inactive

monoamine oxidase (MAO) inhibitor: drug that prevents the enzyme monoamine oxidase from breaking down norepinephrine (NE), leading to increased NE levels in the synaptic cleft; relieves depression and also causes sympathomimetic effects

monoclonal antibodies: specific antibodies produced by a single clone of B cells to react with a very specific antigen

mononuclear phagocyte system (MPS): system composed of the thymus gland, the lymphatic tissue, leukocytes, lymphocytes, and numerous chemical mediators; previously called the reticuloendothelial system

mucolytics: drugs that increase or liquefy respiratory secretions to aid the clearing of the airways

muscarinic receptors: cholinergic receptors that also respond to stimulation by muscarine

myasthenia gravis: autoimmune disease characterized by antibodies to cholinergic receptor sites, leading to destruction of the receptor sites and decreased response at the neuromuscular junction; it is progressive and debilitating, leading to paralysis

mycosis: disease caused by a fungus

mydriasis: relaxation of the muscles around the pupil, leading to pupil dilation

myocardial infarction: end result of vessel blockage in the heart; leads to ischemia and then necrosis of the area cut off from the blood supply; it can heal, with the dead cells replaced by scar tissue

myocardium: the muscle of the heart

myosin: thick filament with projections that makes up a sarcomere or muscle unit

myxedema: severe lack of thyroid hormone in adults

narcolepsy: mental disorder characterized by daytime sleepiness and periods of sudden loss of wakefulness

narcotic agonists–antagonists: drugs that react with at some opioid receptor sites to stimulate their activity and at other opioid receptor sites to block activity

narcotic agonists: drugs that react at opioid receptor sites to stimulate the effects of the receptors

narcotic antagonists: drugs that block the opioid receptor sites; used to counteract the effects of narcotics or to treat an overdose of narcotics

narcotics: drugs, originally derived from opium, that react with specific opioid receptors throughout the body

negative feedback system: control system in which increasing levels of a hormone lead to decreased levels of releasing and stimulating hormones, leading to decreased hormone levels, which stimulates the release of releasing and stimulating hormones; allows tight control of the endocrine system

nematode: a roundworm such as the commonly encountered pinworm, whipworm, threadworm, *Ascaris,* or hookworm

neoplasm: new or cancerous growth; occurs when abnormal cells have the opportunity to multiply and grow

nephron: functional unit of the kidney, composed of Bowman's capsule, the proximal and distal convoluted tubules, and the collecting duct

nerve gas: irreversible acetylcholinesterase inhibitor used in warfare to cause paralysis and death by prolonged muscle contraction and parasympathetic crisis

nerve plexus: network of nerve fibers running through the wall of the GI tract that allows local reflexes and control

neuroendocrine system: the combination of the nervous and endocrine systems, which work closely together to maintain regulatory control and homeostasis in the body

neuron: structural unit of the nervous system

neurotransmitter: chemical produced by a nerve and released when the nerve is stimulated; reacts with a specific receptor site to cause a reaction

nicotinic receptors: cholinergic receptors that also respond to stimulation by nicotine

nitrates: drugs used to cause direct relaxation of smooth muscle, leading to vasodilation and decreased venous return to the heart with decreased resistance to blood flow; this rapidly decreases oxygen demand in the heart and can restore the balance between blood delivered and blood needed in the heart muscle of patients with angina

nocturia: getting up to void at night, reflecting increased renal perfusion with fluid shifts in the supine position when a person has gravity-dependent edema related to CHF; other medical conditions, including urinary tract infection, increase the need to get up and void

nondepolarizing neuromuscular junction (NMJ) blocker: no stimulation or depolarization of the muscle cell; prevents depolarization and stimulation by blocking the effects of acetylcholine

nonsteroidal anti-inflammatory drugs (NSAIDs): drugs that block prostaglandin synthesis and act as anti-inflammatory, antipyretic, and analgesic agents

nucleosides: drugs that inhibit cell protein synthesis by HIV, leading to viral death

nucleus: the part of a cell that contains the DNA and genetic material; regulates cellular protein production and cellular properties

nursing: the art of nurturing and administering to the sick combined with the scientific application of chemistry, anatomy, physiology, biology, nutrition, psychology, and pharmacology to the particular clinical situation

nursing diagnosis: statement of an actual or potential problem, based on the assessment of a particular clinical situation, which directs needed nursing interventions

nursing process: the problem-solving process used to provide efficient nursing care; it involves gathering information, formulating a nursing diagnosis statement, carrying out interventions, and evaluating the process

off-label uses: uses of a drug that are not part of the stated therapeutic indications for which the drug was approved by the FDA

oncotic pressure: the pulling pressure of the plasma proteins, responsible for returning fluid to the vascular system at the capillary level

opioid receptors: receptor sites on nerves that react with endorphins and enkephalins, which are receptive to narcotic drugs

organelles: distinct structures found within the cell cytoplasm

orphan drugs: drugs that have been discovered but are not available for use by those who could benefit from them, usually because they are not financially profitable

orthopnea: difficulty breathing when lying down, often referred to by the number of pillows required to allow a person to breath comfortably

osmosis: movement of water from an area of low solute concentration to an area of high solute concentration in an attempt to equalize the concentrations

osmotic pull: drawing force of large molecules on water, pulling it into a tubule or capillary; essential for maintaining normal fluid balance within the body; used to draw out excess fluid into the vascular system or the renal tubule

OTC drugs: see *over-the-counter (OTC) drugs*

ova: eggs; the female gamete; contain half of the information needed in a human nucleus

ovaries: female sexual glands that store ova and produce estrogen and progesterone

over-the-counter (OTC) drugs: drugs that are available without a prescription for self-treatment of a variety of complaints

oxytocics: drugs that act like the hypothalamic hormone oxytocin; they stimulate uterine contraction and contraction of the lacteal glands in the breast, promoting milk ejection

Paget's disease: a genetically linked disorder of overactive osteoclasts that are eventually replaced by enlarged and softened bony structures

pancreatic enzymes: digestive enzymes secreted by the exocrine pancreas, including pancreatin and pancrelipase, which are needed for the proper digestion of fats, proteins, and carbohydrates

paralysis: lack of muscle function

parasympathetic nervous system: "rest and digest" response mediator that contains CNS cells from the cranium or sacral area of the spinal cord, long preganglionic axons, ganglia near or within the effector tissue, and short postganglionic axons that react with cholinergic receptors

parasympatholytic: lysing or preventing parasympathetic effects

parasympathomimetic: mimicking the effects of the parasympathetic nervous system: bradycardia, hypotension, pupil constriction, increased GI secretions and activity, increased bladder tone, relaxation of sphincters, bronchoconstriction

parathormone: hormone produced by the parathyroid glands; responsible for maintaining calcium levels in conjunction with calcitonin

Parkinson's disease: debilitating disease, characterized by progressive loss of coordination and function, which results from the degeneration of dopamine-producing cells in the substantia nigra

passive immunity: the injection of preformed antibodies into a host at high risk for exposure to a specific disease; immunity is limited by the amount of circulating antibody

penile erectile dysfunction: condition in which the corpus cavernosum does not fill with blood to allow for penile erection; can be related to aging or to neurological or vascular conditions

peptic ulcer: erosion of the lining of stomach or duodenum; results from imbalance between acid produced and the mucous protection of the GI lining, or possibly from infection by *Helicobacter pylori* bacteria

peripheral resistance: force that resists the flow of blood through the vessels, mostly determined by the arterioles, which contract to increase resistance; important in determining overall blood pressure

peristalsis: type of GI movement that moves a food bolus forward; characterized by a progressive wave of muscle contraction

pernicious anemia: megaloblastic anemia characterized by lack of vitamin B_{12} secondary to low production of intrinsic factor by gastric cells; vitamin B_{12} must be replaced by intramuscular injection or nasal spray because it cannot be absorbed through the GI tract

petit mal seizure: see *absence seizure*

phagocytes: neutrophils that are able to engulf and digest foreign material

phagocytosis: the process of engulfing and digesting foreign material

pharmacodynamics: the science that deals with the interactions between the chemical components of living systems and the foreign chemicals, including drugs, that enter living organisms; the way a drug affects a body

pharmacokinetics: the way the body deals with a drug, including absorption, distribution, biotransformation, and excretion

pharmacotherapeutics: clinical pharmacology, the branch of pharmacology that deals with drugs; chemicals that are used in medicine for the treatment, prevention, and diagnosis of disease in humans

phase I study: a pilot study of a potential drug done with a small number of selected, healthy human volunteers

phase II study: a clinical study of a drug by selected physicians using actual patients who have the disorder the drug is designed to treat; patients must provide informed consent

phase III study: use of a drug on a wide scale in the clinical setting with patients who have the disease the drug is thought to treat

phase IV study: continual evaluation of a drug after it has been released for marketing

phenothiazine: antianxiety drug that blocks the responsiveness of the chemoreceptor trigger zone (CTZ) to stimuli, leading to a decrease in nausea and vomiting

pheochromocytoma: a tumor of the chromaffin cells of the adrenal medulla that periodically releases large amounts of norepinephrine and epinephrine into the system with resultant severe hypertension and tachycardia

photosensitivity: hypersensitive reaction to the sun or ultraviolet light, seen as an adverse reaction to various drugs; can lead to severe skin rash and lesions as well as damage to the eye

pinworm: nematode that causes a common helminthic infection in humans; lives in the intestine and causes anal and possible vaginal irritation and itching

pituitary gland: gland found in the sella turcica of the brain; produces hormones, endorphins, and enkephalins and stores two hypothalamic hormones

placebo effect: documented effect of the mind on drug therapy; if a person perceives that a drug will be effective, the drug is much more likely to actually be effective

plasma: the liquid part of the blood; consists mostly of water and plasma proteins, glucose, and electrolytes

plasma esterase: enzyme found in plasma that immediately breaks down ester-type local anesthetics

plasminogen: natural clot-dissolving system; converted to plasmin (also called fibrinolysin) by many substances to dissolve clots that have formed and to maintain the patency of injured vessels

Plasmodium: a protozoan that causes malaria in humans; its life cycle includes the *Anopheles* mosquito, which injects protozoa into humans

platelet aggregation: property of platelets to adhere to an injured surface and then attract other platelets, which clump together or aggregate at the area, plugging up an injury to the vascular system

platyhelminth: flatworm or fluke such as the tapeworm

Pneumocystis carinii **pneumonia (PCP)**: opportunistic infection that occurs when the immune system is depressed; a frequent cause of pneumonia in patients with AIDS and in those who are receiving immunosuppressive therapy

pneumonia: inflammation of the lungs that can be caused by bacterial or viral invasion of the tissue or by aspiration of foreign substances

poisoning: overdose of a drug that causes damage to multiple body systems and the potential for fatal reactions

polydipsia: increased thirst; seen in diabetes when loss of fluid and increased tonicity of the blood lead the hypothalamic thirst center to make the patient feel thirsty

polyphagia: increased hunger; sign of diabetes when cells cannot use glucose for energy and feel that they are starving, causing hunger

positively inotropic: causing an increased force of contraction

posterior pituitary: lobe of the pituitary that receives ADH and oxytocin via neuraxons from the hypothalamus and stores them to be released when stimulated by the hypothalamus

postmenopausal osteoporosis: dropping levels of estrogen allow calcium to be pulled out of the bone, resulting in a weakened and honeycombed bone structure

preclinical trial: initial trial of a chemical thought to have therapeutic potential; uses laboratory animals, not human subjects

premature atrial contraction (PAC): caused by an ectopic focus in the atria that stimulates an atrial response

premature ventricular contraction (PVC): caused by an ectopic focus in the ventricles that stimulates the cells and causes an early contraction

Prinzmetal's angina: drop in blood flow through the coronary arteries caused by a vasospasm in the artery, not by atherosclerosis

proarrhythmic: tending to cause arrhythmias; many of the drugs used to treat arrhythmias have been found to generate arrhythmias

progesterone: hormone produced by the ovary, placenta, and adrenal gland; promotes maintenance of pregnancy

progestin: female sex hormone; important in maintaining a pregnancy and supporting many secondary sex characteristics

prophylaxis: treatment to prevent an infection before it occurs, as in the use of antibiotics to prevent bacterial endocarditis or antiprotozoals to prevent malaria

prostaglandin: any one of numerous tissue hormones that have local effects on various systems and organs of the body, including vasoconstriction, vasodilation, increased or decreased GI activity, and increased or decreased pancreatic enzyme release

prostate gland: gland located around the male urethra; responsible for producing an acidic fluid that maintains sperm and lubricates the urinary tract

protease inhibitors: drugs that block the activity of the enzyme protease in HIV; protease is essential for the maturation of infectious virus, and its absence leads to the formation of an immature and noninfective HIV particle

proton pump inhibitor: drug that blocks the H^+,K^+-ATPase enzyme system on the secretory surface of the gastric parietal cells, thus interfering with the final step of acid production and lowering acid levels in the stomach

protozoan: a single-celled organism that passes through several stages in its life cycle, including at least one phase as a human parasite; found in areas of poor sanitation and hygiene and crowded living conditions

puberty: point at which the hypothalamus starts releasing gonadotropin-releasing factor (GnRF) to stimulate the release of FSH and LH and begin sexual development

pulmonary edema: severe left-sided CHF with backup of blood into the lungs, leading to loss of fluid into the lung tissue

pulse pressure: the systolic blood pressure minus the diastolic blood pressure; reflects the filling pressure of the coronary arteries

pyelonephritis: inflammation of the pelves of the kidney, frequently caused by backward flow problems or by bacteria ascending the ureter

pyramidal tract: fibers within the CNS that control precise, intentional movement

pyrogen: substance that resets the thermoregulatory center in the hypothalamus to elevate the body temperature, thus speeding metabolism; some pyrogens are released by active neutrophils as part of the inflammatory response

ratio and proportion: an equation in which the ratio containing two known equivalent amounts is on one side of the equation and the ratio containing the amount desired to convert and its unknown equivalent is on the other side

reabsorption: the movement of substances from the renal tubule back into the vascular system

rebound congestion: occurs when the nasal passages become congested as the effect of a decongestant drug wears off; patients tend to use more drug to decrease the congestion and a vicious circle of congestion, drug, and congestion develops, leading to abuse of the decongestant; also called rhinitis medicamentosa

receptor sites: sites on cell membranes that react with specific other chemicals to cause an effect; a drug may be effective because it reacts with a specific receptor site on particular cells in the body

recombinant DNA technology: use of bacteria to produce chemicals normally produced by human cells

releasing hormones or factors: chemicals released by the hypothalamus into the anterior pituitary to stimulate the release of anterior pituitary hormones

renin–angiotensin system: compensatory process that leads to increased blood pressure and blood volume to ensure perfusion of the kidneys; important in the day-to-day regulation of blood pressure

repolarization: return of a membrane to a resting state, with more sodium ions outside the membrane and a relatively negative charge inside the membrane

resistance: ability of bacteria over time to adapt to an antibiotic and produce cells that are no longer affected by a particular drug

resistance system: the arteries; the muscles of the arteries provide resistance to the flow of blood, leading to control of blood pressure

respiration: the act of breathing

respiratory distress syndrome (RDS): disorder found in premature neonates whose lungs have not had time to mature and who are lacking sufficient surfactant to maintain open airways to allow for respiration

respiratory membrane: area through which gas exchange must be made; made up of the capillary endothelium, the capillary basement membrane, the interstitial space, the alveolar basement membrane, the alveolar endothelium, and the surfactant layer

reticulocyte: red blood cell (RBC) that has lost its nucleus and entered circulation just recently, not yet fully matured

reverse transcriptase inhibitors: drugs that block the transfer of both RNA- and DNA-dependent DNA polymerase activities; prevents the transfer of information that allows the virus to replicate and survive

rhinitis medicamentosa: reflex reaction to vasoconstriction caused by decongestants; a rebound vasodilation that often leads to prolonged overuse of decongestants; also called rebound congestion

ribosomes: membranous structures that are the sites of protein production within a cell

risk factors: factors that have been identified to increase the risk of the development of a disease; for CAD, risk factors include genetic predisposition, gender, age, high-fat diet, sedentary lifestyle, gout, hypertension, diabetes, and estrogen deficiency

roundworm: worm such as *Ascaris* that causes a common helminthic infection in humans; can cause intestinal obstruction as the adult worms clog the intestinal lumen or severe pneumonia when the larvae migrate to the lungs and form a pulmonary infiltrate

rubor: redness, one of the four cardinal signs of inflammation; caused by activation of the inflammatory response

salicylates: salicylic acid compounds, used as anti-inflammatory, antipyretic, and analgesic agents; they block the prostaglandin system

saliva: fluid produced by the salivary glands in the mouth in response to tactile stimuli and cerebral stimulation; contains enzymes to begin digestion as well as water and mucus to make the food bolus slippery and easier to swallow

sarcoma: tumor that originates in the mesenchyme and is made up of embryonic connective tissue cells

sarcomere: functional unit of a muscle cell, composed of actin and myosin molecules arranged in layers to give the unit a striped or striated appearance

schistosomiasis: infection with a blood fluke that is carried by a snail; it poses a common problem in tropical countries, where the snail is the intermediary in the life cycle of the worm; larvae burrow into the skin in fresh water and migrate throughout the human body, causing a rash and then symptoms of diarrhea and liver and brain inflammation

Schwann cell: insulating cell found on nerve axons; allows "leaping" electrical conduction to speed the transmission of information and prevent tiring of the neuron

seasonal rhinitis: inflammation of the nasal cavity, commonly called hay fever; caused by reaction to a specific antigen

secretion: the active movement of substances from the blood into the renal tubule

sedation: loss of awareness of and reaction to environmental stimuli

sedative: drug that depresses the CNS; produces a loss of awareness of and reaction to the environment

segmentation: GI movement characterized by contraction of one segment of small intestine while the next segment is relaxed; the contracted segment then relaxes, and the relaxed segment contracts; exposes the chyme to a vast surface area to increase absorption

seizure: sudden discharge of excessive electrical energy from nerve cells in the brain

selective serotonin reuptake inhibitor (SSRI): drug that specifically blocks the reuptake of serotonin and increases its concentration in the synaptic cleft; relieves depression and is not associated with anticholinergic or sympathomimetic adverse effects

selective toxicity: property of a chemotherapeutic agent that affects only systems found in foreign cells, without affecting healthy human cells (eg, specific antibiotics can affect certain proteins or enzyme systems used by bacteria but not by human cells)

self-care: tendency for patients to self-diagnose and determine their own treatment needs

seminiferous tubules: part of the testes that produce sperm in response to stimulation by follicle-stimulating hormone (FSH)

sensitivity testing: evaluation of bacteria obtained in a culture to determine to which antibiotics the organisms are sensitive to and which agent would be appropriate for treatment of a particular infection

serum sickness: reaction of a host to injected antibodies or foreign sera; host cells make antibodies to the foreign proteins, and a massive immune reaction can occur

shock: severe hypotension that can lead to accumulation of waste products and cell death

sinoatrial (SA) node: the normal pacemaker of the heart; composed of primitive cells that constantly generate an action potential

sinuses: air-filled passages through the skull that open into the nasal passage

sinusitis: inflammation of the epithelial lining of the sinus cavities

sliding filament theory: theory explaining muscle contraction as a reaction of actin and myosin molecules when they are freed to react by the inactivation of troponin after calcium is allowed to enter the cell during depolarization

sneeze: reflex response to irritation in the nasal passages; results in expelling of forced air through the nose

soma: cell body of a neuron; contains the nucleus, cytoplasm, and various granules

spasticity: sustained muscle contractions

spectrum: range of bacteria against which an antibiotic is effective (eg, broad-spectrum antibiotics are effective against a wide range of bacteria)

sperm: male gamete; contains half of the information needed for a human cell nucleus

spinothalamic tract: nerve pathway from the spine to the thalamus along which pain impulses are carried to the brain

Starling's law of the heart: addresses the contractile properties of the heart: the more the muscle is stretched, the stronger it will react, until it is stretched to a point at which it will not react at all

status epilepticus: state in which seizures rapidly recur; most severe form of generalized seizure

stomatitis: inflammation of the mucous membranes related to drug effects; can lead to alterations in nutrition and dental problems

stroke volume: the amount of blood pumped out of the ventricle with each beat; important in determining blood pressure

substantia nigra: a part of the brain rich in dopamine and dopamine receptors; site of degenerating neurons in Parkinson's disease

sulfonylureas: oral antidiabetic agents used to stimulate the pancreas to release more insulin

superinfections: infections caused by the destruction of bacteria of the normal flora by certain drugs, which allows other bacteria to enter the body and cause infection; may occur during the course of antibiotic therapy

surfactant: lipoprotein that reduces surface tension in the alveoli, allowing them to stay open to allow gas exchange

swallowing: complex reflex response to a bolus in the back of the throat; allows passage of the bolus into the esophagus and movement of ingested contents into the GI tract

sympathetic nervous system: "fight or flight" response mediator; composed of CNS cells from the thoracic or lumbar areas, short preganglionic axons, ganglia near the spinal cord, and long postganglionic axons that react with adrenergic receptors

sympatholytic: a drug that lyses, or blocks, the effects of the sympathetic nervous system

sympathomimetic: mimicking of the sympathetic nervous system (SNS) with the signs and symptoms seen when the SNS is stimulated

sympathomimetics: drugs that mimic the effects of the sympathetic nervous system

synapse: junction between a nerve and an effector; consists of the presynaptic nerve ending, a space called the synaptic cleft, and the postsynaptic cell

syncytium: intertwining network of muscle fibers that make up the atria and the ventricles of the heart; allows for a coordinated pumping contraction

synergistic: drugs that work together to increase drug effectiveness

systole: contracting phase of the heart, during which blood is pumped out of the heart

T cells: lymphocytes programmed in the thymus gland to recognize self-cells; may be effector T cells, helper T cells, or suppressor T cells

tachycardia: faster than normal heart rate (usually >100 beats/min)

tachypnea: rapid and shallow respirations, seen with left-sided CHF

teratogenic: having adverse effects on the fetus

testes: male sexual gland that produces sperm and testosterone

testosterone: male sex hormone; produced by the interstitial or Leydig cells of the testes

thiazide: type of diuretic acting in the renal tubule to block the chloride pump, which prevents reabsorption of sodium and chloride, leading to a loss of sodium and water in the urine

thioamides: drugs used to prevent the formation of thyroid hormone in the thyroid cells, lowering thyroid hormone levels

threadworm: pervasive nematode that can send larvae into the lungs, liver, and CNS; can cause severe pneumonia or liver abscess

thromboembolic disorders: disorders characterized by the formation of clots or thrombi on injured blood vessels with potential breaking of the clot to form emboli that can travel to smaller vessels, where they become lodged and occlude the vessel

thrombolytic drugs: drugs that lyse, or break down, a clot that has formed; these drugs activate the plasminogen mechanism to dissolve fibrin threads

thyroxine (T_4): a thyroid hormone that is converted to T_3 in the tissues; it has a half-life of 1 week

tinea: fungus called ringworm that causes such infections as athlete's foot, jock itch, and others

tocolytics: drugs used to relax the gravid uterus to prolong pregnancy

tonic–clonic seizure: type of generalized seizure that is characterized by serious clonic–tonic muscular reactions and loss of consciousness, with exhaustion and little memory of the event on awakening; formerly known as a grand mal seizure

trachea: the main conducting airway leading into the lungs

trichinosis: disease that results from ingestion of encysted roundworm larvae in undercooked pork; larvae migrate throughout the body to invade muscles, nerves, and other tissues; can cause pneumonia, heart failure, and encephalitis

trichomoniasis: infestation with a protozoan that causes vaginitis in women but no signs or symptoms in men

tricyclic antidepressant (TCA): drug that blocks the reuptake of norepinephrine and serotonin; relieves depression and has anticholinergic and sedative effects

triptan: selective serotonin receptor blocker that causes a vascular constriction of cranial vessels; used to treat acute migraine attacks

trophozoite: a developing stage of a parasite, which uses the host for essential nutrients needed for growth

troponin: chemical in heart muscle that prevents the reaction between actin and myosin, leading to muscle relaxation; it is inactivated by calcium during muscle stimulation to allow actin and myosin to react, causing muscle contraction

trypanosomiasis: African sleeping sickness, which is caused by a protozoan that inflames the CNS and is spread to humans by the bite of the tsetse fly; also, Chagas' disease, which causes a serious cardiomyopathy after the bite of the house fly

tumor: swelling, one of the four cardinal signs of inflammation; caused by activation of the inflammatory response

tyramine: an amine found in food that causes vasoconstriction and raises blood pressure; ingesting foods high in tyramine while taking an MAO inhibitor poses the risk of a severe hypertensive crisis

unconsciousness: loss of awareness of one's surroundings

upper respiratory tract: the conducting airways, composed of the nose, mouth, pharynx, larynx, trachea, and upper bronchial tree

urgency: the feeling that one needs to void immediately; associated with infection and inflammation in the urinary tract

urinary frequency: the need to void often; usually seen in response to irritation of the bladder, age, and inflammation

uterus: the womb; site of growth and development of the embryo and fetus

vaccine: immunization containing weakened or altered protein antigens to stimulate a specific antibody formation against a specific disease; refers to a product used to stimulate active immunity

veins: vessels that return blood to the heart; distensible tubes

ventilation: the exchange of gases at the alveolar level across the respiratory membrane

ventricle: bottom chamber of the heart, which contracts to pump blood out of the heart

vestibular: referring to the apparatus of the inner ear that controls balance and sense of motion; stimulus to this area can cause motion sickness

virus: particle of DNA or RNA surrounded by a protein coat that survives by invading a cell to alter its functioning

volatile liquid: liquid that is unstable at room temperature and releases vapors; used as an inhaled general anesthetic, usually in the form of a halogenated hydrocarbon

vomiting: complex reflex mediated through the medulla after stimulation of the chemoreceptor trigger zone (CTZ); protective reflex to remove possibly toxic substances from the stomach

whipworm: worm that attaches itself to the intestinal mucosa and sucks blood; may cause severe anemia and disintegration of the intestinal mucosa

xanthines: naturally occurring substances, including caffeine and theophylline, that have a direct effect on the smooth muscle of the respiratory tract, both in the bronchi and in the blood vessels

Young's Rule: a method for determining pediatric drug dosage based on the child's age and the usual adult dose; it states

$$\text{dose (child 1--12 y)} = \frac{\text{child's age (y)}}{\text{childs age (y)} + 12} \times \text{average adult dose}$$

PARENTERAL AGENTS

Parenteral preparations are fluids that are given either intravenously (IV) or through a central line.

Therapeutic Actions and Indications

Parenteral agents are used for the following purposes: to provide replacement fluids, sugars, electrolytes, and nutrients to patients who are unable to take them in orally; to provide ready access for administration of drugs in an emergency situation; to provide rehydration; and to restore electrolyte balance. The composition of the IV fluids needed for a patient depends on the patient's fluid and electrolyte status.

Parenteral nutrition (PN) is the administration of essential proteins, amino acids, carbohydrates, vitamins, minerals, trace elements, lipids, and fluids. PN is used to improve or stabilize the nutritional status of cachectic or debilitated patients who cannot take in or absorb oral nutrition to the extent required to maintain their nutritional status. The exact composition of the PN solution is determined after a nutritional assessment and must take into account the patient's current health status, age, and metabolic needs.

Contraindications and Cautions

PN is contraindicated in anyone with known allergies to any component of the solution. (Multiple combination products are available, so a suitable solution may be found.) PN should be used with caution in patients with unstable cardiovascular status, because of the change in fluid volume that may occur and the resultant increased workload on the heart. These preparations also should be used with caution in patients with unstable fluid and electrolyte status, who could react adversely to sudden changes in fluids and electrolytes.

Adverse Effects

Adverse effects associated with the use of PN include IV irritation, extravasation of the fluid into the tissues, infection of the insertion site, fluid volume overload, vascular problems related to fluid shifts, and potential electrolyte imbalance related to dilution of the blood. PN also is associated with mechanical problems related to insertion of the line, such as pneumothorax, infections, or air emboli; emboli related to protein or lipid aggregation; infections related to

nutrient-rich solution and invasive administration; metabolic imbalances related to the composition of the solution; gallstone development (especially in children); and nausea (especially related to the administration of lipids).

Clinically Important Drug–Drug Interactions

Some IV drugs can be diluted only with particular IV solutions to avoid precipitation or inactivation of the drug. A drug guide should be checked before diluting any IV drug in solution.

Nursing Considerations

Assessment: History and Examination

Obtain a nutritional assessment. Screen for any medical conditions and drugs being taken.

Evaluate insertion site; skin hydration; orientation and affect; height and weight; pulse, blood pressure, and respirations; blood chemistries, complete blood count with differential, and glucose levels.

Nursing Diagnoses

The patient receiving a parenteral agent may have the following nursing diagnoses related to drug therapy:

- Acute Pain related to administration of the fluid
- Risk for Infection related to invasive delivery system
- Risk for Imbalanced Nutrition related to fluid composition
- Deficient Knowledge regarding drug therapy

Implementation

- Assess patient's general physical condition before beginning test, *to decrease the potential for adverse effects.*
- Monitor IV insertion site or central line regularly; consult with prescriber *to discontinue site of infusion and treat any infection or extravasation as soon as it occurs.*
- Follow these administration guidelines, *to provide the most therapeutic use of PN with the fewest adverse effects:*
  Refrigerate PN solutions until ready to use.
  Check contents before hanging to ensure that no precipitates are present.
  Do not hang bag for longer than 24 hours.
  Suggest the use of on-line filters to decrease bacterial invasion and infusion of aggregate.

- Discontinue PN only after an alternative source of nutrition has been established, *to ensure continued nutrition for the patient;* taper slowly *to avoid severe reactions.*
- Provide comfort measures *to help the patient tolerate drug effects* (e.g., provide proper skin care as needed, analgesics, hot soaks to extravasation sites).
- Include information about the solution being used in a test (e.g., what to expect, adverse effects that may occur, follow-up tests that may be needed), *to enhance patient knowledge about drug therapy and promote compliance with the drug regimen.*

Evaluation

- Monitor patient response to the drug (stabilization of nutritional state; fluid and electrolyte balance, laboratory values).
- Monitor for adverse effects (local irritation, infection, fluid and electrolyte imbalance).
- Evaluate effectiveness of teaching plan (patient can name adverse effects to watch for, specific measures to avoid adverse effects; patient understands importance of follow-up that will be needed).
- Monitor effectiveness of comfort measures and compliance with regimen.

TABLE A | Parenterals

Solution	Caloric Content (cal/L)	Osmolarity (mOsm/L)	Usual Indications
IN SOLUTIONS			
DEXTROSE SOLUTIONS			
2.5% (25 g/L)	85	126	Provide calories and fluid
5% (50 g/L)	170	253	Provide calories and fluid, keep vein open for administration of IV drugs; frequent choice for dilution of IV drugs
10% (100 g/L)	340	505	Hypertonic solution used after admixture with other fluids; provide calories and fluid
20% (200 g/L)	680	1010	Hypertonic solution used after admixture with other fluids; provide calories and fluid
25% (250 g/L)	850	1330	Hypertonic solution used after admixture with other fluids; provide calories and fluid; treatment of acute hypoglycemic episodes in infants to restore glucose levels and suppress symptoms; sclerosing agent for varicose veins
30% (300 g/L)	1020	1515	Hypertonic solution used after admixture with other fluids; provide calories and fluid
40% (400 g/L)	1360	2020	Hypertonic solution used after admixture with other fluids; provide calories and fluid
50% (500 g/L)	1700	2525	Hypertonic solution used after admixture with other fluids; provide calories and fluid; treatment of hyperinsulinemia; sclerosing agent for varicose veins
60% (600 g/L)	2040	3030	Hypertonic solution used after admixture with other fluids; provide calories and fluid
70% (700 g/L)	2380	3535	Hypertonic solution used after admixture with other fluids; provide calories and fluid

Solution	Sodium Content (mEq/L)	Chloride Content (mEq/L)	Osmolarity (mOsm/L)	Usual Indications
SALINE SOLUTIONS				
0.45% (½ normal saline)	77	77	155	Hydrating solution; may be used to evaluate kidney function; treatment of hyperosmolar diabetes
0.9% (normal saline)	154	154	310	Replacement of fluid, sodium, and chloride; flushing lines and catheters; dilution of IV medications; priming of dialysis machines; neonate blood transfusions
3%	513	513	1030	Hypertonic solution to treat sodium and chloride depletion; emergency treatment of water intoxication or severe salt depletion
5%	855	855	1710	Hypertonic solution to treat sodium and chloride depletion; emergency treatment of water intoxication or severe salt depletion

COMMONLY USED COMBINATION FLUIDS*

Solution	Na Content (mEq/L)	K Content (mEq/L)	Cl Content (mEq/L)	Ca Content (mEq/L)	Mg Content (mEq/L)	Lactate (mEq/L)	Acetate (mEq/L)	Osmolarity (mOsm/L)
Plasma-Lyte-56	40	13	40	—	3	—	18	111
Ringer's Injection	147	4	156	4	—	—	—	310
Lactated Ringer's	130	4	109	3	—	28	—	273
Normosol-R	140	5	96	—	3	—	27	295

TYPICAL CENTRAL PARENTERAL NUTRITION SOLUTION*—1 LITER
(Actual concentration of solution and components of any particular solution will be determined by the assessment of the patient's current status and nutritional needs.)

TABLE A | Parenterals (Continued)

Component	Purpose	Dosage	Special Considerations
10% Amino acids	Provides 50 g protein for growth and healing	500 mL	Monitor BP, cardiac output, blood chemistries, urine to determine effect of intravascular protein pull.
50% Dextrose	Provides 850 calories for energy	500 mL	Monitor blood sugar; evaluate injection site for any sign of infection, irritation.
20% Fat emulsion	Provides 500 fat calories, ready energy	250 mL	Monitor for any sign of emboli (e.g., shortness of breath, chest pain, deep leg pain, neurological changes). Carefully monitor patients for any sign of increased vascular workload, especially very young and geriatric patients.
Sodium chloride	Provides sodium and chloride needed for various chemical reactions within the body	40 mEq	Monitor cardiac rhythm, serum electrolytes.
Calcium gluconate	Provides essential calcium for muscle contraction, blood clotting, numerous chemical reactions	4.8 mEq	Monitor cardiac rhythm, muscle strength, serum electrolytes.
Magnesium sulfate	Provides magnesium for various chemical reactions within the body	8 mEq	Monitor BP, deep tendon reflexes, and serum electrolytes.
Potassium phosphate	Provides needed potassium for nerve functioning, muscle contractions, etc.	9 mM	Monitor P, including rhythm, muscle function, and serum electrolytes.
Multivitamins	Provide a combination of essential vitamins to maintain cell integrity, promote healing	10 mL	Monitor for signs of vitamin deficiency or toxicity.
Trace elements	Provide small amounts of elements essential for numerous chemical reactions in the body and maintenance of cell integrity and healing		Periodically monitor blood chemistries to determine adequacy of replacement.
Zinc		3 mg	
Copper		1.2 mg	
Manganese		0.3 mg	
Chromium		12 mcg	
Selenium		20 mcg	

Total non-protein calories: 1350
Total volume of solution: 1250 ml
Dextrose concentration: 25%
Amino acid concentration: 5%
Osmolarity: 1900 mOsm/L

TYPICAL PERIPHERAL PARENTERAL NUTRITION SOLUTION*—1 LITER

(Actual concentration of solution and components of any particular solution will be determined by the assessment of the patient's current status and nutritional needs. Solutions used for peripheral therapy are usually less concentrated and less irritating to the vessel.)

Component	Purpose	Dosage	Special Considerations
8.5% Amino acids	Provides 41 g protein for growth and healing	500 mL	Monitor BP, cardiac output, blood chemistries, urine to determine effect of intravascular protein pull.
20% Dextrose	Provides 340 calories for energy	500 mL	Monitor blood sugar; evaluate injection site for any sign of infection, irritation.
20% Fat emulsion	Provides 500 fat calories, ready energy	250 mL	Monitor for any sign of emboli (e.g., shortness of breath, chest pain, deep leg pain, neurological changes). Carefully monitor patients for any sign of increased vascular workload, especially very young and geriatric patients.
Sodium chloride	Provides sodium and chloride needed for various chemical reactions within the body	40 mEq	Monitor cardiac rhythm, serum electrolytes.

Table A continues on page 830

TABLE A   Parenterals (Continued)

Component	Purpose	Dosage	Special Considerations
Calcium gluconate	Provides essential calcium for muscle contraction, blood clotting, numerous chemical reactions	4.8 mEq	Monitor cardiac rhythm, muscle strength, serum electrolytes.
Magnesium sulfate	Provides magnesium for various chemical reactions within the body	8 mEq	Monitor BP, deep tendon reflexes, and serum electrolytes.
Potassium phosphate	Provides needed potassium for nerve functioning, muscle contractions, etc.	9 mMoles	Monitor P, including rhythm, muscle function and serum electrolytes.
Multivitamins	Provide a combination of essential vitamins to maintain cell integrity, promote healing, etc.	10 mL	Monitor for signs of vitamin deficiency or toxicity.
Trace elements	Provide small amounts of elements essential for numerous chemical reactions in the body and maintenance of cell integrity and healing.		Periodically monitor blood chemistries to determine adequacy of replacement.
Zinc		3 mg	
Copper		1.2 mg	
Manganese		0.3 mg	
Chromium		12 mcg	
Selenium		20 mcg	

Total nonprotein calories: 840
Total volume of solution: 1250 mL
Dextrose concentration: 10%
Amino acid concentration: 4.25%
Osmolarity: 900 mOsm/L

*Note: Multiple combination preparations are available commercially. Each preparation varies in the concentration of one or more components and should be checked carefully before hanging.

DIAGNOSTIC AGENTS

Some pharmacological agents are used solely to diagnose particular conditions. Diagnostic tests that use these agents include

- In vitro tests, which are done outside the body to measure the presence of particular elements (eg, proteins, blood glucose, bacteria)
- In vivo tests, which introduce drugs into the body to evaluate specific physiological functions (eg, cardiac output, intestinal absorption, gastric acid secretion)

Therapeutic Actions and Indications

In vitro tests are often performed as part of the nursing evaluation of a patient, or they may be done at home by the patient as part of a medical regimen. These drugs can include reagents that react with specific enzymes or chemicals, such as glucose, blood, or human chorionic gonadotropin (HCG). Drugs used for in vivo tests may stimulate or suppress normal body reactions, such as a glucose challenge to evaluate insulin release or thyroid suppression tests to evaluate thyroid response. Specific tests of blood, urine, or other bodily fluids are often needed to evaluate the body's response to these drugs and to make a diagnosis. Drugs given as part of in vivo tests are administered under the supervision of medical personnel who are either conducting the test or making the diagnosis. They are usually given only once or used over a short period of time. Their use is part of an overall diagnostic plan to determine the underlying source of a particular problem.

Contraindications and Cautions

The use of any of the in vivo drugs is contraindicated in cases of allergy to the drugs themselves or to the colorants or preservatives used in them. Specific agents may be contraindicated in conditions that could be exacerbated by the stimulation of particular body responses. These drugs should be used cautiously during pregnancy or lactation.

Adverse Effects

The adverse effects seen with diagnostic agents are usually associated with the suppression or stimulation of the response they are being used to test. Because these drugs are given as only part of a test, the adverse effects usually last for a short period and can be tolerated by the patient.

Clinically Important Drug–Drug Interactions

Drug interactions vary with the particular agent that is being used. Consult a drug guide for specific information before giving any diagnostic agent.

Clinically Important Drug–Food Interactions

Because these tests are designed to elicit very specific responses, there is often the possibility that food will interfere with the actions or sensitivity of the test. Consult a drug guide for specific information about drug–food interactions before giving any diagnostic agent.

Nursing Considerations

Assessment: History and Examination

Screen for the following conditions, which could be contraindications to use of the agent: presence of known allergy to any of these drugs or to the colorants or preservatives used in these drugs.

Include screening for baseline status before beginning therapy and for any potential adverse effects. Assess the following: skin and mucous membrane condition; orientation, affect, and reflexes; pulse, blood pressure, respirations; abdominal examination; bowel sounds; blood and urine tests required for the particular test being performed.

Nursing Diagnoses

The patient receiving a diagnostic agent may have the following nursing diagnoses related to drug therapy:

- Acute Pain related to effects of the drugs
- Fear related to the test being done and possible test results
- Disturbed Body Image related to testing procedure and related tests that must be done
- Deficient Knowledge regarding drug therapy

Implementation

- Assess patient's general physical condition before beginning test, *to decrease the potential for adverse effects.*

- Provide comfort measures *to help patient tolerate drug effects* (eg, give drug with food to decrease gastrointestinal upset, provide proper skin care as needed, administer analgesics for headache as appropriate, provide privacy for the collection and storage of urine samples).
- Include information about the drug being used in a test (eg, what to expect, adverse effects that may occur, follow-up tests that may be needed), *to enhance patient knowledge about drug therapy and promote compliance with the drug regimen.*

Evaluation

- Monitor patient response to the drug (adverse reactions, collection of diagnostic information).
- Monitor for adverse effects (neurological effects, gastrointestinal upset, skin reaction, hypoglycemia, constipation).
- Evaluate effectiveness of teaching plan (patient can name adverse effects to watch for, specific measures to avoid adverse effects; patient understands importance of follow-up that will be needed).
- Monitor effectiveness of comfort measures and compliance with regimen.

TABLE B Diagnostic Agents

IN VITRO TESTS

Test Object	Brand Names	Usual Indication	Special Considerations
acetone	Acetest, Chemstrip K, Ketostix	Test for ketones in urine, blood, serum, or plasma	Most frequently used to test urine; Acetest is the only product that is also used for blood products
albumin	Albustix, Chemstrip Micral	At-home urine test for the presence of proteins	Advise patient to follow product storage instructions
urine bacteria	Microstix-3, Uricult, Isocult for Bacteruria	Test for urine nitrates, uropathogens, gram-negative bacteria	Most accurate if used with a clean-catch urine sample
bilirubin	Icotest	Test for urine bilirubin levels	Most accurate if used with a clean-catch urine sample
blood urea nitrogen	Azostix	Estimate of BUN	Used as a reagent strip with whole blood
Candida tests	Isocult for Candida, CandidaSure	Culture paddles or reagent slides for testing vaginal smears	Rapid test for presence of Candida with vaginal examination
Chlamydia trachomatis	Amplicor, Chlamydiazyme, MicroTrak for Chlamydia, Sure Cell Chlamydia	Kits and slides for testing urogenital, rectal, conjunctival, nasopharyngeal specimens for the presence of Chlamydia	Kits are specific for testing specimens
cholesterol	Advanced Care Cholesterol Test	At-home cholesterol test	Kit includes audio cassette with instructions; patients should be cautioned to seek medical care and advice
glucose, blood	Chemstrip bG, Dextrostrip, Glucostix, Glucometer Elite, Accu-Check Advantage and others	At-home testing of blood glucose levels	Patients should be taught how to calibrate the machine, proper blood drawing technique, and importance of seeking follow-up medical care
glucose, urine	Clinitest, Clinistix, Diastix	At-home testing of urine glucose levels	Patient should be taught how to read strips, proper storage of products and importance of seeking follow-up medical care
gonorrhea	Biocult-GC, Gonozyme Diagnostic, Isocult for Neisseria gonorrhoeae	Kits, culture paddles for the detection of Neisseria gonorrhea on endocervical, rectal, urethral, and oropharyngeal specimens	Test kits containing reagents, preservatives as needed for detection of Neisseria gonorrhea during physical examination
mononucleosis	Mono-Spot, Mono-Diff, Mono-Sure and others	Kits, reagents, slides for the testing of serum, blood for mononucleosis	Rapid tests for suspected cases of mononucleosis; all necessary reagents and preservatives included in kit
occult blood	ColoCare, EZ Detect, Hemoocult II and others	Kits and slides for the testing of fecal swabs for the presence of occult blood	Card forms can be used by patients at home in routine screening programs
ovulation	Answer, OvuQuick Self-Test, First Response Ovulation Detector and others	Kits to determine the levels of LH in the urine as a predictor of ovulation	Used at home by patients as part of fertility programs; patients may need instruction

TABLE B Diagnostic Agents (Continued)

IN VITRO TESTS

Test Object	Brand Names	Usual Indication	Special Considerations
pregnancy	*Advance First Response Pregnosis* and others	Kits or urine strips to detect the presence of HCG (human chorionic gonadotropin) as a predictor of pregnancy	May be used at home; patients may need instruction and should be advised to seek follow-up medical care
rheumatoid factor	*Rheumatex Rheumaton*	Slide tests for the presence of rheumatoid factor in blood, serum, or synovial fluid	An aid in the diagnosis of auto-immune diseases
sickle cell	*Sickledex*	Kit for the testing of blood for the presence of hemoglobin S	Diagnostic for sickle cell anemia
streptococci	*Sure Cell Streptococci Culturette 10 Minute Group A Strep ID Bactigen Strep B* and others	Kits, slides, culture paddles for the identification of streptococcal infection in blood, serum, urine, throat, cerebrospinal fluid	Early detection of streptococcal infection to facilitate beginning of treatment before culture and sensitivity results are known

IN VIVO TESTS

Drug	Brand Names	Usual Indication	Special Considerations
aminohippurate	*PAH Aminohippurate Sodium*	Estimation of renal plasma flow and to measure the functional capacity of the renal secretory mechanism	Injected as a 20% aqueous solution; requires careful urine collection
arbutamine	*GenESA*	Diagnosis of CAD in patients who cannot exercise adequately	Causes stress to evaluate body response; must be given with its own delivery device
arginine	*R-Gene 10*	Diagnostic aid to assess pituitary reserve of growth hormone	IV infusion, followed by blood tests to monitor response
benzylpenicilloyl-polylysine	*Pre-Pen*	Skin test to evaluate sensitivity to penicillin and safety of administering penicillin in potentially sensitive individuals	Intradermal or scratch test is used; positive reaction is usually seen within 10–15 minutes
gonadorelin	*Factrel*	Evaluation of gonadotropic capacity of the pituitary gland	Given IV or SC; monitor closely for potential hypersensitivity reactions
histamine phosphate	*Histamine-Phosphate*	SC—to evaluate ability of gastric mucosa to produce HCl IV—diagnosis of pheochromocytoma	May cause severe symptoms, including shock, cardiovascular collapse, even death; monitor patient closely
indocyanine green	*Cardio-Green*	Determining cardiac output, hepatic function, liver blood flow; also used for ophthalmic angiography	Use caution with known allergy to dyes
inulin	*Inulin injection*	Measurement of glomerular filtration rate	Requires blood tests and urine collection
methacholine chloride	*Provocholine*	Diagnosis of bronchial airway hypersensitivity in patients without documented asthma	Inhaled with pulmonary function test immediately; may cause hypotension, chest pain, GI upset
pentagastrin	*Peptavlon*	Evaluation of gastric acid secretory function	Given SC; may cause abdominal pain, flushing, nausea, vomiting, diarrhea, tachycardia
protirelin	*Thypinone Relefact TRH Thyrel TRH*	Diagnosis and assessment of thyroid function	Give IV over 15–30 seconds; patient should remain supine for at least 15 minutes because of risk of hypotension
secretin	*Secretin-Ferring Powder*	Diagnosis of pancreatic exocrine disease Diagnosis of gastrinoma	Requires a 12–15 hour fast; passing of a radio-paque tube for pancreatic function or repeated blood samples for gastrinoma diagnosis
sermorelin	*Geref*	Evaluation of pituitary ability to secrete growth hormone	Single IV injection; follow-up blood tests will be needed to determine response
sodium iodide	*Sodium Iodide I^{123}*	Diagnosis of thyroid function or morphology	Handle with care; oral capsules are radioactive, dispose of properly; thyroid can be evaluated for radiation content within 6 hours of dose

Table B continues on page 834

| TABLE B | Diagnostic Agents (Continued) |

IN VIVO TESTS

Drug	Brand Names	Usual Indication	Special Considerations
thyrotropin	*Thytropar*	Differentiation of thyroid function to estimate thyroid reserve	Given IM or SC qd for 10 days; follow with radioactive iodine test—no response shows thyroid failure
tolbutamide	*Orinase Diagnostic*	Diagnosis of pancreatic islet cell adenoma	Given IV after 3 days of high-carbohydrate diet; prepare to support patient if severe hypoglycemia occurs
teriparatide acetate	*Parathar*	Distinguish between hypo-parathyroidism and pseudo-hypoparathyroidism in patients with hypocalcemia	Given IV over 10 min; patients may experience GI distress, metallic taste

TOPICAL AGENTS

Topical agents are intended for surface use only and are not meant for ingestion or injection. They may be toxic if absorbed into the system, but they have several useful purposes when applied to the surface of the skin or mucous membranes. Some forms of drugs are prepared to be absorbed through the skin for systemic effects. These drugs may be prepared as transdermal patches (eg, nitroglycerin, estrogens, nicotine), which are designed to provide a slow release of the drug from the vehicle. Drugs prepared for this type of administration are discussed with the specific drug in the text and are not addressed in this appendix.

Therapeutic Actions and Indications

Topical agents are used to treat a variety of disorders in a localized area. Table C describes the usual uses for the many different types of topical agents. Because these drugs are designed for topical application, they are minimally absorbed systemically and, if used properly, should have minimal systemic effects.

Contraindications and Cautions

The use of topical agents is contraindicated in cases of allergy to the drugs and in the presence of open wounds or abrasions, which could lead to the systemic absorption of the drugs. Caution should be used during pregnancy if there is any possibility that the agent might be absorbed. Caution should also be used in the presence of any known allergy to the vehicles of preparation (creams, lotions).

Adverse Effects

Because these drugs are not intended to be absorbed systemically, the adverse effects usually associated with topical agents are local effects, including local irritation, stinging, burning, or dermatitis. Toxic effects are associated with inadvertent systemic absorption.

Nursing Considerations
Assessment: History and Examination

Screen for the presence of any known allergy to the drug, which would be a contraindication to its use.

Include screening for baseline status before beginning therapy and for any potential adverse effects. Assess the following: condition of area to be treated.

Nursing Diagnoses

The patient receiving a topical agent may have the following nursing diagnoses related to drug therapy:

- Risk for Injury related to toxic effects associated with absorption
- Acute Pain related to local effects of the drug
- Deficient Knowledge regarding drug therapy

Implementation

- Ensure proper administration of drug *to provide best therapeutic effect and least adverse effects* as follows:
  Apply sparingly. Some preparations come with applicators, some should be applied while wearing protective gloves, and others are dropped onto the site with no direct contact. Consult information regarding the individual drug being used for specific procedures.
  Do not use with open wounds or broken skin.
  Avoid contact with the eyes.
  Do not use with occlusive dressings, which could increase the risk of systemic absorption.
- Monitor area being treated, *to evaluate drug effects on the condition being treated.*
- Provide comfort measures *to help the patient tolerate drug effects* (e.g., analgesia as needed for local pain, itching).
- Provide patient teaching *to enhance patient knowledge about drug therapy and promote compliance with the drug regimen:*
  Teach the patient the proper administration technique for the topical agent ordered.
  Caution the patient that transient stinging or burning may occur.
  Instruct the patient to report severe irritation, allergic reaction, or worsening of the condition being treated.

Evaluation

- Monitor patient response to the drug (improvement in condition being treated).
- Monitor for adverse effects (local stinging or inflammation).
- Evaluate effectiveness of teaching plan (patient can name drug, dosage, adverse effects to watch for, specific measures to avoid adverse effects; patient understands importance of continued follow-up).
- Monitor effectiveness of comfort measures and compliance with regimen.

TOPICAL CORTICOSTEROIDS

These drugs enter cells and bind to cytoplasmic receptors, initiating complex reactions that are responsible for the anti-inflammatory, antipruritic, and antiproliferative effects of these drugs. They are used to relieve the inflammation and pruritic manifestations of corticosteroid-sensitive dermatoses and for temporary relief of minor skin irritations and rashes. These agents should always be applied sparingly because of the risk of systemic corticosteroid effects if they are absorbed systemically. Occlusive dressings and tight coverings should be avoided. Prolonged use should also be avoided because of the risk of systemic effects and local irritation and breakdown. These agents are applied topically two to three times daily.

TABLE C Topical Agents

Drug	Brand Name	Dosage	Usual Indication/Special Considerations
EMOLLIENTS			
boric acid ointment	Borofax	Apply as needed	Relieves burns, itching, irritation.
dexpanthenol	Panthoderm	Apply qd–bid	Relieves itching and aids in healing for mild skin irritations.
glycerin	generic	Combined with other ingredients—rose water	Moisturizing effect for dry skin.
lanolin		Ointment base, applied generously	Allergy to sheep or sheep products—use caution; base for many ointments.
urea	Aquacare Carmol Gordon's Urea Gormel Lanaphilic Nutraplus Ultra Mide 25 Ureacin	Apply two to four times per day to area affected	Rub in completely. Used to restore nails—cover with plastic wrap; keep dry and remove in 3, 7, or 14 days.
vitamin A & D		Apply locally with gentle massage bid–qid.	Relieves minor burns, chafing, skin irritations. Consult health care provider if not improved within 7 days.
zinc oxide		Apply as needed	Relieves burns, abrasion, diaper rash.
GROWTH FACTOR			
becaplermin	Regranex	Apply to diabetic foot ulcers bid–qid	Increases the incidence of healing of diabetic foot ulcers as adjunctive therapy; must have an adequate blood supply.
LOTIONS AND SOLUTIONS			
Burow's solution aluminum acetate	Bluboro Powder Boropak Powder Domeboro Powder Pedi-Boro Soak Paks	Dissolve one packet in a pint of water; apply q15–30 min for 4–8h	Astringent wet dressing for relief of inflammatory conditions, insect bites, athlete's foot, bruise, sores; do not use occlusive dressing.
calamine lotion	Calamox Calamatum Resinol	Apply to affected area tid–qid	Relieves itching, pain of poison ivy, poison sumac and oak, insect bites, and minor skin irritations.
hamamelis water	Witch Hazel A-E-R	Apply locally up to 6 times/day	Relieves itching and irritation of vaginal infection, hemorrhoids, postepisiotomy discomfort, post hemorrhoidectomy care.
quaternium-18 bentonite	Ivy Block	Apply at least 15 minutes before exposure to poison ivy; q4h for continued protection	Barrier lotion to prevent poison ivy/sumac/oak reactions.
ANTISEPTICS			
benzalkonium chloride	BAC Benza Oxy-Clean Zephiran	Mix in solution as needed; spray for preoperative	Thoroughly rinse detergents and soaps from skin before use; add anti-rust tablets for instruments stored in solution; dilute solution as indicated for use.

TABLE C Topical Agents (Continued)

Drug	Brand Name	Dosage	Usual Indication/Special Considerations
ANTISEPTICS			
chlorhexidine gluconate	Bacto-Shield Betasept Dyna-Hex Exidine ibistat Hibiclens	Scrub or rinse; leave on for 15 seconds; for surgical scrub—3 minutes	Use for surgical scrub, preoperative skin preparation, wound cleansing; preoperative bathing and showering.
hexachlorphene	pHisoHex Septisol	Apply as wash	Surgical wash, scrub; do not use with burns or on mucous membranes; rinse thoroughly.
iodine	generic	Wash affected area	Highly toxic; avoid occlusive dressings; stains skin and clothing. Iodine allergy is common.
povidone-iodine	Aerodine ACU-dyne Betadine Betagen Iodex Operand	Apply as needed	Treated areas may be bandaged. HIV is inactivated in this solution; causes less irritation than iodine; less toxic.
sodium hypochlorite	Dakin's	Apply as antiseptic	Caution—chemical burns can occur.
thimersol	Aeroaid Mersol	Apply qd–bid	Contains mercury compound; used preoperatively and as first aid for abrasions, wounds.
ANTIBIOTIC			
mupirocin	Bactroban	Apply small amount to affected area tid	Used to treat impetigo caused by *S. aureus*, *Streptococcus, S. pathogens;* may be covered with a gauze pad; monitor for signs of superinfection, reevaluate if not clinical response in 3–5 days.
ANTIVIRALS			
docosanal	Abreva	Apply qd–bid	Used for treatment of oral and facial herpes simplex cold sores and fever blisters. Caution patient not to overuse.
imiquimod	Aldara	Apply thin layer to warts and rub in 3×/wk at bedtime for 16 wk	For treatment of genital warts and perianal warts; remove with soap and water after 6–10 hours.
penciclovir	Denavir	Apply thin layer to affected area q2h while awake for 4 d	Treatment of cold sores in healthy patients; begin use at first sign of cold sore. Reserve use for herpes labialis on lips and face; avoid mucous membranes.
ANTIPSORIATICS			
ammoniated mercury	Emersal	Apply qd–bid	Protect from light; potential sensitizer provoking severe allergic reactions.
anthralin	Anthra-Derm Drithocreme	Apply qd only to psoriatic lesions	May stain fabrics, skin, hair, fingernails; use protective dressing.
calcipotriene	Dovonex	Apply thin layer twice a day	Monitor serum calcium levels with extended use; use only for disorder prescribed; may cause local irritation; is a synthetic vitamin D_3.
ANTISEBORRHEICS			
chloroxine	Capitrol	Massage into wet scalp; leave lather on for 3 minutes	May discolor blond, gray, bleached hair. Do not use on active lesions.
selenium sulfide	Exsel Selsun Blue	Massage 5–10 ml into scalp; rest 2–3 minutes, rinse	May damage jewelry, remove before use; discontinue if local irritation occurs.
ANTIFUNGALS			
butenafine HCl	Mentax	Apply to affected area only once a day for 4 weeks	Treatment of athlete's foot (intradigital pedia), tinea corporis, ringworm, tinea cruris.
butoconazole nitrate	Femstat 3 Gynazole 1	Apply intravaginally hs for 3–6 days (*Femstat 3*) or apply intravaginally as 1 dose (*Gynazole 1*)	Treatment of vaginal yeast infections; culture fungus, if no response, reculture. Ensure full course of therapy.
ciclopirox	Loprox Penlac Penlac Nail Lacquer	Apply directly to affected fingernails or toenails	Treatment of onychomycosis of the fingernails and toenails in immunocompromised patients

Table C continues on page 838

TABLE C Topical Agents (Continued)

Drug	Brand Name	Dosage	Usual Indication/Special Considerations
ANTIFUNGALS			
clotrimazole	Cruex Lotrimin Mycelex	Gently massage into affected area bid	Cleanse area before applying; use for up to 4 weeks. Discontinue if irritation, worsening of condition occurs.
econozole nitrate	Spectazole	Apply locally qd–bid	Treatment of athlete's foot (intradigital pedia), tinea corporis, ringworm, tinea cruris; cleanse area before applying; treat for 2–4 weeks; for athlete's foot, change socks and shoes at least once a day.
gentian violet	generic	Apply locally bid	May stain skin and clothing; do not apply to active lesions.
naftitine HCl	Naftin	Gently massage into affected area bid	Avoid occlusive dressings; wash hands thoroughly after application. Do not use longer than 4 weeks.
oxiconazole	Oxistat	Apply qd–bid	May be needed for up to 1 month.
terbinafine	Lamisil	Apply to area bid until clinical signs are improved; 1–4 weeks	Do not use occlusive dressings; report local irritation; discontinue if local irritation occurs.
tolnaftrate	Aftate Genaspor Tinactin Ting	Apply small amount bid for 2–3 weeks, 4–6 weeks may be needed if skin is very thick	Cleanse skin with soap and water before applying drug, dry thoroughly; wear loose, well-fitting shoes; change socks at least qid.
PEDICULOCIDES/SCABICIDES			
lindane	G-Well	Apply thin layer to entire body; leave on 8–12 hours wash thoroughly; shampoo 1–2 oz into dry hair and leave in place for 4 minutes	Single application is usually sufficient; reapply after 7 days at signs of live lice. Teach hygiene and prevention; treat all contacts. Assure parents this is a readily communicable disease.
malathion	Ovide Lotion	Apply to dry hair and leave on for 8–12 hours; repeat in 7–9 days	Avoid use with open lesions. Change bed linens and clothing daily; treat all contacts.
crotamiton	Eurax	Thoroughly massage into skin over entire body, repeat in 24 hours. Take a cleansing bath or shower 48 hours after last application	Change all bed linens and clothing the next day. Contaminated clothing can be dry cleaned or washed in hot water. Shake well before using.
permethrin	Acticin Elimite Nix	Thoroughly massage into all skin areas; wash off after 8–14 hours. Shampoo into freshly washed, rinsed, and towel-dried hair, leave on for 10 minutes, rinse	Single application is usually curative. Notify health care provider if rash, itch becomes worse. Approved for prophylactic use during head lice epidemics.
KERATOLYTICS			
podophyllium resin	Podocon-25 Podofin	Applied only by physician	Do not use if wart is inflamed or irritated. Very toxic; minimum amount possible is used to avoid absorption.
podofilox	Condylox	Apply q12h for 3 consecutive days	Allow to dry before using area; dispose of used applicator; may cause burning and discomfort.
TOPICAL HEMOSTATICS			
absorbable gelatin	Gelfoam	Smear or press to cut surface; when bleeding stops, remove excess. Apply sponge and allow to remain in place; will be absorbed	Prepare paste by adding 3–4 mL sterile saline to contents of jar. Apply sponge dry or saturated with saline. Assess for signs of infection. Do not use in presence of infection.
microfibrillar collagen	Avitene Hemopad Hemotene	Use dry. Apply directly to source of bleeding, apply pressure for 3–5 minutes. Discard leftover product.	Monitor for infection. Remove any excess material once bleeding has stopped.
thrombin	Thrombinar Thrombogen Thrombostat	Prepare in Sterile Distilled Water. Mix freely with blood on the surface of the injury	Contraindicated in the presence of any bovine allergies. Watch for severe allergic reactions in sensitive individuals.

TABLE C | Topical Agents (Continued)

Drug	Brand Name	Dosage	Usual Indication/Special Considerations
PAIN RELIEF			
capsaicin	*Capsin* *Dolorac* *Pain-X* *Zostrix*	Do not apply more than 3–4 ×/day	Provides temporary relief from the pain of osteoarthritis, rheumatoid arthritis, neuralgias. Do not bandage tightly. Stop use and seek medical help if condition worsens or persists after 14–28 days.
BURN PREPARATIONS			
mafenide	*Sulfamylon*	Apply to a clean, debrided wound, 1–2 ×/day burns at all times with drug; reapply as needed	Bathe patient in a whirlpool daily to debride wound. Continue debridement with a gloved hand. Cover. Continue until healing occurs. Monitor for infection and toxicity, especially acidosis. May cause severe discomfort requiring premedication before application.
nitrofurazone	*Furacin*	Apply directly to burn or place on gauze; reapply qd	Flushing the dressing with sterile water will facilitate removal. Monitor for superinfections and treat appropriately. Rash is common.
silver sulfadiazine	*Silvadene* *SSD Cream* *Thermazene*	Apply qd–bid to a clean, debrided wound; use ¹⁄₁₆-inch thickness	Bathe patient in a whirlpool to aid debridement. Dressings are not necessary but may be used; reapply when necessary. Monitor for fungal infections.
ESTROGENS			
dienestrol	*Ortho Dienestrol*	1–2 applicators intravaginally for 1–2 weeks; reduce to ½ initial dose for 1–2 weeks maintenance dose 1 applicator 1–3 ×/week	Treatment of postmenopausal atrophic vaginitis and kraurosis vulvae. Lie down for 15 minutes after dose; wear a pad to protect clothing.
estradiol hemihydrate	*Vagifem*	Insert 1 tablet intravaginally qd for 2 weeks, then 1 tablet intravaginally two times per week	Treatment of atrophic vaginitis. Attempt to taper every 3–6 mo.
ACNE PRODUCTS			
adapalene	*Differin*	Apply a thin film to affected area after washing	Do not use near cuts or open wounds; avoid sunburned areas; do not combine with other products; limit exposure to the sun. Less drying than most acne products.
altretinoin	*Panretin*	1% gel; apply as needed to cover lesion bid	Treatment of lesions of Kaposi's sarcoma. Inflammation, peeling, redness may occur.
azelaic acid	*Azelex*	Wash and dry skin; massage thin layer into skin bid	Wash hands thoroughly after application. Improvement usually seen within 4 weeks. Initial irritation usually passes with time.
masoprocol	*Actinex*	Wash and dry area; massage into area morning and evening	Do not use occlusive dressings; may cause transient burning
metronidazole	*MetroGel* *Noritate*	Apply cream to affected area	Treatment of rosacea.
sodium sulfacetamide	*Klaron*	Apply a thin film bid	Wash affected area with mild soap and water, pat dry. Avoid use in denuded or abraded areas.
tarazotene	*Tazorac*	Apply thin film qd in the evening	Avoid use in pregnancy. Drying, causes photosensitivity. Do not use with products containing alcohol.
tretinoin, 0.025% cream	*Avita*	Apply thin layer qd	Discomfort, peeling, redness and worsening of acne may occur for first 2–4 weeks.
tretinoin, 0.05% cream	*Renova*	Apply thin coat in evening	Use for the removal of fine wrinkles
tretinoin, gel	*Retin-A-micro*	Apply to cover qd, after cleansing	Exacerbation of inflammation may occur at first. Therapeutic effects usually seen in first 2 weeks.
MOUTH PRODUCTS			
amlexanox	*Aphthasol*	Apply to aphthous ulcers qid after meals and hs, following oral hygiene; for 10 days	Consult with dentist if ulcers are not healed within 10 days. May cause local pain.

Table C continues on page 840

TABLE C | Topical Agents (Continued)

Drug	Brand Name	Dosage	Usual Indication/Special Considerations
ANTIHISTAMINE			
azelastine HCl	*Astelin*	2 sprays per nostril bid	Avoid use of alcohol and OTC antihistamines; dizziness and sedation may occur.
NASAL CORTICOSTEROID			
fluticonosone	*Flonase Flovent Rotodisk*	Adult: 88–440 mcg intranasal bid; lower dose if also on corticosteroids Pediatric: 500–600 mcg bid via rotodisk	Preventive treatment for asthma, not a primary treatment. May take several weeks to see effects. Pediatric use for children 4–11 years.
HAIR REMOVAL			
eflornithine	*Vaniqa*	Apply to unwanted facial hair bid for up to 24 weeks	Approved for use in women only
SKIN SUBSTITUTE			
graftskin lasting	*Alpigraf*	Apply to wound, keep clean, loose cover	Treatment of venous leg ulcers lasting >1 mo; diabetic foot ulcers lasting >3 wk

TOPICAL CORTICOSTEROIDS

These drugs enter cells and bind to cytoplasmic receptors, initiating complex reactions that are responsible for the anti-inflammatory, anti-pruritic, and anti-proliferative effects of these drugs. They are used to relieve the inflammation and pruritic manifestations of corticosteroid-sensitive dermatoses and for temporary relief of minor skin irritations and rashes. These agents should always be applied sparingly because of the risk of systemic corticosteroid effects if absorbed systemically. Occlusive dressings and tight coverings should be avoided. Prolonged use should also be avoided because of the risk of systemic effects and local irritation and breakdown. These agents are applied topically bid–tid.

Drug	Brand Name	Dosage	Usual Indication/Special Considerations
alclometasone dipropionate	*Aclovate*	Ointment, cream: 0.05% concentration	Occlusive dressings may be used for the management of refractory lesions of psoriasis and deep-seated dermatoses.
amcinonide	*Cyclocort*	Ointment, cream, lotion: 0.1% concentration	
betamethasone dipropionate	*Alphatres, Diprosone, Maxivate, Teledar*	Ointment, cream, lotion, aerosol: 0.05% concentration	
betamethasone dipropionate, augmented	*Diprolene*	Ointment, cream, lotion: 0.05% concentration	
betamathasone valerate	*Betatrex, Beta-Val, Dermabet, Valisone*	Ointment, cream, lotion: 0.01% concentration	
clobetasol propionate	*Cormax, Temovate*	Ointment, cream: 0.05% concentration	
clocortolone pivalate	*Cloderm*	Cream: 0.1% concentration	
desonide	*DesOwen, Tridesiolon*	Ointment, cream: 0.05% concentration	
desoximetasone	*Topicort*	Ointment, cream: 0.25% concentration Gel: 0.05% concentration	
dexamethasone	*D Spray Aeroseb-Dex*	Gel: 0.1% concentration Aerosol: 0.01% concentration Aerosol: 0.04% concentration	
dexamethasone sodium phosphate	*Docadron phosphate*	Cream: 0.1% concentration	
diflorasone diacetate	*Florone, Maxiflor, Psorcon Florone E*	Ointment, cream: 0.05% concentration Cream: 0.5% concentration	
fluocinolone acetonide	*Flurosyn, Synalar*	Ointment: 0.025% concentration Cream: 0.01% concentration	
	Flurosyn, Synalar, Synemol *Fluonid, Flurosyn, Synalar*	Cream: 0.025% concentration Solution: 0.01% concentration	

TABLE C Topical Agents (Continued)

Drug	Brand Name	Dosage	Usual Indication/Special Considerations
TOPICAL CORTICOSTEROIDS			
fluocinonide	Lidex	Ointment: 0.05% concentration	
	Fluonex, Lidex, Vasoderm	Cream: 0.05% concentration	
	Lidex, Topsyn Gel	Solution, gel: 0.05% concentration	
flurandrenolide	Cordran	Ointment, cream: 0.025% concentration	
		Ointment, cream, lotion: 0.05% concentration	
		Tape: 4 mcg/cm²	
fluticasone propionate	Cutivate	Cream: 0.05% concentration	
		Ointment: 0.005% concentration	
halcinonide	Halog	Ointment, cream, solution: 0.1% concentration	
		Cream: 0.025% concentration	
halobetasol propionate	Ultravate	Ointment, cream: 0.05% concentration	
hydrocortisone	Cortizone 5, Bactine Hydrocortisone, Cort-Dome, Dermolate, Dermtex HC, HydroTex	Lotion: 0.25%	
	Cortizone 10, Hycort, Tegrin-HC	Cream, lotion, ointment, aerosol: 0.5%, 1% concentration	
	Hytone	Cream, lotion, ointment, solution: 1% concentration	
hydrocortisone acetate	Cortaid, Lanacort-5	Ointment: 0.5% concentration (OTC preparations)	
	Corticaine (R$_x$), FoilleCort, Gynecort, Lanacort 5	Cream: 0.5% concentration (OTC preparations)	
	Anusol-HC	Cream: 1% concentration	
	Cortaid with Aloe	Cream: 0.5%, 1% concentration (OTC preparation)	
hydrocortisone buteprate	Pandel	Cream: 0.1%	
hydrocortisone butyrate	Locoid	Ointment, cream: 0.1% concentration	
hydrocortisone valerate	Westcort	Ointment, cream: 0.2% concentration	
mometasone furoate	Elocon	Ointment, cream, lotion: 0.1% concentration	
	Nasonex	Nasal spray: 0.2%	
prednicarbate	Dermatop	Cream: 0.1% concentration: preservative free	
triamcinolone acetonide	Flutex, Kenalog	Ointment: 0.025% concentration	
	Aristocort, Flutex, Kenalog	Ointment: 0.1% concentration and 0.5% concentration	
	Aristocort, Flutex, Kenalog, Triacet, Triderm	Cream: 0.025% concentration and 0.5% concentration	
		Cream: 0.1% concentration	
		Lotion: 0.025% and 0.1% concentration	

OPHTHALMIC AGENTS

Ophthalmic agents are drugs that are intended for direct administration into the conjunctiva of the eye. These drugs are used to treat glaucoma (miotics constrict the pupil and decrease the resistance to aqueous flow), to aid in the diagnosis of eye problems (mydriatics dilate the pupil for examination of the retina; cycloplegics paralyze the muscles that control the lens to aid refraction); to treat local ophthalmic infections or inflammation; and to provide relief from the signs and symptoms of allergic reactions.

These drugs are not generally absorbed systemically because of their method of administration. They are classified in Pregnancy Category C, and caution should always be used when giving drugs during pregnancy or lactation.

Contraindications and Cautions

These drugs are contraindicated in the presence of allergy to the specific drug or to any component of the product being used. Although they are seldom absorbed systemically, caution should be used in any patient who would have problems with the systemic effects of the drugs if they were absorbed systemically.

Adverse Effects

Adverse effects of these drugs include local irritation, stinging, burning, blurring of vision (prolonged when using ointments), tearing, and headache.

Clinically Important Drug–Drug Interactions

Because of their actions on the eye or because of the components of the drug, many of these drugs cannot be given at the same time but should be spaced 1 to 2 hours apart. Check the specific drug being used for details.

Dosage

The usual dosage for any of these drugs is one to two drops in each eye or in the affected eye two to four times daily, or 0.25 to 0.5 inches of ointment in the affected eye or eyes.

Nursing Considerations

Assessment

Screen for the following: allergy to the specific drug or components of the preparation; underlying medical conditions that would be affected if the drug were absorbed systemically.

Evaluate eye, conjunctival color; note any lesions. A vision examination may be appropriate.

Nursing Diagnoses

The patient receiving an ophthalmic agent may have the following nursing diagnoses related to drug therapy:

- Acute Pain related to administration of the drug
- Risk for Injury related to changes in vision
- Deficient Knowledge regarding drug therapy

Implementation

- Assess patient's general physical condition before beginning test, *to decrease the potential for adverse effects.*
- Follow these administration guidelines *to provide the most therapeutic use of the drug with the fewest adverse effects:*
  Solution or drops: Wash hands thoroughly before administering; do not touch dropper to eye or to any other surface. Have patient tilt head backward or lie down, and stare upward. Gently grasp lower eyelid and pull eyelid away from the eyeball; instill drops into pouch formed by eyelid. Release lid slowly; have patient close the eye and look downward. Apply gentle pressure to the inside corner of the eye for 3 to 5 minutes to retard drainage. Do not rub eyes; do not rinse eyedropper. Do not use eye drops that have changed color; if more than one type of eye drop is used; wait at least 5 minutes between administrations. Refer to Figure D-1.
  Ointment: Wash hands thoroughly before administering; hold tube between hands for several minutes to warm ointment; discard the first centimeter of ointment when opening the tube for the first time. Tilt head backward or have patient lie down and stare upward. Gently pull out lower lid to form pouch; place 0.25 to 0.5 inches of ointment inside the lower lid. Have patient close the eye for 1 to 2 minutes and roll the eyeball in all directions; remove any excess ointment from around the eye. If using more than one kind of ointment, wait at least 10 minutes between administrations. Refer to Figure D-2.

Inner canthus
Conjunctival sac
Outer canthus

FIGURE D-1. Administration of ophthalmic drops.

Conjunctival sac

FIGURE D-2. Administration of ophthalmic ointment.

- Provide comfort measures *to help patient tolerate drug effects* (eg, control light, analgesics as needed).
- Include the following information—in addition to the proper administration technique for the drug—in the teaching program for the patient, *to improve compliance and provide safety and comfort measures as necessary:* safety measures may need to be taken if blurring of vision should occur; burning and stinging may occur on administration but should pass quickly; the pupils will dilate with mydriatic agents and the eyes may become very sensitive to light (the use of sunglasses is recommended); any severe eye discomfort, palpitations, nausea, or headache should be reported to the health care provider.

Evaluation

- Monitor patient response to the drug (changes in pupil size, relief of pressure of glaucoma, relief of itching and tearing related to allergic reaction).
- Monitor for adverse effects (local irritation, blurring of vision, headache).
- Evaluate effectiveness of teaching plan (patient can name adverse effects to watch for, specific measures to avoid adverse effects; patient understands importance of follow-up that will be needed).
- Monitor effectiveness of comfort measures and compliance with regimen.

TABLE D | Ophthalmic Agents

Drug	Usage	Special Considerations
apraclonidine (*Iopidine*)	To control or prevent post-surgical elevations of intraocular pressure (IOP) after argon–laser eye surgery	Monitor for the possibility of vasovagal attack; do not give to patients with allergy to clonidine
azelastine (HCl) (*Optivar*)	Treatment of ocular itching associated with allergic conjunctivitis.	Antihistamine, mast cell stabilizer. Dosage (≥3 y): 1 drop b.i.d. Rapid onset, 8-h duration
bimatoprost (*Lumigan*)	Reduction of IOP in patients with open-angle glaucoma or ocular hypertension	Used for patients who are intolerant to other IOP-lowering drugs or who have failed to achieve optimum IOP with other IOP-lowering medications
brimonidine tartrate (*Alphagan, Alphagan P*)	Treatment of open-angle glaucoma and ocular hypertension	Selective α_2-antagonist; minimal effects on cardiovascular and pulmonary systems. Do not use with nomoamine oxidase inhibitors. Dosage: 1 drop t.i.d.
brinzolamide (*Azopt*)	To decrease intraocular pressure in open-angle glaucoma	May be given with other agents. Dosage: 1 drop t.i.d. Give 10 min apart from any other agents.
carbachol (*Carbastat, Miostat, Carboptic, Isopto Carbachol*)	Direct-acting miotic; for treatment of glaucoma; miosis during surgery	Surgical dose: a one-use only portion. For glaucoma: 1–2 drops up to t.i.d. as needed.
cyclopentolate (*Ak-Pentolate, Cyclogyl, Pentolair*)	Mydriasis/cycloplegia in diagnostic procedures	Individuals with dark-pigmented irises may require higher doses; compress lacrimal sac for 1–2 min after administration to decrease any systemic absorption
dapiprazole (*Rev-Eyes*)	Miotic: iatrogenically induced mydriasis produced by adrenergic or parasympathetic agents	Not for use to reduce IOP; do not use if constriction is undesirable. Do not use more than once a week.
demecarium (*Humorsol*)	Treatment of glaucoma and strabismus; cholinesterase inhibitor	If response is not adequate in first 24 h, consider another agent. Do not use more often than necessary; 1–2 drops/wk up to 1–2 drops/d have been used.
diclofenac sodium (*Voltaren Ophthalmic*)	Photophobia: for use in patients undergoing incisional refractive surgery	Apply 1 drop q.i.d. beginning 24 h after cataract surgery; continue through the first 2 wk after surgery.

Table D continues on page 844

TABLE D | Ophthalmic Agents (Continued)

Drug	Usage	Special Considerations
dipivefrin (*Propine, AK Pro*)	Control of IOP in chronic open-angle glaucoma	1 drop q12h; monitor closely with tonometry
dorzolamide (*Trusopt*)	Treatment of elevated IOP in open-angle glaucoma or ocular hypertension	A sulfonamide; monitor patients taking parenteral sulfonamides for possible adverse effects
dorzolamide 2% and timolol 0.5% (*Cosopt*)	To decrease IOP in open-angle glaucoma or ocular hypertension in patients who do not respond to β-blockers alone	Administer 1 drop in affected eye b.i.d. Monitor for cardiac failure; if absorbed, may mask symptoms of hypoglycemia or thyrotoxicosis.
echothipate (*Phospholine Iodide*)	Treatment of glaucoma; irreversible cholinesterase inhibitor; long-acting. Accommodative esotropia.	Given only once a day because of long duration of action; tolerance may develop with prolonged use but usually returns after a rest period
emedastine (*Emadine*)	Temporary relief of signs and symptoms of allergic conjunctivitis	1 drop in affected eye up to q.i.d. Do not wear contact lenses if eyes are red; may cause headache, blurred vision.
fluorometholone (*Flarex, Fluor-Op*)	Topical corticosteroid used for treatment of inflammatory conditions of the eye	Improvement should occur within several days, discontinue if no improvement is seen. Discontinue if swelling of the eye occurs.
fomivirsen sodium (*Vitravene*)	Treatment of retinal cytomegalovirus in AIDS patients who cannot tolerate other agents	Injected into affected eye every other week for two doses, then every 4 weeks; do not use if previously treated with cidofivir within past 2–4 wk.
homatropine (*Isopto-Homatropine, Homatropin HBr*)	Long-acting mydriatic and cyclopegic used for refraction and treatment of inflammatory conditions of the uveal tract	Individuals with dark-pigmented irises may require larger doses; 5–10 min is usually required for refraction.
idoxuridine (*Herplex*)	Treatment of herpes simplex keratitis	1 drop every hour during the day, every 2 h at night. May use with corticosteroids.
ketotifen (*Zaditor*)	Temporary relief of itching due to allergic conjunctivitis	Remove contact lenses before use—may be replaced 10 min after administration. An antihistamine/mast cell stabilizer.
latanoprost (*Xalatan*)	Treatment of open-angle glaucoma or ocular hypertension in patients intolerant or unresponsive to other agents	Remove contact lenses before use and for 15 min after use; allow at least 5 min between this and the use of any other agents; expect blurring of vision
levobetaxolol (*Betaxon*)	Reduction of IOP with chronic open-angle glaucoma, ocular hypertension	1 drop b.i.d.; may take up to 2 wk to see results; do not combine with β-adrenergics.
levocabastine (*Livostin*)	Relief of allergic conjunctivitis	Treatment may be needed for up to 2 wk. Do not wear soft contact lenses during use of this drug. Shake well before use, and do not use any discolored solution.
levofloxin	Treatment of bacterial conjunctivitis caused by susceptible bacteria	1–2 drops per day in affected eye
levobunolol (*AK Beta, Betagan Liquifilm*)	Lowering of IOP with chronic open-angle glaucoma, ocular hypertension	1–2 drops b.i.d. Do not combine with β-blockers.
lodoxamide (*Alomide*)	Treatment of vernal conjunctivitis and keratitis	Patients should not wear contact lenses while using this drug; discontinue if stinging or burning persists after instillation
loteprednol etabonate (*Lotemax* (0.5%))	Treatment of steroid-resistant ocular disease	1–2 drops q.i.d.
(*Alrex* (0.2%))	Treatment of postoperative inflammation after ocular surgery	1–2 drops q.i.d. beginning 24 h after surgery and continuing for 2 wk. Shake vigorously before use. Discard after 14 d. Prolonged use may cause nerve or eye damage.
metipranolol (*OptiPranolol*)	β-Blocker; used in treating chronic open-angle glaucoma and ocular hypertension	Concomitant therapy may be needed; caution patient about possible vision changes.
natamycin (*Natacyn*)	Antibiotic used to treat fungal blepharitis, conjunctivitis, and keratitis; drug of choice for *Fusarium sotani* keratitis	Shake well before each use; store at room temperature. Failure to improve in 7–10 d suggests a nonsusceptible organism; re-evaluate.
olopatadine hydrochloride (*Patanol*)	Mast cell stabilizer and antihistamine; provides fast onset of relief of itching due to conjunctivitis and has prolonged action	Not for use with contact lenses; headache is a common side effect.
pemirolast potassium (*Alamast*)	Prevention of itchy eyes due to allergic conjunctivitis	1–2 drops q.i.d.

TABLE D Ophthalmic Agents (Continued)

Drug	Usage	Special Considerations
pilocarpine (*Adsorbocarpine, Akarpine, Isopto Carpine, Pilocar, Piloptic, Pilostat*)	Chronic and acute glaucoma; treatment of mydriasis caused by drugs; direct-acting mitotic	Can be stored at room temperature for up to 8 wk, then discard. May use 1–2 drops up to six times per day, based on patient response.
polydimethylsiloxane (*AdatoSil*)	Treatment of retinal detachments when other therapy is not effective or is inappropriate; primary choice for retinal detachment caused by AIDS-related cytomegalovirus retinitis or viral infection	Monitor for cataracts; must be injected directly into the aqueous humor.
rimexolone (*Vexol*)	Corticosteroid; postoperative ocular surgery for the treatment of anterior uveitis	Monitor for signs of steroid absorption
suprofen (*Profenal*)	NSAID; used to inhibit intraoperative miosis	Local burning may occur; monitor patient for cross sensitivities to other nonsteroidal anti-inflammatory drugs (NSAIDs).
travoprost (*Travatan*)	Reduction of intraocular pressure in patients with open-angle glaucoma or ocular hypertension	Reserve for patients who are intolerant of other IOP-lowering medications or who have failed to achieve optimum IOP with other IOP-lowering medications.
trifluridine (*Viroptic*)	Antiviral; used to treat primary kerato-conjunctivitis and recurrent epithelial keratitis due to herpes simplex virus types 1 and 2	Transient burning or stinging may occur; reconsider drug choice if improvement is not seen within 7 d. Do not administer longer than 21 d at a time.
unorpostone (*Rescula*)	Treatment of open-angle glaucoma ocular hypertension in patients who do not respond to other agents	One drop b.i.d.; not for use in children or during pregnancy or lactation. Remove contact lenses during use.
vidarabine (*Vira-A*)	Treatment of acute keratoconjunctivitis and recurrent epithelial keratitis due to herpes simplex types 1 and 2; superficial keratitis caused by herpes simplex virus and not responding to idoxuridine	Treat an additional 7d after epithelialization has occurred; if no improvement is seen in 21 d, consider other therapy.

VITAMINS

Vitamins are substances that the body requires for carrying out essential metabolic reactions. The body cannot synthesize enough of these components to meet all of its needs, therefore, they must be obtained from animal and vegetable tissues taken in as food. Vitamins are needed only in small amounts because they function as coenzymes that activate the protein portions of enzymes, which catalyze a great deal of biochemical activity. Vitamins are either water soluble and excreted in the urine, or they are fat soluble and capable of being stored in adipose tissue in the body.

Therapeutic Actions and Indications

Vitamins act as coenzymes to activate a variety of proteins on enzymes that catalyze biochemical activity. They are indicated for the treatment of vitamin deficiencies, as dietary supplements when needed, and as specific therapy related to the activity of the vitamin.

Contraindications and Cautions

These drugs are contraindicated in the presence of any known allergy to the drug or the colorants, additives, or preservatives used in the drug. They are categorized as Pregnancy Category C and are used to maintain adequate vitamin levels during pregnancy and lactation.

Adverse Effects

The adverse effects primarily associated with these drugs are related to gastrointestinal upset and irritation, which is caused by direct gastrointestinal contact with the drugs.

Clinically Important Drug–Drug Interactions

Pyridoxine, vitamin B_6, interferes with the effectiveness of levodopa.

Fat-soluble vitamins may not be absorbed if given concurrently with mineral oil, cholestyramine, or colestipol.

Nursing Considerations

Assessment

Obtain a nutritional assessment. Screen for any medical conditions and drugs being taken and for any known allergies. Evaluate skin, mucous membranes; pulse, respirations, and blood pressure. Complete blood count (CBC) and clotting times may need to be evaluated with specific vitamins.

Nursing Diagnoses

The patient receiving vitamins may have the following nursing diagnoses related to drug therapy:

- Acute Pain related to GI discomfort
- Risk for Imbalanced Nutrition related to replacement therapy
- Deficient Knowledge regarding drug therapy

Implementation

- Assess patient's general physical condition before beginning test, *to decrease the potential for adverse effects and assure need for the drug.*
- Advise patient to avoid the use of over-the-counter preparations that contain the same vitamins, *to prevent inadvertent overdose of the vitamin.*
- Provide comfort measures *to help patient tolerate drug effects* (eg, take drug with meals to alleviate gastrointestinal distress).
- Include information about the solution being used in a test (eg, what to expect, adverse effects that may occur, follow-up tests that may be needed) *to enhance patient knowledge about drug therapy and promote compliance with drug regimen.*

Evaluation

- Monitor patient response to the drug (adequate vitamin intake).
- Monitor for adverse effects (GI upset).
- Evaluate effectiveness of teaching plan (patient can name adverse effects to watch for, specific measures to avoid adverse effects; patient understands importance of follow-up that will be needed).
- Monitor effectiveness of comfort measures and compliance with regimen.

TABLE E Vitamins

Vitamin	Solubility Type	Recommended Dietary Allowance	Therapeutic Uses/Special Considerations
A (*Aquasol A, Palmitate-A 5000*)	Fat	1000 μg (male) 800 μg (female) 1300 μg (lactation) 375–700 μg (pediatric)	Severe deficiency: 500,000 IU/d for 3 d, then 50,000 IU/d for 2 wk given IM or PO. Protect IM vial from light. Hypervitaminosis A can occur, including cirrhotic-like liver syndrome with central nervous system effects; gastrointestinal drying, rash, liver changes. Treat by discontinuing the vitamin and give saline, prednisone, and calcitonin IV. Liver damage may be permanent.
ascorbic acid (*Cecon, Cevi-Bid, Dull C, Vita-C, N'Ice Vitamin C Drops*)	Water	50–60 mg (male) 50–60 mg (female) 70–90 mg (lactation) 70 mg (pregnancy) 30–45 mg (pediatric)	May be given PO, IM, slow IV, or SC. Treatment of scurvy: 300–1000 mg daily. Enhanced wound healing: 300–500 mg/d for 7–10 d. Burns: 1–2 g/d. Also being studied for treatment of common cold, asthma, coronary artery disease, cancer, schizophrenia. May be very toxic at high doses.
calcifediol (D_3) (*Calderol*)	Fat		Management of metabolic bone disease or hypocalcemia in patients receiving chronic renal dialysis: 300–350 μg/wk daily or on alternate days. Discontinue if hypercalcemia occurs.
cholecalciferol (D_3) (*Delta-D*)	Fat	200–400 IU (male) 200–400 IU (female) 400 IU (lactation) 400 IU (pregnancy) 300–400 IU (pediatric)	Vitamin D deficiency: 400–1000 IU/d. May be useful for the treatment of hypocalcemic tetany and hypoparathyroidism
cyanocobalamin (B_{12}) (*Big Shot B12, Crystamine, Crysti 1000, Cyanoject, Cyomin, Rubersol 1000*)	Water	2 μg (male) 2 μg (female) 2.6 μg (lactation) 2.2 μg (pregnancy) 0.3–1.4 μg (pediatric)	Deficiency: 25–250 μg/d. (Note: oral route is not for the treatment of pernicious anemia.) Pernicious anemia: 100 μg IM each month for life; given with folic acid; nasal route is preferable.
D	Fat	200–400 IU (male) 200–400 IU (female) 400 IU (lactation) 400 IU (pregnancy) 300–400 IU (pediatric)	Vitamin D deficiency: 400–1000 IU/d. May be useful for the treatment of hypocalcemic tetany and hypoparathyroidism. Encourage balanced diet and exposure to sunlight. Do not use with mineral oil.
dihydrotachysterol (DHT, D_2) (*DHT, Hytakerol*)	Fat		Treatment of postoperative tetany, idiopathic tetany, hypoparathyroidism. Initial dose: 0.8–2.4 mg/d for several days, then 0.2–1 mg/d to achieve normal serum calcium. May supplement with oral calcium.
E (*Aquavil-E, Vita-Plus E Softgels*)	Fat	15 IU (male) 12 IU (female) 16–18 IU (lactation) 15 IU (pregnancy) 4–10 IU (pediatric)	Used in certain premature infants to reduce the toxic effects of oxygen on the lung and retina; do not give IV; report fatigue, weakness, nausea, headache.
ergocalciferol (D_2) (*Calciferol, Drisdol Drops*)	Fat	200–400 IU (male) 200–400 IU (female) 400 IU (lactation) 400 IU (pregnancy) 300–400 IU (pediatric)	Give IM in gastrointestinal, biliary, liver disease. Refractory rickets: 12,000–500,000 IU/d. Hypoparathyroidism: 50,000–2,000,000 IU/d. Familial hypophosphatemia: 10,000–80,000 IU/d plus 1–2 g phosphorus.
niacin (B_3) (*Niacor, Nicotinic Acid, Nicotinex, SLO-Niacin, Niaspan*)	Water	15–20 mg (male) 13–15 mg (female) 20 mg (lactation) 17 mg (pregnancy) 5–13 mg (pediatric)	Prevention and treatment of pellagra: up to 500 mg/d. Niacin deficiency: up to 100 mg/d. Also used for the treatment of hyperlipidemia if no response to diet and exercise: 1–2 g t.i.d. Do not exceed 6 g/d. Feelings of warmth, flushing may occur with administration but usually pass within 2 h.
nicotinamide (B_3) (*Niacinamide*)	Water	15–20 mg (male) 13–15 mg (female) 20 mg (lactation) 17 mg (pregnancy) 5–13 mg (pediatric)	Prevention and treatment of pellagra: up to 50 mg, 3–10 times per day.
P (bioflavonoids) (*Amino Opti-C, Bio-Acerola C, Citro-Flav 2000, Flavons 500, Pan C-500, Peridin C, Quercetin, Span C*)	Water	Unknown	Used to treat bleeding, abortion, poliomyelitis, diabetes, and other conditions. There is little evidence that these uses have any clinical efficacy.

Table E continues on page 848

TABLE E | Vitamins (Continued)

Vitamin	Solubility Type	Recommended Dietary Allowance	Therapeutic Uses/Special Considerations
phytonadione (K) (*Mephyton*)	Fat	45–80 µg (male) 45–65 µg (female) 65 µg (lactation) 65 µg (pregnancy) 5–30 µg (pediatric)	Hypoprothrombinemia due to anticoagulant use: 2.5–10 mg PO, IM. Hemorrhagic disease of the newborn: 0.5–1 mg IM within 1 h of birth: 1–5 mg IM may be given to the mother before delivery. Hypoprothrombinemia in adult: 2.5–25 mg PO or IM.
pyridoxine HCl (B_6) (*Aminoxin, Nestrex*)	Water	1.7–2 mg (male) 1.4–1.6 mg (female) 2.1 mg (lactation) 2.2 mg (pregnancy) 0.3–1.4 mg (pediatric)	Deficiency: 10–20 mg/d PO or IM for 3 wk. Vitamin B_6 deficiency syndrome: up to 600 mg/d for life. Isoniazid poisoning (give an equal amount of pyridoxine). 4 g IV followed by 1 g IM q30min. Reduces the effectiveness of levodopa and leads to serious toxic effects—avoid this combination.
riboflavin	Water	1.4–1.8 mg (male) 1.2–1.3 mg (female) 1.7–1.8 mg (lactation) 1.6 mg (pregnancy) 0.4–1.2 mg (pediatric)	Treatment of deficiency: 5–15 mg/d. May cause a yellow or orange discoloration to the urine
thiamine HCl (B_1) (*Thiamilate*)	Water	1.2–1.5 mg (male) 1–1.1 mg (female) 1.6 mg (lactation) 1.5 mg (pregnancy) 0.3–1 mg (pediatric)	Treatment of wet beriberi: 10–30 mg IV t.i.d. Treatment of beriberi: 10–20 mg IM t.i.d. for 2 wk with multivitamin containing 5–10 mg/d for 1 mo. Do not mix in alkaline solutions. Used orally as a mosquito repellant, alters body sweat composition. Feeling of warmth and flushing may occur with administration, usually passes within 2 h.

CANADIAN DRUG INFORMATION

Presented here is a list of Canadian brand names for frequently used drugs. The brand name appears in italics with the corresponding generic name listed in parentheses.

A

Abenol (acetaminophen)
Acet-Amp (theophylline)
Acilac (lactulose)
Acti-B$_{12}$ (hydroxocobalamin)
Actiprofen (ibuprofen)
Aerosporin (polymyxin B)
Albert Glyburide (glyburide)
Albert Oxybutynin (oxybutynin)
Alcomicin (gentamicin)
Allerdryl (diphenhydramine)
Alti-Acyclovir (acyclovir)
Alti-Diltiazem (diltiazem)
Alti-Doxepin (doxepin)
Alti-Ibuprofen (ibuprofen)
Alti-Ipratropium (ipratropium)
Alti-Minocycline (minocycline)
Alti-MPA (medroxyprogesterone)
Alti-Nadolol (nadolol)
Alti-Piroxicam (piroxicam)
Alti-Ranitidine (ranitidine)
Alti-Sulfasalazine (sulfasalazine)
Alti-Trazadone (trazodone)
Alti-Triazolam (triazolam)
Alti-Valproic (valproic acid)
Amatine (midodrine)
Ampicin (ampicillin)
Anandron (nilutamide)
Anapolon 50 (oxymetholone)
Anexate (flumazenil)
Anturan (sulfinpyrazone)
Apo-Acetazolamide (acetazolamide)
Apo-Allopurinol (allopurinol)
Apo-Alpraz (alprazolam)
Apo-Amoxi (amoxicillin)

Apo-Ampi (ampicillin)
Apo-Asa (aspirin)
Apo-Atenol (atenolol)
Apo-Baclofen (baclofen)
Apo-Benztropine (benztropine)
Apo-Bromocriptine (bromocriptine)
Apo-Cal (calcium carbonate)
Apo-Capto (captopril)
Apo-Carbamazepine (carbamazepine)
Apo-Ceclor (cefaclor)
Apo-Cephalex (cephalexin)
Apo-Chlorodiazepoxide (chlordiazepoxide)
Apo-Chlorpropamide (chlorpropamide)
Apo-Chlorthalidone (chlorthalidone)
Apo-Cimetidine (cimetidine)
Apo-Clomipramine (clomipramine)
Apo-Clonazepam (clonazepam)
Apo-Clonidine (clonidine)
Apo-Clorazepate (clorazepate)
Apo-Cloxi (cloxacillin)
Apo-Cyclobenzaprine (cyclobenzaprine)
Apo-Desipramine (desipramine)
Apo-Diazepam (diazepam)
Apo-Diflunisal (diflunisal)
Apo-Diltiaz (diltiazem)
Apo-Diltiazem (diltiazem)
Apo-Dimenhydrinate (dimenhydrinate)
Apo-Dipyridamole (dipyridamole)
Apo-Doxepin (doxepin)
Apo-Doxy (doxycycline)
Apo-Erythro (erythromycin)
Apo-Erythro EES (erythromycin)
Apo-Erythro-S (erythromcyin)
Apo-Famotidine (famotidine)
Apo-Ferrous Gluconate (ferrous gluconate)
Apo-Ferrous Sulfate (ferrous sulfate)
Apo-Fluoxetine (fluoxetine)
Apo-Fluphenazine (fluphenazine)
Apo-Flurbiprofen (flurbiprofen)
Apo-Fluvoxamine (fluvoxamine)

Apo-Furosemide (furosemide)
Apo-Gemfibrozil (gemfibrozil)
Apo-Haloperidol (haloperidol)
Apo-Hydralazine (hydralazine)
Apo-Hydro (hydrochlorothiazide)
Apo-Hydroxyzine (hydroxyzine)
Apo-Ibuprofen (ibuprofen)
Apo-Imipramine (imipramine)
Apo-Indomethacin (indomethacin)
Apo-Ipravent (ipratropium)
Apo-ISDN (isosorbide dinitrate)
Apo-K (potassium chloride)
Apo-Lisinopril (lisinopril)
Apo-Loperamide (loperamide)
Apo-Lorazepam (lorazepam)
Apo-Lovastatin (lovastatin)
Apo-Mefenamic (mefenamic acid)
Apo-Megestrol (megestrol)
Apo-Meprobamate (meprobamate)
Apo-Metoclop (metoclopramide)
Apo-Metoprolol (metoprolol)
Apo-Metronidazole (metronidazole)
Apo-Nadolol (nadolol)
Apo-Napro-Na (naproxen)
Apo-Naproxen (naproxen)
Apo-Nifed (nifedipine)
Apo-Nitrofurantoin (nitrofurantoin)
Apo-Nizatidine (nizatidine)
Apo-Nortriptyline (nortriptyline)
Apo-Oxazepam (oxazepam)
Apo-Oxtriphylline (oxtriphylline)
Apo-Oxybutynin (oxybutynin)
Apo-Perphenazine (perphenazine)
Apo-Pindol (pindolol)
Apo-Piroxicam (piroxicam)
Apo-Prazo (prazosin)
Apo-Prednisone (prednisone)
Apo-Primidone (primidone)
Apo-Procainamide (procainamide)
Apo-Propranolol (propranolol)
Apo-Quinidine (quinidine)
Apo-Sotalol (sotalol)
Apo-Sucralfate (sucralfate)
Apo-Sulfinpyrazone (sulfinpyrazone)
Apo-Sulin (sulindac)
Apo-Tamox (tamoxifen)
Apo-Temazepam (temazepam)
Apo-Tetra (tetracycline)
Apo-Thioridazine (thioridazine)
Apo-Timol (timolol)
Apo-Tolbutamide (tolbutamide)
Apo-Trazadone (trazodone)
Apo-Triazo (triazolam)
Apo-Trifluoperazine (trifluoperazine)
Apo-Trihex (trihexyphenidyl)
Apo-Trimip (trimipramine)

Apo-Zidovudine (zidovudine)
Aquacort (hydrocortisone)
Asmavent (albuterol)
Atasol (acetaminophen)
Avirax (acyclovir)
Avlosulfan (dapsone)
Ayercillin (penicillin G procaine)

B

Bacitin (bacitracin)
Balminin DM (dextromethorphan)
Barbilixir (phenobarbital)
Barbita (phenobarbital)
Beclodisk (beclomethasone)
Beclovent Rotocaps (beclomethasone)
Benemid (probenecid)
Bentylol (dicyclomine)
Benuryl (probenecid)
Bepadin (bepridil)
Bepen (betamethasone)
Betabloc (metoprolol)
Betacort (betamethasone)
Betaderm (betamethasone)
Beta-Tim (timolol)
Betnesol (betamethasone)
Betnovate (betamethasone)
Bonamine (meclizine)
Bretylate (bretylium)
Bronalide (flunisolide)
Burinex (bumetanide)
Busodium (butabarbital)
Butalan (butabarbital)

C

Calcite 500 (calcium carbonate)
Caltine (calcitonin, salmon)
Candistatin (nystatin)
Canesten Vaginal (clotrimazole)
Carbolith (lithium)
Cedocard SR (isosorbide dinitrate)
Celestoderm (betamethasone)
C.E.S. (estrogens, conjugated)
Charcolate (charcoal)
Chlorprom (chlorpromazine)
Chlorpromanyl (chlorpromazine)
Chlor-Tripolon (chlorpheniramine)
Cibalith-S (lithium)
Ciloxin (ciprofloxacin)
Citro-Mag (magnesium citrate)
Claripex (clofibrate)
Clinda-Derm (clindamycin)
Clonapam (clonazepam)
Clotrimaderm (clotrimazole)
Combantrin (pyrantel)
Congest (estrogens, conjugated)
Corax (chlordiazepoxide)
Creon (pancrelipase)
Crysticillin-AS (penicillin G procaine)

Cyclomen (danazol)

D

Dalacin C (clindamycin)

Dehydral (methenamine)

Deproic (valproic acid)

Dermovate (clobetasol)

Diarr-Eze (loperamide)

Diazemuls (diazepam)

Digess 8000 (pancrelipase)

Dihydroergotamine Sandoz (dihydroergotamine)

Dimelor (acetohexamide)

Diodoquin (iodoquinol)

Diomycin (erythromycin)

Dioptic's Atropine (atropine)

Diphenylan (phenytoin)

Dipridacot (dipyridamole)

Dixarit (clonidine)

Dopamet (methyldopa)

Doxycin (doxycyline)

Doxytec (doxycycline)

Duralith (lithium)

Duretic (methyclothiazide)

D-Vert (meclizine)

E

Eltor (pseudoephedrine)

Endantadine (amantadine)

Entocort (budesonide)

Entrophen (aspirin)

Epimorph (morphine)

Epival (valproic acid)

Eprex (epoetin)

Ergomar (ergotamine)

Erybid (erythromycin)

Erythrocin (erythromycin)

Erythrocin I.V. (erythromycin)

Erythromid (erythromycin)

Estromed (estrogens, esterified)

Etibi (ethambutol)

Euflex (flutamide)

Euglucon (glyburide)

F

Falapen (penicillin G potassium)

Ferodan (ferrous salts)

Fero-Grad (ferrous salts)

Fertinorm HP (urofollitropin)

Fluor-A-Day (sodium fluoride)

Fluotic (sodium fluoride)

Formulex (dicyclomine)

Froben (flurbiprofen)

Froben-SR (flurabiprofen)

Furoside (furosemide)

G

Gen-Amantadine (amantadine)

Gen-Atenolol (atenolol)

Gen-Baclofen (baclofen)

Gen-Captopril (captopril)

Gen-Cimetidine (cimetidine)

Gen-Clomipramine (clomipramine)

Gen-Clonazepam (clonazepam)

Gen-Diltiazem (diltiazem)

Gen-Fibro (gemfibrozil)

Gen-Glybe (glyburide)

Gen-Medroxy (medroxyprogesterone)

Gen-Minocycline (minocycline)

Gen-Nifedipine (nifedipine)

Gravol (dimenhydrinate)

H

Haldol LA (haloperidol)

Hepalean (heparin)

Hepalean-Lok (heparin)

Heparin Leo (heparin)

Hip-Rex (methenamine)

Honvol (diethylstilbestrol)

Humulin U (insulin)

Hycort (hydrocortisone)

Hydromorph Contin (hydromorphone)

Hy/Gestrone (hydroxyprogesterone)

I

Iletin PZI (insulin)

Immunine VH (factor IX)

Impril (imipramine)

Indocid (indomethacin)

Indocid P.D.A. (indomethacin)

Indotec (indomethacin)

Infufer (iron dextran)

Inocid (indomethacin)

Isotamine (isoniazid)

Isotrex (isotretinoin)

K

Kabolin (nandrolone)

Kalium Durules (potassium chloride)

K-Exit (sodium polystyrene)

Kidrolase (asparaginase)

Koffex (dextromethorphan)

L

Lactulax (lactulose)

Lanvis (thioguanine)

Largactil (chlorpromazine)

Laxilose (lactulose)

Levate (amitriptyline)

Lithizine (lithium)

Lopresor (metoprolol)

LoSec (omeprazole)

Loxapac (loxapine)

Lyderm Cream (fluocinonide)

M

Malogen in Oil (testosterone)

Mandelamine (methenamine)

Marzine (cyclizine)

Maxeran (metoclopramide)

Meclomen (meclofenamate)

Medrol Verider m (methylprednisolone)

Megace OS (megestrol)
Megacillin (penicillin G benzathine)
Meprolone (methylprednisolone)
Mesasal (mesalamine)
M-Eslon (morphine)
MetroCream (metronidazole)
Micozole (miconazole)
Minims (atropine)
Minims Sodium Chloride (sodium chloride)
Minox (minoxidil)
Minoxigaine (minoxidil)
Mireze (nedocromil)
Modecate Deconate (fluphenazine)
Moditen Enanthate (fluphenazine)
Monazole 7 (miconazole)
Monitan (acebutolol)
Multipax (hydroxyzine)
Mycifradin (neomycin)
Mycil (chlorphenesin)
Myclo (clotrimazole)
Myrosemide (furosemide)

N

Nadopen-V (penicillin V)
Nadostine (nystatin)
Nalcrom (cromolyn)
Natulan (procarbazine)
Naxen (naproxen)
Neo-Tric (metronidazole)
NidaGel (metronidazole)
Nobesin (diethylpropion)
Norlutate (norethindrone)
Norventyl (nortriptyline)
Norzine (thiethylperazine)
Novahistex DM (dextromethorphan)
Novahistine DM (dextromethorphan)
Novamoxin (amoxicillin)
Novasen (aspirin)
Novo-Alprozol (alprazolam)
Novo-Ampicillin (ampicillin)
Novo-Atenol (atenolol)
Novo-AZT (zidovudine)
Novo-Baclofen (baclofen)
Novo-Butamide (tolbutamide)
Novo-Captopril (captopril)
Novo-Carbamaz (carbamazepine)
Novo-Cholamine (cholestyramine)
Novo-Cholamine Light (cholestyramine)
Novo-Cimetine (cimetidine)
Novo-Clopamine (clomipramine)
Novo-Clopate (clorazepate)
Novo-Cloxin (cloxacillin)
Novo-Cycloprine (cyclobenzaprine)
Novo-Desipramine (desipramine)
Novo-Difenac (diclofenac)
Novo-Diflunisal (diflunisal)

Novo-Digoxin (digoxin)
Novo-Diltazem (diltiazem)
Novo-Doxepin (doxepin)
Novo-Doxylin (doxycycline)
Novo-Famotidine (famotidine)
Novo-Fibrate (clofibrate)
Novo-Fluoxetine (fluoxetine)
Novo-Flurbiprofen (flurbiprofen)
Novo-Flutamide (flutamide)
Novo-Furan (nitrofurantoin)
Novo-Gemfibrozil (gemfibrozil)
Novo-Hylazin (hydralazine)
Novo-Hydrazide (hydrochlorothiazide)
Novo-Hydroxyzin (hydroxyzine)
Novo-Ipramide (ipratropium)
Novo-Levamisole (levamisole)
Novo-Lexin (cephalexin)
Novolin ge (insulin)
Novolin ge lente (insulin)
Novolin ge Toronto (insulin)
Novolin ge ultralente (insulin)
Novo-Loperamide (loperamide)
Novo-Lorazem (lorazepam)
Novo-Maprotiline (maprotiline)
Novo-Medopa (methyldopa)
Novo-Medrone (medroxyprogesterone)
Novo-Meprazine (methotrimeprazine)
Novomepro (meprobamate)
Novomethacin (indomethacin)
Novo-Metoprol (metoprolol)
Novo-Mexiletine (mexiletine)
Novo-Minocycline (minocycline)
Novo-Naddol (nadolol)
Novo-Naprox (naproxen)
Novo-Nidazol (metronidazole)
Novo-Nifedin (nifedipine)
Novo-Oxybutynin (oxybutynin)
Novo-Pen G (penicillin G)
Novo-Pen VK (penicillin V)
Novo-Pentobarb (pentobarbital)
Novoperidol (haloperidol)
Novo-Pindol (pindolol)
Novo-Pirocam (piroxicam)
Novo-Pramine (imipramine)
Novo-Pranol (propranolol)
Novo-Prazin (prazosin)
Novo-Prednisolone (prednisolone)
Novo-Prednisone (prednisone)
Novo-Profen (ibuprofen)
Novo-Propoxyn (propoxyphene)
Novo-Pyrazone (sulfinpyrazone)
Novo-Ranidine (ranitidine)
Novo-Rectal (pentobarbital)
Novo-Rythro (erythromycin)
Novo-Salmol (albuterol)

Novo-Secobarb (secobarbital)
Novo-Sotalol (sotalol)
Novosoxazole (sulfisoxazole)
Novo-Spiroton (spironolactone)
Novo-Sucralfate (sucralfate)
Novo-Sundac (sulindac)
Novo-Tamoxifen (tamoxifen)
Novo-Temazepam (temazepam)
Novotetra (tetracycline)
Novo-Timol (timolol)
Novo-Tolmetin (tolmetin)
Novo-Triolam (triazolam)
Novo-Triphyl (oxtriphylline)
Novo-Tripramine (trimipramine)
Novo-Triptyn (amitriptyline)
Novoxapam (oxazepam)
Nozinan (methotrimeprazine)
Nu-Alpraz (alprazolam)
Nu-Amoxi (amoxicillin)
Nu-Ampi (ampicillin)
Nu-Capto (captopril)
Nu-Cephalex (cephalexin)
Nu-Cimet (cimetidine)
Nu-Clonidine (clonidine)
Nu-Cloxi (cloxacillin)
Nu-Diclo (diclofenac)
Nu-Diflunisal (diflunisal)
Nu-Diltiaz (diltiazem)
Nu-Doxycycline (doxycycline)
Nu-Erythromycin-S (erythromycin)
Nu-Hydral (hydralazine)
Nu-Ketoprofen (ketoprofen)
Nu-Loraz (lorazepam)
Nu-Medopa (methyldopa)
Nu-Metoclopramide (metoclopramide)
Nu-Metop (metoprolol)
Nu-Pindol (pindolol)
Nu-Pirox (piroxicam)
Nu-Prazo (prazosin)
Nu-Ranit (ranitidine)
Nu-Tetra (tetracycline)
Nu-Trazodone (trazodone)

O

Occulcort (betamethasone)
Octostim (desmopressin)
Ocu-Phrin (phenylephrine)
Opium TCT (opium)
Oracort (triamcinolone)
Orafen (ketoprofen)
Orbenin (cloxacillin)
Orcipren (metaproterenol)
Orfenace (orphenadrine)

P

Palafer (ferrous fumarate)
Parvolex (acetylcysteine)

PCE (erythromycin)
PDF (sodium fluoride)
Pedi-Dent (sodium fluoride)
Penbec V (penicillin V)
Penbritin (ampicillin)
Penglobe (bacampicillin)
Pentacarinat (pentamidine)
Pentids (penicillin G)
Peptol (cimetidine)
Peridol (haloperidol)
Phazyme 55 (simethicone)
Phenazine (perphenazine)
Phenazo (phenazopyridine)
Phenytex (phenytoin)
PMS-ASA (aspirin)
PMS Benztropine (benztropine)
PMS Bethanecol Chloride (bethanechol)
PMS-Ceclor (cefaclor)
PMS-Cephalexin (cephalexin)
PMS-Chloral Hydrate (chloral hydrate)
PMS-Cyproheptadine (cyproheptadine)
PMS-Desipramine (desipramine)
PMS-Egozinc (zinc)
PMS-Fluoxetine (fluoxetine)
PMS-Haloperidol (haloperidol)
PMS-Hydromorphone (hydromorphone)
PMS-Ipecac (ipecac)
PMS-Isoniazid (isoniazid)
PMS-Lithium Carbonate (lithium)
PMS-Loxapine (loxapine)
PMS-Mefenamic Acid (mefenamic acid)
PMS-Methylphenidate (methylphenidate)
PMS-Metronidazole (metronidazole)
PMS-Neostigmine Methylsulfate (neostigmine)
PMS-Nortriptyline (nortriptyline)
PMS-Nystatin (nystatin)
PMS-Prochlorperazine (prochlorperazine)
PMS-Procyclidine (procyclidine)
PMS-Promethazine (promethazine)
PMS-Propranolol (propranolol)
PMS-Pyrazinamide (pyrazinamide)
Ponstan (mefenamic acid)
Pressyn (vasopressin)
Prevex B (betamethasone)
Primazine (promazine)
Primene (amino acids)
Procan SR (procainamide)
Procyclid (procyclidine)
Procytox (cyclophosphamide)
Prodox (hydroxyprogesterone)
Progestilin (progesterone)
Propaderm (beclomethasone)
Propanthel (propantheline)
Propoint (diethylpropion)
Propyl-Thyracil (propylthiouracil)

Puregon (follitropin beta)
Purinol (allopurinol)
Pyribenzamine (tripelennamine)
Q
Quinate (quinidine)
Quintasa (mesalamine)
R
Reactine (cetirizine)
Regibon (diethylpropion)
Renedil (felodipine)
Revimine (dopamine)
Rhinalar (flunisolide)
Rhinocort Tubuhaler (budesonide)
Rhodacine (indomethacin)
Rhodis (ketoprofen)
Rho-Fluphenazine Deconate (fluphenazine)
Rholosone (betamethasone)
Rhoprosone (betamethasone)
Rhotral (acebutolol)
Rhotrimine (trimipramine)
Rhovail (ketoprofen)
Riphenidate (methylprednisolone)
Rivotril (clonazepam)
R.O. Atropine (atropine)
Robidex (dextromethorphan)
Rofact (rifampin)
Rogitine (phentolamine)
Roychlor (potassium chloride)
Rylosol (sotalol)
Rynacron (cromolyn)
Rythmodan (disopyramide)
S
Salazopyrin (sulfasalazine)
Salbutamol (albuterol)
Saline from Otrivin (sodium chloride)
Salinex (sodium chloride)
Salofalk (mesalamine)
Sarisol #2 (butabarbital)
S.A.S. (sulfasalazine)
Scheinpharm Testone-cyp (testosterone)
Sotacar (sotalol)
Stemitil (prochlorperazine)
Stemitil Suppositories (prochlorperazine)
Sterine (methenamine)
StieVA-A (tretinoin)
Sulcrate (sucralfate)

Supeudol (oxycodone)
Synacthen Depot (cosyntropin)
Synflex (naproxen)
T
Tamone (tamoxifen)
Tanta Orciprenaline (metaproterenol)
Taro-Sone (betamethasone)
Tebrazid (pyrazinamide)
Teejel (choline salicylate)
Tegopen (cloxacillin)
Tenolin (atenolol)
Texacort (hydrocortisone)
Tija (oxytetracycline)
Topsyn Gel (fluocinonide)
Travel Tabs (dimenhydrinate)
Trexan (naltrexone)
Triadapin (doxepin)
Trichlorex (trichlormethiazide)
Trikacide (metronidazole)
Triptil (protriptyline)
U
Ultracef (cefadroxil)
Ultradol (etodolac)
UltraMOP (methoxsalen)
Urasal (methenamine)
Urozide (hydrochlorothiazide)
Ursofalk (ursodiol)
V
Vamin 18 (amino acids)
Velbe (vinblastine)
Ventodisk (albuterol)
Vivelle (estradiol)
Vivol (diazepam)
Voltaren Ophtha (diclofenac)
Voltaren Rapide (diclofenac)
W
Warfilone (warfarin)
Winpred (prednisone)
X
Xanax-TS (alprazolam)
Y
Yodoquinal (iodoquinol)
Z
Zapex (oxazepam)
Zoladex L.A. (goserelin)
Zonalon (doxepin)

G

CANADIAN IMMUNIZATION SCHEDULES FOR INFANTS AND CHILDREN*

The following is an overview on routine immunization schedules for infants and children. This information is not intended to present a comprehensive review; the reader is encouraged to seek additional and confirmatory information.

---

*Reprinted by permission from Repchinsky, C. (ed.). *Compendium of pharmaceuticals and specialties.* Ottawa: Canadian Pharmacists Association, 2001.

Reviewed 1999 by V. Marchessault.

Few measures in preventive medicine are of such proven value and as easy to implement as routine immunization against infectious diseases. Immunizations carried out as recommended in the following schedules (Tables 1, 2, and 3) will provide protection for most children against the diseases shown.

Both live and inactivated polio vaccines have been used in Canada with equal success in preventing the occurrence of paralytic poliomyelitis, but inactivated vaccine is now preferred.

Following a standard schedule ensures complete and adequate protection. However, modifications of the recommended

---

| TABLE 1 | Routine Immunization Schedule for Infants and Children |

Age/Time	DTaP[a]	IPV	Hib[b]	MMR	Td[c]	Hep B[d] (3 doses)
2 months old	X	X	X			Infancy
4 months old	X	X	X			
6 months old	X	X[e]	X			or
12 months old				X		
18 months old	X	X	X	X[f] or		
4–6 years old Grade 3–7	X	X		X[f]		preadolescence (9–13 yrs)
14–16 years old					X	

[a]DTaP (diphtheria, tetanus, acellular or component pertussis) vaccine is the preferred vaccine for all doses in the vaccination series, including completion of the series in children who have received ≥1 dose of DPT (whole cell) vaccine.

[b]Hib schedule shown is for PRP-T (e.g., Act-HIB) or HbOC (e.g., Hib TITER) vaccine. If PRP-OMP (e.g., PedVax HIB), give at 2, 4, and 12 mo of age.

[c]Td (tetanus and diphtheria toxoid), a combined adsorbed "adult type" preparation for use in persons ≥7 years of age contains less diphtheria toxoid than preparations given to younger children and is less likely to cause reactions in older persons.

[d]Hepatitis B vaccine can be routinely given to infants or preadolescents, depending on the provincial/territorial policy; three doses at 0, 1, and 6-mo intervals are preferred. The second dose should be administered at least 1 month after the first dose, and the third dose should be administered at least 4 months after the first dose, and at least 2 mo after the second dose.

[e]This dose is not needed routinely but can be included for convenience.

[f]A second dose of MMR is recommended, at least 1 mo after the first dose given. For convenience, options include giving it with the next scheduled vaccination at 18 mo of age or with school entry vaccinations at 4–6 y of age (depending on the provincial/territorial policy), or at any intervening age that is practicable.

[g]Delay until subsequent visit if child is <12 mo of age.

[h]Recommended schedule and number of doses depend on the product used and the age of the child when vaccination is begun (see the current *Canadian Immunization Guide* or the product monograph for specific recommendations); not required past age 5 y.

[i]Omit these doses if the previous doses of DTaP and polio were given after the fourth birthday.

DTaP, diphtheria, tetanus and pertussis (acellular) vaccine; Hep B, recombinant hepatitis B vaccine series; Hb, *Haemophilus influenzae* b conjugate vaccine; IPV, inactivated polio vaccine; MMR, measles, mumps and rubella vaccine; Td, tetanus and diphtheria toxoid, "adult type."

Adapted from *Canadian immunization guide* (5th ed.). Health Canada, 1998, with permission of the Minister of Public Works and Government Services Canada, 1998.

TABLE II | Routine Immunization Schedule for Children <7 Years of Age not Immunized in Early Infancy

Timing	DTaP[a]	IPV	Hib	MMR	Td[c]	Hep B[d] (3 doses)
1st visit	X	X	X	X[g]		
2 months after 1st visit	X	X	X[h]	X[f]		
2 months after 2nd visit	X	X[e]				
6–12 months after 3rd visit	X	X	X[h]			
4–6 years of age[i]	X	X				
14–16 years of age					X	Preadolescence (9–13 y)

Footnotes same as for Table I.

schedule may be necessary because of missed appointments or illness. Interruption of a recommended series does not require starting the series over again, regardless of the interval elapsed.

Similar vaccines are now available from different manufacturers, but they may not be identical. It is therefore essential for the user to read the appropriate chapter in the current *Canadian Immunization Guide,* as well as the manufacturer's package insert.

REFERENCE

1. National Advisory Committee on Immunization. *Canadian immunization guide* (5th ed.). Ottawa: Health Canada, 1998.

TABLE III | Routine Immunization Schedule for Children = 7 Years of Age Not Immunized in Early Infancy

Timing	Td[c]	IPV	MMR	Hep B[d] (3 doses)
1st visit	X	X	X	
2 months after 1st visit	X	X	X[f]	
6–12 months after 2nd visit	X	X		
10 years after 3rd visit	X			Preadolescence (9–13 yrs)

Footnotes same as for Table I.

CANADIAN NARCOTIC AND CONTROLLED DRUGS*

Table 1 summarizes the requirements for prescribing, dispensing, and record keeping for narcotic and controlled

*Reprinted by permission from Repchinsky, C. (ed.). *Compendium of pharmaceuticals and specialties*. Ottawa: Canadian Pharmacists Association, 2001.

drugs. This information is not intended to present a comprehensive review; the reader is encouraged to seek additional and confirmatory information (eg, Controlled Drugs and Substances Act, Narcotic Control Regulations, Food and Drugs Regulations).

Reviewed 1999 by the Bureau of Drug Surveillance, Health Canada.

TABLE 1 | Narcotic and Controlled Drugs Summary

Classification and Description	Legal Requirements
NARCOTIC DRUGS • 1 narcotic (eg, cocaine, codeine, hydromorphone, morphine) • 1 narcotic + 1 active non-narcotic ingredient (eg, *Cophylac, Empracet-30, Penntuss, Tylenol No. 4*) • All narcotics for parenteral use (eg, fentanyl, pethidine) • All products containing diamorphine (hospitals only), hydrocodone, oxycodone, methadone or pentazocine • Dextropropoxyphene, propoxyphene (straight) (eg, *Darvon-N, 642*)	• Written prescription required. • Verbal prescriptions not permitted. • Refills not permitted. • Written prescription may be prescribed to be dispensed in divided portions (part-fills). • For part-fills, copies of prescriptions should be made in reference to the original prescription. Indicate on the original prescription: the new prescription number, the date of the part-fill, the quantity dispensed and the pharmacist's initials. • Record and retain all drug sales and purchases in a manner that permits an audit. • Report the loss or theft of narcotic/controlled drugs as well as forged prescriptions within 10 days to your Regional Office, Drug Programme at the address indicated at the back of the Drug Forgery Report or the Drug Loss/Theft Report forms.
NARCOTIC PREPARATIONS • Verbal prescription narcotics: 1 narcotic + 2 or more active non-narcotic ingredients (eg, *Cophylac Expectorant, Darvon-N Compound, Fiorinal with Codeine, 692, 282, 292, Tylenol No. 2* and *No. 3*) • Exempted codeine compounds: contain codeine up to 8 mg/solid dosage form or 20 mg/30 mL liquid + 2 or more active non-narcotic ingredients (eg, *Atasol-8, Robitussin with Codeine*).	• Written or verbal prescriptions permitted. • Refills not permitted. • Written or verbal prescriptions may be prescribed to be dispensed in divided portions (part-fills). • For part-fills, copies of prescriptions should be made in reference to the original prescription. Indicate on the original prescription: the new prescription number, the date of the part-fill, the quantity dispensed and the pharmacist's initials. • Exempted codeine compounds when dispensed pursuant to a prescription follow the same regulations as for verbal prescription narcotics. • Record and retain all drug sales and purchases in a manner that permits an audit.

Table 1 continues on page 858

TABLE 1 | Narcotic and Controlled Drugs Summary (Continued)

Classification and Description	Legal Requirements
	• Report the loss or theft of narcotic/controlled drugs as well as forged prescriptions within 10 days to your Regional Office, Drug Programme at the address indicated at the back of the Drug Forgery Report or the Drug Loss/Theft Report forms.

CONTROLLED DRUGS
• Part I
 eg, amphetamines (*Dexedrine*)
  methylphenidate (*Ritalin*)
  pentobarbital (*Nembutal*)
  secobarbital (*Seconal, Tuinal*)
  preparations: 1 controlled drug + 1 or more active noncontrolled drug(s) (*Cafergot-PB*)
	• Written or verbal prescriptions permitted.
	• Refills not permitted for verbal prescriptions.
	• Refills permitted for written prescriptions if the prescriber has indicated in writing the number of refills and dates for, or intervals between, refills.
	• Written or verbal prescriptions may be prescribed to be dispensed in divided portions (part-fills).
	• For refills and part-fills, copies of prescriptions should be made in reference to the original prescription. Indicate on the original prescription: the new prescription number, the date of the repeat or part-fill, the quantity dispensed and the pharmacist's initials.
	• Record and retain all drug sales and purchases in a manner that permits an audit.
	• Report the loss or theft of narcotic/controlled drugs as well as forged prescriptions within 10 days to your Regional Office, Drug Programme at the address indicated at the back of the Drug Forgery Report or the Drug Loss/Theft Report forms.

• Part II
 eg, barbiturates (amobarbital, phenobarbital)
  butorphanol (*Stadol NS*)
  diethylpropion (*Tenuate*)
  nalbuphine (*Nubain*)
  phentermine (*Fastin, Lonamin*)
  preparations: 1 controlled drug + 1 or more active noncontrolled ingredients (*Fiorinal, Neo-Pause, Tecnal*)
• Part III
 eg, anabolic steroids (methyltestosterone, nandrolone decanoate)
	• Written or verbal prescriptions permitted.
	• Refills permitted for written or verbal prescriptions if the prescriber has authorized in writing or verbally (at the time of issuance) the number of refills and dates for, or intervals between, refills.
	• Written or verbal prescriptions may be prescribed to be dispensed in divided portions (part-fills).
	• For refills and part-fills, copies of prescriptions should be made in reference to the original prescription. Indicate on the original prescription: the new prescription number, the date of the repeat or part-fill, the quantity dispensed and the pharmacist's initials.
	• Record and retain all drug sales and purchases in a manner that permits an audit.
	• Report the loss or theft of narcotic/controlled drugs as well as forged prescriptions within 10 days to your Regional Office, Drug Programme at the address indicated at the back of the Drug Forgery Report or the Drug Loss/Theft Report forms.

Index

Note: Page numbers with "t" denote tables; those with "f" denote figures; those with "b" denote boxes.

PROGRAM LICENSE AGREEMENT

Read carefully the following terms and conditions before using the Software. Use of the Software indicates you and, if applicable, your Institution's acceptance of the terms and conditions of this License Agreement. If you do not agree with the terms and conditions, you should promptly return this package to the place you purchased it and your payment will be refunded.

Definitions

As used herein, the following terms shall have the following meanings:

"Software" means the software program contained on the diskette(s) or CD-ROM or preloaded on a workstation and the user documentation, which includes all accompanying printed material.

"Institution" means a nursing or professional school, a single academic organization that does not provide patient care and is located in a single city and has one geographic location/address.

"Geographic location" means a facility at a specific location; geographic locations do not provide for satellite or remote locations that are considered a separate facility.

"Facility" means a health care facility at a specific location that provides patient care and is located in a single city and has one geographic location/address.

"Publisher" means Lippincott Williams & Wilkins, Inc., with its principal office in Philadelphia, Pennsylvania.

"Developer" means the company responsible for developing the software as noted on the product.

License

You are hereby granted a nonexclusive license to use the Software in the United States. This license is not transferable and does not authorize resale or sublicensing without the written approval or an authorized officer of Publisher.

The Publisher retains all rights and title to all copyrights, patents, trademarks, trade secrets, and other proprietary rights in the Software. You may not remove or obscure the copyright notices in or on the Software. You agree to use reasonable efforts to protect the Software from unauthorized use, reproduction, distribution or publication.

Single-User license

If you purchased this Software program at the Single-User License price or a discount of that price, you may use this program on one single-user computer. You may not use the Software in a time-sharing environment or otherwise to provide multiple, simultaneous access. You may not provide or permit access to this program to anyone other than yourself.

Institutional/Facility license

If you purchased the Software at the Institutional or Facility License Price or at a discount of that price, you have purchased the Software for use within your Institution/Facility on a single workstation/computer. You may not provide copies of or remote access to the Software. You may not modify or translate the program or related documentation. You agree to instruct the individuals in your Institution/Facility who will have access to the Software to abide by the terms of this License Agreement. If you or any member of your Institution fail to comply with any of the terms of this License Agreement, this license shall terminate automatically.

Network license

If you purchased the Software at the Network License Price, you may copy the Software for use within your Institution/Facility on an unlimited number of computers within one geographic location/address. You may not provide remote access to the Software over a value-added network or otherwise. You may not provide copies of or remote access to the Software to individuals or entities who are not members of your Institution/Facility. You may not modify or translate the program or related documentation. You agree to instruct the individuals in your Institution/Facility who will have access to the Software to abide by the terms of this License Agreement. If you or any member of your Institution/Facility fail to comply with any of the terms of this License Agreement, this license shall terminate automatically.

Limited warranty

The Publisher warrants that the media on which the Software is furnished shall be free from defects in materials and workmanship under normal use for a period of 90 days from the date of delivery to you, as evidenced by your receipt of purchase.

The Software is sold on a 30-day trial basis. If, for whatever reason, you decide not to keep the software, you may return it for a full refund within 30 days of the invoice date or purchase, as evidenced by your receipt of purchase by returning all parts of the Software and packaging in saleable condition with the original invoice, to the place you purchased it. If the Software is not returned in such condition, you will not be entitled to a refund. When returning the Software, we suggest that you insure all packages for their retail value and mail them by a traceable method.

The Software is a computer assisted instruction (CAI) program that is not intended to provide medical consultation regarding the diagnosis or treatment of any specific patient.

The Software is provided without warranty of any kind, either expressed or implied, including but not limited to any implied warranty of fitness for a particular purpose of merchantability. Neither Publisher nor Developer warrants that the Software will satisfy your requirements or that the Software is free of program or content errors. Neither Publisher nor Developer warrants, guarantees, or makes any representation regarding the use of the Software in terms of accuracy, reliability or completeness, and you rely on the content of the programs solely at your own risk.

The Publisher is not responsible (as a matter of products liability, negligence or otherwise) for any injury resulting from any material contained herein. This Software contains information relating to general principles of patient care that should not be construed as specific instructions for individual patients.

Manufacturers' product information and package inserts should be reviewed for current information, including contraindications, dosages and precautions.

Some states do not allow the exclusion of implied warranties, so the above exclusion may not apply to you. This warranty gives you specific legal rights and you may also have other rights that vary from state to state.

Limitation of remedies

The entire liability of Publisher and Developer and your exclusive remedy shall be: (1) the replacement of any CD which does not meet the limited warranty stated above which is returned to the place you purchased it with your purchase receipt; or (2) if the Publisher or the wholesaler or retailer from whom you purchased the Software is unable to deliver a replacement CD free from defects in material and workmanship, you may terminate this License Agreement by returning the CD, and your money will be refunded.

In no event will Publisher or Developer be liable for any damages, including any damages for personal injury, lost profits, lost savings or other incidental or consequential damages arising out of the use or inability to use the Software or any error or defect in the Software, whether in the database or in the programming, even if the Publisher, Developer, or an authorized wholesaler or retailer has been advised of the possibility of such damage.

Some states do not allow the limitation or exclusion of liability for incidental or consequential damages. The above limitations and exclusions may not apply to you.

General

This License Agreement shall be governed by the laws of the State of Pennsylvania without reference to the conflict of laws provisions thereof, and may only be modified in a written statement signed by an authorized officer of the Publisher. By opening and using the Software, you acknowledge that you have read this License Agreement, understand it, and agree to be bound by its terms and conditions. You further agree that it is a complete and exclusive statement of the agreement between the Institution/Facility and the Publisher, which supersedes any proposal or prior agreement, oral or written, and any other communication between you and Publisher or Developer relative to the subject matter of the License Agreement.

Note

Attach a paid invoice to the License Agreement as proof of purchase.

Dosage Calc-Challenger CD-ROM

INSTALLATION INSTRUCTIONS

Windows:
1. From Windows 95, 98, 2000, NT Start menu, select Run.
2. Type D:\setup (Where D is the CD-ROM drive letter).
3. Follow the on-screen instructions.
4. Note:
   This software is designed to run with Netscape Communicator or Navigator 4.78 or higher or Internet Explorer 5.0 or higher, and comes with Netscape 6.2.3 and Internet Explorer 5.5. If you do not have Netscape Communicator or Navigator 4.78 or higher or have Internet Explorer 5.0 or higher, choose to install Netscape 6.2.3 or Internet Explorer 5.5.
5. To start the program after installation, select "Dosage Calc-Challenger" from the "Dosage Calc-Challenger" folder in the Programs option in the Start menu.

Macintosh:
1. Double click the "Dosage Calc-Challenger" icon on the desktop.
2. Double click the "Install Dosage Calc-Challenger" icon.
3. Follow the on-screen instructions.
4. Note:
   This software is designed to run with Netscape Communicator or Navigator 4.78 or higher or Internet Explorer 5.0 or higher, and comes with Netscape 6.2.3 and Internet Explorer 5.5. If you do not have Netscape Communicator or Navigator 4.78 or higher or have Internet Explorer 5.0 or higher, choose to install Netscape 6.2.3 or Internet Explorer 5.5.
5. To start the program after installation, double click the "Start Dosage Calc-Challenger" icon in the "Dosage Calc-Challenger" folder on the hard drive.

Patient Teaching CD-ROM to Accompany Karch's Focus on Nursing Pharmacology, 2nd Edition

INSTALLATION INSTRUCTIONS

Insert the CD into your CD-ROM drive.

The program should begin running automatically. If it does not, follow these steps:
1. View the contents of the CD. This can be done in several ways depending on your operating system.
   Windows:
   • Double click on "My Computer."
   • Double click on the icon for your CD-ROM drive
   Macintosh:
   • Double click the "Karch" icon on the desktop.
2. Double click on the file "index.html" in order to begin using the program.